THE
COMPLETE
CANADIAN
HEALTH
GUIDE

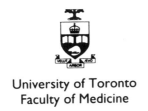

University of Toronto
Faculty of Medicine

The Complete
Canadian
Health Guide
REVISED EDITION

June Engel, Ph.D.
with updates to this edition by
Michael Evans, M.D., C.C.F.P., Assistant Professor,
Department of Family and Community Medicine,
Director of Public Education,
Faculty of Medicine, University of Toronto

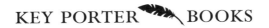

KEY PORTER BOOKS

I dedicate this book to the memory of my father,
a chemist and violist,
who taught me to appreciate the world of science,
and
to my daughter, Stephanie, and her remarkable family

Library and Archives Canada Cataloguing in Publication

Engel, June
   The complete Canadian health guide / June Engel. — Completely rev. and updated / by Michael Evans

ISBN 1-55263-666-6

   1. Medicine, Popular. 2. Family—Health and hygiene. I. Evans, Michael, 1964– II. Title.

RC81.E63 2005   616.02'4   C2005-900133-X

The publisher gratefully acknowledges the support of the Canada Council for the Arts and the Ontario Arts Council for its publishing program. We acknowledge the support of the Government of Ontario through the Ontario Media Development Corporation's Ontario Book Initiative.

We acknowledge the financial support of the Government of Canada through the Book Publishing Industry Development Program (BPIDP) for our publishing activities.

Key Porter Books Limited
Six Adelaide Street East, Tenth Floor
Toronto, Ontario
Canada M5C 1H6

www.keyporter.com

Electronic formatting: Jean Lightfoot Peters

Printed and bound in Canada

05 06 07 08 09 6 5 4 3 2 1

Publisher's Note: The contents of this book are not intended to be used as a substitution for consultation with your physician. All matters pertaining to your health should be directed to a healthcare professional.

Contents

PREFACE *11*

ACKNOWLEDGMENTS *13*

CHAPTER 1: WHAT IS GOOD HEALTH ALL ABOUT? *15*
 What is health? *15*
 Measuring health *17*
 Changing attitudes to healthcare *20*
 How to assess health news *21*

CHAPTER 2: CULTIVATING A HEALTHIER LIFESTYLE *23*
 Preventable illnesses *23*
 Overcoming the risks of smoking *23*
 Weight control is crucial to good health *32*
 Active people are healthier *40*
 Sleep hygiene and sleep disorders *49*
 Preventing needless injuries *54*
 Putting drug use in perspective *60*
 Tackling alcohol abuse *64*

CHAPTER 3: GETTING MEDICAL HELP WHEN IT'S NEEDED *74*
 Improving patient–doctor relationships *74*
 Using medical checkups wisely *79*
 Natural, alternative or complementary medicine *82*

CHAPTER 4: NUTRITION TOWARD HEALTH *89*
 The basics of good nutrition *89*
 Rules for healthy eating *89*
 Improving nutrition in the senior years *94*
 Nutrition for athletes *95*
 Sorting out the cholesterol puzzle *97*
 Choosing the right fat mix *102*
 Dietary fiber is still in *103*
 Make carbohydrates (starches) your dietary mainstay *104*
 Sugars aren't all bad *105*
 Proteins in the diet *105*
 In praise of fish *106*
 Vegetarian diets *106*
 The caffeine story *107*
 Vitamins: most people don't need supplements *109*
 Minerals in the diet *115*
 Water is also an essential dietary component *119*

CHAPTER 5: LOOKING AFTER THE SURFACE *121*
 Caring for your skin *121*
 Remedying dry skin problems *122*
 Help for the anguish of acne *127*
 Psoriasis control *128*
 Shingles is a pain *131*
 Help for aging skin *132*

Avoid skin's number-one enemy   *134*
Protect yourself against skin cancers   *135*
Hair, beautiful hair   *139*
Choose hair-care products wisely   *144*
Getting rid of lice   *145*
Hand and nail care   *148*
Foot care   *148*
Banishing warts   *151*

CHAPTER 6: EYE, EAR AND TOOTH CARE   155
Eye care   *155*
Ear care   *164*
Ear infections   *172*
Tooth and gum care   *174*

CHAPTER 7: SEXUAL HEALTH   179
Developing healthy sexual attitudes   *179*
Tracking key stages in sexual development   *180*
Main sexual development stages   *183*
Combatting sexual exploitation and abuse   *184*
Masturbation   *185*
Sexual dysfunction   *185*
Sex therapy   *187*
Sexually transmitted infections   *189*
Recent trends in birth control   *196*

CHAPTER 8: WOMEN'S SPECIAL HEALTH CONCERNS   205
Different influences on women's health   *206*
Societal influences on women's health   *206*
Sexuality and reproductive health in women   *211*
Menstruation and menstrual problems   *214*
Vaginitis: common and annoying, but curable   *218*
Vaginal yeast infections or candidiasis   *219*
Cervical cancer and genital warts   *220*
Ovarian cancer   *223*
Endometriosis   *225*
Menopause: time of transition   *227*
Hormone replacement therapy: yes, no or maybe?   *230*
Heart disease in women: the leading killer   *233*
Breast cancer   *236*
New genetic tests bring critical choices   *243*

CHAPTER 9: MEN'S SPECIAL HEALTH CONCERNS   246
Trouble with the prostate   *246*
Prostate cancer   *249*
Infertility   *252*
Vasectomy: pros and cons   *253*
Remedying sex problems   *253*
The circumcision controversy   *257*
Male breast cancer: men get it too!   *258*

CHAPTER 10: PRODUCING THE HEALTHIEST POSSIBLE BABY   260
Preconception preparation   *263*
Fertilization and conception   *264*
Reversing infertility   *265*
Pregnancy in the over-thirties   *267*

Modern "windows" into the womb   *268*
The course and care of pregnancy   *270*
Choice of birthplace and birth assistant   *272*
The role of midwives   *273*
Changes in the mother's body during pregnancy   *276*
Charting fetal progress   *276*
Nutrition in pregnancy   *277*
Exercise in pregnancy   *280*
Spotting high-risk pregnancies   *280*
Prenatal classes: preparing for labor   *281*
The three stages of labor   *283*
From fetus to newborn: a leap into the unknown   *284*
Cesarean birth: time for reappraisal   *285*
Newborn child–parent bonding   *287*
Breast is still best   *288*

CHAPTER 11: HELPING CHILDREN GROW UP HEALTHY   *293*

Breastfeeding   *293*
Instilling good eating habits   *294*
Choosing the right baby formula   *296*
Toilet training   *297*
Building in self-esteem   *298*
Preventing avoidable injuries   *299*
Preventing childhood choking   *300*
Recognizing and managing childhood disorders   *302*
Understanding childhood fever   *304*
Allergies   *308*
Asthma   *310*
Autism   *311*
Birthmarks   *312*
Cerebral palsy   *313*
Chickenpox   *314*
Colic   *315*
Common colds   *315*
Croup   *315*
Juvenile, type 1 or "insulin-dependent" diabetes   *315*
Diarrhea   *316*
Diphtheria   *316*
Down syndrome   *316*
Ear infections   *317*
Eczema   *319*
Enuresis (bedwetting)   *320*
Epiglottitis   *322*
Epilepsy (seizure disorder)   *323*
Fifth disease (erythema infectiosum)   *323*
Foot disorders   *323*
Giardiasis   *324*
Haemophilus influenzae type b infections   *324*
Hepatitis A   *325*
Hepatitis B   *325*
Impetigo   *326*
Measles   *326*
Meningitis   *327*
Mumps   *328*
Pinkeye (conjunctivitis)   *328*
Polio (poliomyelitis)   *328*
Rheumatic fever   *329*

Roseola *329*
RSV infections *329*
Rubella (German measles) *330*
Scabies *330*
Sore throats *330*
Sudden Infant Death Syndrome *331*
Teething *333*
Tetanus (lockjaw) *333*
Thrush or candida (yeast) diaper rash *333*
Tonsillitis *334*
Whooping cough (pertussis) *335*
Worms *335*

CHAPTER 12: PUBERTY AND ADOLESCENT CHANGES *337*
The stages of adolescence *338*
The physical changes of puberty *340*
Body-image concerns *341*
The tragic pursuit of thinness: anorexia nervosa and bulimia *343*
Psychosocial development in adolescence *348*
Helping adolescents through the transition *348*
Medical checkups for adolescents *350*
School problems *351*
Adolescent sexuality *351*
Risk-taking behavior *354*
The heavy toll of adolescent suicide *355*
Teenage and student substance use *360*

CHAPTER 13: MODERN ENVIRONMENTAL HEALTH HAZARDS *362*
Allergies *362*
Hay fever can ruin life's pleasures *365*
Insect allergies: what bit or stung you? *367*
Food allergies: one person's meat is another's poison *369*
Latex allergy: a burgeoning environmental problem *373*
Tight-building syndrome *374*
"Total allergy syndrome": twentieth-century disease or multiple chemical sensitivity *377*
How safe is our drinking water? *378*
Getting the lead out *382*
Coping with temperature extremes *384*
Staying fit on the job *385*
Toward healthier global travel *387*
Melatonin update: can it relieve jet lag? *393*

CHAPTER 14: COPING WITH MENTAL AND EMOTIONAL PROBLEMS *395*
Where does stress come from? *395*
Coping with stress *398*
Depression: more than just transient blues *401*
Modern treatments can help: it's worth "sticking with it" *405*
Depressive variants *408*
Holiday blues *411*
Manic depression *412*
Borderline personality disorder *414*
Chronic fatigue syndrome *415*
The disabling effects of anxiety disorders *419*
Schizophrenia *425*
Finding therapy for mental and emotional problems *428*

CHAPTER 15: KEEPING UP THE QUALITY OF LIFE WITH ADVANCING YEARS 430

The aging brain *430*
Caring well for elderly relatives *432*
Incontinence *435*
Parkinson's disease *440*
Osteoporosis *444*
Alzheimer's disease *451*
Caregivers also need respite and support *455*

CHAPTER 16: SOME SPECIFIC DISEASES AND DISORDERS 456

AIDS *456*
ALS or amyotrophic lateral sclerosis *460*
Anemia *460*
Arthritis *463*
Asthma *467*
Athlete's foot *471*
Attention-deficit hyperactivity disorder *473*
Back problems *476*
Bovine encephalopathy and Creutzfeldt-Jakob disease *479*
Bowel problems *479*
Bronchitis *486*
Carpal tunnel syndrome *487*
Common cold *488*
Creutzfeldt-Jakob disease (and links to "mad-cow" disease or BSE) *490*
Cystic fibrosis *491*
Diabetes *492*
Dizziness *500*
Dry eye *503*
Emerging infectious diseases: a new danger *504*
Epilepsy (seizure disorder) *505*
Fibromyalgia *510*
Gallbladder problems *512*
Halitosis: banishing bad breath *512*
Headaches *513*
Heart disease *517*
Heart murmurs *526*
Heartburn: not from the heart *527*
Hemophilia *529*
Hemorrhoids *530*
Hepatitis *533*
Hernias *539*
Hypertension (high blood pressure) *541*
Influenza *543*
Itching or pruritus *546*
Kidney failure *548*
Kidney stones *550*
Leukemia *552*
Liver cirrhosis *555*
Lung cancer *556*
Lupus *557*
Lyme disease *559*
Lymphoma, non-Hodgkin's type *561*
Multiple sclerosis *562*

Peptic ulcers: digesting more than food   *563*
Strokes   *566*
Stuttering   *574*
Thyroid disorders   *576*
Tuberculosis: back with a vengeance   *580*
Urinary tract infections   *582*
Varicose veins   *585*
Voice abuse: remarkably common!   *586*
West Nile Virus infection   *589*
Does your work environment make you sick?   *590*
Ergonomic workplace health   *592*
Zoonoses: disease from pets   *594*

CHAPTER 17: EMERGENCY FIRST AID   *598*
How to help in an emergency   *598*
General principles of first aid   *600*
The ABCs of AR and CPR   *600*
Allergic shock (anaphylaxis)   *602*
Asphyxiation (suffocation)   *603*
Asthma   *603*
Bites and stings   *603*
Bleeding   *605*
Burns and scalds   *605*
Choking: the Heimlich maneuver   *606*
Choking infants need back blows and chest thrusts   *608*
Convulsions   *609*
Dressings and bandages   *609*
Ear injuries   *609*
Electric shock   *610*
Eye injuries   *610*
Fainting   *610*
Fractures   *610*
Frostbite and freezing   *611*
Head injuries   *611*
Heart attack   *612*
Hyperthermia (heat illnesses)   *612*
Hypothermia (cold injury)   *613*
Mouth injuries   *614*
Nosebleeds   *614*
Poisonings   *614*
Seizures   *615*
Shock   *615*
Sports injuries   *616*
Teeth (knocked out)   *618*
Unconsciousness   *618*
Water accidents   *618*
Where to learn first aid and CPR   *619*

APPENDIX: SENSIBLE USE OF MEDICATIONS   *620*
Use and abuse of prescribed drugs   *622*
Use nonprescription medications wisely   *625*

WEB RESOURCES   *632*

INDEX   *634*

Preface

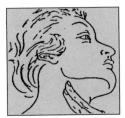 AS WITH PREVIOUS editions of *The Complete Canadian Health Guide*, the third edition aims to translate medical knowledge into clear comprehensible terms, to dispel misconceptions, to help people assess medical news correctly and distinguish truth from fiction (or half-truths). Its goal is to help people manage their well being and healthcare as competently as possible. Despite an ever-growing avalanche of medical news and Internet material, an escalating public interest in health matters and an avid search for reliable information, people often remain confused or worse still, misled.

This third and revised edition of the book has been updated with the help of Dr. Michael Evans, director of public education for the Faculty of Medicine, at the University of Toronto and assistant professor in the Department of Family & Community Medicine. Dr. Evans is leading many initiatives that help the public make more informed health decisions as well as being chief medical editor of Ontario's website for the public that won the 2004 "Webby" as the world's premiere government website. As before, most of the material in the *Health Guide* is evidence-based—that is based on reliable scientific evidence and results obtained through well-conducted, randomized, controlled trials that provide peer-reviewed and trustworthy information.

The book is a concise, readable source of health information, and hopes to arm people with the evidence and practical knowledge needed to sort through the mass of conflicting health pronouncements, enabling them to make sensible, informed healthcare decisions. Any medical terms or jargon used are translated into straightforward language that everyone can understand, and enough background is given to put each topic in context. The book has been prepared with the assistance of health professionals from the University of Toronto and other medical experts across North America.

Rather than simply presenting an encyclopedic compendium of diseases and ailments, the book is divided into various areas of health concern such as lifestyle, nutrition, exercise, sexuality, reproduction, parenting, childcare, helping adolescents, mental health problems and aging. There are sections on the care of various body parts—such as skin, hair, eyes, ears and teeth—and the health problems concerning them. Special sections are devoted to the health concerns of women, men and children, and to contemporary worries such as skin cancer, sexually transmitted infections, depression and suicide. Throughout, the focus is on health promotion, disease prevention and self-care or "care management," which is ideally a collaboration or partnership between healthcare consumers (patients) and their healthcare providers, and should address social, emotional and psychological problems as well as physical ones. We hope the book fosters an inquiring attitude that leads people to analyze the medical information they read, hear, see or seek.

Over the past couple of decades, there has been a significant shift in the way people look after their health. Previously, the doctor acted as the central health-information provider, making all key decisions about patient care. Knowledge about the scientific basis underlying a certain condition was often ignored or available solely from healthcare professionals. Today, the Internet has dramatically changed the dynamics of doctor–patient relationships which have become interactive partnerships. The explosion of on-line medical and health websites, journals and chat-groups has given millions of computer users instant access to masses of health information, much of it previously obtainable only in libraries or from medical specialists. Whereas in the past people might have sought health information from their doctors or friends, they now log on to search for an answer to their symptoms or how to deal with a specific health problem. Studies show that roughly half of Internet information seekers search the Web for answers to their health concerns before consulting their healthcare providers, and that much of the time they find relevant information in the first 3 websites visited. Increasing numbers also seek counsel from alternative medicine sites and from "Tele-Health" phone services where they may receive advice from a nurse, dietitian or social worker.

However, this trend to make Internet-based health decisions and "self-diagnosis" has drawbacks and risks as the cyber health information may not be accurate, valid or up to date. Web-based material from various sites may be biased (based on personal experience or anecdotes) false, incomplete and product-oriented or profit-motivated, easily leading to faulty self-treatment for an ailment that's been wrongly e-diagnosed, while missing the real problem. Studies show that only 1 in 4 Internet users actually takes the time or trouble, or knows how to, evaluate the quality, reliability or sources of the information-provider. Trials also show that consumers assess material or discriminate according to poor criteria such as the site's presenting image, whether it portrays someone well-dressed, wearing a white coat or in a laboratory. Although seemingly sound, information obtained via the Internet may not be trustworthy or true. It should be thoroughly checked out to determine its validity and whether it is peer-reviewed and evidence-based.

Essentially, people still need to consult doctors in order to make the best possible choices for treating or managing a specific health concern. The decision about which treatment or course of action best fits a particular problem should be based on evidence from high quality trials, together with the physician's clinical experience which also plays a crucial role in good medical decision-making. "It's probably best," suggest the experts, "to have your symptoms assessed by a qualified physician, correctly diagnosed, and *then* look up or research the problem on the Net." In the modern Internet age, with its wealth of disparate but not necessarily reliable or trustworthy health information, a book such as ours, which is strictly evidence-based and contains the collected scientific wisdom of many renowned medical experts on each topic, can be a particularly valuable resource with which to check, validate or question health information obtained elsewhere. To help people evaluate medical news on the Net and in the popular press, our book explains how science works, why certain strategies, procedures or treatments are tried and their relative merits and drawbacks. The approach is evidence-based, discussing the latest peer-reviewed evidence for and against various tests, procedures and therapies so that, together with their doctors and other healthcare providers, people can decide whether and why to accept a certain test or treatment. We list the pros and cons of different procedures, treatments and medications used for various conditions, with evidence for their usefulness and drawbacks, so that people can make informed choices. Where medical opinion is sharply divided, both sides of the argument are explained, so that people can discuss the issues more fully with their physicians and know what questions to ask. There's also a comprehensive section on first aid and using medications wisely.

While *The Complete Canadian Health Guide* aims to help readers become more informed about ways to manage their health, it in no way seeks to replace physician care. Specific concerns must still be discussed with medical caregivers. But we hope to facilitate communication with health professionals. The better we all understand what goes on in our bodies—and its relationship to lifestyle habits and to mental, social and emotional influences—the more we can do to keep ourselves well and to recognize and deal with any problems that crop up. How can we take care of our responsibilities in this life, if we cannot first take care of ourselves?

Note: A list of reliable, well-researched websites is provided at the end of the book (see page 632).

Acknowledgments

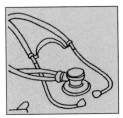

THIS BOOK WOULD never have happened without the wisdom, help and support of scores of medical experts at the University of Toronto's Faculty of Medicine and across North America. In particular, I must thank the successive advisory boards of *Health News*, the Faculty's lay health bulletin which I wrote and edited for 20 years. I would especially like to thank three consecutive chairs of that advisory board—Drs. Gerard Burrow, Fred Lowy and Mary Jane Ashley—for their warm encouragement and contribution. A special thanks also to Drs. Warren Rubenstein, Cornelia Baines and Harvey Skinner for tirelessly helping me to check and revise a never-ending series of health topics, and for being ruthlessly critical in an amazingly constructive manner.

It is a mammoth task to get each section of a book on so many topics checked by relevant specialists. And since some of the material came from *Health News*, I owe thanks to everyone who contributed to the publication and to the medical experts who provided source material and checked what I wrote on various subjects. Much gratitude also to Isolde Prince who excels in hunting down references at a moment's notice, and to Madeline Koch, a computer magician who can speedily input revisions.

For assistance in updating this third edition of the book, I must thank Dr. Michael Evans, assistant professor in the Department of Family & Community Medicine at the University of Toronto, and director of public education at the Faculty of Medicine, who brings to it his clinical knowledge and wide-ranging expertise.

For help with specific parts of the book I'd like also to express my gratitude to those who helped with previous editions, in particular to Dr. Peter Alberti, Dr. Harvey Anderson, Dr.

Margaret Baigent, Dr. Michael Barrett, Dr. Helen Batty, Dr. Karen Binkley, Dr. Anne Biringer, Dr. Claire Bombardier, Dr. Norman Boyd, Dr. Irv Broder, Dr. Joe Bruni, Dr. Robert Buckman, Dr. Ken Cadesky, Dr. June Carroll, Dr. Bob Casper, Dr. Zave Chad, Dr. Roy Clark, Dr. David Cole, Dr. Desmond Colohan, Dr. David Cowan, Dr. Steve Cunnane, Dr. Rosalyn Curtis, Dr. Loretta Daniel, Dr. Raisa Deber, Dr. Christine Derzko, Dr. Diane Donat, Dr. John Dreopoulis, Dr. Isser Dubinsky, Dr. Andy Duic, Dr. John Edmeads, Dr. Richard Ellen, Dr. Stan Epstein, Dr. Michael Evans, Dr. Gail Eyssen, Dr. Roberta Ferrence, Dr. Bill Fisher, Joyce Forster, Dr. Richard Frecker, Dr. Melvin Freedman, Dr. Bernie Fresco, Dr. Paul Garfinkel, Dr. Ron Gold, Dr. Martin Goldback, Dr. David Goldbloom, Dr. Peter Gill, Dr. Dafra Gladman, Dr. Anthony Graham, Dr. Mark Greenberg, Dr. Paul Gully, Dr. Henry Hallam, Dr. Gillian Hawker, Dr. Jenny Heathcote, Dr. Stephen Holzapel, Dr. Keith Jarvi, Dr. Russell Joffee, Dr. Robert Josse, Dr. Kevin Kain, Dr. Harold Kalant, Dr. Debbie Katzman, Dr. Armand Keating, Dr. Sid Kennedy, Dr. Anne Kenshole, Ms. Ann Kerr, Dr. Bernice Krafchik, Dr. Steve Kunns, Dr. Ed Keystone, Dr. Jay Keystone, Dr. Alan Knight, Dr. Anthony Lang, Dr. Donald McLachlan, Dr. William Mahon, Dr. Andrew Malleson, Dr. Aaron Malkin, Dr. Morton Mamelak, Dr. Chuck Leber, Dr. Joel Lexchin, Dr. Arthur Leznoff, Dr. Don Low, Dr. Rena Mendelson, Dr. Linda Mickleborough, Dr. Heather Morris, Dr. Robert Murray, Dr. Tim Murray, Dr. Ted Myers, Dr. Julien Nedzelski, Dr. Marion Olmstead, Dr. John Oreopolis, Dr. Howard Ovens, Dr. Fred Papsin, Dr. David Patrick, Dr. Anita Rachlis, Dr. Stan Reed, Dr. Doug Richards, Dr. Knox Ritchie, Ms. Monika Riutort, Dr. Wendy Roberts, Dr. Michael Robinette, Dr. Walter Rosser, Dr. Miriam Rossi, Dr. Bruce Rowat, Dr. Lawrence Rubin, Dr. Jim Ruderman, Dr. John Rutka, Dr. Diane Sacks, Dr. Daniel

Sadowski, Dr. Issac Sakinofsky, Dr. Russell Schachar, Dr. Richard Schabas, Dr. Ricky Schachter, Dr. Allan Scomovic, Ms. Mary Sharpe, Dr. David Shaul, Dr. Morris Sherman, Dr. Harvey Skinner, Dr. Linda Short, Dr. Ken Shulman, Dr. Allan Slomovic, Dr. Douglas Snell, Dr. Paul Steinhauer, Dr. Leonard Sternberg, Dr. Donna Stewart, Dr. Gordon Sussman, Dr. Donald Sutherland, Dr. Richard Swinson, Dr. William Tatton, Dr. John Trachtenberg, Dr. Joan Vale, Dr. Sarah VanderBurgh, Dr. Hillar Vellend, Dr. Mladin Vranic, Dr. Philip Wade, Dr. Evelyn Wallace, Ms. Earlene Wasik, Dr. John Wherrett, Ms. Joan Wright, Dr. Trevor Young, Dr. Barry Zimmerman, Dr. Stanley Zlotkin.

Finally, I must thank my family and friends for their forbearance during the years that I worked on the book for long hours, seven days a week, devoting too little time or attention to them.

What is good health all about?

What is health? • Measuring health • Changing attitudes to healthcare • How to assess health news

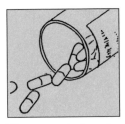

WHAT IS HEALTH?

There is no universally accepted definition of health. The meaning of health has changed through the ages and across different cultures. The term derives from the Anglo-Saxon word "haelth," meaning safe, sound or whole. The term "disease" generally refers to a diagnosable physical or biochemical abnormality, while "illness" means the personal experience of sickness, the perceived suffering and disability due to a disorder. In other words, disease is what the doctors say you have, while illness is what you feel.

Today's public seems to have immense faith in medical technology, believing that whatever ails them will somehow be cured by modern therapeutics. Many people in Western cultures confidently expect medical expertise to provide a cure or "technological fix" for almost every ill. And people seem transfixed by the torrent of publicity accompanying every new medical announcement, no matter how equivocal the research finding, no matter how experimental the treatment. With the help of medical progress, and through personal fitness efforts, people hope to escape disease, conquer life's everyday ailments and even evade the decline of aging.

Although the health improvements seen during the last century are popularly attributed to advances in medical science, historian Thomas McKeown concluded in his 1976 study of the British population that many of the health improvements in the nineteenth and early twentieth centuries actually predated most of the major medical discoveries. Far from being due to medical progress, the improved health status of the British population was the result of smaller family size, a cleaner environment, better hygiene, water purification and improvements in food production and distribution. To this day, the major predictors of health in various populations are things like education, lack of poverty, social networks and positive work experiences.

From the mid-1900s onwards, medical practice has been largely based on a *biomedical* model that has focused more on curing illness than preventing it. During the past few decades, North American medical practitioners have concentrated mainly on identifying diseases and dividing them into categories—for example, targeting a "cirrhotic liver" or "ischemic heart" for treatment. This method tended to separate physical from psychological problems, which were sometimes dismissed as "all in the head." Even today, many tend to focus on the physical aspects of a health concern, rather than recognizing the underlying psychiatric sources of their problem. The reluctance to disclose emotional and psychological distress and the emphasis on physical complaints can confuse care givers, delaying diagnosis and appropriate treatment of mental health disorders. People may hesitate to acknowledge emotional or psychiatric symptoms because of the continuing social and

1

THE BASICS OF HEALTH

Health depends on four essentials: biology—the "genes" or body you're born with; a health-promoting environment—clean air and water, no excessive noise or other pollution; lifestyle—good diet, avoiding smoking or excess alcohol intake; and the quality and accessibility of healthcare.

Putting the WHO definition into more concrete terms, good health demands:

- enough food and shelter; adequate income;
- good hygiene—clean air and water supplies and adequate sewage disposal;
- a stable, secure and health-promoting environment;
- physical fitness;
- lifestyle factors that enhance physical fitness—adequate exercise, sound sleep, not smoking, avoiding excess alcohol and other health-harming drugs; eating a low-fat diet; avoiding needless injuries (e.g., by using seatbelts and bike helmets);
- the ability to meet crises and environmental challenges;
- self-responsibility in looking after health and dealing with illness—together with chosen healthcare providers;
- emotional balance—healthy self-esteem, "feeling good" about oneself;
- mental health—the ability to cope with stress and emergencies;
- social well-being—forging intimate relationships, interacting effectively with other people;
- a nonaggravating interaction with the environment—for example, avoiding contaminants that may worsen personal ailments (such as hay fever, asthma);
- access to adequate medical care when needed.

cultural stigma surrounding mental health disorders, and for fear of being labeled as weak or inadequate. Yet, greater awareness of the fact that optimizing mental well being can help solve many health problems, and even be the complete solution for some, would go a long way in improving our society's health.

Modern views of health

Views of health and illness are now undergoing radical changes in meaning and perception. The idea of health as the "absence of disease or infirmity" is shifting to an image of an "optimal state of well-being for body and mind." The emerging *biopsychosocial* model of health regards mind, spirit and body as one intertwined unit and tries to treat people less mechanistically, as "whole persons," paying more attention to emotional, psychological and social factors. Health is no longer viewed as something that "just happens" by luck, fate, chance or good genes, but as a positive asset that people can work toward. Health promotion and disease prevention are today's mottos. But to achieve health, people need the information necessary to make sensible choices, and they need a supportive,

health-promoting environment. This has become especially important as people live longer but often with such chronic diseases as arthritis, heart disease and/or depression.

In 1948 the World Health Organization (WHO) defined health as a "state of complete physical, mental and social wellbeing, encompassing the ability to achieve full potential, deal with crises and meet environmental challenges." In other words, health—or wellness, to use a trendy term—is the capacity to respond favorably to physical effort, to live within one's own potential and carry out tasks with vigor and alertness, leaving enough energy to meet unforeseen emergencies. Although many health professionals and lay people still adhere to the "freedom from disease" concept, the WHO definition has profoundly altered views of health and healthcare. By implying that health is a positive resource that people can work toward rather than an inbuilt feature in those lucky enough to avoid disease, the new definition suggests that people have a fair measure of control over their health.

The concept of health given in the 1986 Ottawa Charter for Health Promotion goes still further, outlining the fundamentals for health as: "Peace, shelter, education, food, income, a stable ecosystem, sustainable resources, social justice and equity"—prerequisites that go far beyond what has traditionally been considered necessary for health. For example, people can't easily remain healthy if there's a lack of food, or if the air is polluted, or during wartime when they're anxious about being killed. The Ottawa Charter also stressed that health is a means rather than an end in itself: "A resource for everyday life, not the objective of living." Rather than spending inordinate amounts of money on curing disorders that could be prevented, it suggested, we should allocate more funds for education and disease-prevention.

Just being fit isn't it!

In search of good health and longevity, many contemporary North Americans devote endless time and effort to fitness. They jog, do aerobics, watch their weight, restrict cholesterol intake, and get annual medical checkups. The quest for fitness leads them to spend considerable time caring for their bodies—on exercise bicycles and rowing machines, in swimming pools, weight rooms, saunas, whirlpools and massage centers, learning how to breathe, conquer stress, manage low back pain, eat sensibly and erase wrinkles.

To acquire a fashionably lean body, some slavishly follow the latest exercise or diet fads. One only has to look at the current popularity of the Atkins or other "low-carb" diets to see not only individual but cultural obsession. Fixated on the pursuit of thinness, many no longer exercise "for fun," or to enjoy the marvels of the human body. They do their workouts with grim-faced determination devoid of pleasure—not to increase cardiovascular fitness or muscular strength—but merely to become or stay thin. Beyond any health benefits, some people seem to view fitness as a way to purify the soul and become a nobler person. Fitness—equated not only with the sought-after slender look, but also with "success"—is seen as an end in itself, so that any malaise or sign of illness seems like an affront. The slightest tinge of unwellness, even everyday aches and twinges, may seem worrisome and send people scurrying to the doctor.

Yet, as one University of Toronto expert puts it, "Just being fit isn't it!" Although physical fitness—for example, acquiring muscular strength and flexibility and maintaining desirable weight—is a prerequisite for well-being, fitness alone doesn't guarantee good health. Being physically fit when mentally unbalanced, "stressed out," socially isolated or emotionally disturbed doesn't add up to good health. And exercising obsessively not only increases the risk of sports injuries but may jeopardize family and social life.

MEASURING HEALTH

Since the WHO definition of health came out, many researchers have tried to measure its main components—namely, physical, mental and social well-being. Not surprisingly, efforts have concentrated on physical health, the dimension easiest to measure. However even that is an elusive property. For example, some people diagnosed with a disease such as arthritis or diabetes may feel perfectly healthy and function well. Or older people with disabilities such as osteoporosis or atherosclerosis may consider

themselves in "excellent health for someone of their age"—a common viewpoint, especially among those with an optimistic outlook.

People living in various cultures perceive health and disease in various ways, tolerating different degrees of pain and discomfort. And the perception of health and illness also varies vastly from one person to another. Two different people with the same disease may experience it very differently. While one person may express agony from a small cut or splinter, another may stoically put up with a far worse wound, bruise or other ailment.

Take as examples a man who inherited a polycystic kidney disease that destroyed both kidneys by midlife. Even though he requires thrice-weekly dialysis (after two failed kidney transplants), he nonetheless enjoys a "healthy life" in which he swims three times a week, walks to work and pursues an active professional career. Similarly, a woman bank employee considers herself "healthy" even though she lost one breast to cancer 15 years ago, and suffers from arthritis and carpal tunnel syndrome (pinched wrist nerve), for which she wears a wrist splint at night. In contrast, we all know healthy people with no physical disorders who perceive their health to be quite poor. Interestingly, self-perception of one's health (regardless of actual physical health) is a strong predictor of quality of life.

The placebo effect

The discrepancy between objective disease and its subjective experience is well illustrated by the placebo effect, where inert substances known as placebos—"dummy drugs"—provide relief from a wide range of disorders even though they contain no biologically active ingredient against the conditions being treated. For instance, plain sugar or chalk gives relief to many people who think they are taking "real drugs" and believe in their healing powers. Other factors, such as the size and color of the pill, can also predict effect. Medical and surgical procedures can also act as placebos, even if they have no true curative action. In a recent trial for knee problems, surgeons either did the operation they thought would work or they just made a small incision in the knee to make it seem as if

TO ASSESS THE VALIDITY OF A HEALTH REPORT, ASK SOME BASIC QUESTIONS

- **What procedure or therapy is being described, what is the outcome (end-point) and do you care about it? (for example, a slight change in "trabecular bone mass" may be of interest to scientists but you are more interested in interventions that prevent a hip fracture).**

  Are the people in the study like you? If they are not like you, it is difficult to generalize. (Many studies are done on special high-risk populations to prove a point and to increase the likelihood of disease or adverse events occurring so the study needs fewer people).
- **Is the study "randomized," with people selected by chance and similar in both experimental and control groups?**

(The hormone replacement or HRT studies are a good example. Many postmenopausal women were put on HRT because of data from non-randomized trials. When randomized control trials were introduced, they didn't show the big improvements in heart disease and osteoporosis that had been hoped for.)
- **How many test subjects "fell by the wayside"— perhaps leaving too few by the end of the study? (This has become less of an issue, but many early trials didn't mention the people who dropped out of the trial for good or bad reasons and only told us about the people who completed the trial. Results for the total group that started at the begin-**

ning is a better reflection of reality.
- **How well "blinded" was it? Were both doctors and test-subjects unaware which group people were in?**
- **How significant is the effect found? Superior to other treatments? How do the results compare to those of other studies? (Many trials may show some benefit but the extent of this benefit is very small or not worth the side effects or hassle).**
- **Who financed the study—is there any conflict of interest? (The reality is that most drug trials are financed by the pharmaceutical industry which has a built-in desire to show a positive result. This is why the above questions are so important to ask in order to be confident about the results.)**

they had operated. The incision was just as effective as the operation.

Evidence from many studies indicates that about one-third of those treated with placebos obtain symptomatic relief for conditions such as postoperative discomfort, chest pain, stomach upsets and motion sickness. This result can be as high as 50 to 60 percent, in, for example, trials with Irritable Bowel Syndrome. People treated with placebos improve because of faith in the "healer" (physician) and because they expect a pill or procedure to be effective. If it's *expected* to work, the method will likely afford relief. An even more remarkable finding is that 10 percent of people receiving placebos report that the fake drug causes unpleasant side effects such as

skin itching, diarrhea and nausea—effects similar to those found among people taking the chemically active equivalent.

Mental and social health are harder to measure than physical health, although efforts have been made to do so. Given the subjective nature of social health, assessing it can be challenging because there are many diverse but equally satisfactory ways of functioning socially. Just as health is hard to quantify, so is sickness. At one end of the wellness spectrum are "perfectly healthy" individuals with no diagnosable diseases who have a sense of control over their lives, see change as a challenge rather than as a threat, have no significant symptoms of "disease" (unwellness) and feel energetic, satisfied with their social, spiritual, occupational and personal existence.

Elsewhere on the scale are those with recognized and diagnosed disorders. The state labeled "disease" represents conditions with detectable symptoms and abnormalities as well as "silent" diseases such as high blood pressure, which although demonstrably present may not exhibit symptoms or be felt by the sufferers. At other points on the scale are those who feel "vaguely ill" or "out of sorts"—people with a vague sense of "dis-ease" that isn't diagnosable or easily explained by conventional medicine.

Many of us are the "worried well"

Although North Americans on the whole are a remarkably healthy lot, with an increased life expectancy, many of us worry unduly about our health and want to be still "healthier." As U.S. physician Dr. Arthur Barsky writes in his book *Worried Sick*: "Our sense of physical wellbeing has not kept pace with the improvements in our collective health status…there is a pervasive atmosphere of dis-ease. The ability to appreciate good health and achieve a secure feeling of physical well-being eludes us." Dr. Barsky sees us as a society in headlong pursuit of health and medical care. "Wellness," he concludes, "has become something deliberately and consciously sought after. Good health, seen as an end in itself and not just as a means to other goals such as family and professional life, has become an imperative, a sort of supervalue that symbolizes personal achievement, self-esteem, and willpower."

USEFUL TERMS TO KNOW

- A *placebo* is an inactive substance (or procedure) given to a control group to parallel the treatment being investigated. Placebos are necessary to check the efficacy of a treatment being studied. As mentioned earlier, about one-third of test subjects react positively to any treatment, active or inactive, perhaps because of the expectation of benefit. But in time, if the drug or procedure is effective, it will outperform the placebo.

- A *clinical trial* is an investigation of human beings—not animals—done to observe the effect of some kind of intervention (treatment, drug or procedure), often in a hospital.

- *Epidemiological research* is the study of the determinants and distribution of disease. It attempts to discover the risk factors for certain diseases by describing the frequency and distribution of exposures (health-related events) in human populations.

- A *control group* is a group of people used for comparison. The experimental or trial group takes the drug or has the procedure, and the control group gets either the best available current therapy, no treatment or a placebo. Both groups should be very similar in terms of risk for the diseases of study.

- A *randomized controlled trial* (RCT) is the "gold standard" of studies in which decisions about who makes up the trial group and the control group are made *randomly* (the "flip of a coin" method), not by personal choice or preference, to eliminate bias.

- A *case-control* study looks backward in time to compare past exposure to certain factors in people with the problem or disease being studied ("cases") with exposure in people without the disease ("controls"). For example, over the years many studies have found that tobacco smoking is far more common in those with lung cancer than in those without. Case-control studies do not prove anything, but indicate a possible link.

- A *clinical trial or experimental study* (experiment) is done forward in time, and with tight controls, to establish a direct cause-and-effect link—for example, to show that a new drug works better than a currently used one.

- A *survey* examines a limited group of people. Its results can be extended to a larger population only if the sample is representative of the larger population. For example, the results of a survey of young athletes may have little application to the population at large.

- A *meta-analysis* is an analysis of pooled results from many studies to determine whether a procedure, treatment or test really has an effect or alters outcome (health or survival).

- A *double-blind study* is one where neither the participants nor the researchers know which people are in the experimental group and which are in the control group. Double-blind studies are used to eliminate unconscious bias or other psychological effects among the researchers.

- *Anecdotal evidence* is word-of-mouth testimony or hearsay, based on a few cases, rather than statistically significant scientific evidence. However, accumulating anecdotal evidence (such as several people alleging that "something in the office air is making my throat sore") often leads to a hypothesis or theory which can then be tested through a scientific study.

Almost every aspect of daily life is scrutinized for its health implications and labeled healthful or harmful—making everyday actions into a series of "prescribed" and "forbidden" behaviors. In the name of health, foods are dubbed as "good" (life-prolonging) or "bad" (health-harming) according to the latest fad—instead of being regarded as nutrients for the body. Our society's idealization of thinness has made even people of normal weight feel fat and somehow to blame for today's natural biological tendency towards a larger body size (partly because of better nutrition in the Western world). Personal habits, diet and leisure activities are constantly modified in line with the latest publicity about what constitutes a healthy lifestyle and a desirable "look."

New "evidence-based" approach to medical practice

Ironically, while many people are turning to "natural" methods, medical practice is undergoing a radical shift and becoming more "evidence-based," with decisions about patient care being based on the best available current research evidence. The term "evidence-based medicine" (EBM) was coined by researchers at Ontario's McMaster University during the late 1970s, and the idea has since caught on across the world. It sprang from the astounding discovery that only about 20 percent of commonly used childbirth practices were backed by scientific evidence. Some routine obstetric procedures such as pre-delivery enemas and episiotomies were not only useless but often harmful (and since abandoned). Similarly, some common cardiac treatments not

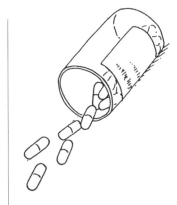

COMMON ERRORS IN EVALUATING MEDICAL NEWS

- Too much readiness to believe the popular press;
- overreliance on the competence and objectivity of the media;
- uncritical willingness to jump to unwarranted conclusions;
- belief that unchallenged information is necessarily accurate;
- too little time spent by reporters checking facts and making sure that they understand them clearly;
- too little background material provided to journalists;
- failure to realize that health stories are often cut, altered and shaped to meet media constraints;
- unawareness among the medical community of the pervasive public faith in "media messages";
- understanding that the need for a high-impact headline that sells is typically more of a driver than a balanced and complete review of a topic.

only didn't strengthen, but in fact weakened, failing hearts.

Past medical practice relied largely on observation, clinical experience and the opinions of accepted "authorities." The way of the future is to base treatment decisions and patient care on solid evidence from well-conducted clinical trials. Evidence-based practice de-emphasizes anecdotal observations and instead calls for trials that have outcomes that people care about. While today's physicians must still acquire clinical and diagnostic "instincts," they also need to develop new doctor-skills to keep up with and evaluate research findings. In order to track down the best current procedure or treatment for a particular problem, physicians must learn how to scan the medical literature and distinguish strong from shaky findings. Essentially, EBM integrates clinical expertise with judicious use of results from good randomized trials.

The *randomized, controlled trial* (RCT) is the "gold standard" of medical studies in which people are assigned to the test (treatment) group, or to the "control" (non-treatment) group, by a completely random process. Using the "play of chance" to decide whether people receive the procedure to be tested—or an alternative (or no) treatment—is the best safeguard against bias. Analyzing the pooled results from many RCTs that are looking at many findings in a "meta-analysis" can be especially helpful in showing doctors what's effective and what isn't. New guidelines founded on meta-analyses are fast emerging (for instance, from international networks such as the Cochrane Collaboration and Oxford's Bandolier) to help with day to-day healthcare decisions.

CHANGING ATTITUDES TO HEALTHCARE

Critics of our healthcare system castigate it as too technological, distant and inhumane. The older traditional model of healthcare is therefore gradually being replaced by a broader more humane and user-friendly model, where the authoritarian attitude is giving way to a more egalitarian approach. This method is often called "patient-centered medicine." The restricted "absence-of-disease" concept is being replaced by a flexible, multidimensional view of health. The patient is increasingly seen as a partner in health transactions rather than as a passive recipient of treatment. Some of the responsibility and decision-making in healthcare is shifting onto the consumer or patient, instead of being put entirely on the professional caregivers. Thus, looking after health or disease is becoming more of a collaboration between consumers and health professionals. This paradigm has become increasingly important as people are now being seen as the "quarterbacks" of their own disease management both for chronic disease and basic self-care.

While some people may still opt for the quick medical fix, preferring to know little about it, many now want to be educated healthcare consumers. They prefer to understand what's wrong with them and what treatments are proposed, to weigh up the options and to participate in their own health management. Studies show that well-informed healthcare consumers who take an active role in discussing and selecting their treatment feel more in control. They generally stay healthier and recover faster from disease and/or surgery, than those who don't share the responsibility.

In some ways, taking responsibility for one's own health is a demanding role that not everyone is prepared for or wishes to accept. In becoming part of the healthcare team, people are expected to read up on their ailments and take an active part in managing them. Some studies investigating the call for greater patient participation in the decision-making process find a duality or mixed reactions. While people want to be informed and welcome the opportunity to participate, they still look to healthcare professionals for a great deal of guidance. The call to be "better informed" and take more part in decisions also has its down side, as some health-conscious people may regard sickness as a slur on their character something that's entirely their own fault. Yet it is absurd to think or expect that all illness will vanish or be avoided simply by one's own efforts. Just as death is inevitable, there will always be diseases that afflict us.

Many medical schools now emphasize the need for physicians to understand the impact of illness, improve their communication skills and become better listeners. Sick people are generally anxious and seek help not only for physical ills but also for social and emotional problems. Ideally, anything that produces distress and affects health—be it physical, emotional or spiritual—should be taken into consideration by the attending physician. In many centers, medical education is emphasizing care by non-hospital, community-based healthcare workers. More and more, healthcare is moving from hospitals and other institutions to care in the home by visiting professionals which is less expensive and often brings swifter improvement.

Consumers seeking medical attention can help to conserve healthcare dollars by learning how to access and use the system appropriately—for example, by finding a trusted family physician to look after minor and everyday health concerns, rather than using expensive emergency services for this purpose, and by altering their lifestyle to avoid illness.

Health and the Internet

The Internet has revolutionized the ability of many people to make informed medical decisions about managing their health and illness. Consumers can rapidly access reams of information about any health topic. Unfortunately, while there is no shortage of health portals, there is certainly a shortage of high- quality resources. Random searches have led many people down the path to "cyberchondria" as they self-diagnose themselves with deadly diseases based on a few symptoms. A collection of excellent websites can be found at www.mini-med.utoronto.ca by going to the site and clicking on "student resources." Of particular note are three sites: /medlineplus (http://medlineplus.gov; a one-stop-shopping site), Hitting the Headlines (http://www.nelh.nhs.uk) a UK service that reviews different headlines for study quality and www.healthyOntario.com (a local health portal). A good general rule is that if the site is trying to sell you something, it is likely unreliable. And while hearing from other individuals with the disease in question is helpful, it is important that you keep this information in perspective and view it as the experience of one person who may be biased. When available, blinded randomized control trials are the most trusted source of information.

BEWARE THE SLIPPERY SLOPE OF WORDS

- **"Doctor" may mean a physician or someone with a Ph.D. in some subject other than medicine, such as chemistry, philosophy, theology or physiology.**
- **"May" does not mean "will."**
- **"In some people" does not mean "in everyone."**
- **"Indicates" does not mean "proves" or "confirms."**
- **"Contributes to," "is linked to" or "is associated with" does not mean "causes."**
- **"Proves" refers to** conclusions based on scientific evidence systematically amassed in several studies. (One study, taken alone, seldom proves anything.)
- **A "breakthrough" is a rare happening— for example, the discovery of penicillin or the development of the polio vaccine are rare events.**
- **"Doubles the risk" may or may not be meaningful, depending on the risk in the first place. If the risk was one in a million and is now doubled,** that's still only one in 500,000. But if the risk was one in 100 and it doubles, it's now one in 50 and a real cause for worry.
- **Studies comparing "before" and "after" effects are not as scientifically valid as controlled studies because comparing past with present treatment introduces too many variables. Two procedures are best compared simultaneously to avoid bias and eliminate coincidental factors.**

HOW TO ASSESS HEALTH NEWS

Beset by medical reports of all kinds, our society is obsessed with health issues. Many of us are intensely curious about medical, health and nutritional news. Newspapers devote entire sections to lifestyle topics, and TV programs regularly cover medical issues. We are deluged with messages and services designed to make us fitter and help us stay young, ward off disease and expunge every complaint. The print and broadcast media are today's main sources of health information. With each passing month, a different disease is highly publicized to explain vague discomforts and afflictions—such as Yuppie flu (chronic fatigue syndrome), candidiasis or 20th-century allergy syndrome. Even the most preliminary research findings may be trumpeted and mislabeled as a breakthrough, spawning a press conference, torrents of publicity and sometimes, cruelly raised hopes. Many of these "announcements" are messages skilfully crafted by the pharmaceutical industry's public relations firms for a particular target market. These messages are often delayed in goodwill to raise awareness of the disorder, but have the net effect of making many of us wonder if we are truly well. There is a famous saying in medicine that a well patient is an "un-worked-up patient."

All too many people bring no critical

appraisal skills to the health news they hear unquestioningly believing whatever they are told. They don't know how to assess medical news and easily jump to false conclusions based on phrases such as "suggests," "increases risks" or "contributes to." In fact, many pay less heed to what they're told in a doctor's office than what they read in the popular press—perhaps because it's easier to absorb information at home than in an anxiety-provoking clinical atmosphere.

Many people don't realize that, on the whole, journalists don't regard themselves as educators but as information conveyors who try to report findings as accurately as possible. Unfortunately, health news is often poorly reported and simplified to the point of distortion. The media tend to "humanize" complex medical topics with personal anecdotes or dramatized images, sometimes sacrificing accuracy. Some of those reporting on health stories have little or no background knowledge of scientific matters. Many a reporter sent to cover medical issues is diverted from a regular sports, crime or entertainment beat. Moreover, the material handed in by journalists is frequently changed by desk editors, producers and others in charge, to fit available space, to adhere to the organization's image or even to please financial backers.

Direct to Consumer Advertising
An emerging area of health media is "direct to consumer" (DTC) advertising. Most of us have seen the ads that touch on a common concern (anxiety, heartburn, acne) and tell us that solutions are awaiting us, but then end with a rapid overview of negative side-effects. The advertising for products for erectile dysfunction are a good example of the pros and cons of this kind of marketing. On the one hand, this is a common problem that men find difficult to mention or discuss, yet for which medication is quite effective. The ads make it easier for men to flag the problem for their doctors. This is all good, but problem is that the ads oversimplify human intimacy and one gets the sense that after a man takes the pill, the couple will have a perfect sex life. As is true with most advertising, key messages are distilled, simplifying a complex health issue that can be misrepresented. DTC advertising certainly improves awareness of important

preventable diseases, but it can also be anxiety provoking for consumers as each campaign increases the public worry about diseases they do not have. Perhaps if we could have unbiased resources giving balanced media reports, we might be able to strike a happy medium between information and scare-mongering.

Bridging the communication gap
For the public to evaluate health stories better and for medical scientists to get their message across more reliably, all must consider the constraints of the communication networks. People must learn to assess medical news more critically, bearing in mind not only the quality of the information but the limits of the medium through which it's being conveyed. The trick is to use a bit of skepticism.

Working within a tight time-frame, reporters can easily distort the facts, especially when trying to render their piece interesting or to make the front page. Moreover, items handed in by the reporter may later be topped by an eye-catching headline—possibly one chosen hours before the item was even handed in. A health story may be truncated again at the last moment and key phrases or qualifying clauses chopped out for space reasons. Even the most assiduous and responsible of news reporters seldom has time to check and recheck the facts. But it's crucial not to over-sensationalize material which could be misinterpreted in the rush of getting a story out.

Health professionals should familiarize themselves with the way in which the different media put together news items, remembering the pressure under which many journalists work, with copy often processed at breakneck speed. They can help to avoid the perils of distortion by capsuling their message in the right way and rehearsing it beforehand. Many successful medical communicators use a succinct "pyramid" style, stating the key message (the discovery, advance or results) first, then explaining why the finding is useful, supporting it with relevant background material. Routinely translating complex jargon into lay terms can help to get the message right, and scientists can make themselves available for last-minute telephone checking.

Cultivating a healthier lifestyle

Preventable illnesses • Assessing your lifestyle • The risks of smoking • Weight control is crucial to good health • Getting enough exercise • Sleep hygiene and sleep disorders • Preventing needless injuries • Putting drug use in perspective • Tackling alcohol abuse • Sensible drinking tips

PREVENTABLE ILLNESSES

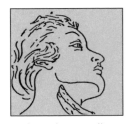

Much disability and early death stems from diseases caused by lifestyle. The foremost causes of death in North America today—heart disease, cancer strokes, liver cirrhosis, diabetes, unintentional injuries and suicide—are largely self-induced. What's needed is more illness prevention, employing strategies to get people not to smoke, to eat lower-fat, heart-healthy diets, to get enough exercise, to moderate alcohol intake, to steer clear of other health-harming drugs, to avoid needless injuries and to foster emotional health.

A *Computerized Lifestyle Assessment* program, developed at the University of Toronto's behavioral science department, provides a quick, confidential way of assessing your lifestyle strengths and weaknesses, giving a printout about activities that upgrade or undermine health. For instance, a woman who thinks she leads an exemplary life—who exercises daily, eats a balanced vegetarian diet, doesn't smoke, drink or take drugs—may be in poor health due to emotional problems stemming from her obsessive traits and lack of social supports. Or a man with good work and social relationships, who doesn't smoke and has a moderate alcohol intake, may endanger his life by being overweight (with high blood pressure, the beginnings of diabetes and a potential heart problem).

OVERCOMING THE RISKS OF SMOKING

2

Tobacco smoking is known to be dangerous, yet 21 percent of Canadians still smoke, and smoking remains the number-one preventable cause of death and disease in North America. In Canada smoking causes 40,000 preventable deaths each year—about 20 percent of all annual deaths. It is responsible for an estimated 30 percent of all cancers, one-third of heart-disease fatalities and 85 percent of deaths due to lung cancer. On a positive note, it appears that the number of smokers is declining. According to the latest results from the Canadian Tobacco Use Monitoring Survey (CTUMS), for data collected between February and December 2003, over 5 million people, representing roughly 21 percent of the population age 15 years and older, were current smokers, of which 17 percent reported smoking daily. Approximately 23 percent of men were current smokers, higher than the proportion of women (18 percent). The decline in smoking among youth 15–19 years continued in 2003 to 18 percent, with 12 percent reporting daily smoking and 7 percent occasional smoking. This is a decrease from 22 percent in 2002 and is a 10 percentage-point improvement from 28 percent in 1999, when CTUMS was first conducted. Slightly more teen girls reported smoking than boys (20 percent vs 17 percent). However, among daily smokers, boys smoke slightly more cigarettes per day (13.0) than girls (11.7). The tragedy is that many young people are still lighting up, usually while still in school. Smoking schoolmates inspire others to try cigarettes. Canadian surveys show that smoking usually begins in adolescence. The earlier someone starts smoking, the greater the danger of addiction and death from a tobacco-related disease. Out of every 100,000 smokers half will eventually die from a tobacco habit acquired in adolescence.

Most teens know that smoking causes lung cancer and aggravates respiratory ills (such as bronchitis and asthma) but are unaware of the grim reality that smoking causes a wide range of other tobacco-related disorders such as heart disease, hearing loss, cataracts, various cancers (of the throat, bladder kidneys and stomach), infertility (in men) and reproductive difficulties in women. Among women, lung cancer has now outstripped breast cancer in North America as the major cancer killer of women. Yet, the tobacco companies continue their relentless portrayal of cigarette smoking as "cool" and "empowering."

The good news is that many former smokers have given up. Faced with the undisputed reality of its health dangers and the inescapable truth that "smoking kills," together with escalating bans on smoking, nearly half of all living North Americans who ever smoked have quit. On another positive note, Canada is a world leader in nonsmoking policies and controls—in establishing smoke-free environments, curbing ads, restricting workplace smoking and issuing health warnings. In fact, smokers have almost become social outcasts—forced to sneak outside and huddle with their cigarettes. They're becoming society's butts for not butting out, and for continuing a practice that's not only self-destructive but also harms others.

Secondhand or environmental tobacco smoke also harms

The adverse effects of environmental tobacco smoke (ETS)—secondhand smoke—have become blatantly clear. ETS is a complex mixture of smoke escaping from a tobacco product plus that exhaled by smokers. It contains 50 known carcinogens (cancer-causing chemicals)

and six developmental or reproductive toxins that affect reproductive health—possibly causing cervical cancer, increasing the risk of spontaneous abortion and decreasing the rate of fetal growth.

Environmental tobacco smoke causes lung cancer—held responsible for 3,000 U.S. cases annually—and it increases the risk of coronary heart disease and nasal sinus cancers. (Spousal smoking increases the risk of death from heart disease or stroke in nonsmoking partners.) Children are at particular risk from ETS. In the year 2000 in Canada, 25 percent of the 2.4 million households with children under the age of 12 reported regular exposure of these children to ETS in the home from cigarettes, cigars or pipes. This appears to be a substantial improvement from 1996/97, when there were smokers in 33 percent of such homes. Nevertheless, this means that approximately 900,000 children under the age of 12 continue to be regularly exposed to ETS at home. Considering that an additional 760,000 children between the ages of 12 and 17 were also regularly exposed to tobacco smoke at home in 2000, this means that over 1.6 million children under the age of 18 have increased risks for health and of taking up smoking. Children living in smoke-ridden households are at increased risk of developing asthma, and of having ear infections and respiratory illness.

Shaking tobacco's addictive hold isn't easy

Stopping smoking is not an event, it 's a process. To anyone who's ever tried to quit smoking or watched someone else try, it's obvious that stopping is no easy task. Nicotine is a psychoactive drug that affects a person's mood, alertness, ability to concentrate and relaxation. Despite tobacco company claims to the contrary, nicotine is highly addictive.

The U.S. Surgeon General's 1988 report stated that "cigarettes and other forms of tobacco are just as addicting as heroin and cocaine, illegal drugs regarded by most adults with scorn and disapproval (if not outrage)." The urge to maintain blood levels of nicotine and stave off withdrawal symptoms is clearly shown by those who brave a snowstorm in the middle of the night to replenish supplies.

KEY STEPS TO BETTER HEALTH

- **Not smoking tobacco;**
- **maintaining a desirable weight;**
- **exercising sufficiently;**
- **getting enough sound sleep;**
- **avoiding accidental injuries;**
- **moderating alcohol use;**
- **avoiding other health-harming drugs;**
- **coping with stress;**
- **fostering family and social relationships;**
- **looking after emotional needs.**

Withdrawal symptoms frequently undermine quitting efforts

Of those who manage to quit, 20 percent succeed at the first try, and 50 percent take six tries to stop. When someone stops smoking, the nicotine deprivation often provokes a swift and unpleasant withdrawal effect that's a common reason for would-be quitters to light up again. While physical withdrawal symptoms, which peak at 48–96 hours, generally subside in about a week and are gone within a month, the psychological dependence may linger on.

Symptoms of nicotine withdrawal include:
- a slowed heart rate;
- difficulty concentrating;
- reduced cognitive (thinking) ability;
- irritability, anger;
- anxiety ("the jitters"), restlessness, insomnia;
- tremors (nervous shaking);
- headaches;
- slight dizziness or "spaced-out" sensation;
- tingling or numbness in the arms and legs;
- greater hunger especially for sweets;
- increased coughing, because smoking paralyzes the hair-like cilia that naturally clean the lungs; coughing occurs as the cilia regain their cleansing action and subsides once normal function returns;
- a craving for and incessant thoughts about smoking. Half of those who relapse say they light up again because of it. Some quitters mourn as though they'd lost an old friend and source of comfort.

Physiological withdrawal symptoms can be reduced by nicotine replacement from chewing gum or skin patches. But nicotine substitution therapy is best used together with counseling. Since psychological dependence may outlast nicotine's physical hold, cessation programs focus equally on overcoming behavior and habits, helping ex-smokers develop a nonsmoking self-image.

Quitting tactics: "If at first you don't succeed—try, try again"

Almost 80 percent of smokers claim they'd like to stop, especially if there's an easy way to do it! Most tobacco smokers have tried to quit at some time in their lives (over 60 percent have tried to quit at least once) and the average smoker attempts to quit 4 to 11 times before achieving success. It's never too late to quit. Of those who succeed, 90 percent quit on their own—often "cold turkey"—just with the support of family and friends. In 2003, the Canadian Tobacco Use Monitoring Survey asked smokers and former smokers who had quit or tried to quit in the past two years what methods they had used to help them quit (respondents could identify one or more methods used in their quit attempts). Of those who attempted to quit (successful or not) most (55 percent) reported reducing the number of cigarettes they smoked. Many (31 percent) used the nicotine patch including 10 percent of 15–19 year olds and 38 percent of those 45 years and older. The next most common method (25 percent) was making a deal with a friend or family member to quit together. As well, many smokers had seen a doctor (71 percent) in the year before the survey. Of these, more than half (53 percent) had been advised to reduce or quit smoking by their doctor and 60 percent of those had been given information on quit-smoking aids such as the nicotine patch or counseling programs.

Treatment methods include self-help guides, behavioral therapy, pharmacotherapy—such as nicotine replacement or Bupropion (Zyban), a medication that helps combat addiction—and many other methods. Most cigarette smokers who quit manage to do so with self-help methods rather than through formal programs. Repeated quitting attempt usually pay off, many smokers "give up" half a dozen times before finally managing to stop for good. Drug therapy effectively doubles your chances of quitting, but not all want to use this method. Combined strategies, such as using nicotine replacement therapy together with behavioral intervention or Bupropion, generally work best. Other methods such as acupuncture, hypnosis, and various electronic aids may work for some, but haven't been shown effective in controlled studies.

Not all smokers find it equally hard to quit. The least dependent or lightest smokers—those who smoke fewer than 10 cigarettes a day—find it easiest to stop. About 30 percent of heavy smokers find it "fairly difficult" and 19 percent call it "very tough" to stop smoking. Those who reach for a cigarette within 30 minutes of

FIGHTING THE FIVE "A's" THAT PERPETUATE SMOKING

- **Addiction.** Nicotine in tobacco is among the most powerful and rapidly absorbed psychoactive (mood-altering) substances known, at least as addictive as heroin. It is now formally listed as an addictive substance, and nicotine addiction is labeled the "Tobacco Dependence Disorder." Tragically, the incentive to quit often comes only after a heart attack or other serious tobacco-related illness. Even then, it's hard for many to stop—witness the post-bypass patient who surreptitiously escapes to light up in the visitors' room.
- **Advertising** by tobacco companies is a major contributor: a powerful campaign against good sense and good health, promoting a habit that kills millions annually. With so much bad press about smoking, tobacco companies are seeking new markets for their dangerous products, especially in developing countries, where consumption—even among children—is rising rapidly. The tobacco industry spends billions to associate tobacco with glamour, success and sophistication. In its battle to seduce recruits, the industry must strive incessantly to counter evidence that cigarette smoking is unhealthy.

- **Acceptance** of tobacco use, in contrast to other addictive drugs such as alcohol or heroin, supports the popular view of smoking as a pleasurable and tension-releasing pastime with which to "fill lonely hours," "mark occasions," "solve problems" or "be companionable." Paradoxically, while society deplores the use of illicit drugs—which kill a couple of dozen Canadians annually—it tends to ignore the 30,000-plus annual deaths from smoking.
- **Apathy**—the "I've heard it all before" or "It won't happen to me" or "I'll never manage to quit anyway" syndrome—keeps many people smoking, as does neglect by physicians in not stressing the dangers of smoking or not assisting people to quit. Many smokers don't bother to try stopping because they believe that "nothing works" and quitting is just too tough.
- **The Awareness Gap** is the persistent ignorance about what smoking does to the body. As one official from Canada's Laboratory Centre for Disease Control says: "Many smokers still remain unconvinced that inhaling tobacco smoke—either their own or that of others—harms health."

awakening, or before getting out of bed, are usually the most addicted. They need more quitting determination and support than those who can wait until after breakfast for their first cigarette! Having once stopped, many ex-smokers relapse at times of crisis.

Recognizing the dangers of smoking helps many quit

While most people are vaguely aware that smoking is bad for their health, many don't know just how it damages the body. Surveys reveal that close to half of all smokers are totally unaware that smoking shortens life expectancy by 10 to 15 years and that, as well as lung cancer smoking is a major cause of emphysema, heart disease and stroke; it also increases the risk of stomach ulcers and cancers of the colon, kidney, mouth, throat, pancreas, bladder vulva and cervix. Nor do most people realize that sharing a home with a smoker for several years increases their chances of dying from lung cancer or heart disease. Women smokers often don't realize that the habit can harm their repro-

ductive system, damage an unborn child—by stunting its growth—put babies at increased risk of sudden infant death syndrome, and possibly diminish a child's future learning capacities. Few smokers know (or they may deny) that second-hand smoke damages children, increasing their risk of respiratory illness as well as encouraging them to smoke later on.

Physicians can play a major role in helping smokers overcome the addiction by actively supporting those who want to quit. Quitting advice from a healthcare professional (perhaps listing the damaging effects of smoking) carries more weight than what's heard elsewhere. Trials of smoking-cessation programs find that physician counseling improves success rates by 6 percent. But many doctors don't know much about cessation techniques, and aren't set up to assist quitters. The family physician can personalize the situation by referring to the smoker's health status, family background and medical history. Physicians can also prescribe nicotine substitutes to help smokers through the early withdrawal stages.

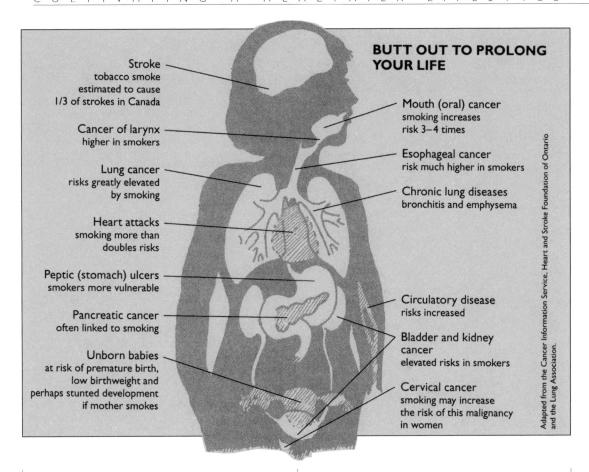

BUTT OUT TO PROLONG YOUR LIFE

Stroke
tobacco smoke estimated to cause 1/3 of strokes in Canada

Cancer of larynx
higher in smokers

Lung cancer
risks greatly elevated by smoking

Heart attacks
smoking more than doubles risks

Peptic (stomach) ulcers
smokers more vulnerable

Pancreatic cancer
often linked to smoking

Unborn babies
at risk of premature birth, low birthweight and perhaps stunted development if mother smokes

Mouth (oral) cancer
smoking increases risk 3–4 times

Esophageal cancer
risk much higher in smokers

Chronic lung diseases
bronchitis and emphysema

Circulatory disease
risks increased

Bladder and kidney cancer
elevated risks in smokers

Cervical cancer
smoking may increase the risk of this malignancy in women

Adapted from the Cancer Information Service, Heart and Stroke Foundation of Ontario and the Lung Association.

Smokers sometimes believe that changing brands or switching to "light" cigarettes will lower their health risks. But switching to lighter brands won't guarantee lower exposure to nicotine or tobacco's toxins, because those who smoke "light" or "ultra light" cigarettes often unconsciously alter their smoking habits (e.g., puff harder or cover vent-holes) and absorb just as much nicotine and tar. By taking a "deeper drag" they may actually increase the risks of lung cancer because they inhale more deeply.

Success in conquering tobacco addiction requires motivation, serious commitment, planning and the "right moment." Those who just idly think about "stopping sometime" are less likely to succeed than those who find definite reasons and set a specific time for doing so. Finding a strong personal reason for quitting, whatever it is, is a critical step in making the choice to become a nonsmoker. Those who succeed are fully aware why they chose to stop. Remember—it can take six to eight tries, but it's worth it!

Stop "cold turkey" rather than tapering down

The ability to quit is highly individual. Some people stop "cold turkey" while others taper off slowly. Although millions have succeeded with either approach, studies indicate that withdrawal symptoms subside faster for smokers who stop completely than for those who gradually cut down.

Cutting down is often self-defeating, unless it's a preparatory step to quitting. Studies show that those who taper off may find it extra hard to quit, and will generally change their smoking manner to get more from each drag. A Canadian study on smoking which used blood tests to measure nicotine levels before and after reducing the number of cigarettes found that participants who smoked an average of 37 cigarettes a day achieved only slightly lower blood levels of nicotine when they cut down to 10–15 cigarettes daily. Their blood-nicotine levels went down less than expected because they took more puffs from each cigarette and inhaled more deeply to compensate for the smaller number smoked. Most smokers didn't

BASIC QUITTING STAGES

- **Pre-contemplation:** At this stage you are not actively considering change. You are not prepared to plan for change, often feel that you are unable to do so, and may rationalize your reluctance by concluding that the cons outweigh the pros. You are often in a state of *denial.*
- **Contemplation:** You are now considering changing your behavior, but are not ready to do so. You have conflicting feelings and thoughts about making changes in your life. This ambivalence is often uncomfortable. You may have a low sense of self-confidence regarding accomplishing the task that prevents you from making a commitment.
  - Consider and discuss fears, concerns and potential roadblocks to change
  - Identify potential risks and rewards associated with change
  - Observe patterns in your behavior , e.g. make an eating diary
- Let your friends offer you support and assistance when you feel ready to change.
- **Preparation:** At this stage you are seriously considering changing and are often willing to commit to starting the process. You are generally anxious about your ability to change. This is when you start making small changes and develop strategies to avoid or overcome your addiction cues.
- **Action:** You are ready to set a quit date and choose the quitting strategy. You need positive reinforcement and likely some quitting aid (e.g. Zyban, nicotine replacement, and/or gum). As well, you build on your preparations by implementing strategies to manage your own smoking patterns and the cues that spark the smoking urge, identifying difficult moments and likely lighting-up temptations and planning to avoid them. Problem-solving with professionals or friends is key.
- **Maintenance, maintaining cessation:** You need to be aware of your previous reasons for resuming addiction. Typically, this involves a "slippery slope" issue where you "just have one cigarette" when out with friends or at a stressful time. It should be noted that **relapse** is extremely common and is in fact another stage to learn from.
  Note: knowing the stages of change are especially helpful when counseling a friend or loved one. It is highly unlikely that you can get somebody to move two stages at once, but if you can get somebody to move even one stage, you will certainly deserve a sense of accomplishment.

difficult to generalize, people who smoke less than 10 cigarettes a day may have less need for nicotine replacement and other smoking cessation aids. Often the focus for these people is to see or imagine themselves as "non-smokers."

Set a target quit date

Casting off the smoking habit takes energy, attention and scheduling, plus all the support a would-be quitter can muster. Smokers must change their habitual response to countless daily cues and plan ahead how not to smoke when having a cup of coffee, reading the paper or dealing with a crisis. Timing is critical: choose a convenient time to stop smoking, preferably during a nonstressful period. Trying to break the habit during a difficult time at work or at home will only make it harder. Having said this, it is unlikely that there will ever be a "perfect" time.

Discuss the intention to quit with a sympathetic, knowledgeable person, preferably someone who really understands the problems and wants you to succeed. Check out the resources and cessation guides beforehand. Countless aids and stop-smoking programs are now available from many health agencies and hospitals. Surveys reveal that 90 percent of smokers prefer to quit on their own—perhaps aided by pamphlets, books, guides or videos. On the appointed day, either stop altogether or cut back according to your personal agenda. On the big day, keep very busy—plan an outing or shopping spree, go to a movie or attend a favorite sports event.

Nicotine-substitution therapy tides many over withdrawal pangs

Substitution therapy using nicotine in various delivery systems, from chewing gum to skin patches, or from inhalers and nasal sprays, is a crucial part of many quitting plans. There are two key aspects to addiction: 1) the actual nicotine addiction and 2) behavior patterns. This second aspect might involve a social trigger or just the fact that you are used to bringing your hand to your face many, many times a day. While addictive, most of the negative health impact of a cigarette is not the nicotine— it is all the toxic ingredients in the tobacco (about 4,000 in all, 50 of which are known cancer-

mind cutting their daily intake by about half, but complained bitterly when asked to smoke less than that. The remaining cigarettes were not only more avidly smoked, but offered greater pleasure, increasing the chance of backsliding to full smoking.

Smokers who gradually reduce their blood nicotine level may live in a state of constant withdrawal. The longer the body goes without a cigarette, the lower the blood nicotine drops and the more pleasurable the next smoke becomes. After cutting down to 12 or fewer cigarettes daily, many reach a point beyond which they just can't reduce. This is why experts urge people to quit "cold turkey" once they've cut down to 12–15 cigarettes a day. Although it is causers). The amount of substitute nicotine supplied by gum or patch is more consistent than the nicotine supply from cigarettes because it goes into the blood stream more slowly, avoiding the peak "highs." The first rule in substitution therapy is not to smoke at the same time that you are using it. By easing the impact of the nicotine withdrawal, smokers can tackle the behavioral aspects of smoking and then slowly wean themselves off the nicotine by using substitutes of increasingly lower strengths.

Nicotine gum

Nicotine chewing gum is available in 2- and 4-mg formulations (with the latter needing a prescription). The 2-mg formulation is recommended for those who smoke fewer than 25 cigarettes a day, and the 4-mg formulation is for those who smoke more. The scheduled dosage of 1 or 2 pieces of gum per hour gives better results than as-needed usage. The manufacturer's usual recommendations are to use the gum for 6 weeks and then taper use over another 6 weeks. However, much longer usage has not been associated with any increase in adverse effects. Nicotine gum may taste odd at first, but many chewers quickly get used to it. Since each chew releases a little nicotine, chewing must be slow, with pauses of a few seconds between chews. This is called "chew and park" and the gum should not be used for more than 30 minutes. Chewers carry the nicotine gum with them at all times, perhaps keeping it where they formerly stored their cigarettes. Side effects of the gum—a bad taste, upset stomach, hiccups and a sore mouth—are usually mild enough to allow continued use.

Patching up smokers

Nicotine skin patches overcome some of the side effects of nicotine gum and provide an easier way for some to get replacement nicotine into the bloodstream. The patches, such as the Nicoderm, Habitrol, ProStep and Nicotrol brands, deliver nicotine through the skin. Prescribed by a physician, the nicotine patch looks like a square or round Band-Aid. Usually prescribed for a 10–12-week course, patches should be applied to hairless areas of the skin, and the site changed daily to prevent irritation.

Habitrol, Nicoderm and ProStep are changed every 24 hours, whereas Nicotrol is applied first thing in the morning and removed at bedtime (16 hours of use). Nicotrol is not available in Canada. The patch comes in strengths of 21, 14, 11 or 7 mg. The strongest patch achieves blood nicotine concentrations equivalent to about half that supplied by smoking a pack to a pack and a half a day. Nicotine patches are used in a gradual, step-down fashion, starting with the highest strength for four to six weeks, then the 14 mg dose for a few weeks and lastly the weakest patch. Success rates improve if nicotine substitution is used together with supportive therapy, especially if given by a health professional.

The inner membrane or control system of the patch releases nicotine steadily into the bloodstream, avoiding the highs provided by cigarettes. While 24-hour use may stave off early-morning craving, some users experience insomnia, vivid dreams or nightmares, so many decide to leave it off at night. The patch may cause skin itching or burning in some, or (less often) a rash, inflammation and an occasional allergic reaction. The commonest side effects are minor skin irritation (reddening and itchiness) at the application site and insomnia for those patched overnight.

Those who still feel edgy or desperately want to smoke may supplement with nicotine gum or an extra 7 mg patch for especially stressful occasions. For someone on one of the weaker patches, an extra 7 mg patch can safely be used in times of need. But since the patch contains a potent drug, it must be kept away from children, pets and nonusers. Always discard patches (folded up) after use, and trash safely. Report any side effects noticed.

Many studies confirm that wearing the patch diminishes the symptoms of nicotine withdrawal. It decreases the craving for tobacco and the restlessness, irritability, anxiety and loss of concentration frequent in those who quit. With the physical distress lessened, quitters can concentrate on overcoming the behavioral aspects of their addiction. Eventually, users are weaned off the drug, and ideally they remain both smoke- and patch-free. But when users ultimately give up their patches, some "grieve" over the loss of their nicotine fix.

GETTING THE MOST OUT OF NICOTINE PATCHES

- **Put the patch on every day at the same time.**
- **Put it on at quit day or the night before (as this may reduce early-morning craving).**
- **If wearing the patch for the full 24 hours causes insomnia, consider removing it at night, although this may lead to greater early morning cravings.**
- **Change the site daily to avoid skin irritation.**
- **Wear the patch in the bath or shower or while swimming.**
- **Carry nicotine gum to prevent relapse in stressful situations.**
- **Remember that the patch is not suitable for people with serious heart problems, pregnant women or those with chronic skin disorders.**

RUNDOWN OF SMOKING-CESSATION AIDS

- Self-help print materials and manuals for "going it alone" provide a simple approach for the many smokers who prefer to quit on their own. For publications, consult local health units, local branches of the Lung Association, Heart and Stroke Foundation and Cancer Society, local drug-abuse services, Ontario's Addiction Research Foundation and the Non-Smokers' Rights Association.
- Formal cessation clinics, programs and classes are run by local health agencies, hospitals, work-site or other organizations—on either a profit or a nonprofit basis. Many include pre-course activities, such as charting smoking patterns, scheduling a quit date and practicing stress-coping techniques. Most cessation programs also teach behavior-modification techniques, such as cue-extinction (to avoid smoking triggers), stress management, a self-reward system and relapse-avoidance training.
- Nicotine substitution therapy—with nicotine supplied by a less harmful delivery system, such as chewing gum, skin patch or inhaler (just becoming available)—helps many smokers give up tobacco. It's best used as part of an overall cessation program.
- Smoke Stoppers, run by the National (Canadian) Centre for Health Promotion, is a program designed by formerly smoking healthcare professionals. Participants quit cold turkey partway through the five-week program.
- Smokenders Canada Ltd. is a six-week program to help smokers reduce their cigarette intake gradually while learning to change habits, reactions and behaviors associated with smoking.
- Acupuncture, an ancient Oriental art, may suppress the desire to smoke. Needles are put into the outer ear and left in place between treatments, to be stimulated whenever the smoking urge surfaces. Acupuncture may make cigarettes taste odd and dull the wish to smoke. Acupuncturists usually perform three to five treatments and may refuse to do more if it doesn't work. There has not been any high quality research showing that acupuncture is better than placebo-.
- Laser therapy (or laser acupuncture) is a method that claims high success rates, but hasn't yet been scientifically validated. Using laser beams on acupuncture points may reduce nicotine craving.
- Hypnosis, a popular smoking-cessation aid, is sometimes called the "quick route to behavior modification." It is offered in individual or group sessions, on a once-only or repeat basis. Prices and credentials vary widely and don't necessarily correlate with expertise or success rates. Hypnotic suggestion makes smoking seem so undesirable that people develop headaches or become nauseated if they light up. Positive reinforcement helps people feel virtuous for not lighting up. Hypnosis won't help everyone but may be worth a try for those who fail with other methods. However, anybody can practice hypnosis, so get a professional referral. Again, there have been no high quality trials showing evidence that it is better than placebo.
- "Magic" filters are not that magical! Some cigarette filters claim to help smokers "taper down" to zero. Available in drugstores and supermarkets, kits usually cost under $20. For instance, One Step at a Time (produced by Teledyne) has four reusable filters that eliminate 20, 50, 70 and 90 percent of the tar and nicotine. The filters are used over an eight-week period. One serious flaw is that smokers may simply smoke more cigarettes or inhale more deeply to compensate for the decreased tobacco products. Studies show that many who try Teledyne filters get stuck at the fourth filter stage, unable to quit completely.
- There are also over-the-counter antismoking medicines: certain lozenges aim to make cigarettes taste bad by causing an unpleasant body reaction to nicotine. (Unlike Nicorette gum, they do not contain nicotine.) For example, silver acetate, ammonium chloride and carboxylase (an enzyme) in such products as Healthbreak lozenges or BanSmoke gum interact with nicotine to make it taste foul. Although widely promoted, none of these products has been scientifically proven effective.
- Local hotlines or buddy-calling systems can help smokers quit at low cost; hotlines give callers quitting information and a reading list. One Ontario hotline found that of callers who attempted to stop, 21 percent had quit for at least a week and were also abstinent at a six-month follow-up.

Success rates for the patch are good—up to 40 percent remaining nonsmokers. Placebo-controlled trials find the nicotine patch to be about twice as effective as dummy patches in helping people to quit. Quit rates averaged 17 percent for one year 12 percent for two years. The patch can be combined with Bupropion (Zyban) or Nortriptyline.

Medications for quitting

Bupropion (Zyban') has now been shown to be very effective in helping with smoking cessation. The bupropion molecule is the same as that of Wellbutrin ' and therefore they should not be taken together. We are not totally sure how Zyban works, but it affects dopamine production. Nicotine stimulates the release of dopamine in the brain and it is the effect of this neurotransmitter than leads to "feeling good" after a cigarette. A 7-week course of sustained-release bupropion in doses of either 150 mg once a day or 300 mg a day (in two 150 mg doses daily) given to smokers with no history of depression resulted in abstinence rates at 1 year of 23 percent compared with 12 percent among control subjects. In this study weight gain among abstainers was greatest for those taking a placebo and least for those taking 300 mg of bupropion daily. Another study compared bupropion (150 mg twice a day), the nicotine patch alone, the nicotine patch plus bupropion (150 mg twice a day) and placebo over a 9-week period. At the end of 1 year, abstinence rates were 30 percent in the bupropion-only group, 36 percent in the bupropion plus patch group, and about 16 percent in the placebo- and patch-only groups. Bupropion has been found to be effective in smokers not intending to quit as well as those with COPD (lung disease) and those who previously relapsed to smoking after nicotine replacement therapy (NRT) or bupropion.

SOME QUIT TIPS FOR BUTTIN' OUT

- Recognize that nicotine in tobacco is addictive.
- Realize that it's difficult but not impossible to quit.
- Find a personal motive for choosing not to smoke.
- List reasons for stopping and post in a prominent spot—near phone or desk pad.
- Put cigarettes in new, inaccessible places; buy one pack at a time, preferably least-favored brands.
- Limit smoking to outdoors until ready to quit.
- Be skeptical of those who say they gave up "completely alone" or just "walked away from it"—a huge understatement for the complex behavior involved in combating nicotine addiction. They probably got much support from family, friends, colleagues, a persuasive physician and the rising cost of cigarettes.

  Don't just think of why you shouldn't smoke, but why you do (e.g., to improve concentration, take a break at work, for camaraderie, etc.). Awareness of the reasons for smoking can help people develop a more pragmatic quit-strategy.
- Feel good even about buying no more cigarettes or throwing out all ashtrays—a gigantic step forward.
- Congratulate yourself on the decision to liberate yourself from smoking.
- Publicize your intention to quit.
- Recruit support from family, workmates and friends.
- Choose a definite target date and select a method that suits your needs, starting with the simplest. easiest, and cheapest—understanding that no approach is likely to be effortless.
- Celebrate each smoke-free day, week or month. Reward the accomplishment.
- Focus on the immediate benefits of butting out—improved blood circulation, reduced heart-attack risks, better exercise tolerance, sweeter smell, whiter teeth, money saved, social acceptance.
- Expect to overcome hurdles but anticipate possible relapses. Repeated tries improve coping skills and raise the odds for ultimate success.
- Practice cue-extinction to overcome smoking triggers and arm yourself in advance to cope with crisis situations that could sabotage quitting plans.
- Plan how to avoid relapses at stressful or socially tempting times—especially in the first weeks after quitting.
- Don't dwell on a single failure—rejoice for even a few smoke-free days; next time will be easier.
- Try not to be overly judgmental or hard on yourself if goals aren't reached. Instead of saying "I failed," tell yourself "It didn't work this time around," or "I am one step nearer to success."
- Analyze the reasons why a method didn't work.
- Try any new strategy, unless it's hazardous or outrageously over-priced.
- Remember that the only real failure in smoking cessation is the failure to try again.
- Above all, keep trying!

The antidepressant, nortriptyline (Aventyl, Pamelor), in doses of 50 to 100 mg/day, has also been shown to increase abstinence rates among smokers with and without a history of depression.

Fears of post-quitting weight gain are exaggerated

Some smokers go on smoking for fear of gaining weight. Some quitters actually lose weight, but most do gain an average of about 4.4 kg (10 lbs). To offset possible weight gain, quitters can exercise more and replace fat-rich snacks with less calorific items, fulfilling the desire for oral satisfaction by chewing sugarless gum or crunching carrot sticks. In any case, a bit of extra weight is far less of a health risk than smoking. It is also important to recognize that by stopping smoking you will increase your exercise capacity and, therefore, your long-term ability to manage your weight by more activity.

The benefits of quitting start almost at once

The immediate benefits of not smoking can fortify a smoker's resolve to stop. The cardiovascular benefits and reduction in heart attack risks begin within 30 minutes of the last smoke: the pulse rate slows down and blood pressure drops toward normal. Within hours of the last smoke, the blood's carbon monoxide levels go down, reviving its oxygen-carrying capacity. A couple of days later nerve endings begin to recover revitalizing the sense of smell and taste. Within 72 hours of smoking cessation, the lung's bronchial tubes expand, enhancing exercise capacity. In the months after quitting, shortness of breath noticeably decreases. In both men and women, heart-attack risks decline markedly in the year after quitting and are largely back to nonsmoking levels two to three years later. The greatest benefits occur within the first 3 to 5 years of giving up tobacco. And 15 years after quitting, the increased cancer risks due to smoking revert to normal levels. The survival benefits of *not* smoking also hold true after age 65. It's worthwhile even for seniors to quit.

Where to get quitting help

A dizzying array of smoking-cessation aids, pro-grams and guides is now available, varying from ways to make cigarettes seem undesirable to stress management, nicotine fading (using progressively stronger cigarette filters), pharmacotherapy—which includes nicotine substitution by gum or skin patch and dopamine-modulators to overcome the pleasurable stimulus—acupuncture, laser therapy and hypnosis. There are formal programs run by companies and nonprofit groups, costs varying from zero to $500; many hospitals now offer free quitting information. Although some programs allege that paying good money makes quitters try harder; cost does not predict whether or not an antismoking program will be effective. The higher price may simply attract more motivated quitters. Programs that tackle psychological as well as physical problems usually work best.

It's wise to ignore touted success rates and select a method that seems appealing. Cited success rates for quit programs range from 15 to 30 percent (except for programs that also use Nicorette gum or nicotine patches—which may have higher success rates). In selecting a quit-smoking program, remember that no single quitting method suits everyone. Smokers often do best with several cessation approaches. Women, for example, often prefer group therapy while men tend to opt for physician advice. If one method doesn't work, try another!

Useful websites include:
- quitnet.com
- quitsmoking.about.com
- gosmokefree.ca/cessation
- stopsmokingcenter.net/
- surgeongeneral.gov/tobacco/default.htm

Health Canada Quit Tools:
http://www.hc-sc.gc.ca/hecs-sesc/tobacco/ quitting/index.html#tools

For more information, call the Health Canada toll-free telephone line: 1-877-513-5333.

WEIGHT CONTROL IS CRUCIAL TO GOOD HEALTH

Second to tobacco smoking, obesity is now the leading cause of preventable illness and death in North America. The number of overweight people in the developed world has risen dramatically in the last decade, to the point where obesity is called an "epidemic," even dubbed a "pandemic" (worldwide disorder) by the World Health Organization.

"Cosmetic obesity," which confers no health risks, differs from "medical obesity," which endangers health and increases risks of diabetes, hypertension, cardiovascular disease and several cancers. In the U.S., 33 percent of the population—about 60 million people—are sufficiently overweight to qualify as medically obese. Similarly, about one-third of Canadians aged 18 to 74 are overweight. The reasons for the excess weight are complex, but add up to an excessive calorie intake and a sedentary lifestyle that burns too little energy. Modern urban life, with people using cars for even the shortest shopping trip, means that less and less energy is used while food becomes ever more calorie-dense, palatable and easily available.

Changing medical approach to obesity

In the past, obesity was generally thought to result from weakness, lack of self-control and the irresponsible choice to "overeat and under-exercise." It's now recognized as a consequence of genetic, environmental, behavioral and social influences. Modern medical experts call obesity "a chronic disorder of multifactorial origins that responds poorly to treatment and needs long-term therapy and attention." As one University of Toronto expert puts it, "Obesity remains one of the world's most intractable disorders and the difficulty of reversing it is as well known to physicians as to their discouraged patients." Only about five percent of the obese manage to shed unwanted pounds permanently; the other 90 to 95 percent regain or pass their starting weights within a year or two.

Given the difficulty of losing weight, the slightly overweight—who consider a few extra pounds cosmetically undesirable and strive to lose them—are urged to accept a few extra pounds. According to international experts such as the late Dr. Hilde Bruch and Dr. John Garrow, we've carried our obsession with slimness to absurd extremes, forcing even moderate fatties to aim unrealistically for a shape that's unnatural to their biological makeup. The current view is that obesity needs aggressive treatment only if it

threatens health. Those in whom the excess weight doesn't endanger health are advised to "live comfortably with a slight degree of excess weight rather than subject themselves to the stress of repeated dieting."

What weight is overweight?

People are considered medically obese if they are 20 percent or more above their "ideal" weight as stated on standard weight/height tables. This can be measured by the *body mass index* or BMI which is the weight in kilograms divided by the height in meters squared. A BMI of 20–25 is considered within the healthy range; a BMI of 25–27 is the "gray area" with possible weight-linked health risks, and a BMI over 28 qualifies someone as "obese." A chart to plot your weight and height is often available at your doctor's office. A BMI over 28 gives a fourfold increase in the risks of diabetes, stroke and heart attack; and a BMI of 29 to 30 gives a 50 to 60 percent higher risk of early death than in those with BMIs of 25 to 27. People who are muscular can be falsely called obese, and those who have large stomachs but skinny legs ("potato-on-a-toothpick" bodies) can be falsely labeled with a low BMI. To assess BMI, the metrically challenged can take weight in pounds and multiply it by 703 and divide it by the height in inches squared. Therefore for a 180 lb. person who is 5 foot 5 inches tall (65 inches) – 180 × 703 = 126, 540, divided by 65 × 65 (4,225) = 29.9.

Waist circumference (WC) and the waist–hip ratio (WHR)

New ways of measuring obesity and the risk that comes with it are the waist circumference and waist–hip ratio. These measure "truncal obesity," the size of the belly or tummy, which is a key predictor of cardiac risk.

- Measured at the end of normal expiration, while the person is standing with feet hip width apart, find smallest measurement below the rib cage and above the belly button. For WHR, compare it to the widest part around the hips.
- The World Health Organization states that more than 102 cm or 40 inches in men and over 88 cm or 35 inches in women indicates a

KNOWN HEALTH RISKS OF OBESITY

- **hypertension (elevated blood pressure)**
- **glucose intolerance (build-up of blood sugar)**
- **insulin resistance (failure of body cells to use insulin normally)**
- **diabetes (non-insulin-dependent diabetes mellitus)**
- **gall bladder disease**
- **disturbed blood lipid (fat) profile**
- **arthritic and other joint problems**
- **cancer (increased risk of breast and uterine cancer in post-menopausal women, risk of prostate and colon cancer in men)**
- **sleep apnea (obstructed breathing)**
- **psychological problems such as depression and low self-esteem**
- **social stigma, difficulty finding jobs.**

DIET THERAPISTS ADVISE A MULTIPRONGED APPROACH, INCLUDING:

- a sound food plan to meet all nutrient needs;
- development of self-management skills for changing eating behavior;
- avoiding total fasting—now considered dangerous because it alters the enzyme pathways, which catalyze and regulate fat buildup or breakdown; 70 percent of the loss through fasting is fluid, protein and muscle, which are all regained when the fast ends.
- possibly trying a brief course of drug therapy with appetite-reducing medication, under doctor supervision. These tactics rarely provide a long-lasting

solution, but they can help people kick-start their program.
- daily planned exercise using large muscle groups (legs, arms), such as walking, cycling, skiing or swimming, to encourage weight loss and, as an added bonus, to reduce appetite;
- self-acceptance at a weight slightly above that suggested by reference tables;
- understanding that at times overeating lapses will occur, and that this is not a catastrophe;
- no pressure to reach impossible weight goals;
- a positive support system, enlisting help

from physicians, relatives and friends;
- no illusions about "quick" cures that promise rapid reduction;
- rejecting the dieting concept, since this implies "going on" and therefore eventually "going off" a regime;
- recognition that the main goal is not just to lose but to keep weight off, by aiming for gradual (i.e., 0.5–1 kg, or 1–2 lb, weekly) loss with permanent changes in eating habits;
- behavior modification, whereby an eating-disorder specialist helps the person relearn eating habits and revamp lifestyles.

high risk for diabetes, hypertension and coronary heart disease. The renowned U.S. Nurses' Health Study reported that women with waist circumferences of 76.2 cm (30 inches) or greater had over twice the risk for coronary artery disease compared with thinner women.

- According to the appropriately named Lean and Associates, health risks are significant for waist–hip ratios of more than 0.95 for men and 0.80 for women. The Nurses' Health Study found that women with a waist–hip ratio greater than 0.75 had over double the usual risk for coronary artery disease.

Currently, 31 percent of Canadian adults are obese, with a BMI over 27. The health risks of obesity include raised blood pressure, blood lipid changes (high cholesterol), heart disease, diabetes (which increases risks of premature death from cardiovascular disease) and various cancers (prostate and bowel cancer in men, breast and uterine cancers in women). Analysis

of the Framingham Heart Study data showed a 3–7 year decrease in life expectancy among obese individuals compared to persons of normal weight. Obesity is also linked to psychological disorders such as depression. In addition, it's a social handicap leading to discrimination, reduced educational opportunities, difficulty finding jobs, poverty and failure to enjoy family life.

Where and how fat is deposited also counts

Fat over the abdomen (shown by the waist-to-hip ratio) is most likely to increase health dangers. When men put on weight, the fat accumulates largely around the trunk or belly giving an "apple shape." In women, fat stores tend to increase all over the body, and in particular on the thighs and buttocks, giving a tapered "pear" look.

Why are we getting fatter?

The simple answer is more calories in (through eating) and fewer calories out (by activity). However, many influences contribute to obesity, including social, genetic and cultural factors. For example, twin studies suggest that about 70 percent of the influence on body weight is genetic, while about 30 percent is environmental. Twins brought up in different eating environments have strikingly similar BMIs. Another example would be the technological changes in our society that diminish activity, such as power windows, computers, food processors, and escalators. One estimate puts the loss of activity from these "advances" at 11 lbs. a year, which would explain why so many of us find ourselves on the home jogging machine. Other more insidious causes of obesity include suburban planning (no sidewalks), computer and video games. Many American and Canadian children watch 4 or more hours of television daily, and two-thirds watch at least 2 hours a day. These figures don't count the time spent playing video games, watching videos, and working or playing on computers.

Having said this, one key reason for the rise in obesity is an increased consumption of high-energy/calorie foods. Many of the obese cling to the false belief that they have low metabolic

SOME PRACTICAL TIPS FOR WEIGHT CONTROL

- Reduce food intake (but not below 1,000–1,200 calories daily for women, and 1,200–1,600 for men and adolescents), relying on low-fat foods and emphasizing grains, fruit and vegetables. Recent studies suggest that the body transforms dietary fat into fat stores more smoothly than starches and sugars, so be especially wary of high-fat foods.
- Go for a gradual weight loss not exceeding 1 kg (2.2 lb) weekly.
- Plan an increase in daily and weekly physical activity.
- Choose a weight-loss regime that offers variety and fits your lifestyle—preferably one planned by someone with good nutritional credentials (e.g., a registered dietitian, hospital nutritionist or physician knowledgeable about eating disorders). Weight Watchers is often recommended by professionals.
- Be supervised by a trained nutritionist or physician if substantially restricting your food intake.
- Aim for permanently improved eating patterns. Remember that changes must be forever—you can't revert to your old ways once the weight is lost.
- Realize that obesity is due to many factors, some biological, some psychological, each needing attention.
- Remember to eat slowly, avoid packaged fatty snacks, go easy on salad dressings and processed foods, bake or poach rather than fry foods.
- Find enjoyable treats to replace food, such as gardening, walks, movies, visits to friends.

rates, reduced energy needs or hormonal disorders, although investigators don't find such disorders to be more common in the obese than in lean individuals. "Considering that most people put one and half tons of food into their mouths each year" notes one nutritional scientist, "it's amazing that they don't pay more attention to its composition and impact. There's a crying need for better nutritional advice and more medical school training about the causes, risks and treatment of obesity, and more empathetic management." Simply put, we are getting fatter because we eat too much and exercise too little. Stated scientifically, we take in more energy (calories) than is given out in activity. A person who regularly takes in more energy than is expended—even as little as two percent more—will gain about 2.3 kg (5 lb) of fat tissue per year. The average North American gains 9.1 kg (20 lb) of weight from age 20 to 55.

Self-deception or "underestimating the calories consumed" may also contribute. In one study, 60 percent of the obese claimed to be "small eaters" but grossly under-reported their energy (food) intakes. Many of the overweight eat a scanty breakfast and lunch, but consume large amounts at and after dinner which can add up to thousands of extra calories. Some are night bingers who don't count the snacks or binges eaten as a "meal." Controlling obesity is more than just saying "no" to food. It means altering lifestyle, eating behavior and exercise habits.

Genes contribute but aren't the primary cause

Research has recently uncovered some 20 genes that contribute to obesity. Not surprisingly, given the difficulty our ancestors had in finding food, fat genes tend to be energy-conserving. But the changing environment of the modern developed world, with its abundance of cheap, palatable, highly calorific foods and increasing inactivity, means that genes which predispose us to lay down fat might be "maladaptive." One Quebec expert explains that "genes alone aren't to blame for the obesity epidemic. The human gene pool hasn't changed in thousands of years, so environment and behavior must be the main reasons." Today's increasingly low activity rates play a key role.

Our bodies may be programmed to defend a "set weight"

The "set-point" theory holds that the body naturally settles to a stable weight, as if programmed for it (much as a thermostat keeps the heat in a house steady). If valid, the set-point idea may help explain why most dieters fail miserably in their reducing efforts as the body struggles to defend its weight plateau.

In studies on prison volunteers where men were fed vast amounts of food (up to 10,000 calories a day), some became obese while others on identical fare consumed four times their usual dietary intake but gained less than expected. People vary in their ability to burn off extra calories. During the overfeeding phase, metabolic rate and body-heat produc-

CASE STUDY: SUCCESS AFTER AN UPHILL DIETING BATTLE

Janet grew up as the only child of immigrant parents who were proud of her early chubbiness. Her father, survivor of a concentration camp in Poland, also tended to be stout, and as his business expanded, so did his waistline. He had little time for Janet and was often traveling, secretly resentful of his daughter, as he'd wanted a son. Janet's mother, a slim social-climber occupied with her bridge club, volunteer work and cocktail parties, plied Janet with cookies and candy to keep her quiet, giving her little real attention. As Janet grew into a moon-faced, impassive schoolchild, she seemed to pick up every cold and other minor infection around. Now 47 and a mother of three, she recalls that "food had an overwhelming power over me. I'd be sitting eating in a cafe with no idea how I'd got there. My stomach owned me. I felt condemned by others—as I incriminated myself—for lack of willpower, for the inability to melt away my mounds of flesh."

When Janet was ten years old and weighed 58 kg (128 lb), the family doctor convinced her parents that she should reduce under medical care. Insulted at the mention of psychiatric counseling, her parents ignored his advice and continued to tempt her with strudel and cream. The pounds crept on until finally her parents realized that the plumpness which had seemed so endearing in early childhood was now shameful. After years of pressing food upon her, they suddenly began to watch her every bite. Defiant at the sudden reversal, Janet ate more than ever, becoming a grossly obese teenager. She was humiliated by the jeers of her peers. Her mother began to drag her from doctors to beauty parlors to reducing clinics.

"She badgered me to stop eating and moaned that no man would want so ugly a creature," recalls Janet. Like nearly all the obese, Janet hid behind her fat, using it as an excuse for failure, to explain why she gave up piano and had no friends. "As long as I stayed fat," she says, "I could avoid facing deeper issues, remain blameless, steer clear of sex and avoid possible rejection. The fat hid any feminine curves I might have had, helping me rationalize that if men didn't like me it was because of my size. My fat kept them away, preventing people from getting to know or reject the real me." In a way, she felt that her fat made her more important, more like her Dad, from whom she craved approval. "I was afraid that if I got thin I'd be shown up as a sham, a nothing."

In her twenties, however, Janet tried every dieting trick. No matter how stunning the temporary losses, the weight crept back. After a briefly slimmer phase at age 24, she gained some confidence, started to make friends and married. "But even after I married—partly to spite my mother, who'd said I'd never find a husband—the old food habits took over." Despite her happy marriage to an accountant, she still felt a complete flop, abandoning one university course after another, going from one weight-reducing strategy to the next. At age 32, she was more than 30 kg (70 lb) overweight for her 170-cm (five-foot-seven) height and delicate frame. Her husband tried to help but couldn't curb her binges.

As Janet once told her group reducing session, her two children, then five and seven, were mortified by her appearance but didn't dare mention it. "It took the children's disapproval for me to realize that I was in big trouble," she admits, "to see that I needed psychological help." Finally, the children's embarrassment, the aggravation of being fat, the leg chafing, the hindrance to job advancement, the need for two seats on the bus drove Janet to seek help from a sympathetic physician. Ultimately, she knew she had to tackle the deeper reasons for overeating. After a thorough medical examination, the doctor prescribed a supervised 1,000-calorie-a-day diet to bring her 96 kg (212 lb) down to manageable size and a walking program. Janet used a pedometer and aimed for 7,000 steps a day.

Janet kept a food diary, recording every morsel eaten, along with its caloric value. Like many other dieters, she got a rude shock to discover how she'd

tion went up in most of the volunteers so they burned more energy. When normally lean individuals became fat, they required more calories to maintain the excess weight than did the previously obese. By the same principle, when we diet, the body reacts as if starved and lowers its metabolic rate to conserve energy. These metabolic changes may persist even when the weight is lost and the diet ends. A formerly obese person requires about 15 percent fewer calories to maintain body weight than someone of similar build who was never obese.

What should be my target?

The amount of weight loss to aim for depends on the individual, but, in general, people set unrealistic goals such as their "wedding weight." Many aim to lose 30 percent or more of their weight, whereas the health and cardiovascular benefits are already achieved at 5–10 percent of initial weight loss.

kidded herself about the calories in that piece of cherry pie (about 400 calories) or handful of peanuts (440 calories per half cup). Her therapist cautioned her against gulping down food or compulsively clearing her own or her children's plates. "It's far better," she suggested, "to eat slowly, put less in the mouth and take time over a meal, because the brain's hunger receptors don't respond for 20 minutes or so."

Therapy helped Janet untangle her poor childhood relationships and boosted her ego. Her now aging mother was asked to stop nagging, and the family was advised that reproaches were counterproductive. They were asked instead to emphasize her good points—her quick wit, high intelligence and cheerful nature. Janet's children were asked to help themselves to dessert rather than putting it on the table, and to prepare their own meals for a while so Janet wouldn't get the urge to nibble.

About six months into her reducing program, Janet returned to college. Her exercise routine expanded to include swimming and more energetic aerobics. Janet won her battle against obesity in 18 months, to plateau at 65 kg (142 lb). For a while, her body image lagged behind her weight loss—she would be amazed that there was room for someone else to sit beside her on the bus, that she could get into a size 14 dress. Her changed self-image allowed her to pursue her career. She earned her B.Sc. and, at age 37, her Ph.D. A year later she was lecturing at the university, and at age 45 she became a full professor.

In bringing up her own children and looking after her grandchildren, Janet took special care not to repeat her parents' mistakes. She never overstuffed them, and didn't use food as a bribe or substitute for attention. She instilled in them a sensible attitude toward food—so that they would eat when hungry, not for attention—and a love of exercise. In other words, she practiced prevention—the best obesity cure of all.

Treatment: diet alone isn't enough

Treatments vary, but therapists agree that diet alone is not likely to keep weight off. The solution lies in comprehensive lifestyle changes and medical treatment when obesity threatens health. The best idea is to attack on several fronts—improve eating patterns, increase activity, have professional behavior therapy, and, if medically advised, try a session of doctor-supervised drug therapy. Surgery is a last resort.

Most physicians believe in actively treating obesity only if people have signs of weight-linked disorders such as diabetes or high blood pressure. Before suggesting therapy, they assess the family background (are mother, father or both obese?), the cardiovascular and blood lipid (fat) profiles, insulin action and glucose tolerance, thyroid hormones and fat distribution— whether it's mainly on the belly or more evenly distributed. Losing weight is hard, but keeping it off is the real battle, and modern therapy focuses on sustaining weight loss.

Why crash diets are such dismal failures

Very low-calorie diets (below 1,000 calories a day) can be hazardous, especially if prolonged. No diet with an energy content less than 1,000–1,200 calories should be undertaken without medical guidance. Once crash diets are stopped, the weight comes back fast, perhaps exceeding the previous amount.

Going on a diet is a false concept, since to lose weight successfully people must make life-long changes. Instead, many put their lives "on hold" until they've lost a planned amount, and then enthusiastically resume their old eating habits. Most dieters have a high relapse rate, with a resultant sense of failure. In one 1994 U.S. survey, dieters gained back on average two-thirds of the weight lost within a year, and five years later 95 percent had regained the entire lost weight or were even heavier. One reason for failure is that the initial weight loss is mostly water; also, dieters eating less than 1,200 calories a day may lose muscle (protein) before fat, thus weakening rather than thinning down their bodies. Moreover, in a crash diet the body adapts to restricted food intake, regarding it as a crisis that threatens survival. Given "starvation rations," the body lowers its metabolic rate and reroutes enzyme pathways to conserve energy, so that a little food goes farther. Once the diet stops, the enhanced energy-conserving pathways make weight gain faster than before. "Yo-yo dieting" might permanently reduce the body's metabolic rate and encourage fat storage.

Another argument against stringent diets is that they set up false expectations and impose monotonous eating patterns that cannot be kept up. The very idea of a "diet" suggests something short-term. Once the diet stops, bad

OBESITY IS UNDER COMPLEX REGULATION WHICH INVOLVES

- genes (family background)
- activity levels and energy expenditure
- energy intake—calories eaten
- food composition (relative amounts of carbohydrate and fat)
- sex hormones (such as estrogens, testosterone)
- corticoids and other "stress" hormones
- insulin and blood sugar regulation
- appetite-regulating signals from the gastrointestinal tract such as *cholecystokinin* (which reduces appetite) and *somatostatin* (which boosts appetite)
- central nervous "neurotransmitter" signals from the brain's hypothalamus—via substances such as "neuropeptide Y" (an appetite-stimulant) or "glucagon-like peptide I" (an appetite-suppressant)
- biochemical signals from fat tissue (e.g., leptin)
- childhood rearing patterns and psychological make-up

eating patterns return. Instead of strict "calorie counting" and "forbidden foods," many lose more easily on unrestricted low-fat, high-carbohydrate regimes. Eating more frequent small meals may also help. The exclusion principle—forbidding certain foods—leads to failures: no food should be taboo or it will become irresistible. Better to have a few mouthfuls of ice cream in the regime than to go on a binge.

Diets

U.S. studies demonstrate that at any one time 40 percent of women and 20 percent of men are on a diet. However, in most studies, one- to two-thirds of any initial weight loss is regained within a year and almost all of it within 5 years. There are no well-done diet trials showing long-term weight reduction. Recent work has focused on low-calorie (LCal) versus low-fat (LF) versus low carbohydrate diets (LC) such as the Atkins diet. In general, the LC show slightly better outcomes at the beginning, but the results tend to even out at a year. There are still concerns about the adverse effects of low-carbohydrate diets on other health parameters such as heart disease. The likely bottom line is that all diets work and none of them work. All diets work by giving us a "system" (e.g. reducing calories, regular weigh-ins), but most are hard to maintain over the long haul.

The Mediterranean Diet that is high in fruits, vegetables, legumes and whole grains has been examined for its impact on health outcomes rather than just weight loss. It includes fish, nuts and low-fat dairy products and emphasizes the use of olive oil. A recent Greek study showed that every 2-point increase (on a scale of 0–9 where 9 is perfect adherence to the diet) in the Mediterranean Diet score was associated with a 25 percent reduction in the risk of death from any cause, a 33 percent reduction in the risk of death from coronary heart disease, and a 24 percent reduction in the risk of death from cancer. The benefit was greater in women, in people older than 55, in never-smokers, in heavier folks, and in sedentary people.

Behavior therapy is often useful

Behavior modification, in which a therapist helps the overweight person restructure eating patterns and revamp his or her lifestyle, helps many people control obesity. The approach focuses on relapse training—anticipating and coping with lapses in the reducing program. Counselors teach people how to handle occasions such as dining out, parties, anniversaries and events of special culinary temptation, and help them get back on the rails if they break the diet. The key is to avoid the "all or none" attitude that makes dieters give up if they touch a morsel of forbidden food. On average, behavior therapy can give losses of 8.5 kg (20 lb) after 20 weeks, in combination with good nutritional efforts. "The successful management of obesity," according to one specialist, "is the result of a knowledgeable sympathetic physician or therapist with the time and concern to plan therapy and set realistic goals."

Move it! More activity crucial to successful weight loss

Increasing activity is essential to combat obesity "Exercising is better than counting calories," comments one expert from Buffalo University, "but it need not be the huffing and puffing form—no need to run marathons, join aerobics classes or jog. Brisk walking will do." Ideally activity should be incorporated into the everyday lifestyle. Intermittent high-intensity exercise, alternating with lower-energy movement, seems to work best. "Take every opportunity to move," advises one physiologist. "Climb stairs instead of taking the elevator, park the car a block away from work; go down the corridor to consult a colleague instead of phoning." Every bit of energy expenditure counts.

Pharmacotherapy or drug treatment helps some

Medications are likely no magic bullet, but they may be useful for some people. Previously, dieters used stimulants or appetite suppressants such as fenfluramine as weight-loss aids. These have largely been taken off the market for safety reasons. Two new medications have emerged: orlistat (Xenical) and sibutramine (Meridia). Xenical works by reducing the amount of fat absorption in the gut and when you use it with a fatty meal, some of the fat remains unabsorbed. This can make for unpleasant side effects such as diarrhea and flatulence. However, the discomfort can be a powerful motivator not to eat fat! Meridia, which inhibits uptake of the neurotransmitters, norepinephrine and serotonin, is more mysterious but works on the satiety center and makes us feel full. A systematic review of long-term results with Xenical taken three times a day showed that people lost 2.7 kg and those on daily Meridia experienced 4.3 kg greater weight loss compared to placebo. The number of people achieving 10 percent or greater weight loss was 12 percent higher with orlistat and 15 percent higher than placebo with sibutramine therapy. Weight-loss maintenance results were similar with both drugs. Xenical caused gastrointestinal side effects and Meridia was associated with small increases in blood pressure and pulse rate. In most studies, weight creeps back once the medication is stopped .

Surgery is a last resort

For the very obese, who find it impossible to lose any other way, surgical stomach stapling or jaw-wiring (plus a waist-cord to monitor gain) may be an ultimate option. Surgery reduces the size of the stomach from about one quart to a few ounces so that people feel full and nauseous if they eat more than a small amount. A Swedish study is examining the benefits of stomach stapling in reducing the health risks of obesity in a group of very obese patients with BMIs over 35.

Summing up the weight-loss message

Would-be reducers must abandon fad diets and the notion of a "quick fix." What's needed are long-lasting lifestyle changes. Weight-loss medications don't eliminate the need to change nutrition and exercise habits, but they help people get started and stick to the necessary changes. People often finally lose weight when they stop dieting, don't watch the scales, eat prudently with good portion control, and learn to accept themselves as they are. Anyone who is less than 20 percent overweight (and has a BMI under 27), with no weight-related illness, probably needn't bother to reduce. People with BMIs over 28 usually do need to lose for health reasons, especially if they're "apple-shaped" (with abdominal fat). But there's no magic bullet.

Obesity is curable only by a lifelong commitment to correcting faulty eating and exercise patterns. But remember that even a small weight loss of 2 to 5 kg (5 to 10 lb) can improve health. The obese need a great deal of support: in organizing and sticking to a long-term reducing plan, and reassurance that they'll manage it. A good friend or supportive relative can help reinforce a dieter's resolve by removing food temptations, and by suggesting a walk, movie or some other activity instead of dining out. Examining the National Weight Control Registry, a longitudinal prospective study of individuals 18 years and older, who have successfully maintained a 30-pound weight loss for a minimum of 1 year, we find the following:

- Registry members report that weight loss has led to significant improvements in self-confidence, mood and physical health. Surprisingly, 42 percent of participants report that maintaining their weight loss is less difficult than initially losing the weight.
- Successful weight-losers report making substantial changes in eating and exercise habits to lose weight and maintain their losses.
- Two-thirds of successful weight-losers were overweight as children and 60 percent report a family history of obesity.
- Approximately 50 percent of participants lost weight on their own without any type of formal program or help.

How did they lose weight?

- Successful weight-loss strategies were indivual and varied, possibly including some of the following methods: 90 percent utilized diet *and* activity; 88 percent restricted food intake and 44 percent controlled their food portions. Forty-four percent counted calories and 33 percent focused on a low-fat diet while 22 percent exchanged foods in their diet (e.g. replacing sugar with Equal, Splenda or other artificial sweeteners).
- Individuals exhibited high levels of physical activity (2800Cal/wk or 60 min/day), but simple walking was the most frequently cited exercise.
- Most had a feedback system that involved weighing themselves weekly.
- Ninety percent were breakfast-eaters. Most

ate regular meals, had fewer than three meals out and less than one fast food meal per week.

ACTIVE PEOPLE ARE HEALTHIER

The message is loud and clear: exercise benefits body and mind and should be an integral part of everyone's life. Studies on postal and transit workers found a third fewer heart-attack deaths among those who were active than among those who sat still at work. Sedentary British bus drivers had more heart disease than conductors, who moved about Washington letter carriers suffered fewer heart attacks than sedentary postal clerks; inactive Israeli kibbutz workers had more than double the heart-attack rate of those doing physical labor. A study of over 6,000 U.S. longshoremen, aged 35–74, showed that the vigorously active (unloading boats) had half the coronary death rate of the inactive (clerks and foremen). A British study that followed the pursuits of 18,000 middle-aged civil servants showed that 30 minutes a day of physical activity in chosen sports—walking, hiking, jogging, swimming—at rates using 7.5 kcal (kilocalories) a minute, halved the risks of heart attacks. (Note: 7.5 kcal is the amount of energy used in one minute of brisk walking, at a rate that burns 450 kcals per hour.) Another study, of 1,700 Harvard alumni aged 35–70, found fewer heart attacks in those expending more than 2,000 kcal (equivalent to about 32 km, or 20 miles, of brisk walking by an average-weight man) per week. In sum, any *sustained* activity—walking, running, dancing, rowing, mountain climbing—that burns 2,000–3,500 kcal weekly will help protect the heart. Lower energy outputs probably do not protect the heart.

Although activity also helps seniors stay agile, only one-third of Canadians over age 65 even take recreational walks, let alone regular exercise. Yet many an elderly person who keeps on exercising has a lower heart rate than an inactive youngster who sits eating chips in front of the TV. Age is no barrier to fitness—regular exercise can't necessarily cure ailments, but it improves mental outlook, enhances body image and makes life more enjoyable. It's never too late to start!

Aerobic exercise is the cornerstone of fitness

The purpose of aerobic exercise, which literally means exercise "with oxygen," is to enhance oxygen availability throughout the body, by creating a demand on the cardiovascular system (lungs, heart and blood vessels). Aerobic exercise should consist of continuous, steady, rhythmic movements of large muscles. Done at the correct pace, intensity and duration, aerobics strengthen the heart, allowing it to pump more blood for less effort.

Among the best, most convenient and easiest of aerobic activities are brisk walking, running, jogging and cycling, done at sufficient speed and for long enough. Swimming is also highly recommended, provided it is not too leisurely. It doesn't jar the legs or abuse the feet and suits people of all ages. Less effective aerobics are tennis, golf and volleyball, which are stop-and-start activities. Workouts involving mainly the upper body and isometrics (strength exercises) increase muscle power but have little significant effect on cardiac health because they do not work the cardiovascular system hard enough. Once aerobic muscle energy is exhausted, an anaerobic (without oxygen) enzyme pathway comes into play, allowing a short burst of extra muscular

OVERALL HEALTH BENEFITS OF REGULAR VIGOROUS ACTIVITY

- The pleasure of movement;
- a sense of well-being—greater vitality and zest for life;
- less fatigue;
- a healthier appearance;
- increased physical and mental efficiency;
- less need for medical care and lower medical costs;
- better weight control and body composition;
- better sleeping patterns;

- improved ability to handle stress and crisis situations;
- possible delay in the outward signs of aging;
- psychological benefits, e.g., reduction of mild anxiety. Researchers suggest that physical activity may be as good as psychotherapy or medication in relieving mild to moderate depression;
- mood elevation—a euphoric lift experienced after at least

20 minutes of steady running ("runner's high") or equivalent activity, owing to release of the body's natural, opiate-like chemicals (endorphins);
- reduced risks of osteoporosis—especially through weight-bearing activities (walking, jogging);
- possible protection against coronary heart disease;
- possible lowering of blood pressure.

THE FIVE BASIC COMPONENTS OF FITNESS

• *Cardiovascular endurance.* Also known as cardiorespiratory or aerobic endurance, cardiovascular fitness enables the heart to withstand sudden exertion—such as fast stair-climbing, jogging or snow-shoveling—that calls for an increased oxygen supply to the working muscles (and faster removal of wastes such as lactic acid and carbon dioxide). Since both oxygen and wastes are carried by the blood, the heart must pump harder and move blood faster to meet muscular demands. A fit heart, with a slower resting beat (pulse rate at rest), can pump more forcefully, expelling more blood per beat than an unfit one. Many physically fit people have resting heart rates as low as 40–50 beats per minute, making them well able to cope with sudden physical exertion.

• *Muscular (isotonic) endurance.* The ability of a large muscle group to apply repeated force over a period of time is essential in many jobs. Bricklayers and typists need good shoulder, arm and back endurance. Weight-lifting and workout machines are popular ways to increase muscular endurance. For correct muscular training techniques, consult Fitness Canada.

• *Muscular (isometric) strength.* The ability of a muscle or muscle group to exert force against resistance provides efficiency for everyday tasks.

• *Flexibility.* Flexibility depends on a full range of movement for the body's joints. Stretching exercises, each held for a minimum of 10 seconds—preferably longer—develop and retain flexibility, especially crucial to maintain mobility with advancing years and to reduce injury risks from sudden bursts of movement (such as running for a bus).

• *Body composition.* Body composition depends on the ratio of fat to lean muscle and bone. Less fat and more muscle improves overall fitness. But some body fat is essential for insulation, protecting vital organs and—in women—carrying female hormones. Women ideally have 13–18 percent body fat, men 10–13 percent by weight. The amount of body fat can be gauged by skin-fold measurements (pinching skin with calipers)—more than 2.5 cm (1 in) is too much—or more accurately by the water displacement method. (Or try the mirror test: do you like what you see?)

energy, as in sprints to the finish line. But after the extra endeavor—the final sprint, shoveling snow or a narrow escape—the oxygen debt must be repaid.

Throughout exercise sessions, the emphasis should be on control, not how high or how fast. It's better to exercise at half the speed, in the correct position, than flailing madly. Remember, you do not have to "burn" (a term formerly used by misinformed fitness instructors) or overuse a muscle to attain the desired toning effect. Pain is not gain for sensible exercise.

How much exercise does it take to protect the heart?

All too often, physicians vaguely tell patients to "get more exercise" without specifying how much or what type. Yet, much as medications are individually prescribed, so too exercise routines should be tailored to a person's age and lifestyle. It's wise to consult a fitness instructor about your own needs and ask for advice on how best to start. Experts tell you to begin with a medical checkup and fitness test, especially if you are over age 35 or have disorders such as dizziness, high blood pressure, diabetes, arthritis or signs of cardiovascular disease. An appropriate test may spot weaknesses in lungs, heart or blood circulation that could make over-arduous exercise dangerous. Also, you should start gradually and work up to full workouts. A sudden plunge into unaccustomed exercise invites injuries, disillusionment and dropouts.

Current medical opinion holds that for the full aerobic heart-protecting benefits, people must exercise at least three times a week, steadily for at least 20–30 minutes, with movements that involve the large muscles (arms and legs). The activity should be regular and done at the right intensity (heart rate). Ideally, never let more than four days go by without a workout. The cardiovascular system must work vigorously enough to improve the heart's pumping capacity but not so hard as to strain it. If you exercise at the right intensity, the effort will bring on a sweat and should increase your pulse to the "training range," i.e., 60–85 percent of the heart's maximum pumping capacity.

To calculate the correct training heart rate, estimate your own maximum heart rate (heart

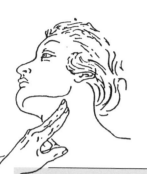

rate at exhaustion) by subtracting your age from 220. The target range for your exercise sessions is 60–85 percent of that. (Note: 220 beats per minute is the exhaustion rate of a young child.) A 50-year-old man, for example, has a maximum heart rate of 220 – 50 = 170 beats per minute and he should exercise at 60–85 percent of that rate, which means between 102 and 144 beats per minute. And don't suppose that, if 85

FINDING YOUR PERSONAL TARGET HEARTRATE ZONE

AGE	MAX.	60%		85% (cut-off)	
		Beats/10 secs.	Beats/min.	Beats/10 secs.	Beats/min.
25	195	22	132	30	180
30	190	19	114	27	162
40	180	18	108	26	156
45	175	18	108	25	150
50	170	17	102	24	144
55	165	17	102	23	138
60	160	16	96	23	138
65	155	16	96	22	132
70	150	15	90	21	126
			or less		or less

Monitor your heart rate by taking your pulse (on wrist or neck) about five minutes into the aerobic routine, then again at peak exercise intensity, keeping the legs moving while doing so.

The easiest way to take your pulse is by placing your middle two or three fingers on the carotid artery in the neck (see diagram), but not so tightly that you suppress it! Or, take the pulse with the middle two fingers (not the thumb) on the wrist. Start at zero and take the pulse for 10 seconds, then multiply by six to obtain your heart rate per minute. Also take the pulse rate after completing the aerobic component, then assess the speed of recovery—the time taken to reach the resting heart rate.

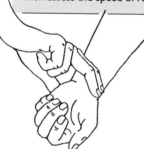

percent of the maximum rate improves cardio-vascular fitness, 90 percent is better. It's not necessary or even safe to exercise above that 85 percent mark. Above the cut-off level, the body's activity may become "anaerobic"—done without oxygen—and not benefit but even perhaps harm the body.

A more simple answer is that if you don't do anything currently, then *just walk more*. Studies show that there are significant benefits when people walk a mile a day, whereas the benefits of doing another 1–7 miles a day are minimal. Using a pedometer is a good way to document the number of steps taken or amount of walking and to get competitive with your

partners and friends. Most people report that on days when they don't move very much they feel tired and sluggish and on days when they walk more they have much more energy.

New guidelines emphasize benefits of moderate exercise

Recent research shows that although vigorous aerobic exercise protects the heart best, lower intensity or "moderate" exercise can also reap cardiovascular rewards. New guidelines call for moderate exercise on most days of the week, but not necessarily all in one go. You can do 5- to 6 minute bouts of moderate exercise and accumulate enough for a 30-minute training effect. Nor is it essential to take your pulse. Instead, try the "breathing and voice" test to check if you're within the target zone. This test is based on a general rule established by British climbers to "climb no faster than you can talk." At the minimum training rate, breathing should be clearly audible and you should be able to talk while exercising (able to converse, but not necessarily to sing!). If barely able to speak, the exercise is fully aerobic. If you can't talk while exercising, it's time to slow down. A personal perception of "exerting oneself to the fullest but not to exhaustion" also helps gauge whether you're in the right exercise mode, not working too hard or exceeding aerobic tolerance.

The breathing test
Lower limit training: should clearly hear breathing.
Upper limit training: breathing heavily but no wheezing.

The talk or "voice" test
Lower limit training: can easily carry on a conversation.
Upper limit training: just able to talk while exercising.

Use it or lose it
Regular exercise enhances the lungs ability to absorb oxygen, increases the amount of blood pumped by the heart with each beat, increases the number of mitochondria that keep the muscle cells working, expands the network of capillary blood vessels which carry oxygen to

the muscles and raises the activity of respiratory enzymes—no mean feat! But the benefits drop precipitously once habitual exercise stops.

Some training benefits are gone after even two weeks of inactivity, and significantly more in four to ten weeks. After twelve weeks about 70 percent of the muscular strength and endurance built up by regular exercise is gone. The heart puts out less blood with each beat and the ability of the working muscles to burn fat fades. The agility and coordination needed for sports such as tennis, skiing or swimming also decline. After long abstinence from activity, former regulars may have to start training from scratch.

Unfortunately, the largest drop in cardiovascular health comes quickly: half vanishes within two to three weeks of diminished activity. The body's oxygen-absorbing capacity drops in the first month of inactivity, as does the heart's pumping capacity. The increased mitochondrial (energy-producing) activity in the muscles falls in a couple of months. The expanded blood-capillary network may persist through several months, but if it isn't put to much use, the body becomes like a railroad that's lost most of its traffic—the tracks are there but not used enough.

Don't omit warm-ups and final cool-downs

A warm-up of seven to twelve minutes is essential before starting an exercise routine—to warm up the muscles slowly and prevent injury. Warm-ups should use movements similar to the intended activity, done slowly. They should also stretch the muscles of the back and extremities, start increasing the heartbeat, raise blood pressure and body temperature, increase elasticity of tendons and joints and trigger biochemical pathways that supply energy for movement. A proper warm-up may also protect the heart from irregular beats which can occur with sudden, vigorous exercise.

A cool-down of five to ten minutes allows a slowdown of physiological activity and gradual return to resting levels. During the cool-down, do not drop the head below the heart (to avoid dizziness). The cool-down helps to avoid the transient giddiness, lightheadedness or chills that can occur when exercise stops too abruptly. During vigorous exercise, the heart pumps

blood fast to the working muscles. Stopping suddenly lessens the pressure on the valves of the leg veins so that less blood is pushed back to the heart. The blood may temporarily "pool" in the extremities, depriving the heart and brain of oxygen, producing dizziness or fainting.

A few precautions

Try not to exercise after a heavy meal. When the stomach is full, much of the blood supply is diverted to the digestive system, and exercising may compromise the blood supply. The heart and working muscles will then have less than their full oxygen supply. You could also vomit and choke.

To avoid heatstroke, don't exercise under a hot sun, or in excessive heat. Prevent dehydration by replacing fluids lost during exercise. Drink plenty of liquid—preferably water, not alcohol, which only dehydrates you further!

After exercising, avoid steam, hot saunas or very hot showers until the body is well cooled down. Sudden heat makes surface blood capillaries dilate (widen) and may keep blood away from the heart.

Try not to regard recreational activity as a competition to the death. If exercise becomes obsessive, it can worsen health problems. Some grim-faced, lip-biting exercisers look more stressed out than hard-driving executives. For them, exercise is not the healthy, relaxing therapy it should be but a situation where they are pitted against themselves or others. Someone who starts each day with a pre-breakfast run—striving for a better speed each morning—then has a daily lunchtime squash game and a vigorous evening workout may be overdoing things, and increasing rather than relieving tension.

A few athletes and exercisers exhibit such a compulsive approach to their activity that it has

---

THE EXERCISE PRESCRIPTION

Frequency:	**at least three times a week.**
Intensity:	**in target heart rate zone (60 percent of maximum heart rate = lower limit; 85 percent = upper limit).**
Duration:	**minimum of 20–30 minutes (at target heart rate).**
Type:	**continuous, steady and rhythmic, using large muscle groups (legs and arms).**

Note: There is little training effect if exercise is less than three times a week or is done below 60 percent of the maximum heart rate. Listen to your body: if it tells you the time's ripe to work out more vigorously, act accordingly; if it signals a need to slow down, do so!

TYPICAL SIGNS OF HEART ATTACK

- **chest pain or heaviness**
- **pain spreading to left shoulder, arm or jaw**
- **Profuse sweating, nausea**
- **pallor (paleness)**
- **dizziness**
- **swollen ankles, feet**

SAFETY SUGGESTIONS FOR SUMMER SPORTS

- *Remember that exercising in the heat* strains the heart more than similar activities done in cool conditions, so ease up in summertime. It takes two to three weeks to become acclimatized to warm-weather exercise.
- *Always warm up and cool down*, even in hot weather.
- *Avoid running or other vigorous exercise* during the hottest time of the day (11:00 a.m.–3:00 p.m.).
- *Try not to be in direct sunlight* all the time. (See Chapter 17, Emergency medicine, for ways to recognize and treat heat stress/heatstroke.)
- *Use sun-protection/sunscreen* to avoid excess exposure to UV rays (see section on skin cancer in Chapter 5).
- *Wear loose clothing* in a material that breathes—cotton is best in hot weather—so that air can circulate over the skin, allowing sweat to evaporate. Light colors reflect the sun's rays better than dark colors.
- *Use a well-ventilated, wide-brimmed hat* to shade the head and neck in sunny conditions.
- *Allow for water-stops* every 20 minutes or so.
- *Watch for hypothermia* (excessive body cooling) in water sports. A dangerously low body temperature can result from exposure to cold water or windy conditions, and Canadian waters rarely warm up, even at the height of summer. The main signs of hypothermia (cold injury) are: shivering (although it stops when people are overchilled), slurred speech, stumbling, weakness, confusion, drowsiness, shallow breathing, weak pulse, loss of consciousness (maybe). Treatment for hypothermia is to keep the person warm and dry, seek medical attention, never give alcoholic beverages. (See Chapter 17, Emergency medicine, and following section on winter exercise.)

FOR WINDSURFING:

- *Always wear a personal flotation device* (PFD) or lifejacket (it's required by law).
- *Know your own limits* and stick within them.
- *Windsurf with a buddy* for support and assistance.
- *Have a friend ashore* who knows where you plan to go and is on the alert for rescue if necessary.
- *Check the weather forecast* before setting out—put ashore before thunderstorms hit.
- *Be on the alert for shipping hazards*—give large vessels a wide berth.
- *If a novice, avoid overchilling* from dumps into cold water.
- *Head for shore* if tired.

FOR SAILING/BOATING:

- *Learn to handle the boat*; keep rigging and equipment in good order. Know and respect your own limits and those of the crew.
- *Ensure that all boaters wear a lifejacket or PFD*—you are required by law to have one for each passenger. (About one-third of all drownings occur through people not wearing PFDs.) Approved lifejackets automatically turn people who fall overboard face up for air; PFDs only keep them afloat.
- *Take good care of your PFD*—do not use it as a cushion or fender. Dry in open air and keep dry.
- *Be sure children have lifejackets* of the right size. A too-small jacket will not float a child high enough to breathe, a too-large jacket can slide right off.
- *Practice capsizing*, man-overboard and self-rescue techniques.
- *Get weather forecasts;* watch for signs of impending storms. Shorten sail well ahead of time.
- *Check and obey local boating guidelines* and regulations.
- *Sail sober!* Avoid alcohol until landing safely; many boating deaths are linked to alcohol. It is illegal for anyone to consume alcohol on a boat unless it has overnight facilities and is moored for the night.

FOR WATER-SKIING:

- *Learn technique* from a certified instructor.
- *Check all equipment* before setting out.
- *Always have an observer* in the boat—it is the law.
- *Use common sense* if driving water-skiers: go slow for beginners.
- *Wear an approved lifejacket or PFD.*
- *Be sure that the skier, boat-driver and observer all use the same hand signals* for "go" and "stop"!
- *Stay away from docks*, boats and shallow areas; avoid swimmers.
- *If fallen into the water, lift ski* to signal position.

FOR SWIMMING:

- *Never dive into unknown waters* that could be shallow or rocky and cause a head injury/unconsciousness.
- *Don't swim too soon after eating.* Stomach cramps can lead to vomiting, even drowning. Wait half an hour to an hour after eating a full meal before swimming.
- *Take out contact lenses* before swimming—they easily get contaminated (especially soft contacts) and can get lost!
- *Stay close to shore or to a boat* if not a strong swimmer.
- *Get out of the water in thunderstorms.*

FOR BIKING:

- *Ensure that the bicycle functions properly*, especially the brakes.
- *Make sure the bike fits* the rider—many accidents happen to people on oversized bikes, especially children.
- *Obey the rules of the road,* stop at all intersections, marked or unmarked. Use the correct hand signals.
- *Never ride two abreast.* Keep hands available for the bike; carry parcels in fixed holders.
- *On long trips, carry a water bottle*—dehydration is common in summer bikers.
- *Be visible at night*: use lights on bike, or reflectors on bicycle or clothes. Children should not ride at dusk or in the dark—it's very risky.

- *Above all, wear an approved helmet*; it can significantly reduce the frequency and severity of brain damage from cycling accidents. Get a helmet approved by the CSA (Canadian Standards Association) or an equivalent one.
- *Let children choose their own helmet*; never trade safety for style, but make sure the child likes the selected model.
- *Select a bike helmet with adjustable straps* and a quick-release buckle that doesn't pinch: adjust straps for a snug fit.

FOR HIKING:
- *If hiking, always carry waterproof matches, compass, knife*, snare wire, fishhook, first-aid kit, high-calorie snacks.
- *Learn wilderness survival* if hiking in isolated areas. Don't wander aimlessly if lost—fix position relative to a hillock, lake, other landmark or the sun. Follow downhill slopes—they may lead to a recognizable trail or lake.
- *Make camp during daylight* on an elevated spot in a clearing (more visible to rescuers). If lost, build three fires in a triangle (a recognized "distress signal"), preferably on rocky ground (in order not to start a forest fire), adding green boughs for extra smoke.

FOR TENNIS:
- *Warm up beforehand*, being sure to include good calf stretches and Achilles tendon (heel) stretches to reduce risks of Achilles tendon injuries—common in tennis players.
- *Avoid incorrect arm posture* during the swing, strike and follow-through.
- *Aluminum tennis frames aren't advised for novices*; fiberglass or the newer vibration-dampening materials provide greater flexibility.
- *Beginners should take lessons* to ensure proper techniques that lessen chances of injury.
- *"Tennis elbow"*—painful swelling from racquet vibrations—arises from incorrect form and a faulty grip that increases the

vibrations traveling up the arm. Consider buying a strap that reduces vibration, resting, stretching, and learning better technique.

FOR GOLF:
- *Do warm-ups before the game*, with special attention to stretching the lower back and hamstring muscles.
- *Lessons ensure that the body moves* correctly during swing, strike and follow-through.
- *Even golfers can suffer dehydration* and heat stress—so drink enough and be vigilant!
- *Back problems are common* among golfers, although golf seems to be a leisurely game unlikely to cause injury. Back-strengthening exercises are a good idea. And don't forget the post-golf stretch to prevent lower-back tension.

Golfers get a different type of painful elbow in which the pain is on the inside of the elbow (golfer's elbow). It benefits from the same interventions as tennis elbow.

FOR ROLLER-SKATING OR ROLLER-BLADING:
- *Wear splint-type wrist guards*, knee and elbow pads.
- *Helmets are a must.*
- *Stick to quiet, level streets* until able to stop!

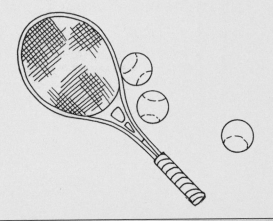

AVOID "OVERUSE": PAIN IS NOT GAIN FOR SPORTS

Pain signals something wrong and should never be ignored. It's an urgent message to slow down and attend to what's causing the discomfort. If someone continues to exercise—trying to "run off" the pain—further damage will occur. The only way to combat the inflammation due to muscular overuse is to rest when there is pain and resume exercise when it subsides. Overuse injuries typically cause stress fractures and/or inflammation.

Stress fractures—hairline bone breaks —occur if repeated exercise creates such intense muscle fatigue that the muscles can no longer adequately support the skeleton. "Continuous loading" that exceeds the bone's inherent elasticity may bend the bone and eventually produce a hairline crack. The treatment of stress fractures involves rest until bone healing is complete—up to eight weeks—with limited exercise during recovery that won't aggravate the injury (try swimming or stationary bicycling for leg overuse problems).

Inflammation, the body's natural response to tissue injury, often affects muscles and tendons, especially where they attach to bone. The inflammatory pain may disappear between activity and during pre-exercise warm-ups but reappear during or following activity. The condition is termed *tendonitis* if it affects a tendon, *bursitis* if the inflammation affects a joint bursa—the fluid-filled pouch near the joint. Treatment is simple: remove or stop the movement that causes the pain, cool with ice, elevate the painful part and follow with stretching and strengthening exercises (preferably advised by a physiotherapist).

SAFETY TIPS FOR SPECIFIC WINTER SPORTS

FOR TOBOGGANING:

- *Recognize that while tobogganing is an excellent family sport*—the best of aerobic exercise, as it entails hill climbing and carrying a load (the toboggan)—it takes a heavy injury toll.
- *Wait until the ground is covered with a thick layer of soft snow*. A thin layer often conceals logs, rocks or chunks of ice. Hitting a chunk of ice can be as dangerous as striking a hard rock.
- *Make sure the hill isn't too icy or steep*. An icy hill makes the toboggan go faster and it is harder to control.
- *Wear a helmet*. About half of all tobogganing injuries are to the head, sometimes serious.
  Avoid collisions! Watch for benches, trees and other structures, as well as other tobogganers.

FOR CROSS-COUNTRY SKIING:

- *Dress appropriately*. Remember that this sport requires more exertion than downhill skiing, and wear lighter clothing. But watch out for hypothermia and frostbite, which are distinct risks when out on the trail, especially when the temperature drops at day's end. Layering is key.
- *If skiing across a frozen lake or pond, beware of cracks* in the ice. Stay within 6 m (20 ft) of shore, and steer clear of rocks or docks where the ice may be thin.
- *Eat and drink enough before setting out* to stock up on energy and prevent dehydration.
- *Take along snacks of complex carbohydrates* (e.g., dried fruit, granola bars).
- *Stick to well-traveled trails and ski in pairs*. For maximum safety never venture alone onto isolated trails.
- *Plan the route ahead* and stick to it, calculating expected return time and leaving the information with someone who's not going out. Tell people where you are going.
- *Leave enough time to get back before dusk*, unless the trails are well lit.
- *Carry a first-aid kit* and light plastic blanket—they easily fit into a backpack.
- *Fall backwards*, if you must fall!

FOR DOWNHILL SKIING:

- *Remember that there are an estimated 10 injuries per 1,000 downhill skiers per season*, half of them severe enough to need medical care, mostly the first time people venture onto their skis each year. The most frequent ski injuries are to the knees and head.
- *Helmets are a must, especially for children*. A collision with another skier or a tree is a distinct possibility!
- *Get in shape beforehand*, perhaps with "ski-fit" classes. Include workouts to build strong leg muscles. (Nowadays, with the ankle locked into place, torsional forces go to the knee instead of the ankle during a fall.) Knee injuries are frequent among alpine skiers, so work the quadriceps (the muscle on the front inside of the thigh) and the calf muscles ahead of time to help avoid injuries.
- *Start each ski day with warm-up exercises*. A cold, unstretched muscle is prone to injury.
- *Increase carbohydrate intake* before a ski day to maintain stores of glycogen (for muscular effort).
- *Make sure that all equipment is in proper working order*. Have skis checked by a reputable dealer in the fall to ensure that bindings will release when needed. Bindings must be adjusted to the skier's weight, height, age and skiing ability. (Novices may prefer looser bindings that easily release.)
- *Stop skiing before fatigue sets in*. Most downhill skiing injuries occur in the late afternoon, after enthusiasts have already been at it for several hours.
- *Dress warmly enough* in layers, as this is not a "high activity" sport. Protect the hands, legs, face and feet from the cold (the latest boots contain battery warmers!).
- *Watch for soft snow* where skis can get stuck without release of bindings.
- *Beware of ice!* The bindings may release in time, but ice is hard to fall on and an outstretched arm easily fractures.
- *When night skiing*—an option at many resorts—recognize your limits and stop when tired or cold. After warming up by the fire with a cup of hot chocolate or soup, you can always return to the slopes!

FOR SKATING:

- *Get skates with firm ankle support and a snug fit. Break in new skates slowly.*
- *Before going out on the ice*, check that the skate blades haven't become dull or rusted.
- *Many skating clubs and rinks insist that beginners and all skaters under age 16 wear helmets*, but others feel that only pair skaters need the extra protection for the twists and throws.
- *Padded pants provide protection* in a fall, but some instructors believe that wearing pads makes skaters too dependent on them, so that they never learn to fall properly.

FOR ICE HOCKEY:

- *Make sure all equipment is in good repair*. About one-third of hockey injuries are due to equipment failure, because players wrongly consider themselves invincible in their protective gear. While hockey gear is expensive and children grow out of it fast, it is vital to replace it regularly. Older players in particular should consider replacing old equipment. It is not uncommon for older players to have equipment that is 15 years old. This will not protect you.
- *Replace cracked shin pads or helmets* and brittle equipment where the foam is damaged.
- *Make sure helmet padding* is adequate.

FOR SNOWMOBILING:

- *Be in sufficiently good shape* to lift the machine if necessary!
- *Watch for frostbite* and other signs of excess body cooling.
- *Carry a first-aid kit*.
- *Wear a jacket with built-in flotation capacity* (e.g., Mustang type), if going over ice.
  Check with local experts before traveling over ice.

HOT TIPS FOR COOL SPORTS: SAFETY TIPS FOR WINTER EXERCISE

- *Never overdress*. A common mistake among winter exercisers is wearing not too little but too much clothing.
- *Keep clothing loose*. Tight socks, shoes or gloves can cut off the circulation, leading to frostbite.
- *Protect the head and neck*. Up to 40 percent of the body's heat can be lost from the head. The best bet is a wool or polypropylene cap or hood which also covers the ears. A balaclava or a cap with a fold-down face mask is useful on very cold days, in falling snow or gusting wind—but be sure it doesn't reduce vision or hearing.
- *Wear a scarf or neck tube* that can be put over the mouth to warm cold air before it's breathed in (carry a neck tube in your pocket—it can cover the ears, mouth and most of the face).
- *Use light, thin clothing to maintain the body's "microclimate."* Have good ankle and wrist closures to trap the heat generated. Remove layers if too warm (tying garments around the waist or putting them in a day pack). Don them again if cold.
- *Dress in layers to vary insulation*. One should feel chilly in the first five minutes of winter exercise and comfortable after that.
- *Choose underwear—closest to the skin—*for absorption, to draw sweat away from the skin so that it keeps the body drier. Modern "thermal" underwear often has an inner layer (usually synthetic) that absorbs perspiration and "wicks" it to the outer layers, keeping moisture off the skin. (Pure cotton tends to hold in sweat and become cold and clammy.)
- *Make at least one layer wool*, either the middle or second- to-top layer—for optimal warmth. Wool retains body heat even when wet,
- *Make the top or outer layer windproof*, preferably of fabric that "breathes" so that moisture isn't trapped inside. Gore-Tex, and nylon fit the bill. Nylon provides better protection from strong winds than most woven fabrics and is also water-repellent.
- *Turtlenecks are good for cold days* to protect the back of the neck (a high heat-loss area).
- *Zip 'em up!* Jackets should be fastened in *two* ways—with both zips and buttons or Velcro—to make them fully windproof. Choose clothes for ease of removal, i.e., clothes that unzip or unbutton to let you cool off or close swiftly again if you're cold. (Tie a small loop of string or fabric to zippers so you won't have to search for the ends or remove gloves.)
- *Pants can be cotton with a nylon covering*, wool or Gore-Tex—waterproof for skiers. Use tights, leg warmers or thermal long johns underneath in really cold weather.
- *Wear goggles* to protect the eyes. Leave no area of the face exposed in severe cold.
- *To keep the hands warm, mittens are better* than gloves since they keep the fingers together, with less surface area for heat to escape. In very cold weather the warmth of mittens is worth the loss in dexterity. Mitten or glove liners are excellent for very cold days.

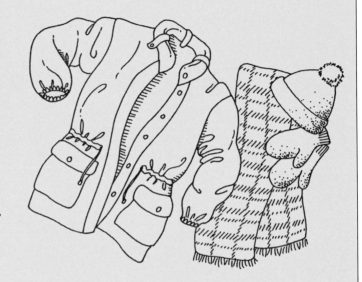

- *Protect the feet well*. Thick-soled rubber boots with lace-ups and a removable felt liner (that can be dried out) are ideal for snowy, icy or slushy conditions. They can be removed and exchanged for other footwear when getting into the car. (Snow boots can cause accidents if worn while driving!)
- *Footgear should be loose enough* to allow the toes to wiggle, and to trap warm air and allow room for an extra pair of socks.
- *Don't go out on an empty stomach*. Food provides energy to combat the cold. It may even prevent hypothermia if you are lost, stranded or injured.
- *Increase carbohydrate intake*. Choose the complex variety, avoiding too many sugary sweets. Take snacks along if planning to be out for more than an hour or two.
- *Never push yourself to exhaustion*. Overdoing it may leave the body uncoordinated and vulnerable to injury. (Don't expect to have the same stamina in winter as in summer; even a one-degree drop in temperature reduces endurance.)
- *Be on the defensive against fog, mist, twilight and darkness*. When planning a hiking or cross-country ski trip, remember that the days are much shorter in wintertime. And listen to the weather forecast!
- *Beware of ice!* While some people manage to exercise in the worst weather without injury, exercising on ice is often risky unless the pace is slowed (take smaller steps and wear footwear with good traction). For safety, carry a rope and ice awl if trekking on ice. If starting to fall through ice, throw the body forward, hands outstretched, and try to propel yourself to safety with your legs.
- *Develop an emergency or "injury action" plan*. Deal promptly with minor injuries to stop them from becoming major problems, and watch for frostbite.

(See chapter 17 for frostbite and cold injury treatment.)

been likened to anorexia nervosa, the condition common in adolescent girls where dieting is carried to the point of starvation. Preoccupation with diet and exercise can lead to excessive weight loss, emaciation or even death.

Although people can exercise until a ripe old age, frequency and duration of exercise, rather than high intensity, usually bring greater rewards for older people. Moderate exercise can upgrade heart health, if done most days of the week, at a minimum training level—in the "talk" zone where breathing is clearly audible and people can still talk easily while exercising. Walking is great exercise; done regularly at the target pace it increases cardiovascular fitness, lowers blood pressure and strengthens the spine, hip and leg bones (reducing fracture rates). Even a brisk, 20-minute daily walk might help protect against death from heart attack. Ordinary activities such as gardening, vacuuming, shopping, climbing stairs, mowing the lawn or dancing also count as exercise.

If just starting an exercise program, begin slowly and don't push yourself too hard; get a medical checkup to assess your physical fitness. Don't hold the breath while working out—it can cause a brief rise in blood pressure which may be risky in those with hypertension or heart conditions. Know the signs of heart problems.

Alerting signs of heart trouble

If you experience any or several of the following symptoms, go to the nearest emergency unit or call your physician: chest discomfort or pressure; pain down the arms (especially the left shoulder or arm); pain in the neck and into the left jaw; swelling of ankles or hands; purple fingertips; lightheadedness; profuse sweating; anxiety.

Any suspicion of unexpected heart trouble demands urgent medical attention. If you wait to make sure, it may be too late. (For more on heart problems see the section on heart disease in Chapter 16 and emergency action for heart attacks in Chapter 17.)

General tips for sensible exercise

• *Plain water is the safest drink.* Caffeine and alcohol should be avoided—both are diuretics that flush water out through the kidneys. Drink two to three cups of water two or

three hours before engaging in strenuous activity, another cup 15 minutes before the start and then one cup every 15–20 minutes. Take plenty of fluid after exercise to rehydrate the body (Strongly colored urine signals dehydration and the need to replenish liquids.)

• *Alcohol should be avoided* because it impairs judgment and coordination (easily leading to mishaps such as falls overboard when boating) and gives an illusion of warmth, although it speeds up body cooling/heat loss (by allowing the blood vessels to expand, speeding up heat loss) so that body temperature drops faster. It's also a diuretic.

• *Drink plenty!* One needs ample fluids before, during and after exercising, particularly in hot weather. To maintain a safe core (inner) body temperature, the body must sweat profusely to cool the body. During strenuous exercise the body can lose up to 2 litres (0.5 gal) of water per hour, which seriously decreases the circulating blood volume. Dehydration is a major danger in ardent exercisers.

• *Drink as much in cold weather as in hot.* It's easy to become dehydrated in cold weather because of the water lost by sweating and because the cold air inhaled must be moistened as well as warmed.

• *Be extra vigilant when exercising in windy conditions.* Wind can increase or mask the onset of sunburn or hypothermia (body-chilling).

• *Make footwear comfortable and supportive.* Shop for shoes in the afternoon, when feet are hot and possibly swollen. The shoe sole should be flexible, for easy push-off, and an extra layer of shock-absorbent foam helps to protect the toes. Beware of a stiff and uncomfortable midsole. The heel should be well cushioned for shock absorption, especially in runners. A padded collar topping at the back protects the Achilles tendon. Leather is increasingly used for sport shoes, although those whose feet tend to get hot may prefer a leather and mesh mixture.

Key steps in managing sports injuries

Protection, rest, ice, compression, elevation (PRICE) plus controlled or limited motion are the basic tenets for managing sports injuries, whatever their causes. One University of

Toronto specialist prefers the term MICE meaning "movement (limited), ice, compression and elevation"—to downplay the idea of extended rest and immobility for sports injuries. The primary goal is to reduce the inflammation that follows injury in the first 72 hours or so. The body may overreact, allowing too much fluid to collect, prolonging healing time. Once the swelling goes down, gentle controlled movement should begin, with gradual return of the injured area to full function.

General principles for sports injuries:

- *Consult a physician* about any but the mildest of sprains, strains or other injuries.
- *Never disregard pain.*
- *Wrap the injured part in ice* (well-crushed, or a package of frozen peas, wrapped in a towel or old woolen sock, to prevent frostbite) and apply for 15–20 minutes every two hours for severe injuries, every six hours for milder injuries. Deep-seated injuries will require the full 20 minutes, one to four times daily. Apply ice for briefer periods if injury is close to the skin. (Do not use ice if you have circulatory problems.)
- *Apply pressure* (compression) with an elastic bandage that's moderately tight but does not press on nerves or reduce blood circulation. Always wrap from the point farthest away from the heart toward the heart (e.g., wrist to elbow). The tensor bandage should not usually be worn at night, to prevent circulation problems. *Tip*: if the far end of the limb turns blue, the bandage is too tight!
- *Elevate the injured part* above your heart to prevent pooling of accumulated fluid in inflamed tissues. Prop legs at rest above hip level. Injured hands and forearms can be supported in a sling with hands at shoulder level. For upper-arm injuries, raise the arm above the head at regular intervals.
- *To reduce swelling/inflammation*, try ASA; for pain, take acetaminophen.
- *Begin limited gentle exercise during recovery* to regain strength and flexibility, preferably guided by a trained physiotherapist.
- *Return to full activity only when well healed* and pain-free—usually ten days to eight weeks for a sprain, depending on severity.
- *Go easy on the use of heat* (often improperly used to treat exercise-induced injuries). Never apply heat to an acute bruise, strain or soft-tissue injury (That means no hot baths and no heating pads following such injuries.) Heat may make the injury feel better but will also increase local inflammation and worsen the swelling. It's generally best to opt for ice in the short term. Heat should only be used, if at all, once the swelling has gone down. "Contrast baths"—alternating cold with hot water—may be useful for stimulating blood circulation to the injury, but only several days after the acute injury phase. (See also Chapter 17.)

SLEEP HYGIENE AND SLEEP DISORDERS

Most adults average seven and a half to eight hours of sleep per night but need more sleep when they're stressed and less when untroubled. Some individuals can do with as little sleep as five hours nightly or less, historic examples being Napoleon, Thomas Edison and Chou En-lai. Others require nine or more hours. Studies show that bed-sharing couples sleep less than singles but couples in separate beds sleep more soundly!

Sleep requirements are greatest in infancy (16–18 hours a day), and gradually decrease. The soundest sleep is typically that of ten- to twelve-year-olds, who effortlessly slumber nine to ten hours nightly and remain fully alert all day long. During adolescence sleep patterns approach the adult average, later decreasing to about six hours a night in the elderly. Sleep patterns in older people are variable, generally more fragmented with more nocturnal awakenings, possibly due to inactivity and daytime naps.

In very young children, bedtime fears, nightmares and bedwetting are the commonest sleep problems, while adolescents typically find it hard to get up. Young adults most often complain of difficulties in falling asleep, but sleep peacefully once they have dropped off. In contrast, the elderly, who tend to turn in early and fall asleep fast, awaken often and have difficulty getting back to sleep, sometimes because of arthritic pain or other health problems. Over a third of our population complains of insomnia, and in desperate attempts to get a good nights rest many turn to alcohol, sedatives or tranquilizers.

Curiously, sleep experts report frequent discrepancies between the way people think they sleep and their actual sleep patterns, as is shown when they are wired up to EEG (electroencephalographic) machines, which record brain-wave patterns, with electrodes on the scalp. Many people who call themselves poor sleepers and complain of hardly sleeping a wink all night actually fall asleep quickly in sleep labs and slumber soundly. For some reason—often unknown—their sleep is non-restorative and fails to give them the desired freshness.

Sleep is a dynamic, rhythmic process

Sleep used to be considered an inactive state, but modern science sees it as an active, cyclic process regulated by various neurotransmitters (chemicals that affect nerve impulses). Some sleep phases are as busy and alert as wakefulness, although in different ways. Essentially, sleep begins with relaxed wakefulness, which is a drowsy period lasting a few minutes to half an hour, before people drop off. It progresses into two main states described as non–rapid-eye-movement (non-REM) and rapid-eye-movement (REM) sleep. REM sleep is thought to reflect dreaming periods. Normal sleep begins as non-REM, deep or "delta-wave" sleep, with EEG readings showing a slow wave. The first REM episode occurs some 70 to 90 minutes into sleep and lasts perhaps five minutes, with the EEG registering faster waves of brain activity. Subsequent cycles of non-REM and REM sleep continue through the night at roughly 90-minute intervals, with later REM episodes averaging 15–20 minutes. Morning naps tend to have more REM cycles and more dreams than afternoon naps.

During REM sleep there are recognizable physiological changes—an increased and variable heart rate, a rise in blood pressure and respiration, increased cerebral blood flow and oxygen consumption, reduced body-temperature control, marked loss of postural muscle tone (prohibiting movement) and, in men, penile erections. Most of us experience three to six REM periods a night, and if we are awakened abruptly from them we recall vivid dreams that are often later forgotten or repressed. Basically we are the same personalities in dreams as during wakefulness: creative people report more creative dreams, schizophrenics experience bizarre dreams and depressed patients dream of helplessness, hopelessness and escape. Dreams emphasize aspects of our personality that may be less apparent during wakefulness.

REM sleep and dreaming are suppressed by various sedatives (such as barbiturates), antidepressants and alcohol. When deprived of REM sleep, many people become agitated and aggressive. By contrast, people deprived of non-REM sleep become very withdrawn; a few develop symptoms resembling fibrositis—now called the arthritic pain modulation disorder—with musculoskeletal tenderness and increased pain sensitivity at specific body points.

A 24-hour biological clock, or circadian rhythm, controls our wake–sleep patterns. It explains why we tend to sleep better at some times of day than others. In a cave lit only by artificial means, a normal person given plenty of food but no clock or set mealtimes will still maintain a circadian rhythm, usually somewhat over 24 hours (if not forced to adhere to 24-hour routines). Our normal sleep-wake routine, harmonized with the sun's 24-hour cycle, is reinforced by day-time checkpoints such as mealtimes, work or school timetables and regular retiring and rising times. Shift workers classically find it hard to sleep when their circadian rhythm is at odds with their work hours. At night, the biological clock "turns down" many functions that enhance daytime alertness—such as cortisone (adrenal hormone) release, certain transmitter levels and the heart rate. Studies show that workers at the start of a night-shift are slower and less efficient than usual at many tasks. That may explain why so many trucking mishaps and accidents (such as the Three Mile Island nuclear leak and the London, England, underground crash) happen between 1:00 and 4:00 a.m. at the circadian low point. Some airlines and other organizations try to arrange night shifts so that the natural circadian rhythm isn't too drastically undermined. (Jet lag is atypical case of disturbed circadian rhythm and disrupted sleep-wake cycles.) (See Chapter 13 for more on shift work.)

Occasional sleeplessness is not unhealthy

In healthy people, even long periods of sleeplessness produce no permanent detrimental changes. People with some rare brain diseases never sleep yet survive for months. Young, healthy volunteers, kept awake for 24–48 hours or even longer, show remarkably little deterioration in task performance. Despite fatigue and mood changes, bodily reserves can rally to bring performance up to par for short periods. But as sleep deprivation continues, little "microsleeps" occur with lapses in brain function that may cause driving errors or endanger people in other ways. Short-term sleep losses can be harmful to epileptics, in whom they trigger seizures, and to those with jobs that demand focused attention, such as air-traffic control.

Surprisingly, in some clinically depressed people a sleepless night actually elevates mood and performance for a few days. Some European medical centers use sleep-deprivation therapy in depressed patients to reset skewed circadian clocks. Its mechanism is still a mystery, but sleep loss may normalize a disturbed circadian rhythm and improve neurotransmitter balance.

Insomnia—an abnormally prolonged inability to sleep—comes from a disruption of either waking or sleep patterns. Most of us suffer the odd sleepless night when we stay awake due to excitement, worry, jet lag, overuse of caffeine or shift work. But many chronic insomniacs always sleep poorly and feel perpetually fatigued. Of the main types of insomnia, by far the commonest is situational or transient, caused by something like an impending exam, emotional stress, job worry, certain medications, overwork or pain. Sleeplessness that lasts no more than three to four weeks requires no therapy; once the stress or distress passes, so does the insomnia. Some experts recommend the brief use of a sleep remedy, perhaps one of the benzodiazepines (for example Valium, Dalmane, Halcion or Xanax), to provide much-needed rest and prevent short-term sleeplessness from becoming a chronic complaint. These anti-anxiety medications also act as sedatives and are useful for short-term use. Disorders of the sleep-wake cycle (due to abnormal circadian rhythms or biological clock dysfunction) are newly recognized sleep disorders, requiring special therapy.

Sleep medications should never be regularly taken without specific medical advice. The use of most sleep medications, especially short-acting benzodiazepines, leads to tolerance; i.e., the drug is no longer effective unless the dosage is increased. Withdrawal can lead to hangover-like symptoms, blurred vision, disorientation, daytime drowsiness and "rebound insomnia," after even brief use. Once hooked, many people need professional help to kick the habit of a nightly sedative fix. Therefore experts warn strongly against unnecessary or prolonged use of sedating medications—particularly for the elderly, who should take only half the usual prescribed dose or use a shorter-acting drug. (The cumulative effects of long-acting sedatives may leave the elderly in a constantly confused state.)

The use of alcohol at bedtime is likely to be more troublesome than helpful. Although it facilitates sleep onset, it also suppresses the initial REM episode. As the alcohol breaks down, its depressant effects are followed by cerebral excitation and more REM sleep than usual, and the sleeper may be aroused frequently by vivid or distressing dreams. Thus, although alcohol first lulls you to sleep, as its sedating effect wears off it leaves your mind restless and disturbed.

Persistent insomnia—a vicious cycle

Emotional and psychological conflicts, as well as psychiatric disorders, often cause long-term sleeplessness. Insomnia is frequent in the introverted, who tend to mull over problems at night. Among schizophrenics and the depressed, insomnia waxes and wanes with their condition; it is often a sign of depression. A self-perpetuating cycle of insomnia can be set off by some event or illness in people who previously slept perfectly well. The sleepless nights create anxiety about insufficient rest, cause fatigue and lead to more insomnia. Worry about not sleeping often lessens the ability to fall asleep. In trying to combat their insomnia, many people start taking more and more sedatives. They may also take several alcoholic drinks at bedtime, if other drugs no longer put them to sleep. As the cycle continues and drug dependence builds, desperation creeps in.

The management of chronic insomnia

depends on uncovering the underlying reasons for it, through a thorough medical evaluation, physical exam and analysis of psychosocial, alcohol and drug history. Treatment of persistent nonmedical insomnia usually attempts to improve sleep habits and break the vicious cycle. Counseling and psychotherapy may be useful, depending on the extent of anxiety. Sedative drugs may occasionally be used to carry people through an especially troubling time, but never for more than a few days each week.

Daytime sleepiness can be risky

People who sleep too much can be worse off than those who sleep too little. Although less common than sleeplessness, excessive daytime drowsiness is more dangerous. People may fall asleep on the job or at the wheel of a car and cause accidents. Excessive sleepiness, which sometimes goes undiagnosed, is heralded by dozing off without apparent cause, irresistible napping and uncontrollable bouts of sleep at inconvenient moments—while at work, making love, chatting on the phone, eating or driving. If attacks occur during potentially risky circumstances, the affected person is strongly advised to obtain treatment, and to desist from potentially hazardous activities until the condition is under control.

Sleep labs may be able to pinpoint the reason for excessive sleepiness, which has three main causes: narcolepsy, sleep apnea and nocturnal myoclonus.

Narcolepsy is a rare syndrome affecting about one in 2,500 people, which is possibly inherited and first surfaces in adolescence or young adulthood. It is defined as excessive daytime sleepiness with abnormal REM sleep patterns. Symptoms include brief sudden loss of muscle tone with involuntary collapse of the limbs (cataplexy), eye twitching, facial immobility, sleep paralysis (inability to move during sleep) and dreamlike hallucinations. Although narcoleptics appear fully alert, many remain sleepy at all times and most suffer psychological disorders due to the disability.

Narcoleptics typically fall asleep at inappropriate times despite a full night's sleep. Intense emotions such as laughter, surprise, anger and excitement can trigger muscular collapse.

Classic stories about narcoleptics tell of an angry mother who collapses as she swings at her child, a sergeant who falls to the ground motionless as he shouts commands, a fisherman who buckles at the knees while reeling in a fish. Narcoleptic episodes occur because the onset of REM sleep—whether at night or in daytime—occurs suddenly and unexpectedly, or at once after dozing off, instead of following a period of non-REM sleep. The result is immediate vivid dreaming, fragmented sleep and sudden loss of muscle tone.

Since narcolepsy is a lifelong condition without a cure, treatment depends on controlling its symptoms. It includes scheduled daytime naps, suitable stimulants to overcome the daytime drowsiness and antidepressants to suppress sleep paralysis. A new remedy, gammahydroxybutyrate (a natural constituent of the human brain), developed by researchers at the universities of Ottawa and Toronto, not only helps muscular control but can consolidate sleep into coherent periods. It acts as a kind of "sleep-glue" that encourages narcoleptics to sleep at night rather than in daytime snatches.

Other Causes of Insomnia

The following problems such as apnea and night terrors, are often not diagnosed by the person affected but rather noticed by a sleeping partner. Once they are remedied, however, many sufferers experience a significant increase in restorative sleep. The problems listed below are often officially diagnosed in a sleep lab.

Sleep apnea

In *sleep apnea*, breathing ceases for 10–60 seconds from time to time during sleep, sometimes many times a night, momentarily cutting off the body's oxygen supply. The sleeper often remains unaware of the countless nocturnal breathing lapses, accompanied by snoring, which bed partners find unbearably disturbing. The lapses in breathing—an interval of silence followed by a mighty heave, snort or gasp and then resumed snoring—are both annoying and scary. Reasons for sleep apnea include anatomical obstructions (such as a jaw abnormality, enlarged tonsils or adenoids), nasal polyps, sleeping on the back, loose dentures and flabby throat muscles (in the elderly). It is typically a condition of the obese—especially middle-aged men. Telltale features of this rare but hazardous disorder include a slowed heart rate, abnormal leg kicking and flailing movements, falls from bed and sleepwalking. Some apnea sufferers complain of choking sensations that interrupt their sleep, and report memory problems, hallucinations, irritability, mood or personality changes and waning sex drive.

Treatment of apnea includes weight loss (for the obese), decongestants, sleeping on the side (perhaps with a tennis ball fixed in the pajama back to prevent rolling onto the back), avoidance of alcohol and medications (such as sedatives and tranquilizers) that depress breathing, mask-like devices to improve airflow and surgery to correct anatomical impediments. Many apnea sufferers will benefit from a device that provides Continuous Positive Airway Pressure or CPAP. Although it looks somewhat daunting, a trial often, but not always, improves daytime energy.

Restless Legs Syndrome and Periodic Limb Movement Disorder

Restless leg syndrome (RLS) and periodic limb movement disorder (PLMD) are two separate but related intrinsic disorders of sleep that are often diagnosed because of partner complaints. While the sufferer may be unaware of the movement, it can still prevent him or her from entering a deep sleep. RLS typically involves a conscious urge to move the legs usually accompanied or caused by uncomfortable or unpleasant sensations in the legs. The urge or sensation is relieved or reduced by movement but returns quickly when movement stops. It is worse in the evening or during the night than it is during the day.

PLMD is diagnosed on the basis of clinical history plus the recorded evidence of periodic limb movements in sleep. This entails rhythmic leg-jerking that can awaken the sleeper and/or the partner. Episodes of twitching last from five minutes to two hours and alternate with peaceful sleep. The restless night produces extreme daytime drowsiness. The affliction appears mostly in middle-aged men and women, and is of unknown cause, but it is often seen in kidney

patients who are on peritoneal dialysis, and in people with fibrositis. The treatment is with drugs that suppress the leg jerks. Alcohol and caffeine should be avoided, and leg-stretching exercises are sometimes recommended.

Night terrors and sleepwalking

Predominantly a problem of the young, night terrors and sleepwalking start around age four and usually vanish by adolescence. The sleeper partly awakens from deep slumber and is simultaneously asleep and semiconscious. In night terrors, a terrified child may sit up in bed and scream while still seemingly asleep; the episode of fear usually occurs an hour or two after bedtime, and the youngster usually cannot be awakened. Night terrors are more common when schedules are erratic or when children are stressed or overtired, so regular schedules may diminish the

---

TIPS TO PROMOTE HEALTHY SLEEP

Avoid:
- daytime naps;
- heavy meals late at night;
- arguing or working in bed;
- alcoholic nightcaps (which fragment sleep);
- drinking too much fluid in the evenings;
- caffeine-containing products such as coffee, tea, colas, chocolate;
- evening hunger—eat a light snack. drink a glass of milk or have cereal with milk (rich in tryptophan, a natural food component conducive to sleep);
- smoking tobacco (which is a stimulant);
- regular use of tranquilizers and sedatives;
- trying too hard to go to sleep, which may have the opposite

effect (instead of lying there counting sheep, do something—read a relaxing novel or watch TV);
- self-reproach for inability to sleep: it's not an illness, a crime or even necessarily unhealthy;
- staring at the bedside clock (turn it to the wall);
- overwork or getting too exhausted.

Do:
- have a good daily exercise routine (especially in the late afternoon or early evening), to promote sleep;
- use the bedroom for sleep and sex, not for all general activities;
- provide a quiet, dark, comfortable sleep environment;

- keep the ambient temperature right— not above 75°F (24°C), which disturbs sleep, but not too cold;
- regulate your sleep and awakening times to reinforce your circadian rhythm—go to bed after about 16 hours of nonstop activity and stay there! Have a regular wake-up time;
- sleep as much as needed to feel refreshed the following day, but not more; curtailing time in bed seems to solidify sleep, while staying in bed lightens it;
- allow an hour's relaxing "wind-down time" after the day's turmoil before retiring to bed;
- seek professional assistance if needed.

problem. Waking the child up to discuss the fear usually just aggravates the condition.

Sleepwalking, in which movement is clumsier than normal but still remarkably deft, also occurs in semi-arousal from deep sleep. As they roam, sleepwalkers often perform purposeful actions such as eating, toothbrushing and dressing—usually indoors, although some venture outside. Occasional sleepwalking appears in 5 to 15 percent of children (compared to night terrors in only about 5 percent). Again, stress and emotional tension increase the problem. Should sleepwalking continue into adulthood, psychotherapy may be advisable. Management includes safety measures to prevent the injuries so easily incurred by unprotected sleepwalkers. Doors and windows should be well secured and harmful instruments should be put away.

Before you imagine yourself to be a sleep-disordered person, remember that in most people sleep problems are temporary and harmless. For the small number of people with serious sleep disturbances, new research can help. And finally—sleep is as vital to health as diet and exercise and should be given enough attention.

PREVENTING NEEDLESS INJURIES

Traumatic injuries are a major and little-appreciated health problem in this country. They are the commonest cause of death in those aged one to 34 and rate fourth as a cause of all deaths in North America, behind cardiovascular diseases, cancer and respiratory illness. Since injuries so often kill the young, they pose as serious a health problem as diseases in terms of productive life years lost.

During the 1930s, many people were crushed to death in malfunctioning elevators; children suffered terrible burns when their nightwear caught fire; infants often choked on small toy parts or were strangled in the rails of their crib. Even in the 1970s, countless Canadian deaths occurred among people who motorcycled bareheaded, drivers who didn't use seatbelts and children who rode unrestrained in cars on parents' laps. Thanks to intensive consumer lobbying, legislation, public education and engineering improvements, many dangers once considered part of life have been reduced. Killer elevators and inflammable nightwear are

becoming a thing of the past, and unhelmeted motorcyclists appear suicidal to most onlookers.

Yet death from unintentional injuries still takes an appallingly heavy toll. And death is only the tip of the iceberg. For every trauma death, 45 people with injuries are admitted to hospital. Injury-related death rates in Canada exceed those in Japan, Australia, Sweden and most West European countries. Children are especially vulnerable. One University of Toronto expert notes that "during peak travel times, emergency rooms are filled with children whose injuries could have been minimized or prevented by a little good car sense." In Sweden, for example, simple measures such as introducing bike lanes and arranging routes to school through traffic-free zones have halved the injury rates among children.

"Accident" is a misnomer—most are not random

Too many of us regard injuries as random, chance events that "just happen" through fate, human nature, clumsiness or bad luck. The very term "accident" suggests something unexpected and unavoidable. The fact that the circumstances leading to injury are considered unpredictable may explain why accidents aren't generally considered a health problem.

However, there has been a dramatic shift in medical thinking about so-called accidental injuries. The notion that injuries are unpredictable is now outmoded, replaced by the view that they are both predictable and preventable. The very term "accident" is being abandoned, because injuries—like diseases—arise for definite reasons. While the idea of an accident-prone personality is a myth, certain factors are closely tied to injury—particularly high childhood activity levels, risk behavior and family stresses (such as house moves, job loss or divorce).

Public-health specialists point out that, like diseases, many injuries have clear-cut causes—such as icy sidewalks, insufficient lighting or poorly timed shift work rotation. Car crashes may happen because of poor vision (wrong glasses) or alcohol consumption. People may fall in the shower for lack of a safety mat. Children can get hurt in countless ways: by a television falling on them when they pull on the cord, by being shut in a cupboard, through playground mishaps. It may seem unforeseeable that a preschooler would dart in front of a car and get hurt. However, as a group, five-year-olds living on busy streets are quite likely to be hit by cars, more so than a similar group living in a village. Among teenagers and adults, alcohol use and failure to use seatbelts are as clearly linked to injury as high blood cholesterol is linked to heart disease. The list is endless.

Experts stress that most injuries are predictable, can be anticipated and in many cases could be prevented. Injuries typically occur through lack of awareness, inadequate planning and society's acceptance of unsafe environments. Although there's no entirely risk-free environment, much can be done to reduce the dangers. Once the causes of injury are identified, preventive measures can be put into place— much like marketing low-fat products to combat high blood cholesterol. But unfortunately injuries rarely garner the same attention as cancer heart disease or meningitis. A news story about one meningitis case typically gets greater coverage than a car crash that killed six teenagers the same day.

Who's most at risk?
At all ages, males have more injuries than females. Boys undertake more hazardous activities and have more injuries than girls in every category. Boys drown 14 times more often than girls; they are killed on bicycles five times more often and hit by cars three times more frequently. Injury risks peak in toddlers and in teens—both stages of life when ability and experience are mismatched.

After our highways and roads, home is another frequent site of injuries. Although thoughts of "home" conjure up images of comfort and security, home mishaps account for almost 40 percent of injury and death away from the workplace. Socioeconomic status also affects injury rates. For complex reasons, but mainly because of overcrowding and poor supervision, children of low socioeconomic status have an above-average number of injuries. There are also large variations in provincial injury rates, which are usually higher for Native than non-Native populations.

Children are especially vulnerable
Canada has introduced laws covering child car seats, childproof packaging, flame-resistant nightwear toy labeling, fireworks and a multitude of other hazards. However childproof packaging isn't going to work if parents don't fasten the lids properly; child car seats won't work if they aren't used. Caregivers frequently underestimate dangers to children. A recent survey found that parents were more worried about their child being kidnapped or abusing drugs than about the less dramatic but far more prevalent risk of traffic injuries. Only 6 percent of parents surveyed knew that injury is the leading cause of childhood deaths.

Childhood injuries typically happen when caregivers relax their watchful gaze, become distracted or overestimate a child's skill. They can even occur with parents or other caregivers in the next or the same room. Not everyone realizes that within seconds a child can fall off a high surface (even a bed), drown (even in the bathtub or diaper pail) or get badly burned (by a hot kettle or iron). Anticipating how and where injuries occur is the first step in avoiding them. Childproofing of the home, the car and other surroundings must be geared to each age group's ability, activity and competence levels. The greatest danger arises when activity levels exceed a child's judgment abilities.

Different dangers at different ages
Newborns can't get into much harm on their own, but safety measures include smoke detectors, cribs of safe design and infant car seats (correctly used and properly installed).

Infants/crawlers: A baby a few months old can roll over put things in its mouth, crawl and fall from high places or get burned by hot liquids or cigarettes. Never leave an infant unattended on a high surface—don't wait until your child falls off the table to find out that it can roll over.

Toddlers and preschoolers: Injury risk increases sharply as crawlers become toddlers. As they learn to walk and climb, the home becomes increasingly unsafe. Kitchens, bathrooms, closets and drawers need to be reorganized. The risk of burns increases with toddlers—from tap water stoves, irons and heaters. Toddler reins have not really caught on in this country, but they're a good idea to pre-

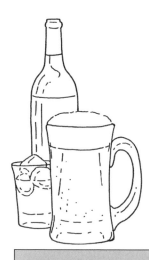

vent small children from darting in front of cars or getting lost in crowds. Besides falls from furniture, stairs and playground equipment, drowning is a special threat at this age. Poisonings also peak in toddlers, being 10 times more frequent than in older children. Grandparents' or other visitors' purses containing medications (such as heart pills—for instance, digoxin—sleep-aids or painkillers) should be kept safely away from exploratory young fingers. It's also wise to childproof the homes of grandparents and other relatives visited.

Schoolchildren are less likely to be injured than younger age groups, but pedestrian and bicycle injuries are common at this age, when children may still lack the skill to negotiate busy streets. Up to age 10 they should not be per-

mitted to cross busy streets unsupervised. Children must be shown (not told) how to stop and look both ways—left and right and then left again—before crossing the street. Tragically, children are sometimes killed by the family car in their own driveway. Watch for children playing behind the car; approach the driver's seat from behind the car and walk around the vehicle to do a safety check before reversing out.

Teenagers: Adolescence is the time of greatest risk, as many teenagers challenge authority, have a sense of invincibility, overestimate their abilities and show off to peers. Statistics show that access to firearms and other means of self-destruction increases risks of teenage suicide—a leading killer of adolescents. (In Quebec, for instance, suicides outdo traffic crashes as a cause of adolescent death.) One in 50 North American teenagers is involved in an auto crash. Drivers under age 21 drive faster and are less likely to wear seatbelts than older people. Substance abuse (liquor and drugs) is an added danger.

Preventing the six major causes of injury

Traffic collisions

Automobiles are becoming safer. Modern cars have shatterproof windshields, collapsible steering columns, headrests, and air bags. Seatbelts have been highly effective in preventing death and injury from traffic mishaps. During a collision, safety belts protect passengers by preventing ejection from the moving car; minimizing the severity of injuries due to impact with the vehicle's hard surfaces. Worn properly, lap and shoulder belts halve the chances of death in an auto crash, often allowing people to walk away from an incident that would otherwise have killed them.

In Canada, all children must legally be restrained in car seats. Properly designed child restraints (seats) not only provide safety but permit children to see out of the window (as they're sitting higher). Small infants should be in seats placed against the dashboard—facing the rear window—so they can see the driver. Older children should be properly secured in an approved child seat facing forward, in the back of the car. Yet sadly, only about one-third of chil-

ALCOHOL AND DRUGS POSE EXTRA DANGERS

Alcohol is often a factor in injuries, especially among teenagers. Everybody knows it is dangerous as well as illegal to drink and drive. Liquor impairs judgment, coordination and balance. Surveys show that 36 percent of teenage males and 17 percent of teenage females involved in traffic fatalities have blood-alcohol levels over the legal limit. If, despite the risk, parents allow their teenage children to drive cars and motorcycles, they must teach them road safety and clearly explain the dangers of drinking and driving. Many adolescents themselves are becoming more aware of drinking-driving hazards, and peer-group organizations, such as Students

Against Drinking and Driving, are very effective in promoting responsible habits. Some authorities promote graduated driving licenses for young drivers, rather than "carte blanche" permission to drive anywhere, anytime. Thus, on first obtaining a driver's license, a teenager might be prohibited from highway driving, as well as driving late at night or with other teenagers in the car.

It's even dangerous to drink and walk. More than one-half of pedestrians over age 16 involved in fatal traffic incidents have blood-alcohol levels over the legal limit. It is equally hazardous to drink and swim or sail, and alcohol consumption is a common factor in boating

mishaps. Likewise, half of all adults who die in house fires are found to have high blood-alcohol levels. Falls, too, are often linked to alcohol ingestion. Besides alcohol, drugs—whether illicit, prescription or over-the-counter (OTC) medications—can increase injury risks. For example, some antihistamines (such as Hismanal and Chlor-Tripolon) increase drowsiness and may impair driving ability. Painkillers and sedatives also impair the ability to drive or operate machinery safely. In one University of Toronto hospital study, 75 percent of those coming in with trauma injuries had high blood levels of OTC or prescription medications.

dren are properly restrained while traveling in cars; many parents only belt in their children on long trips (even though most traffic mishaps happen at busy intersections or close to home). (See also Chapter 11 about preventing childhood injuries.)

Air bags, a newer automobile safety feature, are meant to complement lap and shoulder seatbelts—to give further protection. They inflate on impact, protecting front-seat passengers from injuries to the face and spine in frontal, but not in side, rear or roll-over collisions. Sensors under the hood pick up the impact, producing inflation within milliseconds, so that air bags balloon out to surround the driver and front-seat passenger. Air bags reduce fatal injuries from auto crashes and are credited with saving almost 2,000 lives in North America since 1990. They are now standard equipment in about 60 percent of vehicles sold in the U.S., and in almost half of all new vehicles sold in Canada Air bags do not replace seatbelts but offer added life-saving protection.

Wearing seatbelts remains a must, or people will be thrown forward into the air bag when it deploys, sustaining possible damage from its impact. While seatbelts give adequate protection at speeds under 40 km/h (25 mph), at higher speeds the head usually strikes the dashboard or steering wheel and the brain moves forward in the skull at a swift pace. Air bags prevent the violent forces on neck and head in frontal crashes, so that the brain moves forward less forcefully against the skull and is less likely to be drastically damaged. Moreover, being built into the car air bags work without compliance; unlike seatbelts, worn at will, air bags inflate automatically, their protection not contingent upon voluntary action. Air bags reduce fatalities from motor vehicle mishaps by 10–15 percent over and above the 40 percent injury diminution provided by seatbelts (if worn).

While air bags protect most adults they may endanger infants in rear-facing child seats, small children and very short people—those under 160 cm (62 inches) in height—who may have the seat pulled far forward. Publicity about injuries and some deaths (about 55 in the U.S. and four in Canada) from air bags that burst or forcefully hit car occupants has led to changes in their use. New "smart" air bags are being developed that will be able to detect the vehicle's speed and alter the inflation force accordingly; they're also able to sense passenger size and whether occupants are belted in. Future air bags will have "on-off" switches, so they can be deactivated when an infant is in a rear-facing child seat, or a child under 12, a very short person or someone with a certain medical condition is in the front seat.

In praise of seatbelts
- Make "buckling up" automatic whenever riding in a motor vehicle.
- Remember that seatbelts must be well tethered and correctly adjusted.
- Wear the seatbelt assembly as snugly as possible without being uncomfortable.
- Consult your doctor if you are in an accident, even if you were belted and seem uninjured.

Bicycle and motorcycle safety measures also reduce the traffic-injury toll. Falls from bicycles can be very serious. Parents often buy a bike that is too big for the child, so he or she will grow into it. This is a mistake. Bicycles should fit the child. Because people tend to fall head first, cycling injuries often damage the head and brain causing death. Children should wear bike helmets from the time they get their very first bike. Although bicycle helmets reduce the risk of brain injury by 85–88 percent, fewer than 4 percent of schoolchildren and few adults wear them. Children in bicycle-mounted seats should also wear helmets. Motorcyclists must also wear helmets, especially as they have a 40 percent higher chance of dying in a traffic collision than people traveling in cars.

Helmets work as shock absorbers. Most properly designed and manufactured bike helmets consist of an outer shell, an energy-absorbing liner a layer of soft foam and fabric pads and a good retention system. The helmet distributes the force of impact and its inner foam absorbs the blow, preventing it from crushing the skull and injuring the brain. The foam liner—the life-saving portion—is usually made of expanded polystyrene or more costly but better polypropylene or polyethylene; it shouldn't be too stiff, because if it doesn't bend

WAYS TO PREVENT UNINTENDED INJURIES

- **Wear a seat belt when traveling in motor vehicles**
- **don't "drink and drive" (about half of all car crashes are alcohol-linked)**
- **push for "traffic calming" measures**
- **always wear a helmet when cycling**
- **stop falls by "safe-proofing home"; improve bone strength to reduce fracture risks (take calcium and vitamins as advised)**
- **reduce fire hazards by installing smoke detectors and butting out cigarettes properly**
- **use safety caps on medicine bottles**
- **safeguard pool areas and teach children to swim**
- **always wear life jackets when boating, and limit alcohol intake**
- **don't keep guns at home; store very safely if you do**

PREVENTION IS A MUST

Injury prevention involves:

- education, which includes anti–drinking-and-driving campaigns, bicycle-safety campaigns, home safety education;
- legislation, which includes seatbelt laws and compulsory child car restraints;
- modification of the product or environment, including measures such as childproof medicine containers, flame-resistant toys and nightwear, home smoke detectors.

While they can reduce injury risks, none of the three methods works on its own. Safety tutoring alone will not necessarily alter behavior. Studies have shown over and over again that telling people what to do may not make them comply. On the other hand, passing laws aimed at an uninformed and resistant public is not likely to work either. By contrast, passive injury control (making the environment safer) can be dramatically successful. Childproof medication containers are one example. Deaths from aspirin ingestion dropped in the United States from 144 deaths per year in 1960 to 12 per year in 1973 after childproof-packaging legislation came in. However, passive protection can be expensive, and the public must sometimes be coerced into compliance. Prevention is most successful if done at the community or "grass roots" level, where everyone participates in making the environment safer.

porosis (taking calcium supplements and vitamin D).

Fire hazards

Studies show that deaths from fire are far less common in homes with smoke detectors than in those without them. Being incapacitated by smoke is a major cause of death in house fires, which often start at night. The elderly and the very young are in particular danger; because they can't get out fast enough. Smoke detectors should be installed on each floor; near bedrooms, living rooms and in the basement. They alert people before smoke levels become dangerous. Check smoke-detector batteries regularly. In addition, every family should plan and practice fire drills. In nighttime fires people are drowsy, and those who have practiced beforehand are less likely to panic. Plan to meet at a designated spot outside the house in case of fire, so that you can quickly determine who's missing or still inside.

Burns and scolds, especially from hot coffee, irons and lit cigarettes, endanger young children, who may be scalded/burned even when held on the lap by an adult drinking coffee or smoking. Children can also sustain severe burns by chewing electrical wiring. A child's skin is more sensitive than an adult's and takes less time to sustain heat injury. Electrical devices and outlets should be blocked from young fingers. Check for frayed wiring. Discourage smoking in the home. Make sure hot food is covered or out of reach.

Suffocation

Some 40 percent of all injury-related deaths under age one are due to suffocation or choking on food and toy parts. Small parts from toys and games belonging to older siblings are frequent offenders. Round things are a special danger to tiny throats—such as small balls and round foods. Avoid giving children under age four round hot dog pieces, peanuts, popcorn, hard candy and non–bite-sized pieces of food that require chewing, as well as small toys and uninflated balloons. Swallowing bits of balloon or even whole uninflated balloons has been known to choke children in minutes. Never leave a child alone in a car; as deaths from asphyxiation have occurred when children got tangled in the straps.

or crush on impact, the shock isn't adequately absorbed. Models have become lighter more stylish, and more comfortable. Approved helmets include the older hard-shell types, the newer thin-shell or micro-shell models and the latest, lightest, no-shell types.

"Traffic calming," a strategy pioneered by European city planners, helps reduce injuries by diverting high-speed, high-volume traffic away from the city core and residential areas, reduces permissible speeds to 16 to 32 km (10 to 20 miles) per hour and narrows streets to decrease pedestrian injuries.

Falls

Injuries from falls are especially common in the elderly and young children. Fatal falls often occur on stairways, or from windows, trees, roofs and steep embankments. Older people often fall from ladders or on sidewalks, slippery floors or stairs. A serious hazard in themselves, stairs become still more dangerous if objects are left on them. Death and serious injury from falls in baby walkers are also common; many medical experts consider baby walkers highly dangerous. To reduce injury from falls, the elderly should safeproof their homes, and try to strengthen their bones by offsetting osteo-

Poisonings

Poisoning, the second most common reason for hospitalizing children under age four, becomes a potential danger as soon as a child begins to put things in its mouth. For every poisoning death that occurs, 20,000 toxic ingestions are reported to local Poison Control Centers across the country. Although medicine and poison containers are now usually childproofed, all medications and household cleaners should be stored out of a child's sight and reach. Not all poisons are obvious: perfumes, cosmetics, alcohol, paints and paint thinners can also be toxic. Keep poisons in original containers marked "poison." Never store paint thinner or similar substances in a cup or glass, even for a minute. If it's not something you'd feed a child, don't leave it within the child's reach. Keep ipecac syrup at home to induce vomiting if necessary, but call the Poison Control Center before administering it. Keep the local Emergency and Poison Control Center numbers near every phone.

Drowning

A residential swimming pool is considered an even more likely cause of death for a child under five than riding in the family car. Childproof fencing around swimming pools is the law in Canada, which greatly reduces drowning risks. But toddlers can drown in a small amount of water in a bathtub or a bucket, not just in pools or lakes. Teens are also at risk

GENERAL HOME SAFETY TIPS

- Wipe up spilled liquids or grease immediately— they invite disaster.
- Replace burned-out or inadequate light bulbs; have lights and light switches at both the top and bottom of stairs; install night lights in dark hallways.
- Secure scatter rugs with rubber backing or anti-skid coating, or by tacking them in place.
- Wear well-fitting, well-tied shoes or nonslip footwear when working around the house.
- Repair curled linoleum, broken or loose tiles and loose floorboards promptly.
- Install handrails or handles on the bathtub to aid getting in and out. Also use nonskid bathmats.
- Discourage use of electrical appliances in the bathroom. Be sure bathroom electrical outlets are grounded or on a ground-fault interrupter.
- Clear snow and ice promptly from stairs and porches. Sweep away water to prevent ice patches.
- Make sure that bed lamps are easily turned on and off—for getting up at night—to avoid falls.
- Install a night light in the bathroom.
- Keep water heaters at non-scald low levels.
- Put out grease fires by covering with a large lid. Do not use water or dump baking soda as they may cause worse spattering.
- Do not carry out a pot of grease that's on fire—a slip or trip could be fatal.
- Keep a dry-chemical fire extinguisher in an accessible location and tell everyone where it is and how to use it. Follow instructions for shaking and inspecting it regularly.
- Avoid portable home heaters, which can easily give burns.
- Keep electrical appliances away from curtains.
- Check electrical appliances for defects.
- Clean fireplace and chimney regularly.
- Equip house with smoke detectors and regularly check the batteries.
- Place firescreen around fireplace.
- Put out cigarettes in deep, flat-bottomed ashtrays and never empty them into wastebaskets or garbage until completely cooled.
- If on multiple medications, use a well-marked pillbox to avoid dosage errors. Ensure bottles have safety caps.
- Read labels on household products, noting which are corrosive, toxic or inflammable. Take appropriate precautions when using.
- Work with volatile chemicals in a well-ventilated space.
- Store knives in a proper knife rack on the wall or in a drawer adapted for this purpose.
- Avoid picking up broken glass with the fingers. Sweep it up and wrap it in newspaper before discarding. Pick up bits with wet paper toweling.
- Store power tools away from power source.
- Do not refuel gas-powered equipment when the engine is running or hot, and be extremely careful in cold weather that you do not spill gasoline on your hands—it can cause instant freezing.
- Don't keep guns at home.
- Take first-aid training.

TIPS FOR POOL AND WATER SAFETY

- Do not let children run alongside pool edges, as they are wet and slippery.
- Have a childproof fence surrounding the swimming pool.
- Install a telephone near the pool and use it,, so that supervising adults are not called away. This also provides a quick way to call for help if necessary.
- Make sure safety equipment—rings. buoys and lifejackets—is within reach and undamaged.
- If boating, obey the law by providing lifejackets or personal flotation devices for all passengers.
- Install propeller guards on motorized boats. Propellers are dangerous and a frequent source of terrible cuts and other injuries.

of water-related injuries, and must learn the rules of boating (such as wearing lifejackets), and be aware that alcohol and swimming or boating make a bad mix, regardless of TV ads suggesting the opposite. Learning how to swim does not necessarily decrease the risk of drowning. In fact, novice swimmers are among those most likely to drown, as they're apt to venture out too far be deceived by the distance covered or energy expended and run into trouble when trying to swim back.

PUTTING DRUG USE IN PERSPECTIVE

Illegal drug use, while serious and personally devastating, is not, as is commonly believed, increasing dangerously in Canada. Rather, it is declining, especially among schoolchildren. Statistics show that only a small minority of Canadians use illegal drugs, and an even smaller proportion use drugs with any regularity. Most illicit drug users try them only experimentally or occasionally for recreation. On the other hand, over three-quarters of the normal adult population regularly use legal, socially sanctioned caffeine, alcohol and nicotine (tobacco).

From earliest times, intoxicating substances have been popular; although their legal status has varied from culture to culture. Archaeologists have unearthed evidence of *cannabis sativa* (marijuana) use dating back 8,000 years, and cannabis is still smoked throughout the Middle East. Biblical writings frequently mention wine. Coca leaves are still chewed by many Bolivian and Peruvian Natives as a source of cocaine. East

Indians chew betel nuts, which contain arecoline, a nicotine-like substance. Opium (from the poppy plant) has been used for centuries as a painkiller and inducer of euphoric drowsiness. Many medicines still contain opiates (e.g., codeine and morphine), and before 1912 opiate dependency was common throughout America, with women users outnumbering men two to one. Opium eating and smoking remains an accepted practice in many East Asian countries. Yet some groups and religions—for instance, orthodox Moslems and Mormons—rigorously forbid all drug use.

Rumors of illicit-drug epidemics create a "war-on-drugs" mentality that overlooks the extent to which drug use is a widespread social custom in Western culture. In fact, moderate responsible drug use (of alcohol and caffeine) is actually linked to an active social life, while total abstainers are sometimes regarded as "antisocial." In Canada, caffeine, alcohol and nicotine are so popular that many people don't think of them as drugs. One University of Toronto expert suggests that "instead of labeling drug use as an epidemic we should more accurately call it endemic." In other words, drug use is such an entrenched part of our modern lifestyle (as of most human societies past and present) that it is more the rule than the exception.

Traditionally, substance dependence has been regarded as a social, rather than a medical problem. More recent evidence challenges this view. In many ways, substance dependence is remarkably similar to other chronic illnesses, such as type 2 diabetes mellitus, hypertension and asthma. The impact of individual choice, genetics and environment plays a similar role in the causes and treatment of all these disorders. As with other chronic illnesses, the treatment of substance dependence often requires medication as well as long-term planning, counseling, and follow-up.

Approximately 5–10 percent of all North Americans over the age of 12 are ongoing non-medicinal users of prescription psychoactive medications, illicit drugs and inhalants. Roughly, 25–30 percent of North Americans report having used illicit drugs. The lifetime prevalence of illicit drug abuse and dependence is 6.2 percent.

Substance abuse can have many adverse

health consequences. People who have substance use disorders very commonly also have mental health problems. For example, many people self-treat their anxiety with alcohol or marijuana. Approximately one-third of those with mood disorders have an addictive disorder as well. Domestic violence is more common in households where someone has a substance use disorder. Some regions of North America, including Vancouver, New Jersey and New York, have HIV incidence rates as high as 50 percent among people who inject drugs.

Drug users also suffer a disproportionate number of medical emergencies, something that has been increasing over the last decade. Common medical emergencies associated with illicit drug use include overdose, suicide and acute infections. In addition, more marginalized populations, including Aboriginals, street youth and the inner-city poor are not only more likely to use drugs disproportionately, but they also suffer disproportionate amounts of harm from their use of drugs.

The discrepancy between reality and the public perception of illicit drug use arises partly from mistakenly equating street violence, drug busts, seizures, criminal activities and hospital admissions with the extent of illicit drug use. But drug arrests and detox rates don't necessarily correlate with the amount of drug use. Drug seizures can increase while use remains the same or declines. And the number of people requiring drug-abuse treatment doesn't reflect present use because of the time lag between the development of a specific drug problem and the seeking of treatment by users.

What is a drug?

A drug is any substance other than body constituents or those needed for normal body functioning (e.g., food) which, on ingestion, alters brain and body function. Therapeutic drugs are used—often on prescription—to cure or alleviate health problems. Psychoactive or mood-altering substances—today's most popular drugs—alter the way people think, feel and act, and include most illicit drugs, as well as many legal and socially acceptable substances.

Some drugs (amphetamines, cocaine, caffeine) are stimulants, which increase alertness.

Others (alcohol, barbiturates) are depressants, which dampen brain activity, reduce anxiety and seemingly calm the spirit. Still others (lysergic acid diethylamide or LSD, and phencyclidine or PCP) are hallucinogens, which produce visual and auditory hallucinations. Certain drugs occur naturally, such as psilocybin or "shrooms" (an LSD-like substance from mushrooms), mescaline (from the peyote cactus), cocaine (from coca leaves) and heroin (from poppies). Others are made from plants (e.g., alcohol, from fruit, vegetables or grains). Yet others are synthetics, manufactured legally or illegally (e.g., amphetamine or "speed" and methamphetamine or "ice").

Why people take drugs

Psychoactive substances have a great range of effects. They help people overcome shyness and encourage self-esteem, remove pain, promote joviality (at ceremonies, parties) or create an intense "high" or elation that is a goal in itself. They may be taken for private pleasure—wine with dinner, a cigarette afterwards. Some "do drugs" for fun, mind-expansion or in order to belong to the "in group," or they may be a last resort for people who are at a low point in their lives, those who want to escape from a difficult home or school situation, to rebel, to cope with distress or to alleviate a psychological disturbance such as depression. Some people take to drugs rapidly because of sociopathic (antisocial) tendencies or simply because they mix with drug-taking companions. According to the modern biopsychosocial model, which attributes drug use to biological, psychological and social causes, people may use or become dependent on drugs because of a biological or metabolic predisposition, and a social reason like peer pressure and/or psychological factors (e.g., depression, anxiety).

Whatever the reasons for taking drugs and whichever drugs are used, they feed into the brain's limbic system, stimulating a "reward mechanism" that reinforces drug-taking behavior. The only common feature in the countless reasons for drug use is that the substances somehow reward the user. The same impetus (e.g., anxiety) may lead one person to alcohol, another to tranquilizers, yet another to overeating, depending on which solution seems best, easiest and most accessible.

Most of those who do drugs take several. According to Health Canada, one in 20 Canadians has tried more than one mood-altering drug—mainly hashish (a form of marijuana) and cocaine in the young, sleeping pills and non-medical tranquilizers (not used for the purpose prescribed) in older people. About 10 percent of separated and divorced Canadians use more than one drug; one-third of tranquilizer users also take sleeping pills; nearly all cocaine users also take marijuana; and many heavy alcohol drinkers also smoke tobacco. People with a "pro-drug" mindset will likely experiment with any new substance and add it to their repertoires.

Use is not necessarily abuse

There's no sharp distinction between moderate, responsible drug use and excessive or abusive use. Rather there is a continuum of gradual increase which may lead to dependence.

Drug abuse is defined as use "severe enough to cause health damage, social disruption, financial, workplace and family problems." (However, the term "abuse" is gradually being replaced by "use.") If drugs become someone's main solution for every difficult situation, the habitual manner of coping, there's an abuse problem. The greater the reliance on drugs, the worse problems it creates. Whether substance use becomes abuse also depends on whether the substance is legal or illegal and on cultural values. For example, LSD is nonaddictive, yet even occasional LSD-taking may be dubbed "drug abuse," because it's illegal. On the other hand, while Canadians consume a lot of caffeine, few coffee drinkers would be dubbed drug abusers. But if coffee were illegal—as it was during the Ottoman Empire, when thousands were punished for drinking the forbidden brew—caffeine consumption would be seen as drug abuse.

What is addiction?

Despite repeated efforts to define it, addiction remains poorly distinguished from habit, and the term is loosely used for any compulsion—such as being "addicted" to chocolate. The term "dependence" is now often used instead of or interchangeably with "addiction." Research suggests that drug dependence represents an abnormal response by a minority of people. The clue to dependence lies in whether the habit can be stopped—as one expert puts it: "Can you give up easily or not?" The greater the dependence, the harder it is to quit. Drug dependence includes psychological and physical dependence. The psychological aspects of addiction are at least as critical as physical dependence, and may dominate life to the exclusion of all else. According to social-learning theory, addiction is a pattern of drug use that is largely but not entirely out of the individual's control. People con regain control and give up the drug.

Circumstances can affect drug-taking behavior

People's attitudes can have a lot to do with their drug use. Their mindset is critical. An anxious, insecure person may react differently to a particular drug than someone who's secure, relaxed and confident. Ambitions or lifestyles may determine which drugs are used and how. For instance, an aggressive person who's eager to succeed or dominate may take stimulants (such as amphetamine or cocaine) to boost confidence and overcome inertia. Lethargic types who feel underactive may also choose stimulants but for different reasons—to heighten energy and alertness.

The place of drug-taking is also critical.

THE USUAL EFFECTS OF DRUGS

Most mood- and mind-altering drugs have some or all of the following effects:

• **tolerance**—the body's adaptation to repeated consumption, with ever-higher doses needed to achieve the desired "high." With some drugs such as amphetamines, tolerance builds so fast that before long users may need 20 times the starting dose to obtain any effect. Barbiturate users may become so tolerant that the gap between the amount they need to get high and a lethal dose becomes perilously small;

• **physical dependence**—the body's response to the drug, which means that when it's abruptly stopped there are usually unpleasant (and sometimes drastic) withdrawal symptoms;

• **psychological dependence**—emotional and mental preoccupation with the drug's effects. A substance may become so central to existence that a dependent user will be unable to go for even a day without a "hit," dose or alcoholic drink. The greater the reliance on the drug's perceived benefit, the more effort the user will make to get it.

ADDICTION IS NOT PREDICTABLE

"Once an addict, always an addict" and the "addictive personality" are widely touted myths. Experts stress that there's no such thing as an addictive personality; addicts can and often do give up their substance dependency.

On the other hand, drug use does not always lead to dependence. Given conducive circumstances—the right place, time and surroundings—almost anyone might use drugs, without necessarily becoming dependent. Studies of U.S. soldiers serving in Vietnam, where use of opiates was widespread, showed that ordinary, healthy people of widely varying background became regular heroin users without becoming addicted, and then gave up the habit. The soldiers had easy access to cheap. high-grade heroin, and almost 50 percent used it regularly (once or twice weekly). But for most of them the habit was transient, triggered by heroin's ready availability and the stress of war. Once back home, most veterans easily gave up the drug and only a fraction—about 5–10 percent—lapsed into reuse. This had nothing to do with the soldiers' personalities or the amounts of heroin taken. Once they were removed from the drug-taking ambiance, most simply no longer wished to use heroin. The only significant factors linked to resumption of heroin use were a pre-Vietnam record of drug use, a low academic record and a prior criminal record.

Consumed in lively surroundings such as a party or a trendy bar; alcohol tends to make drinkers feel convivial, but a lonely drinker in a dingy tavern is likely to feel forlorn and depressed.

The administration route is key. Chewed or swallowed substances are absorbed slowly from the gut, diffusing into the bloodstream to produce a gradual high. Sniffing a drug gets it into the bloodstream faster; and smoking it gives a still more rapid effect. Injected into a vein, drugs enter the bloodstream immediately, producing the quickest high of all.

Rituals also play a part. The place and means of administration may have ritualistic significance, giving users heightened expectations, a sense of camaraderie or the exultation of belonging to a special fraternity.

The menace of "designer drugs"

Manufactured cheaply in clandestine laboratories from readily available chemicals, the increasingly popular "designer drugs" are designed to skirt the law through the fact that they have slightly altered chemical structures, although they achieve comparable drug effects. Designer drugs often cannot be detected by current drug tests, and hit the streets faster than regulating agencies can track or restrict them.

"Ecstasy" or MDMA (*3,4-methylene-dioxymethamphetamine*), a current favorite whose effects are a cross between those of mescaline and amphetamine, is a potent hallucinogen synthesized in Germany in the early 1900s. It produces the euphoric rush of cocaine, together with mind-expanding sensations similar to those of LSD. Selling for about $10 a dose, it's been dubbed the "yuppie psychedelic." Taken orally, "Ecstasy" intensifies emotions, causes euphoria, increases energy and raises body temperature. Its action lasts four to six hours and it's commonly used in "raves" or all night parties where some deaths have been reported from dehydration and kidney failure due to the drug's effects. Added concerns arise from the fact that there are no quality checks, and Ecstasy can cause serious disorientation, jaw pain, mouth stiffness, psychotic aftereffects, panic attacks and even Parkinsonism (effects like those seen in Parkinson's disease)—hand tremors, drooling, rigidity and a stooped gait—due to destruction of dopamine-secreting brain cells. The U.S. Drug Enforcement Agency has put it on "Schedule One" (together with heroin and LSD) because of its dangers.

"Ice," or crystallized *methamphetamine*—named for its white crystalline look and touted as an alternative to crack—can be homemade. Purer than the formerly popular methadone—"meth" or "crank"—and now manufactured in California, "ice" came from Japan to North America via U.S. troops in the 1940s. Smoked like crack, "ice" is at least as addictive, pernicious and long-lasting. Prolonged use can cause lung and kidney disorders as well as permanent brain damage. Overdoses are often fatal. Put simply, "ice" can and does kill. Nonetheless, as it is cheaper and more potent than crack or cocaine, some fear that it may replace crack on the street.

Phencyclidine (PCP), also known as "angel dust" or "horse tranquilizer" is a white powder that's a cross between a synthetic stimulant

DRUG DEPENDENCE MAY INVOLVE:

- an overpowering preoccupation with and compulsion to get and take a substance;
- increasing use of the substance;
- development of physical dependence (withdrawal symptoms if stopped);
- the need for an "eye-opener"—a dose of the drug first thing in the morning;
- great difficulty in quitting.

SIGNS OF SUBSTANCE DEPENDENCY

- A change in behavior (often the first sign)—secretiveness, unusual moodiness, unexplained absences from home, cutting classes, workplace absenteeism;
- declining or erratic school or work performance;
- an evasive, less affectionate, hostile or distant manner—no longer intimate with family, friends, schoolmates or workmates;
- apathy, a withdrawn demeanor;
- new companions—joining new groups and adopting their language, clothes and style;
- failure to keep curfew, remember birthdays, maintain friendships, do chores, attend to responsibilities;
- memory loss—concentration or learning lapses;
- change in appetite or altered eating habits;
- less or more sleep;
- an angry or defensive reaction—especially at the mention of drugs—and complaints of being "hassled."

FACTORS THAT ENCOURAGE SUBSTANCE DEPENDENCE

- easy availability;
- low price;
- drug-taking companions;
- looking for "kicks" (fun);
- social acceptance of drug use by family, peers and friends;
- ignorance of precise health dangers;
- depression, stress, a need for escape or comfort or ways to cope;
- genetic, biological or inherited vulnerability (possible with alcohol, opiates and perhaps some other drugs).

and a "dissociative anesthetic." It produces unpredictable, sometimes violent behavior, intoxication, even delirium. A widely used street drug among teenagers (the groups who also use LSD, MDMA and other hallucinogens), it's often sprinkled on marijuana joints. PCP is said to alter body awareness and space perception. It impairs thinking ability and—in large amounts—can produce convulsions or coma. Several deaths (killings and suicides) have been reported from PCP overdosing or as a result of the drug's effect on behavior. Laced with or added to cocaine, it can have added dangers. PCP is often passed off as another drug, such as LSD or mescaline.

Getting off drugs

Many drug takers naturally grow out of or abandon their habit. Others decide to stop with more or less distress, according to the degree of dependence. Those who find it hard to quit even when they realize that a substance is destroying their lives need professional help. Seeking advice is not a sign of weakness, and drug dependence can be beaten. Tackling a drug problem early can reduce its toll, and there are many self-help manuals and quit guides available. It's a myth that people must "hit bottom" before quitting.

Formal treatment programs first address the addiction itself, getting the person detoxified and calmed down. Then, when they are no longer drugged, people can examine the reasons for their drug-taking and find ways to break the habit.

Harm reduction programs help decrease drug use without judgmental attitudes by focusing on damage control, to reduce the drug's health-impairing and social consequences. Strategies include free needle and syringe exchanges, outreach (such as automated syringe-exchange machines—used in many European and Australian cities), access to prescription drugs to help get users off illicit substances and establishment of "tolerance zones" (as in several European cities)—designated areas where users can obtain clean equipment, condoms and medical advice or attention.

Harm Reduction

A newer way to tackle drug use is by the concept of harm reduction. This approach acknowledges that there is a problem, but rather than trying to focus all energies on getting the individual to quit, the emphasis is on creating a safer environment for users. One example of this would be a needle exchange program. The program may not reduce injection drug use, but it may reduce the chance of a user becoming infected with HIV or hepatitis C.

TACKLING ALCOHOL ABUSE

Legally sanctioned, socially accepted and easily obtainable, alcohol is one of our society's most destructive drugs—used more widely than all illicit drugs combined. Indeed, while overall drug use has gone down in recent years, 86 percent of Canadians over age 15 still drink alcohol at least once yearly, 10 percent using enough to qualify as problem drinkers, and 5 percent being classed as heavy drinkers ("alcoholics"). A potent psychoactive (mind- and mood-altering) substance, alcohol is favored for its pleasurable effects and its short-term ability to alleviate anxiety. It is a particularly health-damaging drug because it harms almost every organ in the body, and tends to be consumed in large amounts. In Canada, a quarter of all medical hospital beds are occupied by people with alcohol-related illnesses.

In small amounts, alcohol is a pleasing accompaniment to meals, removing inhibitions and helping people relax. But some use alcohol as a crutch for getting through everyday difficulties or to offset anxiety, disappointment, loneliness, boredom or depression—to "forget" the unpleasantnesses of life.

How much alcohol is too much?

Most people know when their drinking is detrimental. Men who regularly consume between four and six drinks a day and women who consistently have two to three daily drinks may incur some memory loss, dulled mental capacity and impaired eye-hand coordination (all three will be reversed if drinking is reduced). Even moderate drinking may alter the pathways in the brain's *hippocampus* (learning center), *hypothalamus* (control center) and *nucleus accumbens* (reward center).

Sensible, low-risk drinking is drinking that has no negative consequences, does not involve drinking every day and doesn't disrupt daily life, work or duties. Many experts define "hazardous use" as the point at which drinkers themselves recognize the negative effects, try to set limits and make efforts to cut back. There's no unanimously agreed-upon boundary between safe and harmful drinking, but there's tenuous agreement that low-risk consumption ranges from one to four drinks per day to a maximum of 14 a week. Average intakes above six drinks a day are labeled as "heavy" or "seriously harmful to health."

TIPS FOR THOSE WISHING TO QUIT A DRUG HABIT

Pre-understanding (thinking of stopping)

- *With no precise knowledge of drug effects*, but feelings of vague concern, collect information about possible dangers.
- *Note feelings and circumstances that trigger a "trip" or binge*—e.g., stress, hostility, anxiety, anger.
- *Self-administer a Drug Abuse Screening Test (DAST)*—to determine how much is taken and how; whether able to get through a day (week) without drugs or able to cut back or stop; if ever had convulsions, tremors, flashbacks, blackouts.
- *List noticeable problems associated with drug-taking* at work, home or in public (e.g., diminished concentration, memory lapses, reduced performance, accidents, family rows).

Understanding (recognizing one's drug problem)

- *Admit possible health and other adverse effects* (possibly already evident to others).
- *Make a drug diary*—when, with whom, how and in what circumstances are drugs taken? When added up, the amount consumed may come as a surprise!
- *Devise a balance sheet of pros and cons of drug-taking*: e.g., pleasures/rewards vs. negative effects.
- *Determine whether drug consumption is already damaging health* (often sufficient to motivate a serious quitting attempt).
- *Decide that no one else is to blame*: the drug-taking is one's own decision. It can be beaten by one's own efforts.

- *Ask family doctor or other expert for advice.* Medical caregivers can often explain the risks of a particular drug, and motivate and support quitting efforts.
- *Realize that certain symptoms* (e.g., anxiety, sleeplessness, paranoia, phobias, hostility) may have been wrongly viewed as the *cause* rather than the *consequence* of drug use.
- *Check out places to get help*—experts, clinics, detox centers—and how to learn new coping skills.

Action phase—making an effort to stop (or cut back)

- *Set realistic goals for change*, e.g., short-term quit strategies—"a week without drugs," "*not* this weekend." Cut back or abstain for a day, week, month at a time.
- *Try self-help tactics*—often the preferred method—with manuals, quit guides and advice from drug-addiction-counseling agencies.
- *Plan to counter temptation*—list drug-taking "cues" and how to avoid or sidestep them.
- *Adopt an open, frank approach when seeking advice*—this is most likely to enlist maximum understanding and a frank, supportive response.
- *Anticipate relapses*—become wary of feelings, events, places that might trigger a relapse.
- *Do not regard a relapse as a failure* or loss of all that's been gained, but as a learning experience—one step on the way to doing better next time!
- *Be prepared for several tries* before breaking a drug habit.
- *Enlist cooperative support* from family and friends. The families of quitters may also need counseling.

HOW DIFFERENT DRUGS AFFECT THE BODY

	Alcohol	Amphetamines ("speed," "bennies," "black beauties," "uppers")	Cocaine ("crack")	LSD and other hallucinogens
Type of drug (chemical)	• ethyl alcohol (ethanol), a clear liquid (in beer, wine, spirits); • made from grain, fruit, vegetables or synthetically; • favored since antiquity for its relaxing, intoxicating properties; • beers contain about 5% alcohol, wines to 12% and spirits about 40%; • a sedative-hypnotic and central nervous system (CNS) depressant.	• synthetically produced: amphetamine (speed), dextroamphetamine (Dexedrine), methylamphetamine or "ice," methylphenidate (Ritalin), etc.; • used as pills, inhaled or injected (speed); • central-nervous-system stimulants that resemble action of adrenaline (natural body hormone).	• derived from South American coca bush (still chewed in Andes to offset fatigue); • crack is mixture of cocaine and baking soda; • cocaine hydrochloride is white powder ("coke," "C," "flake," "snow"); • formerly used in many medicines (until 1920s); • stimulant action—like amphetamine—but now legally classed as a narcotic.	• derived from mushrooms (psilocybin) or cactus (mescaline) or synthetically—e.g., lysergic acid (LSD or "acid") and phencyclidine (PCP)—"hog," "angel dust"; • structures resemble catecholamines—normal brain neurotransmitters; • hallucinogens—can distort reality and produce severe delusions.
Short-term effects (after a single dose)	• effects vary with size, sex and amount of food in stomach; • initial relaxation and loss of inhibitions; • increased sociability; • impaired coordination; • slowing down of reflexes and mental processes; • attitude changes, increased risk-taking and bad judgment, danger in driving car, operating machinery; • sleepiness.	• nervous system briefly stimulated; • reduces appetite; • increases energy, offsets fatigue; • talkative restlessness, greater alertness; • faster breathing; • rise in heart rate and blood pressure (with risk of burst blood vessels and heart failure); • temperature raised, mouth dry, skin sweaty; • pupils dilated; • alleviates nose stuffiness (original medicinal use).	• short-acting, powerful central-nervous-system stimulant, also a local anesthetic; • effects vary depending on whether drug is "snorted" (inhaled), injected, put in mouth, rectum or vagina, or smoked (as crack); • transient euphoria and increased energy; • appetite loss; • rise in heart rate and breathing; • dilated pupils; • agitation, restlessness, talkativeness; • brief rise in sex drive.	• unpredictable effects—at first like amphetamine; • excitation, arousal; • temperature raised; • altered sense of smell, shape, size, color, distance; • exhilaration, "mind-expansion" or anxiety —depending on user; • rapid pulse, dilated pupils, blank stare; • exaggerated power sense with possibly violent behavior; • later—dramatic perceptual distortions; • occasionally convulsions.
With larger doses and longer use	• blackouts (memory loss); • facial flushing; slurred speech; • staggering gait, stupor; • rise in blood pressure; • pancreatitis, hepatitis, stomach ulcers, injuries (broken bones); • effects magnified by other CNS and brain depressants (e.g., opiates, barbiturates, tranquilizers, antihistamines, sleep-aids, some cold remedies); • alone or combined with other drugs, can increase accident rates; • overdose may be fatal due to respiratory distress.	• bizarre behavior, talkativeness, restlessness, tremors, excitability; • sense of power, superiority, aggression; • illusions and hallucinations; • some users become paranoid, suspicious, panicky, violent; • raised blood pressure; • insomnia.	• permanently stuffy nose (if snorted) and risk of perforated nasal septum; • brief euphoric effect followed by "crash"—depression; • anesthetic effect can depress brain function; • bizarre, erratic, perhaps violent actions; • paranoid "psychosis" (disappears if drug discontinued); • sensation of "crawling under the skin"; • convulsions, disturbed heart action, even death.	• anxiety, panic attacks, paranoid delusions, occasionally psychosis (like schizophrenia); • injury or accidents due to drug-induced delusions or distance misjudgment; • risk of fetal abnormalities; • tolerance develops rapidly but also disappears fast with renewed drug-sensitivity; • with PCP, high fever, muscle spasm, erratic behavior, psychosis lasting weeks or more.
Long-term effects (prolonged repeated use)	• harms many body organs: pancreas, gastrointestinal tract, blood circulation, heart, liver, kidneys, brain; • may produce liver cirrhosis, ulcers, memory loss, impotence; • increased risk of cancers (mouth, larynx, throat, maybe breast); • vitamin depletion; • damages fetus; • dependence frequent.	• malnutrition, emaciation (owing to appetite loss); • anxiety states; • "amphetamine-psychosis" (with schizophrenia-like hallucinations); • kidney damage; • susceptibility to infection; • sleep disorders; • psychological dependence.	• weight loss, malnutrition; • destroyed nose tissues (if sniffed); • restlessness, mood swings, insomnia, extreme excitability, suspiciousness/paranoia, delusions ("psychosis"); • depression; • impotence; • risk of heart attacks; • strong psychological dependence.	• long-term medical effects not known; • may include muscle tenseness, "flashbacks"—brief, spontaneous recurrence of prior LSD (hallucinogenic) experiences; • prolonged, profound depression; • panic attacks; • no physical dependence.
Withdrawal symptoms	• insomnia, headache; • nausea; • shakiness, tremors; • sweating, seizures.	• long sleep, chills; • ravenous hunger; • depression.	• few withdrawal effects; sleepiness; • extreme exhaustion; • possibly "cocaine blues" (depression).	• few withdrawal effects, possible "flashbacks," anxiety.

Nicotine	Caffeine	Cannabis (marijuana, "pot," "grass," hashish)	Narcotic (opioid) analgesics (painkillers)	Solvents (inhalants)
• derived from tobacco; • used medicinally in South America; • tobacco smoke contains over 4,000 chemicals but nicotine is the most addictive; • a typical cigarette contains about one mg nicotine but amount absorbed varies with smoker; • stimulates central nervous system.	• derived from tea, coffee beans, kola nuts, chocolate; • used in many medicines (e.g., painkillers, cold/cough, pain remedies, antihistamines); • average cup of coffee contains 60-75 mg caffeine, colas about 35 mg per 250 ml or I cup, teas 20-60 mg/cup.	• derived from cannabis sativa or hemp plant; preparations vary in potency; "hash" most potent, marijuana least; • smoked in "joints" or chewed (sometimes with food); • medicinally used for epilepsy, glaucoma, against nausea; • classed as hallucinogen.	• poppy derivatives (opium, codeine, morphine, heroin) and synthetics (Demerol, methadone, Dilaudid, Percodan); • smoked, eaten or injected; • ancient painkillers used medicinally; • deaden pain, produce euphoria and drowsiness.	• volatile organic hydrocarbons from petroleum and natural gas (e.g., gasoline, toluene, hexane, chloroform, carbon tetrachloride, nail-polish remover or acetone, lighter fluid, paint thinners, cleaning fluid, airplane cement, plastic glue); • hallucinogenic effects.
• speeds pulse; • stimulates, then reduces brain and nervous system activity; • blood-pressure rise; • sense of relaxation; • reduced urine output; • impairs cleansing action of lung's cilia (hairs); • enhances alertness and concentration abilities.	• stimulates brain, speeds nerve-cell transmission; • elevates mood and alertness; • stimulates mental activity; • speeds up breathing, metabolism; • enhances mental performance; • postpones fatigue; • shortens sleep; • more urine output; • rise in blood fats; • increases stomach acidity; • decreases appetite.	• produces dream-like euphoria, laughter, relaxation; • alters sense of space, time; • increases hear trate; • reddens eyes; • dreamy, "stoned" look; • at later stages, users quiet, reflective, sleepy; • combined with alcohol, increased effects, distorted behavior; • impairs short-term memory, thinking, and ability to drive car or perform complex tasks.	• briefly stimulate, then depress higher brain centers; • give quick pleasure surge (for few minutes), then stupor (which mutes hunger, pain, sex drive); • taken by mouth, effects slower, no initial pleasure surge; • pupils tiny, body warm, limbs heavy; • mouth dry, skin itchy; • users may "nod off," alternately awake or asleep, oblivious of surroundings.	• exhilaration, light-headedness, excitability, disorientation; • confusion, slurred speech, dizziness; • distorted perception; • visual and auditory hallucinations; • muscular control impaired; • possible nausea, increased saliva, sneezing; • reflexes dampened; • recklessness, feelings of power, invincibility.
• lung damage; • damaged blood circulation; • slowed wound-healing; • vitamin-C depletion; • shortness of breath; • increases risk of upper-respiratory infections; • cancer-formation risks.	• nervousness, hand tremors; • delays sleep onset, reduces "depth" of sleep, insomnia; • abnormally rapid heartbeat; • jitteriness; • mild delirium possible; • convulsions (rare); • suspected cancer-causing agent.	• slowed digestive (gastrointestinal) activity: • time misjudgment; • sharpened or distorted sense of color, sound; • thinking slow and confused; • apathy, loss of motivation/drive; • large doses can produce severe confusion, panic attacks; • hallucinations (even psychosis).	• extremities heavy; • permanent drowsiness; • pupils become pinpoints; • skin cold, moist, bluish; • progressively slower, depressed breathing; • supervised pain-killing doses let people remain quite clear-headed and safe; • dangers increase with alcohol intake.	• drowsiness and possible unconsciousness; • severe disorientation; • risks increase with fume concentration; • irregular heartbeat, heart action disturbed; • large doses may cause heart failure—e.g., "sudden sniffing death" (especially with spot removers or airplane cement).
• narrowed blood vessels, risk of heart attack, stroke; • bronchitis, emphysema; • raised risk of cancers of mouth, lung, larynx, throat, bladder, pancreas, possibly cervix; • stomach ulcers; • impairs fetal growth; • strong dependence.	• may raise blood cholesterol level; • risk of stomach ulcers; • suspected cancer-inducing agent; • regular coffee use (over 5 cups daily) can lead to dependence (getting "hooked" on drug).	• loss of drive, reduced energy; • regular heavy use increases risk of bronchitis, lung cancer; reduced sex hormones; impaired learning; memory loss; possible decrease in immunity; • psychological dependence.	• constipation; • moodiness; • risk of endocarditis (heart infection) and other infections (AIDS) from needle-sharing; • hormone upsets (menstrual irregularities); • liver damage; • damaged offspring; • strong dependence.	• pallor, thirst, nose, eye, mouth sores; • irritability, hostility, forgetfulness; • may damage liver, kidney and brain; • nosebleeds, impaired blood-cell formation; • depression, weight loss; • other drugs compound damage; • dependence possible.
• anxiety, jitteriness; • inability to concentrate; • increased appetite.	• severe headache; • irritability; • tiredness.	• withdrawal symptoms mild—possible nausea, insomnia, anxiety, irritability.	• striking withdrawal effects (4-5 hours after last dose), sweating, anxiety, diarrhea, "gooseflesh," shivering, tremors.	• restlessness, anxiety, irritability, headaches; • stomach upsets; • delirium (rare).

**FOR MORE
INFORMATION
ON DRUGS,
CONTACT:**

- a family physician;
- community or vol-
  unteer programs;
- public-health agen-
  cies or nurses;
- crisis or intervention
  centers;
- drug-addiction-
  counseling
  centers/clinics or
  "hot lines," such as
  Ontario's Drug
  Information Line:
  (416) 595-6111;
- Alcoholics
  Anonymous (AA),
  Toronto branch:
  (416) 487-5591,
  or Narcotics
  Anonymous (NA),
  Toronto branch:
  (416) 691-9519;
- the Self-Help
  Clearing House,
  Toronto branch:
  (416) 487-4355;
  CAMH (Centre for
  Addiction and
  Mental Health)
  www.CAMH.net.

The French paradox: Is moderate drinking healthy?

The so-called "French paradox" refers to the puzzling fact that heart attack rates among the French are far below those of most industrialized nations, despite coronary risk factors—a diet rich in fat, high blood cholesterol levels, widespread hypertension (high blood pressure) and more cigarette smoking than in the U.S., Canada or Britain. Death rates from coronary heart disease (CHD) for men and women in Austria, Germany and the Netherlands are twice those in France, and are three times higher in the U.K., U.S. and Denmark. Many experts ascribe the low French heart attack rates to their high wine consumption, in particular red wine—leading to the surging popularity of red wine. (However although heart attack rates are low in France, there is an excess of alcohol-related traffic injuries, violent deaths and liver cirrhosis.)

There's growing evidence that a low to moderate alcohol intake does protect against heart disease and stroke. The effects extend beyond wine to all alcohols. Studies from many countries find that moderate alcohol consumers are at less risk of cardiac death than nondrinkers. Taken in moderation, any alcoholic beverage—whether wine, beer or spirits—seems to be okay. Put another way, one drink a day if you are a female, and two drinks a day if you are a male, is "cardioprotective" but more than that likely has a negative effect on the heart. These rules clearly don't hold if you are an alcoholic, or if you have hepatitis or other liver damage.

Specialists stress that a low-risk "drinking package" should consider both daily and weekly intakes. They suggest a limit of 14 standard drinks a week for men, and 9 drinks a week for women, with no more than two drinks on any one day—to avoid ill effects such as injuries and social harm. Drinking limits for women are set lower than for men because their bodies handle alcohol differently, and their lower body weights, different fat levels and other factors put women at greater risk of alcohol's ill effects at lower intakes. Experts also stress that the heart-protecting effects of alcohol can be obtained with *very small* amounts—as little as one drink every

other day. Adverse effects rise steadily with increasing consumption.

Should abstainers be encouraged to take up light drinking for health reasons? Most healthcare professionals think not. They oppose the idea of urging nondrinkers to start consuming alcohol for heart health. "People who don't drink shouldn't start to protect their hearts," says one specialist. "They can equally well stave off heart disease by not smoking, exercising and eating a diet rich in plant foods." For those who do drink, he adds that "one drink *every other day* is enough to protect the heart—no need for two daily drinks!" As alcohol consumption climbs above low-risk limits, its detrimental effects begin to outweigh cardiac benefits, with a rise in injuries and other alcohol-related problems. Heavy drinkers who consume more than 5 drinks daily have 2 to 5 times higher mortality rates than teetotalers or light to moderate drinkers.

Can alcoholism be hereditary?

While alcohol abuse tends to run in families—children of heavy drinkers seem likelier than average to become alcoholics—experts disagree on the extent to which alcoholism is inherited. Studies in Denmark and Sweden during the 1970s showed that children of alcoholics who were adopted during infancy into nonalcoholic homes were more likely to become heavy drinkers than children of nonalcoholics. The search is on for biological markers that could pinpoint the trait for alcoholism—if it exists.

The tendency toward alcoholism seems to come mainly from the father's side. Controversial and still-debated studies on twins separated from their biological parents before six weeks of age and raised in nonrelated families suggest that children of alcoholic fathers are three to six times more likely to become alcoholics than those of nonalcoholic fathers. A 1980 report in the *British Medical Journal* claimed that 30 to 50 percent of the fathers and up to 20 percent of the mothers of alcoholic children are also alcoholic. "Given that it may take more alcohol for them to reach a high, but that the euphoria may be greater," notes one expert, "sons of alcoholic fathers may be prone to alco-

POSSIBLE WARNING SIGNS OF PROBLEM DRINKING

- Concern about alcohol intake and admission of "drinking a bit too much";
- proclaimed efforts to cut back—to drink "only on weekends" or "only after dinner";
- clear negative consequences—work problems, disrupted social relationships, loss of spouse, job, money,
- reduced interest in work, hobbies, church, friends, family;

- recognition of troubled drinking and suggestions by friends, relatives or co-workers to cut back;
- consorting mainly with other drinkers;
- memory loss or blackouts—the inability to remember anything about the night (or day) before;
- lack of concentration, dulled mental acuity;
- physical signs of impairment—

tremors, shaky grip;
- increased personal injuries (cuts, sprains, bruises, fractures) due to impaired motor coordination;
- binge drinking, especially on weekends;
- usually gulping drinks one after another;
- constantly consuming alcohol, secretly on the job or at home; hiding booze;
- desperate need for a "relief" morning drink to ward off withdrawal

symptoms;
- changed behavior— missed deadlines and appointments, lateness;
- going to work the next day with still-hazardous blood-alcohol levels (indicated by alcoholic breath);
- mistakes on the job, lowered productivity, flawed judgment, unexplained absences;
- complaints by fellow workers

about boozing;
- heavy smoking or other drug use (these often go hand in hand with chronic drinking);
- skipping meals, eating only lightly while drinking;
- belligerent, grandiose attitude;
- violent or abusive actions, starting fights;
- hostility to questions about alcohol use; refusal to discuss the topic.

hol abuse because of genetic differences in their brain." The jury is still out on this topic.

Women and alcohol

Although fewer women than men are heavy drinkers, there's a slew of evidence that women are prone to health damage at lower alcohol intakes (less alcohol per body weight) than men. They are more likely to develop liver disease and mental deficiency with smaller amounts of alcohol. One expert explains that "since women's bodies contain more fat and less water than men's, they have less water with which to dilute alcohol. A woman of similar weight and height will therefore have a higher blood-alcohol content after drinking the same amount as a man."

Women also metabolize alcohol differently. They have less gastric (stomach) ADH enzyme than men, so less alcohol is broken down in the stomach, and more passes through to the bloodstream. Furthermore, a woman's liver produces more acetaldehyde, the liver-injuring product of the breakdown of alcohol.

Female hormones may also play a part. Some studies suggest that in the luteal (second) phase of the menstrual cycle, high levels of the hormone progesterone decrease smooth-muscle activity so that the stomach (which is smooth-muscled) doesn't empty as quickly. This

means that alcohol sits there longer before passing into the bloodstream, and therefore blood-alcohol levels tend to be lower than in the first half of the menstrual cycle. So it may conceivably be less risky for women to drink before rather than just after a period. In postmenopausal women, alcohol provokes the conversion of androgens (male sex hormones) into estrogens (female hormones), which some studies suggest may increase breast-cancer risks. On the other hand, increased estrogens offset osteoporosis (bone thinning).

Men who drink heavily become demasculinized because alcohol lowers the level of testosterone (male hormone), diminishes sex drive and effectively castrates them, causing impotence. In men, alcohol also triggers conversion of androgens to estrogens, which may cause breast enlargement, hair growth and other effects, as well as liver damage.

It's well known that babies born to heavily drinking mothers may have *fetal alcohol syndrome* (brain damage), but very recent evidence shows that the male offspring of alcoholic mothers may *also* be demasculinized. The fetal brain of male babies is programmed for masculine behavior long before birth by exposure to testosterone from the embryonic testes. Since alcohol reduces testosterone

DEFINING ALCOHOL DEPENDENCE

Today, alcohol problems are more precisely defined. The latest U.S. Diagnostic and Statistical Manual of Mental Disorders (DSM-IV) and the World Health Organization's "Classification of Diseases" distinguish alcohol dependence from alcohol abuse (harmful use). Alcohol dependence ("alcoholism") is a chronic disorder with recognizable symptoms such as physical withdrawal, loss of control, tolerance and continued drinking despite knowledge of its dire effects.

HOW ALCOHOL MAY PROTECT THE HEART

Moderate, low-risk alcohol intakes increase levels of "good" or HDL cholesterol, thereby improving cardiovascular health. About half the beneficial impact of alcohol on the heart is ascribed to its HDL-raising action. Alcohol may also benefit the heart by decreasing the blood's clotting ability—by reducing platelet "stickiness" or aggregation. The French custom of drinking with meals may further protect the heart by slowing absorption of alcohol, prolonging its anti-clotting effect. Recent studies suggest that alcohol may also protect against heart damage due to non-insulin-dependent diabetes. Some also postulate a "stress reduction" mechanism.

production, male babies exposed to alcohol in a mother's womb may later fail to develop the full range of male behavior. Rats born to alcohol-fed mothers show distinct female instead of male behavior.

Advice from a physician often helps to curb alcohol intake

Paradoxically, while doctors may not ask about alcohol intake and alcohol-troubled people may not mention it for fear of being labeled "alcoholic," most welcome medical advice. Many troubled drinkers don't ask for medical help until they finally realize (or are forced to do so by family and/or employers) how drastically it's undermining their lives. People frequently haven't the faintest idea how much alcohol is damaging their health. Yet even a few words of advice from a physician about the injurious effects of alcohol can curb alcohol intake dramatically. Studies from Britain and Sweden convincingly demonstrated a substantial drop in alcohol use when doctors simply asked about drinking habits at routine medical visits, and informed people that tests showed they were consuming too much for their own good.

INTERNET RESOURCES FOR ADDICTION

Alcoholics/Cocaine/Families/Narcotics/Pills
 Anonymous
 **www.AA.org; www.CA.org;
 www.FamiliesAnonymous.org;
 www.NA.org;
 www.PillsAnonymous.com**
 International, patient-focused
 information
Centre for Addiction and Mental Health
 www.CAMH.net/addiction/index.html
 Canadian health care provider and patient
 information
Harm Reduction Coalition
 www.HarmReduction.org
 U.S.-based site
 Patient-focused information
www.motherisk.org
 Evidence-based information for health care
 providers and patients.
 Reliable information on the safety and risks of

drugs during pregnancy and lactation
National Institute for Drug Addiction
 www.NIDA.NIH.gov
 Broad range of information for patients and
 health providers

Getting help early increases chances of a cure

Traditional treatments for alcohol disorders focused on specialized care for the minority (5 percent) of heavily dependent drinkers with clear signs of alcoholism. The old way was inpatient clinic or hospital treatment, often with lengthy stays of three to six months. But follow-up programs show that 10 years later 30 percent of those treated were still drinking heavily, and 18 percent in one study had died—two and a half times the rate for non-drinkers. It seemed that, because the huge numbers of mildly troubled drinkers were disregarded, people were not getting help until it was too late.

The new approach gears therapy to the whole spectrum of problem drinkers. Moderate problem drinkers who want to kick the habit can often manage with brief outpatient therapy that stresses self-help. Even minimal advice from a family doctor or other health professional, or a few sessions of outpatient sociobehavioral counseling, often helps drinkers cut back.

The decision to reduce alcohol intake is typically triggered by several bad experiences rather than one traumatic event. Drinkers come to realize that the positive aspects of alcohol are outweighed by its costs—hangovers, missed work days, interpersonal difficulties, diminished mental capacity. Among the new treatments for problem drinking, two innovative approaches have been developed at Ontario's Addiction Research Foundation (ARF).

The brief method for encouraging sensible drinking is meant for well-motivated "early stage" problem drinkers who have definite reasons to quit or reduce alcohol consumption and want to change their drinking behavior. Treatment involves three short counseling sessions aided by self-help handouts.

The brief intervention method:
- identifies current drinking patterns to show the role of alcohol in everyday life and the sit-

uations that trigger an urge to overdrink;
- motivates drinkers to maintain two weeks of abstinence before deciding on the longer-term drinking goal (initial abstinence tends to improve health and thinking abilities dulled by heavy drinking):
- decides on a suitable goal—either abstinence or controlled drinking;
- teaches strategies for maintaining the chosen goal by keeping records of daily drinking, mak-

ing plans to avoid overdrinking in risky situations, not using alcohol to cope with everyday difficulties and finding constructive ways to fill time formerly spent drinking.

Women tend to do better than men with self-help methods. About 65 percent of women, compared to 30 percent of men, manage to reduce consumption. Men require more therapy sessions (typically 5 to 6) and more "hand-holding" than women. One

TIPS FOR SENSIBLE DRINKING

- If you currently abstain from alcohol do *not* start drinking to lower risks of heart disease—there are many other ways to protect your heart, including exercise and dietary changes.
- Healthy adult men should drink no more than two standard drinks in any day, and no more than 14 drinks a week.
- Healthy adult women should limit intake to no more than two standard drinks a day, and not more than 9 drinks a week.
- Remember that risk increases with rising alcohol consumption for injuries, liver, pancreas and nervous system diseases, and various cancers. For motor vehicle crashes, every extra drink puts you at greater risk.
- Consume drinks slowly and with food.
- Leave gaps of an hour or so between drinks.
- Never drink to intoxication.
- Plan your drinking—decide when, where, and how much. Consider potential dangers such as driving, tiredness, health complications, medications or social pressure.
- Pace your drinking—measure the amount, count the drinks and never drink from the bottle!
- Make the first drink of the evening nonalcoholic, particularly if you're thirsty.
- Alternate nonalcoholic and alcoholic beverages.
- Have diluted drinks, not straight ones, or drink beverages with how or very low alcohol content (e.g., light or very light beer or dealcoholized beverages).
- Sip slowly; remember that a man's body can only handle about a half to one standard drink (8–13 g alcohol) per hour, and a woman's even less, as women are generally smaller and more sensitive to alcohol.
- Don't gulp. Put the glass down between sips.
- Don't refill the glass until it's empty and don't let others (waiters, hosts) do it either.

- Don't drink on an empty stomach—eat while drinking.
- When entertaining, always supply nonalcoholic drinks; don't buy too much booze.
- Prepare ahead by anticipating situations which may increase the pressure to drink. Plan suitable strategies and excuses such as "I'm at my limit" or "I'm driving."
- Learn to say "no thanks" without feeling guilty.
- Never have "one for the road"—it can easily push your blood-alcohol level above the danger (and legal) limit.
- If you regularly drink more than you want to, ask for expert help and develop activities that don't involve alcohol; find alternate interests or hobbies to take you away from your drinking.
- Don't use alcohol as a crutch for getting through tough decisions or difficult everyday situations, or to relieve boredom, loneliness, anxiety or depression, or to aid sexual activities.
- Never use alcohol as a sleep-aid (it disturbs rather than encourages sleep).
- Try to be a good role model for your children by demonstrating restraint.

Never drink:
- while swimming, boating, engaging in other water sports or responsible for others;
- when in a cold environment (alcohol gives a false sense of warmth);
- during domestic quarrels (because alcohol reinforces impulsive, irrational responses, rather than problem-solving techniques);
- if operating complex or dangerous machinery, or driving a vehicle;
- while on medication that interacts with alcohol, such as cough and cold remedies, painkillers, sedatives (if in doubt consult a pharmacist).

MEDICATIONS HELP MANY STOP DRINKING

In controlled trials, several medications have been shown to reduce the frequency and intensity of binges and increase abstinence rates in alcohol-dependent people. These drugs include Naltrexone, Acamprosate and Ondansetron. We don't fully understood how these drugs work, but they likely reduce the body's built-in (bio-chemical) "reward system" for drinking and thus reduce the pleasure.

Disulfiram or antabuse makes people ill when they drink alcohol. Although evidence for the effectiveness of disulfiram is equivocal, it is sometimes useful in highly motivated, stable patients who take it under the supervision of a spouse. Disulfiram inhibits the breakdown of the enzyme, acetaldehyde dehydrogenase, thus causing a toxic accumulation of acetaldehyde, with side effects such as vomiting, flushed face and headache. Disulfiram can cause death through hypotension and arrhythmias. Patients who have severe heart disease, psychosis, severe depression or severe liver disease should avoid it. Other than disulfiram, the above medications are safe and non-addicting, and are probably under-prescribed.

expert surmises that women may do twice as well as men because of their greater vulnerability: clear signals of health disturbance may strengthen their resolve.

A longer treatment model, the guided self-management approach, is also designed for troubled drinkers willing to take responsibility for handling their problem. This program emphasizes relapse prevention and views recovery as a gradual uphill climb. The key is to see slips not as catastrophes but as minor setbacks on the path to recovery. Guided self-management draws on the drinker's inner resources, identifying weaknesses that could undermine resolve. The program includes brief counseling, relapse prevention, advice and homework to uncover personal risk situations and identification of drinking cues. The aim is to help people analyze their drinking pattern and develop coping strategies to change it. Therapists remain on tap for more counseling if needed. Studies show that even brief therapy often helps drinkers lower intakes.

Severely dependent alcoholics may need more intensive treatment

Intensive residential treatment may still be the answer for those with entrenched alcohol dependence, and many clinics are staffed by former drinkers who have "been there" and managed to conquer their dependence. But liv-ing in (other than a brief stay) isn't necessarily best, as it's an artificial situation, with the drinker isolated from family, friends, job or studies. Acute alcohol poisoning (intoxication) and withdrawal is tackled before underlying psychological or social problems are combated. Detoxification starts by clearing all alcohol from the body. At the same time, medications such as benzodiazepines are given as needed, to ease withdrawal. A multilevel withdrawal reaction may occur, including trembling, exaggerated reflexes, sleeplessness, muscle cramps, cold, sweaty skin, nausea and insatiable thirst. Severely dependent users may experience further symptoms several days later—delirium, hallucinations, fever, blood-vessel expansion, tachycardia (racing pulse) and seizures. An alcoholic who quits too suddenly can suffer cardiac arrest (heart failure).

Once the physical aspects of alcohol dependence are under control, psychosocial therapy aims to restructure the drinker's lifestyle, social and work patterns—with the patient "unlearning" the behavior that leads to drinking and learning new coping skills. Some experts favour an *integrated* approach, using counseling combined with medication instead of older methods that use medication as a last resort. Concurrent counseling gives personal advice, homework and goals, and reviews risk situations.

What about AA and other support groups?

Alcoholics Anonymous (AA), Women for Sobriety and other support groups can assist drinkers to change their ways. According to the philosophy of AA, which still considers alcoholism a disease, a single drink taken by a recovering addict rekindles the craving and renews the old drinking pattern, inevitably triggering a return to heavy drinking, hence AA's insistence on absolute abstinence. AA groups meet weekly or more often and help people stay off alcohol by getting them to talk about their problem, providing a "buddy" system to give support during difficult times. To avert a relapse to old habits, former alcoholics are encouraged to maintain contact with the support group; there is always the risk that a crisis will precipitate a return to drinking, even after several years, and keeping in touch may prevent this.

Is strict abstinence the only way?

While most therapists and detox centers call for complete abstinence in recovering alcoholics, others suggest that for many drinkers—especially early problem drinkers—controlled drinking is a more realistic goal. Some experts call the AA rule for total abstinence artificial in a society where the majority drink occasionally, and argue that treatment should simply aim to help drinkers reduce their intake. Some reformed drinkers prefer to abstain, while others do better with reduced intakes. But while some problem drinkers can learn to take an occasional drink among supportive friends, the tactic is only suitable for selected people.

In contrast to most U.S. authorities who regard controlled drinking as an unacceptable goal for alcohol-dependent people, many Canadian and British alcohol treatment programs aim for controlled drinking—suitable for about 25 percent of cases.

In the words of one expert, "The dilemma for the future is how to curb alcohol abuse, without revoking privileges that the public expects, industry wants and to which most of us are accustomed." Strategies to reduce drinking involve taxation, penalties for drunk driving, increased awareness of alcohol as a drug and opposition to binge drinking. Other tactics include restrictions on alcohol advertising and enforced attachment of health warnings to bottles.

Getting medical help when it's needed

Improving patient–doctor relationships • Using medical checkups wisely • Natural, alternative or complementary medicine • Herbalism plays a key role in natural medicine

3

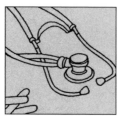

TODAY, PEOPLE INCreasingly want to share responsibility with their physicians for looking after their own health. Many people prefer to know about their medical ailments, understand the treatment possibilities and take a more active role in decision-making. Likewise, healthcare professionals encourage people to become better educated, more involved healthcare consumers. Given today's increasingly complex medical technology, they prefer patients to be "informed consenters" in any tests or treatments undertaken. Looking after health or disease is becoming more of a collaboration between consumers and their medical caregivers. This has become especially true with chronic diseases in which the patient is often the leader of an interdisciplinary team (doctor, nurse, pharmacist, and other allied health professionals) in managing his or her illness over the long haul.

IMPROVING PATIENT–DOCTOR RELATIONSHIPS

Despite the flood of new medical technologies, the patient-doctor relationship—whether with family physician, surgeon, gastroenterologist or other medical specialist—remains an intimate partnership. Trust is of the essence. Both physicians and those they care for must learn how to communicate with each other. More and more,

physicians and medical schools are recognizing the need for better patient-doctor relationships.

Modern medical teaching tries to instruct upcoming doctors in the art of listening, which, together with an empathetic manner can draw out patient concerns and feelings. Exploratory questioning is encouraged, not just about the illness that brought the person to see the physician, but also about lifestyle and hidden concerns or anxieties. Rather than asking questions that require a curt yes-or-no answer, physicians pose open-ended questions interspersed with silences that encourage people to elaborate. Uncovering hidden worries, conflicts and family disputes helps physicians gain a more complete picture and thus propose more effective treatment. Being a competent clinician also means being an empathetic one. "Empathy is not just understanding what the person says, but also what was not said," explains one clinician. "It means bringing out the hidden agenda, things the patient is unconscious of or finds hard to discuss."

During a recent Toronto workshop on doctor–patient communication, the three most common concerns found to come up in patient-doctor interviews were: fear of a serious illness, worry about being abandoned and feelings of guilt or worthlessness. From the doctor's viewpoint, a difficult patient may be someone who provokes uncomfortable feelings—such as anger frustration or inadequacy. From the patient's perspective, a cold, uncaring doctor is one who inspires discomfort or anger (at not being taken seriously), feelings of worthlessness, and who "hurries one along" or makes one "feel stupid." Medical schools these days often employ "standardized patients," usually actors who play a given role with medical students. Experienced clinicians assess these interactions from both a knowledge and empathic perspective and the student receives feedback from the patient as well as from the professor. The key emphasis of this learning experience is that while having knowledge is critical, understanding the patient's problem, fears and expectations are often equally important.

Modern medical schools teach physicians to *understand* what's behind behavior largely by listening attentively to what patients say. When caregivers feed back what the person fears or thinks, the person feels better understood and better able to tackle health problems. It's crucial to establish a trusting patient-doctor partnership in which the physician contributes up-to-date knowledge about the scientific basis for medical treatment and the patient brings his or her own beliefs and life-experiences. Doctor and patient then jointly decide on the best course of action for any particular disorder. This is often called "patient-centered care."

Many people expect (some even pressure) doctors to prescribe medication for every ailment, even though at least 30 percent of all visits to family physicians are for problems that resolve on their own. The newest trend in medical practice, "evidence-based medicine" or EBM, uses tests or suggests therapy only if current research shows they're likely to be beneficial. (Many popular or frequently used tests and treatments have turned out to be not only useless, but downright harmful.) Tests or treatments should be based on solid research evidence, rather than done according to tradition, "expert" opinion, handed-down hearsay or what's in the textbooks (which may be outdated). Doctors are urged to keep up with and apply their knowledge of the latest research findings to each individual patient. Those who practice EBM inform their patients about the known benefits and risks of any proposed procedure—knowing the risks and advantages of any suggested test, drug or therapy makes peo-

ple more likely to follow instructions and benefit from them.

Everyone needs a family physician for ongoing care

Family physicians can handle most day-to-day medical problems. They know the family history, keep charts on hand and make referrals to appropriate specialists or clinics when necessary. At the turn of the century, most doctors were general practitioners who delivered babies, set broken bones and performed minor surgery— procedures now often handled by other specialists. This is partly because the information explosion makes it difficult for physicians to be experts in all areas.

Without a family physician, people may find themselves in a kind of "healthcare limbo," with no specific person to consult in times of need, and no continuity of care. Turning to specialists, walk-in clinics or hospital emergency departments for everyday health matters does not provide optimal healthcare. Specialists such as gastroenterologists or neurologists will refer patients back to their family physician for follow-up.

Similarly, those who go to hospital emergency departments for care—perhaps for an injury or a bout of food poisoning—will be told to "report back" to their family physician for follow-up. Hospital emergency rooms are not geared to everyday health problems, but are set up to deal with acute situations. People who visit the emergency department are seen by different health care providers, who have no access to the person's chart or medical records, no time to track the causes of the problem, nor to discuss it or explain how to prevent it. As well, their objective is not necessarily to help you through your problem, but rather to rule out and resolve any threat of emergency.

Likewise, walk-in or "after-hours" clinics— which bridge the gap between a family physician's office and the hospital emergency unit—don't usually offer consistent follow-up. Walk-in clinics first appeared as "urgent care" centers in the U.S. during the 1970s and have mushroomed across the continent. Offering "no-appointment" care, these clinics are often open 7 days a week for extended hours and are

The newest trend in medical practice, "evidence-based medicine" or EBM, uses tests or suggests therapy only if current research shows they're likely to be beneficial. (Many popular or frequently used tests and treatments have turned out to be not only useless, but downright harmful.) Tests or treatments should be based on solid research evidence, rather than done according to tradition, "expert" opinion, handed-down hearsay or what's in the textbooks (which may be outdated). Doctors are urged to keep up with and apply their knowledge of the latest research findings to each individual patient. Those who practice EBM inform their patients about the known benefits and risks of any proposed procedure—knowing the risks and advantages of any suggested test, drug or therapy makes people more likely to follow instructions and benefit from them.

generally used for some episodic or urgent problem (such as diarrhea, asthma, an infected finger or anxiety attack) for which it's inconvenient or takes too long to see the family doctor. Criticism of walk-in clinics includes the fragmented care, lack of follow-up (needed for chronic conditions such as asthma or diabetes), staff not connected to any particular hospital, and no mechanism for reporting back to the family doctor. If you go to a walk-in clinic about a particular problem for convenience sake, and then follow up with your regular family doctor, make sure you tell the doctor what transpired.

How to choose a family physician

It's wise to find a family doctor who suits your own particular needs and lifestyle. Ideally, a family physician should take an interest in you as a person, not just in your ailment. A good doctor considers emotional as well as physical well-being. Besides dealing with day-to-day complaints, the physician should help you to promote overall wellness, facilitate access to medical specialists when needed, and help in keeping chronic ailments (such as asthma, arthritis or diabetes) under control.

No family physician available?

Unfortunately, the number of Canadian doctors in training was reduced in the 1990s and we now have a shortage, especially in family medicine. It is especially true in rural settings, but is becoming more apparent even in large urban areas. This makes it even more important for you to find a trusted provider. Some tips for getting into a practice include following other family members (doctors often make exceptions for members of families that are already enrolled), contacting the provincial College of Family Physicians as it may have a list of physicians who are taking new patients, and watching out for news of a new practice opening up.

The key question, then, is how to find a family physician who meets individual and family needs. A good start is to ask trusted friends or colleagues for a recommendation. If moving to a new neighborhood, ask the neighbors, local pharmacist or public-health agencies for a good doctor. You may also ask the local medical association, nursing associations, the provincial

College of Physicians and Surgeons or emergency-room nurses (who will know the physicians doing shifts there) about doctors willing to take on new patients.

It's a good idea to find a physician close to home, and preferably one who is willing to provide any special services required—such as obstetric care or home visits (for appropriate situations). Some people prefer a man, others a woman; some a younger others an older doctor. Having found a list of possible physicians, pay an exploratory visit—perhaps for a baseline checkup—to find out whether the person seems to suit your needs. Inquire about the possibility of evening or weekend visits if needed, and ask whether another physician or clinic is on call for nonoffice hours (preferably seven days a week).

The best time to look for a family physician is when you are well. Don't wait until you or someone else in the family is sick! If you've got a serious problem, it's too late to shop around. Family physicians now generally welcome people who introduce themselves as healthy individuals looking for a doctor. If the physician is not willing to discuss the philosophy of care offered, then maybe you should keep looking.

Choose a physician with whom you can communicate and feel free to discuss problems ranging from a bunion to cancer to worries about sex or sick parents. It should be someone who is empathetic, has a "whole person" focus, with whom you feel at ease, who takes into account your life circumstances and beliefs, discusses pros and cons of any procedure in understandable language, involves you in the decisions and doesn't make you feel anxious. Observe the waiting room—is it neat, clean and supplied with up-to-date health information? Is the receptionist polite and helpful? Chat to others in the waiting room. Check out the ambience. Ask whether the practice will monitor pregnancies (if you're of child-bearing age) and whether it is willing to look after the whole family, if desired.

Find out whether the doctor is affiliated with a hospital. Does he or she have admitting privileges? Studies show that physicians with hospital admitting privileges provide the most up-to-date healthcare, because they must meet

DOCTOR CHOICE—POINTS TO DETERMINE

- Is the physician's office within easy reach of home?
- Is parking easy? Is public transportation nearby?
- Is there access for people with canes, crutches or wheelchairs?
- Are there X-ray and lab facilities in the same building or nearby?
- Is the atmosphere friendly and welcoming?
- Is the waiting room clean and neat? Are there toys for kids to play with?
- Is there up-to-date health material around to read?
- Are the office staff helpful? Do they provide useful information and answer questions?
- What are the office hours? Is the office run as a clinic or private practice? Will you always see the same physician or sometimes others in the same practice?
- Is the whole family welcome—if that's what you want?
- Are home visits made if really needed?
- Are community resources and referrals (e.g., to social workers, dietitians, therapists) appropriately arranged?
- Are phone calls promptly returned?
- Who will attend to emergency illness at night, on weekends or at other nonoffice times?
- In case of a real emergency, are you quickly fitted in and seen?
- To which hospital(s) is the physician connected? Does he/she have admitting privileges there?

- Does the doctor listen calmly and attentively while you explain symptoms and feelings?
- Is the atmosphere relaxed?
- Does the physician seem easygoing or is he or she paternalistic and dogmatic? (Some people prefer a more authoritarian approach.)
- Does he or she give you a chance to discuss the problem in your own words or are you interrupted with a barrage of intimidating questions?
- Does the physician regularly ask about your lifestyle and counsel you about smoking, diet and alcohol/drug use, if relevant?
- Is ample time taken to explain the diagnosis and treatment choices, in understandable language?
- Are you involved in decision-making?
- Are medications and their use(s) clearly described?
- How many of the physician's services are covered by the provincial health insurance scheme? Are any extra charges (for filling in forms, phone conversations and so on) clearly explained?
- At the end of the office visit, ask yourself whether you fully understand the medical explanation(s), know what to do, understand the need for test(s) and feel free to call or go back for further clarification. Patients have the right to full disclosure about all suggested treatments or procedures and their possible effects and must give "informed consent" to any proposed treatment or tests.

prescribed standards of care, attend meetings and update their medical education. Family physicians in regular contact with specialists and the full range of hospital services can also facilitate care and arrange hospital admissions more quickly. If seeking a specialist, ask the family physician for the name of one likely to suit your particular situation. If it doesn't work out, report back and ask for another referral.

If it's what you wish, choose a physician you think is likely to tell the truth about any serious disease you or those close to you may have. Before the need arises, it is a good idea to decide how frankly you want to discuss a life-threatening disorder. Be sure all doctors involved know your wishes. You may want a "bottom-line" assessment of your own or a relative's survival chances in order to arrange affairs and power of attorney.

Ask the physician to "be honest about things." While any sickness is troublesome enough, communication about a terminal illness can be tormenting. Bad news inevitably creates stress. Physicians often disagree on how much to reveal about a serious condition, but many now openly explain terminal conditions to patients and/or the family, outlining the options. The goal is to help people retain control and the best possible quality of life.

Making the most of doctor visits

Given the short time allotted per person when you finally get to see the doctor; how can you make the best of it? People don't always use their visits as well as they might Some don't voice real worries (maybe the very problems that drove them to the doctor in the first place),

PEOPLE CAN EXPECT FROM THEIR DOCTORS:

- up-to-date knowledge and skill;
- confidentiality;
- a relaxed, empathetic, nonintimidating atmosphere in which to discuss concerns;
- attentive listening;
- patience and a gentle approach for uncomfortable examinations or procedures;
- a willingness to answer questions clearly (and to acknowledge ignorance, if that's the case);
- prompt return of urgent phone calls;
- availability (of own physician or stand-in) when needed for emergencies;

- referral to other medical specialists if required;
- medications prescribed only if really needed—with an explanation of what each does and side effects to watch for;
- a second opinion from another physician about any suggested diagnosis or treatment, if requested;
- information on how and when test results will be divulged;
- full, appropriate disclosure in understandable language of the diagnosis,

- treatment options and likely prognosis;
- the right to "informed consent"—the right to give or withhold consent for a medical test or treatment after being told of its risks and benefits, without detracting from the doctor-patient relationship;
- no violation (or abuse) of the trusting relationship with the attending physician.

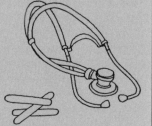

DOCTORS CAN EXPECT FROM THEIR PATIENTS:

- honest communication of all aspects of health—relaying facts about exercise, diet, smoking, alcohol, drug use, known diseases, allergies and medications taken (both prescription and over-the-counter);
- realization that physicians work within certain constraints imposed by the healthcare system and can deal with only one or two problems at any one visit;
- willingness to make special appointments

- for detailed advice if needed;
- willingness to take part in their own healthcare decisions, fully discussing fears and worries;
- willingness to follow instructions (or explain why it's not possible);
- an effort to return for follow-up care when requested;
- an effort to keep appointments for tests or office visits—or to cancel reasonably well in advance;
- careful attention during doctor visits,

- asking questions until what's said is fully understood;
- adherence to medication instructions, remembering that while one pill may be good, two can be harmful;
- an effort to keep track of visits, tests and treatments;
- cooperation in noting the results of treatments (for example, which therapy helped, which had an adverse effect) and to inform the physician of any problems noted.

not mentioning key concerns until about to leave, when they may blurt out questions about some alarming pain or lump.

It's a good idea to compile a list of concerns and questions beforehand. Jot down the points to ask, however trivial they may seem. A list serves as a memory-jogger, saves time and avoids the common mistake of forgetting or neglecting to ask key questions. Try to whittle this list down to two or three key concerns. People who are emotionally troubled or depressed—perhaps after some traumatic experience, such as job loss or bereavement—may request a medical checkup when what they really need is supportive counseling. It's wise to ask the front desk if you can have a longer appointment to allow extra time for discussion, as emotional and psychiatric problems can rarely be covered in a brief appointment. Such issues are not likely to get resolved in one appointment. People with mental health concerns can ask about setting up a few consecutive appointments to resolve issues and inquire about other resources that might be helpful. Many anxious or depressed people imagine they have some fatal illness and need medical reassurance as part of the healing process. This can require a process of ruling out "physical" causes before focusing in on key mental health issues. Emotionally distressed patients will be comforted even if the doctor does not find a physical problem. Astute, sympathetic physicians watch for and give cues for airing underlying concerns, perhaps asking what you suspect "might be the problem and whether you have any other worries to discuss?" The doctor may realize that someone needs extra time to discuss things and suggest a return visit within the next few days or weeks.

Most family doctor practices are very busy and it can be a challenge for clinicians to prioritize the various problems they see on a daily basis. Doctors may also be caught between being the patient advocate ("we need to get a CT scan of this as soon as possible") and gatekeeper ("I am sorry but I cannot order CT scans every week for your headache"). This often involves drawing a "line in the sand," as to how much medical investigation is really necessary. The decision must be made jointly by doctor and patient, which can be challenging when the cause of symptoms remains unknown or unexplained.

Knowing how physicians are paid

Doctors are usually paid a "fee for service," meaning that they are paid according to how many patients they see. Some doctors are paid a salary. Many patients are surprised to find out that doctors in the fee-for-service model are not paid to return phone calls, send e-mails or review lab tests. Many doctors receive 20–40 calls a day and might never see patients if they returned all their calls. And they would usually need to retrieve your chart and review any recent lab tests. This system clearly isn't perfect, but it might explain why you did not receive that call back! The current trend is towards putting doctors on salaries, but debate continues about the best model of service delivery.

USING MEDICAL CHECKUPS WISELY

The shift in medical attitudes means that the annual physical checkup for healthy, nonpregnant adults has been dramatically revamped. The routine yearly battery of medical tests is largely being abandoned in favor of more counseling about lifestyle and health habits.

While some physicians still give their patients exhaustive annual examinations, and many people demand them, the old-fashioned medical checkup is slowly disappearing. In its place are more personalized versions, together with lashings of advice, counseling and exhortations to adopt a healthier lifestyle.

During the 1970s, with the soaring costs of medical care, the Canadian and U.S. governments began to investigate the real value of annual medical exams for all. The Canadian government commissioned the Canadian Task Force on the Periodic Health Examination (CTF)—made up of more than 40 scientists, clinicians and consultants—to evaluate routine medical tests. The aim was to decide which tests should be included, which omitted and which done only for selected "at-risk" individuals. A world leader in the healthcare field, internationally recognized as the first to rigorously assess the value of routine checkups, the Canadian Task Force evaluated 78 different conditions and medical procedures.

Along with many other health agencies, preventive task forces suggest carefully tailoring tests to individuals, and have recommended the abandonment of many routine procedures, such as chest X-rays, electrocardiograms, many

GLOSSARY OF SPECIALISTS

Anesthesiologists decide which type of anesthesia will be used, administer it during surgery and monitor its effects.

Cardiologists specialize in diagnosing and treating abnormalities of the heart and blood vessels.

Dermatologists diagnose and treat skin disorders.

Emergency medicine specialists are trained to work in a trauma center or hospital emergency department.

Gastroenterologists diagnose and treat disorders of the digestive system and liver.

Geneticists specialize in diagnosing and predicting inherited disorders, such as cystic fibrosis, hemophilia and many other disorders.

Gynecologists—see Obstetricians.

Hematologists diagnose and treat blood disorders.

Internists specialize in the internal (but usually nonsurgical)

treatment of adults. Some internists have subspecialties, such as cardiology, gastroenterology or hematology.

Neurologists diagnose and treat disorders of the brain and nervous system, spinal cord and peripheral nerves.

Obstetricians/gynecologists specialize in the treatment of female reproductive systems. An obstetrician also specializes in pregnancy care and delivering babies.

Oncologists diagnose cancer and recommend treatment.

Pediatricians specialize in treating children and adolescents.

Physiatrists specialize in physical therapy and sports medicine.

Psychiatrists specialize in emotional problems and mental illnesses.

Radiologists administer X-rays and ultrasound. A diagnostic radiologist uses radiology to diagnose medical problems. A therapeutic radiolo-

gist uses radiation for the treatment of cancer.

Surgeons diagnose and operate on a wide range of conditions. A general surgeon may specialize further, choosing, for example, thoracic and cardiovascular, pediatric, colon and rectal, or plastic surgery.

Urologists diagnose and treat disorders of the urinary tract and, in men, problems of the reproductive tract.

WHO NEEDS WHAT MEDICAL TESTS, WHEN?

Infants need:
- thyroid function tests (in newborns within first post-birth week);
- the "startle test" to check hearing response;
- immunization at recommended intervals for diphtheria, pertussis (whooping cough), tetanus, polio, measles, mumps, rubella, Hib or Hemophilus influenza B (against infant meningitis);
- well-baby visits, paralleling the immunization schedule, at two, four, six, twelve and eighteen months, and then annually which should include:
  - measurement of child's height, weight and head circumference;
  - a check of the eyes for infection and anatomical defects;
  - a check of hearing—for example, whether an infant can locate sounds as well as would be expected and, later, whether speech is developing normally;
  - a developmental appraisal, to identify mental retardation or learning abnormalities;
  - thorough examination of hips, legs;
  - parental counseling and injury-prevention advice about fire, falls, household poisons and traffic injuries—a crucial part of the well-baby examination. Discussion of parenting problems and advice on home safety and car restraints. Parents are encouraged to ask questions about childcare at every doctor visit.

Growing children need:
- measurement of length, weight and head circumference;
- assessment of parent-child interaction;
- learning/developmental evaluation;
- eye inspection and vision tests;
- injury-prevention advice (such as encouragement to wear bicycle helmets);
- annual dental checkups, after age three, with oral-hygiene advice;
- vaccination booster shots—for diphtheria, polio, rubella (girls), tetanus;
- inquiry about educational progress.

Teens/adolescents need:
- height and weight measurement;
- vision tests;
- checks on sexual health, contraceptive and STD advice;
- smoking-cessation counseling (if appropriate);
- risk-reduction advice.

Healthy adults aged 18–65 need:
- blood-pressure measurement at every physician visit, and at least every three to five years;
- annual dental checkups for gum disease and cavities;
- polio booster immunization (depending on whether live or inactive vaccine was previously used), tetanus and diphtheria booster shots every 10 years;
- quit-smoking advice (if they are smokers);
- cholesterol testing every five years (and more frequently if the levels are raised or if there is any coronary artery disease)
- counseling on alcohol use and traffic-injury prevention.
- there is good evidence to include screening with a Hemoccult test (for blood in the stool) in the periodic health examination of asymp-

tomatic patients over age 50 with no other risk factors. However, there are still concerns about the high rate of false-positive results, feasibility and the small clinical benefit of such bowel screening (over 1,000 individuals must be screened for ten years to avert one death from colorectal cancer). The options for colon cancer screening are threefold (hemoccult testing, that is, looking for blood in the stool, a sigmoidoscopy , and a colonoscopy). A colonoscopy, which looks at the whole length of the colon, can sometimes include removing "precancerous" polyps. "It is typically done every ten years, but is a more invasive procedure. Sigmoidoscopy (examing the lower part of the colon with a fibreoptic tube) is not always available. Hemoccult testing is the easiest procedure, but it has the highest risk of causing a "positive test" that is actually false. So the results would have to be confirmed by a colonoscopy.

Men specifically need:
- testicular exam between 20 and 40 years of age
- discussion about having a rectal exam and PSA testing (for prostate cancer) if over 50, or over age 40 if there is a significant family history. Neither test is very accurate: it can be reassuring if negative, but can cause needless anxiety when the tests produce results that are "false positive" (suggesting disease when none is present).

Women specifically need:
- an annual breast exam;
- mammograms every two years after age 50;
- Pap smear tests at recommended intervals;
- regular pelvic exams to test for cervical cancer;
- chlamydia tests, if sexually active.

The healthy elderly (over age 65) need:
The above tests as appropriate, plus:
- blood-pressure measurement every two years;
- annual anti-influenza shots (to reduce the risk of serious complications that may follow influenza);
- once-only anti-pneumonia immunization—advised in Health Canada's new Canadian Immunization Guide (authorities also suggest pneumonia immunization for high-risk groups such as those with sickle cell anemia, the institutionalized elderly and adults working or living in overcrowded conditions);
- regular dental examinations;
- a full review of all medications being taken;
- those with specific concerns that often trouble the elderly should consider the following when a problem exists:
- eye examination to test for blood-vessel disease, cataracts and glaucoma
- hearing tests—especially for those regularly exposed to loud noise;
- assessment of nutritional status (how well the senior is eating);
- evaluation of the ability to perform the activities of daily living (dressing, bathing, toilet use, cooking, cleaning, shopping)
- cognitive (thinking) impairment tests when a deficit is suspected, especially when noticed by those living with the individual. This is imperative if there is any likelihood of danger or accidents (e.g., leaving the stove on, getting lost)

SOME TIPS FOR DOCTOR VISITS

- Try to schedule the appointment for a time convenient for you.
- If you need a longer consultation, ask for it ahead of time, remembering that doctors can discuss only one or two problems at any one visit. Ask for another visit to discuss less pressing or subsidiary worries.
- On the day of your appointment, phone ahead and ask whether the doctor is on schedule.
- Anticipate delays; take along a good book, work or letter-writing materials.
- Bring a short, clear list of observed symptoms, which might include: new or worsening pain, changes in bowel frequency, appetite or sex drive, or unusual stumbling—anything that may affect physical or emotional well-being.
- Record what the physician says (or, with permission, consider using a tape recorder). Note the name(s) of any disease or disorder diagnosed and any tests ordered.
- Take along all medications—both prescription and over-the-counter—currently being taken, or jot down their names.
- Perhaps bring along a trusted friend or relative—especially helpful for the elderly or those worried about a serious health problem.
- Make sure you understand what the problem or treatment is.
- Ask the physician to repeat any information not fully understood. Keep on asking until any medical jargon is quite clear.
- Remember, there's no such thing as a stupid question! It's all right to call and ask the doctor or nurse a question you left out or only thought of after leaving.

If medications are prescribed:
- Record the generic (scientific) and brand name of each medicine and inquire about side effects.
- Make sure all medications are labeled and kept in original containers to avoid errors.
- Store medicines properly. A bathroom medicine chest may not be the best place because of the high humidity. Unless specifically directed, the refrigerator also is not ideal, as cold temperatures can affect the medication. A locked cabinet in the bedroom is a good place to store medications, beyond the reach and sight of small children.
- Elderly patients or those taking multiple medications, who may have trouble seeing or remembering what medicines should be taken when, can use weekly pill dispensers loaded by a relative or nurse.
- Ask what each drug is supposed to do, how long and when to take it and what to expect in terms of relief and how soon.
- Discard unused and outdated medications; put them down the toilet or, well wrapped, into the garbage.
- Don't reuse old prescribed medication. If the same health problem redevelops, get a new prescription.
- Remind the doctor about other medications being taken—whether prescribed by the same or another physician—and inquire about possible interactions.
- Ask about side effects that may occur with a medication (e.g., drowsiness, nausea, sex-drive alterations). Will it be safe to drive a car or operate machinery? Will the drug action be affected by alcohol, food or sunlight?
- Ask what to do if an unpleasant or seemingly dangerous side effect occurs.
- Never share prescribed medications with others.

blood tests and rectal exams (although some organizations still promote annual rectal exams for prostate cancer in men over age 40). Contrary to popular belief studies show that many of these tests don't work as disease-preventing measures. The most effective are blood pressure tests (to prevent heart attack and stroke) and advice on quitting smoking.

Physicians are urged to give far more advice on the effects of lifestyle on health—whether in the sphere of weight, diet, smoking, alcohol and other drugs, exercise or sex life, rather than spending a lot of time doing complex physical tests.

One U.S. report concludes that "the greatest promise for preventing illness lies in helping people to alter their health-endangering behavior." If a doctor stresses that smoking, a fatty diet or excess alcohol use already shows signs of undermining health, there's a good chance people will change their health-damaging behavior.

Agreement on the need for certain routine tests at checkups

There is wide agreement that the following procedures should be routinely done:
- weight measurement (to help people to keep weight within the healthy range);

- blood-pressure measurements once every two to five years and at each visit in all adults over 18 years old;
- universal childhood immunization against several infectious diseases;
- annual influenza shots for everyone over age 65, and other at-risk groups;
- physical breast examinations by a competent healthcare professional, for all women;
- mammograms (special breast X-rays) every 2 years for women over age 50;
- Pap smears (of the cervix), to detect premalignant or cancerous changes, for all sexually active women, the first two to be done annually and if negative (with no suspicious changes), every three years thereafter (The U.S. Preventive Task Force and many physicians recommend annual pap smears up to age 65);
- tests for chlamydia (a sexually transmitted infection), recommended during first trimester pregnancy (to prevent birthing complications) and for high risk groups (sexually active women under age 25, those who don't use barrier contraceptives, anyone with multiple sex partners or signs of the infection), to prevent spread and complications such as pelvic inflammatory disease and infertility;
- although mass screening for Type 2 diabetes in the general population is not recommended, testing for Type 2 (non-insulin-dependent) diabetes using a fasting plasma glucose test should be done every three years in those 45 years and older. More frequent or earlier testing (or both) should be considered in those with additional risk factors for diabetes, such as a previous high blood sugar or obesity;
- for cholesterol screening, Canadian guidelines recommend screening men over age 40, women who are menopausal or over age 50 for elevated cholesterol. People with risk factors such as a strong family history or any heart disease should have earlier testing;
- colorectal cancer screening: recent guidelines about screening for colorectal cancer recommend that average-risk men and women 50 years and over undergo screening. Although the only screening programs shown by good randomized controlled studies to decrease colon cancer mortality are those using fecal occult blood testing. The new guidelines offer several screening options to be selected by individuals and their physicians. Besides annual fecal occult blood testing (looking for blood in the stool), these tests include flexible sigmoidoscopy (using a short, flexible scope to view the colon) every five years, barium enema (using a dye that can be seen on X-ray) every five to ten years, and full colonoscopy (looking at the entire colon) every ten years.

Controversial, and not universally recommended are:

- screening for osteoporosis. Recent Canadian guidelines suggest there is "fair" evidence to screen postmenopausal women for bone density to prevent fragility fractures. There is no direct evidence that screening reduces fractures. However, there is good evidence for the effectiveness of screening in identifying low bone mineral density (BMD) and good evidence that treating women with low BMD can reduce the risk of fractures.
- tests to prevent or detect prostate cancer include the digital (finger) rectal test,—which only touches a small part of the prostate—and the PSA blood test (for prostate specific antigen) which does detect prostate cancer, but has a high "false positive" rate, leading to many needless investigations and anxiety. The pros and cons of this test are still much debated.

NATURAL, ALTERNATIVE OR COMPLEMENTARY MEDICINE

In their search for relief, ever more people turn to "alternative" therapies—also called unconventional or complementary therapies—to keep themselves healthy or to remedy chronic disorders such as backache, arthritis or cancer. Alternative treatments are not "accepted" standard practice within the medical profession—even though some have a considerable "nonstandard" track record of efficacy.

In fact, estimates show that worldwide only about 30 percent of human health care is delivered by conventional medical practice. The rest includes "folk" cures and alternative methods such as acupuncture, homeopathy, chiropractic, herbalism, "therapeutic touch" and visualization.

Spurred by popular interest in unorthodox therapies, how they work and might augment mainstream treatment, the U.S. Congress has established an office of Alternative Medicine at the National Institutes of Health (NIH) to evaluate the effectiveness and safety of some alternative treatments.

Complementary therapies are growing in popularity, perhaps because the public is increasingly frustrated by mainstream medicine and unconventional therapies give people a sense of "taking personal action" to overcome illness. In giving people a greater sense of control, alternative healing methods may help to decrease symptoms, but most forms have not been objectively evaluated, and practitioners may be legally limited in their ability to treat disease. Most alternative therapies rely on traditional practice (sometimes centuries old) and on testimonials from patients and advocates, and many medical opponents regard them as "dubious." Nonetheless, several unconventional therapies are gaining credence, such as massage, yoga, acupuncture and relaxation, for use alongside conventional treatment.

Who uses complementary therapies and why?

One large American Cancer Society survey revealed that about 10 percent of the U.S. population used unorthodox therapies in the 1990s—generally the better-educated and richer groups (who could afford them). Over 75 percent of advanced (metastatic) cancer patients occasionally use unconventional therapy. When vitamins, diets, relaxation and visualization are included, the number is probably higher

Put off by modern high-tech approaches, many sick people turn to complementary treatments which appear "less intimidating," more "complete," treating people more as "whole persons." Other reasons cited for trying unconventional therapies are that they are "natural," more "person-centered," and less "toxic" than medical treatments. Some people turn to unorthodox therapies because conventional medicine fails them. For example, people with arthritis or advanced metastatic cancer, for whom there is no effective medical treatment,

understandably seek help wherever they can. The focused attention given by some unorthodox therapists can help overcome the feelings of helplessness so common among those undergoing cancer treatments. Unconventional healers tend to allot more time to their clients than many busy medical caregivers.

Calls for more scientific scrutiny of unorthodox therapies

In general, the Western medical establishment has little knowledge of unconventional therapies and tends to dismiss them as "questionable" or "unproven," even as "quackery." Some healthcare professionals oppose alternative therapy because it stops people from sticking to medical treatment or may interfere with it. Some alternative therapies are very costly and some may engender a false hope of cure; a few are considered "dangerous."

Most conventional medical treatments undergo rigorous testing for risks and side effects versus benefits. They have been scrutinized, criticized and debated by other professionals so their dangers are known and benefits quantified. Patients accept medical treatment with "informed consent," having been fully informed about the proposed treatment, its duration, how it works, its probable benefits, possible risks and adverse effects. With standard treatments, the facts may be discouraging but at least they are known: not so with unconventional techniques.

Most physicians feel uncomfortable, therefore, recommending methods for which there's no evidence to prove benefits or harm. Unconventional practitioners may not reveal the percentage of cases that end in failure. Anecdotes claiming improvement do not provide scientific evidence of therapeutic value. For example, cancer cures attributed to untested methods may be supported by stories of people who never even had cancer or went into remission from medical treatment. Even though a cancer is progressing, it may falsely be said to have "gone away"; patients who die and don't return for follow-up might be claimed as a "cure"!

Another argument leveled at unorthodox therapies is the secrecy that sometimes sur-

"WITH" NOT "INSTEAD OF" MEDICAL THERAPY

Most physicians as well as most of those who practice alternative therapy believe that such methods work best alongside or as a supplement to—not instead of—conventional treatment, provided they do no harm. The term "complementary" mirrors the idea that medical care should be the *first-line* approach, with alternative care as an additional choice. Although a few people use unconventional therapy *instead* of suggested medical treatment—like those who give up their prescribed medication and go to Europe or Mexico for treatments not available here—most people use them not to replace but in addition to medical treatment. For instance, some people add yoga, relaxation, massage or herbal remedies to their physician-prescribed regimens. It should be remembered that many herbal medications, although considered benign, actually have significant amounts of active ingredients and can interact with some medications.

CONSUMER TIPS ON HERBAL REMEDIES

- **Use herbal products only as directed, and only for short periods of time.**
- **Do not use them to replace prescribed treatment for serious conditions.**
- **Always tell your physician about herbal remedies being taken.**
- **Purchase from established and reputable suppliers. Some herbalists are knowledgeable and helpful, others less so.**
- **Know what you are buying: are the Latin names of herbs and their quantities listed?**
- **Be cautious in using concentrated oils and teas.**
- **Consult a physician about taking herbs if you have any chronic illnesses, are taking other medications, are pregnant or elderly, and before you consider giving them to children.**
- **Do not give children under age two herbal remedies.**
- **Familiarize yourself with the herbs you're using; inquire about side effects and potential hazards.**

rounds them. Clients may be dissuaded from discussing the "alternative" treatment with their physicians. Secrecy is unscientific; modern medicine progresses by shared information and discussion. It is best to tell the physician about any unorthodox therapy you are trying in case it interferes with your medical treatment.

Happily, there has been a considerable increase in the number of trials examining various alternative approaches. As for allopathic medicine, some have been shown to be no better than placebo while others prove to be effective. Generally speaking, the trials for these interventions have been small with limits regarding the methodology.

Many different alternative therapies

Reflexologists feel the soles of the feet, massaging them to "break up toxic deposits" at specific points in the body. Iridologists claim to assess disorders in every part of the body by looking into the eye's iris, suggesting treatment accordingly. Traditional Chinese medicine considers the interaction of body, mind and spirit, using "pulses" in the wrist to determine where to apply therapy and restore the body's "energy flow." Among the most common are acupuncture, chiropractic, naturopathy, homeopathy, metabolic or "detoxifying" strategies, special diets, herbalism, immune augmentation, imagery and hypnosis. A therapy may have been invented recently or have traditional underpinnings, for instance, stemming from Native American or Chinese medicine—approaches that differ greatly from those of Western medicine. The treatment may have a religious or quasi-philosophical basis, such as the anthroposophy of Rudolph Steiner or homeopathy's doctrine of "like cures like." People may be offered a combination of treatments. For instance, the Gerson method, practiced in Mexico, offers a hodgepodge of a low-sodium diet (consisting of liver extracts and vegetable juices), ozone therapy, clay packs, live-cell therapy and various vaccines.

Examining a few complementary methods

- *Acupuncture*, an ancient Chinese practice, involves direct stimulation of specific points or "energy meridians" by twirling acupuncture

needles, using electroacupuncture, acupressure or moxybustion (burning herbs such as the daisy-like plant, *Artemisia vulgaris*). It works by blocking the transmission of pain by neurotransmitters, possibly also triggering release of *endorphins*—the body's own opiates.

- *Chiropractic methods* focus on musculoskeletal (bone and muscle) disorders, particularly—but not exclusively—spinal disorders such as back, neck and head pain, disc problems, muscle strain and postural abnormalities. Practitioners aren't medical physicians, but need many years of training to qualify and must be licensed by self-governing agencies.
- *Metabolic therapies* use "purifying" agents to "detoxify" the body and eliminate cancer with specific detoxifying agents such as *laetrile*. The U.S. National Cancer Institute failed to show laetrile had any benefits and there have been some laetrile-related deaths, possibly due to the cyanide in apricot pits. Other supposedly cancer-curing methods include antineoplastons (shown by U.S. researchers to be useless, even life-threatening), cancell and "chelation therapy" (which can reduce the body's zinc levels and deplete blood calcium, with possibly serious consequences).
- *Naturopathy*, based on a belief in the body's innate healing power, is practiced by naturopaths (NDs) trained in basic medical sciences (such as physiology, pathology, histology) and the use of botanicals, homeopathy, acupuncture, hydrotherapy and other methods. They try to eliminate the causes of disease with natural remedies, rather than just suppressing symptoms, arguing that interfering with the body's "balance" by taking medication leads to trouble down the road.
- *Homeopathy*, a controversial method, is based on the "law of similars," meaning that a substance that produces a certain set of symptoms in a healthy person can also cure those symptoms in a sick person, the difference being mainly the size of the dose. Homeopaths use the smallest possible dose—micro-doses—which may mean diluting a substance in water dozens or even hundreds of times. (Critics question the efficacy of such very dilute substances.)
- *Physical therapies* include treatments with

electricity, radio waves, magnetism and oxygen (usually administered as peroxide, germanium sesquioxide or ozone). Ozone therapy, very popular and used by thousands in Europe, is based on the premise that cancer cells have different metabolic needs than normal cells and prefer a "low oxygen" milieu; oxygen saturation is hostile to cancer cells. (This therapy can cause kidney damage and has been banned by the U.S. Food and Drug Administration.)

- *Immuno-augmentation therapy* may try to stimulate the immune system by injected protein extracts, *lymphokine activated killer (LAK)* cells or heat-shock proteins (recently produced by genetic engineering). U.S. scientists who investigated the procedure concluded that the materials used were mostly diluted blood proteins, mainly albumin—of no proven use in boosting immune function. Some of the injections provoke severe allergic reactions or hepatitis infection.

Herbalism plays a key role in natural medicine

Herbalism, originating from traditional Chinese medicine, is an ancient form of treatment using plants and animal extracts (often as pills or capsules). Some of our most widely used modern drugs originate from plants, although the healing ingredients are now often chemically synthesized. The heart drug *digitalis*, for instance, derives from foxglove plants; *morphine* comes from the poppy; *quinine* for malaria is made from cinchona bark; the chemotherapy drugs *vincristine* and *vinblastine* come from the periwinkle plant. Sick animals are suspected of consuming plants for their medicinal properties. For example, Harvard anthropologists have documented chimpanzees chewing bitter. Aspilia leaves, which contain active antifungal and antiparasitic agents. But many plants once considered medicinal are now considered weeds.

Many Europeans remain firm believers in herbal remedies, convinced that "natural" is best. A recent U.K. poll revealed that 76 percent of British family doctors study alternative medicine after graduating, and in North America, herbalists command a sizable following. More

and more North Americans are also taking herbal agents. They may be mixed in specific proportions to relieve pain, hormone imbalances, breathing disturbances, heart problems, and gastric upsets. Although most herbal remedies haven't been medically evaluated to Western standards, some have been extensively studied by equivalent methods.

Herbal remedies are available in health food shops and traditional ethnic stores, and from naturopaths and herbalists. Their regulation varies greatly from place to place. In some European countries, they are listed as medications and covered by health insurance schemes; in others they are classed as foods. In Canada, most herbal products are not legally permitted to be sold as medications but only as foods, and warning labels are not required, although a few bear federal Drug Identification Numbers (DIN), approving their sale as drugs. Most occupy a "grey area" between medications and food. While most herbs are harmless when used in moderation, large doses can cause adverse reactions. Problems reported with strong herbal teas—for instance, comfrey and gordolobos—include bleeding, gastrointestinal problems and liver disorders. Pyrrolizidine in gordolobos teas, widely consumed in the southern United States for sore throats, is no longer considered safe as it may cause liver disease, especially in large doses. "In general," according to one expert, "herbal medicinal teas ought not to be consumed in amounts above three or so cups a day."

The most highly toxic plants have already been eliminated from the herbalist's stock-in-trade. Lily of the valley, daffodil, deadly nightshade, foxglove, jimsonweed and hemlock are banned by Health Canada. But occasionally, an amateur herbalist gathers a poisonous plant and mistakes it for a harmless one. In one recent case, a woman mistook oleander for eucalyptus, and died after drinking the tea In another case, an elderly couple died within 24 hours of overdosing on digitalis, mistaking poisonous foxglove for comfrey.

Herbal remedies can also interact with prescription and nonprescription drugs, and with each other. Some plants such as tonka beans, melilot and woodruff, which increase bleeding,

---

POSSIBLE RISKS OF ALTERNATIVE TREATMENTS

- **Absence of safety regulations;**
- **lack of scientific testing—benefits may be uncertain;**
- **interference with conventional treatment;**
- **reliance or overconfidence in a complementary therapy that leads people to abandon medical treatment;**
- **prohibitive costs that could produce financial hardship;**
- **difficulty in distinguishing honest, principled practitioners from those who are not;**
- **sense of personal failure and guilt if an unorthodox regime doesn't succeed;**
- **fruitless pursuit of false "cures" that may prevent the terminally ill from "making the best" of the time left.**

TOP ITEMS FOR THE MEDICINE CABINET

Stocking a medicine cabinet sensibly doesn't mean stuffing it full of remedies for every conceivable ailment, but selecting those items most likely to come in handy for everyday needs and some emergencies. In general, less is better. Any products that have lost their label or passed their expiry date should be thrown out. The following classes of over-the-counter products have been recommended by University of Toronto experts as useful for common problems that may not need medical attention, or as temporary measures to be used before consulting a physician.

• Analgesics such as ASA (acetylsalicylic acid), and acetaminophen are potent painkillers, effective against headaches, backaches and many other aches and pains. Both ASA (e.g., Aspirin) and acetaminophen (e.g., Tylenol, Tempra, Panadol) are antipyretics (fever reducers), but ASA should not be given to children because of the risk of Reye's syndrome—a dangerous liver and brain disorder. ASA (but not acetaminophen) is also an anti-inflammatory agent, able to relieve arthritis and other conditions such as inflamed muscle injuries.

• Syrup of ipecac induces vomiting and is a useful standby, especially if young children swallow a poisonous product Syrup of ipecac can be given at any age and induces vomiting in about 10 minutes. But call the Poison Control Centre or doctor before giving the syrup, as forced vomiting may be inadvisable. Substances such as bleach or lye (Lysol) burn a second time "on the way up" and some floor waxes, kerosene and other volatile materials would be inhaled again while vomiting, possibly causing more harm. However, when a medical expert condones its use, the syrup can give fast, effective treatment and prevent the poison from being absorbed, and may even help to avoid a trip to the hospital.

• Anti-nausea pills or suppositories such as dimenhydrinate (Gravol), available in pediatric and adult strengths, quell nausea, car sickness and mild vomiting. The suppository form is useful when vomiting prevents pills from being kept down.

• Antiseptic agents keep cuts, scratches, sores and scrapes clean. While many physicians promote soap and water as a good "first choice" antiseptic to kill microorganisms, various commercial antiseptics are available: old-fashioned iodine (messy and stinging to use), Betadine (an organic iodine compound that stings less but stains like iodine), pHisoDerm (an antiseptic liquid soap), chlorhexidine solution (Hibitane) and hydrogen peroxide. Weak solutions of plain salt or, better still, Epsom salts are useful for soaking infected wounds. Antibiotic creams and ointments (such as Polysporin and Bactroban) are recommended by many physicians but are of debated usefulness in some cases.

• Oral anti-itch and anti-allergy products usually contain antihistamines of one kind or another. Individuals should select the type that works best for them. In general, the most sedating antihistamines are the most likely to relieve itchiness or allergy symptoms—e.g., chlorpheniramine (Chlor-Tripolon) or diphenhydramine (Benadryl). A note of caution: remember that alcohol used with antihistamines may cause excessive drowsiness or retard reaction times. Other medications may also enhance the impact of antihistamines. Weak hydrocortisone products (now available without prescription as creams, ointments and lotions, in 0.5 percent strength) may relieve an itchy skin but should be used with care on the face because of skin-thinning effects. Calamine lotion is a good antidote for itchiness, sunburn or a mild poison-ivy rash.

• Bowel-disorder remedies are available but should be used cautiously. Most pediatricians advise against the use of such products in children under two years of age, unless specifically prescribed. For an underactive bowel a wide range of laxatives is readily obtainable, but it's generally better to eat a well-balanced, fiber-rich diet to keep the bowel active. For specific constipated occasions, mild laxatives can be selected according to taste, such as products containing magnesia or senna, mineral oil and phenolphthalein, or bowel soothers such as Pepto-Bismol. For an overactive bowel or diarrhea, experts may recommend binding agents such as Kaopectate, or bowel-immobilizing drugs such as Imodium. Ranitidine or Zantac is effective for heartburn. But experts advise against use of Imodium in children, as it may mask the severity of symptoms. Imodium immobilizes the bowel rather than clearing up the diarrhea or its cause. Traditional remedies such as arrowroot and oat bran contain natural bowel-binding ingredients.

• For an acidic stomach or regurgitation problems, such as heartburn or indigestion, a vast array of antacid preparations (mostly aluminum and magnesium hydroxide products) is available, including Gelusil, Rolaids, Maalox, Amphojel, Tums and Riopan. Liquid forms, although messier and less portable than tablets, generally give speedier relief.

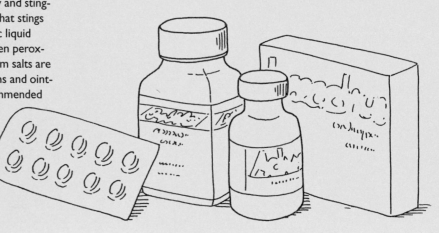

• Cold remedies, taken orally or used as nasal sprays or drops, include decongestants, painkillers and expectorants. Experts strongly recommend products containing one type of ingredient only, not those with a "mixed bag." Single-ingredient products include antipyretics (such as ASA or acetaminophen) to combat fever, analgesics for pain and decongestants against nasal stuffiness. The most effective oral decongestants are pseudoephedrine, ephedrine and phenylpropanolamine, each varying slightly in the strength, speed and duration of its effect and in its stimulating action on the brain (a side effect that may produce agitation or jitteriness). Nasal sprays usually contain similar compounds and/or oxymetazoline or xylometazoline, which have a local vasoconstricting (shrinking) effect on the nasal membranes, easing the congestion. Use of nasal sprays for more than three or four days, at specific intervals, is not recommended because of the rebound effect, which paralyzes the nasal cilia (hairs), preventing them from expelling mucus and thus increasing the stuffiness. Spray decongestants are best reserved for "must clear" occasions, such as air travel. There is limited evidence that these products are effective.

• A good cough medicine is useful for those kept awake by an incessant cough. The most effective cough medicines are prescription products containing codeine. Codeine suppresses coughing by acting on the brain's cough center, not on the throat, and is just as effectively absorbed from pills as from syrups, if not more so, however soothing a syrup may feel to a sore throat! A pediatrician may suggest keeping such a product at home for children with a persistent cough. Dextromethorphan (DM) is a nonprescription cough suppressant, available in single-ingredient formats (e.g., DM syrup, Delfym DM or Sucrets) or combination products (e.g., Benadryl DM, Triaminic DM or Robitussin DM). Physicians advise caution in using cough suppressants as it is not always desirable to suppress a cough. Coughing is the protective mechanism that clears the respiratory tract of mucus (phlegm). Codeine can help suppress the cough center, but needs to be prescribed.

• Skin soothers and softeners are invaluable for scaling, chapped or dry skin, rough hands or sore infant bottoms. Rough, dry skin easily becomes inflamed, and may develop cracks through which infections enter. Effective emollients (skin softeners) include petroleum (petrolatum) jelly, lanolin-based creams and products containing urea, lactic acid or phospholipids. Emollients should be applied to moist skin, to hold in water and keep the surface soft. Calamine lotion is also useful for soothing sunburned or itchy skin but is rather drying.

Safety first at all times

As a "safety first" precaution, experts suggest that even the relatively mild products listed above must be regarded with respect. Some simple rules may avert needless household tragedies or accidents:

• Don't "guess" about the possible severity of symptoms—given even the slightest doubt or uneasiness, check with a physician before using any medication.

• Throw away any product that has lost its label or passed its expiry date (prescription medication should be dated at time of purchase, preferably identifying the person and ailment for which it was bought).

• Mark all potentially poisonous substances with a clear warning sign, such as a red dot.

• Don't share prescription medication or use a medication prescribed for someone else—different people need different products.

Special precautions for children:

• Keep all medications well out of children's reach.

• Show children the symbol for toxicity, which means "Do not touch!"

• Give medicines to children rather than permitting them to self-medicate.

• Try not to let children see adults self-medicating too freely and too often or taking many combined products. Discuss the risks of drug interaction.

(For more on medications, see Appendix.)

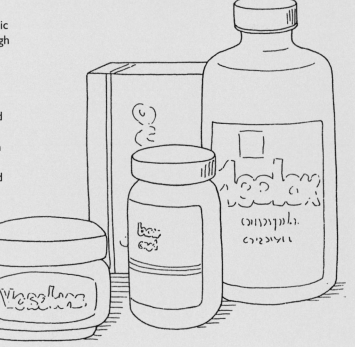

should not be consumed by those with circulatory disorders or those regularly taking ASA. Others such as bearberry and St. John's Wort are diuretics, and shouldn't be taken by those on prescribed diuretics. Recent trials with Kava Kava, an anti-anxiety preparation, have shown that it may be toxic to the liver. In the final analysis, shopping for herbal products is a matter of *caveat emptor*: buyer beware!

Deciding on your complementary therapy

People considering an unconventional method should do a thorough check before starting it. "It's best to tell medical caregivers about the alternative therapy," counsels one family physician as some unorthodox methods can counteract medical treatments. Since it's easy to be misled or taken advantage of by unscrupulous practitioners, find out what's what before accepting treatment. Gather as much information as possible and weigh the risks and benefit. Beware of unpleasant methods and of costly "miracle cures." Ask the complementary healer to explain the theory behind the suggested

therapy, being wary of any that seem excessively expensive. Talk to others who have undergone the same treatment. The American Council on Health and Safety suggest asking whether the method has shown benefits that clearly exceed harm and whether it's been objectively (scientifically) proven effective.

For more information: Consult specialty associations, e.g., the Acupuncture Foundation of Canada (Tel: 416/752-3988); the Canadian Holistic Medicine Association (Tel: 416/485-3071); Read: "Alternative Systems of Medical Practice: A Report from the National Institute of Health, Washington, DC," (Tel: 202/512-1800); "A Guide to Unconventional Cancer Therapies," published by the Ontario Breast Cancer Information Exchange Project (Tel: 416/480-5899). Useful websites are CAMLine (www.camline.ca/), www.herbmed.org/, Office of Natural Health Products (www.hc-sc.gc.ca/hpfb-dgpsa/nhpd-dpsn/index.html), National Center for Complementary and Alternative Medicine (http://nccam.nih.gov).

Nutrition toward health

The basics of good nutrition • New dietary intake standards • Nutrition for athletes • The cholesterol story • The right fat mix • Fiber is still in • Make carbohydrates (starches) your dietary mainstay • Sugars aren't all bad • Proteins in the diet • In praise of fish • Vegetarian diets • Caffeine limits • Beyond vitamins: plant chemicals that fight disease • Most people don't need vitamin supplements • Minerals in the diet • Water is also essential

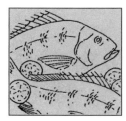

THE BASICS OF GOOD NUTRITION

In the past few decades we've been deluged with fast-changing, often unvalidated rules for good eating. Despite the information overload, many people still don't understand the simplest basics of sound nutrition. Unable to separate fads from truths, they slavishly follow eating slogans or bestseller diets. Nearly every week the announcement of some new study, not necessarily confirmed or medically accepted, sends them scurrying after the latest supposedly life-prolonging diet.

Sensible nutrition—the cornerstone of good health—is neither obscure nor hard to understand. The trick is to regard food not only as tasty and pleasurable but also as a source of fuel for the body's growth, and of *nutrients*—chemicals vital to all life processes. The food you eat is broken down into sugar (glucose), which is the energy source for all the body's cells, and into other chemical building blocks that are reassembled to form the substances needed by the body—such as digestive enzymes (catalysts), muscle-building components, immune agents, blood cells and hormones.

The main nutrient categories acquired from food are: carbohydrates (starches and sugars), proteins, fats, water, minerals and vitamins. Food must provide them all in adequate amounts. Each nutrient class performs a specific task in the body. For example, carbohydrates provide energy; fats become part of cell membranes and transport fat-soluble substances such as some vitamins and some hormones; minerals help regulate key functions such as blood production, respiration and bone and tooth formation; water is an essential part of every cell and serves as a transport medium. If food provides too little of any nutrient, the body cannot function properly.

Balance is the key. Eat a widely varied diet low in fat and rich in complex carbohydrates in amounts that keep you at a healthy weight. The daily diet should average 30 percent or less fat as a proportion of caloric intake and 12–15 percent protein, and about half the food eaten should be carbohydrates, preferably the complex kind (in whole grains, potatoes, pastas, rice, fruits, legumes and vegetables) rather than refined (sugars). Provided the overall meal plan is varied and balanced, there's no need to avoid favorites such as an occasional milkshake, candy bar or hot dog.

Up to date, action-oriented and easy to read, the guidelines stress overall eating behavior and the entire dietary mix rather than giving daily meal plans. People should eat not just to prevent deficiencies but to promote health and reduce the likelihood of today's main killer illnesses: heart ailments and cancer.

RULES FOR HEALTHY EATING

A 1997 report on Dietary Reference Intakes, prepared by a joint panel of Canadian and U.S.

4

experts, has developed dietary standards for the intake of several key nutrients. The new guidelines will ultimately harmonize U.S. and Canadian nutritional recommendations, merging the American Recommended Daily Allowances (RDAs) and Canadian Recommended Nutrient Intakes (RNIs) into a joint set of guidelines. The Dietary Reference Intakes (DRIs) suggest not only the minimum nutrient intakes needed to prevent deficiency diseases, but also the optimal amount necessary for good health—for instance, the daily intakes of calcium and vitamin D needed to build strong bones, or the amount of fluoride for cavity prevention and healthy teeth (0.5 microgram per kilogram per day). In some cases (as for calcium, vitamin D, vitamin B_{12} and magnesium) the new dietary intake standards are higher, in some cases lower (as for phosphorus).

For the first time, the nutritional guidelines also specify a "tolerable" (safe) upper limit for nutrient intakes—the maximum daily dose of any vitamin, mineral or other nutrient that's unlikely to cause adverse effects or damage health. For example, the ceiling for calcium is set at 2.5 grams (2,500 mg) per day; above that level it could interfere with iron absorption, increase the risk of kidney stones and have other hazardous effects. The upper safe level (UL) for vitamin D is 2,000 IU (15 micrograms) per day—higher levels could be toxic. In specifying upper safe limits, the nutritional experts hope to prevent the ill effect of overuse or megadosing.

Variety, balance and fun are key

To banish the view that good nutrition is boring, the federal guidelines emphasize the pleasurable aspects of food, downplaying restriction, elimination or limitation. The guidelines include the Recommended Nutrient Intakes (RNIs)—outlining the whys and wherefores for the suggested daily amount of all nutrient, including trace element such as copper, chromium, cobalt and selenium.

The central nutritional messages are to reach and stay at a healthy weight, enjoy a varied diet and, above all, eat less fat. The amount of fat in the average Canadian diet is well above the recommended 30 percent. We're among world leaders in fat consumption, only slightly behind the United States, Britain, the Netherlands, Denmark, Germany, Hungary and France. The chief changeover in the past few decades is in the *types* of fat eaten—from animal to vegetable types—rather than a reduction in overall intake. There's lots of hidden fat in fast and takeout foods, salad dressings, bakery products, crackers, snacks and restaurant meals.

For growing children, the advice to lower fat intake should be followed with caution. Many experts question fat reduction for children, as it

IN ESSENCE, OUR DIET SHOULD:

- provide energy (calories) that will maintain a healthy body weight;
- include nutrients in amounts specified by the new, harmonized U.S.–Canadian Dietary Reference Intakes (DRIs)—when they exist—or in line with the older U.S. Recommended Daily Allowances (RDAs) or Canadian Recommended Nutrient Intakes (RNIs);

- contain 30 percent or less of the energy (calories) consumed as fat, no more than 10 percent saturated (animal) fat;
- provide 55 percent of energy as carbohydrates, from a variety of sources;
- limit sodium intake (especially table salt);
- include only two alcoholic drinks daily for men, less for women;
- contain no more caffeine than the

equivalent of four cups of regular coffee per day;
- contain enough calcium (at least 1 g a day) to build and retain strong bones;
- provide sufficient fluoride for healthy teeth.

In everyday language, that means we should:
- eat enough to achieve and maintain a healthy body weight, but not less than 1,800 calories a day,

as lower amounts may not provide all essential nutrients. Those who want to lose weight should not go on unbalanced, intermittent or fad diets but should exercise more;
- enjoy a wide range of foods, using moderation and variety as watchwords;
- consume several daily servings of fiber-rich plant foods such as whole grain cereals

and breads, pastas, rice and legumes;
- eat 5 to 10 daily servings of vegetables and fruits, emphasizing orangey-red, yellow and leafy green types (rich in antioxidants);
- limit fat intake and choose lower-fat dairy products and leaner meats, preparing foods with little or no fat;
- moderate salt and alcohol use.

may shortchange youngsters of much-needed calories and endanger their health.

The right food for different ages

While good nutrition is important at every stage of life, the body's needs vary as people age. In adolescence, early adulthood and middle age, the body goes through changes that make special nutritional demands. As people grow older, they become more restricted in what they can comfortably eat. For women, dietary needs change during pregnancy, lactation and menopause. By adapting eating and exercise to the special needs of their age group, people can improve their vitality and their ability to withstand stress and illness.

For infants up to six months of age

Breast milk is the perfect food for infants in the first six months of life. Infants have a high metabolic rate, and their rapid growth makes ample nutrients and water essential. Vitamin D and iron supplements may be recommended. Fat is essential for nerve and brain development. When weaning an infant off milk or formula, gradually add a wide assortment of solid foods, starting with cereals, progressing to nonallergenic foods (e.g., apples, carrots, bananas), and adding other items one by one to achieve a richly varied, balanced diet. (See Chapter 11 also, page 294).

Childhood (age two to puberty)

Pay special attention to sufficient intake of calcium and iron for growing bones and other organs. Teach healthy eating behavior—start children on well-varied diets, offering plentiful fruits, vegetables and whole grains. Limit sugary snacks. Teach children to eat only when hungry and to stop eating when full. Ensure proper nutritional intake by offering a few choices among healthy foods, not by forcing a child to eat everything on his or her plate. (See Chapter 11, "Instilling good eating habits in children.")

Adolescence (about 12–18 years)

With the body's nutritional demands at their peak, erratic meals because of today's teenage lifestyle and the advent of menstruation in young women, food must be "nutrient-dense"—providing adequate protein, vitamins and minerals for their calorie content, not just energy. Iron lost in menstrual blood needs to be replaced. Adolescents need ample protein and vitamins (notably Bs) and higher calorie intakes to cope with the huge spurt in growth (often nearly doubling the body's size). Iron and calcium tend to be too low in teen meals. Dieting, common in girls, tends to deprive teenagers of much-needed nutrients. Serious dieting can stunt teens' growth, prevent the achievement of full height, retard the onset of menstruation in girls, and shortchange calcium needs.

Studies by Nutrition Canada depict female adolescents as a poorly nourished group. They ignore good nutrition, not realizing its role in health and appearance, or understanding that it lays the foundation for healthy childbearing. Many girls go on extreme diets in an effort to stay thin. Nutrition Canada reports a widespread shortage of iron and folic acid (a B vitamin) in adolescent girls, with added risks of calcium and vitamin D lack—slightly worse among the Indians and the Inuit than in the general Canadian population. In a recent evaluation of adolescent diets, a University of Toronto expert found that boys, who consume more total calories and at least get some protein by eating sandwiches, hot dogs and hamburgers, usually have more complete diets than girls, of whom 25 percent were low in iron and vitamins. Studies also show that snacks and soft drinks compose almost a third of the average adolescent's total calorie intake. While snacking was frowned on in the past it's now acceptable provided the snacks include nutrient-rich items (fruit, low-fat yogurt, nuts, whole-grain items) rather than fat-drenched fries, cookies or chips. To ensure adequate teen nutrition, keep the fridge stocked with healthy snacks.

Early adulthood (18–40 years)

Food intake should be matched to activity in order to maintain weight at the desired level. A steady balanced diet of fresh foods that supply essential nutrients in recommended amounts is the key, providing 50–60 percent of calories from carbohydrates (as in whole grains, pastas, potatoes, rice), 12–15 percent from protein and no more than 30 percent from fats (two-thirds

STEPS TOWARD HEALTHIER EATING

1. Avoid food faddism, and replace the concept of "good" versus "bad" foods with the principles of balance, moderation and variety. Shop for nutritional value rather than fashion or trends. Ignore any nutritional news not based on scientific evidence. Never favor or shun a food because of unvalidated rumors about its possible merits or dangers. Diets that make a fetish of single foods (e.g., grapefruit, pineapple, raisins or brown rice) or food groups (e.g., protein or starches) are unbalanced and can cause serious health problems, sometimes far more severe than the disorders they set out to correct.

2. Eat the right amount to maintain a healthy (desirable) weight. When the energy (calories) consumed does not balance energy output, the result is either obesity or malnutrition. Calorie requirements per kilogram and per pound per day for average healthy Canadians are:
   - for infants (two to four months)—119 cals per kg (54 cals per pound)
   - for adolescents (both sexes)—44–53 cals per kg (20–24 cals per pound)
   - for women (aged 23–50)—36 cals per kg (16 cals per pound)
   - for men (aged 23–50)—44 cals per kg (20 cals per pound)
   The average woman is deemed to be 162 cm and 55 kg (5 feet, 4 inches and 120 lb); the average man about 180 cm and 77 kg (5 feet, 11 inches and 170 lb).

3. Nutritionists stress balance and variety as key dietary principles, emphasizing local fresh foods when possible, rather than imported or canned goods. (Frozen foods are also a good source of high-quality nutrients.)

4. Eat a wide range of foods from all food groups, emphasizing plant sources such as grains, seeds, fruit, vegetables and legumes (e.g., chickpeas, lentils, beans). The "phytochemicals" in plant foods may help protect against certain diseases.

5. Aim for 5 to 10 daily servings of varied fruit and vegetables, emphasizing differently colored (red, orange, yellow, dark green) types rich in vitamins, minerals and antioxidants. Natural antioxidants (such as beta-carotene and vitamins A, C and E) and other plant components may help ward off certain cancers. (For example, the red compound in tomatoes has different properties and health benefits than the orange components in cantaloupe, squash or carrots).

6. Make your diet high in carbohydrates, especially the "complex" variety from fruits, vegetables, whole grains, cereals and legumes, to make up 55 percent or more of your total calories. This means becoming more of a plant-food eater, consuming more legumes, cereals, breads, vegetables and fruits, rice and pastas.

7. Abandon the mistaken idea that carbohydrate (starch) is fattening. Starch, sugars and other carbohydrates have only four calories per gram, compared to fats, with nine calories per gram.

8. Eat generous amounts of fiber (e.g., from whole grains, cereals, legumes, seeds, nuts and vegetables). Fiber, or roughage, a partly indigestible component of plant foods, helps to soften and expand stool, speeds elimination and offsets constipation. The World Health Organization (WHO) advises us to eat 24–35 g (0.8–1.2 oz) of fiber a day. Good sources are oat and wheat bran, unpeeled fruit and vegetables (e.g., boiled or baked potatoes, cabbage, broccoli, carrots, unpeeled pears and apples), strawberries, bananas and legumes (dried beans, lentils, chickpeas).

9. Reduce fats to 30 percent or less of all calories consumed. Choose a sensible fat mix, with no more than 10 percent of calories as saturated (animal) or trans fat, 8 to 10 percent as polyunsaturates (e.g., peanut, sesame, sunflower, safflower seed oils), the rest as monounsaturated forms (such as olive, canola, walnut and flaxseed oils). Watch for and avoid unhealthy, cholesterol-raising *trans* fatty acids—in hydrogenated vegetable oils (e.g., many margarines, baked and processed goods).

North American fat consumption is still way above the recommended level of 30 percent or less of overall calories. While many people have cut down on meats, they tend to eat more high-fat cheeses, fat-laden grain mixes and muffins, salad dressings and fluid-creams. While more fat is eaten in the form of vegetable oil, fats and oils have the *same number* of calories wherever they come from—whether it's beef, chicken, mayonnaise or granola. In fact, some popular foods such as croissants contain more fat than the traditional foods they replace, such as toast with butter. We must cut down but not eliminate dietary fat—it's essential for energy and growth, especially in young children, and for the absorption of fat-soluble vitamins. Make the fat eaten a mix of saturated fat (in meats, whole-milk products, butter), polyunsaturated oils (from fish and vegetables, e.g., sunflower, safflower, soya, cottonseed and some nut oils) and monounsaturated fats (such as olive, flax, peanut and canola oils). Olive oil is one of the least hydrogenated edible oils and contains natural antioxidants, which keep it stable and stop it from becoming saturated (hydrogenated) and going rancid for many years.

To reduce fat consumption:
- Steam, bake or poach foods. Deep-fat frying or flaming (flambéing, barbecuing) of foods produces oxidized components known to be toxic at very low concentrations.
- Make sauces with skim, not whole milk, and use low-fat yogurt instead of cream.
- Become a "hidden fat" detective. Watch for saturated fat or trans fatty acids in processed foods such as crackers, pizza crusts, cookies, desserts and dressings.
- Choose leaner cuts of meat and trim off the fat; broil or bake rather than fry. No need to shun meat altogether—besides high-quality protein, it provides many other vital nutrients, such as iron, zinc and vitamins B_6 and B_{12} (to name a few).

• Use skim or one percent milk instead of homogenized or two percent; eat fruit instead of pie or cake for dessert.

10. Don't exceed your protein needs. Protein is essential, but many eat more than they really need. Protein intake should be around 15 percent of total calories, but most Canadian diets currently exceed that amount. Protein needs vary according to age, sex and activity levels. In general, men aged 23–50, of average height and weight, need about 56 g per day, and women of the same age need about 41 g. Our protein consumption averages 83 grams per day—about 50 percent higher than the recommended level. Since protein foods tend to be expensive, it is practical as well as healthy to decrease amounts eaten. Meat or poultry need not be eaten at every meal or even every day. Proteins from fish, low-fat dairy products and plants are also good. Legumes and nuts are excellent protein sources and most whole grains, fruits and vegetables also contain some protein. But vegetarian sources must be balanced to provide complete protein (with all the necessary amino-acid components).

About 20 g of protein are provided by: 85 g (3 oz) of cooked beef, lamb, veal, chicken or fresh fish; 150 mL (two-thirds of a cup) of canned salmon; six sardines; 105 mL (7 tbsp) of cottage cheese; two frankfurters; or 90 mL (6 tbsp) of peanut butter. Therefore, two to three servings of these foods alone fulfill daily protein needs—even though we also get some protein from other dairy products, grains and vegetables. Include soya products (such as tofu, soymilk and miso) as an inexpensive and valuable source of high-quality protein and health-promoting compounds such as genestein and phytoestrogens.

12. Eat fish several times weekly. Cold-water, deep-sea fish such as tuna, herring and halibut are rich in omega-3 fatty acids which may protect the heart and cardiovascular system by reducing the blood's clotting action. Even fattier fish—such as salmon, swordfish and mackerel—are healthy choices. Fish provide high-quality protein and are generally low in cholesterol, although shellfish are somewhat higher. Canned fish is equally healthy.

13. Try not to skip breakfast. A nutritious breakfast helps to improve concentration and enhance mental performance, especially in children, and reduces impulse eating or bingeing later in the day. It should include a fruit or juice containing vitamin C, complex carbohydrates such as whole grains, and protein (milk, low-fat cheese, sometimes an egg).

14. Eat lightly at night. People who save up all day for a large dinner at night may increase the body's conversion of food to fat. Evening snacking may provide as many calories as a second dinner.

15. Shake the salt habit. Excess sodium from salt (sodium chloride) might increase risks of high blood pressure. Most people require only one or two grams per day, an amount easily supplied from a varied diet without added cooking or table salt (unless you are in a very hot climate, or exercising vigorously and sweating profusely).

16. Ensure adequate calcium intake for bone strength. Premenopausal women need one gram (1000 mg) a day (e.g., from 3 to 4 glasses of low-fat milk, yogurt or other dairy sources); teenagers, postmenopausal women and everyone over age 65 need 1,300 to 1,500 mg a day (plus enough vitamin D).

17. Get enough dietary iron from liver, red meat or equivalent plant sources (e.g., lentils, spinach, raisins) to maintain healthy blood cells and prevent iron-deficiency anemia.

18. Watch your B vitamin intake, with special attention to folic acid (also called folate or folacin), needed to protect the heart and cardiovascular system. Adults need 400 micrograms (mcg) folate a day, from organ meats, legumes (e.g., split peas, lentils) and green vegetables (e.g., broccoli, spinach). Women of childbearing age, especially those who may or plan to get pregnant, may wish to take supplements to protect their babies from neural tube defects (such as spina bifida). The upper safety limit for folate is 1000 mcg a day. Vegetarians and the elderly must also make sure they get enough vitamin B_{12} (2.4 micrograms a day). It's only available from animal sources (such as meat, eggs, fish and poultry). Strict vegetarians and older people who absorb this vitamin less efficiently also need supplements. B_{12} deficiency can cause pernicious anemia (lack of red blood cells).

19. Only use dietary supplements if medically advised—they're no substitute for the richly varied mix in real food. Intakes of vitamins and minerals above recommended or tolerable upper safety limits (ULs) may irreversibly damage health. But certain groups such as the undernourished, the elderly, pregnant and lactating women may need vitamin/mineral supplements.

20. Drink enough fluids. Water, a vital nutrient, helps regulate body temperature and acts as a solvent, transport medium and tissue lubricant. An average adult needs about 2.8 liters (3 quarts) per day from all sources, including fruit and vegetables (80 percent or more water), milk (87 percent), juices, soups, coffee, tea and other beverages. Note, however, that alcohol and the caffeine in tea, coffee and colas are diuretics that increase urine output, thus increasing the body's water needs.

If you drink alcohol, consume no more than 27.3 grams (two standard drinks) in any one day. Guidelines suggest that men limit weekly alcohol intake to 14 standard drinks, and women to 9 drinks weekly. Pregnant women are advised not to drink as there may be *no safe level* of alcohol for an unborn child.

Finally, relax and enjoy food! Remember that there's nothing wrong with occasional "junk" food such as chips, candy, donuts, cream cake or chocolates, provided they're not a major part of your diet.

SENIORS NEED "NUTRIENT-DENSE" FOODS

The corollary of eating less in quantity is that the elderly often get less in quality. Although old people may eat less, what they eat must be nutrient dense and as health-promoting as possible. Seniors should choose "nutrient-rich" foods packed with essential nutrients. Some experts see a pressing need for the food industry to develop "nutrient-dense" foods high in or enriched with protein, vitamins and minerals.

from monounsaturated and polyunsaturated forms). Overeating leads to obesity and the accompanying health hazards of raised blood pressure, diabetes and cardiovascular disease. The calorie intake of a normally active woman should be around 1,800–2,100 calories a day, and of a man around 2,700–3,000 calories daily. Since bone density continues to build until age 35, adults need enough calcium to protect the bones from later osteoporosis. Many young women, especially those who are pregnant or lactating, need iron and folic acid supplements to meet their requirements. Women on birth-control pills should ask about the need for vitamin supplements. For the rest, a well-varied diet with lots of fruit and vegetables should provide all needed vitamins and minerals.

Middle age (40–65 years)

After age 40, nutritional needs change with the gradual slowing of metabolic activity. Calorie requirements drop by about 5 percent per decade. Constipation may be a problem and some drugs hinder the absorption of certain nutrients. Women's iron needs diminish when menstruation ceases. By contrast, calcium needs rise at menopause in women, and after age 65 in men, who also suffer osteoporosis in later life. Women approaching menopause need to think about osteoporosis as estrogen's protective effect disappears. To offset bone loss, women need at least 1,000 mg of calcium per day (See Chapter 15, the section on osteoporosis, for other precautions.)

Seniors

In the elderly, altered dietary habits may stem from tooth problems (which lessen the enjoyment of hard-to-chew foods), diminished taste and smell (which reduce appetite) and a sluggish digestive system (which may cause constipation, heartburn and bloating). The elderly require more or less the same amount of nutrients as younger people, except for a small decline in energy (calorie) needs. But many seniors have eating habits and lifestyles that place them at risk of malnutrition. Unless they stay physically active, many older adults find it hard to take in enough food to give them sufficient nutrients, making them "nutritionally disadvantaged."

IMPROVING NUTRITION IN THE SENIOR YEARS

Key nutritional problems among the elderly include excess fat consumption, a shortage of protein, certain minerals and several vitamins. Most crucially, many seniors are short of calcium and vitamin D, putting themselves at risk of osteoporosis and multiple fractures. Many people over age 65—especially those with low incomes—also consume too little vitamin C, E, B_6, B_{12} and folic acid (folate). As people spend less time outdoors in the sunlight, vitamin D stores can be low, and some need a supplement. A low zinc intake is also common because seniors eat less meat, legumes and grains/bread. Reasons for the dietary shortfall include difficulties with shopping or cooking, consuming too little fruit and vegetables, not eating any milk products, diets altered because of illness or dental problems, use of multiple medications, isolation, depression and loneliness.

Seniors must get enough protein

The loss of lean body mass (mostly muscle) so common in seniors may arise partly from eating too little protein. Protein-rich foods include lean meat, poultry, eggs, canned or fresh fish, non-fat or low-fat dairy products, legumes and grains. Eggs are an excellent source of cheap, high-quality protein for seniors, also rich in several minerals and vitamins. Eating 3 or 4 eggs a week is unlikely to drive up cholesterol significantly or endanger health.

Foods high in protein, low in fat

Food	Protein (g)
Cottage cheese (2% B.F.) (250 mL)	33
Tuna, canned in water (125 mL/85 g)	30
Chicken breast, skinless (1/2 breast/86 g)	27
Pork tenderloin, trimmed (3 slices/89 g)	26
Loin chop, broiled (1 chop/87 g)	25
Ground beef patty, lean and broiled (1 patty/88 g)	22
Lentils, cooked (250 mL/209 g)	19
Milk (2% B.F.) (250 mL/1 glass)	9
Yogurt, plain (1.5% B.F.) (125 g)	7

Get enough calcium and vitamin D for healthy bones

Mast experts believe that, "within the limits of genetic make-up," a high calcium intake—from food or supplements—can help preserve bone mass (strength) in older people, men as well as women. On average, menstruating women (with normal estrogen outputs), women on hormone replacement therapy (HRT) and men need about 1,000 mg (one gram) calcium a day. Postmenopausal women not on HRT and *every-one over age 65*, needs 1,200–1,500 mg calcium daily. Older men also need to increase calcium intake and continue weight-bearing exercise to prevent bone deterioration.

Tip: Look for calcium-rich food sources such as milk, low-fat cheese, yogurt, dried raisins, nuts, tofu, broccoli, canned sardines and salmon (eaten with the bones). Add milk or yogurt to mashed potatoes; add skim milk powder to milk-based soups or desserts. Avoid "calcium robbers" such as excess caffeine and phosphate (which bind calcium) in colas and soft drinks.

Tip: Get vitamin D from fortified milk or fortified cereals, eggs and fatty fish (salmon), or take a supplement of 400 U of vitamin D per day—either singly or in a multivitamin preparation (but check with a nutritionist or physician before taking a supplement).

Lack of folate can be a real problem

Folic acid, also known as folate or folacin (one of the B vitamins), is essential for the health of our blood, bones and nervous system. Lack of dietary folate can contribute to a certain type of anemia, mouth ulcers, skin problems, cardiovascular disease and possibly depression. The latest guidelines suggest 400 micrograms of folate daily for older women and men. Good sources include liver split peas, lentils, broccoli, yeast, wheat germ and whole wheat products. Women of child-bearing age should be especially careful to obtain enough folate, as a lack can cause birth defects in unborn babies.

Seniors still need plenty of fiber from food

The walls of the gastrointestinal tract lose strength and elasticity with age, slowing "motility" or the ability to move feces out, so constipation is a common complaint for people over 65. Fiber or roughage, a partly indigestible component of plant foods, helps to soften and expand the stool and move it through the bowel. The experts suggest we eat 20 to 26 grams of fiber a day—but don't increase amounts too quickly as it might cause abdominal discomfort.

To increase fiber intake:
- Choose foods such as brown rice, whole-grain breads, baked beans, peas, lentils, bran cereals, fresh or dried fruits and vegetables;
- Add chopped or grated vegetables, lentils, beans, chickpeas or barley to soups, or salads;
- Start the day with bran cereal. Check nutritional labels—at least 6 grams of fiber per 100 grams is a good balance. Adding fruit will further increase the fiber content.

Seniors must also drink enough water

The body's water content tends to decrease with age and dehydration is a distinct risk for older adults. Declining kidney function and decreased thirst contribute to the water loss. Older adults exposed to hot weather or who have a feverish illness can get easily dehydrated, even to the extent of becoming dangerously confused. Some older adults find it hard to drink enough water or other fluids because of difficulty in getting up from a chair or bed, navigating the stairs or even turning on taps. Seniors with bladder-control problems may be afraid to drink too much since it means more frequent trips to the toilet. Aim for 6 to 8 glasses of fluid a day including water milk and juices. Go easy on alcohol and caffeinated drinks, which are diuretics that increase urine output.

NUTRITION FOR ATHLETES

Varied diets supply the needs of most athletes, which are not very different from those of other people. Contrary to common mythology, vitamins don't build competitive strength! And sodium losses even in vigorous events are generally quite small.

Nutrient overdoses can't improve performance

Good nutrition can maximize the body's athletic potential, but it has never been known to make an average athlete into an Olympic winner. There is a common misconception among sports enthusiasts that "more is better"—more protein, more vitamins, more minerals—but those tempted to overdose on certain nutrients should remember that doing so cannot upgrade performance and may harm the body.

Water, water and more water

Water is the ideal drink for heavy exercisers. Dehydration can occur not only during a race, but over a long heat wave or a prolonged period of training, if fluid replacement does not precede and follow each training session. Accumulated dehydration can even occur in those doing thrice-weekly vigorous workouts. It's not unusual for a runner to lose water amounting to a 225-ml (8-oz) glass every six to eight minutes. Ideally, fluid intake should equal sweat loss. Experts suggest that athletes drink two to three cups of water two or three hours before engaging in strenuous activity, another cup 15 minutes before the start and then one cup every 15–20 minutes. Also take plenty of fluid after exercise to rehydrate the body. Drinking a cup every 20 minutes is wise when competing.

Excess protein can stress the body

Protein requirements of athletes are often wrongly assumed to be greater than those of non-athletes. Many regular exercisers continue to eat far more protein than they need, taking it in as fat-laden meats, or as protein powder, liquid or pills. Yet protein beyond the body's needs is simply stored as unnecessary fat, or converted to glucose. Protein needs may increase slightly in the early stages of training to provide increased muscle mass, enzymes and red blood cells. Although opinions vary, a liberal estimate for protein requirement during the initial phase of training is 1.2–1.5 grams per kilogram (0.5–0.7 grams per pound) of body weight per day. Once the body is accustomed to the demands of heavy exercise, protein requirements can usually be met by supplying 0.8–1.0 g/kg/day (0.4–0.5 g/lb/day). For a 70-kg (155-lb) person, this might be met by: 2 glasses of milk (8 g per 250 ml/1 cup) and two small servings of meat, poultry or fish (85 g each). The average diet provides pro-

tein in amounts that greatly exceed daily requirements. Inadequate protein intake is rarely a problem in our society. Even heavily training athletes can build muscle on the recommended protein intake as long as they also eat enough high energy (carbohydrate) foods. The excess nitrogen produced (by deaminating protein) must be excreted by the kidneys as urea, a process that requires much water. Hence an excessive protein intake may unduly burden the liver and kidneys.

Carbohydrates are good sport foods

Carbohydrates provide most of the energy for intense exercise. Much of the body's glucose is stored as glycogen, most in the liver; the rest in muscle. The supply of glucose from glycogen can be a limiting factor for long-distance or long-lasting athletic events. Any means to spare glycogen or increase its storage will help endurance athletes. When the glycogen is used up, the body switches to other less efficient mechanisms for obtaining glucose. Adequate glycogen stores depend on a diet plentiful in carbohydrates: 43 percent—the average Canadian carbohydrate intake—is too low for the physically active.

Are there merits to carbohydrate loading?

"Carbohydrate loading" has become popular among endurance competitors to increase glycogen stores. Experts emphasize that carbohydrate loading is useless for events less than 90 minutes in duration, as normal glycogen stores are sufficient to tide competitors over events lasting up to two hours. The loading process is also known as glycogen supercompensation, since it stimulates the liver to build up greater-than-normal glycogen reserves. These glycogen stores may delay marathoners from "hitting the wall" or cyclists from "bonking" (becoming confused and unable to continue). In its classic form, carbohydrate loading involves, first, a depletion bout for one day, in which the body's glycogen is used up by exercising to exhaustion; this is followed by three days of a low-carbohydrate diet (consisting mainly of protein and fats); and concludes with three days of a carbohydrate-rich regime to supersaturate the muscles with glycogen.

SORTING OUT THE CHOLESTEROL PUZZLE

The term "cholesterol" conjures up images of looming disaster but despite a deluge of publicity about it, few really know what cholesterol is, nor the extent to which a high blood level can endanger the heart. An elevated level of LDL ("bad") blood cholesterol ranks just behind smoking and high blood pressure as a major risk factor for heart disease. High levels of blood cholesterol contribute to the formation of fatty plaque (deposits) in the arteries and the condition known as atherosclerosis, which leads to coronary heart disease. Studies suggest that almost half the North Americans over age 30 have blood cholesterol levels above the healthy upper limit of 5.2 millimoles per liter (mmol/l) or 200 milligrams per deciliter (mg/dl) (see table). However not everyone with high blood cholesterol will develop heart disease.

What exactly is cholesterol?

Cholesterol is a white waxy fat (lipid) essential to human life that is a natural component of most animal tissues. It is a constituent of cell membranes and nerve coatings and a building block for some hormones, vitamins and bile salts (which help to digest fat). Although North Americans consume on average 400–500 mg per day, cholesterol is not a vital part of the diet. Regardless of amounts eaten, the body manufactures ample quantities for its own use.

Cholesterol is carried around in the blood by special molecules, the lipoproteins—which include chylomicrons, very low-density lipoprotein (VLDL), low-density lipoprotein (LDL), high-density lipoprotein (HDL) and apolipoproteins. VLDL transports mainly triglycerides (fatty compounds that increase with the consumption of sugar and alcohol), which also increase heart disease risks. LDL cholesterol is considered bad because it contributes to the development of fatty deposits (plaques) that clog up and block the arteries. By contrast, the HDL or good type helps to protect against heart disease and stroke by taking cholesterol away from the arteries and delivering it to the liver where it is converted into bile acids and excreted.

Although blood tests may show that someone has a high total blood cholesterol, an

TEST	DESIRABLE	BORDERLINE	UNDESIRABLE
Total cholesterol:	below 200	200–240	above 240
LDL cholesterol	below 130	130–160	above 160
HDL cholesterol	above 45	35–45	below 35
Triglycerides	below 200	200–400	above 400

NB. Levels in milligrams per deciliter, for those with no cardiovascular disease

Equivalent cholesterol numbers

mmol/l	mg/dl	
0.9	35	
3.4	130	
4.1	160	considered "safe"
4.9	190	
5.2	200	
6.2	240	considered "high"

accurate heart-risk assessment can only be obtained by knowing the LDL cholesterol level in blood. To get the true picture, *both* LDL and HDL levels must be measured to obtain the HDL/LDL ratio. Since cholesterol levels vary from day to day, a first "high" count may be unreliable; it takes several fasting blood tests to establish the proper blood-cholesterol level. Even though someone may have a seemingly raised blood cholesterol, if the HDL level is high there may be no real heart disease risk.

Many people mistakenly assume that eating foods rich in cholesterol is the only way to raise blood levels. However eating saturated or animal fat and trans fats also drives up blood cholesterol. For example, the Finns, Hungarians and Americans, who eat lots of animal fat, have the highest national blood-cholesterol levels, while the Japanese, who eat more fish and soya products, have low levels. A high blood cholesterol can also arise through one's genetic make-up, for instance, from an inherited disorder called hyperlipidemia (a propensity to high blood fats). Besides a high LDL cholesterol, other features—some beyond one's control—influence heart-attack risks. For instance, being male and/or having diabetes and high blood pressure are cardiovascular risk factors. Lifestyle activities that endanger the heart include smoking, being overweight, lack of exercise and undue stress.

The first line of attack in lowering blood cholesterol is lifestyle change—reducing intake of cholesterol and saturated (animal) fats, and

FACTORS THAT RAISE LDL ("BAD") BLOOD CHOLESTEROL

- Diseases such as hypothyroidism (under-active thyroid); some advanced liver and kidney ailments; ovarian failure;
- some inherited conditions such as hypercholesterolemia, where a genetic flaw

dramatically elevates blood cholesterol because faulty liver receptors can't remove it;
- certain drugs such as corticosteroids and vitamin A derivatives;
- being obese or overweight;

- eating too much fat, (especially saturated and trans fats), drinking excess alcohol and consuming cholesterol-rich foods (in "responders," whose blood cholesterol rises in tune with amounts eaten).

SO HOW MUCH CHOLESTEROL IS IT SAFE TO EAT?

Some health authorities suggest precise limits to cholesterol intake, but most oppose a "blanket rule," gearing intake to age, lifestyle, genetic background and individual needs. The World Health Organization suggests "restricting cholesterol intake to 250 mg daily" with an "upper limit of 300 mg a day." Many other health agencies also suggest that we try to "reduce consumption toward 300 mg or less" per day, provided infants and children get enough total calories and essential nutrients.

getting more aerobic exercise. While consuming less cholesterol-rich foods (e.g., eggs, cream, liver, shrimps) can modestly lower blood cholesterol, the effect varies widely from person to person. In some ("responders") eating less cholesterol lowers blood levels, while in others blood cholesterol may hardly vary, no matter how little is consumed. Beyond dietary cholesterol, it's the amount of saturated (animal) fat consumed and *trans* fatty acids (in some margarines and many processed foods) that raise LDL cholesterol. So avoiding cholesterol-rich foods isn't enough; it's equally important to reduce your saturated and trans fat intake.

To test or not to test blood cholesterol?

Medical experts still argue about whether when, how and whom to test for blood cholesterol. The debate hinges on the usefulness, cost benefit and number of lives that could be saved by population-wide screening. Not everyone with a high cholesterol will develop heart problems. It's just one of many cardiac risk factors. Many experts oppose cholesterol tests for the entire population (above a certain age) as such screening would not definitely lower cardiac death rates. Instead they focus on cholesterol-lowering lifestyle changes for everyone. As it stands today, screening guidelines vary from country to country. Some health authorities suggest cholesterol blood tests for all men and women over age 30; others, like most Canadian health agencies, favor screening men over age 40 and women aged 50 and over. Yet others propose testing only people with known coronary risk factors such as smoking, abdominal obesity (waist girth above 100 cm), those with

known heart disease, people with a family history of early heart attack or hyperlipidemia (high blood lipids) or people with high blood pressure and those with diabetes or kidney failure. Not only do the different healthcare agencies suggest different screening guidelines, but they also argue about which tests to do: whether to measure just total cholesterol, or—more accurately and usefully—to also check LDL and HDL levels. In general, the advice is that anyone found to have a high LDL cholesterol level should try to lower it in order to protect the heart, first by dietary changes and exercise, and—if that fails—by taking cholesterol-lowering medications.

How much blood cholesterol is too high?

There is no universally agreed blood cholesterol level that threatens the heart; rather there's a sliding scale with a rising risk as cholesterol levels climb. In giving advice about blood cholesterol and the need to lower it, doctors go by the LDL cholesterol figure, not the total blood level. As LDL cholesterol goes up, so do the chances of having a heart attack or stroke.

Cholesterol levels in blood are expressed differently in different countries, either as milligrams per deciliter (mg/dl) or millimoles per liter (mmol/l). Experts have set arbitrary danger points for total blood cholesterol at 240 mg/dl or 6.2 mmol/l, and LDL readings of 160 mg/dl and over are considered "too high" for cardiac safety. LDL levels between 130–160 mg/dl are designated "borderline risk." Individuals in the high LDL-cholesterol bracket (160 mg/dl or higher) or those with one or more additional heart-risk factors should start cholesterol-lowering efforts.

New guidelines push for still lower LDL blood cholesterol levels

Recently revised guidelines in Canada and the U.S. call for more aggressive efforts using cholesterol-lowering medications to lower LDL cholesterol levels (especially for people at risk of cardiovascular disease), in the hope of preventing heart attacks and stroke.

The revised Canadian guidelines, based on the Heart Protection and other studies, suggest new target goals for LDL blood cholesterol, in particular for those with cardiovascular risk factors.

The Canadian guidelines suggest that:

- *People at high cadiovascular risk* should try to reduce:

LDL-cholesterol below 2.5 mmol/L (100 mg/dl)

Total cholesterol below 4.0 mmol/L (150 mg/dl)

- *People at moderate cadiovascular risk* should aim for:

LDL-cholesterol levels below 3.4 mmol/L (130 mg/dl)

Total cholesterol below 5.0 mmol/L (180 mg/dl)

- *People with few or no cadiovascular risk factors* should aim for:

LDL-cholesterol levels below 4.1 mmol/L (160 mg/dl)

Total cholesterol below 5.2 mmol/L (200 mg/dl)

NB: cardiovascular risk factors include: obesity, high blood pressure, smoking, diabetes, hyberlipidemia, strong family history of early heart disease, kidney disease.

The latest (2004) U.S. guidelines from the National Cholesterol Education Program propose still more stringent goals for LDL blood cholesterol, calling for more aggressive cholesterol-lowering drug treatment, especially for people with known cardiovascular risks. Their new guidelines suggest lowering target LDL-levels for people at high cardiovascular risk from 2.58 mmol/L to below 1.81 mmol/L (less than 70 mg/dl): for those at moderate cardiac risk

they suggest lowering the target LDL cholesterol level from 3.36 mmol/L to below 2.58 mmol/L (100 mg/dl).

Following these recommendations, more and more people will likely be advised to take statins and other cholestrol-lowering drugs, with a possible rise in the adverse affects of these medications.

HDL ("helpful" or "good") blood cholesterol protects the heart

Total blood-cholesterol levels may read high because of an elevated LDL (bad) or HDL (good) cholesterol. If the HDL is 25 percent or more of the total reading, that's a good sign, as

---

CHOLESTEROL-LOWERING MEDICATIONS INCLUDE:

- **Resins—such as cholestyramine (Questran) and colestipol (Colestid) —drugs already used for 20 years that tie up bile acids thus using up the body's cholesterol stores. They can cause - bloating;**
- **Triglyceride-lowering agents such as gemfibrozil (Lopid);**
- **Niacin (vitamin B$_3$), which in large doses reduces triglyceride levels. Side effects include flushing and skin irritation;**

- **Statins (HMG-CoA reductase inhibitors) which reduce cholesterol production by blocking the enzyme needed for its manufacture in the liver. Depending on the dose, statins can dramatically lower blood cholesterol and some help to absorb the fatty plaque that clogs up arteries. The statins include atorvastatin (Lipitor), cerivastatin (Baycol), fluvastatin (Mevacor), pravastatin (Pravachol)**

- simvastatin (Zocor) and rosuvastatin (Crestor). Since they can cause myopathy (muscle weakness) and (rarely) damage the liver, those taking statins need frequent medical checkups and blood tests.
- **Cholesterol-absorption inhibitors such as ezetimibe (Ezetrol) are now often also prescribed, along with statins, to achieve still lower LDL-cholesterol levels.**

NON-FAT FACTORS THAT MAY INFLUENCE BLOOD CHOLESTEROL

May lower blood-cholesterol levels:
- **soluble fiber:** from beans, oats, fruits and vegetables;
- **polyunsaturated fats:** help to lower LDL, or "bad," cholesterol. Safflower, sunflower, sesame and soybean oil are good sources;
- **monounsaturated fat.** Olive and canola oil

are good sources;
- **fatty ocean fish:** certain deep-sea fish, such as mackerel, herring, salmon and tuna, contain special polyunsaturated fatty acids called omega-3s, which may lower blood cholesterol;
- **aerobic exercise:** although overall cholesterol remains the

same, regular exercise helps increase HDL ("good") cholesterol.

May raise LDL blood-cholesterol levels:
- **excess weight:** each 1 kg (2 lb) of excess weight adds, on average, one mg/dl to LDL blood cholesterol;

- **foods high in saturated fat:** more than any other factor, a diet high in saturated fat raises blood-cholesterol levels. Sources of saturated fat include beef, butter, whole-milk dairy products (especially cheeses), dark poultry meat, poultry skin and coconut, palm

and palm-kernel oils;
- **foods high in cholesterol:** only animal products contain cholesterol. Eggs and organ meats are the richest sources;
- **smoking:** increases LDL ("bad") cholesterol and decreases HDL ("good") cholesterol.

BEWARE OF "CHOLESTEROL-FREE" LABELS

Scientists raise quizzical eyebrows at the "cholesterol-free" labels on foods that never contained any cholesterol in the first place. "Cholesterol-free" labeling has been aggressively used to market goods, and consumers should examine each claim individually. Read not just the claim but the "nutrition information" with the smaller print! Health and Welfare Canada stipulates that any low-cholesterol item must also be low in saturated fat, and the "low-cholesterol" or "cholesterol-free" label must also declare all types of fat in the product. Many cholesterol-free products (e.g., margarines) are prepared with hydrogenated vegetable oils, obliterating the benefits of the natural polyunsaturated oil. The hydrogenation process converts some polyunsaturated fats to trans fatty acids. For instance, the hydrogenation process used to stabilize vegetable oils, as in making peanut butter or margarine, not only adds hydrogen (making them more saturated) but also rearranges some of the natural chemical bonds to the unhealthy trans fatty acid form. Scientists have shown that trans fatty acids raise LDL ("bad") cholesterol in blood. Thus, food manufacturers who use hydrogenated forms of vegetable oils negate their health benefits. Processed foods containing trans fatty acids include pizza crusts, puddings, crackers, cookies, rolls, potato and corn chips, soft candy, breaded foods, french fries, frozen waffles and most margarines. Displaying the trans fatty acid content of foods on nutrition labels might help consumers make better-informed food decisions. For now, the thing to remember is to *eat less fat overall*.

this form protects the heart. HDL levels tend to be high in the physically active and people who exercise vigorously, and/or in those who consume their fats mainly in poly- or monounsaturated forms. Replacing saturated fat with polyunsaturates (e.g., from safflower, sunflower, corn and flaxseed oils) can help raise HDL levels. The HDL fraction often rises dramatically in athletes and those doing heavy physical work. A high HDL blood cholesterol may even outweigh the detrimental effect of an elevated LDL level. In other words, a high HDL to LDL ratio exerts a heart-protecting influence.

Restructuring diets to lower blood cholesterol is surprisingly easy

Weight loss and dietary changes are the primary tactics in lowering blood cholesterol, and they can be achieved with small, common-sense alterations. Cutting back on saturated fats is a giant step. People can avoid all visible fat, switch from fatty, marbled cuts to leaner cuts, give up bacon and salami (obviously fat-laden), eat fish two or three times a week and use jam alone on bread

DIETS FOR LOWERING CHOLESTEROL

Your guide to healthier eating:
- Variety and moderation are still the Golden Eating Rule—eat a wide variety of fresh foods, emphasizing those in season.
- Bring down fat intake to 30 percent or less of total calories.
- Limit saturated fats to no more than 10 percent of total calories by restricting or eliminating marbled meats, processed luncheon meats, cold cuts, cream, butter, baked goods, sauces, salad dressings and processed products made with animal fat or saturated (hydrogenated) vegetable oils (mainly palm and coconut oils).
- Choose polyunsaturated oils such as safflower, sunflower, corn, soya, walnut oils (with an upper limit of 10 percent of all fat eaten), and balance with monounsaturates (olive, canola, avocado, flax, peanut oils). A ceiling of 8 to 10 percent polyunsaturates in the diet is recommended because animal experiments suggest that eating a higher proportion of polyunsaturates could increase the risk of certain cancers.
- Use soft margarines (containing 40 to 55 percent unsaturates— preferably *nonhydrogenated*), instead of butter or block-style margarines. Watch the labels!
- When choosing margarine, select one with the maximum amount of *nonhydrogenated* (polyunsaturated) and least hydrogenated fatty acids. Watch for trans fatty acids that raise LDL (bad) cholesterol. (Calculate the amount of trans by adding up the saturated, mono- and polyunsaturated fatty acids and sub-

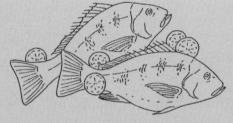

tracting from the total declared fat.)
- Make sauces with skim, not whole, milk; use yogurt instead of cream, and low-fat rather than whole-milk cheese.
- Read the labels on processed foods, particularly desserts, dressings and sauces. Desserts often contain vast amounts of concealed fat.
- Steam, poach, bake or broil instead of frying.
- Substitute fish or poultry for animal meats.
- Switch to low-fat salad dressings, or favor olive oil and plain lemon types.
- Make soups and stocks a day ahead and refrigerate, so hardened fat can be lifted off before serving.
- Eat more complex carbohydrates from fruits, vegetables and cereal grains.
- Eat fish (particularly cold-water oceanic types) two to three times weekly.
- Consume only one alcoholic drink or less per day.
- Avoid buying snacks (chips, peanuts, cookies) ahead "in case of company"; if you don't have them, you'll be less tempted!

without butter or margarine. They can buy low- or no-fat dairy products, omit cream soups, gravies, mayonnaise, fatty dressings and potato chips and cut back on cheese—substitute cottage cheese and use yogurt instead of sour cream. Increasing the amount of soluble fiber eaten (especially from oat bran, beans and other legumes) can also help to reduce blood cholesterol. Do the "visibility" test. Look at the food on your dinner plate and try to see less meat or cheese amid a sea of vegetables and starchy foods. A little piece of meat should be nestled among attractive mounds of multicolored vegetables (peas, carrots, sprouts, tomatoes) and pasta, potatoes or rice. Remember that new eating habits are not emergency measures—they are a diet plan for life.

Aggressive drug treatment increasingly promoted to lower blood cholesterol

While physicians formerly hesitated to prescribe cholesterol-lowering statins for lack of evidence that they saved lives, and because their long-term safety was untested, these medications are now increasingly prescribed to prevent heart attacks and strokes. New studies have shown that lowering LDL cholesterol can reduce cardiac risks and prolong survival. For instance, the "PROVE IT" randomized, double-blind trial (on over 4,000 subjects with heart disease) showed that getting LDL blood cholesterol below the 100 md/dl (2.59 mmol/L) mark with statins (such as Lipitor or Zocor) lessened coronary problems and improved outcomes.

However these drugs are expensive; people have to stay on them for life (as cholesterol shoots up once they are discontinued) and they do have side effects. Moreover, statins can only reduce blood cholesterol by 20 to 60 percent, so to achieve a desirably low LDL measure, a second cholesterol-lowering agent such as niacin (vitamin B3) or ezetimibe (Ezetrol)—which blocks cholesterol absorption—may have to be added.

Although statin medications are generally considered safe and well tolerated, especially at low doses, they can cause myalgia (muscle pain and weakness), occasionally liver problems (due to elevation of the enzyme, aminotransferase) and, rarely, rhabdomyolysis (a flu-like illness).

CHOLESTEROL AND FAT CONTENTS
(per 90 g/3 oz, unless otherwise specified)

	Cholesterol (mg)	Total fat (g/oz)	Saturated fat (g)	Calories
Egg yolk (one large)	221	5.3	1.6	61
Cheddar cheese	92	30.0	18.0	362
Peanut butter (15 ml/1 tbsp)	0	8.0	1.5	95
Tofu/bean curd	0	4.1	0.6	65
Whipping cream (32% fat, unwhipped, 1 cup/250 ml)	290	79.0	50.0	743
Milk (2%, 250 ml/1 cup)	19	5.0	3.0	124
Butter (15 ml/1 tbsp)	32	12.0	7.0	103
Real mayonnaise (per 15 ml/1 tbsp, 65% oil)	9	12.0	1.0	112
Mayonnaise (less than 35% oil per 15 ml/1 tbsp)	4	7.3	0.5	74
Liver (calves, braised)	502	6.2	2.3	148
Liver (beef, broiled)	350	4.4	2.0	150
Fish/Seafood				
Crab (Alaskan, steamed)	48	1.0	trace	85
Steamed clams	29	3.0	0.4	90
Sole (broiled)	61	1.4	0.3	105
Cod (baked)	50	0.8	0.1	95
Trout (broiled)	66	3.9	0.6	136
Lobster (canned)	65	0.5	0	87
Shrimp (steamed)	176	1.0	0.3	90
Oysters (raw)	45	2.0	0.5	59
Tuna (light, canned, in water)	16	0.5	trace	112
Tuna (canned, in oil)	16	7.0	1.3	178
Salmon (pink, canned)	21	6.7	1.5	122
Meats & Poultry				
Beef (lean, roasted)	81	8.0	3.2	192
Veal (lean, roasted)	106	6.0	1.7	176
Pork (lean, roasted)	59	10.0	3.4	200
Lamb (leg, roasted)	78	7.0	2.3	162
Wiener, hot dog (one)	19	11.0	4.0	118
Fresh pork sausage	72	30.0	10.0	330
Chicken (with skin, roasted, light & dark meat)	75	12.2	3.4	219
Chicken breast (no skin, roasted)	70	3.0	0.9	149
Chicken (leg/thigh, no skin)	85	7.6	2.1	172
Duck (with skin)	72	24.3	8.5	303

N.B.: These are not necessarily standard serving sizes but used for comparison. Figures from Health and Welfare Canada's Nutrient File for 1991.

UPDATING YOUR FAT FACTS

- **Saturated fats**, usually solid at room temperature, include dairy fats, lard, shortening, cocoa fat, beef, pork and other animal fats. They contain *saturated fatty acids*, which tend to raise LDL-cholesterol in blood (promoting heart disease).
- **Polyunsaturated fats**, which contain mainly *polyunsaturated fatty acids* (PUFAs) include flaxseed, safflower, sunflower, corn, soybean, sesame and most nut oils. (Safflower oil has about 75 percent polyunsaturates and sunflower oil about 66 percent, compared to corn oil with 59 percent polyunsaturate content and sesame oil with 40 percent). Polyunsaturates tend to lower blood levels of harmful LDL cholesterol.
- **Monounsaturated oils** contain *monounsaturated fatty acids* (MUFAs) and include olive, canola and peanut oils, and some nut oils. (Olive oil contains about 70 percent monounsaturates, sesame oil has 40 percent and canola about 60 percent.) Among the cooking oils, olive oil is the only one that contains natural antioxidants, which keep stop it from becoming saturated (hydrogenated) and going rancid for many years; its reported health benefits may stem partly from its antioxidant properties.
- **Trans fatty acids (TFAs)**—produced by hydrogenating unsaturated vegetable oils—raise LDL-cholesterol as much as, or even more than, saturates, increasing heart disease risks.
- **Unsaturated long-chain omega-3 fatty acids** ("omega-3's") are polyunsaturated fatty acids found in flaxseed oil and many oceanic fish (e.g., salmon, mackerel, sardines, herring). They may exert cardiovascular benefits by reducing the stickiness or clotting power of blood platelets, and stabilizing the heart rhythm.

Therefore, people on these medications need regular check-ups and monitoring; they should report any muscle weakness or discolored urine. In addition, the statins interact with some other drugs—such as verapamil, erythromycin, clarithromycin (Biaxin), cylosporine, ketoconazole (Nizoral), itraconazola (Sporanox) and others—so may have to be discontinued while taking them. Consult your doctor about such interactions.

CHOOSING THE RIGHT FAT MIX

Despite all the publicity about low-fat diets, many people still don't know what's what in the world of fats. Fats—or lipids, to use the scientific term—are molecules made of a glycerol backbone with different fatty acids attached. Fatty acids have varying compositions and carbon chain lengths. Some fatty acids are "fully saturated" (with hydrogen atoms), others "unsaturated" (not fully saturated with hydrogen atoms). They come in a vast array of foods, sometimes lurking, unexpectedly, in crackers, muffins, sauces, dressings, cakes, pizzas, cookies and a slew of processed and ready-made foods.

Fats containing saturated fatty acids tend to be solid at room temperature and are mostly animal fats such as butter lard or bacon. They raise levels of LDL ("bad") cholesterol and are heart-damaging. Fats and oils containing unsaturated fatty acids are more liquid at room temperature—like vegetable oils such as corn, olive, nut, sunflower and safflower oils. They tend to lower LDL cholesterol and raise HDL ("good") cholesterol, protecting the heart. *Trans* fatty acids, rare in nature (although found in some animal fats, such as beef) are made by hydrogenating polyunsaturated vegetable oils to make them harder and more "spreadable" at room temperatures, and to give them longer "shelf life" (less likely to go rancid). Like saturated fats, the trans fats tend to raise LDL cholesterol.

Nutrition labels list the amounts of carbohydrate, protein and the different fats, in grams per serving size. The fat content of food appears as total fat, and amounts of saturated, polyunsaturated and monounsaturated fatty acids. Although the amount of *trans* fatty acids isn't listed, it can easily be calculated by subtracting the sum of saturated, poly- and monosaturated forms from the total.

How trans fats fit into the picture

Trans fatty acids (TFAs) in the diet are produced by hydrogenating polyunsaturated vegetable oils, often to make a variety of margarines and also by deep frying foods. During hydrogenation, some of the unsaturated double bonds are converted from the usual *cis* to the more saturated *trans* form. Trans fatty acids are found chiefly in margarines, spreads, mayonnaise, salad dressings, baked goods, pizza crusts, snack and convenience foods (such as potato and corn chips, cookies, crackers) and deep-fried items (such as French fries).

Hydrogenating polyunsaturated vegetable oils turns them into health-damaging trans fats. During hydrogenation, the structure of the unsaturated fatty acids changes from the natural and "kinky" (bulky) and loosely packed *cis* form to become more like tightly-packed, straighter saturated fatty acids. Although previously thought by most scientists to have no detrimental health effects, it now seems that *trans* fatty acids have the same (or still greater) cholesterol-raising and heart-harming effects as saturated fats. TFAs may also raise blood triglycerides, another blood lipid (fat) that damages the heart.

Use the 10:10:10 rule to balance your fat intake

Amid controversy about individual fatty acids, the *basic dietary message* remains unchanged: lower the overall amount of fat eaten to 30 percent or less of total calories. Too much of *any* fat is bad! Of the fats eaten, make the saturated and trans fat variety no more than 8 to 10 percent of your total food intake, polyunsaturates 10 percent and eat 10 percent monounsaturates. (Since there is some concern that excessive amounts of polyunsaturates may increase risks of certain cancers, nutritionists suggest that polyunsaturate consumption not exceed 10 percent of the total calorie intake.) Replacing saturated fats with monounsaturated forms whenever possible and eating fish frequently make for a heart-healthy diet.

How can we make good dietary fat choices?

"Ideally, we should choose fats according to the fatty acids they contain," notes one nutritional scientist, "because different fatty acids have different properties and varying health effects." In practice, we still have lots to learn about the different fatty acids, but we can follow a few basic principles. Firstly, since we North Americans still eat too much fat, we need to become better "fat watchers" and reduce overall intakes. That means eating less fried and snack foods, less processed foods (which often contain hidden fat) and going easy on margarine, butter, fatty meats and fat-laden dressings. In choosing margarine, substitute softer for harder types. Select one with the lowest percentage of "hydrogenated" fat and the maximum content of *non-hydrogenated* (polyunsaturated) fat.

DIETARY FIBER IS STILL IN

In the last 10 years or so, the popularity of dietary fiber as a health-promoting aid has been

FIBER-RICH FOODS			
Food	**Fiber (g)**	**Food**	**Fiber (g)**
Kidney beans (187 g)	6.7	Potato, boiled without skin (272 g)	2.8
Lima beans (199 g)	6.6	Prunes (5) (42 g)	5.0
Baked beans with tomato sauce, canned (267 mL)	5.8	Pears, canned (262 g)	4.8
Brussels sprouts, boiled (250 mL/1 cup)	5.0	Applesauce, canned and unsweetened (250 mL/1 cup)	3.6
Carrots, boiled (250 mL/1 cup)	5.0	Apple (1 medium)	3.5
Corn, canned (250 mL/1 cup)	4.8	Orange (1 medium)	2.6
Broccoli, boiled (250 mL/1 cup)	4.0	Peach (1 medium)	2.6
Tomatoes, stewed and canned (250 mL/1 cup)	4.0	Banana (1) (114 g)	2.4
Potato, baked without skin (156 g)	3.4	Bran buds cereal (125 mL/1/2 cup)	10.7
Green beans (250 mL/1 cup)	3.4	100% bran cereal (125 mL/1/2 cup)	9.9
Green peas (125 mL/1/2 cup)	3.6	Oatmeal (cooked) (187.5 mL/3/4 cup)	1.6
Lentils (125 mL/1/2 cup)	3.7	Shreddies, whole-wheat (200 mL)	3.2
		Whole-wheat bread (2 slices)	2.8
		Macaroni (250 mL/1 cup)	1.2

Source: Health Canada.

somewhat eclipsed by the emphasis on "low carb" and low-fat items—witness the vast array of "light" and "fat-reduced" products lining supermarket shelves. However, new evidence reaffirms the value of dietary fiber and its many diverse health benefits. Consuming enough of the right types of fiber can combat bowel disease, help lower blood cholesterol, protect the heart and mute swings in blood sugar—thereby improving diabetes management.

Under the less trendy term "roughage," fiber enjoyed considerable respect in past eras, and during the 1970s its image was enhanced by British physician Dennis Burkett, who practiced for many years in rural Africa and attributed Western ailments such as hernias, hemorrhoids, diabetes, bowel disease and heart problems to diets low in fiber. Some of us may remember the heyday of wheat bran during the late 1970s—with the widescale promotion of bran cereals and granolas—or the "oat bran craze" of the 1980s, with oat products in all shapes and sizes massively promoted to lower blood cholesterol. When a few studies showed that at best, oat bran may modestly reduce blood cholesterol, its popularity nosedived. But oat bran is making a slight comeback as the U.S. Food and Drug Administration now permits product labels to claim that, as part of a low-fat diet, oat cereals "may reduce the risk of heart disease."

Nutritional scientists remind us that no single form of fiber is best. Neither oats nor wheat bran are the whole story "People need *many different types of fiber* from varied fruits, vegetables, seeds and grains to obtain maximal nutritional benefits." The old idea of fiber as an inert part of food, passing undigested from mouth to anus and expelled in stool has been dramatically revised. The term "fiber" encompasses many complex carbohydrates, natural polymers such as cellulose and woody plant lignins, pectins, gums (guar arabic, agar carrageen), psyllium, and many other components not yet fully identified. Far from being inert, each exerts different effects on the body.

According to current guidelines, healthy adults should consume 26–35 grams of fiber daily from varied plant foods. The present North American fiber intake averages 11 grams a day. Health Canada and equivalent U.S. agencies suggest doubling this amount by eating more grains and unpeeled (but well-washed) fruit and vegetables, being sure to include both *insoluble* and *soluble* fiber. It is best to increase amounts gradually and it may be wise to consult a physician before greatly increasing fiber intake. Initially, eating large quantities can cause bloating, which generally subsides in a few weeks. Eating 26 grams of fiber daily may seem like a lot but can be done by having two fruits at breakfast (say a banana or orange and some raisins) with whole grain cereal, fruit as between-meal snacks, 3–5 servings of vegetables daily, and several bread and grain servings.

Insoluble fiber, from wheat bran and whole grains, as well as the skins of many fruits, vegetables, and seeds, makes stools bulkier and speeds their transit through the gut. Like a sponge, insoluble fiber absorbs many times its weight in water swelling up and helping to relieve constipation. High-fiber diets have replaced bland, low-residue treatments for many bowel problems.

Soluble fiber includes pectins, gums (such as guar), *betaglucans,* some hemicelluloses and other compounds in oats, legumes (peas, kidney beans, lentils), some seeds, brown rice, barley, oats, fruits (such as apples), some green vegeta-bles (such as broccoli) and potatoes. Soluble fiber breaks down as it passes through the digestive tract, forming a gel that traps certain substances, perhaps reducing the absorption of cholesterol into the bloodstream. Studies find that people on high-fiber diets have lower total cholesterol levels and may be less likely to form harmful blood clots than those who consume less soluble fiber. A recent U.S. report found that soluble fiber reduced heart disease risks in men who ate more than 25 g per day, compared to those who consumed less than 15 g daily.

Soluble fiber may also benefit those with diabetes—both insulin-dependent diabetes mellitus, and non-insulin-dependent forms—by helping to control blood sugar through delayed gastric (stomach) emptying and slowing the entry of glucose into the bloodstream, lessening the postprandial (post-meal) rise in blood sugar. Dietary fiber can help blunt the sudden spikes in blood glucose that occur after a low-fiber meal. (Researchers believe that a lifetime of blood glucose spikes could contribute to Type II or non-insulin dependent diabetes mellitus—which typically strikes after age 40, and more than doubles the risk of stroke and heart disease. The cholesterol-lowering effect of soluble fiber may also help those with diabetes by reducing their elevated heart disease risks.)

MAKE CARBOHYDRATES (STARCHES) YOUR DIETARY MAINSTAY

Simple carbohydrates or sugars (such as glucose, sucrose and fructose) are small molecules which we eat as refined products. They are good "pure" energy sources but provide few other nutrients. By contrast, complex carbohydrates are large molecules made up of simpler sugars that come in a vast range of foods—from potatoes, pears and pasta to cabbages, bread and popcorn—which usually provide other nutrients besides energy. For instance, 15 ml (1 tbsp) of sugar or an average soft drink provides about 50 calories, similar to one slice of wholegrain bread. But the complex carbohydrates in bread come with additional nutrients such as B vitamins, zinc, iron, calcium and valuable fiber. Although dieters trying to shed pounds traditionally considered potatoes, pasta and other carbohydrates fatten-

SORTING OUT THE VARIOUS SUGARS

There are many different sugars with fancy names such as fructose, galactose (in human mother's milk), lactose (in cow's milk), maltose and glucose. Sucrose or table sugar is a molecule composed of two smaller sugar molecules strung together. It is made from sugar beet or sugar cane. Basically sugars are similar; they vary somewhat in sweetness and chemical makeup, but no one type is healthier than another. Chemically, sugars fall into three main groups:

• monosaccharides, simple sugars such as fructose or glucose found in honey, fruits, vegetables, syrups and lactose;

• disaccharides, a chain of two simple sugars linked together—as in sucrose (table sugar);

• polysaccharides, made of many simple sugars strung together —such as starch or glycogen (energy-storage molecules).

Glucose is the form in which the body's cells use sugar for energy. Glucose is stored in the liver and muscles as glycogen and released as needed. Different foods have different effects on the rise in blood sugar that follows eating. Insulin, from the pancreas, is released in response to this sugar rise, and speeds up the absorption of glucose from the blood by the body's cells. A baked potato or white bread elevates blood sugar more than rice or corn. Legumes (peas, beans, lentils) tend to flatten the rise in blood glucose after eating owing to their soluble fiber content— an advantage for those with diabetes who want to prevent large blood-sugar swings.

ing, cutting them out has been shown to work against weight loss.

In fact, carbohydrates are less likely to be converted to body fat than dietary protein or fat, and they also have a beneficial effect on the microflora (bacterial inhabitants) of the human gut. Populations that consume a high-carbohydrate diet have lower rates of cancer and cardiovascular disorders.

SUGARS AREN'T ALL BAD

In recent years, sugar has not only been accused of increasing tooth decay but has also been blamed for obesity, diabetes, hypoglycemia, depression, an alleged "Halloween effect" (obstreperous behavior following the ingestion of sweet treats), aggression and even crime and delinquency. But these claims are based largely on exaggerated reports, anecdotal information and poorly controlled studies. Rigorous scientific scrutiny shows that many of the accusations are false.

The only valid argument against the prudent consumption of sugar is its detrimental effect on human teeth. Sugar is no more fattening than other foods, despite the widespread belief that it causes obesity. Although sugar is often blamed for the weight gained from desserts and candy, it is the fat in them rather than the sugar that's the culprit.

Tests show that sugar is *not* a proven cause of hypoglycemia, which is defined as low blood sugar and is signaled by sweating, shakiness, drowsiness and weakness lasting a few minutes to an hour. Hypoglycemic symptoms vanish soon after ingesting some sugar or injecting glu-

cose, and this prompt relief by eating sugar distinguishes *true* hypoglycemia from conditions such as panic reactions, neurosis and anxiety. Hypoglycemia is a rare condition; contrary to the popular view that it's reaching epidemic proportions, it hardly ever occurs in response to foods eaten by healthy people.

Well-controlled studies demonstrate that, rather than triggering irritability, restlessness or aggression, sugar tends to be calming, possibly due to an increase in the brain transmitter serotonin, which is known to have a sedating effect.

PROTEINS IN THE DIET

A protein is a chain of amino acids that can form many different configurations—like a chain of beads—and can combine with other substances.

PUTTING ENOUGH BALANCED PROTEIN INTO A MEAL

Combination	Amount	Grams of protein
Peanut butter	45 ml (3 tbsp)	12.0
Whole-wheat bread	2 slices	5.2
Lentils	250 ml (1 cup)	15.6
Brown rice	125 ml (½ cup)	2.5
Pasta (e.g., macaroni)	250 ml (1 cup)	6.5
Cheddar cheese	40 g	10.5
Whole-grain bread (or roll)	1 slice (or 1 roll)	2.2
Kasha (groats)	250 ml (1 cup)	8.0
Egg	1	6.5
Potato (baked)	1 medium	4.0
Oats (oatmeal)	250 ml (1 cup)	4.8
Skim milk	250 ml (1 cup)	9.0
Whole-wheat toast	2 slices	5.2

EATING MEAT IS NOT A CRIME

Despite warnings about the dangers of animal fat and "mad cow" disease or *bovine spongiform encephalopathy* (although the disease has very rarely surfaced in North American cattle), many people crave steaks, chops and burgers. Eaten in moderation—ideally no more than two or three 3-ounce servings a week—meat can be part of a healthy eating plan. There is no need to shun it entirely. Lean cuts of beef, pork and lamb provide high quality protein as well as minerals and vitamins. For healthiest effect, choose low-fat cuts, trim off any visible fat, limit portions to 3 ounces or less, and when possible replace red meat with poultry (turkey, chicken), fish or vegetarian foods as your main protein source.

Slight differences in the amino-acid makeup and sequence of the various proteins in our bodies—in our blood, muscle and other proteins—distinguish us from one another and make us what we are. The possible amino-acid arrangements are almost infinite, and thousands of different proteins have already been identified in living creatures. Proteins are constantly broken down in our bodies, and continually built up again and replaced. Without dietary protein, growth and other bodily functions would not occur.

While plants and some bacteria can manufacture all the amino acids they need, the human body can manufacture only 13 of the 22 needed. The amino acids our bodies can manufacture are termed nonessential, while the nine we can't make must come from food, and are termed essential amino acids (EAAs). They are histidine, isoleucine, leucine, lysine, methionine, phenylalanine, threonine, tryptophan and valine.

Protein in food is broken down by the digestive system into its constituent amino acids, which enter the body's pool of amino acids and can be reassembled into vital body substances such as the hormone insulin, the muscle protein myoglobin, the keratin in hair the respiratory enzymes and countless others. Each cell manufactures the proteins it needs using the building blocks available. If, however one or more of the essential amino acids is lacking, others that may be present cannot replace them in forming crucial body proteins.

IN PRAISE OF FISH

A ration of fish or fish oil two or three times weekly may help to prevent high blood pressure and heart disease. Fish oils are also promoted to help prevent some cancers. Omega-3 fatty acids in the fish oils from deep-sea fish may benefit migraine sufferers by altering the release of the brain transmitter serotonin. They may also help arthritics and asthmatics by inhibiting leukotriene formation, which promotes inflammation and some immune dysfunctions common to these disorders. Paradoxically, the types of fish that nutritionists used to brand as "less healthful" because of their high fat contents are the very ones that contain the desirable polyunsaturated, omega-3 fatty acids.

The protective effect of fish oils on the car-diovascular system stems from two particular omega-3 fatty acids—eicosapentanoic acid (EPA) and docosahexanoic acid (DHA)—obtainable from deep-sea fish. A diet high in omega-3s produces cells and tissues rich in compounds that alter blood platelet behavior and reduce the blood's clotting ability.

The benefits of fish oil in lowering heart-disease risks depend on the reduction in blood-clotting due to alterations in the metabolism of prostaglandins and allied compounds which play a key role in blood clotting, and the inhibition of blood-platelet stickiness or aggregation. Consuming deep sea fish rich in omega-3's improves heart health.

Seal meat, as well as fish such as salmon, bluefish, herring, mullet and scad, which inhabit deep, cold waters, tend to have the greatest benefits. Certain shellfish such as conch, oysters and clams also have fair amounts of omega-3. These shellfish are not—as was once believed—particularly high in cholesterol.

VEGETARIAN DIETS

Previously regarded as fads, vegetarian diets have recently gained popularity. Plant foods may offset the risk of certain diseases such as heart ailments and cancer.

Studies show that vegetarians tend to eat less saturated fat and cholesterol and more polyunsaturated fats than the average meat-eater although those consuming eggs, milk and cheese may still eat lots of saturated fat! A vegetarian diet rich in whole-milk products such as cheese is high in saturated fats and could endanger the heart. The Canadian Dietetic Association defines a "prudent" diet—one that offers optimal protection against a variety of diseases—as largely vegetarian, low in fat, with generous and varied quantities of plant foods. Whole grains, legumes, fruits and vegetables may provide several potentially health-protecting substances: fiber; carotene (a precursor of vitamin A which may protect against cancer); vitamins C and E; enzyme inhibitors; and selenium.

Vegetarians differ

The term "vegetarianism" encompasses:
- semi-vegetarians, who eat some fish or seafood, eggs and dairy products; they mimic

the diets of many traditional cultures which use animal products as condiments rather than as main dishes;

- lacto-ovo vegetarians, who eat eggs and dairy products but no meat, poultry or seafood;
- lacto-vegetarians, who consume dairy products but exclude eggs, meat, poultry and seafood;
- pure (vegan) vegetarians, who exclude all foods of animal origin.

Vegetarianism requires careful planning

Healthy vegetarianism entails more than the haphazard avoidance of animal foods. The body's cells don't distinguish between the sources of nutrients, provided they arrive in ample supply. However getting the right nutrients in the right amounts from plants requires more forethought than obtaining them from animal products. A vegetarian diet, with or without eggs and/or milk, can still provide all essential nutrients. With a good cookbook and the advice of a qualified dietitian, even very strict vegetarians can produce healthy meals. But nutritional problems are less likely with vegetarian diets that include eggs and milk. While most essential food elements can be found in plant foods, those on extreme vegan diets may be short on high-quality (complete) protein, vitamins B_{12} and D (especially when there is little sunlight available), calcium, iron and iodine, especially if legumes, dried fruits and iodized salt aren't consumed.

Meeting complete protein needs is crucial

Although we talk about "eating" protein, it's really the amino-acid components in proteins that the body needs as building blocks. During digestion, we break up animal and plant protein into its constituent amino acids, which our cells reassemble into human proteins (e.g., hemoglobin, keratin, muscle-myoglobin, insulin) for normal function and repair. The problem for vegetarians (especially vegans) is not only getting enough amino acids but getting the right kind in the right proportion—especially of the nine essential amino acids (EAAs) that the body can't manufacture for itself. If even one of the nine is low or absent, it can halt the manufacture of a vital body component, such as a particular

---

SOME TIPS TO HELP VEGETARIANS

- **Learn good mixes for complete protein:**
  - Legumes/leafy vegetables plus cereals;
  - Soybeans plus grains (wheat, corn, rice, rye);
  - Soy/sesame produce (e.g., tofu) plus low-fat milk;
  - Nuts plus wheat, oats, corn, rice or coconut.
- **Eat some fruit and vegetables raw,** as cooking destroys some vitamin C.
- **Be vigilant about key minerals,** especially iron and calcium, which are often poorly absorbed from many vegetable foods and can be carried out of the body bound to plant phytates and oxalates.
- **For vegans:** foods that supply the best nutrient value include fortified (check the label) soy milk; soybean products; legumes; hummus (chick peas plus sesame); green leafy vegetables (collards, kale, turnip greens, brussels sprouts, cauliflower, spinach, cabbage, broccoli) and fruits.

---

enzyme or hormone. In contrast to most animal foods, plants contain essential amino acids in ratios different from those the body requires. In other words, while eggs, milk, meat and some fish contain "complete" protein (the appropriate ratio and pattern of EAAs), many plant foods lack one or more EAAs and thus supply "incomplete" protein.

To obtain complete protein from entirely vegetarian fare, people must combine two or more plant proteins, preferably at each meal, e.g., grains with legumes or peas with rice. Grains are low in the amino acid lysine, but combined with legumes (peas, beans), which are rich in this amino acid, they provide the right quota.

In practice, many traditional cultures have achieved a well-balanced protein intake. In India, for example, vegetarians stay healthy on a diet rich in lentils (dahl), chick-peas and rice. Many East Indians use animal products as just a small addition or appetizing condiment, not as a main dish. The Chinese use animal or fish products as a minor addition to beansprout, mixed vegetable, noodle, rice or soy curd dishes. Mexican corn tortillas filled with beans, Middle Eastern hummus and falafel, South American and Mexican tacos with beans and the North American peanut-butter sandwich all provide excellent complete protein.

THE CAFFEINE STORY

Throughout history, humans have ingested caffeine for either a mood lift or medicinal purposes. In earliest times it was obtained by chewing coffee plant leaves, and later by brewing them as a hot beverage. Tea was the first hot caffeinated beverage consumed, a popular drink

ARE YOU GETTING ENOUGH VITAMIN B12?

Vitamin B$_{12}$ normally comes only in animal produce, although bacteria on fecally contaminated plant foods may provide some. Lack of B$_{12}$ can lead to *pernicious anemia* (too few red blood cells) which can cause irreversible nerve damage. (Heralding symptoms of B$_{12}$ shortage may be fatigue, headaches, tingling of hands and feet, balance upsets.) Most North American diets supply plenty, but strict vegetarians who eat no eggs or milk must obtain B$_{12}$ from supplements or fortified foods. Former meat-eaters who become vegetarians may have enough B$_{12}$ stores to last for years before needing supplements. Seniors should pay special attention to B$_{12}$ intake because its absorption declines with age and many seniors are at risk of vitamin B$_{12}$ deficiency. Those who are short need a boost by injection or B$_{12}$ supplements.

in China some 1,600 years ago, later spreading to Japan and ultimately to Europe. Since then coffee has become one of the world's most popular drinks. Although the United States consumes three-quarters of the world's coffee beans, Canadians have a higher per-capita coffee intake. Most North Americans also ingest considerable quantities of caffeine from cola drinks and chocolate.

The current arguments over the safety of caffeine revolve around its possible contribution to heart disease, osteoporosis, cancer birth defects, sleep disorders, stomach ulcers and nervous ailments. The 1990 Federal Canadian Eating Guidelines advise us to "consume no more caffeine than that equivalent to four regular cups of coffee per day because of its possible link to heart disease." One University of Toronto expert, while agreeing that "it's wise to curb excessive intakes," calls the suggested restriction to four cups of coffee a day "needlessly restrictive."

How caffeine affects the body
People differ widely in their response to caffeine. In most, it enhances mental alertness. Doses of 50–200 mg (one or two cups of coffee) increase alertness and decrease drowsiness. Doses above 500 mg may produce symptoms formerly known as "caffeinism"—headaches, tremors, nervousness and irritability.

Caffeine is rapidly absorbed from the intestines, peaking in the blood after about 30 minutes, and being distributed to all tissues of the body. The speed of caffeine absorption is slower when the stomach is full. Smokers tend to metabolize caffeine much faster than nonsmokers.

Like many mood-altering substances, caffeine can be habit-forming, and the habit may lead to overconsumption. To determine whether you are dependent, simply eliminate all caffeine sources from the diet for one day. If a throbbing headache results—relieved only by a caffeine "fix"—chances are that you are suffering caffeine withdrawal.

Beyond vitamins: Phytochemicals that help fight disease
In their never-ending quest for health and longevity, people eagerly seek dietary fixes.

Looking for shortcuts, many swallow supplements. Beyond vitamins, many now also take other supplements such as garlic capsules and broccoli pills to try and stave off disease.

Phytochemical supplements—vegetables in a pill?
For people who know they should eat more vegetables but can't bring themselves to do it, veggie pills might seem to offer promise. But even if supplements provide some valuable compounds (which not all do), taking pills means missing out on other valuable plant nutrients and the taste of food itself. In addition to the expense (one bottle can cost as much as $20), those who take pills may not eat the recommended daily 5 to 10 servings of fruit and vegetables.

Defining the "phytochemicals"—chaos around the new terms
An ever-expanding array of previously unknown plant compounds with hard-to-pronounce names is being uncovered, some thought to ward off disease. With names like *anthrocyanins*, *lycopenes*, *xanthenes*, *isothiocyanates* and *sulphoraphane*, the newly identified plant chemicals seem to belong more in a test tube than in a salad. They are often lumped together under the term *phytochemicals*—*phyto* from the Greek word for plant—denoting their plant origins. But there's considerable confusion from the many different loosely used labels such as "nutrichemicals," "antioxidants," "nutriceuticals" (from "nutrient" and "pharmaceutical"), "designer foods," "pharmafoods" and "chemopreventive agents"—each with a slightly different meaning. Common to all trendy labels is the assumption that certain plant components can prevent or cure a specific disease. In truth, they may alter or mute the *risk factors* that lead to disease, but they do not actually treat it.

Phytochemicals in living color
Many phytochemicals are the very pigments that lend fruits and vegetables their attractive hues, some of them antioxidants that may offset oxidative cell damage. Antioxidants in fruit and vegetables are believed to help prevent formation of "free radicals" that damage DNA, thereby preventing cancer.

Other antioxidants include the pale yellow of potatoes and cauliflower conferred by *anthroxanthins* (Greek for "yellow flower") and the yellow color of corn—from another antioxidant called *lutein*, thought to play a role in preventing macular degeneration (a leading cause of blindness). The red pigment in tomatoes is *lycopene*, another antioxidant that seems to protect against several forms of cancer. In one study, researchers found that people who ate raw tomatoes seven times a week halved their risk of stomach, bladder and colon cancers.

The blue in blueberries, grapes and eggplant arises from the pigment anthrocyanin ("blue flower" in Greek). Anthrocyanins dilate blood vessels which may help lower the risk of heart disease and stroke: their presence in grapes may partly explain why a daily glass of wine helps lower the risk of heart attack.

Probing the antioxidant craze

The recent popularity of certain highly publicized plant "antioxidants" lies in their supposed heart-protecting and cancer-preventing capacity. The theory is that beta-carotene, vitamin C (ascorbic acid) and vitamin E (*alpha-tocopherol*) may protect the heart by blocking the oxidation of LDL cholesterol. Although some studies suggest that antioxidant supplements may reduce cardiovascular disease, critics point out that vitamin-takers tend to be health-conscious people who may have a generally heart-protecting lifestyle. Moreover, plants contain many *other* compounds that could be the active players.

The latest research shows no evidence of cardiovascular benefits from beta-carotene supplements, nor from vitamins A, C and E. In fact, the Finnish "ATBC" study found that taking beta-carotene supplements for 5 to 8 years did not reduce, but actually increased, fatal heart attack rates. It also found that although vitamin E supplements reduced nonfatal heart attacks it did not decrease (but in fact increased) total heart attack deaths. Other reports have further dashed hopes that beta-carotene may stave off heart disease. One trial ended abruptly when results revealed elevated lung cancer risks in those taking supplements. Researchers conclude that high-dose beta-carotene offers no health advantages and may in fact carry risks.

Studies on vitamin C and A supplements also show no clear evidence of cardiovascular benefits. Two new "kids on the block" to watch for are *homocysteine*—which, in excess, may contribute to heart disease, stroke and thrombosis (clots), its ill effects possibly offset by high doses of folic acid and vitamin B_{12}— and *lutein* in spinach and broccoli. Studies suggest that lutein may have strong heart-protecting properties. No harm in eating lots of broccoli!

Real food beats phytochemical supplements

Before jumping onto the phytochemicals bandwagon and rushing out to buy veggie pills, investigate the evidence. Scientists must first demonstrate the health benefits of the newly isolated plant compounds, prove they are not toxic and that they don't interact adversely with other dietary components. So far the evidence for the disease-preventing capacity of supplements is far less convincing than that for whole fresh fruit, grains and vegetables. As one expert cautions, "we abandon the natural mix of compounds in fruit and vegetables at our peril. Ample fresh vegetables and fruit remains your best anti-oxidant, anti-disease cocktail."

VITAMINS: MOST PEOPLE DON'T NEED SUPPLEMENTS

The easy availability of over-the-counter vitamins and the popular view of them as "natural" wonder foods able to ward off disease has made supplements and megavitamin therapy increasingly popular. But studies find no evidence of better health or longevity in regular supplement users. Supplements are not necessary for children or adults who eat a well-varied diet.

What are vitamins?

Vitamins are organic chemicals that are essential to human life. They include 13 substances and some "hangers-on" classed with them (choline, folic acid, inositol, biotin). Vitamins help the body transform food into energy, aid the immune defenses, promote good eyesight, contribute to blood and tooth formation and assist many other body functions. Some vitamins (A, D, F, K) are fat-soluble and the rest

KNOW YOUR VITAMINS

Vitamin	Good Natural Sources	Recommended Nutrient Intake (RNIs)	Toxic Dose (chronic, regular use)	Symptoms of Megadose Toxicity	Signs of Deficiency
A (Retinol Carotene)	liver, dark green and orange-yellow vegetables, milk, margarine, cantaloupe	Infants to 3 years: 400 Retinol Equivalents (RE)/day 4 years to adolescence: slow increase with weight-gain Men: 1,000 RE/day Women: 800 RE/day Lactation: 400 RE extra/day	40,000 IU (adult) 25,000 IU (child)	Headache, nausea, vomiting, double vision, ear-ringing, bone, joint, abdominal pains, hair loss, muscle pain, dry or peeling skin	Xerophthalmia (dry, crusty and inflamed eyes, infections), night blindness
D (Cholecalciferol)	fortified milk, fish-liver oils, egg yolk, butter, liver	Infants: 400 International Units (IU)/day 2–6 years: 200 IU/day 7–49 years: 100 IU/day Age 50+: 200 IU/day Pregnancy and Lactation: 200 IU/day extra	150,000 IU (adult) 10,000–30,000 IU (child)	Hypercalcemia; nausea, appetite loss, weight loss, dry skin	Rickets in children (bow legs, pigeon breast, protruding ribs, curved spine), osteomalacia in adults (bone pain in legs and back, spontaneous fractures)
E (Alpha-Tocopherol)	vegetable oils, eggs, whole-grain cereals	Infants: 3 mg/day Children 2–12 years: 4–8 mg/day Adults: 6–10 mg/day Age 50+: 5–7 mg/day Pregnancy: 2 mg extra/day Lactation: 3 mg extra/day	No toxic dose specified but probably 300–1,500 mg	No specific toxicity syndrome. Individual reactions include blurred vision, headache, nausea, fatigue, muscle weakness, slow clotting	Never seen except in premature infants
K (Menadione)	liver, leafy green vegetables, cauliflower, dairy products	Not established; part of requirement met through synthesis in the intestine	No toxic dose specified	"Spot hemorrhage" on skin, kidney damage	Very rare
B$_1$ (Thiamin)	pork, legumes, bran, dried yeast, oatmeal, enriched bread, peanuts, whole wheat, milk and milk products	0.40 mg/1,000 kcal/day for all age groups Pregnancy: extra 0.1 mg/day Lactation: extra 0.2 mg/day	5 mg	No known toxicity	Beri Beri (numbness in legs, muscle wasting, heart failure, scaly skin)
B$_2$ (Riboflavin)	milk and milk products, calf liver, other organ meats, bran flakes, brewer's yeast, pork, leafy green vegetables, enriched bread	For all age groups: 0.5 mg/1,000 kcal/day Pregnancy: extra 0.3 mg/day Lactation: extra 0.4 mg/day		No known toxicity	Ariboflavinosis (growth retardation, oral inflammation, dry and scaly skin)

Vitamin	Good Natural Sources	Recommended Nutrient Intake (RNIs)	Toxic Dose (chronic, regular use)	Symptoms of Megadose Toxicity	Signs of Deficiency
Niacin	meat, poultry, fish, enriched bread, eggs, avocados, dates, figs, prunes (milk, meats provide tryptophan, a niacin precursor)	7.2 Niacin Equivalents (NE)/1,000 kcal/day for all age groups. Pregnancy: 2 NE extra Lactation: 3 NE extra	100 mg	Face flushing, sweating, hand and foot tingling; liver damage (at 1–3 g/day)	Pellagra (skin rash, inflammation, diarrhea, psychosis, with severe lack)
Biotin	milk and milk products, beef liver, oatmeal, soybeans, clams, eggs, salmon, shrimp, chicken, avocado, beans, bananas, peanuts	Not established; suggested intakes: 1.5µg/kg body weight/day		No known toxicity	Not known, except in rare cases of excessive raw-egg consumption
Pantothenic acid	liver, yeast, eggs, salmon, milk, avocado, chicken, lamb leg, banana, pork, molasses, peanuts, cauliflower, oranges	Not established; suggested intakes 2–3 mg/day for children and adults	10–20 g	Diarrhea with doses greater than 10 g	Not known
Pyridoxine (B$_6$)	organ and muscle meats, whole-grain cereals, legumes, avocado, beer, cantaloupe, cabbage, milk, eggs	Depends on protein intake 0.015 mg/g protein eaten, averages to: Men: 1.8 mg/day Women: 1.1 mg/day	1,000–2,000 mg	Neurotoxicity with numbness and tingling in feet and hands, difficulty walking, imbalance, clumsiness	Muscle weakness, irritability, unstable gait
Cobalamin (B$_{12}$)	beef liver, chicken liver, clams, oysters, tuna, lamb leg, milk, eggs	Infants: 0.1 µg/day Children: graded increase Adults: 1.0 µg/day Pregnancy: 1.2 µg/day Lactation: 1.2 µg/day		No known toxicity	Pernicious anemia (burning tongue, appetite loss, abdominal pain, irritability, depression, delirium, nerve disorders)
Folacin (Folic acid)	raw spinach, romaine lettuce, liver, fish, poultry, legumes, broccoli, bananas, avocado, oranges, cooked beets, apricots	Adults: 3.1 µg/kg body weight/day Infants and children up to age 4: 4 µg/kg/day Children and teens: 3.5 µg/kg/day Pregnancy: 7 µg/kg/day Lactation: 5 µg/kg/day		No known toxicity	Megaloblastic anemia (pallor, fatigue, burning tongue); neural tube defects in fetus of folate-deficient women
C (Ascorbic acid)	citrus fruits and juices, strawberries, green leafy vegetables, green peppers, tomatoes, potatoes, melon, cauliflower	Children: requirement increases with weight from 20 mg/day–30 mg/day (up to 15 years) 15+ years: Males: 40 mg/day; females: 30 mg/day Smokers: Males: 60 mg/day; females: 45 mg/day Pregnancy: extra 10 mg/day Lactation: extra 25 mg/day	1,000–10,000 mg	Diarrhea, intestinal cramps, skin rashes, kidney stones, nausea, vomiting, "rebound scurvy," interference with some diagnostic blood tests	Scurvy (bleeding gums, lethargy, weakness, irritability, weight loss, joint pain)

(the eight different Bs and C) dissolve in water. If one or other of the vitamins is in short supply or absent, deficiency diseases may occur—such as blindness due to a lack of vitamin A, or pellagra (skin problems) due to B-vitamin shortages. The beneficial effect of a vitamin in preventing disease was first shown in 1753 when a Scottish surgeon proved that giving sailors daily oranges or lemons could prevent scurvy on long sea voyages. The antiscorbutic factor was later shown to be ascorbic acid—now known as vitamin C. The last vitamin to be isolated was vitamin B$_{12}$, in 1948.

Each vitamin performs specific tasks in the body. Vitamin A (from liver, eggs, orange and yellow fruit and vegetables) promotes vision and skin health; vitamin D (from fish, fortified milk) is vital to bone and tooth strength; vitamin C

VITAMANIA: PROBING A FEW VITAMIN TRUTHS AND MYTHS

Vitamin C (ascorbic acid) and the common cold

Vitamin C megadoses are widely promoted for the common cold and other ills. A well-conducted University of Toronto study that compared people given a placebo (inactive agent) to those taking vitamin C (one gram a day and four grams at the first sign of cold symptoms), found vitamin C offered no protection against colds. Moreover, regular intake of vitamin C in amounts far above recommended amounts (30–45 mg per day) can produce diarrhea, an acidic urine that favors the formation of kidney stones and (in susceptible people) excessive breakdown of red blood cells or excessive iron absorption.

Examining the vitamin E debate

Vitamin E (alpha-tocopherol) is an antioxidant that protects cell membranes, but its precise physiological role is unknown. It is readily available from leafy greens, nuts, seeds, mayonnaise and vegetable oils; and no deficiency has yet been identified in humans. While it has few known toxic side effects, recent research suggests that large amounts may antagonize the action of vitamin K in blood clotting. The current recommended intake for vitamin E in adults is 7 mg a day for men, 6 mg daily for women (about 30 International Units/IU), but some suggest levels of 100 IU daily, to improve heart-health. Excess can be harmful.

Former claims that supplements of about 100 IU may protect the heart by lowering LDL blood cholesterol have now been disputed. Studies on its benefits have given contradictory results. A Texas study found supplements of 400 IU vitamin E daily effective in reducing oxidation of LDL-cholesterol; the Iowa Women's Health Study on 34,000 postmenopausal women, found no reduction in heart disease with vitamin E supplements, although natural food sources seemed protective. The Cambridge Heart Antioxidant study found large doses (800 IU daily) seemed to reduce heart attack risks, but concluded that more research was needed. Several large, randomized trials are under way in Europe and the U.S. which should provide answers in a few years. The collected results suggest no heart-protecting benefits from vitamin E supplements. Nutritional scientists warn that the safety of large supplements remains unknown.

Niacin (vitamin B$_3$) and its touted benefits

Vitamin B$_3$ or niacin is found in meat, butter and eggs. This vitamin has been promoted for reversing the depression, memory loss, irritability, headaches, hallucinations and paranoid delusions that accompany the formerly widespread deficiency condition known as pellagra (now uncommon in the Western world). While niacin megadoses for the relief of mental illnesses have proved useless, high doses are sometimes helpful in reducing blood triglyceride levels in people at risk of heart disease. The recommended daily level of niacin intake is 13–18 mg. The new Reference Dietary Intake report, prepared by a joint panel of U.S. and Canadian experts, has now set an upper safety level for niacin intake at 35 mg/day. Daily consumption above this level can cause severe flushing, itching and other symptoms. Experts warn that "individuals who take over-the-counter niacin to self-treat themselves for a high cholesterol or high blood pressure are courting trouble. High doses can produce severe side effects such as gout, headaches, liver damage and an upset blood-sugar balance."

Vitamin B$_6$ (pyridoxine) can be dangerous in excess

Vitamin B$_6$ (pyridoxine) is essential to health and amply available from foods such as poultry, tuna, eggs, grains, bananas, nuts and potatoes. Megadoses can cause harm. Huge doses of vitamin B$_6$—as high as 800 mg a day—have been popularly promoted to counteract the bloating, moodiness, irritability and breast tenderness of premenstrual syndrome (PMS), even though studies show no consistent evidence for its efficacy in remedying PMS. A review of the uses of vitamin B$_6$ for PMS concluded that there's no proof that B$_6$ is beneficial for the relief of PMS. The chief danger of B$_6$ megadosing lies not in controlled amounts prescribed by a physician who's on the alert for signs of damage, but with self-administered doses taken on the assumption that it's a harmless nutrient.

Guidelines issued by the joint U.S./Canadian committee for Dietary Reference Intakes (DRIs) set the "tolerable upper limit" or safety level for B$_6$ at 100 mg/day. Amounts above that can trigger a painful (and often irreversible) nerve disorder called sensory neuropathy, with numbness in hands and feet, unsteadiness, gait problems and an inability to walk without a cane. Doses as low as 250 mg a day, on a continued basis, may damage nerve function. Recovery from the nerve degeneration can take months to years.

(from citrus fruits, berries, green peppers) ensures healthy skin and gums and aids wound healing; vitamin F (from nuts, vegetable oils, olives, grains) is an antioxidant that protects the body's cells against damage by oxidation; vitamin K (from cauliflower, broccoli, cabbage, soybeans) aids blood clotting; and the B vitamins (from nuts, liver, mushrooms, dairy products, eggs) assist in a host of vital functions. But we require only tiny amounts of most vitamins, easily supplied by a varied, well-balanced diet.

Besides knowing which vitamins we need and what each does, we should also know how much of each is recommended. The American Recommended Daily Allowances (RDAs) or Canadian Recommended Nutrient Intakes (RNIs), published by federal agencies, spell out the amounts of each vitamin required by healthy

Excess B_6 intake may also block the action of penicillamine (not to be confused with penicillin), L-dopa and certain anticonvulsants.

Higher daily folate intakes advised to protect hearts and babies

Recent evidence shows that a plentiful intake of folic acid (one of the B vitamins)—also called folate or folacin—may not only help to prevent heart attacks but can significantly reduce the risk of birth defects involving a malformed brain or spine. The DRI report suggests a daily folate intake of 400 mcg/day for everyone over age 14 but more for women of childbearing age. For any woman who plans to or might become pregnant, the new guidelines recommend a folate-enriched diet providing 600 micrograms (mcg) of folic acid a day, to reduce the chances of having a baby with neural tube defects. Neural tube defects include *spina bifida* (where the spinal cord doesn't close) or *anencephaly* (where the brain doesn't develop properly—usually fatal before birth). To avoid such defects, women must eat enough folate *before* becoming pregnant and especially in the very first month of pregnancy, when the baby's embryonic brain and spinal cord are just forming. A pre-pregnancy folate supplement, as well as during pregnancy, can help prevent neural tube defects. Foods rich in folate include citrus fruit, most berries, organ meats, dark green leafy vegetables (such as spinach, broccoli, romaine lettuce and legumes (dried peas, beans, lentils). Some grain products such as breads, cereals and pastas are now folate-enriched. The Dietary Reference Intake (DRI) report suggests women who plan to conceive may wish to take a folate supplement, but should ask their physicians about it.

One added advantage of a higher folate intake is that it decreases blood levels of homocysteine, an amino acid which, if elevated, can increase risks of cardiovascular disease and heart attack. Many people who have heart attacks, strokes and venous thromboembolism (vein clots), especially at a young age, have abnormally high blood levels of homocysteine. A high blood homocysteine is often tied to low B vitamin intakes. Recent studies find that people on folate supplements had lower levels of circulating homocysteine. The *Nurses Health Study* found 400 μg/day (0.4 mg/day) of folate protected against heart disease.

Folate intakes should not exceed the upper safe limit of 1,000 mcg per day. Levels above that might mask signs of B_{12} deficiency and pernicious anemia, especially in the elderly. (Older people who eat few or no animal foods are at risk of vitamin B_{12} deficiency.)

Supplements: Avoiding excess or "too much of a good thing" ...

Experts devising the new Dietary Reference Intakes have now added "tolerable (maximum) upper limits" to the nutritional guidelines, to protect people from the dangers of overdosing on vitamins, minerals or other nutrients. The guidelines emphasize that "too much of a good thing" may be far from good.

If, notwithstanding this advice, you do decide to take supplements, choose a balanced multivitamin product that includes iron and contains nutrients in amounts below the upper safe limits. Remember, it makes no difference (except to the wallet) whether the vitamin preparation is synthetic or the more expensive "natural" type. The body can't tell them apart! Treat your supplement as medicine, lock it away from children and take it with meals.

Supplements occasionally advised for certain at-risk groups

*   Pregnant women—usually advised to take supplements of folate, iron and calcium.
*   Stringent dieters or those on inadequate diets with calorie intakes below 1,000–1,200 per day may require supplements.
*   Strict vegetarians and their children who avoid eggs and milk and, especially, the nursing infants of such mothers, as well as their other children, are at risk of deficiencies of B^{12} and other vitamins, and should take supplements.
*   People with certain diseases or on some medications that curtail nutrient absorption may need specific supplements (e.g., heavy alcohol drinkers and aspirin-takers whose body may be depleted of folate and vitamin C).
*   The elderly, who often have little appetite and become undernourished, may benefit from a daily multiple vitamin-mineral supplement.
*   Women with heavy periods may need extra iron (to prevent anemia).
*   Smokers who use up vitamin C at a faster rate than nonsmokers.
*   Breast-fed infants who need vitamin D supplements; formula-feds may need iron-fortified formula.
*   Children over age three who live where water isn't fluoridated may need fluoride supplements.

THE AMOUNT OF IRON ABSORBED FROM FOOD DEPENDS ON:

- *The body's iron status.* **When iron stores are low or if people are iron-deficient, the body absorbs more from food. Absorption also improves during growth spurts and pregnancy, when iron needs increase.**
- *The form of iron in the foods consumed.* **Iron from animal products is more readily absorbed than iron from plant foods.**
- *The mix of foods eaten.* **People can boost their iron absorption by being careful about the food combinations eaten. For example, vitamin C (in citrus fruits) enhances iron absorption, while the presence of calcium (in dairy products) inhibits it. (See also section on anemia in Chapter 16.)**

people, taking into account age, gender and certain conditions such as pregnancy and lactation. Ultimately, the new DRI (Dietary Reference intake) standards will lead to a new set of uniform U.S-Canadian guidelines for healthy eating.

The new guidelines, issued in 1998, have increased the suggested intake levels for several vitamins, also specifying their safe upper intake limits. For instance, the report advises men and women aged 51 to 79 to consume 10 mcg (400 IU) of vitamin D a day—double the previously recommended intake—and 600 IU/day for those over 80 years old. The safe upper limit for vitamin D is 2,000 IU a day. Vitamin D is produced by the skin in the presence of sunlight, and supplied in foods such as milk, and margarine (usually D-fortified) and fish. A D-vitamin supplement may be suggested for those living in climates (like Canada) where sunlight is sparse during winter months, or for the elderly who may not eat properly or venture outdoors.

Most healthy adults do not need vitamin supplements. Vitamin deficiencies that were common a few generations ago are now very rare in most developed countries, where people eat sufficiently varied diets. Modern methods of preservation, rapid food transport and a diet that includes all essential nutrients ensure that most of us are not vitamin-depleted. Moreover, in North America, the vitamins that could be lacking in everyday diets are often added to fortify commonly eaten items such as milk, cereals and flour.

For vitamins "more" is by no means "better"

Since the 1950s, megavitamin proponents have promoted the use of various vitamins in doses much higher than recommended daily amounts to correct a wide range of disorders. The "more is better" approach has led to the dramatic overuse of vitamins, which are often used as medicines to combat conditions for which there is no satisfactory cure, such as muscle aches, fatigue and stress. Considering that the body cannot efficiently use excess vitamins, it's amazing how many people who eat sensibly still take supplements "just to be on the safe side." Yet, excess vitamins may be neither safe, nor better.

Taking pills instead of food not only deprives you of *other* valuable ingredients, but may also engender a false sense of security and deter people from eating heart-healthy diets and adopting other measures to reduce disease risks. A further downside of relying on supplements is that people may miss out on trace (but vital) nutrients in certain foods, for instance, cobalt and selenium. Or, for example, calcium supplements don't contain the other valuable nutrients provided by natural food sources (such as low-fat dairy products).

In large doses, vitamins act as drugs

In megadoses, vitamins are no longer nutrients but become "pharmacologically active substances" which—like all such substances—may produce harmful effects. "When consumed from sources other than food," notes one U.S. expert, "vitamins and minerals become potent drugs." With more than 40 percent of North Americans now taking supplements, experts warn about the dangers of excess. Single-ingredient supplements may interfere with or compete with the absorption of other vital nutrients. For instance, too much calcium may hinder iron absorption; too much copper can interfere with zinc metabolism. Separate B-vitamin pills may alter the absorption of others. Health may be damaged before someone even notices something is wrong.

In the United States, all vitamins (except folic acid) are classed as nutrients, with no legal restrictions on the dose or potency of products marketed. But in Canada vitamin preparations are viewed as drugs and must be approved by Health Canada's Bureau of Nonprescription Drugs before being offered for sale. When the manufacturer applies for a drug identification number (DIN), Health Canada checks the dosage against existing legislation to make sure it's not too high. (However, authorities cannot control the number of pills someone takes.) One expert at the Health Protection Branch of Health Canada suggests looking for the DIN symbol followed by a 6- or 8-digit number on any vitamin preparation. If the product doesn't bear this mark it is not officially approved and can't be sold legally.

THE NEW PHYTOCHEMICALS

- *Phenolic compounds in tea.* Tea—both black and green—is especially rich in antioxidant phenolics which may help prevent tumor formation. In animal studies, several kinds of black and green tea inhibited cancers of the skin, lung and esophagus, supposedly by blocking DNA oxidation. The evidence in humans is mixed, but some studies report a low incidence of cancer in tea-drinking populations. Evidence also suggests that heavy tea-drinkers have reduced blood pressure and lower blood cholesterol levels. Both green and black tea seem equally effective.

- *Isoflavones: the benefits of soya.* Isoflavones, found in soya beans, garbanzo beans, chick peas, and liquorice have effects that mimic those of the female hormone estrogen and may help protect against heart disease. In Eastern cultures, soya is considered a healthy and nutritious food as well as a medicinal agent. In China, the word for soybean, *ta tou*, means "great bean" and according to ancient folklore it helps fight heart disease. Recent research has shown that diets rich in soya help to reduce high blood levels of LDL ("bad") cholesterol by an estimated 12 to 15 percent. The isoflavones in soya are converted in the gut to phytoestrogens ("plant estrogens")—among them quercetin and genistein—compounds thought to reduce blood cholesterol. Phytoestrogens are also said to alleviate menopausal hot flashes and night sweats.

- *Sulphur compounds: The "promise of garlic."* Besides its established gastronomic value, garlic has long been promoted as a medicinal agent against ailments ranging from headaches to cancer. The *allylic sulphides*, in garlic and other allium vegetables—onions, chives, leeks and scallions—may stimulate enzymes that inhibit bacterial growth. Researchers suggest that a high garlic consumption reduces risks of stomach cancer; others claim it lowers blood pressure and strengthens immune defenses. However, claims for the health benefits of garlic remain to be substantiated.

- *Indoles and isothiocyanates: the broccoli connection.* Antioxidant compounds in *cruciferous* vegetables—such as broccoli, Brussels sprouts, cabbage and cauliflower—are thought to inhibit the DNA damage that triggers some forms of cancer. The *indoles* and isothiocyanates in these vegetables retard the growth of malignant tumors in rats; *phenylethylisocyanate* in broccoli may blunt the carcinogenic effects of cigarette smoke. But these effects remain to be proved.

- *The flax seed link.* Lignin and *alpha-linolenic acid* in flax seeds are thought to reduce the risks of heart disease, breast and colon cancers.

- *Monoterpenes,* such as *D-limonene* (in orange peel, citrus oils) and similar compounds in cherries have some anti-tumor properties—usefulness to be confirmed.

Even water-soluble vitamins can be toxic in megadoses

Whereas the dangers of megadosing with fat-soluble vitamins, especially vitamins A and D, are quite well known, many assume that any surplus of water-soluble vitamins will be harmlessly flushed out of the body in urine. However, even water-soluble vitamins can be harmful in large doses. For example, in 1998, the joint U.S.–Canadian dietary DRI report set new maximum limits for the intake of several B vitamins. The "tolerable" upper limit for vitamin B_6 is 100 mg a day; above that level it can be neurotoxic (nerve damaging). The ceiling for folate intake is 1,000 micrograms daily; for niacin (B_3) it's 35 mg/day, and for choline (another B vitamin) intakes should not exceed 3.5 g/day. (Above that level, excess choline can trigger a blood pressure drop and cause a fishy body odor.)

Doses of vitamin C over one and a half grams a day may cause diarrhea, increase the risks of kidney stones and even lead to "rebound scurvy" (when megadosing stops, the body may falsely react as if short of vitamin C).

The key to safe vitamin taking is to limit intakes to levels below the safe upper limit, and to choose preparations with labels bearing a DIN (Canadian) number or "USP" sign (meaning the product meets U.S. pharmacological standards). Remember that large amounts act as drugs and that both high doses taken for a short time and lower doses ingested over the longer haul may be risky.

MINERALS IN THE DIET

Minerals are inorganic elements that occur widely in the earth's crust. Although the body's mineral content totals no more than about 4 percent of its weight, minerals play a crucial part in many body functions and are vital to growth and efficiency. Our bodies contain over 50 different minerals, and a crucial 22 are essential to our well-being. These key minerals fall into two categories:

- seven macro or major minerals required in large amounts—calcium, chloride, magnesium, phosphorus, potassium, sodium and sulphur;
- fifteen micro or trace elements, required in only trace amounts—including chromium, copper, fluorine, iodine, iron, manganese, molybdenum, selenium and zinc.

KNOW YOUR MINERALS

Macro or Major

Mineral	Function	Food Source and RNI
Calcium (Ca)	Vital to tooth and bone formation, blood clotting, nerve and muscle action. Absorption depends on sufficient intake of vitamin D and phosphorus. Deficiency causes rickets, poor growth, bone deterioration, muscle cramps. Excess may cause kidney stones, spastic muscles.	Milk products, sardines, salmon, oysters, soybean curd, broccoli, spinach, lentils, beans (dried and green). RNI: Infants: from 250–400 mg/day; 1–9 year olds: 500–700 mg/day; 10–18 year olds: 700–1,100 mg/day; Adults: men: 800 mg; women: 700 mg; up to 500 mg extra for pregnancy and lactation and after menopause. (250 ml/1 cup skim milk—317 mg; 85 g canned red salmon—100 mg; 125 ml/½ cup cooked spinach—88 mg.)
Chlorine (Cl)	Essential to water balance, acid-base regulation, digestion. Deficiencies rare.	Fish; salt. RNI: not clearly established.
Magnesium (Mg)	Vital to bone structure, nerve transmission, muscle action, protein metabolism, energy production, heart action. Deficiencies common among heavy drinkers, excess sugar users, long-term diuretic takers, occasionally in people on birth-control pills or taking excess vitamin D.	Whole grains, green vegetables, bananas, apricots, milk, nuts, seafood, hard water. RNI: Infants: 20–30 mg/day; Children: 3.7 mg/kg body weight per day; Adults: 3.4 mg/kg body weight per day; pregnancy additional 45 mg/day; lactation additional 65 mg/day. (1 medium banana—58 mg; 250 ml/1 cup 2% milk—40 mg.)
Phosphorus (P)	Essential to bone formation, fat transport, nerve action, overall energy metabolism. Intake should balance calcium intakes (body needs same amounts). Deficiencies may cause poor growth.	Meat, liver, milk, tuna, poultry, soybeans, bran, eggs, peas, broccoli, potatoes. RNI: Infants (0–4 mo): 150 mg/day; (5–12 mo): 200 mg/day; Children: gradual increase with age; Adults: men: 1,000 mg/day; women: 850 mg/day; pregnancy and lactation: 200 mg extra/day (85 g liver—400 mg; 250 ml/1 cup skim milk—232 mg; 125 ml/½ cup cooked soybeans—161 mg.)
Potassium (K)	Involved in body's water balance, acid-base regulation, protein synthesis, muscle and heart action. Deficiencies likely with prolonged diarrhea, vomiting, kidney disease, frequent diuretic use, severe dieting (water loss may flush out potassium to levels low enough to endanger heart function). Excess may also impair heart function.	Bananas, milk, oranges, tomatoes, potatoes, spinach, broccoli, fruits, whole grains. RNI: not established. (250 ml/1 cup skim milk—428 mg; 1 medium orange—360 mg; ½ avocado—857 mg.)
Sodium (Na)	Regulates water balance, acid-base levels; involved in muscle action, skeletal structure and transport of materials such as glucose across cell walls. Deficiencies rare since most foods have ample amount. Imbalance upsets water retention; excess may raise blood pressure, increase cardiovascular risks.	Meat, eggs, cheese, ham, bacon, sausages, dried fish, nuts, butter, table salt, canned and processed foods, salty snacks, baking soda, antacids, bran. RNI: not established. (1 large egg—69 mg; 30 g cheddar cheese—186 mg; 250 ml/1 cup bran flakes—270 mg.)
Sulfur (S)	Found in almost all body cells, a component of many amino acids (used in protein building). Deficiencies rare.	Eggs, lean beef, lentils, kidney beans. RNI: not established.

Micro or Trace

Mineral	Function	Food Source and RNI
Chromium (Cr)	Vital to body's correct insulin use. Deficiencies may increase risk of diabetes.	Scarce in most foods – amounts depend on soil conditions; some in brewer's yeast, whole wheat. RNI: not established.
Cobalt (Co)	Crucial component of vitamin B_{12}; may be lacking in strict vegetarians; extreme lack can cause pernicious anemia.	Exclusively of animal origin—liver, clams, meat. RNI: not established.
Copper (Cu)	Crucial to blood formation, skeleton, nerve action, many enzymes (body catalysts). Deficiencies (rare) cause anemia, bone damage; excess may be linked to certain mental ailments.	Oysters, lobster, liver, bran, pecans, walnuts, bananas. RNI: not established. (85 g liver—2 mg; 250 ml/1 cup bran flakes—0.5 mg; 1 medium banana – 0.26 mg).
Fluoride (F)	Promotes resistance to tooth decay by hardening enamel. Shortage increases tooth decay; excess mottles teeth, causes bone abnormalities.	Seafood, seaweed, tea; best source is fluoridated water. RNI: not established, but 1 mg/l water (fluoridation) advised.
Iodine (I)	Crucial part of thyroid hormone, thyroxine, which regulates body metabolism. Insufficiency causes thyroid problems such as goiter (enlargement of thyroid), poor mental and physical growth.	Iodized salt, seafood, kelp, seaweed, dairy products near the sea. Content in plants varies according to soil conditions. RNI: Infants and children: 5 µg/100 Kcal/day; adolescents and adults: 160 µg/day; pregnancy and lactation: 25 µg extra/day.
Iron (Fe)	Central core of red blood-cell pigment, hemoglobin, which carries oxygen to tissues; vital part of some enzymes. Shortages common, especially in women—lack occurs after blood loss. Deficiencies cause fatigue, weakness, iron-deficiency anemia. Absorption by body requires enough dietary copper and is improved by vitamin C.	Liver, red meat, egg yolks, poultry, leafy green vegetables, raisins. RNI: Infants (0–12 mo): 1–7 mg/day; Children (1–11 years): 6–8 mg/day; Adolescents: males: 10 mg/day; females: 13 mg/day; Adults: males: 9 mg/day; females: 3 mg/day (8 mg/day after menopause) (85 g liver—8 mg; 85 g hamburger—2.9 mg; 40 g raisins—1.5 mg.)
Manganese (Mn)	Works with zinc in some metabolic actions, activates enzymes, vital to nerve transmission.	Raisins, tea, spinach, broccoli, peas. RNI: not established. (40 g raisins—201 µg; 125 ml/½ cup cooked broccoli – 119 µg.)
Molybdenum (Mo)	Body use unclear; possibly linked to enzyme function.	Legumes, whole grains, organ meats. RNI: not established.
Selenium (Se)	Function unclear; thought to help prevent heart and cardiovascular diseases.	Meat, egg yolks, seafood, wheat germ, milk. RNI: not established.
Zinc (Zn)	Contributes to insulin action, enzyme activity, carbohydrate metabolism, blood circulation, absorption of vitamin A, wound healing; key role in child growth. Deficiencies retard physical and mental growth, impair appetite, hinder learning.	Meat, oysters, liver, wheat germ, yeast, bran. RNI: Infants (0–4 mo): 2 mg/day; Children: increasing requirements with age; Adults: women: 9 mg; men: 12 mg; more after illness; pregnancy and lactation: 6 mg extra. (85 g liver—3.3 mg; 250 ml/1 cup bran flakes—1.3 mg.)

GOOD SOURCES OF IRON*

Meat, poultry and fish (mg)

Calf's liver (3 small slices, 95 g)	13.5
Chili con carne with beans	9.2
Beans with tomato sauce and pork	8.8
Hamburger (4 oz) with bun	6.3
Baked trout (1 serving, 93 g)	4.7
Spaghetti with meat balls and tomato sauce	3.9
Chicken pot pie (1 serving)	3.6
Dark turkey meat (86 g)	1.9
Lean roast beef (90 g)	3.1
Broiled steak, lean (88 g)	2.7

Cereals, fruit and vegetables

Cooked lentils (1 serving, 250 mL)	7.0
Fresh, boiled spinach	6.8
Whole wheat shredded wheat (200 mL)	5.9
Bran flakes with raisins (200 mL)	5.6
Raisins (1 cup)	3.6
Snow peas	3.3
3 licorice sticks (33 g)	2.6
1 bagel (medium, 9 cm diameter)	1.6
2 slices of whole wheat toast	1.6
1 slice cheese pizza (65 g)	1.4

* Portions equal 1 serving or 250 mL, unless otherwise stated.

Source: Health Canada. *Nutrient Value of Some Common Foods.*

A well-balanced, varied diet supplies enough minerals for most people, although pregnant or lactating women may need supplements prescribed by their physician. Minerals regulate intricate biochemical functions such as heart action, molecular transport across cell membranes, muscle activity, water balance, nerve conduction and immune defenses. If one or another is low or missing, the body's function may be impaired. For instance, a low calcium intake hinders bone formation, too little iron can lead to anemia, a lack of iodine is linked to thyroid problems and zinc deficiency slows wound healing and diminishes the sense of taste.

New guidelines boost calcium requirements

In order to build strong bones from an early age, and to offset the risk of osteoporosis and bone fractures later in life, the latest guidelines suggest higher calcium intakes at all ages. Calcium is crucial not only for bones and teeth, but also for nerve and muscle action and for regulating blood pressure. It plays a key role in transporting materials across cell membranes and for communication between and within body cells. A drop in blood calcium will trigger secretion of parathyroid hormone to mobilize calcium from the bones. Since calcium is lost in urine, feces, tears and sweat, the body must continually restore losses with calcium from food. If food

does not provide enough, the body will take what it needs from the bones. Low-fat dairy products are good sources of calcium, especially milk or yogurt (which contain about 300 mg calcium per cup).

Since maximum bone mass is laid down in adolescence, teenagers need about 1,300 calcium a day (obtainable from 3 to 4 servings of milk products) but many consume far less. Adults aged 19 to 50 need at least 1 gram (1,000 mg) calcium daily, and those over age 50 should consume at least 1,200 mg per day, either from food or supplements. Calcium needs rise during pregnancy and lactation to about 1,300 mg/day, but any lost from the bones during pregnancy and breast feeding is quickly and naturally made up after weaning.

The DRI panel set the ceiling for calcium intake at 2.5 g (2,500 mg) a day—taking into account mineral interactions and physiological effects. Intakes of calcium above that limit can impair health by interfering with iron absorption, disturbing bone remodeling and causing "milk alkali syndrome" (constipation and impaired kidney function).

Making sure you get enough iron

It's easy to forget that iron deficiency and anemia are still widespread problems. Infants, children and women are at particular risk for iron deficiency and anemia. Young children are often low in iron—as many as 10 percent of 18-month-old children in North America from low-income families are iron-deficient. About 25 percent of adolescents and young women have a low iron status and are at risk of iron-deficiency anemia. Those with low iron stores may need supplements. (See also Chapter 16.)

Different amounts of iron are absorbed from different foods. Although we tend to link spinach with iron, the mineral is poorly absorbed from most vegetables. In general, "heme" iron from animal products is better absorbed than "non-heme" or inorganic iron in plant foods. But the *mix of foods* eaten is a crucial influence—the presence of other foods that enhance or reduce iron absorption. For example, vitamin C increases the amount of iron that can be absorbed from plant foods. The inclusion of vegetables or fruits rich in vitamin C at a vegetarian meal may double iron absorption. The presence of "heme" iron from animal foods also enhances absorption. Eating a little meat, fish, liver or poultry with vegetarian foods can raise iron absorption.

Conversely, certain compounds such as *tannin* (in tea) reduce the "bioavailability" of iron. Other iron-inhibitors include *phytates* (found in unprocessed whole grain cereals and bran) and certain spices (such as oregano). Calcium also blocks iron absorption. As little as one glass of milk (about 165 mg of calcium) halves iron absorption, so many experts suggest people taking calcium supplements avoid taking them at the same time as an iron-rich meal, and not when taking an iron supplement.

Tips for getting more iron in your diet

- Eat a little meat, fish or poultry several times a week, but choose low-fat forms.
- Have some citrus fruit or juice with your breakfast cereal.
- Drink tea *between* rather than with or right after a meal.
- When eating vegetables or cereals high in iron, include foods rich in ascorbic acid.
- If you are a vegetarian, include ascorbic acid (vitamin C) sources such as citrus fruits, green peppers or cabbage at most meals.
- Take calcium supplements not with but between iron-rich meals.
- Don't sprinkle raw wheat bran on foods, as it reduces iron absorption.
- Keep iron tablets well away from children who may mistake it for candy with dire consequences.

WATER IS ALSO AN ESSENTIAL DIETARY COMPONENT

Rarely listed among required nutrients, water is the most vital substance to life. While human beings can survive prolonged fasts without any food, several days without water usually means death. We can tolerate a loss of half our fat or protein reserves, but even a 10-percent depletion in body fluid is serious, and a 20-percent loss can be fatal. An average adult needs about 2–2.8 liters (2.8–3 quarts) of water a day, including amounts ingested from food. Many vegetables and some fruits are 80 percent or more water; milk has 87 percent and beef 55 percent water.

Although you may consider yourself a "solid person," the human body is mostly water. Newborn babies are 75 to 85 percent water, women are 55 to 65 percent water and men 65 to 75 percent. The sex difference is due to a higher proportion of fat in a woman's body; fat holds less water than lean muscle. If the body is dehydrated, the kidneys will cut back on water lost through urine, and the urine will become dark and concentrated.

Water carries nutrients and waste products to and from the body organs through the bloodstream and lymphatic system. It lubricates the joints and mucous membranes and is the solvent in which nutrients are carried, digested and absorbed. Without water, the body couldn't get rid of toxic wastes through urine and feces. Nor could it cool itself. Water regulates body temperature through sweat; the reason obese people have a harder time cooling off is because fat under the skin acts as an insulator.

Water from food and drink is released inside the body by the metabolic breakdown of proteins, carbohydrates and fats. Babies need proportionately more water than adults, and should be offered bottles of water between feedings in hot weather. Drinks containing concentrated nutrients, such as milk, sugar-sweetened soft drinks and salty tomato-based juices, count more as food than as drink since they increase the body's water needs. Contrary to widespread belief (especially among weight-conscious women), drinking water does *not* cause bloating or weight gain.

In hot weather or during workouts the amount of water lost through sweat can rise dramatically. Exercisers may lose up to two or more liters (over two quarts) of body water in one hour of vigorous exercise, resulting in extreme thirst, giddiness and a possibly dangerous rise in core body temperature. The water loss may seriously decrease the circulating blood volume and endanger the heart. That's why it's essential to drink lots of water in hot weather and during and after prolonged activity. Sports medicine specialists urge athletes to "force liquids" in the summer heat, advising them to tank up with water before as well as during and after vigorous activity.

Although some people claim warm liquids cool you faster because they increase perspiration, that's no help on humid days. Exercisers should avoid sweet drinks, because sugar slows the absorption of water into the blood and draws water from the body tissues, where they really need it. Beverages containing caffeine or alcohol are not recommended to replenish body water because they're diuretics which increase water loss. Electrolyte drinks are not advised unless people lose more than 2.8 liters (three quarts) of water (2.5 kg, or 6 lb of weight) during prolonged activity such as marathons.

Water intoxication a possible but rare event

Compulsive or excess water drinking has been recorded for people with certain psychiatric disorders. It has also been reported in those about to be subjected to urine drug tests in the workplace (aviation industry) or after athletic events—in an effort to dilute the urine and avoid detection. Water toxicity can occur if someone rapidly drinks a large amount of water in a few minutes or has impaired renal function where the kidney can't excrete fluid fast enough. In one recently recorded case a worker told to have a urine drug test drank a great deal and exhibited clear signs of water intoxication: confusion, slurred speech, unsteady gait, a rapid pulse and seizures due to severely diluted blood plasma and a consequently disturbed sodium balance. The excess water and diluted circulation to the brain results in cerebral dysfunction and mental confusion. A 40-year-old flight attendant who exhibited typical water toxicity was reported in California. Her body retained excess water after she was told to "drink several cups of water" for a random urine test ordered by the U.S. aviation board. Anxious and stressed in the crowded room and fearing a laboratory error she just couldn't urinate despite the consumption of three liters (over three quarts) of tap water in two hours. She couldn't void and was sent home, later becoming dizzy and confused, with a severe headache and suffering a seizure.

Hyponatremia or low blood and body sodium levels may follow excess fluid ingestion. This is seen in some compulsive water drinkers—mainly psychiatric cases—who may suffer seizures and be put on drugs for years without the reason for their excess water malady being uncovered.

For further information on nutrition the following three booklets can be obtained from Health and Welfare Canada:
- *Nutrition Recommendations, The Report of the Scientific Review Committee*, 1990 ($18.95, available by mail from Canadian Government Publishing Centre, Supply and Services Canada, Ottawa, Ont. K1A 0S9);
- *Call For Action* (summary of SRC and CIC reports), 1990 (available by mail from Branch Publications Unit, Health Services and Promotion Branch, Health and Welfare Canada, 5th Floor, Jeanne Mance Bldg., Ottawa, Ont. K1A 1B4).
- *National Institute of Nutrition* (Ottawa) (613) 235-3355; website: www.hc.sc.gc.ca, or www.min:ca.
- Call the U.S. Institute of Medicine at 1-800-624-6242 for information on the new DRI guidelines; website www.nep.edu

Looking after the surface

Caring for your skin • Remedying dry skin problems • Help for the anguish of acne • Psoriasis control • Shingles is a pain • Help for aging skin • Avoid skin's number-one enemy • Protect yourself against skin cancers • Hair, beautiful hair • Choose hair-care products wisely • Getting rid of lice • Hand and nail care • Foot care • Banishing warts

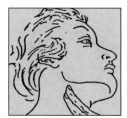

CARING FOR YOUR SKIN

Pride in one's appearance starts with the skin, the body's largest, most visible organ. The skin's appearance portrays a social and sexual image to the outside world, and humans generally lavish more care on the skin of the face and neck (and perhaps also the arms and legs, in women) than on other parts of the body. Anyone who's had an unsightly pimple on the nose or chin on the night of a prom or heavy date knows how acutely embarrassing even a small facial blemish can be. By comparison, most of us pay scant attention to the skin on parts of the body not usually displayed in public. However, far from being mere vanity, looking after the body's wrapping also improves its health.

Keeping skin clean is a good start
Skin that looks, feels and smells attractive enhances self-esteem, hence the millions spent each year on cosmetics. But steering a sensible course through the countless skin products is no easy matter. One young woman recently complained that she couldn't decide on the "right way" to clean her skin, or between the merits of soaps versus cleansing creams, because everyone offered different advice. Her esthetician warned her never to touch her face with soap, but to clean it with cleansing lotion and astringents and to apply special day and night creams, especially under the eyes. Her dermatologist told her the opposite: to wash her face with mild soap and warm water, to use creams sparingly on her oily skin and not to lather on anything under the eyes. (Eye creams can cause puffiness if left on overnight; if used at all, they're best applied for 10 minutes or so and then wiped off.) Most dermatologists consider expensive cleansing creams hardly worth the cost. Cheaper ones, or even plain mineral oil, do an equally good job for those who are not prone to acne.

Each stage of life requires a slightly different skin-cleaning routine. During childhood, adolescence and young adulthood, most dermatologists suggest washing with gentle soap and warm water—not hot or cold—and rinsing well to remove the soap. (Hot water isn't advised because it's very drying.) In young infants and the elderly, who have extra-sensitive skins, soaps should be used sparingly and washing should be less frequent. Overwashing makes the skin dry and flaky.

The right skin cleanser also depends on the skin type. One evaluation found that cleansing creams were not necessarily less drying than soaps. Any soap is fine unless you have dry skin, in which case mild, superfatted types (such as Neutrogena, Dove, Caress, Petro-phylic, Allenbury's and Lowila) are best. One University of Toronto dermatologist recommends "avoiding deodorant and antiseptic soaps unless a physician prescribes them."

5

STRUCTURE OF THE SKIN

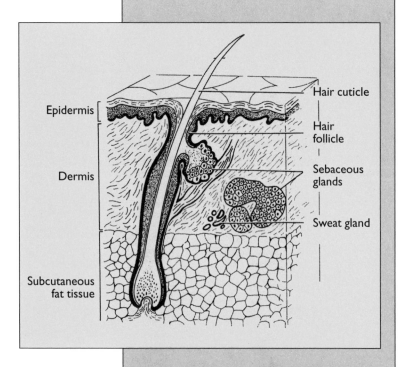

The skin basically has two layers: an outer epidermis, and an inner layer or dermis which includes the hypodermis. Men generally have thicker skins than women, but as people age the skin of bath sexes becomes thinner and more fragile.

The top stratum corneum ("horny layer") of the epidermis is composed of flat, colorless cells, arranged like overlapping roof shingles, that are constantly shed and replaced by fresh cells. Anyone who has acquired a tan knows how quickly it fades as the outer epidermal layer is replaced by new cells. The epidermis is coated with an oily liquid called sebum, which gives skin its suppleness, smoothness and sheen, and helps to retain moisture. The skin's color is produced by pigment-forming cells (melanocytes) in the epidermis that produce a pigment (melanin) that protects it from sun damage by deepening its hue.

The underlying layer or dermis, is largely composed of connective tissue, made up of collagen and elastin fibers which give skin its elasticity and firmness. The dermis contains blood vessels, which supply nutrients, as well as nerves, hair roots and nail roots, and three types of glands: the sebaceous oil glands, eccrine sweat glands and apocrine scent glands. The sebaceous glands produce sebum. Excess sebum production can backfire, causing greasy hair and plugged oil ducts, possibly contributing to acne. The amount of oil produced by the sebaceous glands determines whether a person has dry skin (underactive sebaceous glands), oily skin (overactive sebaceous glands) or normal skin (sebaceous glands working just right).

Astringents containing alcohol may be useful for the oily-skinned but will further dehydrate dry skin. If used at all, astringents should be dabbed on lightly with cotton balls (not paper tissue, as it irritates the skin). Despite claims that various astringents "close the skin's pores," none fulfills this promise.

Many dermatologists suggest replacing tub baths with showers, as showers are less drying and more hygienic. The constant stream of clean water removes dirt and bacteria more efficiently. However as a relaxant after a hard day or to soothe aching muscles, a warm (not hot and drying) bath can do wonders. A pumice stone can be used while showering or bathing to remove tough, dead skin from the soles of the feet and elbows, but rub gently to avoid harming the skin. Bubble baths and bath oils should be used sparingly. Bubble baths may appear harmless but can trigger skin irritation and may provoke urinary-tract infections in children (especially girls). While bath oils may soothe dry, itchy skin, they also make the tub slippery and increase the risk of falling. It is safer to apply creams or oils directly to damp skin after showering than to add them to the bathwater. Always use a non-slip mat in the tub, and add hand-rails to the tub or shower enclosure for seniors.

REMEDYING DRY SKIN PROBLEMS

Turning up the thermostat alleviates winter's chill, but also dries out the indoor air making us susceptible to dry, itchy skin. This irritating problem starts off as a tight, dry feeling, but can lead to cracked, chapped, inflamed and oozing skin, known as eczema or dermatitis. The commonest causes of dry skin are centrally heated homes and workplaces, lack of room moisture, cold, dry air and too much bathing or showering. The best antidotes are to humidify the indoor surroundings well and, as one dermatologist puts it, "to moisturize, moisturize, moisturize," to trap water in the skin's surface. The application of a simple moisturizer should take place right after bathing.

John, a radio technician who lived in a small, stuffy apartment, proves the point. He rarely opened the windows and his "sealed" office was overheated. He habitually took two daily showers—one every morning, the other after his evening workout. Every year come November he'd become very itchy, particularly on his shoulders and arms, sometimes scratching until he drew blood. Finally a colleague persuaded him to see a specialist. The dermatologist took a careful history to determine whether there were any chemical irritants at work—there were none, except perhaps the photocopier fluids—and then told him to buy a humidifier for the apartment, to shower only once daily, to wash with mild, superfatted soap and to apply moisturizer to his damp skin right after showering. The dermatologist also prescribed a menthol/camphor lotion for the itchy areas. The itch soon vanished, and John keeps it at bay by repeating the same treatment when needed. Anyone with scaling, itchy skin that doesn't respond to moisturizers should seek medical advice.

While the combination of oil and sweat normally keeps human skin soft and supple, various factors—such as lack of humidity or overexposure to water, sun, chemicals and soaps—can dehydrate it. If the skin loses water more rapidly than the deeper cells can replenish it, the upper layer dries out. Dry skin may also be linked to dermatitis (skin inflammation and irritation) or allergies and skin diseases. Characteristically, dry skin ("xerosis") starts out as small, whitish scales, possibly with some reddening and cracking. Many sufferers complain that their faces feel taut to the point of cracking. Although scratching may momentarily alleviate the irritation, the friction can lead to further breakdown and infection. Although considered useful for muscle strain and arthritis, the increasing use of hot tubs can play havoc with your skin. The combination of very hot water and multiple chemicals can lead not only to dry skin, but may also produce allergic reactions (to chemicals in the water) and folliculitis (infection of the skin).

Untreated dry skin can develop into eczema, with soreness, inflammation, and perhaps bleeding and swollen, oozing, crusty patches. Dermatologists often use the terms "dermatitis" and "eczema" interchangeably to denote badly inflamed, scaling, weepy skin. Once eczema is entrenched, it's difficult to reverse except with topical steroids such as hydrocortisone creams.

Skin itchiness can arise from innumerable causes

In tracing the causes of skin itching, physicians consider not only winter's cold and indoor dryness but allergic or drug reactions, cosmetic acne (triggered by commercial skin products), contact and noncontact dermatitis, exposure to poison ivy or other plants, insect bites and the effect of chemical irritants, as well as certain skin diseases such as psoriasis.

Contact dermatitis is an inflammatory skin irritation, sometimes due to an allergy or to direct contact with specific substances. The irritation produces inflamed, itching, red patches, and perhaps oozing blisters—especially on prolonged exposure. Typical cases are a long-time bricklayer who suddenly developed sensitivity to the chrome in cement at age 50 and had to give up his job and take early retirement, and a hairdresser whose skin was suddenly irritated by the hair products she used on clients, forcing her into a career change. Strong irritants such as acid can blister the skin within minutes or hours; weaker irritants such as soaps or cosmetics may take some weeks to cause the dermatitis.

The skin on some parts of the body is more likely to develop dermatitis than others. The eyelids in particular are more prone to contact dermatitis than thicker-skinned areas such as the scalp, soles and palms. If the rash spreads rapidly to areas of skin not originally in contact with the irritant, it can take time to track down the causative agent. It helps if people remember the area of skin first involved as a pointer to the substance(s) causing the reaction. Sometimes the irritated patch has clear margins. It isn't always easy to distinguish allergic from other dermatitis.

A long list of substances can provoke contact dermatitis, including dyes, metals (such as mercury or nickel, in jewelry), rubber, topical medicines (such as neomycin or streptomycin creams), commercial fabric finishes, laundry products, shoe leather, perfumes, shampoos, makeup, some local anesthetics, sulfas and tars. Cosmetic ingredients, such as PPD (paraphenylenediamine) in hair dyes, preservatives (in creams), local anesthetics and lanolin, often cause dermatitis and should be avoided by those sensitive to them. Occupational dermatitis is common among hairdressers, shrimp-peelers, furniture-makers, bakers and many others daily exposed to irritating chemicals.

Ear-piercing is an often unsuspected cause of contact dermatitis, in which the itching arises due to nickel used to harden the earring metal. (Gold or stainless steel earrings usually avoid the problem.) Once the nickel allergy is entrenched, any jewelry containing nickel will irritate the skin.

For self-treatment of mild dermatitis, a 0.5 percent hydrocortisone topical ointment, cream or lotion—now available without prescription— can relieve the itching, redness and scaling. But if symptoms persist or worsen after five to seven days, a doctor should be consulted. In that case stronger cortisone preparations or oral products may be prescribed, after the cause of the dermatitis has been established and eliminated.

Atopic dermatitis, or skin itchiness is often linked to inherited allergies, but almost anything can trigger it rapid changes in temperature, sweating, wool, polyester or nylon clothing, heavy and greasy ointments, soaps, detergents and emotional stress. In infants and children, atopic dermatitis may begin on the cheeks a few months after birth and spread to the elbows and knees, possibly provoked by crawling. During childhood, the dermatitis often moves to the creases of the arms and legs, possibly also the neck, scalp, wrists and ankles. Atopic dermatitis can be aggravated by foods given in infancy, such as eggs, milk, wheat and citrus fruits, but after two years of age, foods no longer seem to play a dominant role. The condition often clears up in adolescence, although it may continue into young adulthood. Kids and adults who have a personal or family history of asthma are more prone to this kind of dermatitis. Think of your lungs or your skin as a "filter system" between you and your environment; asthma or atopic dermatitis results from an overwhelmed filtering system that starts to swell or overreact.

Hives, or *urticaria* with large red patches and severe skin itchiness, can result from allergies and numerous triggers that release histamines in the body, such as drugs, chemicals, foods, inhalants, fungi, bacteria, insect stings, dust, feathers, molds, fumes, pollens, metals, heat, cold and light. The reddened, swollen skin blotches are usually evanescent—they last only a short time in the same place—but they may occur elsewhere the next day. Occasionally hives persist a month or more, a condition known as "chronic urticaria," but fortunately they too eventually burn out. Occasionally internal disorders such as thyroid disease, cancer or ulcerative colitis cause hives. Emotional stress can aggravate hives, although stress is often unfairly blamed. For instance, one dermatologist describes a woman who always broke out in itchy hives at her mother-in-law's house and attributed it to their tense relationship. The dermatologist later discovered that the parents-in-law had feather pillows that triggered the skin problem; after her in-laws changed to foam pillows, the woman no longer got hives when she visited them. Treatment of hives means avoiding the triggers or allergy-provoking substances to prevent the histamine release. Antihistamines and anti-inflammatory creams may help once the condition arises.

Impetigo is a highly contagious skin infection due to staphylococcal or streptococcal bacteria that enter the skin through small scratches. Usually seen in infants and young children, it typically starts off as small red, itchy macula (spots) that turn into blisters that soon rupture and develop thin yellow or golden, oozy crusts. Left untreated, the sores may last for weeks, can be passed on to others and may occasionally lead to complications such as rheumatic fever and kidney disease in children. However impetigo is usually easily managed (once the causative bacteria are pinpointed) by gently removing the crusts, washing well with an antibacterial soap, applying topical antibacterials and giving antibiotic tablets. For more widespread cases, oral antibiotics are often indicated. Parents looking after children with impetigo should take precautions to avoid catching or passing on the infection—by washing the hands after touching the child and making sure each family member has a separate towel. (For impetigo in children, see Chapter 11.)

Choose moisturizing skin products wisely

A cream or moisturizer's price and scientific-sounding ingredients are no guarantee of effectiveness. For good moisturizing ability, there's really no need to get any fancier than plain old petrolatum or petroleum jelly. But petroleum jelly is sticky, which makes other face products seem more appealing. However any cream or oil that holds moisture in the skin will do. Inexpensive products such as cocoa butter mineral oil and lanolin are as effective as expensive creams (although lanolin may cause allergies in some). One dermatologist calls the choice simple: "Never pay for the name." She adds, "Beware of the cosmetic claims! The right cream or moisturizer is a matter of cost and personal preference."

Whatever their price, moisturizers, hand and body creams, face, eye and night creams all work by trapping water and providing a protective layer on top of the skin. All are basically oil and water mixtures, with emulsifiers added to keep them well mixed, and sometimes perfumed as well. They coat the skin with oil and block evaporation of the moisture. While they can't cure dry skin, moisturizers provide protection, relieve the dry, itchy feeling and reduce the tendency to crack. Although most of the water in the cream or moisturizer evaporates, the oil stays on as a lubricant making the skin more pliable.

Despite their various forms—ointments, creams, lotions, foams, gels and oils—all moisturizers contain roughly similar ingredients: occlusives (which block the evaporation of water), humectants (which attract water) and emollients (oils such as mineral oil) that smooth the skin by filling in the spaces between dry skin flakes. The thickness of moisturizing creams varies according to their oil-water ratio. The thicker the product, the more oil it contains; the thinner the cream, the more water it contains. "Vanishing" or day creams have more water than night creams. The heavier or greasier it is, the greater the cream's lubricating qualities.

As a rule, the drier the skin, the thicker the cream to use. For dry or sensitive skins, choose any affordable moisturizer that is rich in oil. One inexpensive way to moisturize is simply to soak the skin in warm water for a few minutes, pat off the excess and apply any oil or cream of choice to the damp skin. As mentioned above, light mineral oil, cocoa butter and petroleum jelly are just as effective as costly commercial products, and because they contain no perfume or preservatives they are unlikely to irritate the skin or cause allergies. However, many dislike the texture of these plain, simple products.

Watching for allergic reactions to skincare products

Face creams rarely cause allergic reactions, but certain ingredients can act as irritants or provoke allergies, particularly perfumes, preservatives, salicylic acid, resorcinol, oxidizing agents and lanolin. Sometimes this happens because products are used on parts of the body for which they were not intended. A body cream suitable for the arms or legs may induce puffiness if used under the eyes. Skin-bleaching creams are among those most likely to cause allergic reactions. They should not be used by dark-skinned people except with medical supervision, as they often cause an inflammatory reaction and permanently lighter skin patches.

Hair products may cause skin allergies, especially those containing paraphenylene diamine or thioglycolates. Hair-removers containing barium or calcium sulphide or calcium thioglycolate can also cause allergic skin reactions. Nail polish can produce not only nail splintering and yellowing, but also allergic reactions if it touches the skin. A trace of nail polish on the eyelids can make them red and swollen, yet many of those with an allergic eyelid reaction don't realize that nail polish was to blame.

Deodorants and antiperspirants

Perspiration from the eccrine glands helps to regulate the body's temperature and cool it down after exercise or during a fever by evaporation from the skin's surface. But if accumulated sweat stays on the skin for a few hours, especially in the body folds or on clothing, a strong body odor develops. The bacterial breakdown of sweat in the underarm or groin areas causes the most offensive odors. To counteract the smell, modern folk tend to use deodorants. Although deodorants decrease body odor they don't reduce sweating, so many people prefer products containing both a deodorant and an antiperspirant. (Shaving off underarm hair also decreases the odor.)

The earliest deodorants were merely perfumes used to mask body odor and were introduced by the high priests of ancient civilizations as part of their religious rituals. Only in the twentieth century did scientists discover that the bacterial breakdown of sweat is mainly to

TIPS FOR PREVENTING SKIN DRYNESS AND WINTER ITCH

- Keep room temperature low but comfortable— not overheated.
- Humidify indoor air as much as possible (clean humidifiers to avoid contamination by molds).
- Keep skin clean and well moisturized.
- Use warm water for washing—not too hot or cold.
- Favour a mild soap or soap substitute, such as Dove, Petro-phylic or Neutrogena.
- Limit use of soap, detergents and solvents in wintertime.
- Favor showers and sponge baths—they are less drying than sitting in a tub of water.
- Apply moisturizers to damp skin.
- Use moisturizers recommended by University of Toronto experts, including white petroleum jelly, Dormer 211 baby oils, Nivea products, Moisturel and any personally chosen lubricants that work!
- Avoid too much friction from harsh washcloths and abrasives.
- Use lotions containing menthol, camphor or lactic acid for itchy areas, provided there's no cracking or inflammation (as it may sting); apply lotions to moist skin.
- For skin that is inflamed, red, cracked and scaling use a steroid anti-inflammatory cream or lotion such as hydrocortisone—but only with a doctor's advice and for about six weeks. Seek medical advice if skin problem persists.
- Soothe dry, itchy skin with cool compresses using Burow's solution (diluted one in 20) or Epsom salts in water—but use no menthol/camphor anti-itch products until cracks are well healed.
- Try oatmeal baths to soothe mildly inflamed skin. Place 60 ml (4 tbsp) of oatmeal in a sock and run the bathwater through.
- Try short-acting oral antihistamines (such as hydroxyzine) to relieve skin itching.

- Wear soft natural fabrics (jersey cotton, silk) next to the skin and avoid wool, nylon and polyester.
- Beware of pure lanolin skincare products, which cause allergic reactions in a few.
- Don't use paper tissues to apply oils or astringents or to remove makeup, as they are made from wood pulp and can irritate the skin: instead, use cotton balls (stored in a container to avoid contamination).
- Wear protective, cotton-lined rubber gloves when immersing hands in water or doing household tasks, and wear gloves in cold weather.
- To avoid chapped, sore lips, especially in children, apply roll-on lip balm or plain petroleum jelly (Vaseline); tell children not to lick their lips too often, and protect them from the cold.
- For severely dry, flaky scalp or dandruff (which can be fungal, due to *P. ovale* infection), try tar shampoos or get a doctor's prescription for Nizoral (ketoconazole 2 percent) or some other shampoo that reduces flakiness.
- Remove face makeup with cleansing cream or lotion (depending on skin type) or wash with mild soap and warm water; pat dry.
- Remove oil-based eye makeup with gentle oils or remover pads, and remove water-based products with water; wipe away from the eyes.
- Wash hairbrush, comb and makeup brushes at least once a week to prevent bacterial contamination.
- Always close cosmetic containers when not in use, to minimize the entry of bacteria.
- Discard old, dry, caked or rancid makeup.
- When engaging in outdoor winter activities, remember to protect the face from cold injury; cover the ears, head and neck; be alert for signs of frostbite; apply a protective face cream and a wide-spectrum sunscreen.

blame for body odor. Today's deodorants come as antibacterial or antiseptic-containing soaps (e.g., Dial, Irish Spring), roll-ons, sprays, sticks and creams. The antibacterial agents used in deodorants include: benzalkonium chloride, hexachlorophene and salicylanilides. Some of these can cause photosensitization, an exaggerated inflammatory response to sun exposure. One safe, inexpensive deodorant recommended by a University of Toronto der-

matologist is Aqueous Zephiran, or benzalkonium chloride, which is a clear colorless, odorless liquid, easily applied with cotton balls.

Products labeled as antiperspirants must reduce normal sweating by at least 20 percent. Many contain metals, particularly aluminum, but experts suggest avoiding aluminum-containing antiperspirants for fear of adverse health effects. Some antiperspirants may also block the sweat glands and cause an irritation or rash.

Antiperspirants containing perfumes, hexa-chlorophene and zirconium can also irritate the skin. (Those containing zirconium should be avoided because a few people develop small lumps, or granulomas, in their armpits from zirconium products.) Do not put antiperspirants on inflamed, wet or recently shaved skin as they may irritate it.

HELP FOR THE ANGUISH OF ACNE

Acne affects many teenagers, and in severe cases leaves permanent, disfiguring scars. Although it's regarded primarily as an affliction of youth, many people continue to have acne into their thirties and forties. Acne is present in over 80 percent of adolescents, 12 percent of women and 3 percent of men aged 25–44. It develops earlier in girls than boys but affects boys more frequently and more severely. Acne should be treated as soon as it strikes, before it

scars the skin and diminishes self-esteem. Improvement can be dramatic with modern therapies. Most people can manage their acne perfectly well once they know what to do.

Basically, acne involves a skin structure, the pilosebaceous follicle or unit, which contains tiny hair remnants, and a sebaceous gland that secretes the oily substance known as sebum. Acne varies from mild (grade one) occasional pimples to severe or cystic (grade four) eruptions. Symptoms range from a few hardly noticeable blackheads (comedones) and the occasional whitehead (pimple) to extensive, pus-filled, scarring cysts that cover the face and extend to the chest, arms and back.

Acne begins with a tiny plug (the comedo) in the sebaceous gland made of excess sebum, dead cells and keratin (a hard, tough protein). If the plug opens to the surface and darkens, it is an "open comedo" or blackhead, caused by accumulated oil and melanin pigment (not dirt).

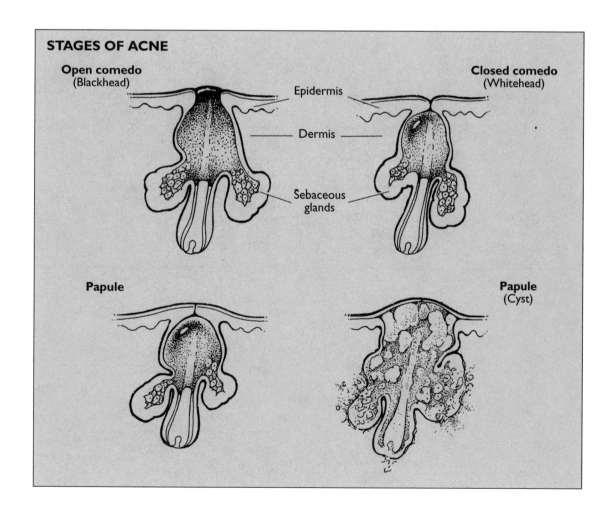

STAGES OF ACNE

Open comedo (Blackhead)   **Closed comedo** (Whitehead)

Epidermis

Dermis

Sebaceous glands

Papule   **Papule** (Cyst)

ACNE TREATMENTS

Note: the acne treatments described below prevent the next "crop" of acne and typically take at least 4 weeks to work.

For mild acne:
• clean the skin well to keep down oil, dirt and bacteria. Do not irritate the skin;
• wash with soap and water, and dry well;
• try to avoid stress and excess tension (acne aggravators);
• do not squeeze or pick pimples;
• shampoo the hair frequently—once a day—and keep the hair off the face;
• change washcloth, pillowcase and shirt frequently;
• drink plenty of water;
• don't use moisturizers, creams or oily cosmetics;
• apply topical tretinoin 0.01–0.05% gel (vitamin-A acid cream or Retin-A creams) if prescribed by the doctor;
• special cleansers and peeling lotions (containing salicylic acid) may be advised;
• 2.5–20% benzoyl peroxide gel (Panoxyl, Benzac) can help mild acne;
• acne medications applied to the skin are drying and can irritate if used too much, so use them cautiously.

Further steps for papulo-pustular (grade two) acne:
• use benzoyl peroxide alternated with topical clindamycin or erythromycin (local antibiotics);
• possibly try oral or topical antibiotics (medically prescribed);
• wear hair off the face, wash hair daily, drink plenty of water, avoid stress and get enough sleep.

Further steps for nodulo-cystic (grade three and four) acne:
• use oral antibiotics (e.g., tetracycline); if they fail, consider oral Accutane or an injection of triamcinolone (steroid);

• if using oral antibiotics, be sure to take the full dose (at least six to eight weeks) before changing treatment, watch for side effects (e.g., sun sensitivity if taking tetracycline);
• topical tretinoin in a cream or lotion can dramatically alleviate acne, either alone or in combination with other treatments. It corrects the processes that plug up the sebaceous gland channels, altering the cycle that forms blackheads and whiteheads. Tretinoin comes in three strengths: the gel, the most drying form, is for people with very oily skin; the lotion is less drying, and the cream dries the skin the least. Other than being expensive, causing some initial local redness and increasing sun (UV) sensitivity, it is a relatively innocuous remedy. Later it may be used alternately with other acne treatments (e.g., benzoyl peroxide). Topical retinoid therapy requires close supervision by a physician;
• oral anti-acne retinoids like Accutane (also called 13-cis-retinoic acid, or isotretinoin), taken by mouth as capsules, can relieve severe or cystic acne, which doesn't respond to conventional treatment. As opposed to the years often required for antibiotic treatment, a short four- to five-month course of Accutane often clears up acne, sometimes for long periods, even forever. But although considered a "breakthrough" for severe acne, this drug has some potentially serious side effects—especially the risk of birth defects and elevated blood cholesterol levels. Its use in women of childbearing age *must* be accompanied by effective birth control. It can also cause initial skin-chapping, dry lips, palms and soles, eye problems, headaches, joint pains and blood disorders. So Accutane must be taken with care under steady medical supervision and many doctors require monthly pregnancy tests.

With progression to grades two and three acne, the follicles become swollen with trapped sebum, cells and bacteria, producing an inflamed red bump—the familiar acne pimple, pustule or papule. Deeper rupture of a follicle may produce the painful cysts and abscesses that typify grade-four acne, with the risk of permanent scars.

The newly developed anti-acne products tretinoin (vitamin-A acid cream) and oral 13-cis-retinoic acid (Accutane), now approved in Canada, have helped countless young people who suffer from this emotionally devastating affliction.

PSORIASIS CONTROL

Psoriasis, a common skin disorder that afflicts 1 to 3 percent of our population—an incidence similar to diabetes—ranges from mild to severe and is usually worst in winter. The two peak ages of onset are the late teens to early twenties and the late fifties to early sixties. The natural history

TIPS FOR CONTROLLING PSORIASIS

- good skincare—patting instead of rubbing skin dry, trying not to scratch or irritate the psoriatic patches;
- basic hand care—washing only when necessary; drying well; using medicated creams on red, scaly areas (but not leaving them on too long);
- wearing cotton-lined rubber gloves when doing laundry or dishes; avoiding activities such as pottery, sanding and furniture-polishing, which involve contact with irritants; delegating jobs that chafe psoriatic areas to others;
- caring well for psoriatic feet, keeping the feet clean and dry to prevent bacterial or fungal growth, wearing cotton socks and well-fitting or open shoes or sandals whenever possible;
- good scalp care—avoiding injury or scratches; special shampoos and topical creams may help;
- regularly using lubricants such as hand lotion or white petroleum jelly to stop the skin from scaling. For hand psoriasis, many people like to wear light plastic gloves to bed to help seal in the lotion or steroid cream;
- medicated ointments such as salicylic acid, steroid (cortisone) and tar products can be very effective;
- crude coal tar and its derivatives, an old standby for psoriasis control, often alleviates psoriasis, especially in combination with UV light therapy;
- anthralin (an alternative to tar) can be applied to affected skin for several hours at a time, but can be hard to manage, because it harms normal skin. An alternative is short-contact anthralin treatment, using a higher dose on affected spots for 5 to 15 minutes only;
- steroid creams or intralesional steroid injections help mild cases with small areas of psoriasis (cover with Saran Wrap to increase steroid absorption). Steroid skin products come in different strengths and ointments are more powerful than creams. Usually patients rotate their use of steroids with other medications to help prevent long-term side-effects and maximize the effectiveness of the medications. In general, medium-strength corticosteroids are used on the torso and extremities and low-potency drugs on the face, genitals and flexural areas;
- the vitamin D analogue calcipotriene, also called calcipotriol (Dovonex), has recently been show as quite helpful in combatting psoriasis;
- ultraviolet light, an old and simple remedy, slows down the skin's over-rapid proliferation. But psoriatics should only expose themselves to sunlight until the skin reddens very slightly, avoiding sunburn, since it will stimulate rather than curb skin growth;
- cyclosporine is proving useful for very recalcitrant psoriasis, but needs care because of possible kidney damage;
- sulfasalazine, an inexpensive drug with few side effects, is considered for oral therapy in some patients;
- capsaicin is a natural chemical derived from hot pepper plants; when used topically as 0.025% cream (Zostrix), it moderates the itching often associated with psoriasis within four to six weeks. The main side effect is burning and stinging, which diminishes with continued use;
- "PUVA" therapy (psoralen pills plus UVA rays) is a new treatment that's had dramatic success (without messy creams or potentially hazardous medications) for severe psoriatics. Psoralen is a plant extract that increases skin pigmentation. Taken orally two hours before UV exposure, psoralen penetrates the skin and is activated by UVA rays. PUVA needs careful supervision, especially shielding of the eyes with special glasses that screen Out the UV rays. Only about 3 to 5 percent of those treated by PUVA fail to respond; side effects include accelerated skin aging and a possibly increased susceptibility to skin cancer. However, the incidence of skin cancer (30 in 1,373) is still low enough to be considered a tolerable risk for patients with disabling psoriasis who don't do well on other treatments;
- "Retinoids" such as tazarotene (Tazorac) or etretinate (Tegison) can be a great help for severe psoriasis, often bringing improvement within days to weeks. Some people require longer use to keep symptoms at bay. But it cannot be used in women of childbearing age because of its fetal-deforming side effects. Side effects include: lip chapping; dry nose, eyes and mouth; joint soreness; a possible rise in blood fats (needs monitoring); and altered liver function. These side effects may fade after a few weeks of therapy and vanish once the treatment stops.
- New biological agents that show promise include etanercept, infliximab, alefacept and efalizumab. They are expensive, but especially effective for "plaque" psoriasis.

is one of exacerbations and remissions. Although its causes remain elusive (it has an immune-system component), new treatments can keep most psoriasis under control. Untreated psoriasis can produce disfiguring, scaling skin patches. Neither an allergy nor an infection, and not contagious, its psychological impact can be devastating. It is responsible for much personal distress, embarrassment and lost work hours. Sufferers try to hide their affliction by avoiding summer clothes and social events or refusing to go out in public. Children may find that other schoolmates refuse to hold hands, swim, attend gym classes or play with them because of the blemishes. Getting appropriate therapy and sharing the heartache of a chronic disease that's part of their lives helps sufferers come to terms with psoriasis.

Psoriasis varies widely in severity

Known since biblical times, psoriasis tends to run in families and hits people of both sexes, and all

FACTORS THAT AGGRAVATE PSORIASIS

- Local injury (rubbing, friction, abrasion) or repeated irritation at a skin site most often sets off the problem.
- Environmental factors—such as pollutants, stress, emotional upsets—may exacerbate or cause psoriatic flare-ups.
- Infection plays a part, mostly in childhood, where streptococcal throat and other infections may produce acute psoriasis that returns during adulthood in a different form; viral infections can also cause flare-ups.
- Certain drugs, such as antimalarials, lithium and beta blockers (e.g. propranolol), can induce a psoriatic attack, as can withdrawal of steroid medication.
- Alcohol may worsen the condition, and alcoholics often fail to comply with the treatment plan.
- Obesity is a possible aggravating factor. While being overweight doesn't cause the condition, it makes psoriasis hard to treat because the plaques tend to "hide" within skin creases.

races and social classes. It can be so mild that it goes undiagnosed (a few small scaling skin patches or sore areas on the elbows or scalp), or severely disabling. It's a recurrent disease that flares up from time to time, often starting in young adulthood. The outer skin cells grow and multiply about 10 times more quickly than required—turning over every four or five days instead of every 28 days. The rapidly dividing cells produce raised, roundish, scaly patches and sometimes red, inflamed eruptions that may become cracked and sore, called plaques. Once they have formed, the plaques tend to recur again and again in the vulnerable areas.

Psoriasis typically occurs in areas of the body exposed to friction, irritation, infection or any other trauma, especially at pressure points such as elbows and knees. In the past, it was most prevalent on the knees (from praying and scrubbing postures), and it's still common there among tile-layers! Psoriasis sometimes affects areas such as the nails and scalp (at the back of the head), where it may be confused with seborrheic dermatitis. In its mild form psoriasis is easy to miss—it may first be noticed by the barber or hairdresser. Diagnosis is by clinical appearance and skin biopsy (or sample) for lab confirmation. While the majority of sufferers have a mild form, about 10 percent of psoriatics have serious skin involvement and/or accompanying arthritis.

Psoriasis was previously thought to be just skin-deep, but it's now known that very severe psoriasis can affect the whole body. If the condition is erythrodermic (inflammatory), it may diminish the body's heat regulation, dilate blood vessels in the skin and cause heat loss and cold-sensitivity. At the extreme end of the spectrum, under 3 percent of psoriatics have severe pustular psoriasis (inflamed lesions or pustules)—a condition that may suddenly flare up, necessitating hospital treatment. Very rarely there is a general erythroderma (total body peeling and redness, with moisture loss and high fever) that can be life-threatening.

Psoriasis treatments—new and old
Physicians now treat not just the affected sites but the whole person. There is no single, effective remedy, although for many patients the plaques spontaneously fade during long periods of remission. People with psoriasis must think "control" or "management" rather than cure. For the obese, losing weight may reduce the problem; for the overbusy, relaxation may help. One doctor found that his psoriasis cleared up when he downsized his hectic practice.

Treatment usually starts with a family physician, who refers patients to a dermatologist if necessary. For mild cases, people often manage successfully by themselves. More severe cases, with ups and downs, need close professional supervision.

Dietary theories for curing psoriasis abound, although there is no evidence that food plays any role in the disease. Some health-food stores promote lecithin, vitamins or other supplements for psoriasis—substances that have not lived up to their promise. Although stress is sometimes considered to be a factor in provoking flare-ups, its precise role remains uncertain.

The best management is achieved at specific centers, such as the University of Toronto's PERC (Psoriasis Education and Research Centre at 416-323-7505), which help to educate people and keep the disease under control. This is most useful for those who might otherwise need hospitalization. Such units not only teach self-care but also provide the opportunity to meet and talk to others about a common handicap.

SHINGLES IS A PAIN

Shingles, or *Herpes zoster*, is an adult reactivation of a childhood chickenpox infection. However instead of covering large parts of the body as in chickenpox, the shingles rash appears on only a small area of skin, often in rows like shingles on a roof. A typical shingles rash is a group of reddish blisters. It follows the path of certain nerves on one side of the body only—generally on the trunk, buttocks, neck, face or scalp—usually stopping abruptly at the midline.

The incidence of herpes zoster is low in children and adolescents, about 0.5 to 1.6:1000 for persons under 20, rising 11:1000 in adults over 80, afflicting both sexes equally. Most people suffer only one attack, although repeat bouts occasionally occur, usually at the same site as the first eruption.

An attack of shingles generally begins with feverish discomfort (chills, headache, upset stomach). A preliminary itching or burning sensation may precede the rash by a few days (occasionally mistaken for a heart attack, lung infection or back problem). But the discomfort is more commonly felt only during and/or after the rash. Pain that persists after a shingles attack is particularly troublesome in people over 60.

The shingles rash starts as a series of raised red spots that turn into clear blisters, which later become cloudy, dry out and crust over. The spots are surrounded by a swollen area and may bleed and become very itchy and painful. In a few people, especially those with defective immune systems, attacks are severe and the rash covers a wide area. The rash may take three to four weeks to heal and may leave whitish-silver or brown scars.

Treatment consists mainly of antiviral agents such as acyclovir—best started within 48 hours of the rash appearing—or use of newer, possibly more effective agents such as famciclovir or valacyclovir. Lingering post-shingles pain is often the worst aspect of the condition because even though the rash generally vanishes, leaving little or no discomfort, pain may continue long after the skin heals.

Post-zoster pain is a continuous itching, burning sensation with bouts of stabbing and shooting or lacerating pain. It is often set off by touching the sensitive area and can last for years. This condition

is called post-herpetic neuralgia (PHN) and is defined as "unrelenting pain that persists for four or more weeks after the acute shingles phase." Some find it agonizing, never letting up except perhaps during sleep, and indeed it's often bad enough to hinder sleep. Many people complain of allodynia (pain on contact with certain stimuli such as the touch of clothing) and hyperpathia (prolonged, radiating pain superimposed on the continuous itch). Fortunately, the pain tends to fade with time, often vanishing in a year or so.

MANAGING THE SHINGLES RASH

- Do not scratch the blisters.
- Apply cold compresses of Burow's solution, Betadine, other antiseptics, drying agents (cornstarch or baking soda) and bandages impregnated with petroleum jelly, with or without topical antibiotics.
- Try a drying lotion containing calamine, alcohol, menthol and/or phenol to speed healing.
- "Splinting" the area—e.g., covering it with cotton and wrapping with an elastic bandage—may relieve active and post-shingles pain.
- Interferon (an extract of the natural defense substance present in all cells) helps some people.
- Acyclovir, given by mouth or intravenous infusion in the first 72 hours of the appearance of the rash, may reduce the severity of shingles and aid healing in both normal and immunosuppressed people, and may, but does not necessarily, lessen post-shingles pain. Some clinicians reserve this treatment for people over 50 as they are more likely to benefit. Newer, similar antivirals such as famciclovir and valacyclovir may be as effective in reducing the sores and pain of shingles and simpler to take.
- Early prescription (within 72 hours of the start of symptoms) of systemic (oral or injected) steroids are occasionally prescribed for sufferers with severe or widespread shingles. This is controversial, with some evidence of less pain in the first month but no effect on postherpetic neuralgia.

REMEDIES FOR LINGERING POST-SHINGLES PAIN

- Older antidepressants (e.g., amitriptyline) help many, not because of their antidepressant effect but because the medication affects the neurotransmitters (chemical messengers) and relieves pain (in doses lower than those normally used for depression).
- Evidence from a smaller number of studies supports the use of topical capsaicin (Zostrix),or hot pepper cream, gabapentin (Neurontin) a new anti-seizure drug, and controlled-release oxycodone an opioid painkiller.
- Sympathetic nerve blockade or local anesthetics may be helpful. But since these methods are elaborate and expensive, and have given little evidence of long-term benefit, anesthetic remedies are not strongly supported.

TO FIGHT OFF THE EXTERNAL SIGNS OF AGING SKIN, TRY TO:

- reduce sun exposure—there is no healthy tan;
- avoid certain facial expressions, such as pursing lips, arching eyebrows or grimacing, which can increase wrinkling;
- stop smoking cigarettes—young smokers often have facial wrinkles akin to those of nonsmokers in their sixties. Years of inhaling cigarette smoke give the cheeks a gaunt look, and nicotine cuts blood flow to the face, causing a leathery, gray complexion;
- avoid rapid weight loss—frequent "yo-yo" dieting can permanently wrinkle the skin;
- get an expert opinion about use of dermabrasion—with a wire wheel or other device to gently "sand" off the top skin layer (this process can leave depigmented areas);
- consider a chemical peel—"painting" an abrasive product over wrinkles near the eyes and mouth, as well as on the cheeks and chin—which slightly wounds the skin and produces a transiently smoother skin. An expert should advise you about this procedure;
- consult a dermatologist about using Retin-A (vitamin-A like) or alpha-hydroxy acid creams or lotions to remove sun-damage spots and smooth the skin;
- Botox, which neutralizes the nerve supply to the skin and thus makes it less likely to wrinkle is another option. A treatment typically lasts 3 months, but can be repeated.

A study done in Iceland followed 421 patients with an episode of herpes zoster for 7.6 years to determine the natural history of pain following the acute episode. Post-herpetic neuralgia was uncommon in patients younger than 60 years, with only 2 percent reporting pain 3 months after the outbreak, all of the cases mild. The severity and frequency increased in patients older than 60, with 13 percent reporting pain and 4 percent reporting moderate to severe pain. In patients over age 70 years, 29 percent had pain at three months. After 12 months, 3.3 percent of patients reported pain, and most of these reports were of mild pain. Six of these patients had pain that was still present 2 to 7 years following the initial outbreak.

If shingles occurs on the face, nose, ears or cornea of the eye, it is known as *zoster keratitis*. This condition can lead to blindness if left untreated. Anyone with shingles on the upper face, no matter how mild, should see a physician at once. A tingling at the tip of the nose may herald eye involvement. When the trigeminal facial nerve and the eyes are affected, people are more likely to experience prolonged post-shingles pain.

What causes shingles?

The *Herpes zoster* (HZV) virus is responsible for both chickenpox in children and shingles in adults. This virus belongs to the same family as the *Herpes simplex* organism responsible for cold sores. Shingles occurs almost exclusively in those who had chickenpox as children and have some but not total immunity to the virus. While chickenpox is highly contagious, caught by inhaling infected droplets, shingles is not generally transmitted from one person to another. But children or adults who haven't yet had chickenpox may catch it if they touch wet shingles blisters.

About 80 percent of North Americans have had chicken pox, usually a mild illness, by age 10. Although childhood chicken pox generally runs its course in a week or two, the virus may linger in the body, hidden within nerve ganglia (centers in the spinal cord). Most of us go through life maintaining an "armed truce" with zoster viruses that have remained in the body after a juvenile bout of chicken pox. If reactivated for some reason, the virus travels along affected nerves, causing a skin eruption as it goes. Once it's widely used, the new chicken pox vaccine (Varivax) may help curb the spread of HZV.

There is some evidence, not proven, that shingles may be precipitated by excessive exposure to sunlight (UV radiation), stress, trauma (wounds, surgery or inflammation) and other events that lower immune resistance. Shingles is more common in older people because immune defences get weaker with progressing years. It also often afflicts AIDS patients.

HELP FOR AGING SKIN

Aging skin normally becomes thinner and drier than younger skin, hence the need to moisturize extra well with advancing years. There's no way to grow older without getting some wrinkles and skin blotches, but avoidance of the sun's harmful rays and protection with good sunscreens go a long way toward preserving the skin's youthful look.

The diminution in sweating and sebum production among the elderly increases the need for regular moisturizers. A good face massage can stimulate the blood flow and reduce dryness, but without lasting benefits. Those with dry, aging skin should avoid harsh soaps, abrasive washcloths, rough towels and grainy cleansers. They should wash less often and, above all, moisturize consistently. Cleansers for the over-65s should be mild (e.g., Cetaphil, Aquanil or Dove), and without astringents. In using makeup for older skins, less is often more.

The elderly may develop discolorations such as senile angiomas (red or bluish patches on the trunk and scrotum), pruritis (itching), and rosacea, which gives a reddish and slightly bulbous look to the nose. One small advantage to aging is that sweating decreases, so there's less need for deodorants, and some conditions such as psoriasis improve. But as sweating decreases, the elderly must watch their body temperature to avoid heatstroke.

Lasers and liquid nitrogen can now lighten some unsightly skin discolorations, but so-called "rejuvenating" and hormone creams are not usually worth the cost, and can be harmful. Most products touted for "skin-renewal," such as bee-extracts, aloe vera, estrogens, mink oils and placental extracts, work no better than plain mineral oil. Exercise, however can help by toning the muscles and increasing the circulation. For the coarse facial hair that sometimes afflicts older faces, a good electrologist can help. But be sure to choose a well-trained technician.

Retinoid (vitamin A–like) products revolutionize skin care

Retinoic acid, or Retin-A (a synthetic derivative of vitamin A), a successful acne remedy, has been found to have certain antiwrinkling effects, and is now prescribed for some elderly faces. A commonly used version is Renova. Retinoids can do marvels for skin disorders such as acne (tretinoin is used topically and Accutane is taken by mouth) and for psoriasis (through Tegison

pills). (For more, see the entry for psoriasis.) The anti-acne products can also lighten sun-damaged skin and smooth light wrinkles. But it takes about four months of regular use to see any antiwrinkle benefits, and the products are costly, available only by prescription. Buyers must beware of imitations containing vitamin A, with deceptively similar labels. The success of synthetic retinoids has prompted manufacturers to add nonprescription vitamin A and its byproducts, such as retinyl palmitate, to moisturizers, which can easily trap the unwary into thinking these products will do the same thing. But although some announce that nonprescription vitamin A can also reduce fine skin lines, neither vitamin A nor any of its currently used derivatives has the antiwrinkling effects of the synthetic, prescription retinoids.

The wrinkle-removing benefit of retinoids was discovered at the University of Philadelphia, where dermatologists noticed that, after a few months of retinoid application for acne, many faces showed a subtle anti-aging effect. Wrinkles were smoothed and brown sunspots lightened. The anti-aging effect may be partly due to a renewed collagen buildup which provides fresh skin support. Experts stress that retinoids are pharmaceutical products which need cautious use and must be geared to individual skin types. One University of Toronto dermatologist warns that "far from offering swift wrinkle removal, retinoid creams must be diligently applied daily, for some months, before any noticeable benefits appear." The products are expensive and erase only the very fine, almost invisible wrinkles, not the crow's-feet around the eyes or mouth. Once the retinoids are stopped, the wrinkles creep back. Since retinoids exaggerate sun sensitivity, those using them must use an extra-protective sunscreen.

Apart from smoothing out some wrinkles, the retinoids herald a new era of successful treatment for several drastic skin problems, including severe acne and psoriasis. The retinoids have radically improved the outlook for those with certain skin disorders and have been hailed as a breakthrough for the treatment of disorders that involve abnormal keratinization (skin turnover). More than 1,000 different retinoids have been produced since the 1940s,

THE NEW SKIN PEELS

Chemicals or laser "peels" take off dead and dry surface cells. While superficial peels and creams only tone skin quality and texture, deeper chemical peels and laser contouring may improve wrinkling and remove discolorations and growths. Alpha-hydroxy acids in strong concentration act as chemical peels, but for quicker results, chemical peels are applied by a plastic surgeon or dermatologist. Deep peels with _phenol_ or _trichloroacetic acid_ can dramatically improve appearance leaving the skin noticeably less wrinkled and blotchy. Side effects of deep peels may be permanent loss of pigmentation, especially in dark-skinned people, creating light patches; there can also be some permanent scarring. After a peel, the skin is _extremely_ sun sensitive, so sunscreens are a must.

Many dermatologists now prefer CO_2 laser "resurfacing," which produces a slight burn, said to be especially effective for wrinkles around the upper lip and eyes, but it's a recent technique, with little known about how long the effects last.

RATING THE NEW ALPHA-HYDROXY ACID CREAMS

Sour milk, in which Cleopatra bathed, contains lactic acid, an alpha-hydroxy acid— prototype of agents now touted as skin rejuvenators in a new range of cosmetics. Alpha-hydroxy products (AHAs)—which include *tartaric acid from many fruits, glycolic acid* from sugar cane, *citric acid* from citrus fruits and *malic acid* from apples—are said to decrease blocked and thickened skin patches. Their effects mimic those of Retin-A—giving some superficial skin smoothing, but improvement may take months to appear and lasts only as long as the preparation is used. While not thought to be harmful, long-term effects are unknown.

and while all behave in a roughly similar manner; each has a slightly different therapeutic effect. Safe retinoid use depends on good patient-doctor communication and close supervision.

But while retinoids are recognized as a valuable treatment for several skin problems, they have come under fire owing to their deforming effects on unborn babies.

In Canada, the retinoids now available are:
• tretinoin or retinoic acid (Stieva–A or Vitamin-A acid)—in three strengths as gels, lotions or creams—used topically as creams or lotions for acne, to repair sun-damaged skin and to abolish light wrinkles. (The topical form is relatively safe and causes no fetal malformations or serious side effects, but the forms taken by mouth deflect fetal development);
• isotretinoin or 13-cis-retinoic acid (Accutane) capsules, taken by mouth, used for severe acne (with caution in younger women);
• etretinate (Tegison), taken by mouth, used mainly for severe psoriasis.

Since the oral retinoid drugs can cause serious fetal malformations, they must NOT be prescribed for; or even contemplated for; anyone who is, or may become, pregnant. Accutane, which is more rapidly excreted than Tegison, may be given to women who practice absolutely reliable, effective birth control for one month before taking the drug, while on it, and for at least one month after discontinuation. Tegison, which is cleared very slowly from the body, is generally not prescribed for any woman of childbearing age unless she's had her tubes tied. Both Accutane and Tegison can be freely prescribed for males, as the retinoids do not affect male reproductive function.

AVOID SKIN'S NUMBER-ONE ENEMY

The sun's ultraviolet rays are essential to human beings in moderate amounts for forming vitamin D by their action on the skin. But in addition, ultraviolet (UV) rays, whether from the sun, a tanning parlor or other sources, can damage and age human skin. Thus sunlight is enemy number one to human skin. Although the sun makes us feel good, it is one of the most injurious environmental agents human skin ever encounters. Solar radiation speeds up wrinkling

and other external signs of aging, and can induce skin cancer and exacerbate allergies. Damage is worst with short, repeated, intense sun exposure—as with trips south when people try to soak up a year's sunshine in a brief vacation. To retain a youthful look and prevent skin cancer protect the skin from excess sun exposure. Close inspection of a habitually tanned person's arms, legs, neck or face reveals a mass of brown spots, mottled white patches, horny bumps, finely etched lines, scaly plaques, rough (premalignant) keratoses, enlarged blood vessels and perhaps small cancerous growths.

To understand how the sun's ultraviolet rays harm human skin, think about what sunlight is: intense electromagnetic radiation emitted from the sun's inner core by the nuclear fusion of hydrogen to helium. The spectrum of emitted sunlight ranges from the long-wave radio and infrared rays through all colors of visible light to the short-wave or high-energy ultraviolet, gamma and cosmic rays. Although they make us feel hot, infrared rays do not injure human skin unless they are intense enough to burn. The brown pigment, melanin, absorbs infrared rays, which explains why black- and brown-skinned people often feel hotter than those with white skins.

The amount of skin damage from UV rays depends on cumulative lifetime exposure. The greater the UV exposure, the more the injury. The shorter the wavelength, the greater the danger. For practical purposes, dermatologists divide ultraviolet rays into three types: UVA, UVB and UVC. The longer UVA rays can penetrate glass and produce some tanning—both immediate and delayed. UVA rays were formerly considered harmless, but dermatologists now know that these rays, including those from tanning lamps, do as much damage as the shorter rays.

The UVB band, often termed the sunburn spectrum, cannot pass through glass but is the principal cause of sunburn, wrinkling and aging.

UVC rays are filtered out by the ozone layer before sunlight reaches the earth.

To counter the sun's assault, the skin's outer layer thickens and darkens. The outer cells divide to form a covering that scatters and bounces back the impinging rays. Pigmentation increases via manufacture of the brown pigment, melanin, which reduces UV penetration. People who tan easily are better protected than those who merely burn or freckle. Especially at risk of skin cancer are the Celtic races with red hair and pale, freckly complexions. Those who inherit dark, olive skins can take more sun exposure with less damage than fair-skinned types.

Sunburn: the immediate damage

When UV radiation hits human skin, some is reflected, some absorbed, some scattered. Damage may be acute (immediate and short-lived) or chronic (long-term and lasting). Sunburn may not show up at once, but peaks 15–20 hours later when a burning, beet-red color appears. Any sunburn, however slight, adds to the risk of getting skin cancer. But with constant exposure, even without any telltale reddening, some skin damage occurs—a few lines etched in, a little cellular degeneration. The lag between the time damage is inflicted and the point at which it shows may be 20 years. By the time obvious skin blemishes appear much irreversible harm has already occurred. Nevertheless, it is worthwhile to prevent further sun damage at any age.

To treat sunburn, take painkillers to ease the pain and soothe the hot skin with calamine lotion. The ensuing blisters should not be broken but simply treated with cool-water compresses. A mild vinegar and water bath may make people feel cooler. A very severe sunburn may require use of topical steroid cream.

PROTECT YOURSELF AGAINST SKIN CANCERS

Skin cancer is on the rise, having doubled in incidence over the past 10 years. One in seven Canadians now develops skin cancer over the course of a lifetime. If sun exposure continues, no amount of defensive action can ward off the wrinkling, color flaws and other irreversible changes that may ultimately lead to cancerous growths. Some skin flaws, seborrheic keratoses that look "stuck on," are benign and have no malignant potential. But other blemishes (actiner keratoses) may develop into premalignant horny patches and ultimately into frank malignancy. Cancerous tumors usually form in the parts that get the most sun—hands, neck, back, face and lower legs.

The danger signals of skin cancer are:
- any ulcer, sore or patch that won't heal;
- a spot that scales persistently;
- any enlarging spot or lump.

Basal cell cancer, the commonest of skin cancers, now affects 30,000–50,000 Canadians each year. It usually occurs on the face, and although it's potentially serious it almost always remains localized and is quite easily treated. Squamous cell cancer, a less common form, may spread more easily. But caught in time, these types can be removed with a 95 percent chance of total cure. People who have had one skin cancer should get regular follow-ups to check for repeats.

Melanoma—a deadly skin cancer

Malignant melanoma is the deadliest of skin cancers. It arises from melanocytes (pigment-producing cells), often from already existing

PEOPLE MOST AT RISK FOR MELANOMA

- "Frecklers"—those who freckle easily, especially when young;
- children who sunburn easily and tan poorly;
- people badly sunburned in childhood;
- "moley" individuals—people with many moles (the more moles, the greater the risk of melanoma);
- redheads, blonds, blue-eyed and fair-complexioned types;
- those who've had one melanoma, or other types of skin cancer or who have family members who've had melanoma;
- people who spend much time outdoors—working or playing;
- people with "peculiar-looking" moles, dysplastic nevi, which are precursor moles quite likely to become cancerous,

RECOGNIZING THE ABCDs OF MELANOMA

ASYMMETRY; **B**ORDER IRREGULARITY; **C**OLOR VARIATION; **D**IAMETER.

- **A**symmetry: an irregularly shaped brown spot or mole with tails and jagged edges may be cancerous; or a skin patch that changes in surface texture—that scales or oozes. A scab that keeps coming off, bleeds incessantly or becomes "velvety" may denote skin cancer and should be investigated.
- **B**order irregularity: scalloped, splayed or perhaps notched edges of a pigmented (brown) spot may be danger signals.

- **C**olor variation: uneven color is a distinct feature of melanoma. Moles may become lighter or darker or acquire black flecks or various shades of gray or pink, or pigment may spread from the mole into skin that otherwise looks normal, with color patches that are next to, but not a direct part of, the mole ("satellite pigmentation").
- **D**iameter: most melanomas exceed six mm (0.2 in) across (wider than a pencil eraser), while ordinary, benign moles are generally smaller.

THE WARNING SIGNS OF MELANOMA
How to distinguish ordinary moles or brown spots from melanomas and their precursors

	Normal moles (common nevi)	"Dyplastic" nevi: possible precursor or marker moles (Unusual-looking, bigger than average, may give rise to melanoma)	Malignant melanoma: cancerous moles/pigmented spots (Recognize by the ABCDs of change: **A**symmetry (one side looks different from the other), **B**order irregularity, **C**olor variation, **D**iameter enlargement (typically bigger than an eraser on a pencil). It should be noted that many skin spots fit these individual criteria, however, the more criteria that fit the more crucial it is to consult a skin specialist (dermatologist).
Color and appearance	• Uniformly tan or brown • Tend to look alike • Regular outline	• Varied mix of tans, browns, blacks, reds/pinks • May differ from each other • Sometimes look like fried egg, with central color blob and flat edges	• Possible darkening, more brown, black and bluish hues • Appearance of multiple shades of pinks, reds, blue; possible depigmentation and white patches in mole; part may vanish (although melanoma is still there)
Size (diameter)	• Usually less than 6 mm or 0.2 in (smaller than a pencil eraser)	• Often 5–10 mm (0.2–0.4 in) across or larger	• Continuing or gradual expansion over time—varies from months to years, slow or fast
Surface, shape and border	• Rounded, with sharply defined edges • Flat or elevated	• Mostly flat with some raised parts • Often merge into surrounding skin • Irregular notched, scalloped and indistinct edges	• Development of notched, irregular margins • Surface may elevate, darken (including surrounding skin—rare) • May develop a new bump that looks like a blister
Number	• Typical adult has 10–30 scattered over body	• Wide variation; few to over 100	• Person usually develops just one at a time • If already had one, another may occur elsewhere
Age of appearance	• Infancy to fourth decade	• Childhood to old age	• Any age—12–70 years (rare in children)
Incidence	• Most people (95–99%) have some normal moles	• In 5–10% of the population • Often run in families (may be due to inherited gene)	• 15 per 100,000 persons
Location on body	• Anywhere, but typically on sun-exposed skin • Rare on nonexposed (covered) sites	• Can occur anywhere but most frequent on back and trunk • Also occur on *unexposed* skin (e.g. scalp, breasts, buttocks)	• Any part of skin (most common on back in men and women, and on lower legs in women)
Sensation	• Not noticed (unless rubbed by garments or movement) • Do not inflame, redden or ooze	• Usually not felt or noticed	• Most are not felt or noticed • Some start to itch, hurt, ooze, inflame, ulcerate, swell, soften or crust over; bleeding a very late sign
Malignant? (Cancerous?)	• No, absolutely not	• No. But increased chance of becoming malignant	• Yes! Melanoma is a skin cancer that can spread (metastasize) to other tissues, e.g., lymphatics, liver, spleen
Malignant potential	• Ordinary moles may turn into melanomas (large congenital nevi, present since birth are especially likely to become cancerous)	• Increased, in comparison to ordinary moles	• Already cancerous

moles, but also anywhere on the body, including the eyes and mouth. In contrast to other skin cancers, malignant melanoma spreads fast and dangerously if not caught early. Untreated, melanoma can kill within a few months to a couple of years. Yet early detection and removal offer an excellent chance of a cure.

Worldwide, there's a sharp rise in melanoma, especially among the fair-skinned. Melanoma rates in Canada have almost doubled since the mid-seventies, an upward shift attributed mainly to greater sun exposure, more outdoor recreation, skimpier clothing and an ardent pursuit of tanning. The much-publicized thinning of the earth's ozone layer (attributed partly to chlorfluorocarbon emissions) is also contributing to the melanoma rise. Mortality from this type of cancer is increasing faster than death from any other malignancy. If the current increase continues, experts predict, this cancer will soon be more common than breast or lung cancer. By the year 2000, an estimated one in 90 Canadians will get at least one melanoma in a lifetime. (At present, about 500 Canadians die annually from it.)

Although melanoma may form in nonexposed areas, the sun's ultraviolet rays are most to blame for its development. There is no such thing as a good tan, yet too many of us link sunlight to a glamorous look, rather than to cancer! Each year's tan adds a little more damage. Short, intense recreational UV exposure, rather than steady low-level exposure, may pose the most serious threat.

The good news is that there's a high chance of curing melanoma provided it is detected early and removed before it penetrates too deep. Pathologists predict an excellent cure rate for those less than 0.8 mm (0.03 in) thick. The deeper the tumor, the greater the likelihood it has metastasized (spread).

Moles may turn into deadly melanomas

Most experts believe that while melanomas may arise on mole-free skin, from melanocytes, some develop within the pigment cells of already existing moles. Research suggests that "moley" people are at an above-average risk for melanoma, especially from occasional excessive sun exposure. There may be a critical period in the evolution of a mole when it can be "promoted" to form melanoma (rather than regressing in the normal manner).

Congenital nevi (birthmarks) occur in 1 percent of newborns, and those bigger than a pencil eraser have a somewhat increased chance of developing into melanoma.

Giant or "garment" nevi—unusually large, hairy moles that are very conspicuous, sometimes over 20 cm (8 in) across and occupying a large area (e.g., from neck to buttocks)—unquestionably have an above-average tendency to become malignant. These moles need not necessarily be removed, but require careful watching.

Solar lentigo ("liver spots") are pigmented spots that appear late in adulthood on sun-damaged skin and are unlikely to become malignant, but a biopsy is suggested to make sure there is no malignant tendency.

"Peculiar" precursor moles may precede melanoma

Dysplastic nevi (odd-looking, multicolored notched moles) were first recognized in 1978 as possible markers or "predictors" of melanoma among 37 patients in six melanoma-prone families, and were dubbed B-K moles. Scientists have since found that dysplastic nevi are possible forerunners of melanoma. About 5 to 10 percent of the population have one or more of these strange moles. Sometimes, but not always, dysplastic moles run in families as a dominant, inherited trait. A certain number progress to malignant melanoma, and the risks are greatest

---

DISTINGUISHING DIFFERENT MOLES

   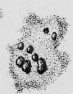

Normal Mole
(smallish, uniform roundish shape, sharp edges)

Dysplastic nevus
("pre-melanoma")
(unusual-looking, largish, varied pink, mixed colours, vague border—may merge into surrounding skin)

Frank melanoma
(cancer)
(often jagged, irregular border, large size, mix of dark and light colors)

SUNCARE TIPS

- Don't expose children under 12 months to direct sunlight.
- Protect newborns under a sun umbrella.
- Cover infant heads when in the sun.
- Wear long-sleeved shirt and pants when in strong sunlight—one can still enjoy activities on the beach or in the park.
- Remember that sheer clothing allows the sun's rays through, leaving underlying skin unprotected (apply sunscreen).
- Be especially vigilant with children with red hair and pale skins—they are at greatest risk of developing melanoma.
- Remember that UV light is reflected from sand, concrete, snow or water. Young skiers and waterlovers often sustain serious sunburns from reflected sunlight.
- Get children into good sun protection habits: teach them regular sunscreen application while outdoors. Model sun protection yourself.
- Note that baby oil is not a sunscreen—the oil intensifies the effects of sunlight and burns skin faster.
- Keep sun exposure to a minimum—especially from noon to 3:00 p.m., when sunlight is most intense.
- Beware of cool, cloudy or overcast days when 70–80 percent of the sun's UV rays still get through.
- Remember that sitting in the shade or swimming underwater does not guarantee protection (UV rays go through water).
- Use sunscreens wisely: choose SPFs of 20 and up. Most experts now recommend 20–30 SPF for good protection (unless the product contains Parsol, in which case a lower SPF may give enough protection).
- Apply sunscreen at least 30–60 minutes before going outside so that it penetrates the skin well.
- Pay special attention to sun-exposed areas —ears, face, scalp, neck, shoulders, back.
- Try different products for different occasions/activities: use a higher SPF for vigorous outdoor exertion (e.g., golfing, running), lower ones for milder exertion (e.g., walking).
- On vulnerable spots (such as nose, cheeks) consider adding a total, opaque sun-block or paste (containing titanium dioxide or zinc).
- Select a broad-spectrum sunscreen that blocks out the sun's shorter (UVB) and some of the longer (UVA) rays—such as those containing Parsol, oxybenzones or dibenzoyl methane.
- If swimming or perspiring profusely, reapply waterproof sunscreen after drying off.
- Send kids off to camp or for summer weekends with the right sunscreen in their bag!
- Be especially vigilant at high altitudes and near the equator, where solar radiation is most intense.
- Become a mole-watcher—examine the entire skin regularly for any changes in moles, freckles or discoloration.
- Get skin check-ups if there is a personal or family history of melanoma, or if you are in a known high-risk bracket.

---

in someone who's already had a confirmed melanoma or who comes from a melanoma-prone family.

When should moles be removed?

Wholesale removal of unsightly moles is impractical, unjustified and cosmetically undesirable. But moles that look suspicious or worry someone should always be removed—namely, any that are injured or irritated by movement, shaving, brushing, belts or clothing. Anyone who thinks a mole has changed color or enlarged, or who particularly dislikes a mole, should have it off. Even the best experts can miss a melanoma, and only a biopsy test can confirm one as harmless or malignant. As one University of Toronto pathologist puts it, "If in doubt, cut it out!"

Protect children from sunburn and sun exposure

Severe or frequent sunburns to a child can greatly increase melanoma risks. Studies show that fair-skinned immigrants who arrived in Australia or Israel before age 10 were far more likely to develop malignant melanoma than those who came at later ages. One bad sunburn during childhood can double the chances of developing skin cancer later in life—an avoidable risk. The message is loud and clear: protect children from sunburn.

Scan a buddy's skin for sinister spots

Self-examination and frequent checks of your loved one's moles are a great idea. The back is a place where melanoma often occurs, especially in men. So check for brown spots that are asymmetrical, have scalloped borders, change color or become bigger. Particularly examine the hands, back, calves of legs, upper arms, ears, and back of the neck, where skin cancers commonly form. Note the pattern of moles and freckles and look for any scaliness, change in color or shape, itching or oozing. Remember: prompt surgical excision of early melanoma offers an excellent chance of cure. If in doubt see your family doctor or a dermatologist.

Choosing the best sunscreen

Everyone is advised to avoid suntanning and, when outside, to follow the SLIP, SLAP, SLOP routine: SLIP on a shirt, SLAP on a hat, SLOP on some appropriate sunscreen (SPF 20 or more, preferably waterproof). The SPF (sunburn protection factor) denotes the protection that a certain product provides. For good sun protection, the SPF number must be 30 or more. The only products that provide sun protection are those containing a specific chemical that weakens or blocks the impact of UV light. The concentration of the UV-screening compound must be high enough to protect your skin type. Ideally a sunscreen should protect against both UVB and UVA rays, but very few chemicals screen out all the UVA, so sun-sensitive people may need a total (opaque) sun block such as zinc or titanium oxide. Although many products are advertised as "sun blocks"—especially those with high SPF—most are not total sun blockers; in other words, they do let some UV rays through. Cocoa butter and oils increase the risks of sunburn and offer no protection against UV rays. Some people argue that sunscreen is a bad thing because it encourages people to stay out in the sun.

PABA (para-aminobenzoic acid) and its esters are among the most widely used sun blockers, followed by benzophenones, cinnamates, salicylates and anthranilates. Usually colorless and invisible, they are cosmetically acceptable provided they don't ruin clothes or produce adverse skin reactions. Alcoholic PABA solutions may turn clothes yellow, sting the face or occasionally cause skin irritation. Although PABA is the best of sunscreens, people cross-reactive to benzocaine and procaine (local anesthetics), some hair dyes and sulfa drugs may be allergic to it.

No chemical offers complete UVA protection, but new products, especially those containing Parsol, block some UVA rays. Broad-spectrum sunscreens containing benzophenones, oxybenzones and dibenzoyl methane also screen out some UVA as well as UVB light. Choose a product that is broad-spectrum if possible for maximum sun protection.

Sun-free tanning lotions may be the solution

Products that dye or stain the skin to give a pseudo-tan do not protect the skin from UV rays, but they enable people to attain the hue they desire, providing skin color without cancer risks. Several companies now market self-tanning milks and creams (not to be confused with tan accelerators) which on prolonged contact give a "bottle tan", turning the palest of skins a warm shade of brown—not the bright orange or pumpkin colors produced by earlier products. Two or three nighttime applications may be needed to attain the desired shade. The depth of skin color depends on the amount and frequency of application. Tan-producing chemicals such as dihydroxy acetone (DHA) stain the skin, and the color develops a few hours after application, depending on the skin type and its amino-acid content. People should do a skin (patch) test before use in case of allergies. Trial and error can show which brand is best for you. Remember that sunscreen is still needed for sun protection.

HAIR, BEAUTIFUL HAIR

The value placed on hair as a symbol of beauty, strength and sexuality is reflected in the billions spent annually on shampoos, conditioners, coloring agents, curling treatments and baldness remedies. In fact, when we meet someone, hair style and color are often the first features we notice.

Fine and transparent, human hair is a vestige of our hairier animal forebears. The adult human body averages five million hairs, of which 100,000 to 150,000 are on the scalp. Odd though it may seem to call the tangle of inert protein arising from the scalp a "healthy head of hair," our hair does reflect the overall state of the body's health. The part of the hair seen above the skin surface is a strand composed mostly of keratin—a tough, elastic protein which also makes up human fingernails, birds' beaks and mammals' hoofs. There are three basic types of human hair: *lanugo*—the very fine, transparent hair covering an unborn baby, shed by the seventh month of fetal development; *vellus hair* (from the Latin for "fleece" or "down")—short, soft, sometimes pigmented

THE STRUCTURE OF A HAIR AND ITS FOLLICLES

The hair shaft has three layers: the cuticle (outer protective layer), the cortex (providing strength) and the innermost medulla, which has no known function.

The hair cuticle, made of tightly overlapping layers of flattened cells, like shingles on a roof or scales on a snake, encases the delicate cortex. If smooth and healthy, the cuticle gives hair gloss by keeping the scales non-porous and tight, preventing water loss. But the cuticle is easily damaged by heat, sun, dryness, salt water, harsh chemicals, or overtreatment (e.g., too much blow-drying, perming, or bleaching), which swells and lifts the scales, leaving the hair dry and brittle. The cortex is made up of tiny keratin fibrils twisted together like yarn, which give hair strength, bounce and elasticity—largely determining the extent of its curl.

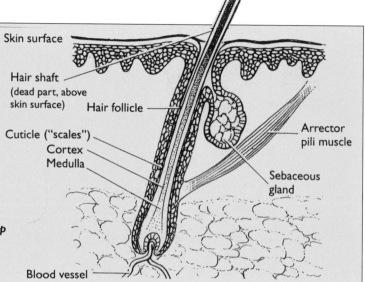

Skin surface

Hair shaft (dead part, above skin surface)

Hair follicle

Cuticle ("scales")

Cortex

Medulla

Arrector pili muscle

Sebaceous gland

Blood vessel

hair covering the entire body except for the soles of the feet and the palms of the hands; and *terminal hair*—the coarse, pigmented, longer hair on the human scalp, face, armpit and pubic regions.

Hair color comes from the pigment melanin, secreted by melanocytes (pigment-producing cells) near the follicle base (see diagram). The more pigment granules there are, and the more tightly packed, the darker the hair. Two kinds of melanin contribute to hair color. Eumelanin colors hair brown to black, and an iron-rich pigment, pheomelanin, colors it yellow-blond to red. Whether hair is mousy, brown, brunette or black depends on the type and amount of melanin and how densely it's distributed. For example, deep-black African hair contains closely packed melanin in the cortex. Black Japanese hair has many pigment granules in the cortex, and a few in the cuticle. Very dark European hair, quite apart from having more melanin granules than lighter or blond hair, has more melanin per granule. When the pigment-producing cells stop working hair loses its color and turns gray, the timing perhaps genetically determined.

Hair grows in cycles

A hair's growth is finite, determined by heredity and the part of the body on which it's growing. The hair follicle goes through alternating anagen (growth) and telogen (resting) phases. On a human scalp the growth phase lasts on average three to six, at most about eight, years. After growing steadily for that period the hair stops

and, after a three- to four-week transition stage, the follicle goes into its resting phase. After three months or so of resting, the same follicle begins to grow a new hair, pushing out the old one, which is eventually shed. A resting hair may stay put within its follicle for a few months, but as a fresh hair grows, the old one is shoved out to make room for its successor. At any one time, about 10 percent of the hair on our heads is in the resting stage, easily shed, while the rest (less easily tugged out) is in the growing phase. Most of us naturally shed 50 to 100 scalp hairs a day.

Given some 100,000 scalp hairs, their growth produces some 30 m (100 ft) of solid protein (keratin) each day—11 km or seven miles per year! Hair cells are among the body's most rapidly dividing cells. Individuals who grow long hair have a long growth period of six to eight years, although their hair may not grow faster than that of those with shorter growth periods. Since healthy scalp hair grows an average of 1 cm (0.4 in) per month, it may take two years to become shoulder-length or six years for uncut female hair to reach the buttocks. (The growth phase of hair is shorter on male scalps than for females.) Scalp hair rarely exceeds a maximum of 750 cm (two and a half feet) in total length. On the eyebrows, the growing phase is only about 10 weeks, so eyebrow hairs never grow very long. Pubic and armpit hair growth rates are roughly similar, while leg hairs grow more slowly and are shorter.

Hair is kept lubricated and shiny by sebum, an oily secretion produced by small sebaceous

COMMON REASONS FOR HAIR LOSS (OTHER THAN MALE BALDING)

- ***Alopecia areata*** (patchy baldness) is a common disorder affecting about 2 percent of the population, where hair on the scalp, eyebrows and beard comes out in oval patches, surrounded by short, broken or frayed thick-tipped club hairs. It usually occurs during childhood or early adulthood, lasting a few months. The small bald patches are sometimes tender and sore. They tend to clear up spontaneously with full hair regrowth, perhaps white or lighter in color at first, then back to the former color. Regrowth may take up to six months, and is sometimes accompanied by hair loss in another patch. Recurrences can occur, especially in those who had the condition as children, or if there are multiple patches. Occasionally the patchy shedding spreads to the hairline, eyebrows and lashes—the more serious *alopecia totalis*—or to the entire body, *alopecia universalis*.

  The reason for this patchy, circumscribed growth stoppage is unknown, but may be partly genetic (in 25 percent of cases), and probably involves an immune-system defect *Alopecia areata* is most common in identical twins, children with Down syndrome, asthmatics, those with eczema, pernicious anemia (a vitamin B_{12} deficiency), hay fever and thyroid disease. *Alopecia areata* can be treated with liquid nitrogen (freezing), phototherapy (light), anthralin (tar), steroid lotions and intralesional steroid injections at the site of hair loss.

- ***Tinea capitis***, popularly known as ringworm—a form of hair loss in children—is due to a fungus often carried by young kittens and puppies. The fungus attacks the hair shaft, causing local areas of hair loss, scalp scaling and possibly inflammation (depending on the site). A scalp sample (biopsy) may be taken to identify the parasite causing the loss, and to rule out other causes, such as psoriasis. Treatment is with antifungals such as oral griseofulvin or ketoconazole (Nizoral) for about six weeks, or a topical antifungal lotion.

- ***Trichotillomania*** (compulsive plucking, twisting, rubbing, pulling or tugging of the hair) is self-inflicted, transient hair loss which produces stubbly patches of short hair in children or psychiatrically disturbed adults—usually on the side of the "dominant" hand. A child may continually but unconsciously twist and pull out the hair owing to frustration or some inner tension (as with nail-biting). The relentless plucking ultimately produces visible hair loss on the scalp and occasionally eyebrows. Treatment includes reassurance for the child and, above all, the parents, and minimizing fuss.

- ***Traction alopecia*** results from too much physical tension on the hair, usually due to tightly pulled hairstyles such as ponytails or braids, or overtight curlers. Excessively rough or overenthusiastic blow-drying can also produce traction hair loss at the tension points.

- ***Friction alopecia*** is due to hats or wigs that are overly tight, the hair literally being broken off or pulled out at the follicle by the tension.

- ***Postpartum hair loss*** can occur one to six months after childbirth; during pregnancy; extra anagen growth produces luxuriant hair, and when the abrupt growth spurt wanes, after delivery, the above-average numbers of resting hairs gradually fall out.

- ***Some illnesses*** can cause temporary hair loss, such as thyroid, adrenal and pituitary diseases; certain forms of diabetes; systemic lupus erythematosus (a connective-tissue disease that may also cause scalp scarring); certain skin disorders,—for instance scleroderma, lichen planus, shingles and herpes. If scalp scarring occurs, the hair loss is permanent.

- ***Acute stress or trauma*** may trigger the sudden shedding of large numbers of growing or resting hairs.

- In ***anogen effluvium***, thousands of growing hairs suddenly fall out within days, for instance, following a catastrophic accident (e.g., loss of a parent or loved person), toilet training (stressful to toddlers), cancer chemotherapy or radiation therapy and fad diets (low in protein or under 1,000 calories a day). Once the cause is removed, rapid hair regrowth is the rule.

- In ***telogen effluvium***, an exaggerated loss of resting hairs typically occurs when a dramatically shortened growth cycle triggers the simultaneous loss of many resting hairs—for example, a few months after a prolonged fever, a severe viral infection, blood loss, serious depression or exposure to toxic chemicals. The birth of a child can certainly be a powerful enough event to trigger this process. Chemicals and drugs known to trigger exaggerated telogen hair shedding include:
  - strong bleaching agents;
  - some high blood pressure or heart medicines (e.g., propranolol);
  - some metals (e.g., arsenic, lead, mercury, thalium);
  - anticoagulants (e.g., heparin, coumarins);
  - antithyroid agents (e.g., carbimazole, thiouracil).

glands near the follicles. A dog can recognize a human being by the typical scent secreted by these glands. Clusters of tiny muscles, the arrector pili, surround and move the hair follicle. Male hormones (androgens) regulate hair growth in both sexes. Pubic and armpit hair are particularly androgen-sensitive and grow at lower androgen levels than hair on the chest or legs. In boys, most pubic hair is grown by age 15, followed by the development of armpit hair two to three years later. In girls, too, an increase in androgens at puberty triggers growth of pubic and armpit hair. Scalp hair is not directly androgen-responsive, but is influenced by local amounts of a testosterone derivative, dihydrotestosterone.

Hair loss worries both men and women

Progressive hair loss begins naturally in both sexes by about age 50, accelerating in the seventies and eighties. About 40 percent of Caucasian men lose some hair by age 35. Hair shedding in males is often due to androgenetic alopecia—genetic/hormonal or "male pattern" balding. But even extensive hair-thinning rarely becomes obvious until 50 percent of the scalp hair has been lost. Many events other than male-pattern balding can make the hair shed, but only rarely do people lose more than half their hair for these other reasons. Hair may fall out because of overtight hairstyles, some illnesses, or excessive coloring and curling. Hair shedding is often noted up to six months after childbirth, following a prolonged fever, surgery, emotional upset, depression or some other traumatic event. Sudden hair loss—all over the head—can also be provoked by crash diets; thyroid, pituitary or adrenal disease; radiation or chemotherapy (for cancer): fungal or other infections; burns; habitual tugging or compulsive hair-pulling; and exposure to certain chemicals and drugs. Except in male balding, hair lost through injury, illness or stress usually grows back within a few months.

Male pattern baldness is widespread and distressing

While baldness isn't a disease, a cure has been avidly pursued throughout history. In the 20 centuries since Julius Caesar reportedly combed his fast-thinning hair over his bald spot, no effective baldness remedy has yet emerged. For most men, including three million or so bald-domed Canadians, losing hair is a fate to be borne with dignity.

A receding hairline reflects age, but not necessarily great age, since some men start balding quite young. With the spurt in androgen secretion at puberty, the hairline moves back a little in 96 percent of boys and 80 percent of girls. Most boys continue to shed hair as they mature. By age 35 to 40, two-thirds of Caucasian men have some signs of balding. There are several patterns of male-type baldness, but it usually follows a characteristic design, starting at the temples, often combined with a balding spot at the back of the head which gradually spreads, leaving a horseshoe-shaped fringe at the sides. The side fringe rarely disappears altogether. Male-pattern balding goes in waves punctuated by periods of stability. The loss may begin at age 20, then stop, only to start up again a few years later. Since male-pattern baldness is largely hereditary, a man can usually, although not always, predict the extent of his future baldness by examining family portraits.

The rate of male balding speeds up with advancing age, or if there is an inherited tendency to bald early or an overabundance of male hormone within the hair follicles. The hormonal link is complex. Eunuchs, who produce no testosterone, never develop male-pattern baldness—even if they inherit a baldness gene. Studies show that while balding men don't have higher-than-average circulating testosterone levels, they do possess above-average amounts of a powerful testosterone derivative, dihydrotestosterone, in the scalp. The hair follicles convert circulating testosterone into dihydrotestosterone, which produces ever weaker hairs. More and more hairs are shed, as the hairs become thinner and thinner until they are too fine to survive daily wear and tear.

People will go to almost any length to regrow thinning hair, but experts stress that, until now, inherited male-pattern balding hasn't responded to most stimulants, applications, injections or other remedies. Specific foods or vitamins don't regrow hair—although good nutrition is essential for healthy hair. A few hormonal remedies may work temporarily; systemic (oral) steroids induce hair regrowth for as long as they are taken, but the associated risks preclude their use; topical female hormones can regrow hair in balding women but have an anti-androgen effect that may feminize male bodies; spironolactone (Aldactone) may help a few men. If women have an endocrine (hormone) imbalance, vitamin-A acid lotions may have the ability to regrow hair in some.

Do any drugs reverse male-pattern baldness?

A medication called finasteride (Propecia) that has been used to treat enlargement of the male prostate gland has recently shown some promise in slowing hair loss. A pill that is taken daily, it blocks the action of an enzyme that transforms testosterone into the dihydrotestosterone form responsible for triggering hair loss. Clinical trials have shown that finasteride prevented further hair loss (as subjectively observed) in 83 percent of men who took the drug for two years (compared to 28 percent who took a placebo!) and increased objective hair counts (72 percent of the placebo group had less hair at two years compared with 17 percent who took the finasteride). These differences were generally not dramatic.

The drug has to be taken continuously for 3–6 months before any benefit becomes apparent, and effects are reversed 6–12 months after the treatment is discontinued. The two most significant side effects of finasteride have been a slightly decreased sex drive and some erection difficulties (in 1–2 percent of men). When the men stopped taking the drug, sex drive and potency returned fully. Manufacturers stress that Propecia should never be taken by women who are or might become pregnant as it can cause fetal defects.

Topical minoxidil (Rogaine) 2 percent, often combined with spironolactone (an anti-androgen, taken orally), has also been used with some success. The idea of using minoxidil for baldness arose because almost all people taking it for circulatory problems unexpectedly found increased hair growth all over the body, sometimes in embarrassing excess. Enterprising researchers ground up minoxidil tablets, put them into a cream and applied the product to balding scalps. The result was hair regrowth in some. Subsequent studies confirmed that minoxidil (marketed as Regaine or Rogaine), regularly applied in the right concentration (a 1 to 2 percent solution), stimulates hair regrowth on some bald heads. But less than 10 percent of men achieve satisfactory results. Regrowth never exceeds 4 cm (approximately an inch and a half).

In about a third of the men who tried it, minoxidil produced a soft, downy fuzz; in the rest, there was no hair regrowth at all! The disadvantages of minoxidil are its high cost, the fact that it only grows hair for as long as it's applied; its unpredictable success; and the fact that it takes at least eight months of daily application to discover if one is among the lucky few whose hair will grow.

Its side effects include local itching and prickling; headaches (in 40 percent of users); dizzy spells or lightheartedness; and heartbeat irregularities. Although the drug appears to be safe when rubbed into the scalp—since little is absorbed into the bloodstream—it is a vasodilator (it expands blood vessels) and is not recommended for anyone with heart disease. An initial burst of enthusiasm notwithstanding, it seems unlikely that minoxidil will improve the fate of most bald heads.

Decision making about anti-baldness treatments

As with other cosmetic concerns, treating baldness is complex and very subjective. Being bald does not endanger health. Having said this, helping people feel that they are more attractive seems to have an effect on their health. Different cultures, of course, have different views on this. In Argentina, plastic surgery for men or women is quite acceptable to many, whereas in North America (outside of Hollywood) most people see it as inappropriate for men. Men need to consider their bank accounts and timing when considering baldness treatments. For example, a professional male might feel that keeping his hair is of paramount concern and well worth the cost and the hassle. Another individual may feel that the cost, the hassle, the likely results, and the reality that the therapy can't continue forever are reasons not to go ahead.

What about hair transplants?

Surgical hair transplantation with scalp reduction (scalp tightening) can be used to regrow hair in both men and women. The ideal candidates are those with thick hair at the donor site (the area from which the hair is taken). Much like shrubs that have been transplanted—roots and all—bits of growing hair transplanted to the bald parts of the scalp may grow well. Punch-graft surgery is performed in successive sessions, usually four months apart, but sometimes spread over years. The procedure is done by taking two to four mm (about 0.1 in) "plugs" of hair-bearing scalp from the still growing parts and trans-

HAIR CARE ADVICE

- avoid binding hair too often or too tightly in styles such as braids and ponytails;
- don't tease or back-comb it too much;
- comb or brush gently;
- dry at low heat or let hair dry naturally without blow-drying;
- massage scalp to enhance blood flow (unless scalp psoriasis exists, in which case never rub the scalp);
- brush hair gently away from the scalp to sweep the natural oils to the ends;
- use a brush with natural or blunt-edged bristles; jagged sharp bristles can damage the hair.

planting them into small holes bored to receive them. It takes 250 to 400 plugs, with 10 to 15 hairs each, to fill a normally receding hairline. In each surgical session, only 75 to 100 plugs are transplanted, so as not to compromise the scalp's blood supply. The plugs are planted in neat rows, back to front, according to a carefully designed plan. Within a couple of weeks the hairs on the transplanted grafts fall out, but, all being well, regrow in a few months. Postoperative complications are few; pain is controlled by painkillers, bleeding is stopped by pressure and hair can be washed within about a week. It's crucial to plant the plugs in the right direction, to avoid a messy look. If done incorrectly, the transplantee may end up with hair going in all directions. One University of Toronto physician recommends that those contemplating hair replacement avoid being "scalped" by looking at pictures of those already treated by the chosen surgeon, before deciding on a hair transplant. It's wise to choose a physician who regularly does the procedure and has the required dexterity!

Women too may bald

In women, baldness is often diffuse alopecia— with hair loss all over the head, rather than just at the top and center. But it too is usually inherited, with progressive diminution in follicle size, and increasingly fine hair. One Dutch study found that 27 percent of women in their thirties and 64 percent of those between 40 and 70 showed some balding. Hair-thinning in women increases after menopause, when estrogen levels drop off, owing to hormonal imbalance. Other causes include: birth-control pills; certain drugs (e.g., danazol, cimetidine, some beta blockers, chemotherapy for cancer); adrenal or pituitary problems. Treatment for female balding includes estrogen therapy, cyproterone acetate, spironalactone, or minoxidil, and a topical solution of estradiol. But in the words of one dermatologist, "A good wig is often the best choice."

Too much hair can be as embarrassing as too little

For some women, too much hair growing in places that shouldn't be hairy can be as distress-ing a problem as male balding. Hirsutism (excessive hairiness), sometimes inherited, can arise from disease involving overproduction of androgens by the adrenal glands or ovaries. Excess hairiness in prepubescent children or during the menopause requires medical and hormonal assessment to rule out an underlying endocrine (glandular) abnormality. Several remedies are available for mild hair overgrowth. Dark hair can be bleached to make it less obvious. Or hair can be removed by plucking, shaving or rubbing with an abrasive such as pumice stone, without making it grow back faster or more stubbly. Waxing—applying hot wax, allowing it to cool and harden and then stripping it off together with the hair—is best done by a trained cosmetician. Depilatories—chemicals that dissolve excess hair on contact—must be used with care in order not to irritate the skin. (It's wise to test a small patch of skin first to check for sensitivity or allergy to the chemicals.) Electrolysis, the only permanent method of destroying hair follicles by an electric current, is a time-consuming procedure which may cause temporary irritation. It leaves tiny, pit-like scars, and if incompletely done results in regrowth. Newer methods using high-frequency current (electrocoagulation) give good results. A skilled operator can destroy 100 hairs in half an hour. But the process must be repeated frequently.

CHOOSE HAIR-CARE PRODUCTS WISELY

A "good" shampoo leaves hair manageable, easy to comb and glossy. It is untrue that washing hair often makes it oilier. Whether dry or greasy, hair should be washed as often as required to look good (even every day). Most experts recommend washing at least once a week to prevent dandruff. Very dry hair may be improved by massaging with a little olive or almond oil, covering and leaving on overnight, before washing next morning. Despite the exaggerated claims for countless products, studies show little difference between one shampoo and the next. Most contain the same basic ingredients with slightly more or fewer unnecessary extras (perfumes, fruit extracts, protein, herbs). Many modern hair technologists recommend acidic shampoos for all types of hair as they don't aggravate the scalp, which is normally acidic (with a pH of 4.5 to 5.5). Acidic products help to tighten the cuticle scales, keep in moisture and enhance shine. More alkaline types (with a higher pH) that claim to suit oily hair may in fact swell the cuticle, bleach the color and be too drying and overly harsh. Protein shampoos do not repair split ends, and although they may coat the hair shaft, making it smoother they cannot "nourish" hair because their molecules are too large to enter the cortex.

Most modern hair conditioners contain cationic quaternary ammonium compounds, providing a positive charge that reduces static and makes hair less "fly-away." Some products, particularly those containing benzalkonium chloride as the active ingredient, are good conditioners. Those with added polymers, collagen, balsam, silicones or resins that bond with and coat the hair shaft, may provide a protective film and smooth out the cuticle, reducing snarls and tangles. Conditioners that give "extra body" may contain waxes that, when dry, make it look fuller; some contain oils/fats (e.g., lanolin, mineral oil) to smooth hair and a few have humectants that supposedly hold in water. Price and exotic ingredients bear little or no relation to efficacy. As with shampoos, most conditioning products that claim to nourish hair do nothing of the sort, as the ingredients cannot enter the hair unless they contain transformants—molecules small enough to penetrate the cortex.

Permanent-waving solutions open up the hair shaft and rearrange the inner hair molecules, breaking and reforming the sulphur bonds by a process that gives off the familiar sulphide odor. Modern perming solutions (mostly ammonium or sodium sulphite) are more flexible, safer and more controllable than former types. They have a gentler hair-reforming action and can be used on fragile or colored hair. Wound on rollers of varying sizes, hair gets a permanent curl of the desired tightness. The extent of the wave also depends on the kind of hair (finer hair curls faster) and the time the solution stays on. To finish, a neutralizing agent or oxidizer is put on to halt the curling process. The perming action must be stopped at the right time to avoid overprocessing. A perm should never be done on hair dyed with metallic products, and only with

extreme care (with gentler lotions) on hair that's recently been bleached or permanently tinted. Dual processing could disintegrate hair made porous by tinting. Perming after hair coloring requires extreme care—as any trained hairdresser well knows.

Straightening hair uses the same solutions as a perm, but is far harder on hair as it must be constantly pulled straight during the procedure.

Combating dandruff

Although many individuals are plagued by dandruff all year round, dry, cold winter air as well as less sunlight, worsen the problem. Dandruff results from the scalp's normal peeling process, and if it is excessive it may be a form of seborrhea. Large, dry, persistent flakes could be due to psoriasis. Medical studies suggest that dandruff may be linked to the fungus *P. ovale*, which is found on everyone's skin. In dandruff sufferers this fungus may be more abundant. While there are differing viewpoints on whether *P. ovale* is the primary cause of dandruff or merely a secondary infection, most dermatologists agree that it plays some role. Even if *P. ovale* is a cause, other factors also influence the development of dandruff. Special shampoos such as those containing selenium (e.g., Selsun), as well as tar shampoos can help to subdue the flaking. It has recently been shown that an anti-fungal shampoo called ketoconazole (Nizoral) can make a considerable difference for many people. Some dandruff sufferers have to resort to cortisone shampoos. People can apply these shampoos as they need to or twice weekly depending on the severity of their condition.

GETTING RID OF LICE

Despite the best efforts of health authorities, head lice continue to plague human beings, especially school-age children. Getting rid of them is tedious, but new medications and a little understanding of louse biology go a long way in eradicating these unwelcome visitors. Anthropologists report signs of lice in most societies, recording their presence on Egyptian mummies and in ancient Greece. When Thomas à Becket was murdered in Britain's Canterbury Cathedral in 1170, a contemporary wrote that "to the horror and amusement of

SORTING OUT DELOUSING PRODUCTS

• *Permethrin* (Nix)—considered the most effective and safest delousing product—is a chrysanthemum product (rinse) that kills mature lice, eggs and hatching nymphs. (It should not be used for people allergic to ragweed or chrysanthemums.) After the area is shampooed, rinsed and dried, the permethrin solution is applied in sufficient quantities to saturate the area and is left in place for ten minutes before being rinsed off with water.

Although a single treatment is sufficient to kill both the nits and the adult lice, many experts recommend a second treatment 7 to 10 days later as insurance. Unfortunately, there is evidence that lice in the United States are becoming resistant to permethrin.

• *Malathion* (Prioderm), a pesticide rinse that's both a louse and nit (egg) killer, has an unpleasant odor and can inflame the eyes (so is not much used).

• *Lindane (Kwellada) shampoo*, the best known and cheapest on the market, needs a repeat 7 to 10 days after the first delousing shampoo to kill emerging nymphs and new adult insects. Not recommended for children under age four; excess use can cause seizures.

• *Step Two* (Step II), containing *formic acid*, comes with a steel nit-comb; the rinse plus combing may loosen nits, but its usefulness remains unproven.

spectators, the lice boiled over like water in a simmering cauldron," escaping from his thick clothing as his body cooled. Lousiness remained widespread in Europe up to the last century, with even the upper classes so notoriously louse-ridden that some observers wondered whether such a constant parasite might not benefit humankind. Not so: the human body louse carries several diseases, including epidemic typhus and trench fever.

The lice that feed on human blood include the body louse, *Pediculus humanus*; the "crab" louse, *Pediculus humanus pubis*, and the head louse, *Pediculus humanus capitis*.

Body lice live primarily on coarse body hair and hidden in the seams of clothing, especially collars—which makes them very hard to detect. But thanks to improved sanitation, frequent bathing and changing of clothes, body lice are rarely found in our society any more. When seen in Canada, body lice infest mostly the very poor, the homeless and the mentally ill.

Pubic lice (known as "crabs") are still with us, and are transmitted by sexual contact, mainly among adolescents and young adults. They may spread to the beard, mustache, eyelashes and eyebrows. If lice of the pubic variety are found on the eyelashes or eyebrows, petrolatum

(petroleum) jelly may be used to suffocate them (it cuts off their oxygen supply).

Head lice, which infest the scalp and head hair, cause no serious health problems. The human head louse is a grayish-brown, blood-sucking parasite about the size of a sesame seed. Although the term "lousy" conjures up images of filth and outbreaks of lice are commonly greeted with disgust, head lice carry no diseases. Despite popular myths equating lice with uncleanliness, these insects infect clean heads as often as dirty ones. Head lice cannot survive at or below room temperatures but thrive in warm conditions—behind the ears or close to the hairline being cosy spots. A louse-ridden human head may give hospitality to about 24 lice at one time. The mature female louse lays minute, teardrop-shaped, whitish eggs close to the scalp, and they are securely attached to individual hairs by a tough, gluey cement. Popularly called "nits," louse eggs hatch in a week to 10 days, and in another week, when they reach maturity, the reproductive cycle begins again. Once a louse egg hatches, its casing or "nit" is left empty. In contrast to the glistening pearly look of live eggs, nit cases are a dull gray. The duration of a louse infestation can be calculated by observing the distance of the eggs or nits from the scalp surface. Hair grows about five to six mm (0.2 in) a week so any nits found farther than that from the scalp are more than seven days old and have already hatched. Both live and hatched eggs remain so firmly attached to the hair that they're hard to remove by ordinary shampooing.

How head lice spread

Human head lice tend to spread among children crowded together in urban daycare centers and primary schools. The louse has no wings, nor can it jump from host to host. It moves by grasping a shaft of hair with its tiny front claws and swinging from hair to hair, so it can't wander far from the scalp. Lice often travel by direct head-to-head contact (as when children sit or play with their heads close together), or indirectly, via shared items such as hats, coathooks, scarves, bike helmets, headphones, hairbrushes, toys or bedding.

Head lice are more common in girls than boys, although not necessarily more common in

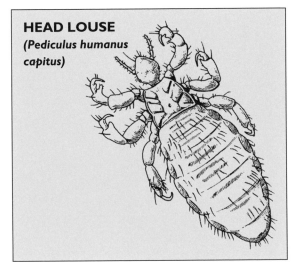

HEAD LOUSE
(Pediculus humanus capitus)

those with long hair. Possibly girls tend to have closer physical contact with each other than boys, making it easier for lice to get around, although boys do switch baseball helmets and other gear. Why lice are uncommon among adolescent boys remains a mystery. Some experts speculate that the male hormones secreted in adolescence may be a louse "turn-off," or that boys have less close physical contact after puberty.

Most large urban schools identify a few children with lice every year. The problem usually surfaces in the early fall when children return to school. Occasionally, a lice epidemic forces a school to close for a couple of days until all the children have been deloused. Health departments and schools are now switching from a "hands-on" head-searching policy to better lice-spotting education for teachers and parents. Each school and education authority sets its own regulations.

How to find head lice

The major sign of head lice is itchiness and scratching, particularly around the hairline and ears. As the itching only starts up a week or two after infestation, there may be no symptoms at first. Some people never feel itchy at all! But scratching may lead to secondary infections, and some louse-ridden people develop scalp scabs and enlarged neck nodes.

Confirmation of head lice means sighting a louse and/or its eggs—just visible to the naked eye. But spotting a louse and detecting the eggs isn't easy, especially on blond hair where they hardly show up at all. Look behind the ears,

close to the scalp, at the back of the neck and top of the head. Parents should check their children from time to time for lice, by parting the hair and examining it in good light, close to the scalp. The best way to see if a child has lice is to look for the eggs: tiny, white, glistening objects (or little gray hatched ones) cemented to the hair shaft, usually close to the scalp. Louse excrement looks like flecks of brown dust. In contrast to nits, dandruff or hair casts (bits of dead hair) are easily dislodged with a fingernail.

The standard treatment for head lice is an extra-thorough hair wash with a medicated, pediculicide (louse-killing) shampoo, or application of an anti-louse lotion once (and possibly again a week later). Effectiveness varies with the product and thoroughness of application. Most shampoos (except for Nix and Prioderm) will not abolish the eggs, and a repeat treatment may be needed. (Nix is a well-recommended cream rinse.) Lindane (Kwellada), an old standby used for 30 years, is primarily a louse-killer and is not as good a nit-killer—it is gradually being replaced by newer products. Some pharmacies store louse-killers behind the counter although no prescription is needed. Once the eggs are dead, they still have to be removed, and they can't just be flicked off. A long-standing infestation with matted hair louse discharge and a scalp infection can make a dreadful mess of hair and take ages to clean up.

"Nit-picking" is usually the worst of a lice problem. Getting rid of all the nits left after a delousing shampoo, by using a fine-toothed metal nit comb or tweezers, is a time-consuming, tedious procedure that can take hours per head, depending on the length of hair and the number of nits. Although nit combs are effective for thick hair they are useless for the very fine hair of a young child. The policy of some schools that children must be free of nits before returning is not based on scientific evidence and should be discouraged. However, if the school insists on this policy, nits can be removed by applying a damp towel to the scalp for 30 to 60 minutes (or by applying a mixture of equal parts water and white vinegar to the scalp, which is then covered with a damp towel soaked in the same material for 15 minutes), followed by combing with a fine-toothed comb. Each egg-

LAYING TO REST SOME LOUSY MYTHS

MYTH: Head lice attack people of poor social standing.
FACT: No! Head lice indiscriminately infest all levels of society.
MYTH: Head lice only infect unhygienic people.
FACT: No! Lice feed equally well on blood from dirty, clean, short- or long-haired human scalps.
MYTH: People often get head lice from animals.
FACT: No! Human head lice do not live on other animals— you can't catch them from a dog, cat, hamster or other pet.
MYTH: People who get head lice should have their heads shaved.
FACT: No! While shaving the head may help in getting rid of lice, it is need-lessly drastic. Several medications can now safely remove head lice.
MYTH: Once treated, head lice never return.
FACT: No! Repeat infestations can occur; no available treatment prevents reinfestation.

PREVENTIVE ANTI-LOUSE STRATEGIES

- **Teach children not to share hats, headphones, combs, brushes or bicycle helmets, and to report any head itching.**
- **Check children's hair regularly for tell-tale signs of nits and lice, especially if a child is scratching a lot.**
- **Wash all clothing and sheets in use at the time of a louse outbreak in very hot water (above 55°C or 130°F) and dry in a hot dryer for 20 minutes at least. (Lice and their eggs are** killed by high temperatures.)
- **Recently used clothing, such as shoes, that are difficult to wash can simply be stored for 24 hours, as head lice can only live 15-20 hours away from their host..**
- **Alternatively, coats, hats and clothing can be left outside all day or overnight in winter (the cold kills lice and eggs), or put into a plastic bag and left overnight in the freezer.**
- **Soak all brushes and combs in hot water** containing pediculicidal shampoo or 2 percent Lysol solution for a couple of hours.
- **Vacuum items such as rugs, furniture, mattresses and pillows thoroughly; don't forget the car seats. Public health authorities agree that there's no need to fumigate.**
- **Certain anti-louse sprays can also be used on furniture, pillows and mattresses.**
- **Report lice in schoolchildren to the school nurse or principal.**

bearing hair can be cut out with scissors, or one may end up using the fingernails! A short haircut may make nit removal less time-consuming, but stigmatizes children. If someone in the family has lice, check all parts of the head on all the rest of the household members.

HAND AND NAIL CARE TIPS

- **Use cotton-lined, vinyl gloves for wet work, but remove them frequently to let hands air out.**
- **Apply hand creams frequently (e.g., Aquatain, Prevex, Glyzerone, Lachydrin, urea-containing types or any chosen moisturizer) after washing.**
- **Try cool compresses to soothe irritated hands.**
- **Use steroid creams prescribed by a physician (eg., Betnovate,** Halog) for badly cracked or inflamed hands.
- **Use nail clippers to remove rough edges of nails, instead of nibbling.**
- **File rather than cut the nails, don't push the cuticle too far back, and use a flat wooden stick or a piece of terrycloth rather than a metal file—it's less damaging.**
- **When applying nail polish, keep the polish and its vapors** away from the face.
- **Remove polish from nails with as little remover as possible.**
- **Yellowing or brittle nails may need a "polish-holiday" for a week or two.**
- **Try to avoid skin contact with polish or removers; use cotton swabs to remove polish; never dip the fingers into the remover.**
- **After using nail-polish remover, wash the nails and massage in cream.**

All household members with signs of infestation should be treated for lice at the same time. People who've had lice must be rechecked once a week for signs of lingering lice for several weeks.

HAND AND NAIL CARE
Dry, cracked, chapped hands are particularly common among mechanics, outdoor workers, cleaning personnel, nurses, surgeons, those who do housework and anyone whose hands are often wet and cold. Since hand irritation may be due to skin diseases such as psoriasis, herpes, contact dermatitis, impetigo or other disorders, it's wise to seek medical advice before assuming that everyday chores are to blame!

The best way to avoid chapped hands is to keep hands well dried and protected from the cold and wind, to wear pure cotton or cotton-lined vinyl gloves for wet work (rubber can cause allergies) and to frequently apply creams to moist skin. (Remove gloves often to air out the hands.) Dry, brittle nails that easily break are another common wintertime problem, but can also be due to illness, or exposure to chemicals, strong detergents or nail-polish removers. Soaking brittle nails in warm water for a few minutes and then applying olive oil or petrolatum (petroleum) jelly at night can strengthen them and make them more flexible.

Most special nail creams are no better than ordinary moisturizers. Nail hardeners will harden the nails, but may provoke a condition where the nail plate lifts from the nail bed. They can also discolor the nails or cause bleeding under them, so they should be used with caution. The adhesives used to apply artificial nails can cause allergic reactions. Contrary to folklore, gelatin usually does nothing for dry or brittle nails, unless the person is suffering from a protein deficiency, in which case it will take three to six months to get noticeable results!

FOOT CARE
Although most of us pitifully neglect our feet, those hard-working extremities deserve the very best of care. Most of us abuse these precious appendages that support and propel us, allow us to jump, dance and play sports, and, in an average lifetime, carry us some 160,000 km

or 100,000 miles, or several times around the world.

Beautiful is not an apt word for most feet, which are often better described as knobbly, gnarled, callused or deformed. The deformities could be avoided by better attention to a good shoe fit! Despite their importance to our everyday movement, few of us lavish on our feet the care we give our face and hands. One doctor notes wryly that when asked to undress for an examination many "remove everything except their shoes and socks!" Taking their feet for granted, or being ashamed of them, people imagine they need no attention. Similarly, some physicians ignore foot problems and omit foot examinations during a checkup visit. However, even a seemingly insignificant foot ailment—an ingrown nail, an infected corn—can completely immobilize someone!

Foot problems arise from inherited tendencies, biomechanical factors, infections and systemic (general) diseases. The more vigorously feet are used, the greater the likelihood of foot problems. Athletes, soldiers and dancers are among those with the worst foot trouble. "Ballet dancers have the world's worst feet," comments one foot doctor "Their feet take an awful beating with bruises, toe fractures, tarsal inflammation and soft corns."

The penalties of ill-fitting shoes and foot fetishism

Although many foot deformities are due to an inherited predisposition, they are greatly aggravated by ill-fitting shoes. Many shoes not only fail to provide enough support but disfigure feet by deforming toe joints and distorting the gait. Most of us pay too little heed to shoe buying. Even with today's emphasis on fitness, and the helpful acceptance of "running shoes for every occasion," many female shoe fashions seem tailor-made for foot torture.

Shoe fetishism and foot-eroticism are still with us. Women who want to look "smart" may wear strappy, tight, uncomfortable, narrow, dangerously high-heeled contraptions in leather canvas and lucite created neither for comfort nor for sensible walking.

The most mutilating of foot fashions was Chinese footbinding, which stunted a baby girl's

---

FOOT SPECIALISTS

Family physicians can advise on or treat most foot problems, but for more complex disorders, specialists are needed. The providers of specialized foot care in Canada are orthopedic surgeons, dermatologists, chiropodists and podiatrists. Any major foot surgery comes under the domain of orthopedic surgeons, who specialize in bone and joint problems. For serious skin problems of the feet a dermatologist should be consulted.

Podiatrists are excellent for general foot care. They are not physicians but DPMs, holding degrees in podiatric medicine, with several years of specialized training in a podiatry school. Using modern biomechanical analysis, podiatrists can identify specific foot faults and design tailor-made orthotic devices and supports that go inside shoes. Orthotics counteract underlying foot or postural faults and can compensate for a deformity, keeping people as mobile as possible. Although regulations vary, podiatrists in the United States and some parts of Canada are not only licenced to treat all foot ailments but also to do minor surgery, such as correcting a hammer toe, or some bunion removals, under local anesthesia. Podiatrists' fees are partly covered by many health insurance plans.

Chiropodists, have less training and do not do surgery, but they will often remove infected toenails, and are a great help with foot care in hospitals and clinics, interacting with physicians, orthopedic surgeons and rheumatologists.

Many chronic diseases such as arthritis and diabetes have a significant foot care component to them. The prevention of these foot problems in people with diabetes or poor blood flow can decrease rates of amputation significantly. Referral by a physician is not necessary to see a chiropodist, but care of the feet is not usually covered by health insurance plans. Good foot care by any one of the above specialists is especially helpful in looking after seniors' feet.

---

foot by bending the bones, to produce a woman with tiny "lily feet" barely able to hobble. This ancient custom supposedly started with a Chinese empress who had been born club-footed. To disguise the royal impediment, the court ladies bandaged their feet, establishing a norm for upper-caste Chinese women. And the practice, which lasted almost into this century, guaranteed they wouldn't marry below their class, as they couldn't walk without the help of servants. Although her toes might be hideously bent, a Chinese bride's tiny shoe was exhibited as proof of her worth. Foot fetishism also exists in other cultures. Ancient Jewish dress included heavy ankle bells that forced women to take tiny, mincing steps; the tinkle of bells beneath bulky skirts was supposed to act as a powerful male aphrodisiac. The wives of some African chiefs are still laden with iron leg chains reducing their gait to a slow waddle.

The high-heeled pump, most damaging of today's styles, was introduced by King Louis XIV's cobbler as an ingenious ploy to make the short monarch look taller. Foot doctors call high-heeled shoes "human leg corruptors"—forcing women to take twice the normal number of steps and teeter precariously rather than walk as nature intended them to. High-heeled shoes, especially those that are too short or have pointed toes, push the big toe toward the other toes, creating excess pressure on the joint that joins the big toe to the foot—perhaps even dislocating it—with a consequent buildup of tissue and fluid to produce bunions. A very pointed shoe warps and bends the toes into the shape of a claw, deforming them into "hammer-toes." The vamp (top) of a high-heeled shoe may irritate and inflame tissues; a too-shallow heel can create pump bumps—bony out-growths at the heel. The posture produced by high-heeled shoes can overarch the spine, contributing to back problems. But the greatest strain in high-heeled footwear is taken by the ankles, which thicken, and by the calf muscles, which shorten. Continual wearing of high heels can alter the calf muscle so much that some women no longer feel comfortable in flat-heeled shoes. Women accustomed to high heels should not change abruptly to flats—this can strain the leg muscles.

How to buy shoes wisely

The cardinal rule in shoe-buying is to sacrifice fashion for foot health whenever possible. Shoes should be wide enough in front not to cramp the toes, with room for air to circulate, and long enough. Some experts suggest that shoes should be a thumb-width longer than the big toe (to give adequate room and prevent toes banging the end of shoes). Test new shoes by walking around for five to ten minutes in the store before buying to be sure the fit is right. The best time to buy shoes is in the afternoon, when feet may have swelled up—even by half a size—from the day's activities. Most people have one foot larger than the other, so get both feet measured while standing, and choose a size that fits the larger foot. As to material—leather is great: calf-skin is pliable and keeps its shape well so it's probably the best shoe leather. Kid stretches,

and pigskin cracks when wetted and then dried. Rubber or plastic shoes are not porous and are apt to cause perspiration—which may foster maceration (wet, irritated skin). It's essential to change shoes (and socks) frequently. A visit to a specialized running shoe store can help. Individual brands are best for certain types of feet and uses. Often the salespeople in these stores have the training to match a brand with your type of foot.

Aging feet need vigilant care

Older people, who are more prone to circulatory problems and infections, should take good care of their feet and have foot problems checked by a professional. Nails, corns and calluses may best be trimmed by a specialist. Foot problems in the elderly cause much discomfort and immobility. The skin may be thin and sensitive and need cushioning in fleecy slippers. Nails may become dry and thick, requiring good moisturizing and specialized trimming. The elderly may find footcare difficult owing to arthritis, frailty or other infirmities. People with diseases such as arthritis, gout and circulatory problems must be particularly watchful about good foot care and look after their feet well. Proper shoe fitting and frequent changes of footwear and stockings are essential.

Diabetics must practice special foot care, and avoid shoes that irritate pressure points. Foot problems that would be minor in nondiabetics can quickly become dangerous in diabetics, so they should always consider getting professional foot care. A loss of nerve sensation may desensitize diabetic feet, allowing them to be injured without this being noticed. A foot ulcer or infected sore can develop without being felt, so diabetics should examine their feet every day for signs of trouble. Restricted blood circulation makes diabetic feet prone to ulcers that could be catastrophic if they develop gangrene. Because of reduced sensitivity to hot and cold, diabetics should avoid overheated baths, not sit too close to fires or heaters, switch off bed heaters on retiring, use no bed-socks unless loose and dry their feet well before putting on socks and shoes. (See also chapter 16, section on diabetes.)

BANISHING WARTS

Warts are due to transmissible viruses. They can occur at any age but are especially prevalent among children aged 12 to 16—perhaps because of their intimacy and the frequency of open scrapes and scratches through which wart infections gain entry. One British study found that about 16 percent of teenagers had warts on the hands, feet or face. These somewhat distasteful, flesh-colored skin protrusions appear on the fingers, face, feet or other parts of the body, including the genitals (where they may be tiny, flat and almost invisible). Some warts persist for years but should nonetheless be investigated as they can spread, even if not especially uncomfortable or unsightly.

While most warts are harmless and reasonably inconspicuous, some become exceptionally big, growing several centimeters (an inch or so) across. On a prominent part of the body such as the face, they present a cosmetic problem. On the soles of the feet, warts can make walking painful. Venereal or genital warts may lead to cervical cancer in women. They should be removed in either sex, and the sex partner should also be checked for warts.

Viruses cause warts—so most are contagious

Warts are due to viruses known as papilloma viruses. About 50 different subtypes of the human papilloma virus (HPV) family have now been identified, and are responsible for warts at specific body sites. Quite contagious, these viruses can be transferred from one body part to another—say, from hands to feet or face—or from person to person. One can pick up wart viruses from damp towels touched by an infected person or from the floors of changing rooms or showers. Genital warts are spread by sexual contact. Nasal wart viruses can be passed among cocaine users who snort the drug through shared holders.

There may be a time lag or "incubation period" of two to three months between the time of exposure, when the viruses enter the skin, and the time the wart is seen on the skin. Most warts are small, but get larger over a few weeks to months, sometimes becoming flecked with little black spots. If scraped, they may bleed in pinpoint flecks. The wart virus concentration in an infected area is greatest 6 to 12 months after infection, gradually declining thereafter, so that warts usually disappear on their own after a few months to a couple of years.

Many wart "cures" claim to take 12 weeks—a time span within which some warts would disappear without any treatment. But warts can persist stubbornly despite all efforts to obliterate them. How and why some warts regress but others don't isn't known. Possibly the body's immune defenses fight off the infection. Some wart treatments work by irritating the warts slightly so that they release wart antigen (active ingredient) into the blood, stimulating an immune response.

Wart cures old and new

Warts often persist because of low immune defenses. The variety of wart remedies demonstrates the difficulty of ridding the body of this stubborn viral nuisance. Wart cures, charms, incantations and spells date back to antiquity— "I ficky ficky thee" is one ancient charm—and some cures promoted magical transference of the wart to something or someone else. For instance, Sir Francis Bacon, the sixteenth-century scientist, rubbed warts with pork fat which he then hung out in the sun, hoping that his warts would disappear as the fat melted. In some parts of Britain, warts are still said to be removed by applying cow dung or rubbing the wart with a fresh potato and then throwing it away. In the western United States, folklore promotes rubbing warts with a coin and then throwing away the coin. In other parts of the world, warts are said to be abolished by rubbing them onto the father of an illegitimate child. The reputed success of some bizarre wart cures may rest more on the tendency of warts to clear up on their own rather than on any real efficacy. Since many of the lesions resolve spontaneously, no treatment is often the preferred choice.

Cryotherapy, or freezing treatment, may require repeat treatments every two to three weeks until the lesions resolve. Liquid nitrogen is preferred, as other methods may not reach cold enough temperatures. Hyperkeratotic (overgrown) lesions should be pared prior to

A RUNDOWN OF SOME COMMON WARTS

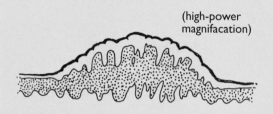

(high-power
magnifacation)

Common warts occur on hands, fingers, face.

Common warts (Verruca vulgaris)

These solitary, raised, "spiky" bumps may grow larger over a few weeks, developing deep, scaly furrows of keratin (a hard protein). They bleed in pinpoint spots when pared or cut. Common warts may occur singly or in groups anywhere on the body, especially on hands, fingers and face—typically on children's hands. Regular treatment with over-the-counter peeling agents (such as salicylic acid and lactic acid in a collodion base) often succeeds in removing common warts, especially if applied after a good wash with soap and water and gentle abrasion with an emery board or callus-file (see "Modern wart treatments").

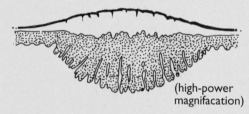

(high-power
magnifacation)

Plantar warts occur on sole (plantar region).

Plantar warts

These foot warts are more common in adults than children. They are stubborn, long-living, deep-rooted, sometimes painful warts on the soles (plantar regions) of the feet. Under the constant pressure of walking they tend to flatten out or be pushed inwards into the foot, becoming very difficult to eradicate. Mosaic plantar warts are made up of several warts amalgamated together, producing large warts that are hard to eradicate. To distinguish an ordinary foot callus (skin thickening) from a plantar wart, the medical test is what happens on cutting or paring the skin: a wart has tiny bleeding points, a callus doesn't usually bleed.

Treatment of plantar warts is usually with a salicylic acid paint, cryotherapy (liquid nitrogen freezing) or lasers. Surgery, X-ray therapy and electrocautery (burning) are not recommended for foot warts, particularly if they occur on weight-bearing surfaces, because of the danger of scarring and permanent discomfort. Gentle planing with an emery board may be all that's needed until they disappear on their own. Foot warts are better left alone than treated harshly, which may irritate the walking surface. A scar on the foot due to rough treatment can end up being a lifetime nuisance—more painful than the wart it was meant to eradicate.

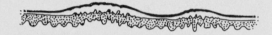

Plane or flat warts

Plain or flat warts

Affecting adults and children, these tiny, flat, flesh-colored or brownish warts usually appear on the face, arms, hands or neck, or occasionally around the eyes. Localized, single flat warts are probably best left alone. Strong wart remedies should never be used on the face as they can cause lasting scars. Multiple severe, flat warts often respond to liquid nitrogen freezing or use of prescribed vitamin A (retinoid) creams that cause superficial peeling. Treatment may trigger the immune system into action by releasing a little wart antigen.

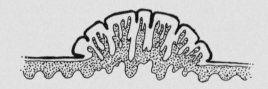

Genital warts:
On females: occur on vulva, cervix, anus
On males: occur on penis and anus

Genital warts (Condyloma acuminata)

The former Greek term for wart, *condyloma*, is now reserved exclusively for genital warts, which occur around the anus and on the penis, vagina, vulva and cervix. They are increasingly common in Canada, both in women and in men. These warts, spread by sexual contact, are often flat, tiny and difficult to spot and diagnose. About two-thirds of women and one-third of men with genital warts also have signs of other sexually transmitted diseases such as chlamydia, gonorrhea or syphilis. There is mounting evidence that certain genital warts may trigger cancer of the cervix in women and, although rare, cancer of the penis in men. (See also chapter 8, section on cervical cancer.)

freezing. For common and hand warts, a single freeze-thaw cycle lasting 5 to 30 seconds with white margins extending 1 to 3 mm beyond the lesion is usually adequate. Plantar warts may respond better to two cycles. Cryotherapy is painful and may cause blistering, but is unlikely to scar.

Modern wart treatments

Salicylic acid is the first line of attack, successful in 80 percent of common warts. Used regularly, salicylic acid will often cure common warts on the hands and feet within 10 to 12 weeks. It can eradicate flat warts, and small foot warts. Salicylic acid is marketed in a collodion base that hardens and covers the area to be peeled. As a solution or paste it is applied nightly from a dropper, or as a plaster (a stronger form). Since these solutions can not only destroy the wart but also damage the surrounding skin, they must not be overlavishly splashed on, but put strictly on the wart, with a toothpick, match or cuticle stick (many supplied applicators are too large). Some physicians will apply Vaseline around the wart to prevent damage of the surrounding area. Wart paints are most effective if applied after the wart has been soaked in water and gently rubbed with a pumice stone or emery board to remove the loose top skin layer, allowing the solution better entry. If the skin gets rough, cracked or painful, salicylic acid treatment should be stopped for a day or two until the skin heals.

Treatments should be repeated every 24 to 48 hours until the skin lines can be seen over the base of the lesion. Examples of the many available products are salicylic acid 17 percent (Compound W gel), salicylic acid 20 percent (Compound W liquid), salicylic acid 30 percent (Compound W plus), salicylic acid 16.7 percent and lactic acid 16.7 percent (Duofilm liquid), and salicylic acid 27 percent (Duoforte 27). Salicylic acid compounds specifically formulated for plantar warts include 40 percent salicylic acid disks and plasters (Carnation Callous and Corn Caps, Clear Away Plantar Wart Remover, Scholl Corn Removers), and salicylic acid 25 percent, lactic acid 10 percent, and formalin 5 percent (Duoplant). Disks or plasters should be purchased or cut to fit the lesion exactly so that normal surrounding skin is not affected. The plaster should then be applied and covered with waterproof tape.

Cryotherapy or freezing (with liquid nitrogen) is typically done at the clinic every 2–3 weeks. Full removal can take weeks to months but for common and hand warts a single freeze-thaw cycle lasting 5 to 30 seconds with white margins (which can sting slightly) extending 1 to 3 mm beyond the lesion is usually adequate. Occasionally, the skin blisters. If too long a gap intervenes between freezings, the warts may regenerate. Done correctly it should not leave scars. It is often the treatment of choice and can be safely used during pregnancy. Plantar warts may respond better to two cycles.

Other wart cures

- *Cantharidin*, available only by prescription, is a mitochondrial cell poison that causes cell membranes to break down and form blisters, getting rid of some especially resistant warts around the nail and other areas, usually without scarring. It should be used with extreme caution, especially in children, and not on the face as it can damage the delicate membranes of nose, mouth and eyes.
- *Duct tape* may also be effective and is cheap and painless. In children, the process of covering the wart with duct tape, wearing it continuously for six days, removing it, soaking and buffing the lesion on the evening of sixth day, reapplying the duct tape the next morning, leaving it on for another six days, and repeating the process for two months may be as or more effective than lightly applied cryotherapy. The acceptability of this treatment may depend on the site of the wart and the families fondness for home improvement.
- *Enucleation* (blunt paring) to remove bulk may be useful for resistant plantar (foot) and other warts, to get rid of a big wart, but needs great care on pressure-bearing surfaces and remains a controversial method.
- *Interferon* and other immune-system stimulants, given systematically, have been tried for difficult warts with good reported cure rates. However, the cost and the risk of skin reactions and other side effects limit their usefulness.

- *Electrocautery* is sometimes used, under local anesthetic, to burn off large warts—but never on the feet. It has had poor results.
- *Laser treatment* is highly successful in eradicating genital and common warts, sometimes as an adjunct to other wart remedies but not on weight-bearing surfaces, as it can produce a painful scar.
- *Surgery* isn't encouraged for treating warts, particularly since the wart virus may spread around the cutting area, leading to recurrence. Surgery may leave a lasting scar or painful lump, particularly uncomfortable on the foot. It's not safe to pare off warts with a razor!

Genital warts can be removed by:

- *Podophyllin*, a natural extract of plants such as the wild flower may apple, arrests cell division and is used in a 25–50 percent solution. Petroleum jelly is put onto the surrounding skin to protect it from the solution, which is precisely painted onto the wart once a week, left on two to six hours, then washed off. As treatment proceeds, podophyllin solution may be left on for progressively longer periods, but some blistering may occur and occasionally severe swelling and inflammation if too much is used. Podophyllin should not be used in pregnant women because it affects fetal development; nor should it be put on the vagina because it can be absorbed into the bloodstream causing vomiting and nausea. Self-treatment is not recommended. If four to six podophyllin treatments fail to get rid of genital warts, other methods such as freezing with liquid nitrogen, laser treatment or electrocautery may be tried. (A biopsy is recommended before starting treatment to check for cancer-causing viral strains.) New forms can be applied by patients themselves.
- *Trichloracetic acid treatment* may help to remove genital warts.
- *Cryotherapy or freezing* is a popular, easy way to remove genital warts. Multiple freezing sessions may be needed, and there is occasionally some local discomfort, although the genital area generally heals easily and fast.
- *Electrocautery* can be useful in removing large areas of genital wart infection, leaving little or no scarring in this area.
- *Laser treatment* is increasingly used to remove genital warts that resist other treatment.
- *Fluorouracil cream* (containing an anti-cancer drug which blocks cell division) is a "last-ditch" method occasionally used for widespread, stubborn genital warts in women, but requires great care.
- *A new therapy is the application three times a week of 5 percent Imiquimod* (Aldara™) cream. In one trial, this immunomodulator cleared lesions in 50 percent of patients who used it three times a week for up to sixteen weeks.

Eye, ear and tooth care

Eye care • Ear care • Ear infections • Tooth and gum care

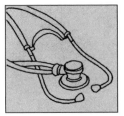

6

EYE CARE

The eyes, said to be "the windows of the soul," can relay clear or blurred images; they may be sparkling or dull, perhaps discolored, red, itchy, squinting or teary, thereby sometimes being a "window on disease." Eyes are sensory organs that give human beings vital information about the world around them. They need to be kept clean and in good working order. Any vision blurring, soreness, redness or other eye problems should receive prompt medical attention in order not to damage these most precious windows on the world.

Eye tests: for whom, when?

Routine eye tests should start in childhood—within the first year of life for conditions such as strabismus (lazy eye), again at age two or three and another upon entering school, at age six or seven. The eyes should be rechecked at age ten or eleven, and again in older teenagers, then periodically through adulthood and annually after age 65.

ANATOMY OF THE HEALTHY EYE

- Retina
- Optic nerve
- Eyeball filled with (clear) aqueous humor
- Lens
- Trabecular meshwork (fluid drainage)
- Iris (colored part)
- Pupil (opening in iris)
- Cornea (transparent "refractive" covering)

The eye functions like a camera. The front is covered by transparent tissue, the cornea. The colored iris opens and closes, like the diaphragm of a camera, controlling the amount of light that enters through the pupil (opening). The lens focuses light onto the retina, which registers images, much like the film in a camera. The retina also contains cells that are sensitive to color. The visual messages go from the retina via the optic nerve to the brain, where they are interpreted.

The front part of the eyeball is full of liquid, the aqueous humor, which carries nutrients to the eye tissues. The aqueous humor has been called "clear blood"—a transparent transport medium. (Obviously it wouldn't be useful to have an eye full of obscuring red blood.) In order for the nerves and other fragile structures within the eye to function properly, the aqueous humor is kept fresh and at constant pressure by fluid inflow from the ciliary body and constant outflow or drainage through the trabecular meshwork.

EYE-CARE SPECIALISTS

Ophthalmologists are physicians who specialize in medical and surgical eye care. In addition to testing vision and prescribing corrective glasses, they diagnose and treat eye disorders, also doing eye surgery for eye disorders when needed. They are graduates of medical schooland are typically consulted when there is a problem. *Optometrists* diagnose, manage, and treat some eye conditions and are licensed to do vision tests, prescribe corrective lenses and fit contact lenses. Although not medically qualified, they have completed a three-year university science course plus a four-year program in optometry. They are excellent at providing basic eye care and can refer you on to an ophthalmologist if there is a concern. *Opticians* are technicians who fill prescriptions for eyeglasses or contact lenses; they are not permitted to test vision or treat eye problems.

Vision is tested by the familiar Snellen chart, with the big E at the top and increasingly small letters below, measuring the ability to see at a distance. A visual acuity of 20/20 means someone can see at 20 feet (6 m) what others with normal vision also see at 20 feet; 20/50 vision is less acute—the ability to see at 20 feet what those with normal sight can see at 50 feet (15 m)—and so on. Other tests assess visual field (side vision), eye-muscle function, intraocular (eyeball) pressure, and the condition of the lens and retina (using an ophthalmoscope) and the cornea (using a slit lamp).

Some diseases that are not ordinarily associated with eye problems do endanger the eyes. For example, 50 percent of diabetics are at risk of eye disorders such as cataracts, glaucoma and retinopathy (retina damaged by flawed blood vessels). People with high blood pressure are also at risk for retinopathy. Rheumatoid arthritis sufferers often develop "dry eye," and people with thyroid disease may have that too, and other ocular symptoms.

Eye-focusing problems

The most common eye trouble that plagues people is faulty eye focusing—refractive errors that occur because light entering the eye isn't precisely focused on the retina by the optic lens and cornea.

In myopia (nearsightedness) nearby objects appear clear and distant ones look fuzzy or blurred. With hyperopia (farsightedness), closeup vision is hazy and distant objects are more clearly seen. Astigmatism is a distortion in the curvature of the cornea or lens. Presbyopia is an impaired ability to focus up close—a problem common in older people. Fortunately, most focusing problems can be remedied simply with corrective lenses.

Refractive laser surgery for myopia removes need for glasses

Quick, relatively painless and increasingly popular, excimer laser surgery can alter the eye's refraction (focusing power) and correct myopia or shortsightedness by changing the cornea's curvature. PRK or "photorefractive keratectomy," suitable for mild to moderate myopia, uses the laser to shave some tissue from the cornea, shaping it to the desired power. The person is left with a large "abrasion" on the cornea. This can cause some haziness in vision as well as some tearing and pain. The eye heals very quickly and so, with the help of a disposable bandage contact lens, such symptoms typically disappear in a few days. Some people experience a surface haze that clouds vision afterwards, but this usually clears within three months. However, post-PRK haze can persist (in about 1 percent of cases), requiring more laser treatment, and some will continue to experience night-time glare. The newer LASIK (laser-assisted in situ keratomileusis) technique, introduced to Canada in 1990, "flaps" back the cornea's top surface with a motorized blade, reshapes the layer beneath to the desired power, then repositions the flap. LASIK can correct more severe myopia, gives immediate, nonhazy vision and less post-operative discomfort than PRK, but is trickier to do, requires greater skill and can produce more serious complications.

PRK and LASIK are outpatient procedures that take only a few minutes to perform. A suitable candidate should be about 18 years of age, in good health, with a stable refractive error. Contraindications are cataract, herpes simplex, retinal disease, diabetic retinopathy, glaucoma and pregnancy. Different surgical techniques are used for people with higher degrees of myopia or hyperopia. In Phakic IOL a lens is inserted into the anterior chamber attached to the iris. In ICL, a soft lens is placed behind the iris and in front of the crytalline lens. Accommodation is preserved and the procedure is highly reversible. However, patients with large pupils and/or shallow anterior chambers are contraindicated.

Contact lenses

Contact lenses are thin plastic (or occasionally silicone) discs, made to prescription, that float on the tears on top of the cornea—the eye's transparent outer covering. The surface layer of oil and tears holds them in place. A good contact lens allows the cornea to breathe (get oxygen) by gas exchange under the lens, or through gas-permeable material. Contact lenses require more care than ordinary eyeglasses because they touch the eyes and transfer onto them whatever is on them—such as pollen, dust or bacteria—possibly causing an infection. Contacts must be kept scrupulously clean with the recommended disinfectant fluids. They are particularly suitable for myopic (nearsighted) eyes. Many people find contacts comfortable, unobtrusive and infinitely preferable to glasses. But not everyone can wear them. Some eyes become irritated by contact lenses. Even satisfied everyday contact lens wearers need a pair of prescription glasses as a standby in case of eye irritation.

Contact lenses now come as soft or rigid (gas-permeable) types, available as either disposable or extended-wear forms (these can be left in overnight, some even up to a week). Hard contact lenses, the first type on the market, have been replaced by gas-permeable forms with superior oxygen permeability. Gas-permeable forms provide better correction for astigmatism than soft contacts, and generally better vision correction, but it takes a few weeks to get used to them.

Approximately 1 out of every 20 contact lens wearers develops a contact lens–related complication each year. Complications range from mild to sight-threatening and can involve the lids, conjunctiva or cornea. Therefore, contact lens wearers need frequent medical eye check-ups.

Soft contact lenses, made of water-absorbing plastics, let oxygen through and are usually comfortable to wear and nonirritating from day one. They are unlikely to be dislodged when playing sports, but they are less durable than rigid types and rip easily. They require meticulous cleaning, overnight disinfectant soaks and are ruined if allowed to dry out. They must always be cleaned with appropriate disinfectant, not with tap water or saline (even if they fall out!) and must *always* be removed at night.

Disposable soft contact lenses are worn for two weeks, then discarded and replaced by a new pair (The latest daily wear forms are worn just for a few days, then discarded.) They are very thin and comfortable to wear reduce the risks of infection and need no special cleaning other than being kept in disinfectant fluid when not worn. Some of the newest soft contacts have built-in ultraviolet protection.

Contact lens care takes time, and it means stocking up on the necessary cleaning solutions and being sure to wash the hands before putting in or removing the lens and before applying eye cosmetics. Wearers shouldn't use old—likely contaminated—eye makeup, or share eye makeup. All contact lens wearers should have a backup pair of regular prescription eyeglasses to wear in case of eye infection or fatigue, and when suffering from a cold, as the contact lens can get coated with secretions, increasing risks of infection and corneal ulceration. As contact lens use increases infection risks, wearers should keep an eye out for and stop wearing them at any hint of infection—such as redness, pain, sticky secretions, blurred vision or light sensitivity.

Sunglasses

Sunglasses are not mere fashion accessories, They prevent eye damage from excess UV light, block glare and are especially helpful when driving, boating, skiing or on the beach. Those who use prescription glasses should have one pair with good-quality tinted lenses. The darkest glasses are not necessarily the best UV blockers. Unless they have a coating that blocks out light in the 290–400 nanometer range, UV rays can still penetrate and harm the eyes. Good dark lenses are usually amber or brown, not purple or gray. Check the labels on sunglasses; look for the proportion of UV-blockage provided. General-purpose dark glasses should screen out 95 percent of UVB (short-wave ultraviolet rays) and 60 percent of UVA (longer-wave UV), and are fine for recreation such as tennis, hiking, skating or everyday boating. Special-purpose sunglasses, recommended for bright situations such as skiing, mountain-climbing and sunny beaches, block 99 percent of UVB and at least 70 percent of UVA, as well as 70 percent of visible light. If the UV-blocking capacity is not marked on the glasses, check with the manufacturer to see how much protection is provided. Never wear dark glasses at night as they compromise vision.

Pay attention to aging eyes

As the eyes age, they undergo normal changes in structure and function that reduce their efficiency. For example, with age the lens loses flexibility, making it harder to focus on nearby

EYEDROPS—CAUTION NEEDED

Most topical eyedrops or ointments tend to concentrate in the eye without getting into the bloodstream and causing side effects. However, some drops affect parts of the body far from the eyes—such as glaucoma medications, which can alter the heart rate and aggravate asthma. Always report any symptoms to the doctor, even if they don't seem related to the eye medication; also report any eye drops used when being medically checked for other problems. Never use someone else's drops; always check expiry date.

SIGNS AND SYMPTOMS OF EYE TROUBLE

- **Eye dryness (grittiness, feeling of "something in the eye");**
- **red or painful eyes;**
- **photophobia (discomfort in bright light);**
- **sudden change(s) in visual function (such as blurriness, decreased side vision);**
- **excess eye secretions, a sticky discharge;**
- **eye swelling and itchiness.**
- **flashing lights**

A RUNDOWN ON SOME COMMON EYE DISORDERS

Dry eye Related to the withering of the lacrimal (tear) glands, this condition predisposes the eyes to infection. True dry eye, or Sjögrens syndrome, is an autoimmune disease—also accompanied by an unpleasantly dry mouth and dry mucous membranes. Lubricating fluids and "artificial tears" can relieve the condition.

Allergies Sensitivity to grass, pollen, animal hair, pollutants or smoke may cause red, burning, tearing, itchy, swollen eyes and eyelids. In addition many soaps, shampoos, perfumes and preservatives, even some contact lens solutions (notably thimerosal), can cause eye sensitivity. To relieve the problem, try cold compresses and/or decongestants and antihistamine eyedrops such as Livostin or Acular. Cromolyn sodium is an alternative eyedrop which, although immediately effective for some, may take days to weeks to work in others. (Remember that eyedrops themselves may cause allergies.)

Eyelid problems Infection of the eyelash follicle is called a sty. A tender lump within the eyelid is called a chalazion. Hot compresses applied several times daily usually relieve the condition. Sometimes a painful or chronic chalazion requires minor corrective surgery.

Blepharitis (eyelid inflammation) This condition, which is most common in the light-haired or people with ultra-sensitive skin, involves itchy, scaly flakes on the lid and lashes. Ulcerative blepharitis is an ulcerating inflammation. Treatment means careful cleansing of the eyelid margins twice daily plus antibiotic creams or ointments.

Conjunctivitis or pinkeye A common infection of the eye's thin mucous membrane (conjunctiva), it produces red, sore eyes and a gritty feeling. The eyelashes are often stuck together in the morning. Antibiotic drops are the usual remedy, along with warm saline rinsing. Pinkeye can be highly contagious and handwashing is essential to prevent its spread, as well as not sharing towels, washcloths or tissues. (See chapter 11, "Childhood problems.")

Conjunctival hemorrhage and episcleritis Conjunctival hemorrhage sounds bad and looks awful but is a harmless, painless red spot on the white of the eye, sometimes brought on by exertion—coughing. or straining at stool or childbirth, for instance—or by bleeding in those taking ASA. The spot usually goes away by itself. Conjunctival hemorrhage occasionally occurs in those with high blood pressure. Episcleritis is a recurring sore or pinkish-red patch on the white of the eye, of unknown cause, possibly related to connective tissue diseases or a prior infection (most often Herpes simplex or shingles (Herpes Zoster).

Corneal scratches Occasionally produced by contact lenses, a fingernail or a bit of grit in the eye, they are extremely painful, with teariness and photophobia (light-aversion). Antibiotics are given, along with eyedrops which temporarily dilate the pupil and paralyze the ciliary muscles of the iris. An eyepatch may be worn for a few days.

Corneal ulcers Resulting from damage to the cornea from an abrasion, or due to diseases such as Bell's palsy (facial paralysis) or infections (such as Herpes simplex), they can lead to corneal ulcers that threaten vision. Treatment is with special eyedrops, or if severe, corneal transplants.

Uveitis An inflammation of the iris (colored part of the eye) and its surrounding area, it causes dull pain, sensitivity to light, teariness and blurred vision. It's not always clear why it arises, but uveitis is serious as it can lead to pupil blockage or glaucoma. Treatment is with topical steroids and dilating eyedrops.

Retinal disorders Damage to the retina includes hypertensive retinopathy—a complication of high blood pressure (with blurred vision), diabetic retinopathy in long-term diabetics and macular degeneration. Retinal problems are now often treated with lasers.

objects. By age 40 most people have to wear reading glasses for close work. The muscles that dilate the pupil also weaken with age, and the pupil becomes smaller so that older people require brighter light than the young for doing similar tasks. Older people may also have trouble adapting from bright to darker places, and increased sensitivity to glare because of reflection in the eye. "Accommodation difficulties" are also common, with a delay in changing focus from distant to nearby objects. Peripheral vision (the ability to see things at the edges of the visual field) and night vision may also diminish.

Age-related macular degeneration

This disorder a common cause of vision blurring which affects about 20 percent of those over 65, occurs because of damage to the macula (from the Latin meaning "spot"), in the retina's central area. Small blood vessels grow into the macular region, harming the retinal cells that control central vision. Developing gradually and painlessly, often in both eyes (either simultaneously or one after the other), macular degeneration distorts images—producing central blurring or dimming while the surrounding vision remains clear. Straight lines or telephone poles may appear wavy or seem to have a missing segment. Because the macula is also responsible for perceiving color hues may look faded.

People with macular degeneration often find it hard to read small print, do close work or navigate stairs. But since side vision remains untouched, they can still walk about and even cross streets unaided, albeit with care and circumspection. The incidence of macular degeneration is about 1 percent in 55-year-olds and rises to 15 percent by age 80. Smoking, hypertension and a family history of the condition are risk factors—approximately 15 percent of people with a family history of macular degeneration will develop it. Macular degeneration is more common in women than men, partly because women tend to live longer. Light-eyed people tend to be more commonly afflicted than dark-eyed. If the condition is diagnosed when central vision is still reasonably intact and before new blood vessels invade the macula, laser treatment may reduce or slow the visual loss.

The two kinds of macular degeneration are the more common *dry* form (85 percent)and the more sight-threatening *wet* (exudative) form that accounts for 90 percent of severe vision loss in the elderly. The less common wet or fast-progressing form of the disease is due to swift growth of abnormal blood vessels that distort the retina and make it bulge, eventually forming scars that destroy central vision. Wet macular degeneration was originally treated with thermal laser photocoagulation but this method was only found to be useful in a select group of patients (10 percent). "Photodynamic therapy," using a nonthermal laser and the photosensitizing drug verteporfin, is more widely applicable.

Unfortunately, laser surgery doesn't work in everyone. Its effectiveness depends on the exact location of the damage. For people who cannot benefit from laser therapy, vision can sometimes be improved with magnifying lenses and other low-vision aids.

Use of vitamin and mineral supplements for macular degeneration is controversial. Some studies have suggested that certain carotenoids, especially lutein and zeaxanthin, which are found in dark green leafy vegetables such as spinach and collard greens, have a protective effect against age-related macular degeneration

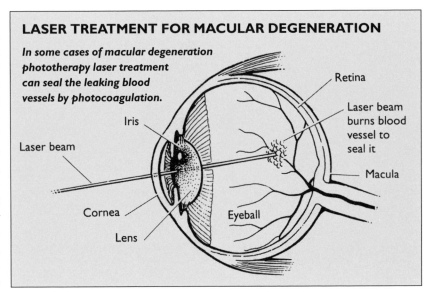

LASER TREATMENT FOR MACULAR DEGENERATION

In some cases of macular degeneration phototherapy laser treatment can seal the leaking blood vessels by photocoagulation.

Retina
Laser beam burns blood vessel to seal it
Macula
Iris
Laser beam
Cornea
Eyeball
Lens

(AMD). Zinc and vitamins may help those who already have macular degeneration, but there is no evidence that it can prevent it. In a four-year randomized placebo-controlled trial of 1,193 healthy volunteers, Vitamin E (500 IU) was not found to prevent AMD.

Glaucoma

Glaucoma is the second-commonest cause of blindness in North Americans over age 50. Left untreated, it inevitably leads to vision loss and blindness. The problem is that glaucoma develops slowly and painlessly, often giving no hint of its presence until it has reached an advanced stage when much sight may already have been lost. People with glaucoma are usually asymptomatic until more than 40 percent of the optic nerve is lost and they begin to experience "tunnel vision" (peripheral field loss) and decreased ability to see. Everyone should have regular eye exams after ages 40–45—even those with no vision complaints.

Glaucoma generally affects both eyes, advancing at varying rates and to different degrees. Most forms of glaucoma progress almost imperceptibly, although some develop quickly. The disorder generally involves a rise in intraocular pressure (IOP) because of drainage or outflow problems in the aqueous humor the watery fluid that bathes the eye. If fluid outflow is hindered, pressure rises and can damage the optic nerve.

Open-angle glaucoma, by far the commonest form, has been dubbed a "thief in the night" because it creeps up stealthily to rob people of their sight. Intraocular pressure builds slowly, producing gradual optic nerve deterioration. Peripheral vision goes first. Tiny blind spots appear at the edges of the visual field, slowly getting larger and spreading. Many people think that the rising intraocular pressure will noticeably swell the eyes. But this isn't so. The visual impairment may only become apparent because of a car accident or may be discovered at a routine eye examination. In serious cases, peripheral vision is altogether wiped out, leaving only central or "tunnel" vision. If this vision also disappears, the result is total blindness. Those with relatives who have glaucoma are at above-average risk, as are diabetics, hypertensives (with high blood pressure) and the strongly myopic (shortsighted).

Whereas, in the past, diagnosis of glaucoma depended primarily on the degree of eye-pressure elevation, IOP is no longer the only criterion. Glaucoma can exist in people with normal eye pressure. Eye-pressure elevation is now considered a risk factor but not proof of glaucoma. Measurement of changes to the optic disc (around the optic nerve) and visual field defects also help to establish diagnosis.

The classic "triad" signaling open-angle glaucoma (seen when the doctor looks in and tests your eyes)
- raised intraocular pressure;
- optic disc changes/abnormality;
- measurable visual field defects (blind spots, peripheral sight loss, "tunnel" vision).

Treatment of open-angle glaucoma aims to lower eye pressure, relieve optic nerve compression and halt sight loss. Therapy usually starts when there's detectable optic nerve damage or dangerously elevated IOP. Most "glaucoma suspects," in whom a pressure rise is the *only* abnormal finding, with no detectable vision loss or damage to the optic nerve, are closely watched for further deterioration. But high-risk groups are treated as soon as eye pressure creeps above normal. Medications (such as eyedrops or tablets) are tried first. If they don't work or are irritating, or if vision worsens, laser or conventional surgery may be advised.

The principle underlying glaucoma treatment is that lowering intraocular pressure will arrest the progression of the disease. Evolving data is showing us that earlier treatment can reduce future problems. Eyedrops, the commonest glaucoma treatment, may decrease eye-fluid production or increase drainage. Some glaucoma sufferers take several kinds of eyedrops as well as anti-glaucoma pills. These may constrict the eye pupil or cause headaches or other minor discomforts, but most learn to tolerate them. Glaucoma medications should be taken as prescribed, not skipped or neglected, because any vision loss that's already occurred can't be restored. Once started, glaucoma therapy is generally lifelong. Yet it's often hard to persuade people with no obvious symptoms to go on taking their medication—especially the elderly, who may be on several other drugs.

Many people don't realize that eyedrops can affect the whole body, as they are absorbed into the bloodstream. Although generally safe, glaucoma drugs drain through the tear ducts and nasal passages and can cause nonocular effects. These can often be minimized by preventing the medication from getting into the tear ducts—for example, by pressing on the side of the nose near the eyelid with a finger or squeezing the eye closed for a few minutes after inserting the drops.

After medical therapy has been tried, the next step is laser or surgical "trabeculoplasty" in which the laser or surgery is used to improve fluid outflow in the eye's drainage system. This procedure is now common for glaucoma, done in about 15 percent of cases. But neither procedure necessarily alleviates the problem permanently. In half the cases, intraocular eyeball pressure may rise again in two years or so, necessitating repeat laser or alternative treatment. Lasers are often used when drops give insufficient control of glaucoma, in the hope of avoiding surgery.

Acute (swift-onset) glaucoma
Fast-progressing but infrequent, the acute or closed-angle form of glaucoma comes on without warning, and accounts for 6 to 10 percent of cases. It occurs when the angle between the iris and the cornea becomes too narrow or

THE MAIN MEDICATIONS FOR OPEN-ANGLE GLAUCOMA

- *Beta blockers* (such as timolol, levobunolol and betaxolol) given as eyedrops decrease fluid production and reduce pressure. Generally safe, they can be absorbed via tear ducts and nasal passages, causing bronchospasm (lung problems)—mainly in asthmatics. They may also lower heartrate and blood pressure, possibly leading to heart failure and sometimes inducing nervous-system changes such as light-headedness, memory loss, lowered sex drive and impotence.

Because of possible cardiovascular effects, these drops should not be used in people with heart problems without specific medical advice and supervision.

- *Miotics* (such as pilocarpine and carbachol) and longer-acting forms (such as phospholine iodide) constrict the pupil, increasing fluid drainage. They may cause headaches and nervous-system changes (sweating, gastrointestinal upsets) if taken in large doses. Pilocarpine can also cause eye burning and vision blurring, reduce night vision (especially in anyone with cataracts), increase myopia, disturb digestion and cause diarrhea and/or appetite loss—mostly a problem in elderly patients.

- *Sympathomimetics* (such as epinephrine, dipivefrin) reduce aqueous inflow and enhance outflow, but can also produce blood-pressure elevation, eye redness and vision blurring. Epinephrine can increase the heartrate and cause heartbeat irregularities. High doses may produce sweating and restlessness as well as blurred vision and teariness. It shouldn't be used in people with heart rhythm problems or after a heart attack. (Propine, a modern form, produces fewer side effects.)

- *Topical Prostaglandin Analogues* (such as Latanoprost or Xalatan) also increase aqueous outflow. They are often used as the first-line treatment now because of their once-daily use and their lack of systemic side effects.

- *Carbonic anhydrase inhibitors* (such as acetazolamide, methazolamide) suppress the eye's fluid production but are less popular than other anti-glaucoma drugs because of longer-lasting side effects—nausea, depression, diuresis (frequent urination) and anemia, and possibly also numbness of the fingers and toes and stomach acidity (acidosis). They should not be used with ASA because of the increased risk of ulcers.

closes up, blocking fluid drainage. It often hits suddenly, with blurred vision, eye pain, headache, nausea and vomiting—symptoms sometimes mistaken for migraine, a digestive attack, stroke or uveitis (eye inflammation). Unlike open-angle glaucoma, which is related to myopia or shortsightedness, this type is linked to farsightedness. Those with small eyes and/or large lenses are at increased risk of closed-angle glaucoma—for instance, the Inuit, with their often small, farsighted eyes. Rare forms of closed-angle glaucoma arise from eye inflammation, a tumor or mechanical damage.

Precipitating factors for acute glaucoma include anything that makes the eye pupil dilate or widen, even emotional events such as weddings, funerals or heart-thumping movies. Acute glaucoma is always an emergency and must be treated quickly. To alleviate the pressure and prevent sight loss, prompt medical treatment and laser surgery are required. Laser iridotomy is a simple, safe, highly effective procedure that relieves closed-angle glaucoma by puncturing a hole in the iris, enabling the fluid to escape. Once someone has had closed-angle glaucoma in one eye, the other is also at grave risk and is often treated preventively at the same time. In cases of known risk, both eyes may get prophylactic (preventive) laser treatment to avoid the onset of acute glaucoma.

Cataracts: new treatments can save sight

Cataracts cloud the eye's transparent lens, diminishing and distorting eyesight. While cataracts can occur at any age, they are most prevalent in people over age 60. Almost half the men and women aged 75 and over develop them. Occasionally young people get cataracts, sometimes because of an inherited predisposition.

Cataracts can arise because of

- metabolic lens changes with advancing years;
- hereditary predisposition (family tendency);
- injuries or blows to the eye ("traumatic cataracts") from, for instance, bicycling falls, hockey injuries or boxing blows;
- excess exposure to X-rays or infrared radiation—hazards avoided by wearing protective goggles. Although the eye's natural lens blocks some UV light, many experts suggest that anyone frequently exposed to bright sunlight should wear special dark glasses;
- microwave radiation in high doses (if insufficiently shielded);

THE EYE WITH CATARACT FORMING

Types of Cataracts

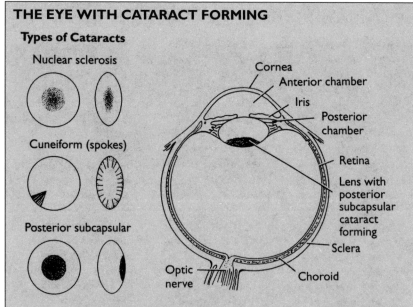

Nuclear sclerosis

Cuneiform (spokes)

Posterior subcapsular

Cornea
Anterior chamber
Iris
Posterior chamber
Retina
Lens with posterior subcapsular cataract forming
Sclera
Optic nerve
Choroid

A cataract is a clouding and/or yellowing of the eye's normally clear crystalline lens due to protein aggregation that makes it too turbid (opaque) to see through clearly. Cataract formation is a gradual process that, in most people, ultimately affects both eyes, although not necessarily at the same time. Some cataracts (nuclear sclerosis or "hard" type) form in the middle of the lens and tend to scatter light rays, producing glare and dimming but not totally obscuring vision. Cuneiform cataracts form as "spokes," affecting only peripheral vision. The type most common with advancing age—"posterior subcapsular"—forms at the back of the lens as an overgrowth of cells, and usually develops quite quickly. Once a cataract begins in a particular part of the lens, it may remain static, but usually spreads. Regardless of type or position, it may require surgery. When a cataract completely obscures vision it is said to be "ripe."

- exposure to toxic chemicals, such as naphthalene or paradichlorobenzene;
- certain diseases such as hypoparathyroidism (underactivity of the parathyroid gland), diabetes, atopic dermatitis (a skin disease), retinal detachment or prolonged eye inflammation;
- certain medications (such as cortisone).

How to know if you have cataracts

The main alerting sign of cataracts is double vision in one eye, vision blurring and perhaps a disturbing glare, especially in bright light (as when facing oncoming headlights). At first the subtle haziness may be hardly noticeable—colors may dull a little, vision may blur when reading with one eye giving a brighter image than the other. As one eye clouds, eyesight seems better with the bad eye closed, but corrective lenses don't seem to improve the foggy vision. One interesting sign that can occur early in far-sighted individuals is "second sight" in

which the cataract may change the refractive index of the lens so that the person can begin to read without glasses.

Only the cataract sufferer can say how much the visual loss impedes everyday life—whether it affects work, recreation, reading or driving. Some find even slightly fogged vision—a 20 to 30 percent diminution in visual clarity—a distinct handicap, while others scarcely notice it. While a cataract does not usually endanger health, the visual blurring may arise from another disorder; careful investigation is needed to exclude other possible reasons for hazy vision. In the presence of an unhealthy macula, even the most technically perfect cataract operation cannot uncloud hazy vision. (See "Macular degeneration.")

Cataracts used to be removed only when they were "ripe." This idea had no scientic basis, and today surgery is scheduled when the person and his or her surgeon agree that the time, not the cataract, is ripe! Since most cataracts progress slowly and they rarely impair eye health, the timing of surgery is flexible and depends on the individual's quality of life and the local wait times for surgery. Often, an early cataract that doesn't interfere with normal activities isn't removed but just periodically checked. Someone whose job is vision-dependent might request cataract removal much earlier than a retired person with a less taxing lifestyle.

About 95 percent of those with cataracts now have plastic lens implants inserted by eye surgery. Thanks to various surgical advances, lens replacement is a relatively simple, painless procedure that can be done at any age. A natural eye lens clouded by cataracts can be removed and replaced with a plastic lens on a "same day" basis, with only a small percentage of sufferers requiring hospitalization.

The type of operation suitable for a given person depends on the cataract's form and size and whether or not other eye diseases are also present. Cataract surgery has been dramatically refined by better microscopes that allow precise surgery with less trauma; a new irrigation/aspiration cutter for phacoemulsification that "squirts" and "sucks" as it cuts, giving the surgeon unhindered movements; use of finer nylon or polypropylene sutures (stitches)—thinner than a single hair—which allow a leak-proof scar; and, above all, intraocular plastic implants inserted during surgery that almost miraculously restore clear vision.

After the cataract operation

After a cataract operation, there is a little discomfort or pain, and that can be allayed with a mild painkiller (such as Tylenol or codeine). There may be some nausea, usually relieved by one or two antinausea tablets. The affected eye may or may not be patched for a day or two after surgery. Some doctors advise their patients to wear a shield taped over the eye at night for a few weeks. The eye may remain irritated for a few weeks, as the incision can be felt upon blinking and moving the eye. Sutures may or may not be used.

Postoperative care is usually minimal, the wound generally being sufficiently healed within three to eight weeks for contact lenses or glasses to be fitted. Strenuous activity must be avoided during recovery and it's imperative to avoid any rubbing, injury or direct blow to the eye. Eyedrops containing an antibiotic and anti-inflammatory agent are generally used. Vision returns quickly in some, but it's more usual for vision to improve slowly. Most people can shop, watch television and socialize within a few days. (Provided the unoperated eye has good vision, driving can also be resumed quite soon.) Most people resume everyday activities within a month or two of the surgery.

No surgical procedure is entirely risk-free, and complications occur in about 5 percent of cataract removals—for example, infection, hemorrhage, retinal detachment, wound breakdown and shifting of an intraocular implant. Warning signs of trouble following cataract surgery are a sudden decrease in vision, pain or discomfort of the eye after a seemingly steady recovery. Such changes should immediately be reported to the surgeon.

Cataract surgery has become frequent and successful, bringing untold joy to those who might formerly have ended their days with hazy vision or total blindness.

THREE OPTIONS FOR REPLACEMENT LENSES

Removal of a cataract leaves the eye very far-sighted and in need of a lens or strong spectacles to focus light onto the retina. Today's cataract spectacles are less bulky. contacts are easier to handle than earlier models, and the plastic lens implant is an enormous improvement.

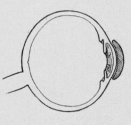

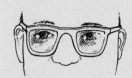

- *Aphakic cataract spectacles,* now lighter and more delicate than they used to be, are the oldest and safest way to achieve vision after eye-lens removal, especially for those who are unable to tolerate contact lenses or who do not qualify for an implant. After a cataract operation in one eye only, a corrective lens may be worn either for that eye or for the unoperated eye to improve vision. Cataract spectacles provide good vision while seated—watching TV, reading and sewing—but not for walking or driving because of poor side vision, abnormal magnification and spatial distortion.
- *Contact lenses* (soft or gas-permeable, daily or extended-wear) can provide more natural perception, giving binocular vision with full central and side vision. But some older patients find even soft contacts difficult to put in, and fragile to handle. Those unduly annoyed by the magnification of a cataract contact lens may also require one in the unoperated eye (to overcome the image disparity). New extended-wear contact lenses can be left in for three months to a year, but must occasionally be taken out and

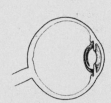

cleaned.
- *The intraocular lens (IOL)* or plastic implant was first tested by a British surgeon in 1979. The plastic implants are made of **PMMA** (poly-methylmethacrylate) because Royal Air Force crews in World War Two did not experience any rejection symptoms to bits of this material that entered their eyes from shattered air-

craft parts. Many of the early problems of these plastic lens implants—such as poor fastening and slippage—have now been overcome, and they have the great advantage of producing vision that's not distorted and that requires no manual dexterity (and no maintenance). In the 30 years since their introduction, implants have been refined to the point where they're now used in up to 95 percent of modern cataract operations.

Each IOL is carefully made, and its focusing power is individually selected according to eyeball length and corneal curvature, which determine the lens power of the implant. Provided the measurements are accurate, an implant can provide almost normal postoperative vision using regular, weak spectacles. Most people with implants need glasses for reading and/or distance vision. If the other eye is also scheduled for later cataract surgery, the implants can sometimes provide normal (even 20/20) vision, provided the eyes are otherwise healthy. Multifocal intraocular lenses that correct near vision as well as distance are

VARIOUS CATARACT OPERATIONS USED

Cataract removal in developed countries uses an extracapsular approach that removes the lens but leaves the posterior lens capsule intact. The lens can be removed by direct extraction or phacoemulsification, in which the cataract is fragmented with ultrasound.

- *Extracapsular surgery*—the more recent method, now used for 95 percent of cataract removals—takes out only the cataract, leaving intact the posterior holding capsule. The advantages of extracapsular cataract extraction are: a smaller incision; better support for the lens implant from the remaining (hind) portion of the capsule; fewer postoperative retinal detachments. Its disadvantage is possible post-capsular clouding after surgery, requiring laser treatment to clear vision in approximately

20 percent of patients within two or three years of extracapsular surgery. High-energy lasers are used to open a postoperatively clouded posterior capsule, rapidly restoring vision with a painless five- to ten-minute outpatient procedure.

- *Phacoemulsification* is a form of extracapsular cataract removal that suits some cases, especially those due to trauma or in young persons who have softer eye lenses than the elderly. In this technique, the surgeon sucks out the lens (with the cataract) using a hollow needle after it has been fragmented (liquefied) by ultrasound. Popular because of the tiny incision required, it has benefits that may be slightly offset by later corneal complications.

Anesthesia for modern cataract surgery may be general or local. A general anes-

thetic may be given to a very young or apprehensive patient, but more commonly the anesthetic is a local "freezing" that numbs sensation (as in dental procedures). Sometimes, to avert anxiety, the patient is briefly sedated by an IV infusion while the local anesthetic is either dropped onto the eye or injected under the eye. The anesthetic requires ten minutes to "take" and the person stays awake for the rest of the procedure. There is no worry about blinking during the operation because the injected medication stops all eye and eyelid movement. The surgery takes about 45 to 60 minutes, including lens removal and eye bandaging. Most patients can get up and walk around within three to twelve hours after surgery. During this time, they can gradually sit up, watch TV and go to the bathroom if they wish. Complete healing takes up to three months.

EAR CARE

The ear is a remarkably precise and versatile piece of sound-receiving and balance-coordinating equipment. It can hear the faintest of sounds and—when one is young—picks up frequencies from 16 to 20,000 cycles per second. However, the ear's capacity to hear and maintain balance often deteriorates with age or exposure to noise or because of certain diseases.

Hearing impairment is an invisible handicap affecting one in ten North Americans. An esti-

mated 50 percent of the population over age 65 experience some degree of hearing impairment. Recent studies by the Canadian Hearing Society noted that over 80 percent of people tested in nursing homes were hearing-impaired. Deafness is disabling more and more people in modern society, not only because of the aging population but also because of widespread noise pollution. Few outsiders realize the impact of hearing loss on someone's everyday life. Besides making conversation difficult, deafness produces isolation and anxiety. The hearing-impaired themselves often don't recognize the problem or take steps to get and use a hearing aid, to help them stay in the mainstream of social intercourse.

Ears don't need washing: they clean themselves

Many people wrongly imagine that ears need regular cleaning to get rid of wax and dirt. In fact, ears need no special washing, cleaning or drying. They have their own inbuilt cleaning mechanism. The external ear canal is lined with thick skin containing sebaceous (oil) glands and ceruminous (modified sweat). Wax or cerumen, composed of glandular secretions, plus dead skin and other debris, forms in the outer part of the ear canal as a natural protection. But it is often impacted by persistent probing of the ear with fingers, Q-tips (cotton-tipped cleaning rods) or assorted instruments—in the mistaken name of cleanliness.

Contrary to popular misperception, ear wax isn't "dirty." It is a protective barrier that prevents contaminants from penetrating the ear canal's skin and producing infection. Enzymes in the wax help to prevent infection. The oil or wax has the added benefit of protecting your inner ear from water. All that's required is gentle washing with a finger in a wet washcloth. Over-vigorous efforts to remove water or dirt from the ears interfere with the body's self-cleansing mechanism, driving dirt farther in. Compulsive ear cleaners who poke their fingers into the ear or roughly or carelessly cleanse it with various cleaning devices such as Q-tips not only remove the enzymes but can damage the delicate skin lining the ear permitting bacteria to enter and produce itchiness, irritation and infection. Q-tips should never be used in the ears. To remove water from the ears it's best simply to tip the head well from side to side and shake gently. A few individuals produce significant amounts of cerumen that can lead to hearing loss. These individuals can attend their local clinic for periodic cleaning when their hearing is affected.

How about ear care when flying?

If air pressure inside the middle ear isn't balanced or if fluid accumulates, the ear can sometimes "pop," causing intense pain—as happens during an airplane descent, when scuba diving or going up fast in an elevator. Even though most modern aircraft cabins are pressurized, it is impossible to maintain exactly the same pressure in flight as on earth. During ascent, as the surrounding atmospheric pressure decreases, the air in the middle ear is at higher pressure and automatically finds its way out of the eustachian tube into the back of the nose, automatically equalizing pressure on either side of the eardrum. Going down, however, is not quite that easy! As air pressure increases upon descent, pressure will be greater outside the eardrum than inside, producing a blocked sensation in the ears. Air cannot enter the middle ear to equalize the pressure, unless the passenger actively swallows or blows the nose. Occasionally, excess pressure can rupture the eardrum, with a bloody discharge.

When one has a cold, the lining of the eustachian tube, like the lining of the nose and sinuses, may be swollen and block the passage of air making pressure equalization impossible. If one must fly with a head cold, it's wise to reduce nasal congestion with decongestant tablets. In addition, a topical nasal decongestant spray such as Otrivin or Dristan should be used liberally when the plane starts its descent. For those who are "stuffed up" with an allergy, antihistamines alone or a combination of decongestant and antihistamine is recommended. Also, because ears tend to block on descent, air should be blown into the middle ear by holding the nose and closing the mouth and forcibly building up

THE STRUCTURE OF THE EAR

The ear is divided into three main parts: the external, middle and inner ear. Sound vibrations travel down the external ear canal or eustachian tube and strike the ear drum, making it vibrate. The air pressure on either side of the ear drum is equalized with every third or fourth swallow (unless the eustachian tube is blocked by a cold, when flying or by large adenoids). Sound vibrations are transmitted across the air-filled middle ear by three tiny, linked bones or ossicles—the hammer, anvil and stapes—then via the foot of the stapes and oval window to the cochlea in the fluid-bathed inner ear. About 3 cm long, the coiled cochlea contains thousands of hair cells that act as sound receptors. As the vibrations hit them, electrical impulses are set up and travel via the auditory nerve to the brain's hearing center. The inner ear also controls the body's equilibrium—balance related to gravity—via three lymph-filled semicircular canals in the inner ear (which are "acceleration detectors" that monitor movement) and the utricle and sacule (static gravity receptors) that relay information about the position of the head at rest. Sensory hairs in these canals orient the body's position in space.

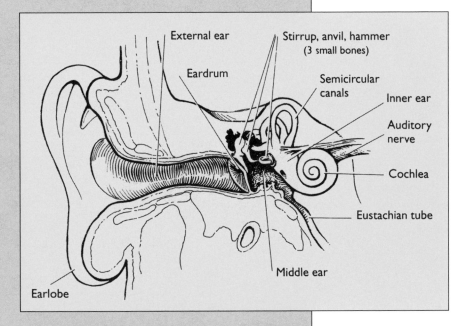

External ear

Eardrum

Stirrup, anvil, hammer (3 small bones)

Semicircular canals

Inner ear

Auditory nerve

Cochlea

Eustachian tube

Middle ear

Earlobe

SOME COMMON EAR PROBLEMS

Hearing loss

Hearing loss can be conductive (faulty transmission of sound waves via the eardrum or failure to transmit sound via the ossicles) or sensorineural (failure in sound reception by nerve cells), or both. Common causes of conductive hearing loss are wax blocking the ear, a perforated eardrum or fluid in the middle ear. Common reasons for nerve or sensorineural deafness are age-related changes (presbycusis), noise exposure, and ototoxic (ear-damaging) drugs. Mixed hearing losses can occur in people with chronic ear disease, who may have conductive hearing loss due to a damaged eardrum and/or injury to the little ear bones as well as infection of the inner ear.

The main causes of hearing loss:

Congenital (present at birth)
- genetic (hereditary);
- environmental causes:
  - prenatal rubella (German measles);
  - infections during pregnancy (which damage the fetus;
  - premature birth;
  - perinatal anoxia (oxygen lack), newborn jaundice, Rh (blood) disease.

Acquired hearing loss
- progressive familial (hereditary) sensorineural hearing loss—usually noted in childhood or adolescence, gradually progressing to severe or profound loss;

Other causes
- presbycusis—age-related hearing loss;
- noise-induced hearing loss;
- ototoxicity (due to drugs that harm the ear);

- head injuries;
- infectious diseases affecting the middle and inner ear.

Some signs of hearing loss in adults:
- trouble understanding conversation in crowded situations or noisy rooms;
- turning the TV or radio up so loud that others are uncomfortable;
- frequently asking for repetition of words and phrases; ignoring people;
- hearing speech but finding the words unclear.

Hearing problems in children

About 4 percent of children have some degree of hearing impairment, which is sometimes mistaken for slow learning or mental retardation. Children should have hearing tests at six months of age, at school entry and again at age ten or eleven.

Normal babies startle, stir or awaken at a loud noise (a dog barking or a jet close overhead). By the age of six months or so, infants will turn their heads toward a familiar voice, even if the speaker is out of sight. By two years, most children can mimic sounds and react to simple commands. Parents should watch for hearing problems.

About one in 1,000 babies is born with a severe hearing defect. By age five, 4 percent of children will have some degree of hearing loss. A recent study showed that in 50 percent of cases there were serious delays in detecting and diagnosing a child's hearing loss. Children suspected of defective hearing need testing and prompt remedial action, particularly since the loss can have a

significant effect on the child's language acquisition and learning and social skills.

Children born with normal hearing may lose it through childhood illnesses such as measles or meningitis, or because of certain drugs. Upper respiratory infections often result in middle-ear infections that need prompt attention to avoid chronic hearing loss.

Some signs of hearing loss in children:
- a newborn baby who does not jump or blink at a sudden loud noise;
- an infant aged three to six months who does not stop crying or stop moving at the sound of a voice or a strange sound;
- a child of nine to twelve months who does not turn toward a speaker;
- a two-year-old who doesn't yet use short sentences. This can be normal, but your doctor may want to have the child's hearing tested if his or her speech is not improving.

Parents should talk to their physician about such symptoms. Conventional audiometry can rarely be performed on children under 4 years of age, but a variety of other techniques can assess hearing capabilities even in infants. Two important tests are otoacoustic emissions (OAE) and auditory brainstem responses (ABR). In response to environmental sounds the cochlea generates very soft sounds of its own that can be detected by a small probe placed in the ear canal (with young infants this is best done when they are asleep). The threshold of hearing loss is then determined by the auditory brainstem response.

---

internal pressure (Valsalva maneuver). This can be done repeatedly as the plane lands.

If able to sleep on the plane, ask the flight attendant to awaken you upon descent. Even without a cold, your ears can be blocked if you are asleep or lying down when landing. That goes for babies, too. Wake them up and feed them to cause swallowing, which helps relieve the pressure. As a last resort, force the baby to cry if it won't feed.

Anyone who dives even a few feet underwater experiences a similar increase in pressure on the outside of the eardrum. Scuba divers are

taught a simple procedure to equalize or "pop" their ears, but sometimes suffer barotrauma or even ruptured eardrums through carelessness or through diving with a head cold or allergies. Diving on decongestants is not recommended, as the medications may impair the diver's ability, or wear off during the dive. Non-divers who want to snorkel might ask the staff who supply the equipment to show them how to "pop" their ears, to avoid discomfort and possible damage.

Ear pain or persistent hearing loss necessitates a visit to the doctor or ear specialist. Any earache or pain, dizzy spells, imbalance, strange ringing in the ears, ear discharge, redness, swelling, or reduced or muffled hearing should always receive prompt medical attention. Treatment with decongestants for two to three weeks may be all that is required. On occasion, however, it may be necessary to lance the eardrum under local anesthetic with the aid of a microscope, to equalize the pressure and reduce discomfort.

Age-related hearing loss

Aging is often accompanied by sensorineural deafness. Presbycusis—literally, "old hearing"—is the term for age-related hearing loss, which affects 50 percent of those over 65 in North America. The hearing tends to become progressively worse with advancing years. Those with presbycusis often complain not only of hearing loss (usually in both ears), but sometimes also of tinnitus (ringing in the ears). It takes only a little hearing loss to make life difficult because, although conversation is audible at low frequencies, it's not easy to hear the high frequencies that go first. Thus, the elderly may have trouble hearing the phone ring. It can also be difficult to distinguish consonants. The problem becomes particularly acute when there's a lot of background noise, as on a bus or at the dinner table. Seniors often accuse others of mumbling! They may say, "I can hear you but I don't understand what you're saying." Conversationalists can help by articulating clearly, keeping the face up so lips can be read and asking if the person has understood.

When hearing loss in the elderly begins, the hard-of-hearing are advised to get immediate counseling about use of a hearing aid, to keep them from becoming socially isolated. Increased hearing difficulties can make a person feel lonely and anxious. Such everyday activities as shopping, banking, attending group gatherings or obtaining simple information can become exercises in frustration, not only for those who have the hearing loss, but also for those who interact with them. Worse yet, hearing loss is often mistaken for senility in the elderly. Anyone who suspects they have some hearing loss should see their family physician and ask to be referred to the appropriate health professional. Given today's sophisticated technology, there is no need for anyone to do without an assistive listening device (hearing aid).

Modern hearing aids

Hearing aids work by amplifying sound, and are most effective in a quiet room with no background noise. The aids are best for one-to-one conversations, watching TV or listening to the radio. Hearing aids are highly individual and are chosen according to the type and severity of hearing loss, the state of the ear canal and the person's ability to manipulate the hearing aid. Hearing aids that don't seem to work properly should be rechecked because many problems are correctable. For instance, some people may have an imperfectly fitted device, while others may need two hearing aids or a different brand.

Today's hearing aids are better smaller and more efficient than yesteryear's and, appropriately chosen and fitted, can greatly improve the quality of life for the hearing-impaired. Traditional hearing aids are behind-the-ear models, but improved technology has allowed the development of models that can be inserted in the ear, partially in the canal, or completely in the canal. Behind-the-ear aids are generally used for children because changes in the canal as they grow would require up to four changes a year for in-canal types. Unfortunately, hearing aids have a bad reputation. Many people remember

SUDDEN SENSORINEURAL DEAFNESS

This condition, in which people suddenly (within days) go deaf, is a rare disorder affecting about 5–20 people per 100,000 per year. It may be mild and temporary or permanent and profound, and may affect one or both ears, sometimes for elusive reasons. Some people aren't aware of a sudden hearing loss in one ear until they go to answer a phone or can't hear a dinner guest on one side. Mumps, measles, influenza or mononucleosis are thought to be possible causes. Sudden deafness can also follow rupture of the eardrum due to a dramatic change in the surrounding air pressure (for instance when diving) or overly strenuous physical exertion. Drugs such as certain antibiotics, diuretics and ASA can affect hearing (in both ears equally)—although with ASA the loss is reversible. Anybody with a sudden hearing problem should consult a physician at once.

HEARING AIDS

Behind the ear

In the ear canal (outer ear)

Within the ear

NOISE-INDUCED HEARING LOSS IS ALL TOO COMMON

We are all painfully aware of the increased noise in modern urban life: sirens, rush-hour traffic, jackhammers, subways. Many of us, attempting to find an escape, walk or drive through the city jacking up the volume on our personal headsets or car radios, compounding problems for the delicate inner ear.

Noise-induced hearing loss is a common cause of tinnitus (ringing in the ears) and of male deafness (more men are occupationally exposed to noise than women). Exposure to continuous industrial noise, snowmobiles, airplanes, power tools and rock concerts may produce temporary partial loss of hearing for a number of hours, called temporary threshold shift (TTS)—a transitory increase in the level sound has to reach to be perceived. Unfortunately, continuous noise over prolonged periods of time may gradually convert TTS into a permanent loss of hearing.

Sound is measured in decibels. A whisper or a quiet countryside averages 30 dB, normal speech 50–55 dB (about 1 m or 3.3 ft away from the source), a vacuum cleaner about 70 dB, the inside of a diesel bus 75 dB, city traffic 80 dB (just under the "hazardous" limit) and a subway 90 dB. A lawnmower, at 90 decibels, is at the "annoyance" level (where regular eight-hour-a-day exposure will cause hearing loss). Acute discomfort is noticeable at about 95 decibels—roughly the sound of an average rock concert, nearby jet plane, chain saw or pneumatic drill. 110 decibels is the danger limit—a level at which even five minutes of steady, unremitting exposure can lead to some hearing loss, the loss increasing if exposure continues for an extended time. At 170 dB, sound can literally blow you off your feet.

Hearing loss builds up at noise exposures above 85 decibels, if experienced daily for an eight-hour day—not an uncommon noise level in many workplaces. Typically, the ability to hear high sounds—birds or women's voices—goes first, followed by loss of low-tone perception. To tell whether your environment is noisy enough to harm your ears, check whether you have to shout to make yourself heard, or whether, when you leave a noisy environment, sound seems muffled. If yes, the noise level is too high and injuring your ears. Excessively noisy environments are nightclubs, bars, busy restaurants and nearby chainsaws, motorboats, motorcycles.

According to the U.S. National Institutes of Health, 20 million North Americans are at risk of hearing loss from noisy work situations, especially farmers, truck drivers, construction workers, policemen and musicians (including classical musicians—playing second bass in the symphony can be an awfully noisy job). The trouble with noise-induced hearing loss is that, while entirely preventable, it's no more curable than other types of deafness. Poor sound perception is compounded when the listener is also exposed to background noise, e.g., a cocktail party or traffic outside an open window.

Those in noisy jobs should wear personal hearing protectors (earplugs, ear protectors)—and turn the volume down during recreational activities! The currently suggested level where hearing protection should begin (on a voluntary basis, no laws about it) is 85 dB, and according to hearing experts, ear protection should be mandatory at 90 dB. It may seem ironic to try to enforce the use of ear protection for industrial work at 85 dB while condoning a 90 dB or higher level for pleasure from discos, rock bands and personal stereos.

If your hearing loss is traceable to work conditions, it may be worthwhile to contact the Workers' Compensation Board to see if you are eligible for a pension or at least rehabilitation with hearing aids. However, workers must have at least a 25-decibel hearing loss in each ear before the Workers' Compensation Board will even consider the case. Presently the board awards a pension of up to 2 percent to those with continuous tinnitus for more than two years, as long as there is a hearing loss of at least 25 percent associated with it.

The message is loud and clear: the more noise we hear today, the less we'll hear tomorrow. Protect your ears from excess noise as much as possible by:

• turning down the volume on radios, TVs and portable sound systems;
• playing personal headsets at lower volumes (not above the halfway setting);
• lodging formal complaints about environmental noise such as too much construction or traffic noise;
• wearing hearing protection when using loud equipment or household appliances;
• avoiding too many noisy concerts, movies, restaurants and lounges (better still, mounting a campaign to have these places turn down the volume);
• keeping noisy toys away from babies and young children.

problems their parents had, expect their hearing aids not to work well and give up too easily. Yet those who don't have hearing aids or who leave them unused in their bureau drawers may benefit from modern advice and a new fitting. In one 1991 London, Ontario, study of 115 elderly patients in a family practice clinic, 30 percent failed a hearing test and most needed hearing aids, yet none had asked for one. Even among those who have hearing aids, many don't make the best use of them. In the same study, ten of eleven elderly who had hearing aids needed to have them updated, replaced or adjusted.

The clumsy old-fashioned hearing aid, worn in a shirt pocket with a long cord to an ear mold, is not often used today except in near-complete deafness. Nowadays, hearing aids can fit inside the ear or even entirely within the ear canal. One type is worn behind the ear. Sophisticated hearing aids are now digitally controlled and programmable (tuning out the hum of low-frequency sounds such as car noises or air conditioners), making them better in noisy situations. Future hearing aids will be even more technologically advanced.

Surgically implantable hearing aids are now being tried. One type for conductive hearing loss has an internal component, a titanium screw implanted behind the ear that fuses with the bone, and an external part, a sound processor with a microphone that picks up sound waves and converts them into vibrations transmitted via the skull and processed by the auditory nerve. More and more types of implant are being investigated.

Ringing in the ears

Tinnitus, an annoying buzzing or ringing sound in the ears, is experienced momentarily by almost everyone at some time—perhaps from a loud, sudden bang near the ear or after a blow to the head. Tinnitus, from the Latin "to tinkle," often accompanies hearing loss. Sometimes it sounds more like a popping noise than a ring. It can be very irritating, even debilitating. Ancient Egyptian and Mesopotamian cures for so-called "bewitched ears" were frankincense and special oils. Modern treatments generally try to improve hearing with assistive devices or use of masking strategies.

Tinnitus is a sign of something amiss in the ear possibly just wax buildup, or damage due to injury, noise or aging. Tinnitus can be subjective or objective. Subjective tinnitus is heard exclusively by the person afflicted. In objective tinnitus the sound can be heard by others. While a nuisance to those who have it, the ear-ringing does not usually signal some dread disease such as a brain tumor or cancer.

Tinnitus can stem from middle-ear infections, multiple sclerosis, injuries such as a bad whiplash, migraines, epilepsy, muscle spasms and exposure to loud noise. People regularly exposed to excessive noise, such as airport employees, often report an unpleasant buzz in the ears. When linked to vertigo (spinning dizziness) and fluctuating, low-tone hearing loss, tinnitus is likely due to an inner-ear disorder such as Ménière's disease. Unfortunately, there is no perfect cure, but for most, tinnitus does improve over time. Background noise such as a fan helps many people. A few may benefit from tinnitus-masking devices that can be worn in or behind the ear.

Tinnitus fluctuates in intensity. It's usually most disturbing at night, and may be worsened by stress or anxiety. A vicious circle can result, where the ear hiss causes annoyance and the irritability in turn worsens the stress and aggravates the tinnitus. Learning to relax and avoid stress may decrease the problem.

Improved hearing through a hearing aid often reduces the annoyance. Special maskers—instruments that produce other sounds of similar frequency to mask the tinnitus—are now available, some combined with hearing aids. However, many people report greater irritation from the maskers than from the tinnitus itself A humidifier or radio turned on low at night can just as well mute the ear-ringing. Biofeedback helps some, by producing carefully monitored relaxation with the help of a therapist.

Medications tried for tinnitus include oral anticonvulsants, which reduce the intensity of tinnitus in some. But these drugs have potentially serious side effects, such as bone-marrow suppression and kidney damage, which limit their usefulness. Antidepressants help some to live with the condition. Despite vast strides in medicine, tinnitus remains a perplexing disorder that's remarkably hard to get rid of.

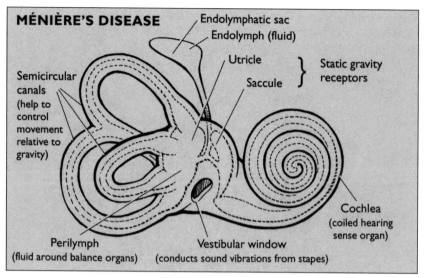

MÉNIÈRE'S DISEASE

Semicircular canals (help to control movement relative to gravity)

Endolymphatic sac
Endolymph (fluid)
Utricle
Saccule
} Static gravity receptors

Perilymph (fluid around balance organs)

Vestibular window (conducts sound vibrations from stapes)

Cochlea (coiled hearing sense organ)

Ménière's disease

This curious disorder affecting two to six out of 1,000 people, takes its name from Prosper Ménière, a former physician-in-chief at the Imperial Institute for Deaf Mutes in Paris. In 1861 he proposed that a common triad of symptoms—vertigo, tinnitus and mild hearing loss—be designated a definite inner-ear disorder. Contrary to the prevailing view, which ascribed such symptoms to brain disease, Ménière attributed them to dysfunction in the inner ear's balancing system. Unfortunately, Ménière died before seeing his theory proved true and his name given to the disease he'd so accurately described.

The disorder generally strikes in mid-adulthood, with a slight preponderance in males. It classically begins with one or more bouts of vertigo. A typical case is Boris, a radio engineer in his mid-thirties, who suddenly felt the room begin to circle dramatically. Nauseated and faint, he sat down, gripping the chair to steady himself. Once the vertigo subsided, he noticed a persistent roaring in his left ear and felt somewhat hard of hearing in that ear. Boris "slept off" the attack and was back at work the next day, but was rather apprehensive because the buzzing in his ear went on for about two weeks. When the same thing happened twice more within the year he began to worry that he had a brain tumor or some other serious illness. Obsessed and fearful that an attack would start at some awkward moment, perhaps even endanger his

life, he became an anxious, overwrought person, quite different from his former confident self.

This case illustrates the hallmarks of Ménière's disease:

- episodic vertigo—typically one or more attacks a year singly or in clusters, lasting minutes to hours, possibly disabling enough to force the person to lie down;
- tinnitus—an incessant hiss or roaring in one ear that may persist, change or disappear;
- fluctuating hearing loss—improving between attacks, but often worsening over time. The hearing loss typically distorts music and voices. The good news is that Ménière's hearing loss may worsen but is never total;
- headaches, sweating, pallor, a slow pulse, nausea and vomiting may accompany acute Ménière's spells, leading the unwary to suspect a stomach upset—until they get to know their illness.

Although the disorder generally includes vertigo, ear-ringing and hearing loss, all three symptoms are not necessarily present together. Between bouts, the disorder usually leaves few or no signs of its presence and hearing often returns to near-normal. Remissions can last for years or, rarely, forever.

The vertigo in Ménière's is distinguished by:

- sudden onset, out of the blue;
- a rotatory sensation with whirling surroundings. On lying down with eyes closed, the person feels as if tossed on a bouncing ship;
- a tendency to stagger from side to side;
- occasionally, vertigo violent enough to throw the person to the ground—known as drop attacks, utricular crises or Tumarkin spells.

The most obvious abnormality seen in Ménière's disease is increased fluid in the inner ear. Known as endolymphatic hydrops, the fluid buildup ruptures a bit of membrane from time to time, allowing the endolymph (fluid rich in potassium) to mix with the outside bathing fluid or perilymph (poor in potassium). This mixing of fluids leads to a biochemical alteration that transiently paralyzes the inner ear's balance (vestibular) system, producing the vertigo. Once the fluid balance normalizes, the vertigo passes.

Ménière's disease tends to engender tremendous anxiety because the vertigo strikes so unpredictably. Sufferers constantly fear

DIZZINESS

Dizziness has many different causes, ranging from trivial to more serious. It quite often accompanies hearing loss, and can arise from a transient or permanent disturbance of inner-ear function. However, dizziness from inner ear problems *must* be distinguished from that due to other conditions such as anemia, hypoglycemia (low blood sugar), cardiovascular ailments, neurological disorders (such as multiple sclerosis) and psychosomatic problems such as anxiety disorders. Dizziness accompanied by blackouts, numbness down one side or difficulty swallowing may indicate a serious nervous system disorder, or stroke.

Dizziness attacks that last only seconds are commonly due to standing up too fast after lying down, or a dysfunction in the inner ear, known as benign paroxysmal vertigo—a problem that usually vanishes spontaneously in a matter of weeks (but may recur). Among those prone to it, paroxysmal vertigo can happen, disconcertingly, several times a day. Simple head exercises can bring complete remission.

Dizziness arising from inner-ear disorders or disturbance of the balance mechanism is true vertigo—with a giddy sensation that the world is "spinning around" or that one is somersaulting helplessly through space—frequently accompanied by nausea. Dizziness lasting from half an hour to a few hours, associated with room-spinning vertigo, ringing in the ear, a feeling of pressure or fullness in the same ear and some hearing loss, is likely due to Ménière's disease (see above). Dizziness without hearing loss lasting from days to weeks may arise from vestibular neuronitis, a viral infection of the inner ear that may permanently injure the balance mechanism.

another attack, making them afraid to continue activities such as driving a car or operating machinery. Reassurance and support are an essential part of therapy, encouraging the sufferers to live, work and drive as normal between episodes. (Although attacks come on unexpectedly, there is usually enough warning to allow sufferers to stop driving or put down a dangerous instrument.)

While nothing reliably stalls an attack, prevents future bouts or slows the progress of this affliction, therapies range from acupuncture and herbal remedies to diuretics, low-salt diets, vasodilators and electrical stimulation. There are various options to consider besides medical therapy, surgery being a last resort for the small number where medical management fails.

Medical therapy reduces symptoms in 80 to 90 percent of cases.

For acute spells, treatment is:
- antinauseants or anti-emetics, e.g., dimenhydrinate (Gravol), or meclizine (Bonamine), as suppositories;
- vasodilators (to widen peripheral vessels and draw fluid from the head);
- sedatives/tranquilizers, to reduce anxiety;
- diuretics (e.g., hydrochlorothiazide) with potassium replacement, to flush fluid from the body;
- dietary salt (sodium) restriction, to reduce fluid retention;

- tinnitus maskers (external sound devices), placed behind the ear. "Masking" distractions, such as listening to the radio or tapes, can minimize the tinnitus.

Surgical remedies, contemplated only if medical treatment brings no relief, have varying success rates:
- labyrinthectomy cures vertigo but also abolishes hearing in the operated ear;
- inserting a "shunt" or plastic drainage tube that lessens fluid buildup is of doubtful value;
- microsurgery to cut the vestibular (balance) nerve removes vertigo but leaves tinnitus untouched, and risks damage to nearby structures (if improperly done).

Chemical strategies include:
- parenteral streptomycin, which may abolish vertigo but leaves varying degrees of imbalance, because it selectively destroys the ear's balancing or vestibular function;
- destruction of the balance/vestibular inner-ear compartment by instilling gentamicin is an effective treatment which destroys some sensory hearing cells, with a usually acceptable risk of some hearing loss.

While Ménière's disease is a most distressing disorder the remissions afford some relief, often for extended periods, and it tends to wane with increasing age.

MIDDLE EAR INFECTIONS ("OTITIS MEDIA")

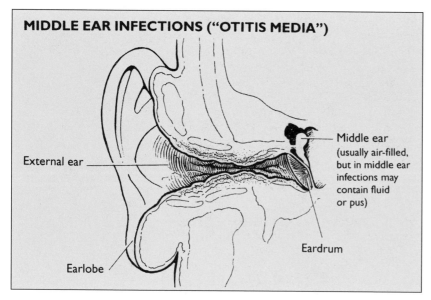

External ear

Earlobe

Middle ear (usually air-filled, but in middle ear infections may contain fluid or pus)

Eardrum

EAR INFECTIONS

External-ear infections

Skin infections of the outer ear canal, popularly dubbed swimmer's ear or tropical ear and medically termed "external otitis," are often due to moisture buildup in the outer ear canal. Dampness trapped in the outer ear sets the stage for infection via small abrasions, cuts or scratches in the skin. Although swimmers are particularly likely to get it, the water need not necessarily come from swimming—showering can do it. Cleaning too vigorously often causes

SWIMMER'S EAR: EXTERNAL EAR INFECTIONS

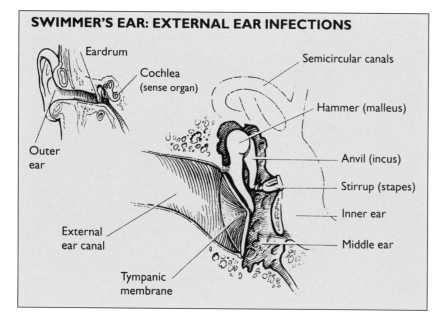

Eardrum

Cochlea (sense organ)

Outer ear

External ear canal

Tympanic membrane

Semicircular canals

Hammer (malleus)

Anvil (incus)

Stirrup (stapes)

Inner ear

Middle ear

the infection because it scratches the skin and allows bacteria to penetrate the ear canal's protective layer of epidermal cells and wax. Dirty fingernails or abrasion with a towel or Q-tip are likelier offenders than swimming in dirty water.

The first sign of external otitis is usually an itching, burning sensation. The ear may be unbearably tender to touch or to the slightest pressure and the outer canal may look swollen and crusty. Movements such as chewing can be agonizing. A foul-smelling, clear or puslike discharge may seep out. Occasionally, the glands behind the ear and in the neck also swell. Fever or generalized body involvement is extremely rare with external-ear infections. However, people should seek medical advice for any earache, as the ears are near to the brain, which could be threatened by spreading infection.

The usual treatment for swimmer's ear is locally applied drops containing a mixture of antibiotics and steroids (to kill the bacteria and suppress inflammation). An acidic rinse of dilute aluminum acetate or Burow's solution (which contains aluminum acetate) may help reduce the swelling. To facilitate entry into a swollen ear canal, the acidic solution can be inserted on a cotton wick, adding more liquid as needed, to trickle down the canal. Painkillers can ease the discomfort.

Most cases heal up after four to five days. Sometimes, the debris must be completely removed by an ear specialist with special cleaning or irrigation, and very occasionally, if an outer-ear infection fails to diminish or shows signs of spreading, drugs are given intravenously in hospital.

Middle-ear infections

Middle-ear infections are almost as frequent as common colds during childhood. Most children have had at least one bout of bacterial middle-ear infection—otitis media—by the time they are three years old. The disorder is more common in boys than girls and most prevalent in winter. The infection usually follows a cold or a bacterial infection. Acute otitis media causes excruciating discomfort, but usually vanishes quickly with the sudden release of pus from the ear.

In middle-ear infections the eustachian tube becomes plugged, air cannot enter and the middle ear fills up with fluid—either clear (serous) or infectious (purulent). Serous otitis media, popularly called "glue ear" is a serious cause of hearing loss in children, typically those aged five to eight. Fluid replacing air in the middle ear deadens sound and can cause hearing loss in one or both ears, perhaps retarding learning in school-age children. Many cases of glue ear resolve on their own or assisted by antibiotics and other drugs. If it does not clear up in three months, ventilating tubes may have to be inserted.

Acute otitis media typically follows a common cold, with symptoms such as sudden pain in the ear; sometimes severe, often starting at night, when a child may awaken howling and pulling at the ears. Or the discomfort may build gradually over 12 to 24 hours. There may also be fever, appetite loss, vomiting and diarrhea. However, some children with otitis media hardly seem sick at all, although the feeling of fullness in the ears (from the fluid) may make them tug at their ears. Since untreated middle-ear infections can also cause other serious complications, such as mastoiditis (infection of the mastoid bone behind the ear) or meningitis, even mild cases need prompt medical attention.

Physicians generally diagnose otitis media by looking at the eardrum with an otoscope (lighted ear-examining instrument). Sometimes it's necessary to remove wax from the outer ear canal in order to see the eardrum clearly.

If the eardrum ruptures, an exudate seeps out and the fluid release usually gives prompt relief. This sounds worse than it actually is—the ear drum is very good at self-repair. Children often wake up with some fluid on their pillows (and less cranky). The vast majority have no long-term hearing problems. Repeat infections, however, can raise the risk of hearing loss. Fluid can remain trapped in the ear even when the symptoms of acute infection are gone, which can affect hearing in the short term. Children may adapt to the slight hearing loss and parents, being unaware of it, may attribute the youngster's slow responses to stubbornness. The first hint of fluid in the ear may be lack of attention in school because a child can't hear clearly or keep up with peers. A child's inexplicable crankiness and fatigue—owing to the emotional toll of not hearing properly—may eventually drive parents to seek medical attention.

The treatment of otitis media is changing. In the past, all kids received antibiotics. Recent reviews, however, show that only about 1 child in 14 does better on antibiotics. This is likely because most infections are viral (and therefore not sensitive to antibiotics), and in part because of the increasing success of vaccines. Keep in mind that the proportion of children who do better on antibiotics is approaching the number who may get a rash or other side effect from these drugs. Having said this, a concerned physician may still decide to prescribe an antibiotic. A researcher named Van Buchem has developed a strategy that dictates that children under 2 years who are otherwise healthy and are likely to be available for follow-up can wait for 24 hours to see if symptoms improve. For children older than 2 years, a wait of 3 days is justified before prescribing antibiotics.

Remember that the symptoms that most irritate your child are pain and fever. Tempra (Tylenol) or ibuprofen (Advil) can reduce both of these. By 10 weeks after a middle-ear infection, approximately 90 percent of children are better without medical therapy. Yet even with antibiotics, some children drag on and on with fluid in the ears. Of those who clear up quickly after a first infection, many get recurrences. Specialists stress the need for frequent checkups and hearing tests in children prone to middle-ear infections.

Myringotomy (putting a small hole in the drum) to drain off the middle-ear fluid may be tried for persistent cases that last three months or more. For children old enough to cooperate, myringotomy can be done under a local anesthetic, but those under age 15 usually need general anesthesia. Some specialists promote myringotomy in the acute phase, since it is a relatively simple procedure, perhaps preferable to continued long-term antibiotics. The rationale for myringotomy with tube insertion is primarily to improve hearing and prevent delays in language development. However, no conclusive evidence has been presented to support or reject this hypothesis. The AAP Clinical Practice Guideline identifies the following as candidates for surgery: children with ear infections lasting 4

THINGS PARENTS CAN DO FOR CHILD-HOOD EAR INFECTIONS

- **If you suspect your child has a middle-ear infection, contact your physician, who will examine the child's ears.**
- **Although ear infections usually get better fast with antibiotics, remember to take all the medication prescribed.**
- **Call the physician if a child shows any of the following:**
  - **a worsening earache despite treatment;**
  - **a high fever over 39°C (102°F) in spite of treatment, or one that lasts more than three days;**
  - **excessive sleepiness, crankiness or fussiness;**
  - **a skin rash;**
  - **rapid, shallow or difficult breathing;**
  - **noticeable hearing loss (doesn't clearly hear noises, tape machine or what's said).**

For more information, contact the Canadian Hearing Society, 271 Spadina Road, Toronto, Ontario M5R 2V3, (416) 964-9595.

months or longer with persistent hearing loss or other signs and symptoms; recurrent or persistent infections in children at risk regardless of hearing status; and structural damage to the tympanic membrane or middle ear.

Tympanotomy—insertion of small plastic ventilating tubes or grommits—is promoted by some specialists for children with persistent, serous otitis media. The tubes are put into the blocked ear under general anesthesia, reventilating the middle ear and preventing or minimizing hearing loss. Randomized trials support the recommendation that tympanotomy tubes be used as initial surgery because the evidence shows a 62 percent decrease in the build-up of middle-ear fluid following the procedure. But "to tube or not to tube" is a much-debated question. Those who favor tubes argue that, although middle-ear infections generally heal without them, tubing helps to avoid a possible developmental lag in learning due to hearing loss. This is particularly critical from age 18 months to three years, when language develops. Missing the critical period may permanently undermine learning ability.

Those against tubing say that time alone (usually three months) makes most children better without any residual hearing loss. They cite surveys showing that with or without tubes, although 20 percent of children still have fluid in their ears and some hearing loss one month after a bout of otitis media, by two months only 9 percent and by the third month only 6 percent are still not back to normal. Opposition to ear tubes is increasing because, although insertion carries no greater surgical risks than average, it is still an operation done under general anesthesia, the tubes often need reinsertion and are a nuisance, as the need to avoid getting water in their ears restricts children's sport activities.

One controversial alternative is continuous low-dose preventive antibiotic therapy given throughout the winter for otitis-prone children whose middle ears predictably flare up at the end of each cold. Use of antibiotics may prevent ear infection. The overall message is to check hearing regularly in all children with chronic or recurrent middle-ear infections.

TOOTH AND GUM CARE

Gum disease, or, to give the condition its correct name, periodontal disease (from the Greek *peri*, around, and *odontos*, tooth), is popularly regarded as an inevitable part of aging, associated with bad breath and lengthy dental treatments. Yet periodontal disease does not need to accompany normal aging. One of the commonest causes of adult tooth loss, periodontal disease is an almost entirely preventable condition. It can usually be avoided or reversed by good oral hygiene and regular dental visits. However, left untreated, the condition will damage the tooth-supporting tissues and may ultimately lead to loss of teeth.

About nine out of ten Canadians experience occasional gum inflammation (inflamed gingival tissues), but the modern approach is to regard periodontal disease as an avoidable infection that can be prevented or kept well under control by good home mouth care and regular, professional cleaning by a dentist or dental hygienist.

Thorough tooth-brushing and, more important, between-the-teeth cleaning (by flossing or other means) go a long way in preventing periodontal disease and helping us keep our teeth to a ripe old age. But estimates show that many Canadians fail to practice even the minimum amount of daily mouth care, and less than half of all Canadians regularly visit a dentist. People are particularly negligent about daily between-the-teeth cleansing/flossing—although periodontal disease usually starts between the teeth.

Bacteria in plaque are largely to blame for gum disease

When the 17th-century Dutch microscopist Antony van Leeuwenhoek examined the whitish matter scraped from the surface of his own teeth under his microscope, he was amazed to see hundreds of tiny creatures, which he described as "small living animalcules that moved very prettily." The substance van Leeuwenhoek had dislodged was dental plaque, and the animalcules were mobile bacteria teeming in it. As we know today, bacteria in plaque are the primary cause of periodontal disease.

Plaque is the soft, gummy deposit that accumulates overnight on teeth, dentures and fillings and makes them feel unpleasantly furry in the morning. Plaque consists of many different bacteria, their nutrients and waste products. Scientists estimate that one gram (0.035 oz) of adult human plaque contains no fewer than 170,000,000,000 (1.7×10^{11}) organisms, of a few hundred different species. Plaque starts to form minutes after the teeth are brushed, and within twelve hours of even the most thorough tooth cleansing, gluey, organized bacterial colonies begin to coat the teeth. After 24 hours the bacteria in plaque already adhere tenaciously to the tooth surfaces—which explains why it's wise to clean the teeth thoroughly more than once a day!

The greater the amount of plaque, the greater the chance of irritating the gingival (gum) tissues. Besides its quantity, the types of bacteria in plaque influence the kind and extent of periodontal disease. While some types of bacteria in plaque live in harmony with the mouth, others are pathogenic (health-damaging) strains that injure the teeth and tissues around them. As plaque accumulates, it gradually acquires more and more destructive bacteria that, together with their toxic metabolic byproducts, attack the oral tissues and trigger the body's inflammatory response. The inflammation can be locally damaging and cause bone resorption (loss). In addition, some bacteria in plaque produce volatile sulphur compounds that smell like rotting eggs, which is why some people with periodontal disease have bad breath.

Calculus, or mineralized plaque—popularly known as tartar—is plaque crystallized into hard, discolored deposits. Like coral in the ocean, calculus provides a rough surface on which bacteria can proliferate. It requires professional scaling (cleaning) by a dentist or dental hygienist.

The two main categories of periodontal disease

Gingivitis (from the Latin *gingiva*, gums) is a relatively common, reversible gum inflammation that affects many, producing at worst no more than a little bleeding, swelling and redness around the gum line. Gingivitis often arises during adolescence, when tooth-cleaning tends to

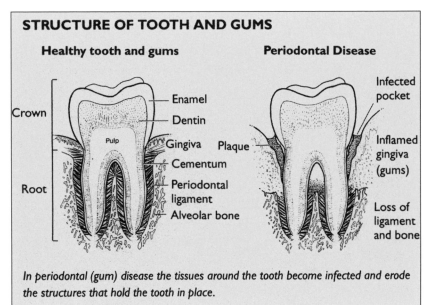

STRUCTURE OF TOOTH AND GUMS

Healthy tooth and gums

Crown

Root

Enamel
Dentin
Pulp
Gingiva
Cementum
Periodontal ligament
Alveolar bone

Periodontal Disease

Plaque

Infected pocket

Inflamed gingiva (gums)

Loss of ligament and bone

In periodontal (gum) disease the tissues around the tooth become infected and erode the structures that hold the tooth in place.

be sloppy, but is usually a disease in name only, causing little "dis-ease"—little pain and discomfort (except for the form once called trench mouth). At present, it's impossible to predict in whom the mere redness and tissue puffiness of gingivitis will progress to the more serious periodontitis. Since there's no easy way to identify those at greatest risk, everyone is encouraged to practice prevention, clean their teeth well to remove plaque, avoid smoking and seek regular dental care.

Periodontitis, a less common but more persistent bacterial infection, affects about 40 percent of adults, ranges from mild to severe and extends deep into the tissues that support the teeth. Advanced periodontitis, which affects

COMMON ERRORS IN MOUTH CARE INCLUDE:

- brushing wrongly, too hard or not thoroughly enough, not up to the gum line, too fast and not for the recommended time—some say three-minute sessions—morning, night and after meals;
- insufficient or no interdental (between-teeth) cleaning—i.e., flossing or using other between-teeth cleaning aids such as rubber-tipped stimulators, toothpicks or stim-u-dents (wooden between-teeth cleaners). Only about 15 percent of Canadians regularly use floss or other interdental cleaning devices;
- overlooking red or bleeding gums—the first signs of periodontal disease;
- waiting until it hurts—seeking dental attention only when a tooth or the gums become painful;
- neglecting regular dentist visits;
- smoking—known to be a strong factor linked to periodontal disease;
- not using fluoride to prevent tooth decay.

about 10 percent of the North American population, can have lasting consequences—including eventual tooth loss. Some forms of periodontitis are rapidly progressive, leading to significant tissue destruction in a few years—especially a type called "juvenile-onset periodontitis," which begins in adolescence and may be hereditary.

The advance of periodontal disease—from a mild inflammatory condition to a deep gum infection—often has few signs until some bone loss in the jaw has occurred, with considerable tooth loosening. Periodontitis advances little by little, down the root of the tooth, taking hold if pathogenic bacteria penetrate deep under the gum tissues (sometimes down to the bone). As the infection progresses, the tissues recede and detach from the tooth surfaces, forming deep pockets (see diagram above). With weakened attachment, the teeth feel jiggly or loose. Dentists use radiographs and a periodontal probe marked off in millimeters to determine the extent of bone loss.

The bacteria responsible for periodontitis cannot be removed by normal tooth cleaning. Severe cases need professional attention to remove the plaque and calculus, a procedure called scaling and root-planing. Together with meticulous home mouth care, this may be all that's needed. But unfortunately, about 15 percent of cases resist such treatment, and should be seen by specialists. For unresponsive cases, finding the right antibiotic would be an invaluable adjunct to therapy.

The modern approach is to try to identify the specific bacteria responsible and to reduce or eradicate them with appropriate antibiotics. There are now a few special commercial laboratories in the United States that use DNA probes to assist dentists in determining the bacteria in the colonizing areas of periodontal decay so that patients may be treated more accurately. The University of Toronto Department of Periodontics runs a consulting service, including limited microbiology, for patients plagued by severe, recurrent periodontal problems who are referred by dentists or specialists.

As in some medical infections, surgery may be needed for extensive periodontal disease, to gain better access for debridement (scraping) to

RATING MOUTH-CARE PRODUCTS

- Plaque removal is best done mechanically by scraping or scrubbing. Meticulous tooth-brushing and flossing should get rid of most of the bacterial film above the gum line.
- Teeth should be brushed at least twice a day, morning and night, and preferably also after meals! The brushing should be thorough and should start young—as soon as the teeth appear (at age two or three). At first, parents can wipe and polish a child's teeth with a washcloth to remove plaque (up to age four or so); later they can supervise brushing until the child becomes adept enough to clean the teeth properly. Tooth-brushing should reach all teeth with short strokes and a gentle rotary motion. (The best way to learn to brush teeth properly is to get a dental professional to show you how.)
- Dental flossing, or between-teeth cleaning, although a bore to many who don't bother, is a must because it is between the teeth that plaque does the most harm. Many dental experts consider between-teeth cleaning or flossing even more important than brushing. It should be done at least once daily, with a gentle scraping motion. Never floss too vigorously or saw at the gums because this can bruise and damage these delicate tissues. Dentists recommend unwaxed or lightly waxed dental floss (waxed frays less). Those who cannot manage floss can use special toothpicks, rubber-tipped devices or interdented toothbrushes.
- The recommended toothbrush is soft, with three to four rows of tufted, polished rounded nylon bristles and a slightly rounded or flat surface. Overly hard toothbrushes can damage the gums. The brush should be changed every three to four months as bristles tend to splay and get dirty.
- Professional scaling should be done regularly (depending on individual needs), as it is not plaque above the gum line but deeper bacterial colonies that cause periodontitis. Only dental instruments used by skilled professionals can remove calculus properly.
- A new generation of power brushes claims superior plaque removal. These are recommended for those whose limited dexterity precludes efficient brushing with conventional brushes.
- Irrigators, or water-spray devices, shoot jets of water between the teeth, which may dislodge food particles and dilute bacterial products but do not remove plaque thoroughly. They are useful adjuncts for people with braces and bridges.

- Toothpastes and mouthwashes are sold with a barrage of anti-tartar, anti-cavity claims. Which toothpaste is best? Does it make any difference? As far as periodontal disease goes, it doesn't matter. Toothpaste is not even essential. Provided the teeth are brushed properly, any toothpaste is as good as any other, although those endorsed by the Canadian Dental Association (CDA) are more likely to provide optimal results. Since toothpaste contains abrasives, it may be a little more effective at removing plaque than tap water alone, but only marginally. Most toothpastes contain about one-fifth to one-third water, a humectant (which keeps it from drying out), binding agents, foaming agents (which make it spread evenly and dissolve in water), abrasives, flavoring and perhaps artificial sweetener. Fluoride-containing toothpastes are highly recommended for fighting tooth decay. Baking soda products are also good tooth-cleansers,

- Claims for antiplaque and antitartar toothpaste and mouthwash abound, and some products contain active ingredients said to fight tartar (calculus). But any antitartar product can only combat calculus buildup after a thorough professional cleaning, and only above the gum line. It cannot remove old deposits but can only block the formation of new calculus. In general, the CDA approval of many products is based more on their fluoride content than on "anti-tartar" claims.

- Among the antibacterials, the more promising ones include *chlorhexidine* (in some prescription mouthwashes), essential oils (in Listerine mouthwash) and *sanguinarine* (in Viadent products).

Sorting out the anti-plaque claims

Whatever a toothpaste or mouthwash promises regarding plaque prevention, it cannot claim to be effective against the diseases of gingivitis and periodontitis, because before any product can make legitimate claims about disease prevention it must undergo rigorous testing. The CDA has recently developed a list of criteria concerning gingivitis control which toothpaste and mouthwash manufacturers must meet before being given the CDA's stamp of approval. So far no commercial product has qualified for approval (the standards are very new), although the American Dental Association has approved Listerine (an over-the-counter agent) and the prescription mouthwash Peridex for controlling gingivitis.

- ***Chlorhexidine***, is an antibacterial substance used in the United States in Procter and Gamble's Peridex and in a number of other mouthwash and gel preparations in other countries. In Canada, some chlorhexidine products can be sold by the manufacturer to dentists for their office use, and dentists can prescribe chlorhexidine formulations that can be dispensed by pharmacists. Chlorhexidine binds readily to the oral tissues, stays in the mouth for some time after rinsing and is the most effective agent in controlling plaque and gingivitis. Over the long term it may transiently stain the teeth and fillings and cause some aberrations in taste sensation. Some acute allergic responses have been reported among hypersensitive individuals.

- ***Essential oils*** (the active ingredients in Listerine) are germicidal agents. Studies show that rinsing for 30 seconds with full-strength Listerine twice a day can decrease plaque buildup on the teeth.

- ***Sanguinarine***, extracted from the roots of the bloodroot (a wild North American flowering plant), has been shown in some studies to reduce plaque buildup and gingivitis. However, the evidence is conflicting—it has not yet been proved to reduce gingivitis over the long haul, although long-term trials are just nearing completion. Viadent, both a toothpaste and mouthwash containing sanguinaria extract, have to be used in combination to achieve the therapeutic effect of the other mouth rinses alone.

- ***A mouthwash called Plax***, containing sodium benzoate, sodium lauryl sulphate and sodium salicylate, has also been claimed by manufacturers to reduce plaque. Recent independent research has not substantiated this claim.

The problem with all these agents is that they do not stay in the mouth long, even the longer-lasting chlorhexidine, so any effect is likely to be transitory, necessitating continued use over extended periods. Furthermore, they do not reach plaque in the pocket below the gingival margin, which is where bacteria do the most damage. Whether these mouthwashes and toothpastes will prove useful at controlling gingivitis in the long run remains to be seen. No study has shown them to be effective in preventing periodontitis.

COSMETIC TOOTH-IMPROVING AIDS

- **Tooth-whitening (bleaching) agents to use at home or in the dental office;**
- **new, light-colored bonding materials to fill in cracks and notches, or use as fillings;**
- **implants screwed into the bone to replace missing teeth;**
- **new orthodontic methods to straighten teeth and adjust the bite;**
- **increasingly, cosmetic tooth improvements are coming on stream. Ask your dentist about them!**

reduce the extent of periodontal pockets and to impede bacterial colonization. Known as flap surgery, the procedure exposes the tooth root for rigorous cleaning and the bone for minor contouring or placement of grafting materials. New forms of periodontal surgery include "guided tissue regeneration," which tries to stimulate new growth of cells over the previously exposed and diseased parts.

Tooth sensitivity a common problem

People whose teeth hurt when exposed to touch, heat, cold, sweet, sour or other stimuli, in the absence of any identified tooth disorder may have a condition called "dentin sensitivity." Previously known as "tooth hypersensitivity," dentin sensitivity sends roughly one in seven North Americans flocking to the dentist for relief, at some time in their lives. If the dentist finds no cavity, abscess, ill-fitting crown or other reason for the pain, it's blamed on "sensitivity" due to excess stimulation of dentin tubules inside one or more teeth.

The primary reasons for dentin sensitivity are enamel loss, gum recession and an exposed root (nerve). Rough toothbrushing often causes it by damaging the gums or eroding the tooth enamel. Those most likely to experience tooth sensitivity are people with receding gums (perhaps due to periodontal disease); habitual night-time tooth grinders—who may fracture their tooth enamel; anyone exposed to acid fumes at work (e.g., battery acids—which erode the tooth enamel); bulimics who habitually throw up (causing tooth erosion from the constant exposure to acidic stomach contents); people who drink vast amounts of fruit juices or carbonated drinks (exposing the tooth enamel to excessive amounts of acid); and over-zealous tooth brushers.

Paradoxically, tooth sensitivity lessens as people age, despite the fact that more dentin is exposed as people get "long in the tooth." The reason for the waning sensitivity is that the tooth pulp (rich in nerves) recedes and secondary or protective dentin, which is denser

and less porous, forms new layers and sensation decreases.

In dealing with tooth sensitivity, a dentist is the first port of call to determine possible causes of the pain—such as cavities, periodontal disease, chipped, cracked or grooved teeth, fractured fillings, damaged crowns or other conditions. If dentin sensitivity is the suspected cause of the problem, the next step is to determine its severity. Often, just explaining that the pain comes from over-vigorous toothbrushing and suggesting a gentler brushing technique and desensitizing toothpastes, solves the problem. Reassurance that the condition is *not* harmful, not a cavity, abscess or periodontal disease, and that it's likely to diminish with time, may be all that's required.

For severe sensitivity, perhaps affecting several teeth, the dentist may suggest trying desensitizers or sealants (protein-precipitating substances, tubule-occluding and tubule-sealing agents)—applied as gels, rinses or toothpastes. Modern self-treatment can be very effective. For instance, potassium nitrate, used as gel or toothpaste (such as Oral B, Sensodyne or Protect), blocks neural pain transmission and relieves many cases within four to six weeks. Fluoride (as sodium fluoride, stannous fluoride or other products) is another effective desensitizer thought to strengthen the calcific barrier (enamel) on the dentin surface. Applied regularly and in sufficient concentration, it can reduce tooth sensitivity in a week or two, although the pain may return in time.

If home treatment with desensitizing agents doesn't work, in-office treatment may be advised. In-office treatments can be rapidly effective, but they require several applications. Methods include occluding the dentin tubules with oxalate salts to prevent the aggravating movement of tubule fluid. If sensitivity is due to notched or cracked teeth, dentists may use sealants such as stannous fluoride that deposit insoluble salts into the dentin tubules, or they may fill the tooth with bonded material, or use varnishes, resins or paints to block the sensitivity.

Sexual health

Developing healthy sexual attitudes • Tracking key stages in sexual development • Combatting sexual exploitation and abuse • The development of sexual behavior • Masturbation • Sexual dysfunction • Sex therapy • Sexually transmitted infections • Recent trends in birth control

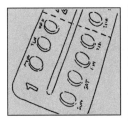

LEARNING TO BECOME a healthy sexual person is a complex process that begins at conception and continues from birth through childhood to puberty, molded by biological, social and cultural forces. Our opinions, beliefs and feelings about sexuality are shaped by a mixture of early childhood learning, religious teachings, social customs, cultural expectations and personal experiences. In turn, these influences determine how, when and what we communicate to our children about sexuality, appropriate sexual behavior and gender roles.

DEVELOPING HEALTHY SEXUAL ATTITUDES

The term "sexual health" has different meanings in various cultures and societies. The World Health Organization (WHO) defines sexual health as "the integration of physical, emotional, intellectual and social aspects of sexual being in ways that are positively enriching and that enhance personality, communication and love." Sexual health involves the capacity to enjoy and control sexual and reproductive behavior, "free from fears, shame, guilt and false beliefs, in accordance with a personal and social ethic." Sexual health is a crucial part of overall health, and since health is a human right, the WHO proposes that sexual health is also a human right.

Canada's *Guidelines for Sexual Health Education* recently published by Health Canada endorse this view. The guidelines describe sexual health as a "major aspect of personal health for people at all ages and stages of their lives." In essence, sexual health depends on a good self-image, comfort with one's body, a knowledge of genital anatomy, being able to communicate sexual thoughts, fantasies and anxieties, feeling free to discuss and negotiate sexual wishes, a sense of dignity and respect for oneself and others.

Despite the upbeat image portrayed by the terms "sexual health" and "healthy sexuality," the guidelines caution that words like "health" and "healthy" might be misused by some to express approval or disapproval under the guise of "medical" authority.

"Nature" and "nurture" jointly script sexuality

Is the script for sexual behavior mainly biological (written in the genes) or due to social conditioning? "The answer," says U.S. gender expert John Money, "is both together, neither alone. The only certainty is that men impregnate, women menstruate, gestate and lactate... Beyond these basic functions, nothing sexual is immutably ordained. We are born male or female, but we're *made* masculine or feminine." The way that adults handle and respond to a child, how they communicate messages about its body and behavior profoundly influence sexual health.

Delineating certain activities as strictly

7

DEFINING SOME KEY TERMS

The terms "sex" and "gender" are often used interchangeably, although each has a slightly different meaning. To add to the confusion, "having sex" is popularly equated with sexual intercourse. Biologists commonly use the word "sex" to identify the sexes—male and female—and their reproductive functions, while "gender" refers to gender-specific behavioral characteristics such as those labeled "masculine" or "feminine."

Gender identity is the internalized or "inner conviction" of being a boy or girl, man or woman. Children learn their gender through countless messages, both verbal and non-verbal, telling them, "You are a boy—you do this" or "You're a girl—you do that."

Gender roles are the *public* expression of our gender (or sexual) identity—depicting to the external world how we want to be viewed as girls or boys, men or women. Sex role displays to others our sense of masculinity, femininity or ambiguity; what we portray to the outside world may or may not coincide with our inner gender identity.

"feminine" or "masculine" can lock people into stereotypes that limit individual expression. Overly rigid stereotyping can condition boys to believe in toughness and girls in submissiveness, producing males who feel compelled to be "in charge" of all sexual moves, and females who think they can't or must not take the initiative. Although gender roles are becoming more flexible, many sexologists warn that male aggression, winning and authority are still deeply ingrained in Western sexual scripts.

Parents provide the background "melody"
Parents act as gender role models, providing values and examples of family, sexual and work relationships. They lay the groundwork for sexual development. Some parents worry about the responsibility of ensuring their child's sexual health in today's sophisticated world, which is pervaded by so much flamboyant and explicit sex information. But while parents lay the foundations for their child's development, they need not feel overwhelmed by it. These days knowledge about sex comes from diverse sources and there are ample guidelines and books to help parents steer their children towards sexual health.

"Parents provide the melody," notes one Canadian Planned Parenthood official and sexual health educator "by their attitudes, the way they answer questions and react to sexual situations. But they don't need to have all the answers on tap, nor need they feel completely at ease about

imparting sex information. The main thing is to keep the channels of communication open." To an awkward question, posed at the wrong moment—perhaps on a crowded subway—a parent can bid for time and say, "That's a good question so let's discuss it tonight," and remember to do so, postponing but *not* dismissing it.

Giving the genitals and reproductive organs correct names such as "penis," "vagina," and "vulva" helps children learn that these body parts are as natural as the rest. Of course, a two-year-old will not understand human anatomy, but it helps to explain things accurately. Parents should remember that they teach as much by facial expressions, gestures and how they react as by what they say.

Children spontaneously explore their genitals as a natural part of growing up and parents who treat toileting, touching the genital area and sexual play with comfort make their children feel natural and positive about their bodies.

School sex education programs can be pivotal
Schools can give young people access to effective sex information, providing them with the knowledge and skills needed to enhance sexual well-being. The goal of sexual health education is to help people achieve positive outcomes such as self-esteem and rewarding relationships, and to avoid negative consequences such as unwanted pregnancy, sexual coercion or sexually transmitted infections.

Since schools are clearly a "vital resource for providing children and adolescents with the knowledge and skills needed to make and act upon decisions that promote sexual health," parents can help their children develop healthy sexuality by finding out about school sex education courses and assessing what and how their children are being taught. It's a mistake to leave this vital part of human education merely to happenstance or chance! Parents can and should play a vital part in their children's sexual health.

TRACKING KEY STAGES IN SEXUAL DEVELOPMENT
The steps that form biological sex, gender identity, sex role and adult sexuality can be considered "critical gates" through which people pass en route to sexual maturity.

The first gate: Fertilization

At conception the chromosomes (genes) of egg and sperm unite. The genes, contained in the DNA molecules inside the chromosomes, are a flexible blueprint and their expression depends upon many influences, both in the uterus and in the outside world. The sex chromosome pair determines the future child's gender: XX makes a female body, XY produces a male. The X and Y chromosomes carry different information in their genes or DNA molecules, and according to this information, different characteristics will develop.

The second gate: Development of immature gonads

Although the early human embryo already possesses the XX or XY chromosomes to guide its gender development, it is not yet *anatomically* male or female. To become male or female the embryo must first develop gonads (reproductive organs). Nature's basic mammalian plan is female. To become a male, the fetus requires "extras"—the Y (male) chromosome to direct the development of a male body and a fetal testis to secrete testosterone (male hormone) at critical fetal stages. (Without these "extras," a human fetus will automatically develop a female anatomy.) An XY (male) fetus normally develops a testis at six to eight weeks of gestation, while XX (female) embryos develop ovaries at 11 weeks after conception.

The third and fourth gates: Production of fetal hormones

Testosterone from the fetal testes triggers development of a penis, scrotum and other male reproductive structures. Females, lacking testosterone, follow the "built-in" pattern to make a clitoris, labia and internal female structures. The male hormone (testosterone) establishes the future male pattern of non-cyclic or acyclic hormone release, also priming brain pathways for male behavior.

The fifth gate: Priming fetal brain circuits

Encoding of neural brain circuits by testosterone (or its absence)—for cyclic hormone release patterns (monthly ovulation and menstruation)

in females, non-cyclic in males—occurs at 11 to 12 weeks of fetal development. As one expert puts it, "not only the male body, but also the foundations of the male mind are created in the womb." Although controversial, some experts believe that fetal hormone (testosterone) levels may drive certain brain areas toward gender-distinctive traits such as greater aggression and visual-spatial ability in males and more verbal fluency in females. But we still do not know exactly how fetal hormones alter brain pathways.

Some researchers suggest that the earlier onset of puberty in girls gives the female brain less time to specialize its two hemispheres—perhaps explaining so-called "female intuition." The closer connection between the two cerebral hemispheres in women may facilitate rapid interpretation of nuances. Males, by contrast, with later puberty and more specialized cerebral hemispheres, may more easily trace logical pathways and zero in on relevant details, excluding extraneous signals. Or so the current story goes!

Modern research has revealed a few gender-specific differences in the development of the cerebral hemispheres, and small anatomical sex differences in certain brain areas. According to Harvard psychologists Eleanor Maccoby and Ruth Jacklin, the only well-founded cerebral sex differences are that girls outstrip boys in verbal skills, and that boys tend to excel at math. Parental attitudes may reinforce or narrow the gap in mental development between the two sexes. Studies show that overprotection may foster intellectual ability in boys, while girls seem to do best when urged to be independent and self-reliant. The details of brain differences in human males and females, and how they arise, is just being elucidated.

The sixth gate: Birth and gender assignment

When a baby is born, the first look is often not at the face but between the legs, assigning the newborn its gender. (Monkeys too inspect their newborn offspring's genitals.) Sex assignment opens the floodgates to the powerful sway of social, religious and cultural influences on the child's gender identity and future sexual behavior.

The seventh gate: From birth onwards—the first four years

After birth, the way that parents, siblings, relatives, friends and others respond to the baby scripts it for "gender-suitable" behavior. Baby girls are supposedly more gently held and cuddled than boys, while boys are bounced around in a more physical way and often less pampered.

By age two, a child can distinguish between "Mommy" and "Daddy." Children notice that their bodies are like that of their mothers and sisters or their fathers and brothers, and identify with the same-sex parent, siblings and others. Around age three to four, children become curious about gender differences. ("Why does daddy have a penis but mommy not?")

Researchers contend that young children learn and enjoy erotic arousal and that early sexual stimulation contributes to normal physical and psychosexual development. Childhood sex play is common and natural. If discouraged from it, children will likely carry on in secret. Playing "house" with friends and siblings may include what's seen at home or on TV, and natural curiosity—"show me yours and I'll show you mine."

Current evidence suggests that most childhood sexual experiences are positive and growth-promoting, unless they involve force or abuse, or trigger negative reactions. Left alone, most children would naturally develop what Canadian sex researcher Bill Fisher and colleagues call "erotophilia"—natural enjoyment of erotic/tactile behavior.

The eighth gate: Middle childhood years and sex play

As children are exposed to new ideas, they learn what adults regard as acceptable or unacceptable behavior. Parents can help by being open to questions and talking about sexuality at "teachable moments"—for instance when bathing a child, seeing a TV sex scene, seeing an ad for tampons, watching a teen mom pushing a stroller or reading a news item about "young boys being molested."

Some children become modest, want to cover up while dressing or bathing, and demand privacy; others are still happy to wander around naked or share a bath with younger siblings. The family should respect a child's wish for privacy and feel comfortable with it.

By age seven to nine, same-sex peer groups become all-important. Teasing and taunting are common. Gender stereotypes can be strong. "Girls don't play football." "Boys are dumb." While peers are a predominant influence, parents still count and they need to tune in to their children's feelings and experiences.

Signs of puberty may appear such as breast swelling and an increase in testicle size. Some girls start their periods. Fantasies, daydreams and crushes on favorite teachers, older teens and adults or media idols are common. At this age, children seek explicit, scientific sex information: "How does the sperm find the egg?" "If a woman killed in a car crash is carrying a baby, will it die too?"

Parents and society can disturb natural childhood responses by negative messages implying that certain sexual feelings or behaviors are taboo and possibly sinful, sometimes building a wall of guilt and shame around sexual activity. If parents punish a child for some sexual expression or behavior they may script the child for erotophobia, fear of things sexual. Those who themselves received childhood messages of guilt and shame about sex may become erotophobic adults, who tend to be limited in the sexual behavior they're willing to try. They may abhor sexual imagery and erotica, suppress sexual fantasies and avoid sexual exploration. Such attitudes may profoundly affect the way their children view sexuality.

The ninth gate: Puberty completes sexual development

Hormonal changes at puberty are a final "gate" in sexual development, with the appearance of secondary sex characteristics. Dating may begin. The mix of sexual fantasies and desire is both exhilarating and confusing. Since sexual "turn-ons" become more evident in adolescence, many believe these feelings are instilled by a first love, a homosexual or locker-room encounter certain movies or some influential older friend. But in reality, adolescence is more a time of revelation than a turning point.

According to U.S. gender authority John Money, the sexual script completed during adolescence is "a love map" of the kind of erotic activities we like to engage in. "Love maps are personalized and unique, each containing innate courtship patterns common to all humans (because of our shared ancestry), also incorporating influences acquired during fetal development and early childhood." In this view, depending on our unique love map, each of us chooses a certain partner and reacts differently to erotic stimuli, replaying a sexual script written in childhood based on the messages received about touching, intimacy, sensuality, erotic play, relationships and connectedness. No amount of later post-adolescent exposure to personal experiences, ads, TV or pornography will alter the basic gender script.

As one eminent therapist points out, "However profound and influential the psychosocial experiences at puberty, earlier forces imprinted during infancy determine sexual health and are responsible for most sexual disturbances, anomalies and ambiguities. The roots of our sexual triggers and fantasies lie far back in our childhood biographies." Each person's sex script, formed by early influences, is consolidated at puberty, and substantiated and replayed through life. This may explain why a second spouse so often resembles the first, or why a homosexual or transsexual stays that way.

The tenth gate: Gender role and sexual orientation

The sexual scripts or love maps engraved through childhood and consolidated at puberty determine sex-partner choice. Partner choice might or might not fit what family, society or religion deem acceptable.

Evidence suggests that in adult relationships, women generally initiate courtship, with subtle signals, while men use more overt styles. In one study asking college men and women how they flirted, researchers found that women recognized and responded to very early stages of courtship, while the young men often seemed insensitive or oblivious to the early flirtatious moves made by women. Men pegged the start of courtship at the first physical contact, women at subtle glances. As one gender expert puts it: "It is as if men are unconsciously blind—or have been blinded by defeminization—to initial courtship moves."

Occasionally, the sex scripting can become badly distorted or perverted if, for instance, a child is sexually abused or receives disturbing sex signals. A distorted sex script may result in "paraphilias": unconventional sexual expressions, perversions or illegal behavior such as pedophilia (sexual desire for children).

MAIN SEXUAL DEVELOPMENT STAGES

From birth to age two, children may:
- explore and touch body parts, including genitals
- begin to develop an attitude (either positive or negative) toward their bodies
- adopt expected behavior for boys and girls

From ages three to four, children may:
- become curious about gender/body differences
- touch themselves and learn to masturbate
- play house, mimic adults, explore sex play with same-age friends and siblings
- establish "gender identity"—inner belief of being male or female
- repeat swear words

From ages five to eight, children may:
- continue sex play
- become curious about pregnancy and birth: "Where did I come from?"
- form strong same-gender friendships
- choose new role models, perhaps teachers, older peers
- compare own situation with peers—identify with peer-groups
- enjoy name-calling, swearing and teasing.

From ages nine to twelve, children may:
- start puberty, especially girls
- become modest and seek privacy when dressing, bathing
- experience emotional ups and downs, become moody
- have romantic crushes on friends, older teens, adults, film and TV stars;
- be strongly influenced by same-gender friends
- feel awkward, develop altered (poor) self-image—girls especially
- have sexual or romantic fantasies
- be forced into decisions about sexual activity and drug-taking.

MANAGING THE MEDIA'S POWERFUL INFLUENCE

"Media literacy"—the ability to assess media messages—is a necessary part of effective sex education. Today's mass media transmit sex information in many formats—TV commercials, soaps, cartoons, talk shows, computers, chat-groups, websites, news, magazines, billboards, video games and movies. Media images often portray unrealistic ideals, influencing children's self-perception, and children may see behavior that they cannot yet comprehend. Links between sex and violence can be most upsetting. Children of all ages need to know their parents are "askable"—available to answer questions and discuss what's heard or seen.

COMBATTING SEXUAL EXPLOITATION AND ABUSE

Sexual abuse is one of the most difficult topics to discuss or explain to children. In doing so, it's crucial to distinguish natural, healthy curiosity and childhood sex play from exploitative behavior. Most early childhood sex play takes place between mixed-gender friends of *similar age*, when both (or all) are willing participants. It's usually lighthearted and untainted by fear or shame. When an older more powerful person forces a child to engage in sexual exploration or activity, this is *not* sex play. It is sexual abuse.

Parents want to know how best to protect their children without scaring them. They want their child to be aware of possible sexual exploitation and know how to deal with it, without becoming unduly frightened or suspicious. There is little point in telling children "don't talk to strangers" when most sexual abusers are someone the child knows and trusts, often a relative or friend of the family.

To help children distinguish normal, playful sex exploration from potentially abusive situations parents can try to explain the difference between "appropriate" and "inappropriate" touches—and what to do if a child encounters unwanted touching or other advances. Children need to recognize their right to privacy. They must learn that they have the *absolute right* to say "no," and know how to reject unwanted touches, kisses, tickling or squeezing.

Playing "What would you do if…" games might help, as well as watching for blurred boundaries, for overly eroticized behavior between an older and younger child. Children should learn to tell trusted adults if anything seems wrong. If age-appropriate sex topics are comfortably discussed at home, a child will likely find it easier to talk about situations that might indicate abuse—such as feeling pressured or bribed into sexual acts by adults or older children.

The benefits of affirming parental hugs

Some psychologists and sex experts fear that our current concern about sex abuse may engender a cold, non-tactile approach to child rearing and parent-child relationships. Many parents, as well as teachers, may avoid touching or hugging a child for fear that their actions will be misunderstood, depriving youngsters of much-needed physical closeness.

Yet, psychologists stress that children thrive both physically and emotionally if cuddled, held and loved, and studies on child-rearing customs around the world reveal a definite link between the capacity for healthy adult sexual intimacy and early love and nurturance. Children who received lots of loving care and caresses became well-adapted, peaceful adults. Those deprived of warmth or given negative messages about their bodies grew into adults prone to violence. We all need plenty of reaffirming hugs throughout life.

Talking about sex with your child

- Teach proper scientific names for body parts, including genitals and reproductive organs.
- Stay "askable"—open to questions—making sure your child knows you're willing to listen and talk.
- Take all questions seriously and answer in age-appropriate detail that the child can understand.
- Keep the information simple, adding detail as the child grows older; ask for feedback to check what's been understood.
- Be honest—if you tell a preschooler that babies are "brought by storks," the child will ultimately learn it's not true.
- Take your time: there's no need to have instant answers to all sex questions. What you don't know you can look up and come back to, but don't dismiss it.
- If you don't know the answer to a question, say so; if you need to think about it, or feel uncomfortable talking about something, say so and discuss it later.
- Reopen the subject if you aren't satisfied with the information you gave or the way you handled a situation.
- Try to treat sexual subjects naturally and clear up misinformation: "I grew in mummy's tummy"; "No dear you grew in the uterus inside mother's body"; "Sperm are swallowed to meet mummy's egg"; "No dear sperm come from daddy's penis and travel up mummy's vagina."
- Remember that children are *always* listening and pick up nuances.

- Check what's being learned at school and what a child knows: "Mummy, what's a condom for?" "What do you think it's for?"
- Avoid generalized, gender-biased foul-mouthing—"she's a slut," or "all men are after just one thing," which can set the stage for self-image problems.
- Remember sex education means more than listing biological facts. Discuss values, feelings and skills to help children become sexually healthy people.
- Be aware that some children ask all kinds of questions, while others aren't question-askers. You may have to seize opportunities to bring up the subject—perhaps when watching TV, seeing a pregnant woman or reading a headline.
- Don't jump to conclusions. If a nine-year-old asks about oral sex, don't presume that he or she plans to try it. These days, children hear about all kinds of things that their parents didn't learn about until much later (if at all).

For more information, consult public health departments; planned parenthood associations; SIECUS (Sexuality Information and Education Council of the U.S.), 130 West 42nd St., Suite 350, New York, NY 10036; the Sex Information and Education Council of Canada (SIECCAN), 850 Coxwell Avenue, Toronto, ON M4C 5R1, Tel: (416) 466-5304; www.sieccan@web.net; the *Canadian Guidelines for Sexual Health Education*, from *Health Canada*, STI control, LCDC, Tunney's Pasture, Ottawa, ON K1A 1B4; and the *Illustrated Series on Sexuality and Relationships* (from SIECCAN). www.sexualityandu.ca

Suggested Reading

When Sex Is the Subject: Attitudes and Answers for Young Children, by Pamela Wilson, Network Publications, 1991.
The New Family Book About Sexuality, by Mary Calderone and Eric Johnson, Harper and Row, 1989.
Where Do Babies Come From? by Angela Royston, Macmillan, 1996.
Canadian Journal of Human Sexuality, published by SIECCAN, 850 Coxwell Ave, North York M5C 5R1. (Tel: 416-466-5304); www.sieccan@web.net.

MASTURBATION

Since sexual intimacy and erotic play are pleasurable, one would expect children to enjoy masturbating and other sexual exploration. The reflex response that produces erections in boys and men may appear as early as 17 weeks of fetal life. Ultrasound pictures reveal erections in the tiny penises of male fetuses. One study of boys 3 to 20 weeks after birth found that seven out of nine had erections as many as 5 to 40 times a day. Girls under a year old have been observed having what to all appearances seems to be a reflexive orgasm induced by pressure on the genitals. The reflexes that result in infant erections and vaginal lubrication are much like the knee jerk and other reflexes, except for the accompanying smiles suggestive of enjoyment.

Masturbation is a normal activity that will not harm those doing it, provided that the individual (or couple) does it in private without disturbing others, and that it's not accompanied by anxiety. But if masturbation generates fears of abnormality, disease (such as "warts on the fingers"), punishment (perhaps because of religious beliefs) or harsh criticism from caregivers who consider it "wicked" or inappropriate, it can engender acute anxiety and cause more harm than good. Occasionally, masturbation is so excessive or even compulsive a preoccupation that it symbolizes some deep anxiety or other psychological problem that needs medical attention and counseling.

Sooner or later, most children learn the pleasures of stimulating their genitals. Two-thirds of the males in one of Dr. Kinsey's early studies reported hearing about masturbation from other boys in their prepubescent or early adolescent years, before trying it themselves. Fewer than one in three males reported rediscovering masturbation entirely on their own. Two out of three females in one sample learned about masturbation by accident, sometimes not until after they were married. Some women reported they had masturbated for some time before they realized what they were doing.

SEXUAL DYSFUNCTION

Almost everyone who is sexually active sooner or later experiences some sexual difficulties. These are often resolved by communicating

SEX AND AGING

With advancing years, many a man anxiously wonders whether his potency will decrease or vanish. The answer is sometimes yes, often no. Many men give up intercourse as they grow older, especially if they encounter occasional impotence or orgasmic problems. But given today's more liberal attitudes, many older men (and women) seek and expect sexual stimulation. In one study of U.S. retirement communities, 20 percent of men and women in their eighties were still sexually active, although their sexual practices were primarily touching/caressing, followed by self-pleasuring to "finish off." Those most sexually active in their younger days were likeliest to remain so as seniors. Unless health problems intervene, people can remain sexually active to a ripe old age. However, a Michigan study found 35 percent of married men over age 60 reported erectile dysfunction, rising to 64 percent by age 80. Curiously, the Michigan study found that drinking coffee increased sexual potency! Men who didn't drink coffee had a less active sex life than coffee imbibers. The authors of the study were puzzled about this link to caffeine—a central-nervous-system stimulant—wondering whether coffee is an aphrodisiac or whether coffee drinkers in general are more "liberal" in their sexual attitudes. The answer remains elusive.

wishes, sharing likes or dislikes, discussing problems and finding ways to become more intimate. While sex problems arise for many reasons— for example, negative parental attitudes to sex, childhood abuse, a bad sex encounter, fear of intimacy—the same roots may produce different sex problems in different people.

Sexual dysfunction may involve recurrent problems with the desire, arousal or orgasmic phases of the human sexual response. Sex problems can be occasional and transient or long-term, depending on their origins. While many sexual disorders arise from some organic cause, most also have psychological dimensions.

Sexual difficulties are remarkably common. One study found that although the majority of North American couples reported "satisfying sex lives," 40 percent of the men reported occasional impotence or erectile dysfunction and 63 percent of the women had some arousal or orgasmic problems. It is difficult to be precise about rates of erectile dysfunction (ED), but the Health Professionals Follow-Up Study revealed erectile dysfunction rates of 12 percent in men younger than 59 years, 22 percent of men 60–69, and 30 percent of men over 70. In addition, 50 percent of the men and 77 percent of the women reported difficulties that were not strictly dysfunctional, such as lack of interest in sex, too little time for it or an inability to relax during intercourse. Another survey found that over half of all North American couples reported some sexual dissatisfaction, such as "lack of enjoyment," "inability to become aroused" or "boring sex lives."

Some couples feel inadequate if they enjoy mutual sexual pleasuring but one or the other doesn't reach orgasm. Many define a rewarding sexual encounter solely in terms of vaginal penetration. Orgasm through intercourse may be the supreme goal, but this is labeled by one therapist as "an obsessive and unrealistic aim when there are so many other ways of enjoying sex."

Failure to live up to expectations (their own or their partner's) may produce profound anxiety. Despite today's more flexible sexual attitudes, some men equate good sex only with orgasm or "going all the way," while women may equate sexual adequacy with the ability to lubricate well and reach vaginal orgasm. Some couples who achieve orgasm by manual or oral stimulation, or with a vibrator think there may be "something wrong" with them. It's a common myth that everyone should be able to become aroused and perform on demand. Many factors influence the human sexual response. Some people experience good sex in a bad relationship, others have bad sex in a good relationship.

Sexual adequacy is defined as "the ability of two people to relate with each other sexually in ways that satisfy and reward both partners." But for many people this simple definition is colored by unrealistic expectations. We are often misled by our own and others' expectations, or by the idealized or distorted media portrayal of sexual relationships. Failure to live up to expectations can create or exacerbate sexual difficulties. When considering sexual health, it can sometimes be helpful to think in terms of "DAO"— that is, the issue of lack of Desire, limited Arousal or no Orgasm. All three are interrelated and each one can cause one or both of the others, but before discussing your concerns try to identify which is cause and which is effect.

Low sex drive and lack of interest in sex are among the most common of today's sex problems. What constitutes a "normal" sex drive is very individual. Our ideas about this can become distorted, especially in the face of media representations that would have us believe that people in a typical relationship have perfect sex every day. Lack of interest in sex may result from a fast-paced lifestyle where overscheduled people don't have the time or inclination to relax and enjoy sex. It can come from being depressed, from being in a poor relationship, or from the way you feel about yourself. It can come from "real life" as couples have kids, try to be successful at work and go through different phases of their lives. Feeling "burned out," couples complain of low sex drive and waning sexual interest. Sex and relationship therapy may help to restore sexual health in such cases.

Sex aversion—an extreme and rare form of sexual disinterest—may involve fear of any sexual intimacy. It usually has deep-seated psychological origins, often requiring intensive therapy. People with the sexual aversion syndrome shun all activities that might lead to intercourse, including petting and kissing. A couple may be in a relationship with no physical contact, and any hint of sexual involvement may trigger strong feelings of disgust or fear in one or the other partner, perhaps violent enough to cause panic. Sexual aversion may stem from a traumatic sexual experience, such as rape or sexual abuse. Therapy plus relaxation techniques may help to eliminate the sex phobia.

Sexual dysfunction in the desire phase of the human sexual response can arise for religious, moral, physical, emotional, marital or occupational reasons. Sexual desire depends on adequate hormone levels and the correct functioning of specific brain circuits. Even when everything is working properly, psychological factors can inhibit or shut down sexual desire. Strong negative messages about sex from parents, family, friends or church, guilt, or fear of pregnancy or infection may quench sexual desire. A recent survey found that 31 percent of couples seeking sex therapy complained of a discrepancy or conflict in their desire for sex. Lack of communication can also undermine sexual desire. Woody Allen's movie *Annie Hall* offers a classic example of different perceptions. When the therapist asks the woman how often they have sex, she answers, "All the time—three times a week." To the same question, the man replies, "Hardly ever—three times a week!"

Occasional low points in sexual desire are natural, but if the indifference persists or becomes troublesome, professional counseling may be the answer.

Sexual dysfunction in the arousal phase means the inability to become sexually aroused. Sexual arousal is swayed by atmosphere, mood, interpersonal conflicts and negative emotions, especially anger. It may be inhibited because of off-putting parental messages about sex, an unpleasant sexual experience, sex abuse, misinformation or performance pressure. Women may be unable to become sexually aroused because the excitement level isn't enough to produce or maintain vaginal lubrication. (The old terms "frigidity" and "impotence" are no longer used because of their negative connotations.) Most healthy men and women experience occasional difficulty in becoming sexually aroused, but if it is a persistent or recurrent problem, sex therapy may be the solution.

Inhibited orgasm can afflict both men and women, but more often women, and is defined as the inability to achieve orgasm and/or ejaculation during intercourse. Men may manage to ejaculate and reach orgasm by masturbation but not with vaginal intercourse, and women too may not reach orgasm during intercourse but may do so with masturbation. Some therapists believe orgasmic problems often stem from fear of intercourse, an unwillingness to perform on demand and anxiety about not satisfying a partner. Therapy often reverses the problem.

For more on specific sex problems in women, see Chapter 8; for specific sex problems in men, see Chapter 9, pages 256, 257.

SEX THERAPY

Sexual dysfunction often vanishes or improves with proficient counseling, usually involving both partners. Sex counselors are trained professionals such as physicians, social workers, psychologists, nurses and psychiatrists skilled in the art of helping people work through the emotions, guilts, hang-ups, worries, anger, myths and misconceptions that bedevil our sex lives. If the sex problem is due to an organic disorder, therapy can still help people accept and adjust to it.

Sex therapy is particularly useful for dysfunctions that involve anxiety, performance fears, stress, ignorance, negative childhood conditioning, relationship conflicts and "spectatoring" (observing oneself and one's responses rather than participating in the event).

A *non-directed "sensate focus,"* in which the goal is sensual pleasure rather than intercourse, is one sex therapy method that helps couples overcome conflicts around mistimed or mismatched sexual desire or a lack of "connectedness." Essentially, this involves taking off the pressure by saying that "we will engage in intimacy but no intercourse this time." The couple learns to approach sexual intimacy as mutual pleasuring without anticipating and focusing on intercourse or orgasm. By concentrating on sensual play—neither partner being pressured or expected to become aroused—the sensate focus exercises can often override performance anxieties and dispel problems due to poor body image, negative sex messages or communication hurdles. The couple learns to relax and playfully explore what gives the other pleasure. Each shows the other what kinds of touching he or she enjoys and where the most erotic places are by communicating verbally or by directing the partner's hand. The exercises work equally well for gay, lesbian or straight couples. Even couples with no sexual difficulties occasionally use the method to enrich their sex lives.

The PLISSIT model of sex therapy, developed about 20 years ago by Dr. Annon, is based on the premise that many people benefit from the very simplest of counseling—even just being permitted to talk about their problems. Reassurance, support and information are often enough to reverse a sex problem without intensive or lengthy psychotherapy. Using a "filter model," sex counselors distinguish people with simple sexual difficulties—who can profit from simple advice—from those requiring more intensive therapy.

The acronym PLISSIT refers to four basic stages:

Permission-Giving—permitting people to talk about their sex troubles, fantasies, fears or wishes;

Limited Information—often used together with permission-giving—providing some basic information (perhaps about erotic zones and genital anatomy) but no specific advice;

Specific Suggestions—given for specific sex problems; for instance, telling a man with premature ejaculation what might slow things down or suggesting how and where a woman afraid of pregnancy can get contraceptive advice;

Intensive Therapy—required by the relatively few with deeply rooted psychological problems who need longer-term psychotherapy.

The first two steps, permission-giving and limited information, are often enough to resolve a sex problem—especially one due to anxiety or misinformation. Many of us occasionally get the feeling that what we are doing sexually, or would like to do, is perverted, deviant or wrong. All we may need is reassurance or someone to say, "If you are comfortable with it, carry on." Once a sex problem has been pinpointed, its solution may be obvious to those versed in human sexual behavior. For instance, a couple in a college dormitory experiencing an orgasmic problem may just be put off by the lack of privacy. One suggestion might be to find a more relaxing place for lovemaking, perhaps a friend's apartment or a nearby motel. Or for a boy worried that masturbation will give him warts, it may be enough to say that masturbation is harmless and normal. Such specific suggestions may seem simplistic, but many sexual problems are in fact relatively simple, superficial and easily remedied.

Unfortunately, there have been cases of irresponsibility and even exploitation among people calling themselves sex therapists. Be sure anyone you consult comes well recommended. A sex therapist should never ask you to take off your clothes, unless for a medical examination, or to engage in any type of sexual activity with or without your partner in the therapist's presence.

If you feel you need a sex therapist, consult your family physician; the Ontario Association of Marriage and Family Therapy, (416) 841-6465 or (toll-free) 1-800-267-2638; local medical associations; BESTCO (Board Examiners in Sex Therapy and Counselling in Ontario); SIECAN: the Sex Information and Education Council of Canada, (416) 466-5304; or psychological associations.

SEXUALLY TRANSMITTED INFECTIONS

Originally termed "venereal" diseases, in reference to Venus, the goddess of love, sexually transmitted infections (STIs) encompass various infections caused by different microorganisms. Some STIs such as syphilis and gonorrhea have been recorded since antiquity. However, many of the 50-plus viruses, bacteria, protozoa and other microorganisms now known to be sexually transmitted have only been identified in this century. Despite the advent of antibiotics, STIs still pose a serious health threat, especially to adolescents and young adults.

Sexually active teens have highest STI rates

The huge increase in STIs among teens is blamed on the ever-earlier onset of unprotected sexual activity, failure to use condoms, a high "pool" of STI infection among young people, plus the fact that STIs so often produce no symptoms and unsuspecting carriers infect and reinfect partners.

STIs are especially common in those who start having sexual intercourse at a very young age, people who frequently change sex partners and those who don't use condoms. At particular risk are young girls who have unprotected sex soon after the menarche (when they start having periods) because the adolescent female genital tract—not yet fully matured—is extra vulnerable to infection, and the cervical mucus hasn't yet built up any immune (antibody) resistance. Women on oral or long-acting hormonal contraceptives are also at great risk because, being protected from pregnancy by other means, they don't "think STIs" or bother to protect themselves (don't insist their partners wear condoms).

Surveys across North America vary, but on average they show that today's adolescents start having sex at age 15 to 19 (with a slight trend among teenage girls to put it off until later). Based on the National Population Health Study, we can assume that in a classroom of 17-year-olds, over half will have had intercourse at least once. If the class is made up of 16-year-olds, about 40 percent will have experienced intercourse. By the time Canadian youths are 15

years old, 1 in 5 will have had sexual intercourse. But although about 50 percent of 15- to 19-year-olds are sexually active—and many report having several partners (some as many as four to eight or even more) per year—70 percent of them never, or only occasionally, use condoms. Condom use is less likely among rural than city dwellers. An Ontario study found that 14 percent of male and 19 percent of female university students had participated in anal intercourse—a high-risk route for HIV and other STI transmission.

Many teens don't realize the high risk of getting STIs, including AIDS, from a single unprotected sexual encounter. (By age 20, about 85 percent of men and women are sexually active, but still equally negligent about protecting their health by using condoms.) Unprotected sex is more likely to occur under the influence of alcohol and other drugs.

Among North American men in their 30s to 40s, AIDS has been a leading cause of death. The use of special medications called retro-virals has made a big difference in reducing the deadly impact of this illness. It should be remembered that those who actually have AIDS represent just the tip of the iceberg: far more are carrying the HIV virus that causes it—able to infect others, and to develop AIDS themselves later on.

Consistent, correct condom use essential to prevent STIs

Most STIs can be prevented by using latex or polyurethane condoms for every sexual encounter—whether it's heterosexual or homosexual, and including oro-genital sex. (For example, the herpes virus can spread from the mouth to the genitals.) The message is simple: if you're having sex with somebody other than a lifetime, monogamous partner—even with someone you know but about whose sex life you're not absolutely certain (a distinct possibility)—use a condom *plus spermicide* for each and every act of intercourse, and make sure it's used properly.

Overcoming teen resistance to condom use

Trying to curb the spread of STIs among adolescents is a huge public health problem. Despite a

WHEN TO GET CHECKED FOR A POSSIBLE STI

- If you know or suspect your sex partner is infected;
- if changing sex partners;
- if there are signs of:
  - a vaginal or penile discharge ("the drip");
  - a rash, warty growths, pimples, itchiness or sores on the genitals;
  - persistent lower abdominal pain;
  - pain when urinating;
  - changes in menstrual flow, unusual bleeding (in women).

N.B.: Women should get regular Pap smear tests to detect and treat early signs of cervical cancer possibly due to an STI infection (e.g., genital warts).

plethora of ads about condom use and free and commonly available samples, appallingly few use them.

There are many complex reasons why so many adolescents have unprotected sex, including discomfort with their burgeoning sexuality, not planning for intercourse, sporadic and unexpected sexual experiences. Some studies find that as few as 2 to 5 percent of young teenagers consistently use condoms.

Teens may be more inclined to use condoms if they see it as a way to improve health, increase control and as the norm or "cool thing to do." Studies find that adolescents are more apt to use condoms if they are perceived as a clean, easy-to-use way to "enjoy sex on the spur of the moment." Adolescent males who think their girlfriends expect them to use a condom (correctly), will do so! Once condoms are successfully used, and girls feel more comfortable, skillful and self-reliant in asking partners to wear them, use would likely continue. (Demonstrating correct condom use can help improve compliance.)

Untreated STIs can have devastating consequences—especially for women

STIs are sometimes called "sexist," as women usually face far more drastic health consequences than men. For anatomical reasons, women are likelier to have "hidden" STIs, for example, internal sores or a cervical discharge, in their internal reproductive organs. These are less obvious and harder to detect. Health complications from STIs are also generally more destructive in women. They include pelvic inflammatory disease (PID), which can scar the fallopian tubes (the tubes that the fertilized eggs travel through on the way to the uterus) and therefore cause sterility and/or ectopic pregnancy (when the egg gets trapped in the scarred tube), and cervical cancer which we now know is directly related to human papilloma virus (genital wart) infections. Women should take as much care to protect themselves from STIs as to avoid unwanted pregnancy.

Some types of sex are riskier than others

Sexually transmitted infections don't respect class or race. They strike men and women of every type, rich or poor gay, heterosexual or bisexual. Any sexually active person who doesn't take proper precautions is vulnerable to STI infection. But on the STI danger scale, some sexual practices are riskier than others. Anal sex is the riskiest, vaginal sex less so and oral sex the least likely to transmit an STI. (But that doesn't mean oral sex is "safe"—it can still transmit infections, including AIDS.) While one encounter is enough to catch a sexually transmitted disease, the risks increase with the number of lovers one has—particularly if they are chosen from groups at high risk of STIs. Epidemiologists have identified certain groups with behaviors that increase this risk—such as adolescents (who often don't take precautions); those with many sex partners; injection-drug users; male homosexuals; bisexuals; anyone who practices unprotected anal sex (especially with multiple partners); those who have unprotected sex with "sex-trade workers" (prostitutes); and those who use nonbarrier contraceptives such as the IUD or "the Pill," unless they also use a condom. Young children can get STIs as a result of sexual abuse.

Carriers often unknowingly spread STIs

One reason for the rampant spread of STIs is their ability to "hide" in symptomless carriers. Many men and women don't know they have a bacterial, viral or parasitic STI because they are asymptomatic, with no sign of infection. Having no symptoms, they don't go to be checked and aren't treated, and if they continue to have sex without condoms they spread the disease. For example, up to 50 percent of men and women with gonorrhea and/or chlamydia may be asymptomatic, although the disease is injuring their reproductive systems. Weeks, months or years may elapse before the serious (and possibly irreversible) complications of an untreated STI become apparent. Moreover, some STIs, such as human papilloma virus (genital warts), AIDS, hepatitis B and herpes infections, aren't curable.

Whether or not they have symptoms, carriers can infect their partners or unborn children. Depending on the particular infection, children born to mothers with some STIs— hepatitis B, serious forms of syphilis, herpes or

HIV (AIDS)—may be endangered by pneumonia or conjunctivitis (eye inflammation, perhaps producing blindness), or other consequences.

Ways to practice "safer" sex

The only sensible approach to sexually transmitted infections is prevention. STIs can be avoided by abstaining from sex, and for some, saying no may be right for a time. Those who do decide to have sex should choose safer options, such as selecting a faithful, noninfected partner (hard to determine) or consistently using condoms. Men and women should carry a packet of good latex condoms to use "just in case." Condoms provide a reasonable barrier against gonorrhea, syphilis, chlamydia, hepatitis B and HIV (AIDS), but not against herpes or genital wart (HPV) infections.

Unfortunately, many women feel embarrassed about condoms, and don't insist that their sex partners wear them, and men may use them inconsistently or incorrectly. Nevertheless, the risk of STI infection should far outweigh minor aversion. Women are urged to take a more "empowering" approach and to insist that male sex partners wear condoms—"No glove, no love." Women and men both need to know that anal sex is particularly dangerous because the delicate anal canal is more easily damaged than the tougher vaginal wall, allowing easier access to microorganisms and exposure to blood. (A woman's risk of STI infection is twice as high by anal as by vaginal intercourse.)

A rundown of some common STIs

Gonorrhea: popularly known as the "clap," gonorrhea is caused by the bacteria *Neisseria gonorrhoeae.* In North America, the incidence is highest among people under the age of 24 in downtown urban centers. Up to 50 percent of men and women with gonorrhea show no symptoms of infection, although they can pass the disease to their sex partners. If any symptoms do occur (usually about one week after exposure) they may include:

In men:
• thick yellowish-green penile discharge;
• sore throat (from oral sex);
• pain on voiding and frequency of urination;
• lower abdominal pain.

In women:
• thick vaginal discharge;
• sore throat (from oral sex);
• lower abdominal pain;
• urinary frequency and pain when urinating;
• increased or painful menstrual periods.

Gonorrhea coexists with chlamydia in up to 50 percent of cases. Untreated, it can result in pelvic inflammatory disease, tubal scarring, infertility and ectopic pregnancy. The bacteria can be passed to newborns, causing a severe eye infection that can lead to blindness. To prevent eye disorders from gonorrhea (or chlamydia), newborns are usually given eyedrops containing silver nitrate or erythromycin.

Gonorrhea is curable with antibiotics but some strains have become resistant to penicillin and tetracycline. Therefore health authorities now recommend other antibiotics such as cefixime, ceftriaxone or ciprofloxacin as a first-line treatment. (Since gonorrhea may coexist with chlamydia, doxycycline or tetracycline is given at the same time.) Those with gonorrhea should inform current and past sex partners, who may have been infected without knowing it.

Chlamydia: far more common than gonorrhea and AIDS, this infection—caused by the bacterium *Chlamydia trachomatis*—is now the most frequently reported STI in North America, and is especially common among sexually active adolescents and young adults.

The chlamydia organism is transmitted between partners through vaginal and penile secretions during sexual intercourse—both heterosexual and homosexual. The bacteria can also travel from infected mother to newborn at birth. Chlamydia is highly infectious (one study showed a 60–70 percent transmission rate). On this basis, it is recommended that all partners should be evaluated and treated within 60 days. If the last act of sexual intercourse occurred less than 60 days prior to the appearance of symptoms or diagnosis, the most recent sexual partner should be treated as well. Symptoms in women include a thick cervical discharge, painful and frequent urination, spotting blood between periods, tubal scarring and lower abdominal cramps. However, in over half the infected women, chlamydia infection produces no symptoms.

METHODS NOT EFFECTIVE IN PREVENTING STIS

• **Washing or urinating immediately after intercourse (this can reduce rates of urinary tract infection but not STIs);**
• **douching;**
• **using nonbarrier birth-control methods, such as the IUD or "the Pill."**

STI CARRIERS OFTEN SYMPTOMLESS

Many women and men with STIs have no symptoms; with no sign of infection, so they don't bother to consult a doctor. Yet they can still transmit the disease to sex partners. When symptoms do appear, they usually surface 2 to 6 weeks following infection by a sex partner of either sex.

PELVIC INFLAMMATORY DISEASE

Pelvic inflammatory disease (PID) is a very serious health threat for women, 17,000 being hospitalized in Canada each year with the condition. But PID is probably far more common than statistics indicate. It affects mainly women under age 25. PID usually results from gonorrheal or chlamydial infections that have paved the way for other invading microorganisms that damage the female genital tract. If an infection ascends from the vagina or cervix, past the endometrium (uterine lining) to the fallopian tubes, pelvic inflammation ensues. PID can cause severe lower abdominal pain, fever, vaginal discharge, bleeding, nausea, pelvic abscess and peritonitis (general abdominal infection). But many PID sufferers have no symptoms other than consequent infertility. About 10 to 20 percent of those with PID become sterile through tubal scarring. Ectopic (outside the womb) pregnancy, in which the fertilized egg begins to grow where it is "stuck" in the scarred tube rather than descending into the uterus causes death of the fetus and can seriously endanger the mother. In Canada there are about 6,000 ectopic pregnancies a year, the majority due to PID. Recent studies suggest that douching is an added risk factor for PID as it spreads the infection. So sexually active women are advised to avoid douching. Early treatment of PID is essential to prevent complications. Antibiotics can eradicate the infecting organisms, but may not reverse the infertility. Women with severe PID need hospital treatment.

In men, chlamydia more frequently produces some symptoms such as urethritis (inflamed urethra) and burning on urination, and is less likely to damage reproductive health, although it may lower sperm counts.

Chlamydia tests can now be done on urine samples. Treatment for men and women is with antibiotics. A new one-time treatment, giving azithromycin in a single dose, works well. The one-dose antibiotic treatment of those infected can help reduce the toll of this disease. People are advised not to have sex for a period of at least 7 days following the start of treatment. Since at least half the sex partners of people with chlamydia are also infected, anyone with this STI should tell any (and all) sex partners, so they too can be treated. (Pregnant women and infants are treated with amoxicillin or erythromycin.) Re-infection with chlamydia most often occurs when partners are not treated, or when someone resumes sexual activity within a network of individuals with a high prevalence of infection. Repeat infection can substantially increase the risk of *pelvic inflammatory disease* (PID) and other complications.

Untreated chlamydia has searing conse-quences. It can spread through a woman's reproductive tract, causing PID—whether or not the woman knows she has the disease (see the box on this page).

In newborns who acquire chlamydia during childbirth, the infection may cause eye infections (conjunctivitis) and lung infections (pneumonia).

Syphilis: caused by the spirochete *Treponema pallidum*, syphilis has been the scourge of many famous people, including King Henry VIII, Oscar Wilde, Van Gogh, Napoleon and Franz Schubert. Although less common than gonorrhea or chlamydia, syphilis is still surprisingly prevalent, with rates rising in some parts of North America. It is passed on via sexual contact and may facilitate AIDS transmission. Untreated syphilis remains contagious for at least one year and possibly up to four. Syphilis is rare in North America, but recently there have been outbreaks in a number of communities. For example, Toronto has experienced a tenfold increase in the number of syphilis cases in the last few years—30 cases in 2001 compared to 308 cases in 2003.

Syphilis develops in three stages, over many years. Stage one, primary syphilis, is a painless red sore or chancre, usually on the man's penis or rectal area, on the woman's cervix, or in the mouth of either sex. This heals in about two weeks, even without treatment. Stage two, or secondary syphilis, occurs one to three months later with a non-itchy rash often on the palms of the hands or soles of the feet, and sometimes also fever muscle aches and swollen lymph nodes. Symptoms disappear without treatment. During stages one or two, syphilis can be cured with a one-shot double dose penicillin injection, preventing progress to stage three, tertiary syphilis, which is rare today. However, tertiary syphilis can occur up to 30 years later damaging heart, bones and brain. Since syphilis can cause fetal defects or be passed on at birth, expectant mothers are screened by blood tests and treated with antibiotics if necessary.

Genital herpes: very common, and acquired through direct mouth-to-genital, anal sex or vaginal-penile contact, genital herpes affects one in five or more North Americans. It can be acquired from someone who has no sign of genital infection and from cold sores on the mouth. (Its increasing incidence is blamed on a rise in oro-genital sex.) Symptoms may be hardly noticeable (especially when first infected) or may be an intense burning or tingling sensation, pain on urination, swollen lymph glands and small blisters anywhere in the groin area (including penis, foreskin, buttocks, vulva or anus, and non-noticeably on the vagina and cervix). Herpes is most contagious when the sores are active, but transmission is still possible (although less likely) when they have healed and become invisible. The herpes virus may lie dormant within nerve tracts for a lifetime, perhaps causing occasional flare-ups. Although a devastating experience for sufferers and highly contagious to others, herpes is not life-threatening unless it's active during pregnancy when it can endanger the newborn during delivery. To avoid this, pregnant women with active herpes at labor may need Caesarian delivery.

Treatment of herpes symptoms is with taking warm sitz baths, practicing good hygiene, wearing loose cotton underwear and taking acyclovir or other antiviral pills. The pills can be taken preventatively or at the very first signs of recurrence. Condoms can help to reduce its spread. A vaccine is in preparation. Genital herpes may jeopardize newborn health if a mother has active sores at the time of birth—which happens in about one per 5,000 births. Any woman who knows (or thinks) she has a herpes infection should be tested shortly before labor for HSV viruses. (For more on herpes in pregnancy, see Chapter 10.)

Trichomonas vaginalis or "trich": this very common, sexually transmitted protozoan infection may produce few symptoms, and both sexes can carry the organism for years without knowing it, transmitting it to sex partners. In some women "trich" causes vaginitis—an irritated or itchy vulva, a malodorous, frothy discharge and perhaps pain on urination. While mainly passed on through sexual contact, trichomonas is hardier (although much less detrimental) than gonorrhea, HIV or syphilis, and can survive on wet towels, washcloths or douching equipment. The infection is treated with oral metronidazole (Flagyl). Partners of infected individuals are also treated, as "ping-

---

WHY STIs SPREAD

- **More permissive sexual attitudes accompanying wide availability of the birth-control pill;**
- **earlier onset of sexual activity among adolescents;**
- **multiple sex partners;**
- **complacency about STIs because of the past success of penicillin and other antibiotics in curing some of them;**
- **the misconception that STIs affect only "high-risk" groups—giving others a false sense of security, as they imagine that they are immune to infection;**
- **lack of knowledge about STI symptoms, and reluctance to be tested by a physician or STI clinic even if infection is suspected;**
- **the insidious nature of STIs, many of which have few or no symptoms;**
- **asymptomatic STI carriers who have no** symptoms but continue to have sex and spread the infection(s);
- **denial of having sexual desire by many adolescents and a resulting unwillingness to "prepare ahead" for possible intercourse;**
- **the teenage belief that "it'll never happen to me," and similar parental beliefs that STIs can't strike their son or daughter;**
- **a "macho" attitude among men, many of whom refuse condoms despite the knowledge that they reduce STI risks;**
- **inadequate medical-school training in the recognition and treatment of STIs;**
- **old habits that die hard—the failure of healthcare professionals who regularly give women Pap smears to "think STIs," do relevant tests, recognize STIs** or give appropriate treatment—perhaps because some don't keep up with medical advances (e.g., they may still use penicillin for drug-resistant gonorrhea);
- **too little effort put into preventive STI education, especially for teenagers;**
- **school boards and teachers who don't discuss sexuality, STIs or contraception adequately, for fear of "promoting promiscuity" or "triggering parental protests";**
- **a hypocritical society willing to condone explicit sex in movies, on TV and in magazines, but downplaying or ignoring risks of unwanted pregnancy and STIs;**
- **a moralistic view that says: "You play, you pay!" and regards STIs as proper punishment for sexuality.**

---

pong" reinfection is common. New "one-dose" treatment for both partners works well. (See also Chapter 8, section on vaginitis.)

Chancroid: relatively rare in Canada, this STI remains common in the southern United States and developing countries, where it has been identified as a co-factor for AIDS. Chancroid produces painful red sores, although it may produce no symptoms if on a woman's cervix. It is treated with erythromycin, ciprofloxacin or a single shot of ceftriaxone.

Human papilloma virus (HPV): very common, these viruses cause genital warts—small, flat, pink or grayish growths found externally on the penis (in men), vulva and vagina and cervix (usually not noticeable to the naked eye) in women. Usually painless but cosmetically displeasing, the warts are sometimes sore, if irritated. They usually appear two to three months after contact, so anyone who has a sex partner infected with HPV or with visible genital warts should be checked for infection. HPV viruses are easily passed on between sex partners and can lead to various cancers including anal and penile cancers in men, and cervical cancer in women. (Smokers are at increased risk.)

Genital warts on the external genitals are removed by podophyllin or trichloroacetic acid, cryotherapy (freezing with liquid nitrogen), cautery (burning) or lasers, but they often need several treatments, and tend to grow back because the surrounding area may still harbor the HPV viruses. Condoms may help to curb transmission.

HPV infections are a huge threat to women as cervical cancer is the second leading cause of cancer deaths in women and HPV is responsible for about 95 percent of cervical cancer. (In 1996 there were almost 400 cervical cancer deaths in Canada.) Regular Pap smears to detect the infection are a must—especially for those with male partners who have genital warts. Regular Pap smears and early treatment of those infected with HPV can halve cervical cancer rates. For HPV-infected women, colposcopy (cervical scraping) can cure the problem and prevent cervical cancer. Newborns of infected mothers are at risk of respiratory papillomatosis, a rare but serious lung disease. See also Chapter 8.

Hepatitis B: passed on mainly by sexual contact, this serious liver infection is also acquired via shared household items such as razors or toothbrushes, or from infected blood products and dirty injection needles. Since there is a very effective vaccine for hepatitis B, all those at risk should get immunized. All teens (12- to 14-year-olds) and many newborns now receive hepatitis B vaccinations. Pregnant mothers should get a blood test for hepatitis B, and babies are immunized at birth if necessary. Infected people should not have sex until their partners are safely vaccinated against hepatitis B.

TIPS FOR PREVENTING STIs (INCLUDING AIDS)

- Always use a condom for sexual intercourse to prevent infection until sure your partner is free of STIs—it's hard to know. Use only recommended latex (not lambskin) condoms. And use them correctly!
- Be selective about sexual partner(s), avoid one-night stands, casual pickups and sexual intimacy with people you hardly know.
- Get to know your sex partner as well as possible.
- Never let sex become a power struggle where one "wins" and the other "loses" (and risks getting an STI).
- Don't assume that STIs can't infect married people, those from "nice" families or seemingly committed sex partners.
- Remember that avowed commitment to a sex partner does not mean freedom from infection and should not engender false security or excuse failure to use condoms.
- Teens might consider postponing intercourse until they feel ready for it—to avoid both unwanted pregnancy and STIs.
- If on the Pill or using an IUD, *also* use a condom to combat STIs, including AIDS.
- Watch for symptoms of STIs: genital sores, rash, discharge, pain on urinating, low abdominal pain. Seek advice.
- Don't be afraid, ashamed or embarrassed to seek medical attention if you suspect you may have an STI. Get tested as soon as possible. If the test is positive, get prompt treatment, tell any sex partner(s) and refrain from sex until cured.

- Avoid sex with anyone who has obvious genital or anal sores.
- Avoid kissing, oral or genital sex when herpes sores are present.
- Remember that past (cured) STIs are no guarantee of protection from reinfection.
- Never engage in anal intercourse without "double bagging," using two condoms and ample lubrication. But remember that even this is not foolproof, as condoms tear easily with the friction of anal sex. Since spermicide irritates the rectum, its use for anal sex is controversial and many now advise against it.
- If using lubricant with condoms for sex, choose only water-based types (e.g., K-Y jelly), not petroleum-based products (e.g., Vaseline), which weaken the condom.
- Women should consider refusing anal intercourse; it is very risky for them, as the anal lining is thinner in women.
- Avoid oral-anal contact, which can greatly increase the risk of STIs and other infections.
- Since STIs can be transmitted by fellatio (penile-oral sex) and cunnilingus (oral stimulation of female genitals), avoid these practices with an infected partner.
- If sexually active with more than one partner, request and get regular STI checkups.

(For a detailed section on AIDS, see Chapter 16.)

COMPARING SEXUALLY TRANSMITTED INFECTIONS

Disease	Symptoms and outlook	Complications	Diagnosis and treatment
Syphilis (the "pox") Spirochete infection. Curable in early stages. Affects mainly those in their twenties. Transmitted by oral, genital, anal contact. After a decline, case numbers rising again in North America, mainly related to drug use or exchange of sex for drugs.	Painless sore (chancre) appears three to six weeks after infection on genitals, mouth or rectal area, most obvious in men, hardly noticed if vaginal. Heals without scarring. About four to ten weeks later, second stage: fever, rash, which disappears but may reappear.	If untreated, chronic, occasionally fatal. Third stage appears up to 30 years later with brain and spinal-cord damage, blindness, insanity. Untreated, can cause miscarriage and birth defects; infants of infected mother may be born with syphilis (congenital syphilis).	Even if no symptoms seen, can diagnose by simple blood test; test results usually positive by the time chancre appears. Antibiotics, taken as prescribed, a dependable cure in early stages (stage one and two).
Gonorrhea (the "clap") Bacterial infection, transmitted by oral, vaginal or anal sex. Prevalent in young women, teens. Untreated, can result in PID and infertility. Up to 50% of infected women and men have no symptoms.	Symptoms (if any) within 7 days of contact: painful urination, thick vaginal or penile discharge, bleeding between periods, sore throat (if contracted via oral sex), rectal pain or discharge (if through anal sex).	May lead to tubal scarring, pelvic inflammatory disease (PID), ectopic pregnancy (outside womb, dangerous for mother). Can cause permanent sterility in both sexes. Eye infection and possible blindness in infected newborns.	Diagnosed by slide-smear and lab culture. Antibiotics a reliable cure but some strains now resistant to standard antibiotics (e.g., penicillin) so require cefixime, cefriaxone or other new drugs.
Herpes Viral infection due to herpes virus types I or II. Spreads via oral, vaginal or anal sex, kissing. Can spread silently, via asymptomatic people. Most easily transmitted by direct contact with active sores or genital secretions.	Symptoms within 10 days; slight fever, tingling, shooting pains, swollen lymph glands, then painful blisters, anywhere on genitals — mainly penis, vulva or anal areas. Subsides without treatment, but can recur. First outbreak usually worst, but sometimes unnoticed.	Virus remains permanently in nerves, stays dormant for months or years. Newborns may get herpes during birth, resulting in central-nervous-system damage or death. Cesarean delivery may be advised for babies of infected mothers.	Diagnosis from blisters (scraping or culture). Acyclovir tablets, not a cure, ease symptoms and reduce length of attack and its severity. Herpes support groups helpful in combating psychological problems.
Chlamydia Bacterial infection—very common in teens, 60–80% without symptoms. Spreads via anal, vaginal or oral sex with infected partners. Often occurs together with gonorrhea.	Like gonorrhea; painful urination, vaginal or penile discharge, abdominal pain, genital itching. But often mild, unnoticed in carriers, can disappear without treatment.	In women, leading cause of PID, ectopic pregnancy, infertility. In men, can produce urinary-tract diseases and prostatitis. Babies of infected mothers prone to eye infections, pneumonia.	Diagnosis by culture or other tests. Antibiotic treatment a reliable cure if caught early.
Genital warts (condylomata) Caused by human papilloma virus (HPV). Highly contagious, spread by intimate bodily contact, especially sexual activity, often accompanies other STIs.	Warts—tiny flat growths on and around genitals—possibly itchy; pinkish, flat, irregularly surfaced, may increase in size. Often undetectable in women in vagina or on cervix, except by physician.	Certain HPV strains linked to cervical cancer in women (and possibly penile cancer in men). Infants born to mothers with HPV may develop warts.	Removal advised—chemically, by freezing or with lasers. Women should have regular Pap smears to detect HPV infection and early cervical cancer changes in time for preventive treatment.
Trichomonas Protozoal infection; most frequent in those with many sex partners; often accompanies other STIs.	Few symptoms: possibly irritated, tender vulva; burning on urination; perhaps copious, possibly foul-smelling yellowish-green, frothy, foamy discharge.	Frequent "ping-pong" reinfection of sex partners. Both need treatment.	Swab/slide examination may reveal twitchy-tailed organisms. Treatment is oral metronidazole (Flagyl)—also for sex partner(s). During pregnancy, use clotrimazole instead.
Hepatitis B Virus passed on via blood, semen, vaginal secretions, saliva, needles, razors, toothbrushes or other objects. Can go from mother to infant at birth. Groups most at risk: those practicing anal sex, those with many sex partners, injection-drug users, babies of infected mothers.	Usually subclinical with few or no symptoms. Possibly flu-like malaise, fever fatigue typically lasting 6 weeks, perhaps jaundice/skin and eye-white yellowing. May linger in body unnoticed. Many of the infected become permanent "carriers." Can make the effects of alcohol on the liver much more devastating.	60–90 percent of infected children and 10 percent infected as adults become lifelong carriers, at risk of cirrhosis and liver cancer. Unsuspecting carriers can infect others. Fulminant, rapidly fatal form in one per 100 cases.	Detected by blood tests for viral markers. No cure. Effective, safe vaccine recommended for all at risk—especially healthcare workers and those living with or close to known hepatitis B carriers.

CONDOMS

Advantages
- **protect against most STIs—if latex or polyurethane and used with spermicide**
- **easily obtained**
- **no prescription needed**
- **low cost**

Drawbacks
- **occasional allergies—to latex or spermicide**
- **interrupts lovemaking**
- **possible slippage, breakage or "spills" (when removed)**

How to curb the spread of STIs

While many people relegate STI education to health professionals and educators, studies suggest that this is hardly enough. Surveys show that Grade 11 students would like to receive sex-related information from their parents but perceive parental knowledge of AIDS and other STIs as "inadequate." Yet many adolescents don't know where else to turn for advice. Parents and educators need to discuss sexuality and STIs candidly and explicitly with youngsters well before they reach adolescence. Teens need advice on both pregnancy avoidance and STI prevention. Physicians can play a major role in helping to prevent STIs by giving teenagers the facts at medical checkups, while taking care to respect their natural urge to explore sexuality. A nonjudgmental approach works best.

Adolescents need to know that they are not alone in having to adopt new sexual practices in the age of AIDS. Today the challenge facing many is how to decline sex while respecting the other person's feelings. Although not an indefinite option for most young people, abstinence from intercourse is increasingly considered an acceptable choice for some.

For more information, contact your local health department; SIECCAN; an STI clinic; your family physician; the revised Canadian "Guidelines for the Prevention, Diagnosis, Management and Treatment of Sexually Transmitted Diseases in Neonates, Children, Adolescents and Adults"—available from Health Canada's Division of STI control at the Laboratory Centre for Disease Control, Ottawa. Sexuality and U is an excellent resource developed by the Society of Obstetricians and Gynecologists (http://www.sexualityandu.ca).

RECENT TRENDS IN BIRTH CONTROL

While the inability to conceive is a searing disappointment to those who want a child, preventing conception remains one of the world's great problems. It is estimated that 41 percent of pregnancies among women aged 35–39 are unplanned and 51 percent among those aged 40–44. Through the ages, women have tried to control fertility by strategies such as putting foreign substances into their vagina or uterus, while men used various animal or plant membranes as sheaths or condoms. Fertility management remains the single most powerful determinant of women's health. Successful fertility control offers women freedom from unwanted pregnancy, a greater likelihood of completing their education, developing work skills and gaining employment, as well as better physical and emotional health.

Today's women are better off contraceptively than their foremothers—with a range of effective, easily available devices—but we still have no ideal birth control method, just a choice of "second bests." Different methods of birth control suit different ages and stages of people's sexual lives, but we continue to demand more of birth-control techniques than of any other drug or device. A good contraceptive must be easily acquired, reliable, safe, morally and physically acceptable and convenient to use.

In the United States and Canada sterilization is now the leading form of fertility control among married people over age 30. The birth control pill remains one of the most reliable and popular contraceptive methods, especially for young women, although its much-publicized cardiovascular side effects (i.e., heart attack and stroke) have put some off it. However, the new low-dose preparations are far safer and the Pill remains a very suitable and safe contraceptive for young, sexually active women. The IUD, or

DIAPHRAGM

Advantages
- **can be inserted ahead—up to six hours before intercourse**
- **insertion conveniently "separated" from lovemaking**
- **possibly some STI protection**
- **no health risks**
- **usable while breastfeeding**
- **within woman's own control**

Drawbacks
- **must be professionally fitted**
- **occasional allergies (to latex or spermicide)**
- **rather messy, needs privacy to insert**
- **should be removed no sooner than 6–8 hours after the last coital act. The maximum wear time is 24 hours**
- **additional spermicide must be inserted into the vagina without removing the device before repeat acts of intercourse when using the diaphragm or Lea's shield.**
- **can dislodge during sex**
- **must be kept clean and dry**
- **must be re-fitted after childbirth or if weight changes (by over 10 lbs)**

intrauterine device, which temporarily lost favor because one particular type—the ill-designed Dalkon Shield—created many problems, still remains a simple, effective contraceptive. Contraceptive users around the world often choose the copper IUD as their preferred method of birth control, especially for "baby-spacing" (use between wanted pregnancies).

New options
New contraceptive options include the hormone "patch" (Evra) and the "ring" (NuvaRing). The patch is applied once a week and is well tolerated, although some women react to the patch itself and some experience more breast tenderness than they do with oral contraceptives. The ring is inserted on or before the fifth day of menses. One vaginal contraceptive ring is inserted into the vagina and kept in place for 3 weeks. It is then removed for a 1-week break, after which a new ring is inserted. Menses will usually occur in the ring-free interval. The ring is available in the US and is being considered for approval in Canada. Despite limited data or experience with either of these options, they may be appealing to some women, especially shift workers.

Some progress but still no perfect contraceptive
The ideal contraceptive would be effective, safe, long-acting, free of side-effects, applied well before intercourse *and* protect against STIs. No available product meets all criteria. Except for condoms with spermicide, most birth control methods do *not* protect against sexually transmitted infections (STIs). And around the world, millions of women remain at risk of unwanted pregnancy. Even in the U.S., about half of all pregnancies are unintended, with over 50 percent of those ending in abortion. In Canada, about one third of all pregnancies are unintended, and 19 percent end in abortion (with over 100,000 abortions annually).

"Although birth control raises many ethical, religious, legal, economical and medical questions," notes the head of the University of Toronto Women's Health Program, "everyone has a right to decide for themselves what contraceptive practices are right for them, and no one has the right to impose their views about fertility control on others."

Teens are still not well educated about birth control
Unfortunately, and with predictable results, a large percentage of sexually active teenagers and young couples use little or no birth control. According to recent estimates, although almost 40 percent of Canadian teenagers are sexually active by ages 14 to 18 (many before age 15), only a third of them use any birth control at first intercourse. Of those who do use birth control, many rely on withdrawal (removal of the penis before ejaculation) or spermicide alone when first having sex. But withdrawal is notoriously unreliable, as the sperm may leak out before orgasm or the man may not withdraw in time, and spermicide (foams, gels or creams) are not enough to prevent pregnancy or STIs. In one U.S. survey, of the teen couples who used birth control at first intercourse, about 18 percent tried withdrawal, 29 percent used a condom and 30 percent were on the Pill, the rest relying vaguely on rhythm methods. Some said they engaged in anal sex "from time to time" (presumably as an alternative way to avoid pregnancy). Curiously, of the teenage girls who were on the Pill, most said their mothers knew about it, but not their boyfriends. When asked about Pill use, many thought that it protected against pregnancy "from the moment the first pill was taken" (in fact, protection may not be effective for a couple of weeks, or even a month), and most didn't know what to do if they missed one pill.

Adolescents tend to shun birth control because of its "premeditated" nature, a reluctance to acknowledge sexual activity, a lack of confidence in themselves, a mistrust about confidentiality, and ignorance or embarrassment in getting supplies. Some feel it's okay to be sexually "swept away" but not to plan for it. One teenage girl who got AIDS said she didn't know her boyfriend "well enough" to discuss safe sex. Yet about 80 percent of women under 30 who use no birth control become pregnant within the first year of becoming sexually active. Many teen pregnancies and STIs occur just after a breakup, when each partner experiments with

BIRTH CONTROL PILL

Advantages
- gives reliable, reversible contraception (if directions followed)
- better regulated, lighter periods
- lowered risk of iron-deficiency anemia (less blood loss)
- fewer benign breast problems
- may lessen risk of ectopic (outside uterus) pregnancy
- diminishes risks of ovarian and endometrial cancers

Drawbacks
- need for daily pill-taking
- nuisance side effects (e.g., headaches, weight gain, nausea, moodiness)
- decreased efficacy if concurrently using some medications (e.g., antibiotics, anticonvulsants)
- slight rise in thromboembolic (clotting) risks—mainly in smokers
- no STI or HIV protection

IUDs

Advantages
- gives long-term contraception (up to 10 years with some copper devices)
- inexpensive
- convenient and unnoticed, once safely fitted
- easily removed and re-inserted if desired
- can be used while breastfeeding

Drawbacks
- increased menstrual flow and cramping (with some IUDs)
- slightly raised risks of ectopic pregnancy if IUD fails and conception occurs
- no STI protection; may exacerbate existing STIs (but doesn't *cause* them)
- chance of slippage or expulsion

CERVICAL CAPS

Advantages
- can be left in for 48 hours
- protect for multiple intercourses
- not felt by partner during sex
- within woman's own control
- can be inserted ahead; do not interrupt lovemaking

Drawbacks
- need professional fitting—harder to insert than sponge or diaphragm
- require careful storage—keep clean and dry
- cannot be used while menstruating
- not always readily obtainable

or establishes a new sexual relationship, using no or inadequate protection.

Recapping contraceptive methods old and new

- **Condoms with spermicide.** Placed over the erect penis, the thin sheath traps sperm and prevents their entry into the woman's cervix, while spermicide destroys them. It's a reasonably reliable method, provided spermicide is also put into the woman's vagina; spermicide-impregnated condoms are not enough. The condom must be made of latex, or more recently, the thinner and stronger polyurethane (*not* lambskin). And it must be used correctly—put on *as soon* as there's an erection (leaving a little space or pouch at the tip), removing the penis right after ejaculation and holding the condom base to prevent spills. (Should the condom break, the woman should *not* douche, but add more spermicide and consider use of the emergency "morning-after" pill, seeking advice from her physician, a family planning or birth control unit.)

  Note: All contraceptives should only be used with *water-based* lubricants (e.g., Astroglide or K-Y jelly), *not* oil-based products (e.g., Vaseline or petroleum jelly).

- **Diaphragms with spermicide.** The latex diaphragm is placed in the vagina with spermicidal gel put inside and around the rim, providing a "holder" for sperm-killing spermicide. More spermicide is added into the vagina at each intercourse. The diaphragm *must be left in for six hours* after last intercourse; it can stay in for 24 hours (longer if intercourse happens at the "24th hour").

Since the diaphragm increases risks of bladder or urinary tract infections (UTIs), it's not suitable for women prone to these infections.

- **Hormonal birth control pills.** The first hormonal oral contraceptive (OC), developed in the 1950s, triggered a revolution in birth control. For the first time women had access to a reliable, inexpensive way of avoiding unwanted conception. The Pill allowed women to space their babies for better health and family life; gave them control over their own bodies; permitted them to decide whether and when to have a baby; and extended many female lives by reducing the toll of unavoidable childbearing. Now used by over 200 million women worldwide, the modern birth control pills give safe, reversible contraception—provided they are taken regularly, *as prescribed*.

  Most oral contraceptives contain both estrogen (which suppresses ovulation) and progestin (which thickens cervical mucus, slows down sperm and stops egg implantation). The combination Pill, containing two different female hormones—estrogen and a progestin—is one of the best-studied drugs ever produced, and provides effective, reversible birth control. It can be safely used by most healthy women up to age 35, including teenagers, once their periods have begun. In pill-taking women menstruation occurs because of "progesterone withdrawal," not true ovarian cycling. Used consistently and on schedule, OCs seldom fail. But although they are 99 percent effective, many women stop using them or forget to take the pills regularly. Also, some medications such as antibiotics and anticonvulsants reduce OC effectiveness.

  Many women who couldn't tolerate the side effects of former high-estrogen forms find the new types acceptable. Today's low-dose estrogen combination pills, with substantially lower amounts of estrogen—averaging 20 to 35 µg (about one-fifth former doses)—have greatly reduced *venous thromboembolic* (clotting) risks such as phlebitis and lung embolism. A recent "meta-analysis" of results from many studies found no increase in clotting diseases with the low-estrogen pill in healthy, non-smoking women. Although the Pill is not advised for *smokers* over age 35, reports suggest healthy non-smoking women can safely stay on it until menopause. Progestin-only forms are useful for women unable to take estrogen—perhaps when breastfeeding or because of hypertension, clotting problems, liver disorders or previous breast cancer—but they have a higher failure rate and cause spotty bleeding.

One lingering worry is the possibly increased risk of breast cancer from Pill use. But a recent summary of 70 studies found no *increased risk of breast cancer* from oral contraceptive use. "Although evidence suggests that the low-estrogen pill won't cause cancer," notes one expert, "it could stimulate growth of an already-existing tumor."

Besides effective birth control, the Pill confers several *non-contraceptive* benefits. It reduces heavy menstrual flow, decreases benign breast discomfort, diminishes risks of PID and protects against ovarian and endometrial (uterine lining) cancers. In fact, some physicians suggest birth control pills for women at high risk of ovarian cancer, once the quest for fertility is oven Changes have even been suggested in U.S. labeling laws to reflect pill benefits in healthy, non-smoking women.

- **IUDs (intrauterine devices).** Inserted by a health professional, IUDs are the most popular contraceptive worldwide, especially favored in China and India. As a "foreign" body in the uterus, the IUD creates an inflammatory reaction in which white blood cells *phagocytize* or "gobble up" sperm and stop egg implantation. (Because there's some risk of expulsion, women must feel for the string to make sure the IUD stays in place.) Most IUDs (e.g., the TCu-200, Nova-T, TCu-380A) contain copper, which increases effectiveness. One new type, the Flexiguard—a copper-covered nylon thread that's free-floating —decreases cramps and heavy periods. Another innovation, progestin-coated copper IUDs (like the Progestasert and norgestrel-impregnated forms), increase efficacy as they halt ovulation.

The IUD best suits monogamous women with healthy reproductive tracts who have already had children and have no STIs or previous PID (pelvic inflammatory disease). It is not advised for anyone with uterine abnormalities, PID, a compromised immune system, a copper allergy or vaginal bleeding of unexplained cause.

- **The cervical cap.** The latex cervical cap (fitted by a health professional but available over-the-counter) resembles a thimble that fits neatly over the cervix, with spermicidal gel put in beforehand. Cervical caps come in various shapes, the "Prentif cavity cap" being the most common. They protect for multiple intercourse, without requiring more spermicide after the first application, but they're not readily obtainable in all areas and may need to be specially ordered.

- **The vaginal sponge.** A non-prescription, spermicide-impregnated barrier product, placed high in the vagina (preferably near the cervix) the sponge is inserted at least 15 minutes before intercourse and remains effective for six to eight (maximum 12) hours, with no need for added spermicide. It must be left in place at least six hours after last intercourse. Newer sponges, such as "Protectaid," have triple spermicide action and protect for multiple coital acts, but have not yet been evaluated for STI protection. (For best results, learn correct use from a health professional.)

- **Female condoms.** Available in the U.S. and recently in Canada, these are non-prescription, polyurethane, disposable pouches, much like an inverted condom, that fit into the vagina, held in place by two rings. Pre-treated with lubricant, most types can be inserted eight hours before intercourse with added spermicide, but many women find them esthetically displeasing and clumsy to use.

- **Advantage 24.** Advantage 24, recently marketed in the U.S. and Canada, is a soluble "bioadhesive" gel, containing nonoxynol-9 spermicide, that's easily inserted into the vagina from the dispenser that holds it. Used instead of other spermicidal foams or gels, Advantage 24 gives stronger and longer-lasting anti-sperm action than other spermicides (which only work for up to 6 hours), with an adhesive that sticks onto the vaginal surface. Advantage 24 can be applied ahead of inter-

SPONGE

Advantages
- **non-prescription and easily available**
- **no fitting needed—one size fits all**
- **"body-friendly" and easy to use (no need for added spermicides)**
- **good for repeated intercourse—up to 12 hours of protection**
- **can be used while breastfeeding**

Drawbacks
- **possible allergies (to spermicide or polyurethane in sponge)**
- **can be dislodged during sex**
- **may exacerbate yeast infections**
- **small chance of tearing on removal**
- **should not be used if there's any known risk of toxic shock syndrome**

ADVANTAGE 24

Advantages
- **non-prescription, pre-measured and easy to carry in purse or pocket**
- **provides some "barrier" as well as sperm-killing action**

Drawbacks
- **occasional burning or irritation when applied—in which case use must be discontinued**

FEMALE CONDOMS

Advantages
- **completely shield the vagina**
- **over-the-counter, disposable product**
- **possible STI protection**
- **give women control (e.g., if partners refuse to wear condoms)**

Drawbacks
- **rather cumbersome and unaesthetic**
- **can be expensive ($3)**
- **take practice to insert**
- **can be dislodged during intercourse**
- **only usable for one sex act**
- **not yet evaluated for efficacy**
- **possible allergic reactions**

course and gives effective sperm-killing action for up to 24 hours, but fresh applications are needed for further acts of intercourse. Advantage 24 might protect against STIs to some extent, but this is still being studied. Experts emphasize that it is designed for use with a condom, not to replace it.

- *Depo-Provera.* Approved in the U.S. and recently also in Canada, Depo-Provera is a long-acting contraceptive, already used by 300 million women around the world. A progestin-only hormone (*medroxyprogesterone acetate*), given by injection once every three months, Depo-Provera prevents pregnancy by suppressing release of ovulation-stimulating hormones, increasing stickiness of cervical mucus, hindering sperm movement and making the uterine lining thin and "hostile" to egg implantation. These progestin-only injections are especially suitable for women who dislike, forget to use or fail with other contraceptives, and for those unable to take estrogen-containing products. About one-third of women on it have no periods, one-third have occasional spotting, and one-third get irregular periods that lessen over time.

  Before having Depo-Provera injections, women need a medical checkup, and the injection is given within 7 days of a menstrual period to make sure the woman is not pregnant. Depo-Provera can exacerbate PMS (premenstrual tension) so it's not recommended for women prone to PMS or depression, as once injected it can't be quickly withdrawn. There are some outstanding concerns about possibly increased risks of osteoporosis if used long-term by young women. Also, it can take five months or more (up to two and a half years) to regain fertility.

- *Emergency contraceptives or "morning-after" pills.* Also called "post-coital contraception, *emergency contraceptive pills* (ECPs) are taken immediately following unprotected or accidental intercourse as a swift "anti-pregnancy" measure. There are two regimens of ECPs currently available: the Yuzpe method and the newer progestin-only method. Both are safe and have no absolute contraindications except known pregnancy. The older Yuzpe method consists of 100 μg of ethinyl estradiol and 500 μg (0.5 mg) of levonorgestrel (two Ovral pills) taken first and then repeated in 12 hours. The progestin-only method approved for use in North America (Plan B®) consists of 750 μg of levonorgestrel taken first and then repeated in 12 hours. ECPs are thought to work primarily by delaying or inhibiting ovulation.

  Randomized trials show that both the Yuzpe and progestin-only regimens taken in time, reduce the risk of pregnancy by approximately 75 and 85 percent respectively, with the progestin-only method producing significantly less nausea and vomiting (5.6 percent vs 18.8 percent). For these reasons, the progestin-only regimen is the preferred method, although its availability and cost may preclude its use in some circumstances. It is wise to take an anti-nausea agent such as dimenhydrinate (Dramamine, Gravol) with the Yuzpe regimen and clinicians usually prescribe an extra dose in case one is lost to vomiting.

  Although standard guidelines state that ECPs should be initiated within 72 hours of unprotected intercourse, recent trials have shown that both regimens continue to have some effect (although diminished) for up to 120 hours afterwards. Maximum protection occurs if they are taken within 24 hours. An analysis of emergency contraception among women using either levonorgestrel or the Yuzpe regimen found that levonorgestrel prevented 95 percent of pregnancies if taken up to 24 hours after intercourse, 85 percent 25–48 hours later and 58 percent if taken after 49–72 hours. The corresponding rates for Yuzpe were 77 percent, 36 percent and 31 percent respectively. There is significant

DEPO-PROVERA

Advantages
- **long-lasting, reliable, highly effective**
- **lighter periods and relief of cramps (in women with painful or heavy periods)**
- **no need to "think" about daily pill-taking**

- or other "on the spot" methods
- **chance for medical checkups when women return for injection**

Drawbacks
- **annoying "spotting" or irregular**

- menstrual bleeding
- **weight gain, headaches, acne**
- **risk of elevated blood lipids (fats)**
- **delayed return of fertility—can take 4 to 31 months**
- **no STI protection**

debate in favour of making these medications available over the counter and an argument can certainly be made for asking your doctor to prescribe them in advance if you have a history of problems with birth control.

Although not available in North America for emergency contraception (but available in Europe), mifepristone (RU 486) a drug with antiprogestational properties has been shown to be as effective as the progestin-only method even at very low doses (10 mg unidose).

The best contraceptive is one that's used

Many women try several methods through their reproductive years, at various ages and life stages. Whatever the chosen method, it must be used consistently and correctly "When evaluating the pros and cons of various methods," notes one specialist, "remember that no birth control method has as high a risk of death as unwanted pregnancy—a risk that increases with age." Mortality due to the complications of pregnancy and childbirth significantly outweigh those from contraceptive use at any age.

Sterilization: considered a permanent contraceptive

For couples who want no more children, permanent sterilization of one partner is a preferred means of birth control. The procedure involves closing off either the vas deferens (through which the sperm travel) or the Fallopian tubes (through which the eggs travel). Female sterilization outnumbers vasectomy by seven to five. When the two procedures are compared, the vasectomy is certainly much less invasive and because of this, its popularity is increasing (especially among female sex partners).

Sterilization of women ("having one's tubes tied") is done by blocking the Fallopian tubes, i.e., tying, burning or mechanically closing (occluding) them with clips or bands. The procedure is normally done as "day surgery" in hospital. Quite often it is done right after childbirth (once a family is completed), or following abortion. After sterilization the average woman is back to normal activities in a few days. The failure rate is less than 0.5 percent.

HOW TO USE A CONDOM

- **Use a new condom for every sex act.**
- **Put the condom on before the penis touches the partner's body; don't wait until the last minute.**
- **Roll the condom onto the erect penis; leave a half-inch space at the top and unroll it all the way to the base. If not circumcised, pull back the foreskin before putting on the condom.**
- **If using spermicide, apply it outside the condom.**
- **Use lubricants for anal sex, but only water-based brands (e.g., K-Y jelly), not greasy types (e.g., petroleum jelly or Vaseline), which**

weaken the latex. **(Some condoms are prelubricated with silicone gel.)**
- **If the condom breaks during intercourse, stop immediately and withdraw. Do not continue until a new condom is on and, if using spermicide, apply more.**
- **After ejaculation and before the penis gets soft, grip the rim of the condom and carefully withdraw. Gently pull the condom off the penis, being careful not to spill any semen. Always remove the condom before the penis becomes flaccid so that it won't slip off and leak.**

- **Handle the condom by the rim.**
- **Wrap used condom in a tissue and throw it in the trash. Because condoms may cause problems in sewers, don't flush them down the toilet.**

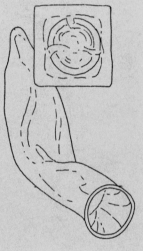

Sterilization of men is a 20-minute procedure (vasectomy) that involves tying or cutting the vas deferens. A few men have unfounded anxieties about impotence and post-vasectomy complications. The failure rate for male sterilization is the same as for females—under 0.5 percent—so it's essential to be tested later, to be sure the procedure was effective. Men often ask if this blocks their semen production and if they can be re-connected. The answer to the first question is that less than 2 percent of semen is sperm so men will not notice the difference. The procedure can be reversed but is not successful in all cases and is a much more invasive and expensive operation than the vasectomy.

Counseling is important for men and women considering sterilization to discuss all options and decide which partner should undergo the surgery. Despite increasing requests for reversal because of the three "D's"—death of a spouse, divorce or disaster (losing children)—sterilization is usually difficult to undo. Since about 5 percent of men and 10

COMPARING BIRTH CONTROL METHODS

Method	How It Works	Suitability	Main Advantages
The Pill Combination low-dose hormone formulation of estrogens plus progestin	Estrogen prevents egg maturation and progestin stops lining of uterus from thickening and preparing to receive egg; cervical plug may impede sperm penetration.	Good for women under age 35 (some say under 40). Not for smokers, especially if over 30, nor for women with high blood pressure, heart problems, diabetes, high cholesterol/blood fats, liver, kidney or gall-bladder disease, epilepsy or jaundice. (See product package list of contraindications.) Does *not* protect against STIs.	• Most effective, reversible method for preventing pregnancy if directions followed; • easy to use; lighter, more regular periods; fewer menstrual cramps; • lower risk of PID (pelvic inflammatory disease) and ovarian cysts; • protects against cancer of the ovaries and uterine lining; • may lessen benign lumpy breast disease; • does not impair fertility; • may reduce risk of ectopic (outside uterus) pregnancy.
IUD Intrauterine device	Mechanism unclear, but foreign body in uterus triggers collection of white blood cells (which kill sperm) and hostile uterine environment impedes implantation of fertilized egg. May prevent fertilization by harming sperm.	Good for monogamous women not exposed to STIs; not suitable for women at risk of STIs, teenagers, women with multiple sex partners; often best suits women who have had all desired children or not allowed for some reason to take the Pill. Does *not* protect against STIs.	• Highly effective; inexpensive; • once fitted, usually unfelt/unnoticed; • needs replacing only once every 2½ years; • convenient, long-lasting; • easily removed and reinserted if necessary; • doesn't generally disturb intercourse; • no daily equipment needed; • no effect on breastfeeding.
Diaphragm with spermicide	Round, flexible rubber cap, smeared with spermicidal foam or jelly, inserted into vagina before intercourse, blocks entry of sperm into cervix (mouth of uterus).	Suitable for women comfortable with touching own genitals; requires expert fitting and instructions for use; not fully reliable for those (e.g., teens) who don't know how, or are likely to use incorrectly. Regular checkups advised; refitting/resizing necessary following pregnancy.	• No health risks; • may help protect against sexually transmitted infections; • may protect against cervical cancer; • no hormonal additives to body; • needn't disturb intercourse (if put in ahead); • no effect on breastfeeding.
Vaginal Sponge	Traps and absorbs sperm, blocks entry of sperm into cervix and chemically kills sperm. Can be worn for up to 30 hours and must be left in for six hours after intercourse. An attached loop facilitates removal.	Suitable for women comfortable with touching own genitals; good for nursing mothers; not fully reliable for women who don't use it consistently and correctly (e.g., teens). NOT suitable for anyone who's had toxic shock syndrome; possibly less effective in women who have already had children (poorer muscle tone).	• One size fits all—no special fitting or prescription needed, available over the counter in most pharmacies; • no hormonal additives to body; • may help prevent sexually transmitted infections; • inserted hours before intercourse; permits spontaneous, repeated intercourse up to 24 hours after insertion.
Condom with spermicide	Thin sheath over erect penis traps sperm, prevents entry into cervix so egg can't be fertilized. Best used with spermicide; newer spermicide-impregnated brands still need water-based sperm-killing foam or jelly (NOT Vaseline or petroleum jelly).	Helps to protect against STIs. Often first method tried by teenagers; good if can incorporate as regular part of lovemaking; not fully reliable for people who are likely to use incorrectly or inconsistently.	• Easy availability in many stores and pharmacies without prescription; • latex brands help protect against sexually transmitted infections (e.g., AIDS, gonorrhea); • gives men an active role in birth control; • offers good protection if used consistently and carefully; • lambskin types not recommended.
Female Sterilization Tubal ligation	Fallopian tubes occluded (clipped), cauterized (burned), or cut to prevent egg from reaching uterus.	Good for women who have completed childbearing; not suitable for those with doubts about future desire for childbearing or fear of infertility.	• Highly effective; one-time, relatively simple procedure, with few complications; • done as "day"/outpatient or in-hospital procedure; • back to work in a few days; • covered by medical insurance.
Male Sterilization Vasectomy	Sperm-conducting tubes (vas deferens) cut, clipped or tied to prevent sperm getting through penis into vagina.	Good for men who have fulfilled desire for paternity; not suitable if anxious about sex life, potency or virility.	• Highly effective; one-time, simple outpatient office procedure, done in 20 minutes; • done under local anesthetic; • less risky than female sterilization; • covered by medical insurance.
Natural Family Planning or **Body Awareness Method**	Requires abstinence from sexual intercourse during female's fertile time. Chart by symptothermal method, recording temperature and changes in vaginal mucus (flow and consistency) to pinpoint day of egg release.	Suitable for stable women, willing to monitor cycles, keep accurate records, and abstain from intercourse for several days each month; instruction course advised; unsuitable for uncommitted women, those with irregular cycles or those who are often ill, do shift work or are unable to keep records.	• Condoned by various religions; • no use of chemicals or devices if used as sole birth-control method; • educates couples about fertility; • can be useful in achieving pregnancy when desired; • enhances body awareness.

Main Drawbacks and Precautions	Convenience, Availability and Cost	Estimated Failure Rate: Among average users:	Among reliable, consistent users:
• Nuisance side effects in 10–12 percent of users: nausea, headaches, weight gain, reaction with other drugs, e.g., antibiotics; and breakthrough bleeding, which may call for brand change. • missed pill requires back-up contraception for rest of month; • slight risk of blood-pressure elevation and possible rise in blood-lipid (fat) levels; • possible rise in cardio- and cerebrovascular risks—far greater with smoking Pill-users; • may aggravate diabetes and epilepsy; • may increase risk of cervical cancer and (rarely) non-malignant liver tumors.	Easy to use for women with regular lifestyle; requires daily pill swallowing, whether or not having regular intercourse. Periodic medical checkups advised while on it. Available by prescription. Discuss benefits vs. drawbacks and drug interaction with physician. Cost: $150-$175 per year.	2–2.5%	0.5%
• Chance of unnoticed slippage or expulsion; • must regularly feel for string to check placement; • increased risk of PID, possibly with resultant infertility (especially in women with many partners); • may increase menstrual bleeding and cramping; • rare chance of uterine perforation during insertion; • possibly higher risk of ectopic pregnancy (outside uterus), miscarriage and septic abortion if conception accidentally occurs with IUD in place.	Inserted by physician. Once in place can remain for 2½ years, often without trouble. Available from physician or family planning clinic. Cost: $25-$50 per insertion, may average $10-$20 per year.	4%	1.5%
• Occasional allergic reactions (to spermicide or latex in diaphragm); • somewhat messy and annoying to insert or remove; • can be dislodged during intercourse; • very rare risk of toxic shock syndrome (less than three per million).	Requires forethought; prescribed and sized by physician or family-planning expert; user must learn correct placement; most reliable for organized, monogamous steady couples; must be left in place six hours after intercourse. Available at pharmacies, family-planning clinics. Cost: $25 each; averaging $8-$10 per year, plus spermicide.	10% with spermicide	2% with spermicide
• Occasional itching, irritation or allergic reactions (to spermicide or polyurethane); • chance of being dislodged during intercourse; • very rare risk of toxic shock syndrome; • possibly annoying to insert and/or to remove; • may contribute to risk of yeast infections; • need water in order to wet the sponge prior to insertion; • a bowel movement or other internal straining may cause the sponge to move, be dislodged, or fall out; • occasional tearing on removal.	Must learn to use correctly (consult physician or family-planning expert before starting use); condoms should be used as well as sponge for first few months (added protection); must be left in place for at least six hours after intercourse. Cost: about $6 for three; might average about $300 a year for three sponges weekly.	14%	10%
• Inhibits spontaneous lovemaking; • unaesthetic; may reduce pleasurable (erotic) sensation; • possible allergy to latex or other condom material and/or spermicide; • can break (1–3 tears per 100 untested brands); • may slip off; • requires care on removal to avoid spills.	Readily obtained in many stores and any pharmacy; must be put on before any genital contact; shop around for best brand; must use with spermicide. Advice available from family-planning centres, family doctor. Cost: around $5 for three (including spermicide); might average $250 yearly for thrice-weekly sex.	14% +	2–8%
• Usual risks of surgery and anesthetic (very few); • irreversible in most cases.	Minor operation done by physician in hospital, often as "day surgery"; woman usually back to work (fully active) in a few days. Cost: $150, covered by medical insurance.	Very low: 0.015%–0.04%	Very low: 0.015%–0.04%
• Some post-operative pain; • occasionally infection (cleared by antibiotics); • usually irreversible; • sometimes (unwarranted) fears of post-vasectomy impotence.	Minor operation done by physician on request; usually in doctor's office or as hospital "outpatient." Cost: about $100, covered by medical insurance.	Very low: 0.15%	Very low: 0.15%
• Uncertain method if periods irregular, or menstrual cycles easily upset; • requires motivated dedication; • disturbs natural sex life; • may cause tension, stress, worry; • requires abstinence from sex for more than a week each month; • high rate of failure if improperly used; • effectiveness dependent on body awareness and knowledgeable use, tracking signs of ovulation.	Reliable only in well-instructed, motivated women; requires cooperation and commitment; advice available from family-planning centers. Cost: computerized cervical thermometers: about $150 each; regular ovulation thermometer: about $15; charting materials: $20 yearly.	20%–40%	2–8%

percent of women suffer post-sterilization regrets, it's wise to get advice beforehand. (For more on vasectomy, see Chapter 9.)

Periodic abstinence

Couples who opt for periodic abstinence, popularly called the "rhythm method," "natural family planning" or "fertility awareness," must limit intercourse to days when conception is deemed unlikely. To be successful, couples must precisely identify a woman's fertile days and avoid intercourse a week before and a few days afterwards. Since sperm can survive for five days or longer in the female genital tract, the "safe" or infertile time is hard to predict. Ovulation generally occurs 12 to 16 days before the onset of menstruation. To distinguish fertile from infertile days, the "symptothermal" method employs three techniques: daily temperature charting, body awareness and observation of mucus flow. Daily temperature charting relies on the peak usually observed just before ovulation. The mucus-watching (or "Billings method") depends on changes in the cervical mucus, which becomes more copious and slippery at ovulation: sexual abstinence is necessary for at least three days after the slippery "show." Intercourse is considered safest immediately after a period, on "dry days" when there's no vaginal dampness. Failure rates vary widely, ranging from 6 to 35 percent. Experts warn that female cycles can be disrupted by emotional upsets, illness or extreme diets. For women not having regular intercourse, the stimulation of a new sexual encounter may itself trigger ovulation outside the normal fertile time.

Women's special health concerns

Different influences on women's health • Societal influences on women's health • Sexuality and reproductive health in women • Menstruation and menstrual problems • Vaginitis • Vaginal yeast infections or candidiasis • Cervical cancer and genital warts • Endometriosis • Menopause • Hormone replacement therapy • Heart disease in women • Breast cancer • New genetic tests bring critical choices

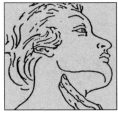

UNTIL RECENTLY women's health was viewed mainly in terms of reproductive concerns—menstrual cycles, birth control, fertility, childbearing, menopause and various disorders of the uterus, ovaries, cervix, vagina and other regions "down there." Today's concept of women's health includes gender-specific influences (such as sexism, violence against women, societal pressures, women's multiple roles and diseases more common in or unique to women) as well as the broader modern view of health—encompassing not only physical components (fitness, nutrition and freedom from disease) but also emotional, social and psychological well-being. Healthcare providers are finally acknowledging that women are not simply smaller men, or men with menstrual cycles, but that their health depends on different biological, metabolic, lifestyle and psychosocial forces, and different risk factors.

"The context and shape of women's lives has changed dramatically during the past few decades," explains the chair of women's health at the Toronto Hospital and University of Toronto. "Besides fulfilling domestic, childbearing and childcare duties, most women (including many mothers of young children) now work outside the home. They are taking on multiple roles as wage earners, homemakers and caregivers to children and aging relatives." Yet despite women's increasing presence in the workforce, society still expects women to be attractive, sexy, nurturing, passive, compliant and unassertive.

Any examination of women's health must consider not only physical but also psychosocial influences—how society's expectations and attitudes affect behavior (for example smoking, self-image and eating disorders)—and the impact of homelessness, isolation and poverty. The majority of North America's poor are women, many of them single mothers, deprived of good nutrition and proper housing, unable to access education and good medical care, at risk of violence and abuse.

One key problem in managing women's health effectively is that women are rarely included in health and pharmaceutical research studies and are therefore given drugs and other therapies that have been tested entirely, or primarily, in men. For instance, although angina (heart pain) is more common in women than in men, women represent only 15 percent of test subjects for most anti-anginal drugs. Similarly, although women are frequently prescribed cholesterol-lowering drugs, most good randomized trials examined their effects only in middle-aged men! Yet women react differently to many therapies; their bodies are smaller and tend to have more fat and less muscle than those of men, and they metabolize many substances differently. "Extrapolating from results found in male subjects," notes the chair of Women's Health at the

8

University of Toronto, "is not good enough—witness the tragedies of DES and thalidomide, drugs prescribed without adequate testing and follow-up in human females."

The good news is that gender-issues and ethics committees are gradually producing a more gender-sensitive attitude and insisting that women be included in studies on any test or procedure that may be used on them, and that information on women's health issues be included in medical school training. Governments, universities and health agencies are setting up special organizations, clinics and research units to develop more knowledge, education, research and guidelines for dealing with women's needs. For instance, an Office of Research on Women's Health has been set up by the National Institutes of Health in Washington to study conditions unique to women. Women themselves also need to become better-informed healthcare consumers, so that—in partnership with their physicians—they can ensure that any test, procedure or treatment offered to them is based on reliable, up-to-date, scientific evidence of its benefits.

DIFFERENT INFLUENCES ON WOMEN'S HEALTH

Women's health can be looked at under several subheads or sections—rather like the portions of a pie. These categories include:

- *Societal influences on women's health and behavior*—multiple roles, stress, fatigue, self-image and self-esteem, eating disorders, tobacco and alcohol use, caregiving, poverty.
- *Reproductive health concerns*—menstruation, premenstrual syndrome, contraception, sexually transmitted diseases, fertility, pregnancy and lactation, reproductive technologies, sexuality and sex problems, vaginal infections, endometriosis, cervical cancer menopause, hormone replacement therapy.
- *Diseases more lethal in women*—e.g., heart disease, lung cancer and AIDS. Heart disease is the number-one cause of death among North American women (eight times more likely to kill them than breast cancer)—and women with a first heart attack are more likely to die of it than men. Lung cancer has overtaken breast cancer as the leading cancer-killer of women,

largely because of the large numbers of young women who smoke, but it's more swiftly lethal than the same disease in men. HIV infections that cause AIDS are now the leading cause of death among 25- to- 44-year-old women in many American cities, and rapidly spreading among teenage girls. (See Chapter 16 for more on lung cancer and AIDS.)

- *Disorders more common in women*—exerting a heavy toll, these include depression, anxiety, eating disorders, arthritic and autoimmune diseases (e.g., lupus, fibromyalgia, polymyalgia, bursitis, Sjogrens syndrome) and breast cancer.
- *Violence and physical abuse*—e.g., rape, battering, trauma—affect women's health not only with bruises, cuts and broken teeth but also with psychological disturbances such as depression, post-traumatic stress disorder somatization disorders and sexual dysfunction, which undermine their ability to work and function. According to recent Canadian surveys, at least 51 percent of women have experienced some form of violence in their lifetimes.
- *Access to healthcare, treatment and research studies*—gender bias still permeates our healthcare system, limiting women's access to tests, treatments, medications, transplants and research results, leading to missed diagnoses and inadequate testing and treatment. Women are still under-researched and under-investigated for some key killers, such as cardiovascular disease, lung cancer and cervical cancer.

SOCIETAL INFLUENCES ON WOMEN'S HEALTH

Studies across the U.S., Canada and Britain show that women routinely report more stress and fatigue than men, and are twice as likely to suffer from depression and anxiety. Many women experience extreme time-pressure from juggling outside jobs, household duties, childcare and perhaps also caring for elderly relatives, with too little time to look after themselves. "Overwhelmingly," says the head of the Women's Health Program at the Toronto Hospital, "women list social factors as key sources of stress and fatigue. Typically, they are tired and stressed because of a combination of home duties and outside work, housework,

DEALING WITH FATIGUE: WHY ARE WE SO PERPETUALLY TIRED?

Many North American women, especially during the child-bearing years, feel so exhausted that the sound of the alarm jolts them wearily awake to the start of another frantically harried day—the need to get children to school, focus on the job, deal with the boss, do the shopping, complete household chores and visit an ailing aunt. British surveys report that 20 percent of men and 25 percent of women feel "continually tired." A recent community survey reported at a Toronto hospital women's health symposium found that fatigue ranks among the top 10 health complaints voiced by women. They consider fatigue a primary health concern and feel "worn out" at least half the time, although they don't consider themselves ill.

Fatigue is a "subjective sense of weariness" not measurable by lab tests. It's defined as a "sustained sense of exhaustion lasting at least six months," reducing the energy for everyday activities and eroding the ability to enjoy life. Being perpetually tired doesn't mean you have a disease, nor that you're suffering from "chronic fatigue syndrome" (a rare disorder often linked to psychiatric problems). But some medical conditions have fatigue as a symptom, including anemia, cancer, thyroid problems, sleep disorders, infections, anxiety and depression. Since fatigue can be a sign of illness or a side effect of medications (such as beta-blockers, tranquilizers, antihistamines and antianxiety drugs), check it out with your doctor. If no medical cause is found, assess your lifestyle, goals, schedule and sleep habits. Ask yourself a few key questions. Are you tired because of "role stress"—juggling the demands of work, family and home? Are your self-generated goals unrealistic—could they be scaled down? Do you go to bed at regular times? Is your bedroom a sleep-inducing environment? Are you exercising enough? Is your tiredness a symptom of depression, which needs to be professionally treated?

child care, lack of sleep, financial worries, relationship problems, emotional causes (which includes anxiety or depression), caring for ill relatives, lack of support, too little time for self and insufficient exercise. Regular exercise is a good antidote to stress and fatigue, if only women can find time for it!"

U.S. psychologist Carol Gilligan claims that women develop a care-focused morality, in contrast to the more justice-focused morality of men. "But men have their own sets of stressors," she notes, "some of which they share with women, others being unique to males. At present, we're undergoing dramatic changes in male-female roles, and change is inherently stressful even if it promises a better life."

Older women often have problems exacerbated by societal prejudices and ageism, which popularly hold that "men mature" while "women age." The health problems of elderly women include osteoporosis, arthritis, heart disease, increased risks of breast cancer and nutritional deficiencies due to poverty, waning appetite, difficulties in going out to shop for food and isolation ("no one to cook for"). Over one million of Canada's unattached elderly women live below the poverty line—at risk of malnourishment, isolation, rejection and under-stimulation.

Women's own expectations of themselves, their perfectionist or self-imposed goals—of being a successful career-woman, perfect homemaker, nurturing mother, sexy lover, gourmet cook and charming hostess—add to the stress. Another key stressor in women is lack of exercise and "no time for oneself." Women often meet all other demands, and look after everyone else before thinking of themselves; and by then they're dead tired and drop into bed. Finding time to exercise is a real dilemma for overworked women, especially those who are what one psychiatrist calls the "type F woman," trying to be "everything to everyone." To reduce stress, women can try to sort out their own personal stressors, prioritize goals and delegate or shake off duties that aren't absolutely necessary. Getting a partner to share the chores is a number one choice. Although partners increasingly share the burden of housework and childcare, women still usually do the lion's share. Studies show that even women with full-time jobs still do 80 percent of the childcare and housework (at least organizing and planning it).

Low self-esteem and self-image problems can undermine health

Society's emphasis on youth and slimness as ideals of female beauty—ideals unattainable by many women—contribute to depression, eating disorders and anxiety syndromes. Building

SMOKING IS A BEHAVIOR THAT GRAVELY THREATENS WOMEN'S HEALTH

Smoking tobacco is a huge risk factor for developing heart disease and lung cancer—today's leading killers of women. Lung cancer rates in women have gone up by a shocking 400 percent in the past 25 years—almost entirely due to smoking. And the disease is more rapidly lethal in women than in men. Young women who smoke cigarettes often take up the habit for social reasons that differ from those of their male counterparts— perhaps because of low self-esteem, to gain peer admiration and look "cool," to help keep their weight down or out of boredom while caring for young children. (Tobacco companies know how to target their ads—for instance as "slims," to capture weight-conscious young women.) About 25 percent of young Canadian women smoke cigarettes, typically starting at age 12–14, putting themselves at grave risk of heart disease and lung cancer, not to mention mouth, cervical and bladder cancers, some of which may not show up until 10, 20 or 30 years later. The health damage from smoking goes up with the number of cigarettes smoked: the more you smoke, the greater the risk. Women who smoke a pack a day have a six-times-higher risk of cardiovascular disease than non-smokers. (See Chapter 2 for the health effects of smoking and ways to quit.)

self-esteem and a good body image are key issues for adolescent girls and young women. Those with a poor self-image are likely to have low career or job aspirations and shaky relationships. "The challenge for today's young women," notes one sociologist, "is to cope with a culture still largely based on male power with an exaggerated emphasis on women's bodies and looks rather than their intrinsic value." Even the recent so-called "reality" TV shows depict highly attractive people competing for unrealistic financial rewards. While some of the pressure on women is self-generated, much of it comes from the media and societal values.

The 1991 Premiers Council on Health Strategies identified self-esteem as a key determinant of good health. Experts stress the need for women to value themselves more highly, to take better care of and nurture themselves The first crucial step is to recognize and overcome lifestyle habits that endanger health—including poor nutrition, smoking tobacco, lack of exercise, insufficient sleep, and inattention to sexual safety and reproductive health. Attending to emotional and psychological well-being is equally important—building self-esteem by emphasizing assets and positive qualities, avoiding denigrating or abusive relationships and knowing when and where to go for professional help if needed.

Recent trials show that people with low self-esteem can be helped by a type of psychotheopy called Cognitive Behavioral Therapy (CBT) that reframes negative thinking patterns into a more positive and realistic light. People who are depressed or have poor self-esteem often rely heavily on external sources of affirmation; they tend to see the cup as "half empty" and distort reality. They tend to interpret all mistakes as being their own fault with a sense of denigration and low self-worth. An interaction with a rude or abusive person makes them assume that they cannot have any meaningful relationships. Individuals with strong social support networks can show greater resilience than those who do not. Social networks can provide women with the means of doing their own CBT, by providing them with an opportunity to vent their feelings with friends and to both give and receive positive and constructive feedback.

Heavy toll of dieting and eating disorders

Efforts to acquire a fashionably lean body are leading more and more young women to diet at the cost of health. Seduced by the slenderness ideal, and coerced by ads suggesting that being slim will make them happier more successful and empowered, many women diet throughout their lives, some foisting the habit on their children at an early age.

Believing that self-control should allow them to achieve the skinny look—despite today's biological tendency to be larger and heavier—many young women restrict calories to 1,000 or fewer a day—too few to supply the necessary nutrients. Dieting is a way in which women with low self-esteem and a poor self-image may try to acquire control; for some it's a substitute for gaining mastery over other aspects of their lives. "Those with low self-esteem may hope to gain approval through

EXERCISE PROTECTS THE HEART AND HELPS WOMEN FIGHT STRESS AND OBESITY

By now most of us are well aware that exercise helps us lose weight, lowers blood cholesterol and benefits the heart. Some of us also know that it helps decrease the risks of diabetes, but fewer realize that exercise can also reduce stress. "Exercise is good therapy for the duress of stress," explains a University of Toronto physiotherapist. "Studies show that aerobic exercise also alleviates depression in both men and women."

How much exercise do you need? The former "exercise prescription"—intense aerobic workouts at least thrice weekly—has now been modified as studies show even moderate activity is good for health; it needn't be the huffing and puffing type—no need to run marathons, join aerobics classes or jog. Brisk walking will do—a brisk two-mile walk every day helps protect the heart. But fewer than one-third of Canadian women exercise vigorously enough to improve cardiovascular health. During the exercise, your breathing should be clearly audible, and you should be able to talk (able to converse, but not nec-essarily to sing!). If you can't talk while exercis-ing, slow down; if you can't hear your breath-ing, speed up.

Women can design a program, tailored to their age and lifestyle, ideally one that includes aerobic (cardiovascular), endurance and weight-training. Aerobic activities include brisk walking, running, cross-country skiing, jogging, cycling and swim-ming—provided it's not too leisurely. Although vigorous exercise best protects the heart, moderate exercise can also reap cardiovascu-lar rewards, as long as it totals about an hour a day. Done on most days of the week, sev-eral less intense exercise sessions, even five-to-six-minute bouts, can improve heart health. It's wise to consult a fitness instructor about your needs and ask for advice on how best to start, and if you have any known heart prob-lem, get the doctor's advice about how much exercise is safe. A sud-den plunge into unaccustomed exercise can cause problems. If you don't do anything, at least walk. If you walk, get a pedometer and walk more. If you walk a lot, get aerobic and consider some mild resistance training (using light weights or rubber-band stretching).

Finally, try not to regard recreational activity as a competi-tion to the death. If exercise becomes obsessive, it can worsen health prob-lems. For grim-faced, lip-biting exercisers, exercise may not be the healthy, relaxing therapy it should be, but a situation where they are pitted against themselves or others. A compulsive approach to activity has been likened to anorexia nervosa, where exer-cise is carried to the point of illness.

---

being thin," notes one expert in adolescent eating disorders, "relying precariously on body size for proof of worthiness rather than on more substantial and enduring qualities." Going further another suggests that "as weight concerns are almost universal, we should no longer consider them pathological but an adaptive response to living in a thinness-obsessed society." Most women can never achieve the idealized shape—no matter how rigorously they diet—because of the body's tendency to maintain a "set-point" and put back lost weight as soon as the diet ends.

Among young women, 2 to 5 percent now develop full-blown anorexia nervosa and bulimia—eating disorders that are 10 times more common among women than men. Anorexia nervosa involves the pursuit of thinness to the point of starvation, sometimes causing devastating health problems, even death. Among severely anorexic women, the mortality rate approaches 20 percent, and few ever recover completely from this devastating illness.

Once regarded as a subset of anorexia, bulimia nervosa is now considered an eating dis-order in its own right, especially prevalent among high school and college girls. It afflicts 2 to 4 percent of 12- to- 25-year-old women (and some adolescent males), who go through cycles of bingeing and purging. The purging doesn't rid the body of unwanted calories, as laxatives work on the large intestine *after* the calories have been absorbed. Likewise, self-imposed vomiting, which may take hours per session, gets rid of only a few calories and is extremely hard on the teeth (eroding the tooth enamel), digestive system, throat and heart. Recent research reveals that many with severe eating disorders have experienced some form of abuse—either sexual or emotional—often engendering feelings of revulsion, guilt, powerlessness and lowered self-esteem. These feelings may translate into an extreme need to "punish the body" through self-starvation.

Besides those with full-blown eating disorders, countless others—not strictly anorexic or bulimic—share some of their characteristics, preoccupied with weight and obsessive exercise. An Australian cohort study found that 8 percent of 15-year-old girls dieted at a "severe level" and 60 percent at a "moderate level." The risk for an eating disorder was increased 18-fold in severe-level dieters and 5-fold in moderate-level dieters compared with nondieters. The nutrient shortages lead to fatigue, an inability to work or learn, disturbed or halted menstruation, anemia (from lack of iron) and low bone density. Many young women's diets fall short of the required quota of calcium (about a gram or 1,000 mg a day) needed to build bones of optimal density. Calcium shortage leads to osteoporosis and fractures later in life. Many young women's diets are also deficient in folate, a vitamin essential for healthy hearts and normal childbearing. Low folate intakes have been linked to increased heart attack risks and a greater chance of having babies with neural tube defects such as spina bifida. Women should be sure to consume the recommended 400 mg of folate daily, from food or suitable vitamin supplements. (See Chapter 4 for more on folate-rich foods.)

Those who start dieting in their teens often fight obesity in midlife. Obesity is an eating disorder that now affects 30 percent of North American women, a big risk factor for arthritis, gallstones, diabetes, high blood pressure and heart disease. (See Chapter 2 for more on obesity.)

For more information, contact the National Eating Disorders Information Centre: (416) 340-4156. (See also Chapter 12.)

The caregivers also need respite and support

Today's caregivers of elderly and frail relatives—90 percent of whom are women—must not forget to nurture themselves. "Becoming a caregiver to elderly or ill parents, spouses or partners is not just a bunch of activities," noted one psychiatrist at a Women's Health symposium. "It has broader emotional and psychological implications. To the receiver care means security and protection, but for the caregiver it may mean endless juggling of conflicting demands and tasks, creating tremendous stress and worry." Caregiving can also impose losses—giving up a job or career and foregoing leisure, recreational and social activities. Informal caregivers tend to be more economically disad-

vantaged, less likely to be gainfully employed and more likely to report physical and mental health problems than non-caregivers. Today's generation will spend on average 18 years looking after their children and 19 years looking after their parents, and much of this burden will fall to women.

Canadian social surveys show that working women still do 81 percent of the domestic chores and childcare, about 46 percent of them also providing eldercare. The so-called sandwich generation is especially hard hit in being mid-life daughters parenting their own parents while still looking after their children—sometimes difficult teenagers. One U.S. estimate finds that women spend about 17 years of their lives in childcare and another 18 years caring for elderly parents (or other relatives). Even in the 1990s, women are still socialized from childhood on to be "carers" as part of their gender-identity formation. In other words, children learn what they live, and they see mainly females in nurturing roles—as baby-sitters, daycare workers, home helpers and kindergarten teachers.

Curiously, studies show that family legacies and tradition tend to designate one member as the caregiver while others remain relatively unencumbered, often offering no or little help. Women caregivers are less likely than their male counterparts to complain or ask for help. Instead, they may just cut back more on their leisure or personal pursuits, leaving no time for self-replenishment. When men undertake caregiving—usually because there's no woman to do it—they tend to focus on practical tasks such as banking, driving and house-fixing. Moreover, they're often applauded for doing things we take for granted if a woman does it!

The assumption that caregiving is "natural and normal" for women allows government and social agencies to undervalue their immense contribution. Women's health advocates say it's high time to change these patterns—to place more value on informal caregiving, to provide more easily available support networks and resources, to set boundaries and limits on what's expected. Above all, it's crucial to remember that not only the old, disabled and ill but also their caregivers need support, love and nurturance.

SEXUALITY AND REPRODUCTIVE HEALTH IN WOMEN

Throughout their adult lives, women are concerned with sexual health and, during the childbearing years, with reproductive issues—birth control, fertility, conception, pregnancy, childbirth and perhaps reproductive technology. (See Chapters 7 and 9 for more on these topics.)

Not so long ago, women were raised to believe they were non-sexual beings not meant to enjoy sexual activity, and that intercourse was mainly for procreation. Even today, the details of women's genital anatomy, their sexual desire and its fulfillment remain largely shrouded in mystery, prejudice and ignorance. "Exactly what turns women on and gives them sexual pleasure is still largely unknown," comments a renowned sexologist from New York's State University at Stony Brook. "For many health professionals, as well as for the public, a woman's genitals are just 'down there,' preferably not mentioned." The work of Masters and Johnson and of Alfred Kinsey tried to shed some light on human sexuality, suggesting that men and women had roughly similar responses, except that men got more sexually aroused by fantasy and psychological factors (now disproved).

With the advent of Viagra, and suggestions that it might enhance not only men's but also women's sexual enjoyment, female sexual function is finally being explored in more detail. (But a recent trial showed no improvement in sexual function for women taking Viagra.) Just recently, the clitoris—the tiny organ crucial to women's sexual pleasure, which engorges much like a penis—has been shown by Australian researchers to be far more extensive than previously thought (or described in anatomical texts).

On the whole, more women than men complain of sexual problems, some due to anxiety about self-image or their relationships. Women, like men, can experience problems in the desire, arousal or orgasmic phase of the human sexual response. Female sexual dysfunction can be subdivided into desire, arousal, orgasmic and sexual pain disorders. Sexual problems are highly prevalent, affecting 30–50 percent of women, but are recorded in less than 2 percent of interviews with primary care physician. Causes include hormonal and medical

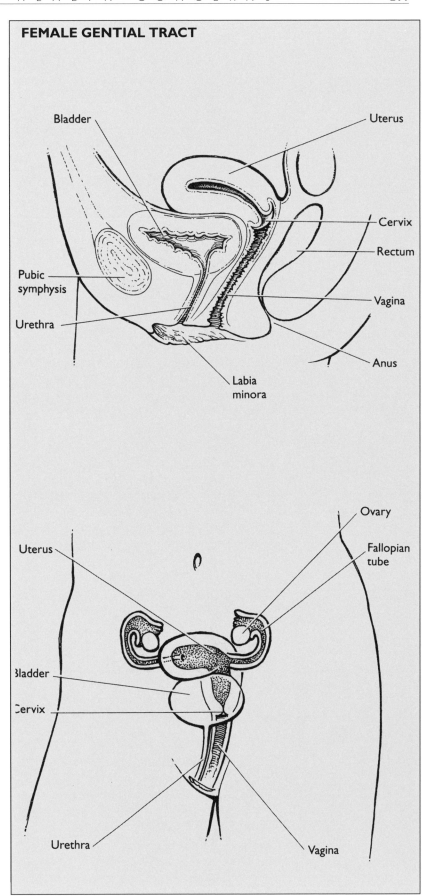

FEMALE GENTIAL TRACT

Bladder

Uterus

Cervix

Rectum

Pubic symphysis

Vagina

Urethra

Anus

Labia minora

Uterus

Ovary

Fallopian tube

Bladder

Cervix

Urethra

Vagina

conditions (eg. diabetes), local physical(gynecological) factors, medications and psychological and partnership factors. A Canadian survey reported in the 1997 *Canadian Journal of Human Sexuality*, found that most men and women (85 percent of women and 71 percent of men) have one or more sexual concerns that reduce sexual satisfaction. The two most frequently reported concerns were "I like to do things my partner doesn't," and "I'm not interested in sex." Sex therapists are now reporting more desire problems—no interest in sex and being "unable to relax"—in both men and women than the previously predominant arousal and performance problems (e.g., lack of lubrication in women, trouble with erections in men).

Today's men and women, both young and old, frequently complain that there's no time for sex. As their lives become ever more rushed and overscheduled, sex easily gets pushed to the back burner. Therapists remind couples that sex requires relaxation to make the feelings flow. Mini-vacations, planning leisure time and talking about good sex can improve sex lives. Part of the problem is that we continue to think that the best time for sex is the same as it was when we first start a relationship—late at night after a date. Making time in the afternoon or going to bed early are the only ways that busy modern couples can make time for a satisfying sex life.

Talking about sexual concerns, preferences and problems can often dramatically improve sex life for both partners. Better communication between partners—both general (nonsexual) communication and disclosure (discussion) of specific sexual likes and dislikes—overcomes many sex problems. Couples who openly discuss their personal sexual likes and dislikes may find both their sexual and nonsexual lives more satisfying.

No need to give up sex at menopause

There's still a pervasive misconception that sex is mainly for the young, and that middle-aged and post-menopausal women are no longer sexual beings. Such attitudes lead some older women, especially those who feel less attractive because of a dry vagina or a few skin wrinkles, to give up on sex, even though many of them admit they feel just as sexually alive and zestful after menopause as before, or even more so. Retirement homes find older people quite interested in sex, even if it's more fondling than intercourse. In a recent survey that asked older women how menopause affected their sexuality, 65 percent maintained there was "no noticeable effect"; others said sexual activity became "less important." But many reported that sexual relations were "more enjoyable" because the fear of pregnancy and need for contraception were gone.

In some older women, performance anxiety, self-image worries and lack of vaginal lubrication diminish sexual satisfaction. But women who continue to be sexually stimulated two or three times a week—by a partner or by self-pleasuring—often retain better-lubricated vaginas than the sexually inactive. However, vaginal dryness can be remedied by estrogen creams (to enhance natural lubrication), plus lubricants such as Astroglide or I.D. lubricant. Also, revamping ideas of "sexual perfection" and accepting different ways to enjoy sex—other than simultaneous orgasm or the need for intercourse—can help improve an older couple's sex life.

Common sex problems in women

Women's sex problems today typically affect the desire phase ("no interest in sex"), but some also have arousal and orgasmic difficulties—"can't get sexually excited" or "never reach orgasm." Women may have trouble getting aroused because of sex-negative messages received in childhood. Some are conditioned to think they must always please the man, ignoring or suppressing their own sexual desires, which can lead to sexual dysfunction. Key sex problems reported by women include:

• *Lack of sexual desire*, which usually arises because one or both partners are overscheduled and rushed, with no relaxed time together to make love, or through lack of privacy (maybe owing to children's constant presence). However, the lack of sexual desire can happen for other reasons such as depression, experiencing pain during sex or relationship issues. Often, the couple finds that interest in sex and sexual satisfaction returns in full force when they take a vacation or go off for a quiet weekend.

- *Sex arousal problems* such as an inability to become excited, hence poor lubrication—often for lack of enough gentle and pleasurable foreplay or tactile stimulation of the right kind. Poor lubrication can easily be remedied (see below), and once comfortable intercourse resumes, natural lubrication may be restored.

- *Dyspareunia*, or painful intercourse, second only to anorgasmia (inability to have orgasm) is experienced by many women occasionally, and is more obvious than anorgasmia (not as easily concealed). Dyspareunia can be primary (starting at first intercourse) or secondary (following a time of pain-free intercourse). It may be complete (occurring at all times) or situational (only with certain partners and in some lovemaking positions), superficial (with pain only at the *introitus* or vaginal entrance) or deep (with pain in the vagina, especially on deep penetration). Pelvic pain may continue after intercourse. Dyspareunia may have anatomical, pathological or psychosomatic causes. It may arise because of endometriosis, PID, birthing scars, a dry vagina, insufficient arousal or other causes.

Since many women are willing to put up with some pain or discomfort during intercourse, mistakenly considering it an unavoidable part of the sex act, there are few reliable statistics on the incidence of dyspareunia. Recent studies suggest it is far more prevalent among women of all ages than hitherto suspected. When reported, it often turns out to stem from an easily treated condition such as a vaginal infection, irritation from contraceptive foam or a dry vagina (too little lubrication). Vaginal dryness alone rarely accounts for painful intercourse, and if it is the reason it can be remedied with good water-based lubricants or even vegetable oils (but not Vaseline, which forms a painful crust), or with vaginal estrogen creams. If medical examination reveals no physical cause, the dyspareunia is attributed to psychological reasons—perhaps due to disapproving parents, or a belief that sex is sinful. Interpersonal conflicts, lack of communication or an unpleasant sexual experience (such as

---

MALE HORMONES TURN ON WOMEN'S LIBIDO

Curiously, it's the male hormone, testosterone, that stimulates libido or sexual interest in both men and women. Libido or desire means thinking about, wanting and fantasizing about sex, while arousal is the actual response to sexual stimulation that sends blood rushing to the clitoris in women (to the penis in men) and causes vaginal lubrication, helping to make intercourse pleasurable. In women, a little testosterone is secreted by the ovaries and adrenal glands with a powerful effect in making them sexually interested and arousable. With aging and after menopause, testosterone output may become inconsistent, and some experts now suggest prescribing male hormones (or combining them with postmenopausal estrogen therapy) to keep women sexually happy. However, long-term use of male hormones by women may produce unwanted side effects such as voice deepening and facial hair. Recent trials on women who had their ovaries removed have shown some improvement with testosterone. However, the women had the most significant rise in function from placebo, with only a slight improvement when testosterone was added.

---

incest or date rape) can turn off vaginal lubrication. Although many women who experience painful intercourse discuss it with their sex partners, they may not mention it to medical caregivers, who could find a solution. (And physicians frequently fail to ask about a woman's sex life.) The essence of treatment is progressive muscle relaxation and vaginal dilatation. This includes Kegel exercises (contraction of the levators) and reverse Kegel exercises (relaxation of the levators), eventually progressing to vaginal penetration with lubricated fingers, commercial dilators or tampons. Once the woman can accomplish these exercises effectively, she may get her partner to participate first by introducing fingers and then, gradually, by working up to penile insertion.

Treatment is with medication, surgery or psychotherapy, or a combination. Anatomical problems such as hymenal tags (remnants) or vulval obstructions are easily removed; lubricants can reduce the discomfort. Sex or couple therapy and special exercises can help to eliminate dyspareunia due to intercourse fears or phobias. The woman can dilate the vagina gently with her finger until it feels comfortable, allowing her partner to participate when she is ready.

- *Vaginismus*—vaginal muscle spasms that interfere with intercourse—may arise because of relationship problems, a sex-negative upbringing, a post-birth episiotomy scar an unpleasant sexual experience or a history of sexual abuse. A woman may be so fearful of having sex that her nervous system automatically causes vaginal spasms, preventing penile insertion. Therapy is with Kegel exercises (to strengthen the vaginal muscles) and using dilators of increasing size to flex the vagina.

- *Anorgasmia*, among the most common of female sex problems, is the apparent inability to achieve orgasm. This problem has sparked much debate about what constitutes the female orgasm. Is a woman sexually dysfunctional if she can't reach orgasm through intercourse but reaches it when her clitoris is manually stimulated by her partner (or by self-pleasuring)? Women experience different degrees of orgasm at different times, with different sex partners. Many women who get neither a superficial nor deep orgasm during intercourse nonetheless enjoy sexual intimacy with a man, although some find it hard to convince their partners that they're sexually satisfied—usually because the man is worried about not performing well enough. (Women may fake orgasm in order to soothe the male ego, a practice deplored by sex therapists.) Most agree it's primarily clitoral stimulation that produces the woman's orgasm but arguments swirl around its variations. The "Big O," or vaginal orgasm, is said to occur in less than 20 percent of women during intercourse, but is quite common through masturbation by the woman or her partner.

Orgasmic failure in women is usually psychological in origin, but can also arise from organic disorders such as multiple sclerosis and other neurological conditions, circulatory diseases (which impair vaginal circulation) and hormonal imbalances, as in Addison's disease (adrenal gland malfunction).

Short-term sex therapy can often help previously anorgasmic women learn how to have orgasms. Successful therapy may include some basic education about female anatomy and human sexuality, teaching women how to stimulate themselves to discover what they find erotically pleasing.

Finding better ways to communicate with a partner can often overcome sex problems and increase sexual satisfaction for both partners.

Counseling to build trust with the partner and group therapy can also be helpful. Couples may be encouraged to share erotic fantasy trips, do sensate focus exercises (pleasuring each other without expecting intercourse) or use a vibrator to increase stimulation. The "tease technique" is often helpful: slow thrusts of the penis until arousal increases, then halting and starting again, in stop-and-go stimulation.

(For more detail on sex therapy, see Chapter 7.)

Reproductive health concerns
Around the world, reproductive concerns—menstruation, fertility, contraception, pregnancy, childbirth, menopause and gynecological disorders—play a huge part in women's lives, although they continue to be underresearched and to receive far too little attention. Pregnancy-related death and illness are still leading killers in developing countries, not to speak of the introduction of bottlefeeding, which still kills millions of babies each year (from diarrheal illness). In the Western world, women still have to deal with menstrual problems (e.g., cramps, heavy or no periods), and with decisions about STD-prevention, birth control, conception, genetic screening and menopause management.

MENSTRUATION AND MENSTRUAL PROBLEMS
Many cultures surround the menarche (onset of menstruation) with taboos, rituals and myths. Some societies consider menstruating women "unclean," think they might turn food bad or damage crops, and isolate them for the first three to five days of menstrual flow each month. While Western society ignores those myths, modern folklore still perpetuates the idea that women should avoid showering, abstain from intercourse or refrain from swimming while menstruating. (While there are no absolute medical indications against it, some studies show increased risks of endometriosis, RID and STDs in women who have sex while menstruating.)

The normal menstrual cycle
The age at which menstruation starts ranges from nine to 16.5 years, but it usually begins by age 14. With improved nutritional standards in

Western society, the average age of menarche has become progressively younger (three months earlier per decade) though it has plateaued in the last decade. In North America today, the average age of menarche is 12.8 years. The onset of menstruation marks the official entry to womanhood, the beginning of the ability to bear children.

The basis of a woman's reproductive capacity—the ovaries and their supply of eggs—is determined before birth, in the developing female embryo. The ova (eggs) destined for fertilization and the production of future human beings are already in place 20 weeks after conception in the tiny fetal ovaries. The miniature ovaries start out with five to seven million immature ova each, but by birth only about two million eggs remain in the newborn girl's ovaries. More eggs disintegrate during childhood, leaving only about 300,000 eggs by the time monthly menstruation begins. More eggs disintegrate and die during the childbearing years, before ever ripening, let alone being fertilized.

After the menarche, one egg a month normally ripens inside one of the ovaries, within an ovarian follicle (sac), under the influence of female hormones. The ovum is released and travels down the Fallopian tube to the uterus. If it's not fertilized, menstruation ensues, the uterine lining and egg are sloughed off and the cycle begins again. The normal menstrual cycle varies from short (21 days) to long (35 days), the norm being 28 days, with blood losses averaging 30–60 ml (2–4 tbsp), sometimes more with a heavy period.

Very heavy periods should not be ignored; they need to be medically checked out. Excessively heavy periods can be due to fibroid growths in the uterus, endometriosis, hormonal abnormalities (low progesterone levels), dysfunctional uterine bleeding or possibly cancer. If menstrual bleeding is frequently heavy, or has clots in it, women may become anemic and need an iron supplement. Menstruating women should pay attention to iron in their diet and eat enough meat, liver, eggs, raisins or iron-rich vegetables.

Some women experience painful periods, known as dysmenorrhea, which can be spasmodic (sharp pelvic cramps at the start of menstrual flow) or congestive (with a deep, dull ache); either type requires medical consultation. Hormone supplements or other remedies may be advised according to the cause.

Amenorrhea

Amenorrhea, the cessation, absence or irregularity of periods, can be primary (if a girl gets to age 17–18 without starting her periods) or secondary (if periods stop after having once begun). Periods may cease or become irregular because of dysfunctional uterine bleeding, fibroid growths, thyroid disorders, blood problems such as thrombocytopenia (low blood platelets), infection, stress, emotional upsets, severe dieting, sudden weight loss or excessive exercise.

In young girls, as the hormonal balance becomes established, periods are often irregular and easily disturbed. According to one U.S. report, women entering the military academy in West Point found the stress of army training rigorous enough to disturb menstrual patterns. Among the 1976 class of normally menstruating women, 73 percent ceased to menstruate within two months of starting their army training, although six months later only 42 percent remained amenorrheic. After 18 months, all but 7 percent had resumed normal cycles. A British private girls' school reported a similar stress effect, with many girls experiencing irregular periods on entering the school but returning to regular cycles once the regimen became familiar. One intriguing aspect of the hormonal control of menstrual cycles is the synchrony often observed in girls' boarding schools, where those sharing a dormitory gradually have their periods at about the same time each month!

PMS: premenstrual syndrome

Premenstrual syndrome, or PMS, has become a popular largely self-diagnosed complaint that's attracted much publicity, even though its existence, duration, onset, prevalence and severity remain scientifically hazy. PMS is defined as a cyclical set of complaints that come on a few days before the start of a menstrual period, typified by symptoms such as headache, breast tenderness, backache, bloating, irritability, depression and fatigue, sometimes debilitating enough to disrupt work and other activities.

Unfortunately, PMS remains poorly understood. The nature or even the existence of premenstrual syndrome has been hotly debated. Since over 200 symptoms of the disorder have been described in the medical literature, such uncertainty is understandable. More rigorous studies have recently shed considerable light on the issue. Premenstrual syndrome does exist and is characterized by both emotional and physical symptoms that recur cyclically during the luteal (second) phase of the menstrual cycle. Symptoms are behavioural (fatigue, insomnia, dizziness, change in sexual interest), psychological (irritability, depressed mood, anxiety) and physical (headache, breast tenderness and swelling, back pain, abdominal pain and bloating, water retention). Women with more severe affective (mood swing) symptoms are classified as having premenstrual dysphoric disorder (PMDD), which is thought to affect about 5 percent of menstruating women. It must be distinguished from the less severe disturbances of cognition, behaviour and mood that affect 20 to 80 percent of women during the premenstrual phase.

PMS is more common in women whose mothers were affected and in those with a history of depression. To meet the criteria for the diagnosis of PMS, symptoms must be severe enough to interfere with social and occupational functioning, occur during the second half of the menstrual cycle and remit completely at the time of menstruation. For PMDD, mood changes smust be marked and cause severe disturbance in work or social functioning. To confirm the diagnosis, the timing of symptoms should be documented in symptom diaries over two or three cycles.

A few studies have linked PMS symptoms to a premenstrual rise in serotonin (a neurotransmitter) and high levels of the hormone progesterone just before menstruation, but without corroboration. To date, no consistent hormonal abnormality has been detected in PMS sufferers. Well-conducted research offers no proof that PMS is consistently accompanied by aggression, violence or psychiatric changes, and no support for the notion of a link between PMS and crime, accidents or family rows. Some experts propose psychological explanations for PMS, such as underlying depression or anxiety disorder. One specialist suggests that PMS is "much overdiagnosed and sometimes not even linked to the menstrual cycle. It may be a learned response or reflect some underlying mood instability." In fact, careful surveys show that some women even report *positive* changes, such as more energy and improved concentration, just before menstruation.

Good nutrition, regular exercise and reassurance that nothing is wrong generally help to allay PMS. Treatments such as progesterone, vitamin B$_6$, diuretics, oil of primrose, gammalinoleic acid and bromocriptine aren't generally helpful and studies show them to be no better than placebos (dummy remedies). The general management of PMS includes a thorough history, checking menstrual regularity, ovulation and hormonal fluctuations and also looking for possible underlying psychiatric disorders. If PMS appears to be severe, support and understanding are a first step, as is a full explanation of the normal female hormone cycle.

"Taking charge of one's life," notes one gynecologist, "seems to be a generally recommended relief strategy." Changes that give women more control over their lives often relieve PMS—for instance, changes in lifestyle: improved diet, more regular exercise and extra time for recreation.

Medications that may alleviate PMS include:
- *antidepressants* known as SSRIs—for women with moderate to severe symptoms, selective serotonin reuptake inhibitors (SSRIs) are the drugs of choice. A systematic review found the SSRIs to be highly effective in treating both physical and behavioural symptoms, with similar efficacy for continuous and intermittent therapy. Sertraline (Zoloft) in doses of 50–150 mg, paroxetine (Paxil) 10–30 mg, fluoxetine (Prozac) 10–20mg and citalopram (Celexa) 10–30 mg have all proved effective in reducing PMS symptoms. Interestingly, citalopram was more effective when used only in the luteal phase than with continuous use.
- *mefenamic acid or an over the counter anti-inflammatory (e.g. ibuprofen)*, started 10–12 days before the menstrual period, but not advisable for those who plan pregnancy or suspect they might be pregnant;

- *alprazolam (Xanax)*—an anti-anxiety drug—taken daily for a week before the period, then tapered off, but concerns about possible addiction limit use of this medication;
- *low-dose danazol (Cyclomen)*—which opposes ovulation—if no pregnancy is anticipated or desired;
- *Gonadotropin-releasing hormone (GnRH) agonists*, as a spray or patch, can be helpful (again, if no pregnancy is wanted).

For severe PMS, physicians may offer hormonal agents to halt ovulation and periods, provided no pregnancy is anticipated.

Excessive exercise disturbs menstrual cycles

In ever-growing numbers, women swell the ranks of morning joggers and take up competitive sports formerly regarded as all-male domains. They participate in marathons with endurance levels at least as high as men's, and a third of all North American high school athletes are now girls. Some women who exercise ardently experience menstrual problems—most of which are no cause for alarm. Typically, excessive exercise leads to a delayed onset of periods, oligomenorrhea (few periods) or amenorrhea (cessation of periods).

For the most part, the menstrual disturbances are transient and totally reversible by reduced training levels and upgraded diets. Exercise-linked menstrual troubles are most frequent in women who commence the intense activity before the menarche.

Although arduous exercise upsets menstrual rhythms, physical exertion is not usually the sole reason. Accompanying factors, such as stress, anxiety and reduced body fat also play a part. The dividing line appears to be at 64–80 km (40–50 miles) of running per week, or equivalent exertion. Almost all women who run over 80 km (50 miles) weekly have menstrual irregularities. A large University of New Mexico study showed 12 percent of women athletes to be menstrually irregular compared with only 3 percent of nonexercisers. All runners covering 90 km (55 miles) or more per week were amenorrheic. The American College of Sports Medicine reports that a third of female long-distance runners have menstrual disturbances.

The exact hormonal mechanism whereby exercise alters menstrual rhythms isn't known. Vigorous activity may affect the brain's hypothalamic regulation of hormone outputs and increase levels of prolactin, growth hormones, androgens and beta-endorphins. One study of female athletes and runners found them amazingly adept at timing their menstruation by controlling body weight, knowing that below a definite point on the scales, periods would stop. The hormonal disturbances caused by excess exercise may produce early-onset osteoporosis, with consequent stress fractures.

Older women, whose periods are already well established when they take up strenuous exercise, are less likely to have menstrual upsets. In fact, older female marathoners often have increased menstrual flow. Women who had menstrual irregularities before going in for exercise may find the disturbances magnified.

Ballet dancers are often beset by menstrual upsets. Ballet dancers usually start menstruating at age 15.4 years—well behind the norm of 12.8 years. Classical ballet ranks second only to football in terms of physical demand, stress and energy costs, with figure skating and gymnastics coming close behind. Current ideals demand that ballerinas be light and easy to lift, fit the costumes and have the right "look." Some dancers try deliberately to delay their menarche by stringent dieting in the hope of retaining a slim, prepubescent shape.

On a warning note, do not assume that all gynecological problems in physically active women stem from their sport. Other reasons, such as endocrine diseases or anatomical defects, must also be considered. If it is the sport that has triggered the problems, a less vigorous training schedule may be all that's needed to regain normal cycles. A gain in body fat and suitable hormone therapy (for instance, estrogen replacement) can also help restore ovulation and fertility.

Many sportswomen with menstrual difficulties have subsequently had successful pregnancies. Women with reproductive cycles altered by exercise can rest assured that normal ovulation will likely recur once exercise is reduced, body fat regained and stress minimized. It's also high time to lay to rest the old

DISTINGUISHING THE DIFFERENT FORMS OF INFECTIOUS VAGINITIS

- A strong, fishy odor signals infection with "mixed" bacteria, producing a milky-gray, runny discharge with a foul odor (worst at mid-cycle and right after intercourse). Adding potassium hydroxide to a sample of the vaginal discharge releases a fishy odor. The standard treatment for this form of vaginitis is metronidazole (Flagyl), taken for seven days. Together with alcohol, this antibiotic causes nausea and vomiting, so those on it should avoid alcoholic drinks until 24 hours after the last dose. The medication should not be used during pregnancy (amoxicillin is an alternative). Occasional douching with dilute vinegar may help to acidify the vagina and get rid of the infection.

- Trichomoniasis vaginalis is due to a tiny, almond-shaped, unicellular protozoan that often produces infection with little or no discomfort and may be discovered only during a routine gynecological examination. Sometimes, however, trich causes vulvar irritation (less bothersome than with candidiasis), and a watery, greenish-yellow, sometimes frothy, bad-smelling discharge that may feel as if one has wet her pants. Urination may be painful. Trich infections are generally sexually transmitted, with frequent reinfection between partners. But trich can survive outside the body for up to three hours and may also spread in bubble baths, hot tubs, whirlpools and via wet towels or facecloths. A look down the microscope at a discharge sample reveals the whip-tailed trich organism. Treatment is a single or seven-day course of metronidazole—for the woman and any sexual partner(s). Treating the sex partner(s) is crucial to avoid reinfection.

notion that women cannot or should not exercise during their menses—belied by the many Olympic records set by menstruating athletes. Sports physicians assure women that unless they are deterred by menstrual cramping, there is no reason to stop exercising or avoid gym classes during a period.

VAGINITIS: COMMON AND ANNOYING, BUT CURABLE

Although rarely serious, vaginitis afflicts women of all ages, even young girls and babies. The term "vaginitis" lumps together several conditions that inflame and irritate the lower female genital tract.

Basically, vaginitis is due to a disturbance in the vagina's internal balance. Most adult women have some vaginal discharge, which fluctuates with age, monthly cycle, sexual activity and stress. The normal discharge varies from clear and slippery to thick and sticky, sometimes staining the underpants yellow. Some women have a profuse vaginal flow just before and during ovulation, but many who complain of a copious discharge simply have an above-average but perfectly normal amount.

Changes in vaginal discharge reflect alterations in the vagina's ecosystem—the balance of microorganisms that normally inhabit its folds. Within the vagina's ridged lining, many bacteria and other organisms dwell in friendly coexistence, or symbiosis. The relative numbers of vaginal microinhabitants fluctuate according to estrogen and other hormone levels; varying amounts of glycogen (a storage carbohydrate); and use of oral contraceptives and other drugs, especially antibiotics.

The healthy vagina is usually kept slightly acidic by harmless lactobacilli—acid-producing bacteria—that live in harmony with most other vaginal microorganisms and keep harmful organisms in check. But in the absence of sufficient lactobacilli, other infectious microorganisms can flourish and irritate the vagina. Symptoms of vaginitis include:

- a change in odor and consistency of vaginal discharge; the discharge may increase, change color smell foul or become blood tinged;
- vaginal inflammation and soreness, and possibly painful urination;
- vaginal itch, and spreading discomfort if the inflammation reaches the vulva (inner and outer folds of the external female genitals).

Tracking down the causes of vaginitis

The main causes of vaginitis are atrophy or vaginal thinning, dryness (as happens in older women), infection and, rarely, mechanical problems (foreign objects in the vagina). Some women have such delicately balanced vaginal ecosystems that even small, temporary changes in acidity can upset them. For instance, semen makes the vagina briefly alkaline for a few hours after intercourse, generally not long enough to cause symptoms, but a few women complain of vaginitis after each coital act. The vagina's inner environment can also be upset by douching, bits of tampon accidentally left in or small objects pushed in by exploratory young girls.

Infectious vaginitis is usually due to one of several microorganisms: mixed bacteria (*nonspecific vaginosis*); yeasts (*Candida albicans*); and *Trichomonas vaginalis*, "trich," a protozoan. Each type has distinct features, but the three vaginal infections may coexist. Occasionally, symptoms similar to vaginitis arise from sexually transmitted diseases such as gonorrhea or chlamydia.

Accurate diagnosis is the key to curing vaginitis

To diagnose the cause of vaginitis, doctors examine the vaginal discharge and may order a lab test culture (growth) to identify the infecting organism. Very often, a quick look down the microscope at the discharge ("smear") on a slide, plus a simple acidity test is enough to reveal what's causing the vaginitis. For instance, women with yeasts, or candidiasis, have thick acidic vaginal secretions; those with trich and/or mixed bacteria have an alkaline discharge. Treatment is chosen according to the type of infection, with follow-up to make sure the chosen medication was correct and to adjust it if necessary. Cure of vaginitis may include treatment of any sexual partner(s), to avoid "ping-pong" reinfection.

However, vaginitis is often poorly managed, and some physicians prescribe "shotgun" therapy based only on vaguely described symptoms, without doing a thorough physical examination or getting proper evidence of what's causing it. Treatment may even be prescribed over the phone! A recent survey found that only one-third of the women given medication for a presumed vaginal yeast infection were ever examined. Physicians frequently didn't take smears or send samples for lab analysis, neglecting the easy office tests that could have given evidence of the cause.

VAGINAL YEAST INFECTIONS OR CANDIDIASIS

The yeast *Candida albicans* is a fungus that often inhabits human intestines and vaginas. As early

PREVENTIVE MEASURES AGAINST YEAST INFECTIONS

- **Daily washing of the genital area with mild, unperfumed soap, especially after intercourse (preferably minimizing use of soap);**
- **rinsing with a 10 percent solution of baking soda or diluted vinegar;**
- **wiping with toilet paper from front to back (this may help avoid fecal contamination);**
- **not staying in wet swimsuits or tight-fitting clothes for long spells;**
- **cutting back on prolonged antibiotic use, if possible and medically advised;**
- **wearing pantyhose with a cotton crotch liner, or all-cotton undergarments;**
- **avoiding excessively long, hot, bubble baths (children too!);**
- **not using vaginal douches unless medically recommended;**
- **avoiding "feminine deodorant" products and perfumed soaps;**
- **taking care to remove tampons in their entirety;**
- **avoidance of sexual intercourse during treatment;**
- **ensuring that all things entering the vagina—penises, diaphragms, tampons—are scrupulously clean!**

as 400 B.C., Hippocrates noted yeast infections, or thrush, as whitish patches on the gums and tongue. Over 50 percent of adult women suffer at least one attack of candida vaginitis, and some have repeat episodes. Ordinarily harmless, candida yeasts produce symptoms if the vaginal ecosystem is disturbed. The less acidic the vagina, the more prone it is to yeasts. Candidiasis occurs most often in young women, less postmenopausally (except in those on estrogen therapy).

The usual signs of vaginal yeast infections are intense genital itching (often severe enough to disturb sleep); sore, swollen, possibly reddened labia; and a thick, white, curdy, cottage-cheese-like discharge. A few women with candidiasis detect a yeasty odor like fermenting dough. There's often also painful urination and discomfort during sex.

Susceptibility to yeast infections increases during pregnancy and with prolonged use of antibiotics or, sometimes, birth-control or hormone replacement pills. Wearing tights or tight jeans traps the candida organisms against the vulva, exacerbating the infection. Other predisposing factors include postmenopausal thinning of the vaginal wall; diabetes; cuts or abrasions in the genital area; too much douching, poor hygiene and soiled underwear (which transfer yeasts from feces to the vagina); and an immune system weakened by HIV/AIDS or other disorders. Eating too much sugar or having a defect in milk sugar (lactose) metabolism may predispose

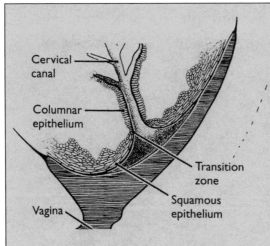

DETECTING CERVICAL CHANGES EARLY TO AVOID CANCER

The cervix, or neck of the uterus, is one of the body's most easily accessible internal organs. The columnar epithelium, which lines the canal leading from the inside of the uterus, changes to the squamous (skin-like) epithelium of the vagina, and this junction between the two types of cells is the transition zone where most cervical cancers begin. Many cervical cell abnormalities subside and vanish on their own, with-out treatment, never becoming a cancer. And the few that do go on to become cancer usually take five, ten, fifteen or more years to do so. The simple Pap or cer-vical smear test can detect abnormal changes in this

Cervical canal

Columnar epithelium

Vagina

Transition zone

Squamous epithelium

some women to yeast infections.

Effective treatment for candidiasis combines antifungal drugs with scrupulous hygiene. Wearing loose cotton underwear may combat but not prevent a yeast infection.

• Antifungals such as miconazole (Monistat), clotrimazole (Canesten), Terazol—as tablets, creams or suppositories, some of them over-the-counter products—halt yeast growth. Newer antifungals such as fluconazole (Diflucan) work well as one-dose tablets. But since many women stop taking the antifungals once symptoms disappear although the yeasts may linger on, a single-shot clotrimazole injection may be best.

• A more recent antifungal, oral ketoconazole (Nizoral), is 90 percent effective against severe candidiasis, but symptoms often return once it's discontinued, and this drug requires close medical care as it can damage the liver. It should never be used during pregnancy or when conception could occur.

• A trusted older remedy—gentian violet—may still be worth a try, although it can produce allergies and is a bit messy!

• Betadine douches are sometimes prescribed for mild cases.

• Sexual intercourse and tampons are discouraged while trying to clear up yeast vaginitis.

• Some women get repeat yeast infections that resist all therapy. Although antifungals clear up 90 percent of vaginal yeast proliferation, the infection comes back again and again, despite efforts to eliminate all possible predisposing factors (such as antibiotics or oral contraceptives). Recurrent candidiasis is sometimes ascribed to self-reinfection, poor hygiene or anal sex—although no scientific studies have proved this transmission route. Applying antifungals to the entire genital area can minimize recurrence.

Very occasionally, yeasts invade other organs besides the vagina, seriously threatening health. But the claims that attribute a host of illnesses to yeast invasions are unsubstantiated. Allegations that candidiasis has reached epidemic proportions owing to carbohydrate-rich diets, birth-control pills, pollution and repressed immune systems do not stand up to scientific scrutiny.

Home remedies for candidiasis are generally considered of dubious help, but one "natural" therapy—inserting yogurt into the vagina—often works, perhaps because yogurt contains lactobacilli that reestablish the vagina's normal acidity and deter growth of harmful organisms. Although messy and of no proven benefit, local yogurt insertion isn't harmful! But excess vaginal douching does more harm than good for yeast flare-ups.

CERVICAL CANCER AND GENITAL WARTS

Next to breast cancer, cancer of the cervix (uterine opening) is the second leading cause of cancer deaths among women aged 25–39, responsible for the deaths of 7,000 American women (and about 600 Canadians) each year. Yet it is an easily prevented cancer because abnormal cellular changes at the mouth of the cervix allow it to be found and treated early. Modern laser and other treatments make this type of cancer eminently preventable if caught early. While Pap tests to screen women for early cervical changes have greatly reduced deaths from this disease, the tragedy is that many women who still develop and die of cervical cancer have never had the simple test, which can detect changes in time to prevent this cancer from becoming lethal.

Cervical cancer usually takes several years to develop, progressing from slightly abnormal precancerous changes, or dysplasia ("dys" meaning abnormal), at the mouth of the cervix to more serious but still noncancerous stages, to early and then full invasive cancer. Before becoming invasive, the localized, noncancerous changes at the cervix can easily be located and destroyed. Left untreated, they may go on to become invasive cancer penetrate the lining of the cervix and invade nearby organs.

The most significant risk factor for cervical cancer is Human Papillomavirus (HPV). The most common high-risk oncogenic (cancer-causing) strains are types 16, 18, 31 and 45. Risk factors for HPV are early onset of sexual intercourse, multiple partners, a partner who has had multiple partners, and lower socioeconomic status. Other significant risk factors for cervical cancer are HIV infection and smoking. Cervical cancer may be asymptomatic, however signs or symptoms include intermenstrual, post-coital or post-menopausal bleeding, unusual vaginal discharge, rectal/bladder bleeding and leg or pelvic pain.

A study by British Columbia's Cancer Control Agency found that cervical *carcinoma in situ* (localized precancerous changes) in women aged 20 to 29 years has trebled since the 1970s. The upswing is ascribed to greater sexual permissiveness and the younger age at which girls now begin their sex lives. There is a clear link between cervical cancer, teenage onset of sexual activity and the number of sex partners a woman has. Cigarette smoking increases the risk of cervical cancer as does the presence of genital warts (and the HPV viruses that cause them) in a sex partner.

Cervical cancer is a sexually transmitted disease

Cervical cancer is very rare in women who don't have sex, but the more male partners a woman has, the greater her risk. Wives and lovers of promiscuous men are also at high risk. For more than 150 years, scientists puzzled over the link between sexual intercourse and cervical cancer especially in women with many sex partners. The suspicion that a transmissible agent might trigger this cancer arose as early as 1842, when a physician reported that the nuns in an Italian convent never developed cervical cancer, a disease then very common among married Italian women. These findings were later confirmed by a Canadian study of 13,000 Quebec nuns, among whom cervical cancer was also conspicuously absent. Any woman who is or has ever been sexually active—even with one man—is at risk and should get regular gynecological checkups for genital wart (HPV) viruses.

Genital-wart viruses prime suspect as cause of cervical cancer

The latest scientific thinking incriminates genital-wart or human papilloma virus (HPV), often transmitted from the penis during sexual intercourse, as the chief cause of cervical cancer. Genital-wart viruses, carried by about one percent of the sexually active North American population, can cause cervical cancer even though many of those who have them aren't aware they are infected. Genital warts are often so tiny they're invisible, and they rarely cause symptoms other than some itching. In men, genital warts occur mostly on the foreskin, head of the penis, scrotum and anal area; in women their most common location is the vulva, perineum (between vulva and anus), cervix and vagina.

Besides those who actually have genital warts, another 15 percent of the population—especially sexually active 18- to- 25-year-old men—carry HPV viruses and can transmit them to sexual partners. HPV-infected women might endanger their newborn babies by passing on the infection at birth. A new vaccine is being developed in the U.S., which might one day help protect women against HPV infection.

Through the years, many agents have been thought to cause cervical cancer. At first trichomonas was suspected, then smegma (collected debris under the foreskin)—both subsequently cleared of suspicion—and later

---

RATING CERVICAL CANCER RISKS

High risk:
- **any woman who has ever been sexually active and had intercourse with men;**
- **those who start having sex as teenagers;**
- **those with multiple sex partners;**
- **those with HPV or genital-wart infections (and possibly genital herpes);**
- **cigarette smokers and those substantially exposed to secondhand smoke;**
- **those with low immune defenses (e.g., transplant patients and others on immunosuppressants);**
- **those whose male sex partners have HPV-caused penile warts, multiple sex partners or ex-partners with cervical cancer;**
- **those who have had a previous positive Pap smear.**

Lowest risk:
- **women who have never had sexual intercourse;**
- **women over age 60 whose Pap smears have always been negative.**

genital *herpes simplex II* (the cold-sore virus) became the prime suspect. But while genital herpes may play a part in cervical cancer studies show that the human papilloma virus (HPV, or genital-wart) virus is the main culprit.

Although genital warts—tiny, flat, almost invisible growths—are hard to see, mild acetic acid (vinegar) put on the genitals of men or women often makes them visible under a magnifying glass. The modern technique of "viral fingerprinting" (analyzing molecules within cells) can identify which HPV strains are in the warts. Estimates suggest that the number of people infected with HPV in North America has more than doubled in the past 10 years and is on the rise, posing a grave health problem, greatly increasing cervical cancer risks.

Take the case of a recently married woman in her early thirties who was told her annual Pap test that revealed small warts on the rim of her cervix. The gynecologist said they should be removed to stop cancer from developing, advising laser treatment, telling her not to have sex with her partner until the genital warts had been cured. Her initial panic and the discomforting thought of being "unclean" were quickly replaced by a flood of relief at having found the condition in time to prevent cancer. A quick, painless office laser treatment removed the genital warts. Apart from a few days of vaginal soreness and the need for sexual abstinence while healing, the episode was soon forgotten. However, the message was clear: get regular Pap tests and gynecological pelvic exams.

Prenatal exposure to diethylstilbestrol (DES), previously given to avert miscarriage, is another high-risk factor for specific forms of cervical cancer. The American College of Obstetricians and Gynecologists strongly recommends that all women exposed to DES before birth should have frequent gynecological checkups, starting at age 14.

Removal of genital warts is encouraged in both men and women

Although the experts suggest removing genital warts whenever detected, their removal doesn't always rid the body of HPV viruses, because the viruses may have infiltrated the whole genital region. If you're concerned about genital warts, consult a family physician, dermatologist or gynecologist, who may first try painting them with a wart remover such as podophyllin or trichloroacetic acid. If that doesn't work, warts can be removed by cryotherapy (freezing), electrocautery (burning) or laser vaporization. However, the warts tend to return, as the infection often lingers. New treatments on the horizon include imiquimod—an immune-system enhancer applied directly to the warts several times a week—and use of interferon (a natural antiviral agent) or the antitumour drug 5-fluorouracil (5-FU), which shows some promise.

While barrier contraceptives (such as condoms) prevent transmission of AIDS and other STDs, they don't fully protect against HPV,

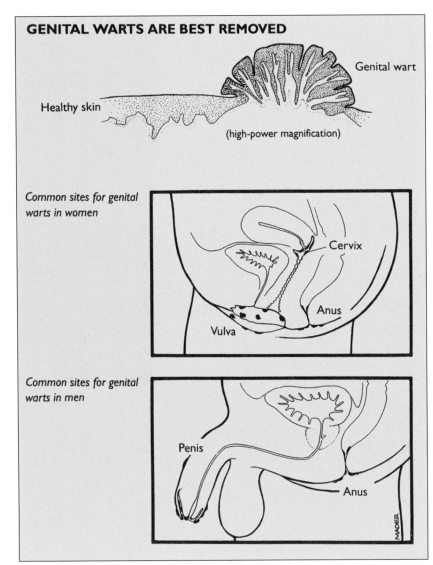

GENITAL WARTS ARE BEST REMOVED

Genital wart

Healthy skin

(high-power magnification)

Common sites for genital warts in women

Cervix

Anus

Vulva

Common sites for genital warts in men

Penis

Anus

MADER

because the viruses permeate the entire genital area. Nonetheless, using a condom may lessen risks of infection.

In men, long-term HPV infection and sub-clinical (hard-to-see) genital warts may produce dome-shaped, glistening "Bowenoid papules," spots that look and test like precancerous lesions but are usually considered harmless. Since these spots contain HPV viruses that could endanger any sex partner they're best removed.

Future approches to genital warts

A number of treatment modalities are available for anogenital warts. One of the newer ones is thrice weekly application of 5 percent Imiquimod (Aldara™) cream. One clinical trial showed that this immunomodulator cleared lesions in 50 percent of patients who used it 3 times a week for up to 16 weeks. However it is expensive and other modalities for HPV treatment include the topical agent podofilox (Condylox), available as a 0.5 percent solution or gel, that is applied to the lesions twice daily. Cryotherapy (liquid nitrogen "freezing") in the office, electrodessication and surgical excision are other options. Cryotherapy is a good starting point as it is easier for the clinician to detect the warts and apply treatment. The clearance efficacy of these methods ranges from 60–90 percent. The latest advance in the approach to preventing cervical cancer is the development of an anti-HPV vaccine. Although no vaccines are currently approved for use, trials are underway. Encouragingly, one study of HPV-16 vaccine demonstrated good protection against pre-invasive disease (100 percent), persistent infection (100 percent) and transient infection (91 percent).

Regular Pap tests can save lives

Named for its inventor, a Greek-American physician, Dr. George Papanicolaou, the Pap smear is a quick, simple, painless test used to pick up pre-cancerous and early malignant cervical changes. A little surface tissue is gently scraped from the cervix with a blunt scraper smeared onto a glass slide and examined under the microscope. Cellular abnormalities can be seen, evaluated and graded. (Abnormal cells have larger nuclei that take up more stain and look darker than normal ones.) Women going for a Pap test should avoid douching, use of tampons and vaginal creams for a day or so beforehand.

If a Pap test result comes back positive—showing precancerous changes—more tests are done. Using special stains and a magnifying colposcope (a large viewing lens), the physician examines the cervix more closely and evaluates the extent of suspicious changes. A biopsy (removal of some abnormal cells) will be done to rule out the existence of cancer.

When told of a positive Pap result, many women panic and think they have cancer. But a few abnormal cells in the cervical smear don't necessarily herald cancer or even an elevated risk of cancer. Modern technology offers simple, quick ways to remove the patch of abnormal cervical cells, by cryotherapy, electrocautery or laser vaporization.

Pap tests can pick up many gynecological infections and abnormalities, including HPV or genital-wart infections, yeast invasions and pre-cancerous and early cancerous changes in the cervix or uterus—giving plenty of time to eradicate them before they develop into invasive, life-threatening cancers. Given the life-saving capacity of Pap smear tests, why do so few women get them—allowing hundreds of Canadian women to die of cervical cancer each year? The answer is that far too many women are unaware of the need for, or bother to go for, regular Pap tests—which are recommended for all sexually active women. How often Pap smears should be done is still a debated matter. Many physicians like to do them every year; the official recommendation is for an annual test in sexually active women, or every two years if a woman has had three consecutive "negative" results, showing no abnormalities. Sexually active postmenopausal women should not dismiss the need for Pap tests as they too may develop cervical cancer.

OVARIAN CANCER

Ovarian cancer accounts for 4 percent of all new cancers, and has the highest death rate among gynecological cancers, ranking fifth as a cause of cancer deaths in Canada. Incidence has remained steady for almost half a century, with only slight improvement in cure rates. Although it can occur at any age, ovarian cancer rates rise after menopause, peaking from age 60 to 75. The hereditary form, found in families where many close relatives have or had ovarian cancer, tends to occur at an earlier age. At present, early detection and treatment before spread are the best ways to increase survival chances. But, unfortunately it is an insidious disease that rarely heralds its presence until an advanced stage when it may already have spread. Only about a quarter of cases are diagnosed before it has metastasized and affected other pelvic and abdominal organs.

The lifetime risk for a woman getting ovarian cancer is about 1 per 100. But about 8 percent of all ovarian cancers are hereditary due to gene mutations (changes) acquired from one or both parents. The inherited susceptibility to cancer arises from changes in breast cancer (BRCA) genes. Mutations in the BRCA1 gene on chromosome 17, and BRCA2 on chromosome 13 increase the risk of both breast and ovarian cancer. A family history of breast or ovarian cancer in close relatives (for instance mother, sister, daughter) may alert a woman to the possibility of being a BRCA-gene mutation carrier. Genetic testing in a specialized clinic can confirm whether someone carries a cancer-susceptibility gene. However, carrying a BRCA1 or BRCA2 gene does not inevitably mean that the carrier will develop ovarian cancer; 20 per cent or more of mutation carriers will **not** develop either breast or ovarian cancer. The decision to seek genetic testing requires careful consideration. Before being tested, women must receive counseling to fully understand the complex feelings and possible consequences of being a mutation carrier, know their possible preventive options and ensure their right to confidentiality.

Other risk factors that increase the possibility of getting ovarian cancer include an early menarche (starting periods before age 12), never having borne any children and late menopause. Protective factors that reduce risks of ovarian cancer are those that suppress ovulation (allowing "the ovary to rest"), such as having multiple full-term pregnancies, breast-feeding for many months, taking estrogen-containing birth-control pills—especially for 6 or more years—and tubal ligation.

Failure to find the disease in its early stages is partly due to lack of detection tests and to the fact that it is a "silent" disease, giving few and only subtle signs of its presence. Moreover, both women and their care providers tend to ignore alerting symptoms such as bloating, "gas," altered bowel habits and unexplained appetite loss, falsely attributing them to other conditions such as stress, irritable bowel disorder or digestive problems. Since the ovaries hang loose in the abdominal cavity, spread is common, especially to the bowel and bladder. Chances of cure depend on the cancer's degree of spread and its grade (aggressiveness or speed of growth) when diagnosed. The prognosis or outlook is best if the cancer is detected and treated while still localized to the ovaries.

Screening for ovarian cancer is unreliable, but there are a few tests used to detect it early. Tests for ovarian cancer include:
- a pelvic exam done by a trained health professional;
- transvaginal ultrasound, with a vaginal probe that can visualize the size and shape of the ovaries, revealing abnormalities;
- a blood test for the tumor-associated antigen marker (CA-125) which, although not specific for ovarian cancer, may suggest its presence if levels are high.

If these tests suggest the presence of ovarian cancer, a laparoscopic biopsy (removing tissue samples through the navel) may be advised to examine the cells and check for malignancy.

Although widespread screening for ovarian cancer is not recommended as current tests are far from perfect, and may lead to needless biopsies, annual screening is advised for women whose family history suggests a high risk of ovarian cancer. These women should have a yearly pelvic exam, an annual CA-125 blood test and a transvaginal ultrasound test.

Today's treatment for ovarian cancer is surgical removal or "debulking" of the cancer—removing all visible traces of malignancy—followed by chemotherapy with a mixture of anti-cancer drugs. New anti-cancer agents are constantly coming on stream to prolong survival, *topotecan*, for example now being widely used. Chemotherapy commonly produces side effects such as nausea, fatigue and hair loss—

effects that are reversible once chemotherapy ends, although it may take some time. Radiation therapy may also be used.

To date, there is no widely applicable way of preventing ovarian cancer although use of oral contraceptives and oophorectomy (removing both ovaries) are options for high-risk women. Using oral contraceptives for 6 or more years reduces the risk of getting ovarian cancer by 70 per cent. Even 1 year's contraceptive use diminishes risks. Prophylactic oophorectomy is a measure sometimes adopted by high-risk women, especially BRCA1 or BRCA2 mutation carriers. Ovary removal not only protects against ovarian cancer but also helps to prevent breast cancer (by removing the source of estrogen). But ovary removal in premenopausal women precipitates sudden menopause, with many attendant drawbacks, therefore needs very careful evaluation.

ENDOMETRIOSIS

Endometriosis is a common, sometimes incapacitating, gynecological problem of menstruating women. It affects mostly women in their 20s and 30s, less frequently teenagers, rarely post-menopausal women. The disorder can lead to much needless suffering because of underdiagnosis—failure to recognize and treat the condition correctly. But the past decade has seen great strides in understanding and treatment.

Endometriosis currently strikes 6 to 15 percent of North American women in their childbearing years. It occurs if bits of the endometrium (tissue lining the uterus) spread to and lodge in other sites—most frequently the ovaries or Fallopian tubes, but sometimes also more distant sites in the pelvic cavity such as the bladder, colon and appendix. Uterine cells found at remote sites probably reached them via the lymphatic system or bloodstream.

How endometriosis arises

In most women, small amounts of menstrual fluid flow backward into the Fallopian tubes and thence into the abdominal cavity, carrying uterine lining cells that may become attached to other organs. These cells may persist and grow as displaced patches of endometrial tissue. Just

as the lining of the uterus expands cyclically and is shed each month during menstruation, endometrial tissue outside the uterus also proliferates and bleeds in tune with monthly hormone cycles. But waste material from the abnormally situated endometrial tissue outside the uterus cannot escape. It accumulates and may form adhesions and scar tissue, with accompanying inflammation, pelvic pain, dysmenorrhea (painful menstruation) and other complications. The adhesions can interfere with normal function—for example, impeding fertility by displacing the Fallopian tube(s). The abnormal endometrial tissue may also form cysts on the ovary, which slowly fill with blood—known as "chocolate cysts" because of their brown color.

The symptoms of endometriosis vary according to the sites affected, ranging from hardly noticeable—many women with the disorder being asymptomatic—to severe and debilitating. Even if painful, the condition often goes unrecognized, as the discomfort may be mistaken for menstrual cramps. Sometimes endometriosis is only detected when women try to become pregnant but can't, and tests reveal adhesions around the Fallopian tubes. On discovering they have endometriosis, many women panic, think their childbearing potential is blighted and rush into efforts to conceive.

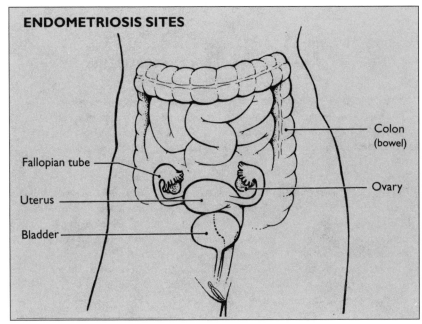

ENDOMETRIOSIS SITES

Colon (bowel)

Ovary

Fallopian tube

Uterus

Bladder

THE MAIN SYMPTOMS OF ENDOMETRIOSIS

- **Premenstrual spotting, menstrual irregularity;**
- **pain—with a period, when urinating, with a bowel movement or during intercourse. The pain typical of endometriosis often starts a few days before a period (when the islands of abnormal ti`ssue swell and release chemicals such as prostaglandins), but it may continue** throughout the menstrual period. The amount of pain by no means correlates with the extent of endometriosis, which can occur with little or no discomfort;
- **dyspareunia, or pain during intercourse, sometimes relieved by a change of position during lovemaking. The pain is most likely with deep penetration, and worst just before a period;**
- **low back pain, if the abnormally situated endometrial tissue attaches to or presses on nerves in the lower back;**
- **infertility, because of the inflammation and adhesions around the uterus and tubes—frequent among women with endometriosis. But not all infertile women have endometriosis.**

confirms endometriosis by identifying it as glandular uterine-lining tissue.

For laparoscopic investigation, carbon dioxide is pumped into the abdomen, providing a cushion of gas that separates the organs and makes them clearly visible. Although it requires general anesthesia, laparoscopy doesn't usually necessitate an overnight hospital stay. Through the laparoscope, endometriosis is often seen as purple, blue, raspberry red or brownish spots on the pelvic organs. In very severe cases, there may be many scars, adhesions and abnormal thickenings. But the amount of discoloration and scarring does not necessarily indicate the severity of endometriosis. What's actually seen may be no more than the tip of the iceberg. Up to 15 percent of women who have endometriosis look normal during laparoscopy, although even small endometrial implants can cause discomfort. Considerable effort has gone into developing noninvasive tests for endometriosis—such as ultrasound and magnetic resonance imaging—but so far none is accurate or sensitive enough.

Many women with endometriosis manage to become pregnant and carry babies to term.

How is endometriosis diagnosed?
The family physician or a gynecologist may detect masses (lumps) or nodules during a routine examination, or a vaginal, pelvic or rectal exam may reveal tender spots. Occasionally endometriosis is discovered by ultrasound exams, but chiefly it's by laparoscopy—looking into the pelvic area with a fiber-optic viewing tube. The laparoscope, inserted via a tiny incision near the navel, allows physicians to see organs inside the pelvis. Analysis of biopsy (tissue) samples taken from suspicious areas

Modern management of endometriosis
A frank discussion with sufferers can often put to rest the anxiety and insecurity. One University of Toronto expert explains that "a key step in treatment is to reassure women and de-dramatize the effects of this progressive but essentially benign disorder." Treatment is tailored to age, childbearing potential or plans and the desire for pregnancy. It may involve minimal intervention and a wait-and-see approach.

The pain may be relieved with painkillers (ASA or acetaminophen). For those with mild endometriosis, medications often diminish the symptoms to tolerable levels, so no further intervention is required. Relief at knowing what the problem is often minimizes the pain. Therapy with anti-estrogen preparations may be the next step. Alternatively, laparoscopic surgery may be recommended, the physician removing as much of the abnormal tissue as possible. Endometrial patches on the ovaries or tubes can be vaporized off with carbon-dioxide lasers or cauterized electrically. Laser techniques lessen damage to adjacent tissue, allowing swifter recovery than with traditional surgery.

CAUSES OF ENDOMETRIOSIS REMAIN ELUSIVE

Endometriosis is an enigmatic disorder, and why only some women get it remains a mystery. In part, the disorder may be linked to menstrual cycle length and flow. It can also occur after abortions and after laparoscopic procedures. The condition may also be genetic—passed on from mother to daughter.

Women who have had several pregnancies or have been on low-dose oral contraceptives for a long time appear to have reduced risks of endometriosis. It has little cancer forming potential. Some gynecologists believe that the more exercise a woman engages in and the earlier she starts athletics, the less the chance of developing

endometriosis. (Vigorous exercise can diminish or abolish ovulation and menstrual periods.) One study suggested that women who exercise more than seven hours a week have one-fifth the usual risks of endometriosis, but only if regular workouts began before age 25.

But large endometrial lesions may still need surgical excision. For women with persistent disabling endometriosis, hysterectomy (removal of uterus and ovaries) may be the best solution.

Medications used for endometriosis

Anti-estrogens used for endometriosis include low-dose birth-control pills, danazol and GnRH agonists (e.g., Synarel), all of which suppress gonadotropin secretion from the pituitary gland, reducing estrogen release. There is good evidence to support the use of anti-inflammatories (e.g. ibuprofen) as a first-line management strategy for women with painful periods.

- *Oral contraceptives* (OCs), especially forms high in progestin, prevent estrogen accumulation in blood platelets, thereby shrinking the patches of endometriosis. While OCs may relieve symptoms and prevent the spread of minimal endometriosis, they are no cure.
- *Danazol* (Cyclomen), a male hormone derivative given by mouth, turns off ovarian estrogen production. Since endometrial tissue is estrogen-dependent, blocking estrogen release can shrink the patches and relieve the pain. Danazol has some anti-inflammatory benefits, but also masculinizing side effects, including worsening acne, hirsutism (excess body hair), skin oiliness, breakthrough (between periods) bleeding and altered fat metabolism. Side effects are usually well tolerated, especially at low doses—but may make women reluctant to use danazol.
- *Gonadotropin-releasing hormone (GnRH) agonists*—also known as luteinizing hormone-releasing hormone (LHRH) agonists—are the newest weapon in the fight against endometriosis. These agents can reduce the size and number of endometrial lesions, often relieving the pain. Given by nasal spray (self-administered), injection or implants, they inhibit estrogen production, temporarily producing a near-menopausal state. These drugs also produce side effects, particularly insomnia, altered bone metabolism (leading to osteoporosis) and menopausal symptoms such as hot flashes, sweats and vaginal dryness. One advantage of GnRH agonists is that long-term use (even for several years) can now be safely accomplished by adding back a low dose of estrogen and progestin when endometriosis symptoms abate. So-called add-back therapy can also stop hot flashes and prevent bone loss without reactivating endometriosis. Although several GnRH agonists have been developed, only nafarelin (Synarel) and leuprolide (Lupron) are so far approved by Health Canada for treating endometriosis.
- *Combination therapy with danazol plus GnRH agonists* is also sometimes tried.

MENOPAUSE: TIME OF TRANSITION

Menopause, long known as the "change of life" or climacteric, marks a transition from the reproductive to the non-reproductive phase of a woman's life. Originating from two Greek words: *menos,* "month," and *pausis,* "halt," it signifies the cessation of menses—no more periods. Scientifically it's said to have occurred after the final menstrual period. When a woman hasn't menstruated for one year she's said to be menopausal. Biologically, menopause occurs when all the eggs in the ovary have gone, halting estrogen secretion. The perimenopause or lead time that precedes it—with some noticeable changes such as more sporadic or unusually heavy periods, and perhaps hot flashes and night sweats—can last several years. It's during this time that women who have them often experience the worst hot flashes.

The average age of menopause in North America is 51.4 years, even though some women go through it in their late 30s or 40s and some continue menstruating into their late 50s. Women who have both their uterus and ovaries surgically removed, or those who have only the ovaries removed, become prematurely menopausal. If only the uterus is removed, periods stop, but the ovaries continue to secrete estrogen until natural menopause. Today's increased longevity means that many women have 30 years or more of active existence after menopause, spending perhaps a third of their lives postmenopausally.

The experience of menopause differs for each woman, varying from those who hardly notice it—except for the cessation of periods—to those who have distressing symptoms that seriously disrupt their lives. Many menopausal symptoms—such as hot flashes, night sweats and insomnia—blamed on the drop in estrogen, are reversible by replacing the missing female hormone. Hormone replacement therapy has been much publicized and promoted for what physicians call a "deficiency" state. But the pendulum is starting to swing back as many question the wisdom of taking hormones for a natural stage in a woman's life, especially as recent studies show HRT does more harm than good.

Once past menopause, many women reach a kind of pleasant plateau—a new phase, a time to enjoy freedom from periods, contraception and baby care, and look ahead to some independent years of health and vigor. For many women, the menopause heralds a profound sense of liberation that may lead to an increased interest in all aspects of life—what anthropologist Margaret Mead called "post menopausal zest."

Recapping common menopausal effects

- *Hot flashes:* sudden rushes of warmth, with reddening of the face and neck and upper chest, accompanied by a wave of sweating that lasts two to four minutes, (sometimes longer) due to changes in the *noradrenergic* (nerve) pathways that control body temperature. Although unpleasant, flashes are not life-threatening—they arise from temporary vasomotor instability (overreactive blood vessels) that send blood rushing to the surface. Fifty to 85 percent of perimenopausal women experience hot flashes, although only 6 percent experience flashes that last longer than 6 minutes. The fact that only 10–20 percent of Indonesian and merely 10–25% of Chinese woman report experiencing hot flashes suggests (compared to far more Western women) that there is a cultural component. Night sweats are common and can interfere with sleep.

- *Vaginal dryness:* Estimates are that 18–21 percent of women experience dryness that can cause pain on intercourse, diminish sexual enjoyment and predispose the affected women to vaginal infections. The vagina becomes less elastic, perhaps dry and itchy, but an active sex life helps maintain vaginal suppleness and lubrication. (Vaginal estrogen creams and lubricants are a great help.)

- *Variable sexual interest:* Waning sexual interest is sometimes reported. For example, the majority of women in an Australian sample reported no change, but 31 percent indicated a decrease and 7 percent reported an increase in sexual interest. This change is obviously multifactorial and may be related to the physiologic changes.

- *Urinary incontinence (UI):* Some studies have found an association between declining estrogen levels and UI and others have not. The prevalence of UI in middle-aged women is 26–55 percent.

- *Depressed mood:* The general consensus is that while menopause might make moods more unpredictable, it does not raise the risk of a Major Depression Episode. Although not necessarily causative, North American and British cohorts reveal higher rates of depression among menopausal women who have previously suffered from bouts of depression.

- *Age of mother's menopause:* Women with premature (younger than 40 years old) and early (younger than 45 years old) menopause report that their mothers also experienced menopause at significantly younger ages.

- *Cigarette use:* Evidence is conflicting: some data suggests no difference whereas other research indicates that women who smoke likely experience menopause 1–2 years earlier than matched controls.

- *Hysterectomy status:* Evidence from a few studies suggests that women who have had a hysterectomy (uterus removal) that pre-

---

HOW TO TELL IF YOU'RE IN OR APPROACHING MENOPAUSE

A simple Pap smear or hormone (estrogen) test on cells taken from the woman's cervix can reveal how close a woman is to menopause. Periods slowly cease over two to three years, gradually becoming less regular as estrogen levels decline. When menopause begins, periods become sporadic, with one or two occasionally missed. Bleeding may be spotty, irregular, occasionally heavy. The periods eventually come to a complete halt.

The first obvious symptoms might be:
- a hot flash or night sweat;
- more frequent need to urinate;
- vaginal drying (noticed as discomfort during intercourse).

N.B.: irregular bleeding or changes in menstrual flow can have other causes and should be investigated.

served their ovaries experience more severe menopausal symptoms.

Lab tests for menopause:

- *Follicle Stimulating Hormone*: High FSH levels indicate menopausal changes in the ovary, however these levels can fluctuate considerably each month depending on whether ovulation has occurred.
- *Estradiol*: Late or post-menopausal women experience a decline in estradiol, but, as with FSH, the values can be highly variable.
- *Inhibin A or B*: a declining levels of inhibin B leads to a rising FSH.

Cultural attitudes to menopause powerfully sway its impact

Menopause occurs in context of the society women live in and what's happening in their personal lives—with relationships, parenting, careers, goals, health and social lives. The culture they live in—the attitudes to femininity, sex appeal and aging—also plays a powerful role. Responses to menopause may have less to do with declining estrogen than with women's and society's anticipation of the changes. In many non-Western societies, menopause is regarded as a natural transition that's not unduly bothersome. Japanese and other Asian women report far fewer menopausal discomforts than those in North American women; some don't even know what a hot flash is. Cross-cultural studies find that Mayan women, for example, report no hot flashes, and Greek women consider them trivial. On the other hand, in patriarchal societies where women's reproductive capacity rates high, its loss is considered a major trauma. In rural Jamaica, where menstruation is called a woman's "house of flowers," its loss is mourned, and menopausal women even report false labor pains and psychiatric disturbances.

A study conducted by the Boston Women's Health Collective found that 90 percent of American women felt either neutral or positive about menopausal changes. Most were more concerned about looking older losing a husband or getting cancer than about menopause. In a recent European survey, when asked whether menopause means the end of sexual appeal, 85 percent of British women said no, but 64 percent of the French said yes. In cultures where women's roles are valued and where the opinions of grandmothers are respected, menopause is considered a minor event. Among the Rajput caste of northern India, a woman who no longer menstruates can finally leave purdah (confinement to the home) and socialize, gaining status.

Generally not as bad as it's made out to be

Although many women experience some discomfort when passing through menopause, some make the transition smoothly, without any need for medical advice. After the event, many say they've never felt better more energetic and relaxed. Some who dreaded it find the experience not nearly as bad as they'd anticipated. Menopause is an intensely personal event, new and uncharted territory for each woman who goes through it. Since lack of knowledge easily produces anxiety, many women claim that, in retrospect, the worst part was not knowing what to expect. Surveys show that in fact under 15 percent of women ever consult a doctor about hot flashes or other menopausal discomforts, which many regard just as a transient nuisance.

The slower the fall in estrogen levels, the less severe menopausal symptoms are likely to be. Chubby women who store some estrogens in their fat tissues often find menopause less troublesome than thin women. For those with distressing symptoms, a few years of estrogen replacement can be useful to tide them over the hot flashes, night sweats, insomnia and other problems that upset them.

The key experience with menopause seems to be its unpredictability. Whether it is bleeding, mood, temperature or other symptoms, many women say that they do have to make changes to adjust to the unpredictability of this stage of their lives; these can often be positive changes.

Menopause is often unjustly blamed for depression

Although women are popularly thought to become depressed at menopause, the idea that menopause causes depression and other emo-

> ### CAN GET ESTROGEN FROM SOY PRODUCTS
>
> **Soy products may provide an alternative, non-pharmacological way to alleviate menopausal complaints and offset osteoporosis. *Phytoestrogens*, found in soya beans, licorice, flaxseed and date palm, are weakly estrogenic and may help protect the bones. In addition, eating soya products such as soymilk, tofu and soya flour may improve the blood cholesterol balance and offset vaginal dryness. Their full potential remains to be investigated.**

MANY REMEDIES TO ALLEVIATE MENOPAUSAL DISCOMFORTS

To alleviate hot flashes women can try:
- a cold drink at the first sign, and for night sweats, a thermos of ice water or an ice pack kept near the bed;
- a strong room fan in summer or winter;
- a cool shower;
- cotton lingerie and sheets that permit perspiration to escape;
- a layered look that allows clothes to be peeled off discreetly;
- avoidance, if possible, of situations that produce hot flashes—unpleasant encounters, overly vigorous exercise, hot-weather sunning, spicy food, gulping meals or alcoholic beverages (especially wine);
- medications—non-hormonal drugs such as belladonna derivatives (Bellergal), an antispasmodic, and clonidine (Dixarit) that may diminish the frequency of flashes; these drugs tone the blood vessels and may keep them from dilating.

To counter vaginal dryness in those not on estrogen:
- many excellent hormone creams are perfectly safe to use; vaginally applied creams (Premarin or Dienestrol), used about twice a week, can retain vaginal elasticity and moisture; some estrogen is absorbed into the bloodstream;
- discomfort during intercourse can also be lessened by over-the-counter water-based lubricants such as K-Y jelly or Astroglide.

To help control urine leakage:
- Kegel (pelvic) exercises can help strengthen a woman's bladder control.

tional upsets is not borne out by scientific studies. The vast numbers of women who never seek medical advice for the changes of menopause show no greater incidence of depression than nonmenopausal women or men. In fact, depression tends to be more common among adolescent and young women.

Women are more likely to be depressed or worried before menopause starts—scared about its possible consequences—than during it. In one large U.S. study, many women, far from being despondent, voiced pleasure at the cessation of periods and an end to childbearing.

Rather than menopause and the loss of reproductive capacity, it's the complex events of middle age—children growing up and leaving home (or being difficult teenagers), changing appearance, fears of fading sex appeal, career decisions and/or retirement (for self and partner), caring for aging parents—that may produce depression or anxiety. But of course those who have frequent night sweats can be constantly fatigued from the loss of sleep.

Is menopause overmedicalized?

Today's tendency to regard menopause as an unnatural state of estrogen deficiency has led to fierce arguments about the way it's handled. At menopause the body's estrogen output by the ovaries declines by 80 percent, although some is still produced by the adrenal glands and fat tissue. Those who favor hormone replacement therapy argue that the loss of estrogen endangers women's hearts—by altering levels of blood cholesterol (and other lipids)—and makes bones fragile and prone to fractures. Replacing estrogen with hormone supplements can reverse these unfavorable changes.

However, many healthcare providers, ethicists and women's groups strongly oppose the medicalization of menopause and labeling it as ovarian failure or an estrogen deficiency syndrome—a condition requiring hormonal replacement. The very terms "deficiency" and "replacement" are seen to medicalize a natural event. Notes one physician, "Women who have *naturally* depleted estrogen levels may not need or benefit from supplements." Some critics go so far as to say that "the current biomedical view of menopause results from an intimate collaboration between estrogen manufacturers and its prescribers, with oral contraceptives first setting the stage for the intense marketing of estrogen products to healthy women."

HORMONE REPLACEMENT THERAPY: YES, NO OR MAYBE?

Whether healthy menopausal or postmenopausal women should take hormones has been highly controversial and confusing. The confusion arises because until recently the large trials being done suggested that HRT can reduce heart disease and offset osteoporosis with only a small increase in breast cancer risks, and that women should take it. These cohort trials, however, were not as dependable as randomized control trials (RCTs). Recent RCTs show that HRT does not really reduce heart disease and has a minimal effect on osteoporosis. So, whereas HRT was strongly promoted for decades, not only to combat menopausal discomfort but also to protect the heart and bones, today's bottom line is that its risks outweigh benefits. While short-term use (for a year or two) may be alright, longer-term use is not recommended for most women. The evidence against HRT comes from several well-designed trials.

The Women's Health Initiative

The Women's Health Initiative (WHI) is the largest preventative study ever mounted to look at hormones in healthy post-menopausal women. It began in 1995 and was slated to run to 2008. Subset arms of the study that specifically looked at HRT in a randomized double-blind trial were the estrogen-progesterone arm, which recruited 16,608 women, and the estrogen-only arm that recruited 11,000 women who had already had a hysterectomy. The regimens being studied were continuous oral conjugated equine estrogen (Premarin)

0.625 mg and medroxyprogesterone (Provera) 2.5 mg daily or 0.625 mg Premarin daily or placebo. The study was formulated to compare risk and benefit simultaneously in a schema that ranked major and minor events postulated to be affected by hormone replacement therapy. Invasive breast cancer and coronary heart disease were the major diseases being measured and deep vein thrombosis, pulmonary embolism, endometrial cancer, stroke, hip fracture and colorectal cancer were the minor. In July 2003, the estrogen-progestin arm of the WHI was halted at the 5-½-year mark when the Data and Safety Monitoring and Review Board determined that the overall risks of HRT outweighed the benefits. Put simply, the risks outweighed the benefits so that if 1,000 women took HRT for 5 years, 2 or more would have a

---

HORMONE REGIMENS FOR HRT

Oral estrogens:
- *Premarin* (conjugated equine estrogen), usual dose 0.625 mg per day;
- *Ogen* (estrone sulfate), 0.75 mg daily;
- *Estrace* (micronized 17 beta estradiol), 1 mg daily;
- *Synthetic estrogens*, such as ethinyl estradiol.

Non-oral estrogen preparations:
- *Skin patches*—e.g., *Estraderm* (transdermal estradiol) or *Estracomb* (combined estrogen-progestin), applied on specific days to certain body sites. It can be useful for women who suffer nausea or other effects from the tablets, but occasionally it irritates the skin.
- *Injectables*, e.g., Delestrogen (estradiol valerate), Climacteron (mixture of estradiol and the male hormone, testosterone);
- *Vaginal creams*—Premarin or Dinestrol.

Progestin preparations:
- *Provera* (medroxyprogesterone acetate);
- *Micronor* (norethindrone);
- *Micronized* ("natural") progesterone.

Different HRT regimens suit different women:
- *Cyclic HRT regimens* use tablets (or a patch) to deliver continuous daily estrogen (at a dose of 0.625 mg a day), with a progestin (usually Provera) added for the first or last 12 days of each month, usually with a withdrawal bleed a day or two after the progestin is stopped. The most usual cyclic regimen is estrogen for days 1 to 25 of each month, with Provera added from days 14 to 25, followed by a withdrawal

bleed or period at the end of each month. (But the monthly bleeds can be erratic and bothersome.)
- *Continuous combined HRT* (Contin) provides daily estrogen and low-dose progestin, with no periods in about 75 percent of women, although some have sporadic (and annoying) breakthrough bleeding in the first year, generally diminishing later. (This regimen may not be as good at maintaining bone mass as the cyclic method.)
- *Estrogen with progestin once every three months* is another option, resulting in four periods a year (which may eventually cease), favored by women who hate the monthly bleeds of the cyclic regimen or the erratic spotting on continuous HRT. However, this system may not suit newly menopausal women, in whom it can cause very heavy periods.
- *A more recent method* uses continuous estrogen (estrone sulfate) with intermittent progestin (given for three days, every three days). This three-days-off, three-days-on progestin regimen produces little or no withdrawal bleeds. It may be especially useful for women who start HRT several years after menopause.
- *Androgen (male) hormones* such as testosterone are sometimes also given, especially to women who have a sudden, premature menopause after ovary removal. Given postoperatively, androgens make women feel more energetic and help reinstate sexual desire. An estrogen-androgen mixture, given as pills or an injection every four to six weeks, can enhance well-being, heighten sex drive and improve cognitive (thinking, concentration) powers. Post-menopausal women who experience loss of libido may also benefit from androgens.

WHO CANNOT OR MUST NOT USE HORMONE REPLACEMENT?

The list of contraindications to HRT has dwindled, and in recent years many groups formerly denied it—for example, women with diabetes, high blood pressure, previous blood clots or heart disease and even some who have had breast cancer—are now permitted to use it, provided they are carefully selected, advised and monitored.

HRT cannot be used by women who have:
- unexplained uterine bleeding (of unknown cause);
- active liver disease;
- active or past breast cancer (with some exceptions).

Women who must use HRT with caution include:
- those with migraine headaches;
- those who have gallbladder disease or liver dysfunction;
- women who have had previous uterine cancer.

cardiac or other problem. The increased risks for coronary heart disease, stroke, breast cancer, and deep vein thrombosis outweighed the benefits of possible decreases in colorectal cancer and hip fracture.

In 2004, the estrogen-only arm of the WHI study was also closed prematurely at the 7-year mark because it failed to show any overall benefit of HRT. The results showed that estrogen increased the risk of stroke, decreased the risk of hip fracture, and did not affect heart disease incidence over an average of 6.8 years.

Quality of life

The estrogen/progestin arm of the WHI study examined several quality-of-life issues that had also been the subject of much anecdotal reporting. Between the treatment group and the controls there was no significant effect on general health, vitality, mental health, depressive symptoms or sexual satisfaction. One year's use of estrogen plus progestin was associated with a statistically significant but small and not clinically meaningful benefit in terms of sleep disturbance, physical functioning and bodily pain. It is important to recognize that women who entered the trial were generally free of major menopausal symptoms. Nonetheless, some women might decide that the benefits of HRT (reduced hot flashes and less vaginal atrophy) are worth the risks and continue to take HRT.

As an alternative, in order to strengthen hearts, women can eat low-fat, high-fiber diets, exercise at a heart-training pace, quit smoking, keep their weight within healthy limits and reduce blood pressure if it's high. To maintain bone density and decrease fracture risks, they can do weight-bearing exercises, eat food containing enough calcium and vitamin D, take care to avoid falls as they age, and possibly take bone-building medications such as Fosamax, Actonel or Calcitonin.

HRT and cognitive (thought) functions

There has been considerable conjecture about the role of estrogen in improving cognitive or thinking abilities. Recent trials have dampened the enthusiasm of those who postulate a positive effect. In one U.S. trial (the HERS—Heart and Estrogen Replacement Study), there was no difference in cognitive function between the treated and placebo groups (average age 71 years). In the WHI Memory Study of women aged 65 or older, estrogen plus progestin did not improve cognitive function, compared to placebo. Although most women receiving estrogen/progestin did not experience adverse effects on cognition compared with placebo, a small increased risk of clinically meaningful cognitive decline occurred in the treated group. The increased risk would result in an additional 23 cases of dementia per 10,000 women per year. Preliminary data from the estrogen-only arm of the WHIMS show that participants who were on estrogen alone had a trend toward increased risk of probable dementia and/or mild cognitive impairment when compared to the women who were taking placebo.

Different ways of taking HRT

Postmenopausal hormones may be given in different doses and by various means—as tablets, injections, through a vaginal device (ring) or a transdermal skin patch that delivers the hormones into the bloodstream. The hormones from the patch bypass the liver so women formerly denied HRT, such as those with gallbladder or liver disease, can now go on HRT. It's also an alternative for those who are nauseated by the oral form. The patch seems less effective in improving blood lipid profiles and its long-term effects on heart disease are not known.

HEART DISEASE IN WOMEN: THE LEADING KILLER

If asked what disease women are most likely to die of, many would list breast cancer as the number-one killer. Yet cardiovascular disease kills eight times more women than breast cancer. It accounts for 41 percent of all deaths among Canadian women, compared with 37 percent of all deaths in men. Across North America, 500,000 women die each year of heart disease, and the myth that heart disease is a man's disease is gradually fading as clinicians realize that women are equally prone to heart attacks—albeit at an older age—and more likely to die of them than men. Yet women are generally unaware of their high cardiovascular risks, know too little about their endangered hearts or how to protect them.

Since most research on heart disease has been done in men, and because symptoms of heart trouble differ in women, both doctors and their female patients may miss or fail to recognize and treat it promptly. Experts claim that women have been underrepresented in heart studies, are underinvestigated for heart symptoms, underdiagnosed and, some say, given less modern, lifesaving treatments. Most studies that explore heart disease have enrolled only men, excluding women and older subjects of both sexes. Even some recently publicized large cholesterol trials were done on men only "High time to reverse the inequity," says one cardiologist at a new Canadian center for women's heart disease.

Heart attacks more often fatal in women

Women usually develop heart disease, for instance coronary artery disease (CAD), about 10 years later than men, often with slightly different symptoms, and often in a more severe form. Until menopause, women's hearts are protected by the female hormone estrogen, which keeps their blood lipids (fats, such as cholesterol) at healthier levels. Protected by estrogen, women start to develop heart disease about 10 years later than men. But at menopause, as estrogen production drops, women begin to catch up to men in heart attack rates, and they're twice as likely to die during or soon after a first heart attack. Also, more women than men suffer a second heart attack soon after the first.

Overall, women generally ask for, or receive, treatment for coronary heart disease at a later or more advanced stage than men.

Gender differences in managing heart disease

Despite the fact that after a certain age both sexes are equally prone to coronary heart disease, there are many gender differences in the way women are investigated and treated. Both women and their doctors are slow to recognize and respond to preliminary signs of heart trouble. For starters, women rarely get the same battery of cardiac tests as men during midlife medical exams, and their chest pain may be dismissed as due to indigestion or anxiety. Chest pain in men is usually taken more seriously and triggers physicians to think "heart" and order tests such as an exercise stress test, perhaps followed by an angiogram (dye test to outline the coronary arteries) and, if necessary, prompt treatment. In contrast, women with chest pain are less swiftly investigated, have fewer cardiac tests, are less often referred to cardiologists for investigation and receive less bypass surgery and other treatments than men. Women with chest pain or other coronary symptoms are half as likely as men to be given an exercise stress test for heart function, but more likely to be treated with a wait-and-see approach.

Women themselves are often unaware of the possible signs of a heart attack and more likely to ignore, dismiss or deny them. Whereas

---

CLASSIC SYMPTOMS OF HEART ATTACK

- **Persistent chest pain, often mid-chest, perhaps radiating to neck, jaw, left shoulder or arm;**
- **sense of tightness or "squeezing" in the chest;**
- **"heaviness" that may feel like indigestion;**
- **sweating, nausea and vomiting;**
- **pallor (pale skin);**
- **shortness of breath;**
- **denial—refusal to believe anything is seriously wrong. In women, symptoms may be chiefly:**
- **shoulder, back or neck pain;**
- **shortness of breath;**
- **nausea, heaviness, sense of indigestion;**
- **sharp pain on breathing in cold air.**

RECAPPING HOW A HEART ATTACK HAPPENS

A heart attack or *myocardial infarction* (MI) usually occurs because the coronary arteries, which lie on the heart's surface and supply it with oxygen, become narrowed or blocked by fatty deposits (plaque) and calcium, producing *atherosclerosis*. Progressive atherosclerosis reduces blood flow to the heart and **the consequent ischemia, or oxygen lack, causes symptoms such as angina (chest pain) and shortness of breath. If the blood flow and oxygen supply are cut off, parts of the heart muscle can be irreversibly damaged in less than one hour. Getting to hospital quickly and starting treatment at once are crucial to** **save a life—as much for women as for men.**

Women's hearts are generally smaller than men's, beat faster both in motion and at rest, react differently to stress—for instance, during a treadmill stress test—and have smaller coronary blood vessels that are harder to work on.

TESTS FOR CORONARY ARTERY DISEASE

- *Electrocardiogram (ECG)*—heart-pattern test using electrodes placed on the chest to delineate the heart's rhythm and electrical activity during contraction (pumping);
- *exercise stress test*—to measure heart function while people walk against elevation on a treadmill to detect oxygen lack under stress (i.e., during vigorous exercise);
- *thallium scan*—with injected radioactive thallium as a tracer; it goes into the heart and indicates myocardial blood flow (to the heart muscle) during treadmill exercise;
- *angiogram*—dye injected via a catheter (fine plastic tube) into a blood vessel in the arm or groin, which reaches the heart and precisely locates blockages in the coronary arteries;
- *exercise echocardiography*—an echogram of heart action taken during exercise;
- *myocardial perfusion imaging*—using technetium labeling to visualize the heart's blood flow—better than an exercise ECG for ruling out CAD in women.

a man with chest pain is apt to take it seriously, and get to hospital fast, women are likelier to call their doctor or a friend about it first, wait to see if the pain vanishes or tidy up before going to the emergency department, arriving later than their male counterparts. The delay can have fatal consequences because it may be too late to use life-saving medications that can dissolve artery-blocking clots within the first 6 to 10 hours of a heart attack.

In addition, *revascularization* treatments to restore coronary bloodflow—bypass surgery or angioplasty (ballooning)—are often less successful in women than in men. Women do less well after bypass surgery, with lower survival rates than men, possibly because their disease is more advanced by the time they are treated, and because their smaller arteries make certain procedures trickier to do. "Although at our center angioplasty and bypass operations have equal success rates in men and women," explains one cardiac surgeon, "women tend to feel less improved afterward, perhaps because their heart disease is different, or more advanced by the time it's treated."

Heart symptoms differ in men and women

In men, a heart attack is often the first (perhaps final) clue to heart trouble, while women tend to get angina as a preliminary symptom. Angina pectoris—from the Greek "to strangle"—is chest pain or heaviness due to lack of oxygen in the heart muscle, often brought on by exertion or stress. The famous Framingham studies found that two-thirds of men first "present" with a heart attack and only one-third have previous angina, while among women about two-thirds first present with angina and only one-third with a sudden heart attack. The typical pattern for female heart disease is a long history of angina—perhaps with chest, shoulder or back pain and shortness of breath—often ignored by both women and their caregivers. "Any chest pain that feels heavy, constricting, strangling, like a heavy pressure or large animal sitting on the chest, should send women straight to the hospital emergency unit," suggest one eminent U.S. cardiologist.

One problem in recognizing angina in women is that it tends to differ from that in men.

When men do complain of it, angina tends to be classic or *retrosternal* pain—an easily recognized pattern felt as squeezing or "crushing pain," a heaviness in the center or left side of the chest (perhaps radiating to the shoulder or left arm)—often brought on by exercise or stress. By contrast, angina in women is often atypical, with no easily recognizable pattern. It may be described as a little neck-ache, occasional pains in the back or shoulder or tingling in the fingers, or as a sharp pain on exertion or in very cold air or be accompanied by nausea. Women may therefore be misdiagnosed and sent home or not properly tested for coronary disease. Since women have atypical angina, and as nonspecific chest pain is fairly common in women (especially young women), physicians may not link chest pain with heart disease but might first look for *other* causes—such as anxiety, a panic attack, heart valve prolapse (heart murmur) or heartburn (acid reflux). Besides coronary disease, acute angina in women can arise from Syndrome X—a condition unique to women, due to microscopic changes in heart vessels not detected by routine cardiac tests.

"It's essential," warns one cardiologist, "that physicians do *not* ascribe chest pain in women to psychological origins or other causes before doing a thorough check for coronary disease. The trick is to diagnose CAD in women, but once diagnosed it should be as vigilantly followed and treated as in men."

Cardiac tests less reliable in women

Diagnosing heart disease in women can be difficult not only because of the atypical angina, but also because the treadmill and other heart function tests were developed from studies done exclusively in men and are less reliable and accurate for women, often giving false results. Even if the treadmill stress tests do indicate possible heart trouble, fewer women than men are sent for further tests with an angiogram. Since the angiogram is invasive and carries a one per 700 risk of major complications, physicians may hesitate to suggest it unless the woman is at known risk of CAD. Newer imaging methods—for instance, perfusion scans and stress echocardiography—are improving diagnosis in women.

Current treatments for coronary heart disease

CAD may be treated medically, with drugs or by mechanical or surgical interventions that offset ischemia (oxygen lack) by *revascularization*—restoring the heart's blood and oxygen supply.

The most common medications used for heart disease are nitrates to quickly relieve angina by dilating the blood vessels (e.g., nitroglycerin as tablets, patches or sprays to put under the tongue); beta-blockers that lower the heart's demand for oxygen; and calcium channel blockers that prevent spasms in the coronary arteries by inhibiting the entry of calcium into the heart muscle. In addition, women may be advised to take a cholesterol-lowering drug, ASA (aspirin) or other anticoagulants to lessen blood clotting, and anti-arrhythmics to stabilize erratic heartbeats.

Besides medication, treatment may include:

- *Thrombolysis*—infusion of clot-dissolving substances during, or right after a heart attack to reestablish blood flow and prevent heart-muscle damage (so-called myocardial salvage). Thrombolytic or clot-buster drugs such as the enzymes *streptokinase* and *tissue plasminogen activator* (tPA) are only helpful within the first 6–12 hours of an attack, so time is of the essence.
- *Coronary percutaneous transluminal angioplasty, or ballooning*, a procedure that inserts a thin plastic catheter with an inflatable balloon at its

---

WOMEN'S RECOVERY SLOWER BECAUSE FEWER ATTEND CARDIAC REHABILITATION PROGRAMS

After a heart attack, women's recovery may be hampered by the fact that they are less likely than men to attend cardiac rehabilitation programs—the cornerstone of recovery for both sexes, involving exercise, conditioning and education about risk management. Women may be less inclined to attend cardiac rehab because they are less often referred, may be less motivated, have more caregiving duties and fewer supports—which leads them to feel guilty—or the need for "permission" to take the time off. Specialists are now creating programs better oriented to women's needs.

WAYS TO PREVENT OR REDUCE YOUR RISKS OF HEART DISEASE

- *Analyze your coronary risks* and try to reduce them.
- *Know the symptoms* of heart attack and what to do.
- *Insist on thorough investigation* of possible heart disease symptoms.
- *Quit smoking*: after five years, former smokers lower their cardiac risks by 50–70 percent.
- *Achieve and maintain* desirable weight.
- *Have regular blood pressure* checks and reduce blood pressure if it's high.
- *Exercise daily*—at a pace discussed with your physician or other healthcare provider—to maintain desired weight, reduce risk of diabetes, lower blood pressure, raise HDL cholesterol, reduce stress and improve fitness. That brisk daily walk may do wonders for your heart and overall health!
- *Reduce fat in the diet* by avoiding fatty meats, snacks and processed foods; favor polyunsaturated and monosaturated oils and eat oceanic fish (e.g., salmon, cod, herring, tuna), which contain omega-3 fatty acids that may protect the heart.
- *Eat a high-fiber diet* with 25–35 gm fiber a day. Dietary fiber helps lower levels of blood cholesterol (and also stabilizes blood sugar in diabetics). Consume lots of legumes (dried peas, beans, lentils), fruit and vegetables, whole grains, flaxseed, nuts (especially walnuts) and soya products. (Experts say that 20 grams of tofu daily or its equivalent in soya milk can significantly protect the heart.)
- *Lower blood triglycerides* by exercise and limiting intake of simple sugars (as in candies, honey, jams).
- *Consider regular low-dose ASA* (Aspirin) as a preventive. Several studies find that "a baby Aspirin a day"—one 160 mg tablet of acetylsalicylic acid—can reduce the incidence of heart attacks in men. However, ASA's effectiveness as a preventive in women is uncertain. (ASA users should take entero-coated products and watch for side effects such as gastrointestinal bleeds and stomach ulcers.)
- *Consume enough (400 mg per day) of dietary folate* (a B vitamin), either in your diet or a supplement as it offsets the heart-damaging effects of homocysteine in blood.
- *Consider trying coenzyme Q-10* or ubiquinone (a product pioneered in Denmark) said to improve heart function and counter angina, with no serious side effects.
- *Try to reduce life-stresses*, to relax and avoid excessive time urgency; take vacations yearly if possible.
- *Have family members learn CPR* (cardiopulmonary resuscitation) to be prepared for emergency treatment until help arrives.

For more information, consult your local Heart and Stroke Foundation, and read the American Heart Association's booklet *Silent Epidemic: The Truth About Women and Heart Disease*.

tip into the blocked coronary artery to stretch the vessel wall and crush any clots, plaque or other obstructions.

• *A stent*—a small device to hold open narrowed arteries—is sometimes inserted during angioplasty.

• *Coronary bypass surgery*, to bypass severely blocked coronary arteries by grafting in new vessels, usually veins taken from the leg or chest, in order to restore the heart's oxygen supply and alleviate angina. Women can receive bypass operations with as good long-term results as men, although they are harder to operate on and face higher surgical risks. (See chapter 16 for more on bypass surgery.)

Male and female heart risk factors roughly similar

• *Family history of heart disease:* having a father who suffered a heart attack before age 55, or a mother who had one before age 65, increases the risk.

• *Diabetes* increases CAD risks about three times above those of nondiabetic women, even at a young age.

• *High blood cholesterol levels* increase coronary risks in both sexes, but total blood cholesterol levels are less critical than the type of cholesterol measured. Women seem better protected by HDL ("good") or high-density lipoproteincholesterol levels, which should be above 45 mg/dL (1.16 mmol/L) than men. Their levels of LDL ("bad") cholesterol should not be higher than 130 mg/dL (3.36 mmol/L).

• *Elevated triglyceride levels* are a separate risk factor in women and should be below 200 mg/dL (2.26 mmol/L).

• *Smoking:* tobacco multiplies risks, depending on amount smoked, and is an escalating health threat in women. Taking birth control pills and smoking can be an especially dangerous duo.

• *Hypertension*, or high blood pressure, is a major risk factor for heart disease in both sexes. Men with hypertension are usually given blood pressure medication, but it's still uncertain whether giving women the same drugs to reduce blood pressure will similarly reduce heart attack deaths. Some studies show a reduced risk through blood pressure reduction, but less so than in men.

• *Obesity*, especially an apple-shaped weight gain (on the belly) is a cardiac danger and women at risk should make every effort to reduce through sensible nutrition and exercise.

• *Stress* can elevate risks of heart attack. (See earlier sections on stress reduction.)

• *Type-A behavior*—in people who are impatient, highly ambitious, aggressive and time pressured (take few relaxing vacations)—is strongly predictive for heart disease.

• *Isolation, poverty, loneliness* and lack of medical care are added heart risk factors for women. (In one study, socially isolated women with many life stresses were at five times greater risk of heart attack than socially supported and non-stressed women.)

BREAST CANCER
Information overload about breast cancer often inaccurate and needlessly scary, has aroused intense anxiety in today's women. Apprehension and the crossfire of differing medical opinions may deter those who find a breast lump from seeking medical advice and prevent women at risk from getting breast checkups. Tragically, despite a blitz of media publicity and efforts to promote breast health, many women still come to their doctors with breast cancers in an advanced and hard-to-cure stage. What's the solution? Still greater breast surveillance and regular screening for those who need it could possibly curb the toll of this disease.

Breast cancer *isn't* a death warrant. Despite the negative "politics" surrounding the disease, there are thousands of women leading perfectly normal lives 10, 20 or even more years after removal of a malignant breast tumor. Survival can be long term, provided the cancer is detected and treated before it spreads. To lessen the risks, women should have their breasts regularly examined and practice breast self-examination, and those over age 50 should have regular mammograms (breast X-rays). Women should remember that although breast cancer is the most commonly dianosed cancer in women, chances of dying of it are less than for lung cancer.

Who needs regular breast screening?
Breast screening uses various methods to look for signs of breast cancer in healthy women in

order to find it at an early stage when treatment can save lives. To date, we have three useful but far from perfect ways to screen for breast cancer:

- breast self-examination (BSE);
- clinical breast examination by a trained health-care professional;
- breast imaging by mammography (X-rays). None of the three techniques is foolproof. BSE, clinical exams and mammography all miss some cancers, but together they are our best method yet of screening for breast cancer. All women should watch for breast changes and get regular breast exams by a trusted healthcare provider. In addition, women over age 50 (possibly even those aged 40 and up) need regular mammograms. The majority of breast cancers are still found by women themselves, either through BSE or by happenstance—perhaps when washing or while being caressed by a partner.

Some key facts and figures about breast cancer

- Breast cancer affects one in nine women in Canada during a normal life span of 80 or more years.
- Increasing age is the greatest risk factor—for instance, at age 30 a woman has a one in 700 chance of getting breast cancer rising to one in 200 by age 40 and one in nine by age 80.
- Most (70 percent) of breast cancers occur in women over age 55.
- Men get it too—about 1 percent of all breast cancers occur in males, with an incidence around one per 1,000. (See chapter 9 for more on male breast cancer)
- If breast cancers are removed when less than 1 cm (0.4 in) across and no cancer cells are found in the underarm lymph nodes, survival chances are excellent.

Mammography remains today's most accurate screening tool

The collected results of many randomized studies conclusively show that regular mammographic screening of women aged 50 and over detects breast cancer at an early, treatable stage and reduces mortality from the disease by about 30 percent. It's important for women to realize that mammograms can be used either to screen

DIFFERENT TYPES OF BREAST CANCER DEVELOP DIFFERENTLY

Breast cancer covers a wide spectrum of disease, in which some tumors metastasize (spread) fast, while others grow very slowly. Some breast cancers rapidly penetrate nearby tissues—sometimes within months, especially in young women—while others take 10, 20 or more years to become invasive, or never spread. (The term "invasive" doesn't necessarily mean that the cancer has already spread to other tissues, just that it's penetrated through the basement membrane of the breast cells.) And although many equate small-

ness with early cancer, small is not the same as early. The early changes are termed carcinoma in situ— meaning "in place" and not invading adjacent tissue. A 1 cm (0.4 in) breast cancer has usually been growing for several years before detection. Even a 0.5 cm (0.2 in) tumor, just detectable on a mammogram, has already doubled its cell numbers about 30 times, and scientists know that spreading can occur within the first 20 doublings of tumor cells. However, the risk of spread is generally less for small tumors.

Breast cancers are

staged by size, the presence or absence of "positive" (cancerous) underarm nodes and biochemical markers that help to distinguish aggressive, fast-growing from milder, slow-growing cancers. The growth of breast cancers with estrogen receptors is stimulated by the female hormone. Very early, premalignant breast changes (cancers in situ) often appear in mammograms as tiny calcifications that might later become cancerous, but if removed in time, never develop into cancer.

(look for) cancer in someone who has no symptoms or as a diagnostic tool to confirm or rule out the suspicion that a breast lump is cancer.

Screening mammography is used to detect disease in otherwise healthy, asymptomatic breasts (with no lumps, nipple discharge or other suspicious signs). It is a routine measure advised for certain groups of women to detect small tissue abnormalities that might indicate latent disease—occult (hidden) cancers lurking inside the breast—too small to be felt even by the most expert of probing fingers.

Diagnostic mammography, by contrast, is used for women who already have signs or suspicions of cancer to make a diagnosis. Diagnostic mammography is often more extensive than screening mammography, using extra "spot" or magnification views to show up abnormalities.

While experts agree that mammographic screening of women over age 50 probably saves lives, they argue about its benefits in younger women. Many U.S. cancer agencies and one Canadian province (British Columbia) recom-

THE ADVANTAGES OF SCREENING MAMMOGRAPHY

- It is the best available early-detection tool with which to fight breast cancer.
- It can spot very early cancers two years or more before they're felt by physical examination.
- Early mammographic detection can reduce breast cancer deaths by 30 percent in women over age 50.
- Benefits clearly outweigh risks for women over age 50.

THE DISADVANTAGES OF SCREENING MAMMOGRAPHY

- Some find the procedure uncomfortable and inconvenient, but this is not significant in most women—rarely rated worse than "a trip to dentist" or "having an injection."

- Mammograms miss 10 to 15 percent of cancers found by clinical exam or biopsy in older women, more in pre-menopausal women, giving false-negative results.
- It can give false-positive results, which create needless anxiety and diagnostic work-ups (with no cancer present). In a study of New England mammography services (where they do mammography every year on women over age 50), the risk for women of having a false positive test result (that recommends further testing because of a supicious result) was 1 in 2 false results;
- It can give a false sense of security in those told their mammograms are clear (of cancer), discouraging them from examining their breasts or getting clinical exams, perhaps leading them to ignore symptoms of fast-growing interval cancers that appear between scheduled mammograms.

mend routine mammograms for women aged 40 to 49. But screening women younger than 50 years old remains controversial as mammography in the 40–49 age group has not been proven to improve survival to the same extent (nor as promptly) as for women in the 50-plus age range. Some trials have shown that for women at risk, especially those who have the BRCA1 gene, and are at high risk for breast cancer, an MRI of the breast may be the better option.

Well-conducted mammography is safe and reliable

The radiation received during a breast mammogram with modern, well-maintained equipment is no more than during a routine lung X-ray. But women having a mammogram can check with the unit or their doctors (if possible) to make sure that the equipment used is up to date and conforms with standards set by the U.S. and/or Canadian radiological societies. Having mammography at special breast-screening centers or clinics helps to ensure that the equipment is safe and the mammograms are accurately interpreted. Apart from some discomfort, there's no need to fear mammograms these days. The brief X-ray examination may save a breast, even a life.

Properly done breast self-examination (BSE)

Most breast cancers are still found by women themselves, not through BSE but by happenstance—perhaps when showering or being caressed. However, for those who wish to practise BSE, it's best learned by a "hands-on" lesson from a trained health professional and should be done at the same time every month.

Do it right to improve the odds

After being strongly promoted for 20 years, BSE is now under fire, mainly because of Russian, Chinese, British and Canadian studies showing that women who do BSE survive no better than whose who don't. Moreover, breast self-examination reveals many benign lesions, leading to anxiety and, perhaps, needless surgery. Nonetheless, many women wish to do BSE and they need to know how. The three key components in doing BSE properly are:

- to examine the breasts visually in the mirror (looking for any changes such as dimpling, asymmetry or discoloration);
- to use the three middle fingers in a rotary motion;
- to use the finger pads when feeling for changes.

For more information, consult your local breast screening center branches of the Canadian Breast Cancer Foundation or the Canadian Cancer Society.

What happens when a suspicious breast change or lump is found?

If a woman (or her partner) feels a lump, nodule or unusual thickening in either breast, she should report it to her family physician or go to the nearest women's health clinic or breast-screening center for a thorough checkup. If there's any suspicion of cancer a mammogram will be done. A biopsy will be ordered if either the physical exam or the mammogram suggests the possibility of cancer.

If the examination indicates a cyst, the liquid may be drawn out by fine-needle aspiration, a swift, painless procedure done in a physician's office. Cysts are virtually always benign, but the fluid is sent for laboratory testing.

When X-ray and other tests suggest the presence of breast cancer the next step is to remove some tissue from the suspicious area and examine it for malignancy. Biopsy—the removal of tissue samples for examination under the microscope—remains the "gold standard" for diagnosing cancer. Only a biopsy can confirm the presence of breast cancer.

New biopsy methods easier and quicker to do

Better biopsy methods, often done with imaging (X-ray or ultrasound) guidance in the radiology or imaging department can now often avoid the need for two surgical steps in breast cancer: one to detect or diagnose the cancer the second to remove the tumor and also some axillary (underarm) lymph nodes. Since the vast majority (75 percent) of breast abnormalities investigated turn out to be benign, clinicians prefer to avoid the discomfort and costs of surgical biopsy whenever possible. The newer methods are just as accurate but quicker, cheaper less invasive, less disfiguring and less nerve-racking than surgical biopsy. They are especially useful for small, nonpalpable (not felt by hand) abnormalities seen on mammograms. The procedures are quick and painless enough to be done in the doctor's office or imaging department, without anesthetic. Following a short rest, the woman can usually carry on with her daily activities after having the biopsy.

Newer biopsy methods include:
• *fine-needle aspiration or FNA*—a painless procedure that takes only a few minutes and is done in the doctor's office using a very fine needle to withdraw some cells from the suspicious area for examination. If the cells are found to be cancerous, there's no need for more biopsy sampling. The next step is surgery to remove the tumor and surround-

---

TIME YOUR MAMMOGRAMS RIGHT TO IMPROVE ACCURACY

A recent University of Toronto analysis of results from over 8,000 women who participated in the Canadian National Breast Screening Study (NBSS) showed that the rate of false negatives in menstruating women varies according to the phase of the menstrual cycle when the breasts are X-rayed. For healthy women who had ever used hormones (mainly birth control pills), there were fewer false-negative results when mammograms were done in the *follicular* (first) half rather than in the *luteal* (second) half of the menstrual cycle. Therefore, premenopausal women who need mammograms might improve their accuracy if— given the choice—they schedule them in the first half of the menstrual cycle. Their breasts are less swollen, less tender and more easily compressed, giving a clearer X-ray image. The precise reasons why there's less chance of false-negative mammograms in the first part of the cycle remain uncertain, but the difference may stem from the effects of hormone levels on the density of breast tissue and the clarity with which small changes show up.

---

ing margins. The type of surgery, its timing and follow-up can be jointly planned with the woman's medical advisors. However, FNA has several drawbacks: it often obtains too few cells for reliable analysis, its results are uncertain and if the needle penetrates a benign area around a cancerous nodule it may miss cancers later identified by surgical biopsy. Many clinicians therefore consider FNA unacceptable because of its high false-negative rate.

• *large-core biopsy*—done by radiologists—the latest and more reliable method. It uses imaging devices (X-rays or ultrasound) to guide the biopsy needle to the suspicious breast area, quickly and painlessly removing cores of tissue for analysis. Cores or plugs of tissue are taken from the target zone, using a large-bore needle or spring-loaded device (gun) under X-ray or ultrasound guidance, for histological (tissue) examination by a pathologist. Large-core biopsy overcomes most failings of FNA, providing enough tissue for accurate evaluation. After the procedure, the woman has a steristrip over the biopsy site, and perhaps an ice pack for a few minutes to stop bruising. Normal activities can often be resumed the same day (but no very strenuous activities for a week).

If the result is no cancer core biopsy has avoided the need for surgery; if the lump is cancerous, the woman and her caregivers

---

WARNING SIGNS OF BREAST CANCER

• A new lump or thickening felt in the breast;
• changed size, shape or contour of one breast or nipple;
• inversion (drawing in) of one nipple;
• nipple scaling (flakiness);
• skin *erythema* (redness), or ulceration;
• lump or swelling in the armpit;
• dimpling/puckering of breast skin;
• spontaneous bloody discharge from one nipple (rare).

plan subsequent surgery and other treatment. The next step is usually lumpectomy to remove the tumor and some axillary (underarm) nodes to test for malignant spread and to stage the cancer.

The advantages of core biopsy are that it's non-invasive, quick and painless, avoids the need for surgical biopsy, provides larger specimens than FNA—enough for a full histological workup by the pathologist and often enough to type and stage the cancer. The drawback is that core biopsy samples are still quite small, and if no cancer is found, surgical biopsy may still be needed.

Surgery for breast cancer

Previously, a woman with a suspicious breast lump or mammographic abnormalities was told that the area would be cut out and scanned for malignancy while she remained asleep on the operating table. If the lump was found to be cancerous, the whole breast would probably be removed. This one-step procedure meant that women would often be put under not knowing whether they'd awaken from the anesthetic with a small biopsy scar or with their entire breast gone. Nowadays things are different. The woman has the biopsy, awaits results and then decides together with her medical caregivers on the best treatment plan. The biopsy tissue sample is analyzed to stage the tumor and determine its features— whether it's aggressive (fast-growing and invasive) or less so, whether it is sensitive to hormones (has receptors for estrogen and/or progesterone) or other biochemical markers that predict the possibility of recurrence and spread. The tumor's stage and characteristics help determine the right treatment. Delaying treatment by a few days does not worsen the outcome, and women need time to think over and discuss treatment options.

If the biopsy reveals cancer further surgery may be needed to excise more tissue and remove the axillary (underarm) nodes to test them for malignancy.

Negative nodes are a good sign

Modern experts prefer to do the axillary removal as a separate procedure after sewing up the first incision, for a better cosmetic result. If the underarm nodes test negative, showing no signs of malignancy, the chances are good for long, disease-free survival. Statistics show about 85 percent of node-negative patients are alive and well five years after removal of a cancerous breast lump, and 70 percent are doing well 10 years later.

Sentinel node biopsy is a new method, less invasive and more precise, for cancer staging, sometimes replacing axillary dissections (which removes 4 to 30 lymph nodes for testing). In sentinel node biopsy (SNB), surgeons use a dye to locate and remove just the "primary" or sentinel lymph nodes draining the tumour.

A radioative tracer may be added to the dye to aid node-mapping. Removing just the sentinel nodes to check for cancer is less invasive, but it is a still-experimental tecnique that awaits results before being universally adopted.

Modern breast-cancer treatment choices

Modern breast-sparing operations are far less drastic than the traditional, radical or Halsted mastectomy, which removed the entire breast and a large section of underlying muscle, leaving the chest sunken and the arm possibly swollen and weakened. Today's cancer operations include:

• *extended simple or modified radical mastectomy*—removing the whole breast and some underarm lymph nodes, but no underlying muscle;

• *simple total mastectomy*—removing breast only (but no underarm nodes);

• *partial mastectomy or lumpectomy*—removing just the tumor and its surrounding margins; lumpectomy, with removal of underarm nodes, followed by postsurgical radiation, is now increasingly the norm.

The choice depends on the size and type of tumor the breast's shape and size, the stage of the cancer and its position in the breast.

Survival rates are the same for lumpectomy and mastectomy

Recent studies show no difference in survival times between total breast removal and lump removal only, for very early cancers. Lumpectomy is considered just as effective and is now

RECAPPING KNOWN RISK FACTORS FOR BREAST CANCER

Unmodifiable risk factors:

- being female and increasing age;
- family history: having two or more first-degree relatives (e.g., mother, sisters, grandmothers) who had early breast cancer (before age 45), especially in both breasts, approximately doubles the risk;
- carrying predisposing genes for hereditary breast cancer (BRCA1 or BRCA2), which increase susceptibility (also to ovarian cancer) giving a 56–83 percent chance of developing breast cancer by age 80 (compared to the average);
- ethnic origin—rates are high among North Americans and Europeans, and especially in Ashkenazi Jewish women
- having unusually dense breast tissue (as shown on a mammogram) or atypical hyperplasia (breast tissue overgrowth containing atypical cells);
- very early menarche (onset of menstruation before age 12) or late menopause (over age 55);
- already having had cancer in one breast.

Modifiable risk factors:

- having no children or bearing them late (after age 30);
- obesity (after menopause);
- eating a high-fat diet (although the precise diet-cancer link remains unclear);
- lack of vigorous physical activity (especially at a young age)—regular exercise may protect against breast cancer;
- long-term use of estrogen-containing birth control pills at a young age;
- long-term hormone replacement therapy (more than 5 to 10 years);
- moderate alcohol consumption (more than three to five drinks a day).

N.B.: Two-thirds of breast cancers occur in women with no identifiable risk factors. And the majority of breast cancers are not inherited but "sporadic"— arising randomly for a variety of reasons, both biological and environmental. But those in a high-risk category—for instance, with several close relatives who had early breast cancer— need extra careful surveillance starting about 10 years before the earliest age at which breast cancer was detected in the family. Surveillance includes annual mammograms, clinical breast examination every six months and monthly BSE.

---

increasingly replacing mastectomy, with radiation applied to the operated breast afterward to minimize local recurrences.

Postoperative drug (adjuvant) treatment, formerly reserved for advanced metastatic disease, is now routinely offered to all node-positive women with breast cancer and very often also to node-negative cases. The treatment suggested depends on the woman's age (whether she's pre- or postmenopausal), and on the stage and type of the cancer—for instance whether or not it has hormone receptors or other "markers."

After surgery, women are often referred for further advice to a medical oncologist (cancer specialist) and/or a radiation oncologist, or to a specialized cancer center. A thorough discussion determines the most suitable follow-up. Since treatment strategies vary from center to center women with breast cancer should seek advice from the most knowledgeable, up-to-date experts around, and above all from someone they trust. If not satisfied, get a second opinion.

The chief problem in breast cancer is not local recurrence but distant spread. That's why breast cancer is now regarded as a potentially systemic disease that can affect the whole body and must be treated accordingly. Since only systemic therapy can stop distant cancer cells from growing into tumors, postoperative drug therapy is now increasingly used. Many women with breast cancer can thus expect to get chemotherapy to kill distant cancer cells.

Although the diagnosis of breast cancer is a devastating experience, most women face up to it well and cope with it. In fact, studies show that many respond with renewed enjoyment of life and stronger interpersonal ties. There's an inevitable period of adjustment, but it's usually improved by knowing as much as possible about the disease. British studies have shown that the more accurate information women are given, in a supportive manner, the better they can face and adapt to this condition, and the better able they are to make acceptable decisions with which they can live. Women given sparse information in a curt, abrupt manner and who don't partake as much in the decision-making, are less able to deal with what happens than those given ample information.

Postoperative treatments: who needs what?

- *Radiation* is now usual in women who have lumpectomies, generally five days a week for three to five weeks. Each session lasts a few minutes, with an initial planning session to determine the suitable site and dose of radiation. There are few aftereffects of radiation apart from a little skin redness (like a sunburn) and possible fatigue toward the end of the course.

- *Chemotherapy* uses various cytotoxic (cancer-killing) agents in an attempt to eradicate cancer cells that have spread. Since anticancer drugs also affect not only nearby healthy tissue but also the whole body, side effects may include transient nausea, hair loss, insomnia, sexual disturbances, fatigue, a lowered white-blood-cell count and, understandably, anxiety. Newer drugs produce fewer side effects. Many women can go on working and exercising through their chemotherapy course.

- *Hormonal therapy* has been tried for many years to impede the growth of certain breast cancers. Strategies include removal of the ovaries, adrenals and/or pituitary glands, as well as administration of competitive anti-hormonal agents or anti-estrogens, such as LHRH (luteinizing-hormone-releasing hormones) analogues and anti-progestins (e.g., RU-486).

- *Tamoxifen*, a powerful synthetic anti-estrogen, is a mainstay of modern hormone therapy. It's well tolerated, with few side effects, and is increasingly used even for node-negative cases. Studies have convincingly shown that tamoxifen can improve disease-free and/or overall survival in postmenopausal women with hormone-sensitive tumors. Although its exact mechanism isn't clear tamoxifen seems to act as both a weak female hormone and an anti-estrogen, blocking the hormone's cancer-promoting effects. Trials with tamoxifen are also looking into its ability to prevent the development of breast cancer in those at high risk.

- *New "designer" anti-estrogens* coming onstream for treating breast cancer include the specific estrogen receptor modulators (SERMS), such as Raloxifene, with effects similar to tamoxifen but fewer undesirable side effects.

- *Aromatase inhibitors* such as anastrozole (Arimidex), letrozole (Femara) and exemestane (Aromasin) reduce estrogen production and work as well or slightly better than tamoxifen, with fewer side-effects.

- *New hormones for advanced breast cancer* include *toremifene* (Fareston), an antiestrogen with effects similar to Tamoxifen.

- *Genetically engineered drugs* such as trastuzumab (Herceptin) show promise for metastatic breast cancer in some women.

Support by family and friends is a key element in helping those with breast cancer the influence being strongest with support from friends, colleagues and health professionals. "Above all," advises one specialist, "women should ask many questions, select medical advisors they trust and be prepared to seek a second opinion, as therapy varies from place to place." If they remain uneasy even though preliminary tests—the physical exam and mammogram—suggest that a breast lump or abnormality is benign (non-cancerous), they should press for a biopsy to be sure.

Breast reconstruction

Breast reconstruction, using either a woman's own tissues or synthetic silicone implants, has become increasingly popular for life after mastectomy. Breast restoration can even be done many years after mastectomy. Any woman contemplating breast replacement should have a full, frank discussion about its merits, including a complete rundown of the techniques available, their failings and advantages, and should recognize that the results aren't predictable. While some surgeons do breast removal and reconstruction at the same time, others rebuild the breast after a delay of six months to two years following mastectomy. The interval allows the incision to heal well, gives time to complete any postoperative radiation or drug therapy and permits any local recurrences to be more easily detected. One plastic surgeon notes that in his experience, "After the recommended wait, about half the women contemplating breast reconstruction decide against it, having come to terms with their disease, gotten used to living without a breast, feeling good about themselves and unwilling to face more surgery. Many women learn to live happily with only one or half a breast, feeling quite at ease with a removable form worn under their clothing."

Women vary widely in their wish for breast reconstruction. Some, knowing the many drawbacks of postmastectomy implants (those still on the market!), refuse to buy in to the myth equating beauty with breasts. After weighing the odds, they decide against reconstruction. They may find that the brush with mortality clarifies their priorities, diminishes the importance of superficial appearances and heightens the awareness that a woman's attractiveness stems not so much from breasts as from innate qualities. However, other women urgently desire breast replacement. The loss of a breast may trigger feelings of being less than whole and of despair at having to wear a prosthesis—a depression known as the postmastectomy syndrome. Some women consider themselves less sexually attractive without an intact breast. For them, breast reconstruction reinstates their body image, immensely improving their lives.

One increasingly popular and successful restoration technique, which overcomes the many drawbacks of silicone implants, is the TRAM flap method, which uses the woman's own tissue to fashion a new breast from muscle and skin taken from the chest wall, buttocks or more usually, from the lower abdomen—by the "tummy tuck" or abdominal flap operation. A flap is removed from the abdominal wall (from the "roll" often seen when seated) and placed into the chest area, providing the skin, fat and muscle to model a new breast. A new nipple may later be created using tissue from the unoperated side (or other skin flaps) and tattoo dyes to get the right look. Very lean women, smokers and those with chronic lung or heart ailments aren't suitable candidates for this type of operation.

NEW GENETIC TESTS BRING CRITICAL CHOICES

Genetic or DNA tests can now identify people in cancer-prone families who are carrying mutations (alterations) in two recently discovered genes—BRCA1 and BRCA2—which predispose them to breast and other cancers. The genetic tests should allow people with these genes to watch for early signs of disease and perhaps treat it in time for cure, or take preventive steps. But the tests raise many practical, ethical, social and legal dilemmas. Knowing that you are carrying a gene predisposing you to breast cancer does not mean that there is an effective therapy for it, let alone a cure or way to prevent it.

A gene is a specific segment of DNA inside the cell's chromosomes. A mutation or change in the DNA may mean that the gene no longer functions properly, making things go wrong or cause disease. Until now, genetic tests looked mainly for genes that would definitely and inevitably produce heritable diseases—such as hemophilia, cystic fibrosis, Huntington disease and sickle cell anemia. Prenatal genetic testing for such diseases before birth allows the detection of fetal abnormalities at an early stage, giving parents the option of terminating the pregnancy—should they so wish—to avoid bearing a baby that's destined to become ill.

However, genetic testing for susceptibility to disease—checking for mutations (gene changes) that are likely but *not certain* to trigger disease later in life—is a matter that raises thorny issues and highly charged questions: Do people want to know they're carrying genes for a cancer that *might* (but won't definitely) develop years, perhaps decades, later? Do their sisters, brothers, children, nephews, nieces and cousins need to know they're also at risk?

Formal genetic counselling is recommended for any woman with a personal or family history that suggests hereditary breast cancer, in order to evaluate the likelihood of a BRCA mutation and to facilitate genetic testing, if appropriate. Pertinent family history may be either maternal or paternal, but should be on the same side of the family. If genetic testing is undertaken, it normally starts with the highest-risk *affected* individual in the family.

Factors that might persuade someone to consider genetic testing for breast cancer include:

- multiple cases of breast cancer (particularly if diagnosed under age 50) and/or ovarian, fallopian tube or peritoneal cancer in the family.
- breast cancer diagnosed under age 35.
- a family member with both breast and ovarian cancer.
- breast and/or ovarian cancer in Ashkenazy Jewish families.
- a family member with bilateral breast cancer—especially if diagnosed under age 50.

POSSIBLE WAYS TO REDUCE THE RISK OF DYING FROM BREAST CANCER

- **Report any visible changes in the size, contour or shape of the breast, any changes in the color or texture of the nipple(s), also any nipple discharge and any new skin dimpling promptly to a health professional.**
- **Have regular clinical breast exams by a qualified health professional, perhaps at a local breast screen-** ing or diagnostic center.
- **If over age 50, get regular mammograms.**
- **Learn BSE from a qualified expert and practice monthly if comfortable with it.**
- **Maintain normal body weight, eat a diet low in animal fats and limit alcohol intake to two drinks a day.**
- **Exercise regularly,** preferably starting before adolescence.
- **Breastfeed your babies—which may reduce risks if done for at least two cumulative years (and is good for the baby).**
- **Remember that, while having breast cancer may be bad, it's worse to have it unidentified and growing bigger without knowing about it.**

- a family member with serous ovarian cancer.
- male breast cancer in the family.
- known BRCA 1 or 2 mutations in the family.

If a mutation in BRCA1 or 2 is identified in someone, other relatives may decide to be tested. If the test is negative, then this person is considered to be at no greater risk of developing cancer than the general population. If no BRCA1 or 2 mutation is found in a family with several known cases of breast cancer, the genetic test could be giving a false negative result, as testing does not identify 100 percent of BRCA1 and 2 mutations. Or it may denote an as yet unidentifed gene, common environmental factors or chance as the reason(s) for beast cancer development.

The benefits and harms of screening for mutations in BRCA1 and 2 remain unclear, as the long-term outcomes of screening and risk-reducing strategies have not yet been determined. Nonetheless, the potential benefits of genetic tests include less aggressive treatment of cancer if it is found at an earlier stage and/or improved survival. Harms include increased anxiety and possible insurance implications (harder to obtain life or health insurance). Again, proper genetic counseling is key.

Those carrying the BRCA1 gene have a 56 to 83 percent chance of developing breast cancer by age 80—compared with the average woman's risk of one in nine if she lives to be 80 or more years old. Carrying the BRCA1 gene also confers a 21 percent chance of developing ovarian cancer by age 70. "But," warns one British geneticist, "remember that even those with the BRCA genes have a 15 percent chance of not getting breast cancer. Moreover, the BRCA1 gene is very large, with many different mutations along the length of its DNA, some weakly predisposing, others strongly predisposing to breast cancer so it's hard to work out any one person's risk." Men carrying the mutant BRCA2 gene have a six-times-higher-than-average chance of getting breast cancer (and greater risks of prostate and pancreatic cancers), and they can pass the genetic susceptibility on to their daughters and sons.

People carrying the BRCA mutations—either men or women—have a 50 percent chance of passing the altered gene to their offspring. But it's only an average risk, and in any one family, all, none or some of the children may inherit the BRCA gene. It's crucial to note that although people born with a faulty gene are at above-average risk, they will not inevitably develop cancer. It will only emerge if other environmental events or genetic "hits" occur during their lifetimes.

Difficult dilemmas for those at risk of genetic breast cancer

In trying to reduce the dangers, those who carry one or other of the BRCA mutations face tough decisions. They need expert genetic counseling and guidance to develop a personalized risk management plan. The problem is that people carrying a cancer-susceptibility gene *do not know* whether it's a weakly or strongly predisposing cancer gene, or whether they will ever develop the cancer. They could be among the 15 percent who won't get the heritable cancer or among the unlucky ones who will.

Genetic testing may be useful for people in highly cancer-prone families, but it has risks and costs. The chief advantages of having a genetic test for cancer susceptibility—even if the result is positive—are that it resolves some of the uncertainty and fear and it may encourage screening and preventive steps (although some of those who test positive deny the danger and stop all surveillance). Drawbacks are the acute anxiety while awaiting results, the chance of wrong (false) results and, if the result is positive, not knowing when and if the cancer will strike, with consequent anger and depression, worries about confidentiality and discrimination by employers and insurance agencies, concern about passing on the "bad" gene to children and strained family relationships. Even a negative test result, which usually elicits a sigh of relief, doesn't mean freedom from breast cancer as sporadic forms can still occur by chance or from environmental causes. Moreover, people who test negative may feel guilty about being spared the "family gene."

Possible "action" choices for women carrying breast cancer susceptibility genes

- Surveillance with a wait-and-see approach, which means six-monthly physical breast exams, doing monthly BSE (learned from a trained expert) and regular mammograms for early signs of the disease. To check for ovarian cancer women need regular transvaginal ultrasound tests and CA-125 blood tests.
- Taking drugs to prevent breast cancer from developing, for instance anti-estrogens such as tamoxifen or raloxifene. Ongoing trials are examining the effectiveness of these drugs in preventing breast cancer so far giving contradictory results. One U.S. trial found tamoxifen can help prevent breast cancer from developing in high-risk women; European studies suggest the drug does not prevent its development.
- Having prophylactic (preventive) bilateral mastectomy—surgical removal of both breasts, with or without breast reconstruction—which reduces but does not obliterate the risk, as cancer can still develop in the chest wall.
- Having oophorectomy (removal of both ovaries) to stop ovarian cancer from developing—also reduces but does not entirely eliminate the risk, because cancer could develop in the residual tissue.
- Taking birth control pills to reduce risks of ovarian cancer.
- Warning other (perhaps unsuspecting) family members that they too might be carrying the cancer-susceptibility gene—a highly charged decision that can cause great psychological distress and family conflict.

One woman from a BRCA1 family says she'd "rather have both breasts off and ovaries out before than after they develop cancer." But even this drastic step isn't foolproof, as noted above. "Having surgery to remove both breasts and ovaries could be overreaction," explains one British geneticist, "especially for those with a *weakly predisposing* version of the BRCA gene."

Men's special health concerns

Trouble with the prostate • Prostate cancer • Infertility • Vasectomy • Remedying sex problems • The circumcision controversy • Male breast cancer

9

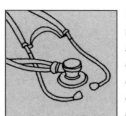

FOREMOST AMONG men's health problems are cardiovascular diseases and cancers—lung cancer is the number-one killer, prostate cancer next. Men are often less informed about health issues than women, less willing to voice their health concerns. Yet early recognition of problems and open discussion of them with health professionals are essential for prompt and effective treatment. Few people are aware that prostate cancer is as common for men as breast cancer for women, affecting 1 in 10 men over 65, and up to 40 percent of the 80-plus group, causing over 4,000 deaths a year in Canada. Following the example of the women's breast cancer movement, men are now beginning to catch up on prostate cancer awareness, forming support groups and fund-raising organizations.

TROUBLE WITH THE PROSTATE

Of men's health concerns, prostate troubles are among the least known but most common. Yet most men may hardly know where their prostate is, remaining barely aware of its presence until it becomes painfully inflamed or enlarged, and obstructs urination or causes other problems.

Found only in males, the prostate gland is a walnut-sized organ situated like a collar under the bladder directly above the scrotum. The gland surrounds the urethra—the tube that carries urine from the bladder out of the body. It can be beset by three disorders: prostatitis—inflammation and/or infection; prostatic hyperplasia—overgrowth or enlargement; and cancer. The chief known function of the human prostate is its contribution to seminal fluid; it produces enzymes that help to liquefy semen and keep sperm moist, mobile and healthy. It also secretes antibacterials such as zinc spermine and spermidine, which give seminal fluid its characteristic odor.

Prostatitis

Often of unknown origin, prostatitis (prostate inflammation) affects about 50 percent of men at least once in a lifetime. It can occur at any age, but usually afflicts men aged 19 to 40. Myths about prostatitis abound. The condition was once blamed on celibacy and dubbed the "priest's disease." Sexual activity was, and often still is, falsely viewed as an antidote that "prevents semen from stagnating." In fact, the disorder strikes sexually active and inactive men alike. While scientific proof is lacking, prostate inflammation has also been linked to prolonged inactivity, long periods of sitting and too much alcohol and coffee.

Prostatitis is typically acute or chronic with the latter often being divided into two sub-categories: chronic bacterial and chronic prostatitis/chronic pelvic pain syndrome. Although prostatitis is occasionally due to a bacterial infection, the majority of cases are non-bacterial (sterile) inflammations with no traceable cause, making the condition hard to treat. Diagnosis involves analysis and culture of a mid-stream urine sample containing some semen (obtained by stroking or massaging the prostate via the rectum to release some into the bladder).

Men with nonbacterial prostatitis have vague discomfort in the groin, ejaculatory pain, erectile problems and perhaps abdominal pain and backache. Complaints are often voiced as "a pain down there" or "crotch ache." Sufferers report burning on urination, a need to urinate often—especially at night—and occasionally a discharge. (The discharge frequently sends men to see their physician.) On examination, the prostate may be slightly sore. Although there's no identifiable infection, men with this ailment are understandably worried about their potency, sex life and fertility. The trouble is that

nonbacterial prostatitis may linger on for long periods. Some experts suggest this is because of low zinc levels, but zinc supplements do not alleviate the condition. Although laboratory tests and cystoscopy (looking into the bladder with an instrument put through the penis) find no infective source, some men may be "silent" carriers of chlamydia, yeasts or other undetected infections (for more information on these, see Chapter 7). Others may have mechanical bladder dysfunction, perhaps a reflux of seminal fluid back into the prostate. Some may have "psychogenic" prostatitis caused by stress, anxiety or depression.

For the acute bacterial prostatitis, antibiotics are prescribed. Men typically need to take them for 4 to 6 weeks as the prostate is difficult to penetrate. Chronic bacterial infections, which typically happen more in elderly men and may present as recurrent urinary tract infections,

MALE REPRODUCTIVE ORGANS

The urethra, a single tube running from the bladder through the penis, conveys both urine and semen out of the body, but not at the same time! When semen is ejaculated, the muscles surrounding the bladder contract and close off its opening so that urine cannot escape during intercourse (or masturbation).

The testes inside the testicles produce sperm, but it takes time for the sperm to mature through several complex processes. Mature sperm gather in the epididymis (tubes located behind the testicles in the scrotum that are amazingly long, about 6 m [20 ft] in length each, but twisted into a small area). Sperm cells take several weeks to work their way through the epididymis, traveling into the vas deferens—one for each testicle—and from there to the seminal vesicles for storage. Small ejaculatory ducts, running through the prostate gland into the urethra, carry sperm out of the body during ejaculation.

The prostate gland surrounds the urethra and produces some seminal fluid.

The paired, sac-like seminal vesicles behind the prostate produce 70 percent of the seminal fluid or semen, which contains sugars that supply the energy that allows sperm to swim through the female reproductive tract. Both the seminal vesicles and the prostate gland continuously secrete fluid into the ejaculatory duct, but more is produced during intercourse. Scientists believe that semen contains other chemicals that help sperm swim vigorously.

Cowper's glands, a pair of pea-sized glands at the base of the penis, secrete some clear, alkaline fluid into the urethra during sexual arousal to neutralize the acidic environment of the female genital tract, which can harm sperm. (Even without vaginal penetration, secretions from Cowper's glands may leak from a partially erect penis, carrying enough sperm to cause pregnancy if the secretions touch the vagina or moist vulva.)

DIFFEREN-TIATING NON-BACTERIAL FROM BACTERIAL PROSTATITIS

• **Nonbacterial (sterile) prostatitis is without any traceable infective agent; it's more a nuisance than a noticeable illness;**
• **acute bacterial prostatitis is a rare, feverish, flu-like infection, causing an acutely tender prostate.**

receive the same treatment but for longer periods of time (4–6 months). Chronic prostatitis/chronic pelvic pain syndrome is the most common but least understood form of prostatitis. It is found in men of any age, its symptoms come and go, and it may be inflammatory or non-inflammatory. Chronic pain in the perineum (the space between the testes and rectum), scrotum, penis, pelvis or lower back is often associated with urinary urgency, urinating at night, weak stream, dribbling, dysuria, sexual dysfunction such as painful ejaculations, post-ejaculatory pain and blood in the sperm. The prostate may or may not be tender. Treatments that are often tried include antibiotics, nonsteroidal anti-inflammatory drugs, diazepam, hot sitz baths, avoidance of spicy foods or excessive alcohol, and even transurethral microwave thermotherapy. Such a smorgasbord of therapeutic recommendations is clear evidence that no treatment has been shown to be particularly effective. Having said this, a 2003 trial using terazosin (Hytrin) showed significant improvement at 14 weeks.

Prostate enlargement is very common with aging

Prostate growth depends on male hormones, mainly testosterone. When testosterone levels are low, during childhood, a boy's prostate remains small—a weight of about 1 gram (0.04 oz). But with the increased release of testosterone at puberty, the prostate gland enlarges. By age 20 it normally weighs about 15 grams (0.53 oz), staying that size until middle age. After age 45 to 50, the prostate often undergoes a growth spurt and swells to three times its previous size—sometimes even becoming lemon-sized. By age 50, almost 20 percent of men have an expanded prostate; by age 70 the figure is 50 percent, and by age 80 enlargement is almost universal.

Since the urethra, which drains the bladder, runs through the prostate, a bulky, enlarged or inflamed prostate can obstruct urination. And if the bladder does not empty completely, it means that men have to urinate more frequently, which is especially noticeable at night. Rarely, the trapped urine may remain in the bladder creating a stagnant buildup that predisposes the bladder to infection and may lead to incontinence. If the prostate really inhibits outflow it may affect the kidneys, producing temporary malfunction and, in extreme cases, renal (kidney) failure. Occasionally, complete obstruction halts all urination. Known as acute retention, this is a painful emergency situation that requires immediate hospital attention and catheterization (removal of urine with a tube). Prostate expansion can also cause cystitis (bladder infection), requiring antibiotic treatment matched to the bacteria responsible.

Prostate enlargement is detected by a digital (finger) rectal examination, X-rays, ultrasound and blood and urine tests. If no difficulties occur the condition may be left untreated, but still carefully monitored for obstruction, cancer or urinary backflow. The enlargement can wax and wane. Interestingly, the signs of Benign Prostate Hyperplasia (BPH),—such as peeing too often, dribbling, retention—are often found with small as well as large prostates, indicating that some prostates grow (enlarge) inward, pressing on the urethral tube.

Modern methods to shrink enlarged prostates

Until recently, surgery was the only known way to relieve problems due to an enlarged prostate. The standard treatment for prostatic enlargement used to be simple: cut away the excess tissue. Although prostate surgery remains a leading operation among older men, an array of alternative treatments is now available to shrink the prostate, including radiation, drugs, balloons and even microwaves.

If surgery is needed, it can now often be done through the urethra itself by transurethral prostatectomy (TURP)—a method that removes the obstruction but not the entire gland. This surgery is not trivial, although it is usually quick and carries no undue risks. A thin tube with a telescopic viewer is passed through the urethra to the prostate and a cauterizer (attachment for burning tissue) removes pieces of the obtruding prostate. This procedure, now employed for over 90 percent of enlarged prostates, spares men the trauma of a full surgical incision, allowing swift recovery. A desk-worker may be back at the job within a week.

However, there are some drawbacks to

TURP—namely, postoperative infection, erectile failure (in about 5 to 10 percent of men operated on) and sterility, a frequent postoperative complication. Another postoperative complication is incontinence, in 1 percent of cases. While prostate reduction or removal often makes men sterile, it need not make them impotent, since the nerves that regulate erections can remain untouched. Potency generally returns within a few weeks or months.

Oral medications to shrink enlarged prostates are increasingly used instead of (or alongside) surgical prostate reduction. Such drugs are preferable whenever possible, as they avoid surgical complications such as erectile dysfunction, incontinence and retrograde ejaculation. Two classes of prostate-shrinking medication are hormone-suppressors such as finasteride (Proscar), which blocks the stimulatory action of testosterone on prostate growth, and the newer "alpha blockers" such as terazosin (Hytrin), doxazosin (Cardura) and tamsulosin (Flomax), which relieve symptoms by relaxing smooth muscle in the prostate and bladder. Tamsulosin just relaxes the bladder, whereas terazosin and doxasozin also relax the blood pressure system. Possible side effects of Proscar include erectile and ejaculation problems, but on the plus side it may stimulate hair regrowth. Possible side effects of Hytrin, Cardura, and Flomax are minimal, but Hytrin and Cardura may cause transient dizziness or fatigue. Proscar takes longer to work and is therefore often used as second-line treatment in combination with one of the alpha blockers, especially in men with large prostates.

PROSTATE CANCER

Prostate cancer, arising in the outer portion of the prostate gland, is stimulated by the male hormone, testosterone, and affects 8 to 10 percent of North American men. The current lifetime risk of prostate cancer is 12 to 16.7 percent, and 20 to 25 percent of men with prostate cancer die of the disease. The incidence of prostate cancer has been increasing since the 1970's—perhaps because of more common and easier diagnosis via PSA screening and incidental discovery of cancer following TURP surgery for enlarged prostates. It is now the second leading cause of cancer deaths in men (after lung cancer). About 200,000 American and 20,000 Canadian men are diagnosed with it each year, leading to fatalities in about one-fifth of cases—mainly in those over 70. The number appears to be rising because of an aging population and a decrease in deaths from heart disease and stroke—allowing men to live longer and develop this cancer. Also, new tests, such as the PSA (prostate-specific antigen) test are detecting it at earlier, symptomless stages.

The good news is that prostate cancer is usually a slow-growing, non-aggressive cancer. Autopsies of men who died of other causes reveal the presence of prostate cancer in 20 percent of 50-year-olds, half of those over age 70, and in 90 percent of men over 90. Only about 8 percent have an aggressive prostate cancer with a rapid downhill course that leads to death within a few years. In other words, men are likelier to die *with* prostate cancer than of it.

The causes of prostate cancer remain unknown, but there may be a genetic component—risks increase for those with close male relatives who had prostate cancer (doubled if one close family member had it, and 10 times higher if two close relatives suffered from it). Its incidence is especially high among black Americans and low among Chinese men—for reasons unknown. Diet is thought to play a part; a high consumption of animal fats is a suspected cause, while high-fiber diets (rich in green vegetables and cereals) lower risks. Sexually transmitted viruses may increase risks.

THE ALERTING SIGNS OF PROSTATE ENLARGEMENT

- **Urgency (an urgent, intense need to urinate);**
- **increased frequency (need to urinate often);**
- **nocturia—a need to urinate at night;**
- **a weak, sluggish urine stream;**
- **difficulty in getting urination started;**

- **"stuttering"—a dribble of urine that starts and stops;**
- **residual leakage and/or dribbling;**
- **reduced ability to hold urine (incontinence);**
- **buildup of urine in the bladder, which may harbor bacteria;**

- **cystitis (bladder infection);**
- **acute urinary retention (if urethra is completely blocked);**
- **formation of calcium stones in the bladder;**
- **kidney problems due to the backup of urine, with possible renal (kidney) damage.**

WARNING SIGNS OF PROSTATE CANCER

- **Frequent, difficult or painful urination;**
- **dribbling urine;**
- **blood or pus in the urine;**
- **pain in the lower back, pelvic area or upper thighs;**
- **painful ejaculation;**
- **bone pain (in advanced cases).**

The numbers for PSA tests: On average, if we take 100 men between the ages of 50 and 70 and give them the PSA test approximately 90 will have a normal result; of these 90, 2 will actually have prostate cancer. Of the 100, 10 will have a high result and will go on to further testing, 7 will be fine (cancer-free) and 3 will have prostate cancer.

Prostate cancer often gives no sign of its presence

Prostate cancer varies greatly in its aggressivity, producing no symptoms in its early stages. Any symptoms that do appear mimic those of benign prostate hyperplasia (enlargement): trouble urinating, perhaps some blood in the urine. Quite often prostate cancer has spread to the lymph nodes, bones or other areas by the time it's found, and bone pain, typically in the back or legs, may be its first alerting sign.

The cancer is often discovered incidentally by a physician during a routine rectal exam—felt as a hard nodule—or in the analysis of tissue from an enlarged prostate. The digital (finger) rectal exam is not a good detection tool for prostate cancer with only a 50 percent accuracy rate.

Other tests include transrectal ultrasound, which shows up irregularities or tumors in the prostate gland, but it's a tricky and expensive test likely to produce "false positive" results—showing cancer where none exists. Its accuracy is unusually dependent on the skill of the person doing the test.

The PSA test measures blood levels of prostate-specific antigen, a protein "marker" that's often (but not always) elevated in men with prostate cancer. The cutoff value for further investigation after finding an elevated PSA is controversial. A common PSA threshold denoting the suitability of follow-up is 4 mg/ml; however, values ranging from 3.0 to 10 mg/ml have been proposed. Trans-rectal ultrasound (TRUS) with biopsy is recommended for men with a PSA reading of 4.0 or greater. Despite the increasing use of this test for screening, evidence of its effectiveness in reducing mortality is still lacking. We will likely know the answer once the results of two large, well–designed, randomized controlled trials become available in 2005 to 2008 (the Prostate, Lung, Colon and Ovary Screening trial, and the European Randomized Study of Screening for Prostate Cancer). Meanwhile, the best approach is to inform yourself about the all the pros and cons of the PSA test and make a decision based on what you find out.

The chief "pro" in favor of PSA testing is that many experts believe that early detection will improve outcomes. As mentioned above, the aggression of prostate cancers is highly variable, the majority being slow-growing. Nonetheless, supporters of the PSA test point out that while this might translate into minimal impact when we look at large cohorts of males, the individual man might prefer to make sure he is not not in the more aggressive prostate cancer group. The key "con" is that the test has a high false-positive rate, meaning that, although no cancer exists, the test result comes back high, creating needless anxiety and leading to more testing (e.g., trans-rectal biopsies, which are uncomfortable) that ultimately shows there's nothing to worry about. As well, many of the cancers removed because of a high PSA may well have been harmless. For example, one trial that randomized men over 70 with prostate cancer to surgery or no surgery, found that there was no difference in lifespan between the two groups. However, this study did find that the men who underwent surgery had a worse quality of life following the operation (more incontinence and erectile dysfunction).

Ultimately then, the PSA test detects most prostate cancers but has a high false-positive rate, so is not reliable for diagnosis or screening. Nor does it predict which cancers will develop quickly. At present, this test is not recommended for universal screening in Canada, but is considered useful for men with identified prostate cancer. Causes of elevated PSA other than prostate cancer can include benign prostatic hyperplasia, prostatitis, urinary retention, cystoscopy and prostate surgery. PSA testing should be deferred for 2 months after resolution of reversible conditions. Drugs such as finasteride (Proscar) decrease PSA levels; so PSA readings should be multiplied by 2 for men on this drug. A variety of methods for increasing the specificity of PSA determination are under active investigation. These include PSA velocity, which is a measurement of the rate of change of PSA over time, age-specific PSA ranges, and PSA density, which correlates prostatic gland volume as determined by ultrasound with PSA levels. So, what seems quite simple, is actually quite complicated. There is no right answer as yet about the validity of PSA tests, and each man's own value system must guide him in deciding whether to take the test. If you do decide to undergo the test, it's crucial to know what you are getting into, so that if the test comes back "positive" or "high," you can keep that result in perspective.

Needle biopsy is the "gold standard" for confirming prostate cancer. A core of cells is taken from the suspicious area via the rectum or urethra to be examined under the microscope. Biopsy is simplified by new techniques such as fine-needle aspiration and transrectal removal of tissue (via the rectum).

Treatment—it's usually up to the man to decide

If prostate cancer is diagnosed, there are a number of treatment choices, none of them curative. Therapy is geared to the man's age, overall health and stage of the cancer—whether it's confined to the prostate (stages A and B) or likely to have spread. Finding the right therapy remains a problem as even under the best of circumstances, the treatments can have serious side effects, most notably urinary incontinence and impotence.

Removing the prostate surgically or irradiating it to destroy the cancer cells can cause unpleasant consequences, and neither method necessarily halts cancer growth. Erectile function is impaired in about 80 percent of men and urinary incontinence is found in 21 percent after surgery (versus 45 percent and 21 percent respectively with just "watchful waiting"). Men must weigh the likelihood of cure or prolonged survival time versus the probable side effects of the various treatments and their impact on quality of life. The decision must be taken in partnership with loved ones and a trusted healthcare team.

The standard treatment options for patients with clinically localized prostate cancer (no metastases or spread beyond the capsule) include radical prostatectomy, external beam radiation therapy, brachytherapy (in which seeds with radioactive material are implanted in the prostate) and watchful waiting. More advanced prostate cancer requires "androgen ablation" in which the testosterone in the body is drastically reduced surgically or chemically.

The overall options are:

- "Watchful waiting"—doing nothing while keeping tabs on the cancer's progress—and checking for signs of spread every few months. This is often preferred for prostate cancer that's likely to remain dormant, allowing men to continue living healthy lives. (Signs of spread may include a rising PSA level, a change in urinary habits, excessive fatigue or bone pain.) The crucial question is: Which men with prostate cancer can afford the wait-and-see approach? So far there's no answer although common sense, a careful assessment of the likely survival time gained by treatment and computer models can help profile those with nothing to lose by watchful waiting. Watchful waiting may suit older men (over age 70) with a localized cancer (no spread beyond the prostate) to avoid the distress and possible complications of surgery or radiation.

- Total prostatectomy—surgical removal of the entire prostate and seminal vesicles—may be suggested for tumors limited to the prostate, providing no cancer cells have escaped the capsule and the man is not too old, too sick or too frail to tolerate surgery. The operation carries risks—a 1 percent mortality rate, a 7 percent risk of incontinence (inability to control urination), a 25 percent risk of partial incontinence, a 10 percent chance of damage to the intestines and a 30 percent risk of impotence. Modern techniques may avoid postoperative impotence by saving the nerve that controls erection. And if the cancer is caught early, survival rates are good.

- Radiation therapy may include:

- external beam X-rays directed to the affected site, done daily for about 6 weeks (side effects may include diarrhea and digestive upsets);

- interstitial radiation from radioactive implants put right into the tumor and left there for a year (with high complication rates);

- a recently developed method of "focal radiation," using tiny gold implants in the prostate to guide the radiation beam right to the tumor, done daily for 8 weeks, with low complication rates (side effects may include diarrhea and digestive upsets).

- Hormone treatments may be used in combination with radiation or surgery, or on their own, to suppress the prostate-stimulating effects of testosterone, producing "medical castration." The formerly used female

BLOOD SUPPLY TO THE PENIS

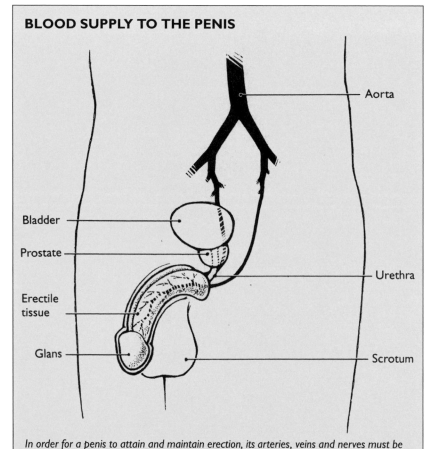

In order for a penis to attain and maintain erection, its arteries, veins and nerves must be in good working order and able to engorge the penis with blood. Psychoerotic or physical stimulation acting on the brain will increase blood flow in the penis, making its spongy (corporal) tissues fill with blood and expand into an erection.

the testes by a process not yet fully understood, although it's known that sperm take about 6 weeks to mature fully. Sperm maturation is controlled by hormones from the brain's *hypothalamus* and pituitary gland (similar to ovulation control in women) and by testicular secretions and the male hormone testosterone. Pituitary FSH (follicle-stimulating hormone) stimulates sperm formation while ICSH (interstitial-cell-stimulating hormone) promotes testosterone production—vital to sperm health, male potency and successful ejaculation.

The path from penis to Fallopian tube is a perilous one for sperm, and millions of sperm per ejaculate (average volume—3 to 5 ml, or less than a teaspoon) are required to achieve fertilization, because so many perish *en route*. They must traverse the vagina—inhospitable because it's acidic, and sperm prefer an alkaline environment—and then go from the vagina through the cervix and uterus and up to the Fallopian tube, where the egg is on its way down the tube to the uterus. Conception can take place in the tubes or in the uterus, but generally occurs in the lower part of the Fallopian tube or just inside the uterus. Only one sperm will usually pierce and fertilize the egg.

The main causes of infertility in men
Other than anatomical abnormalities, the main causes of infertility in men are insufficient or poor quality sperm. Sperm counts vary from 60 to 300 million sperm per ejaculate. (Sperm banks require a minimum sperm count of 100 million sperm per ml [about one-quarter teaspoon], but that is because the freezing process destroys some.) A sperm count below 20 million per ml is considered unlikely to achieve fertilization. But even though they have too low a sperm count to count as "fertile," there are isolated cases on record of men with only 2 to 5 million sperm per ejaculate siring babies.

A low sperm count or sperm of inferior quality may arise because of problems in the testes. If excretory ducts are blocked, damaged or absent there may be plenty of sperm, but they may not be delivered to the woman's vagina. Sometimes the problem is premature ejaculation. All too often the roots of male infertility remain a mystery.

hormones have been replaced by synthetic anti-androgens with less drastic side effects. These include LHRH analogues such as goserelin (Zoladex) given by injection every month or every 3 months. Zoladex has few side effects other than a diminished sex drive, but it attacks only androgen-dependent tumors.

• Orchidectomy, or surgical castration, involves removal of the testes (the main source of testosterone)—occasionally used, but considered psychologically traumatic.

The choice remains agonizingly personal for each man diagnosed with this disease. Support groups are springing up across the continent to provide encouragement and coping skills for men living with prostate cancer.

INFERTILITY
Spermatogenesis (sperm production) occurs in

Various factors may aggravate male infertility:

- excess alcohol consumption;
- post-pubertal mumps (if there is orchitis—painful testicular inflammation);
- undescended testes;
- overheating of the genitals due to tight clothing, long spells of sitting, too many saunas or hot baths (a cool temperature favors sperm survival);
- drugs that diminish sperm count, such as antihypertensives (blood pressure drugs) or marijuana (which reduces sperm quality).

VASECTOMY: PROS AND CONS

Sterilization—vasectomy for men or tubal ligation for women—is today's most popular contraceptive method for those who don't want more children. Since the operation is simpler and safer for men, it is often the male partners who go for sterilization. In North America, over 15 percent of men over age 40 have had a vasectomy. Although it is possible, reversal means major surgery. Success rates can be more than 75 percent, but depend on time since vasectomy was done and individual factors. Therefore, men going for vasectomy should consider it final and realize they'll be infertile afterward.

Candidates are healthy, sexually well-adjusted males over 35 who have fathered at least one child and are in stable relationships. Vasectomy is *not* advised for men who have STDs or undiagnosed bleeding disorders, nor for those who are emotionally unstable or in rocky sexual relationships.

The surgical procedure in vasectomy is simple—it blocks the sperm-carrying tubes, thereby excluding sperm from the male ejaculate. The sperm-carrying tubes are surgically cut and the ends closed. The skin is frozen on the testes and the vas deferens (the tube that carries the sperm) is closed off on each side (with a clip, by sewing or by being cauterized). Afterward, the sperm—which are still produced—are broken down and destroyed by normal bodily processes. After a while the body stops producing sperm. Done under local anesthetic in a physician's office, hospital or clinic, the surgery takes 10 to 20 minutes and requires only a small cut in the scrotum (often with no stitches). There may be some post-operative pain and bruising at the surgical site, reduced by applying ice packs and wearing tight, supportive underwear or a jockstrap for a week or two. Most men are back at work within a few days. Sexual activity can be resumed once the discomfort fades. Since sperm may linger for weeks in the "nozzle" end of the vas, pregnancy may easily result from unprotected intercourse during the immediate post-vasectomy weeks.

Four to 16 weeks are required for sperm to be fully "cleaned out of the pipes" beyond the spot where the surgery occurred. Depending on the number of post-vasectomy ejaculations, sperm are usually cleared from the reproductive tract after about 20 ejaculations. Men should use contraception for at least *3 months*, until semen tests show the ejaculate is entirely sperm-free. This is confirmed by a semen sample and is a critical step before returning to unprotected sex. Vasectomy failures can also occur for technical reasons, and the operation may need to be redone, especially if the cut ends of the vas spontaneously rejoin or "recanalize" while healing.

REMEDYING SEX PROBLEMS

Sexual dysfunction in men may involve transient or recurrent problems with the desire, arousal, erectile or orgasmic phase of the human sexual response. Sex problems can be occasional or long term, depending on their origins. While many sex disorders in men may start with an organic cause, most also have psychological dimensions. An array of new drugs and devices, together with counseling, can often overcome sexual difficulties.

Tests for erectile capacity

For men who can't achieve or keep an erection, the first priority is a complete medical exam and tests to rule out hormone deficiencies, treatable diseases, alcoholism or the influence of medications. In trying to distinguish organic from psychological reasons, physicians also do a psychological work-up insofar as is possible. They ask whether the erectile difficulty came on suddenly (suggesting psychological factors) or gradually (suggesting physical reasons), whether it is always a problem or only sometimes, whether it occurs with masturbation too, only during waking hours or also at night. Specialized tests can determine

NO REDUCTION IN POTENCY OR SEXUAL PLEASURE AFTER VASECTOMY

Vasectomy is *not*—as some men think—castration, nor does it alter the ability to have an erection or enjoy sex. Physiologically, the only difference is that before vasectomy a man's ejaculate contains sperm, and afterward it does not. Sperm accounts for less than 2 percent of semen. The procedure has no effect on hormones (testosterone levels stay the same) and it does not alter arousal, pleasure or the amount of fluid ejaculated. A vasectomy reduces fertility not virility.

whether or not a man is capable of having an erection. (If he can get an erection when intercourse is not the purpose, the problem is likely psychological.) With the advent of new medications for erectile dysfunction, many of these tests are now less frequently done.

- *Early morning erections.* It is not uncommon for men to have erectile problems during sex but be able to have erections at other times. This is reassuring as it shows the mechanics are working.
- *The nocturnal penile tumescence* test is a recent

SOME SEXUAL DISORDERS IN MEN

- **Sex problems in the desire stage** mean an inability to become sexually interested in a partner, sometimes because busy, overscheduled men don't have the time or occasion to relax and enjoy sex. Sex aversion—an extreme form of sexual disinterest—may involve fear of any sexual intimacy, usually with deep-seated psychological origins, often requiring intensive psychotherapy.
- **Sexual dysfunction in the arousal or excitement phase** is the inability to become aroused, perhaps because of negative parental attitudes to sex, an unpleasant early sexual experience, sex abuse, an off-putting relationship, misinformation or performance pressure. Sex therapy is usually the solution.
- **Dyspareunia**—genital pain before, during and/or after intercourse—may be due to penile vascular problems or a tight foreskin that won't retract during intercourse. It can also arise for psychological reasons. The problem needs medical attention and is often easily remediable.
- **Early or premature ejaculation**, afflicting 30 percent of men at some time or other, is an orgasmic disorder where men ejaculate sooner than they wish to. It arises from inadequate control over the precise timing of ejaculation and the responses that trigger it, or because of infrequent ejaculation—if the man hasn't had sex for a while. One sex therapist explains that it often happens if men "lose touch" with their orgasmic sensations: "Timing ejaculation at will is a learned art and takes practice." The disorder is often remedied by more frequent ejaculation (whether by intercourse or masturbation) and appropriate individual or couple therapy. A side effect of some antidepressants (Serotonin Specific Reuptake Inhibitors or SSRIs) is delayed orgasm and these drugs are occasionally prescribed for men who experience premature ejaculation.
- **Inhibited male orgasm** (IMO) is the inability to achieve orgasm during intercourse. Men with IMO often manage to ejaculate and reach orgasm by masturbation but not with vaginal intercourse. Some therapists believe IMO stems from fear of intercourse, an unwillingness to perform on demand or anxiety about not satisfying a partner. A man may

find his orgasm inhibited because he fears loss of control during intercourse, because he's put off by a woman's touch or, in some instances, because he does not want to have sex with one particular woman. This type of sexual dysfunction is more difficult to treat than premature ejaculation, often requiring intensive psychotherapy.

- **Erectile dysfunction**—previously called impotence—is defined as the "inability or waning ability to achieve and sustain an erection for the purpose of sexual intercourse," and afflicts many men at some time or other. (The term "impotence" has now been dropped because of its pejorative connotations.) Accurate statistics on male erectile troubles are elusive. One study reports that as many as 16 percent (another says 34 percent) of healthy young men in their prime have occasional erectile failure. Manufacturing companies who supply erectile devices estimate that 1 in 10 men has erectile difficulties at some point. An array of new drugs, devices and surgical procedures can now help to overcome the problem of achieving an erection.

Once thought to be "all in the head" or, as Sigmund Freud put it, of "psychic origin," erectile dysfunction is no longer considered to be purely psychological. But while organic reasons underlie some types of erectile dysfunction, the problem usually also has psychological overtones. In older men, well over half of the erectile difficulties experienced have contributory physical causes—such as diabetes, atherosclerosis, hormone imbalance, smoking, alcohol consumption, obesity or the use of certain medications (particularly blood-pressure pills). But since sexuality is complex, erectile competence too is complicated. Failure to achieve erection because of a physical cause is often worsened by anxiety. Sometimes what starts out as a sporadic organic dysfunction develops into a psychological hang-up owing to performance fears, and may tip the scales into non-erection. For example, a man with atherosclerotic buildup ("hardening") in his penile arteries may experience occasional erectile failure, which in turn leads to anxiety about nonperformance, exacerbating the problem.

REASONS FOR ERECTILE FAILURE

Physical or organic reasons:

- medical disorders such as kidney impairment, liver cirrhosis, prostate disorders, alcoholism, Peyronie's disease (curvature of the penis), Parkinson's disease, multiple sclerosis and diabetes (many young diabetics experience erectile problems);
- endocrine (hormonal) imbalances such as low testosterone output, thyroid disorders, hyperprolactinemia (excess prolactin hormone), Cushing's syndrome and other adrenal-gland disorders;
- neurological problems such as spinal-cord injury;
- surgery for the prostate gland, bladder or rectum, which may damage the nerves responsible for erection;
- blood vessel disorders that restrict penile blood flow, such as artery-narrowing due to atherosclerosis, or veins that don't clamp off properly to maintain erection (penile veins that don't close off allow blood to drain out and cause penile collapse—a condition sometimes reparable by surgery);
- smoking tobacco—a major reason for erectile failure—because nicotine causes spasms in small penile arteries and also leads to atherosclerosis;
- alcohol—another major cause—because it affects blood flow and acts on brain centers with effects that impede the ability to hold an erection. In addition, alcohol has a "feminizing" effect on the male hormone system so that long-term use may destroy erectile capacity. Heavy drinking lowers testosterone levels, diminishes male sex drive and effectively "castrates" men, causing erectile dysfunction. Alcohol also triggers conversion of androgens (male sex hormones) to estrogens (female sex hormones), sometimes causing hair loss and breast enlargement. Excess alcohol may eventually cause atrophy (shrinkage) of the testes and impair the mechanism that shunts blood into the penis;
- a long list of medications including antihistamines, antipsychotics, antidepressants, marijuana, minor tranquilizers, anticancer drugs, cimetidine (a stomach-ulcer drug), muscle relaxants and especially antihypertensives (blood-pressure medications). As many as 40 percent of men on diuretics and other blood-pressure pills have erectile problems. They should consult their family physician; perhaps other drugs can be prescribed instead. Switching the medication often reverses the problem.

Psychological reasons:

- depression, anger, stress, fatigue, guilt, performance anxiety, job loss or impending exams;
- childhood experiences of parental conflict, sex abuse or disapproving, unjoyful attitudes to sex;
- a negative sex encounter that leaves a man full of self-doubts even though he may be perfectly capable of attaining an erection; feelings of inadequacy may make him hesitate to attempt intercourse. The longer such anxiety lingers, the greater the chance of a persistent sex problem;
- lack of privacy (at home or in student quarters);
- poor communication with a partner, lack of intimacy, fear of causing pregnancy, divergent views on what constitutes a happy sex life and varying perceptions of "normality."

---

innovation that avoids the need for hospital investigation. It tests the occurrence and frequency of nighttime erections. Most men normally have several erections nightly, related to different sleep stages. The nocturnal penile tumescence test simply consists of wrapping a bit of tape with small string binders around the penis while the man sleeps. If the tiny strings holding the tape together break at night, the man is clearly capable of erection.

- *Measuring penile activity in men watching erotic videos*, with devices attached to the penis, can demonstrate erectile competence.
- *Injecting papaverine* is another test for erectile capacity; the drug is injected into the erectile tissue of the penis. In men with normal blood flow, papaverine dilates the blood vessels and induces erection. Its failure to do so may indicate a penile blood vessel disorder. Almost any man capable of erection responds to this drug.
- *Tests for penile blood vessel disorders* and restricted blood flow—an increasingly recognized cause of erectile failure—can be done with ultrasound, arteriography (X-rays used in conjunction with injected dye) and cavernostomy (with saline solution infused into the penis) to examine tissue expansion capacity.

Treatment of erectile dysfunction

If the erectile problem is physical, drugs, hormones or mechanical devices may be the answer. If it's psychological, sex therapy and counseling may help. If it can't be traced to a definite reason, the man may be offered therapy with drugs, devices and counseling. There are now many ingenious methods available to help men regain erectile power. Since drugs and devices won't overcome emotional or intimacy problems, sex or relationship therapy is often also advised. For a variety of reasons, a couple should usually get counseling together. Exercise, yoga, relaxation and a change of environment may also help.

MEDICAL METHODS AND DRUGS TO OVERCOME ERECTILE FAILURE

- *Testosterone-replacement therapy,* GnRH analogues or other drugs can correct some hormone deficiencies. However, despite most media reports to the contrary, there is not much evidence that testosterone improves erectile dysfunction,
- *Corrective surgery* for venous leaks and arterial blockage can sometimes restore erectile ability.
- *Yohimbine,* a plant derivative that stimulates the parasympathetic nervous system and decreases blood outflow from penile tissue, helps about 30 percent of men with mild impotence—which make it about as successful as sex counseling. Side effects of the drug include facial flushing, tachycardia (racing heart), occasional panic attacks, low blood pressure

and tremors.
- *Papaverine,* a self-injectable drug used since 1983, is a smooth-muscle relaxant that increases arterial blood flow in the penis and restricts venous outflow. Injected directly into the side of the penis just before intercourse, it produces an erection in 5–10 minutes, without disturbing ejaculation or orgasm. While some men dislike the idea of needles or drugs, many are enthusiastic about this method and it is gaining popularity. Possible side effects include dizziness, cardiac complications and a painful, prolonged erection lasting several hours—which requires medical relief measures. The effectiveness of papaverine may diminish with repeated injections

and occasionally produces scarring. Papaverine is now often used in combination with phentolamine, and sometimes also prostaglandin E_1—as "triple therapy"— with greater efficacy, smaller doses of each drug and fewer side effects. However, some initial enthusiasts discontinue the method after a while and resort to penile implants.
- Drugs to enhance erections include prostaglandin E_1 and its synthetic versions, alprostadil (Caverject or Edex)— injected into the base of the penis just before intercourse— and MUSE, capsules pushed into the urethra to achieve erection.
- The latest potency-enhancing drugs are taken orally and include the much-publicized sildenafil (Viagra). (See below.)

Mechanical erection-producing devices

Penile prostheses of various kinds can now restore erectile capacity without disturbing libido, ejaculation or orgasm, although they don't enlarge the penis beyond its natural erect size.

Vacuum devices (such as ErectAid), made of silicone rubber and placed on the penis, have a side arm that withdraws air, creating a vacuum around the penis which increases blood flow into the penis. The basic model contains a soft plastic tube that fits over the flaccid penis, and a hand-held pump. A rubber band is wrapped around the bottom of the penis to stop blood flowing out. The cylinder is removed during intercourse and the blood drawn into the penis keeps it erect. "A man can get a good enough erection for penetration, but it's not rock hard," says one University of Toronto expert. "Some love the vacuum devices and others hate them, but many willingly accept them. However, it takes practice to use them deftly." Most are available on prescription for varying sums— some as costly as $500. They are rather cumbersome and may dim sensation, which detracts somewhat from their popularity. The obvious drawback is interference with sexual spontaneity. Also, men must not fall asleep with the rubber band in place.

Permanent penile implants come in inflatable models, or uninflatable models that are semi-rigid (giving a permanent erection). They can be bent down to seem more natural when not in use. One uninflatable model, composed of two silicone rods, is surgically implanted into the penis, providing a natural-looking erection.

Inflatable models—inflated for sex, then deflated afterward—are the more popular type, and operate more like the "real thing." One model is composed of two inflatable tubes put into the shaft of the penis with a fluid reservoir in the abdomen and a pump in the scrotum. Squeezing the pump moves fluid from the reservoir into the penis.

Penile implants are a last resort—and thankfully have become less necessary since the advent of the phosphodiesterase inhibitors (Viagra-type drugs)—as surgical insertion destroys some erectile tissue and the devices tend to break down. The more complex the mechanical device, the more likely it is to malfunction. Advanced models are more reliable, but many still need to be replaced or repaired. A candidate requesting an implant must be in good health, and have a high sex drive and good penile sensitivity; if he has a regular sex partner the partner must favor the idea. It is imperative that the couple be assessed for suitability and well informed about the benefits and risks of implants. The risks include infection—requiring removal—swelling and pain.

Summing up, one urologist notes that "Erection does not equate with good lovemaking, sensuality or happiness," and, "There are many other ways to give and enjoy sexual pleasure." Sex or relationship therapy for both partners together is usually recommended, along with any methods that aim to restore erectile capacity or overcome other male sex problems. (See Chapter 7 for details of sex therapy and how to find a sex therapist.)

THE CIRCUMCISION CONTROVERSY

A bystander to the circumcision debate might feel bewildered by the acrimonious controversy over this tiny scrap of penile skin. The arguments pro and contra circumcision—removal of the foreskin or *prepuce* from the penis, usually done in newborns—continue unabated, with ardent lobbyists on both sides. Those in favor of circumcision say it improves overall health and hygiene. Those against call it barbaric and have joined forces to press for attention to "children's rights," some forming highly visible groups such as the National Organization to Halt the Abuse and Mutilation of Males, the RECAP (Recover a Penis) movement, and in Canada ETHIC (End the Horror of Infant Circumcision).

On the medical side, there's now evidence that circumcision reduces risks of urinary tract infections, decreases vulnerability to sexually transmitted infections CSTIs, including HIV infection or AIDS, and protects against penile cancer. However the benefits are very small. For example, urinary tract infections are reduced by 6 for every 1,000 boys who have the procedure (2 of whom will need hospitalization) and the rate of penile cancer is extremely low.

Critics argue that circumcision has no proven value and that it's a cruel, ritualistic prac-

---

PROBING THE VIAGRA SOLUTION

Sildenafil or Viagra—from a class of enzyme blockers known as phosphodiesterase type-S inhibitors—was originally used to treat angina. It proved useless for angina, although men taking it noticed amazingly renewed erectile vigor. Unlike other erection-enhancing products, which produce erections regardless of sexual desire, Viagra acts on the sexual arousal pathway and works only if the man is sexually excited.

In natural erection, arousal stimulates brain centers to send messages to the penis, releasing nitric oxide, which activates cyclic guanosine monophosphate (cGMP)—a substance that allows the penis to fill with blood. The enzymatic degradation of cGMP later destroys the erection. Viagra boosts erections by stopping the breakdown of cGMP, maintaining the inflow of blood.

Viagra works 30 minutes to 1 hour after being swallowed, the effect lasting about 3 hours; it acts more slowly after a fatty meal. It works best in those whose sex problems stem from emotional causes such as depression, and in men with mild erectile dysfunction.

Side effects include headaches, lowered blood pressure, indigestion, vomiting, nasal congestion, face-flushing and altered color perception (everything "tinged in blue")—side effects being worst with high doses. While most men can safely take Viagra once a day in the recommended dose of 50 mg (up to 100 mg), it must not be used by people on nitrate medications (such as nitroglycerin for heart trouble): the combination could produce a fatal blood pressure drop. It should also not be taken with cimetidine (Tagamet), erythromycin and ketoconazole (Nizoral) or people with the eye disorder retinitis pigmentosa.

Newer versions of Viagra have now come onto the market. There have been no comparative trials done, but the main difference between the various forms seems to be in the half-life of the medication (the time that it remains and works inside the body). Cialis stays in the body longer (30 minutes to 24 hours) than Viagra and hence was nicknamed "Le Weekender" in early trials in France. Levitra is purported to work a little faster, but the instructions are similar to Viagra: i.e., to be taken 1 hour before sexual activity.

---

tice that causes intense pain in newborns, which may leave lasting psychological scars. They claim that circumcision leads to lowered self-esteem, less sexual pleasure and—in extreme cases—a sense of having been castrated. There seems to be no high quality evidence to prove or disprove this theory.

Amid the controversy, all agree on the need for good penile hygiene. Uncircumcised boys must learn to wash their penises well by gently retracting the foreskin until resistance is met (full retraction is not achieved until about age three) and using soap and water. Good

HOW CIRCUMCISION IS DONE, AND ITS CONSEQUENCES

Circumcision is a surgical procedure usually done within a few days of birth (preferably before age 2 months) that removes the foreskin that hoods the end of the penis, thereby exposing its tip, the glans. The operation, which takes 5 to 10 minutes, is done with or without local anesthetic; some practitioners give painkillers such as acetaminophen (Tylenol); others use neither painkillers nor anesthetic. After circumcision, the scar is protected with gauze and petroleum jelly (Vaseline). Complications, which affect 0.2 to 2 percent of cases, are generally minor—maybe some bleeding and superficial infection—although they can be serious and include bacterial infection or kidney failure.

hygiene may help to prevent conditions such as phimosis (unretractable foreskin), balanoposthitis (inflammation of the glans) and posthitis (inflammation of the foreskin), which often necessitate circumcision later on.

Circumcision was introduced to the English-speaking world in the nineteenth century largely for hygienic reasons, and as a possible "cure" for masturbation. But the practice has been declining, and many North American hospitals no longer circumcise babies unless specifically requested. Young physicians often prefer not to do it. Nonetheless, 40 to 60 percent of newborn boys are still circumcised in parts of Canada, and U.S. circumcision figures run around 70 percent.

An exhaustive survey recently reported in the *Canadian Medical Association Journal* concluded that the advantages and disadvantages of neonatal circumcision "cancelled each other out" and were so "evenly balanced" that there are no compelling reasons to support routine circumcision of all newborns. The Canadian Pediatric Society does not recommend routine circumcision of newborns, suggesting the decision be made on personal, cultural or religious grounds, albeit with knowledge of the latest medical findings. When circumcision is performed, experts emphasize the need for careful attention to pain relief.

MALE BREAST CANCER: MEN GET IT TOO!

Male breast cancer makes up about 1 percent of all breast cancer; a certain proportion of it due to the newly discovered BRCA1 and BRCA2 cancer-susceptibility genes. Treatment is similar to that for women, with lumpectomy or mastectomy plus chemotherapy or tamoxifen. As in women, breast cancer in men more often strikes the left breast than the right, less frequently both sides and is most common in those over age 60.

Most types of breast cancer seen in women can also occur in men, but as breast tissue in men consists almost exclusively of ducts, with no lobular (milk-gland) structures, virtually all male breast cancers are ductal. Invasive (spreading) cancers that arise exclusively from the ducts are relatively more common in men than in women. As in women, breast cancer in men may have progesterone or estrogen receptors.

Alerting symptoms in men

Breast cancer in men usually first signals itself as a small, painless lump or nodule under the *areola*—the pigmented area around the nipple—or as a nipple discharge. Since there is usually little glandular or fat tissue to hide a developing cancer; many male breast cancers are quite easily detected. However; men are less likely to look for breast lumps or to recognize the risk if they find one. Since men don't think breast cancer; they may ignore a breast lump for 1 or 2 years, so the cancer can be quite advanced by the time it's diagnosed. Diagnosis of breast cancer in men, as in women, is by needle aspiration (removing some tissue with a needle), or by a "core" or surgical biopsy.

Main risk factors for breast cancer in men

- *A family history of breast cancer* and a genetic predisposition to the disease. Men who carry the altered (mutant) BRCA1 or BRCA2 cancer-susceptibility genes can pass on the predisposition to breast cancer to their daughters and sons. Men with hereditary breast cancer are at higher risk of colon and prostate cancer. New research is uncovering how changes in the BRCA genes cause cancer; holding out the promise of earlier detection and ultimately a cure.
- *Gynecomastia* or breast enlargement, which is not a premalignant state but carries increased risk.

- *Klinefelter's syndrome* (a disorder with an extra X chromosome in all body cells) raises male breast cancer risk 20-fold. However, this is a rare syndrome and accounts for only a small proportion of all male breast cancer. Men with Klinefelter's syndrome have shriveled testes, high levels of the hormone gonadotropin (secreted by the pituitary gland), low levels of androgen (male sex hormone) and normal to low levels of estrogens (female hormones). Most men with Klinefelter's syndrome also have gynecomastia (enlarged breasts), considered a risk factor. The increased risk in men with Klinefelter's may also arise because male hormones used to treat it are converted to estrogens in male fat tissue.
- *Testicular dysfunction*—for instance, undescended testes, congenital groin hernias (present at birth), testicular injuries, mumps orchitis (inflammation of the testes) and testicular infections—can increase the risk of male breast cancer.
- *Occupational factors*, such as exposure of the testes to high temperatures, are thought to increase the risk of male breast cancer. Butchers handling estrogen-treated meats are at above-average risk from exposure to the female hormone. Researchers also report a significantly higher incidence of breast cancer among men employed in the newspaper or newsprint industry. In one study, male journalists in Sweden were found to have greatly increased breast cancer risks. Whether similar exposures occur among journalists in other countries is unknown but warrants further study.
- *Obesity* may be a predisposing factor because of increased estrogen production in fatty tissues.
- *Estrogens*, used to treat some medical disorders, have not yet been evaluated for their impact on male breast cancer. However, an elevated risk of breast cancer was observed in one U.S. study of men treated with estrogens, and a Swedish study found an eightfold increase in breast cancer risk among men working in the soap and perfume industry with creams containing estrogens. In addition, three transsexual men who developed breast cancer after castration and high-dose estrogen treatment provide anecdotal evidence that estrogens may induce male breast cancer.
- *Chronic liver disease* in alcoholic men reduces the capacity to break down estrogens and elevates female hormone levels, also raising male breast cancer risks. In some studies, the risks of breast cancer in men were elevated in tune with the amounts of alcohol consumed (and the extent of liver cirrhosis). Schistosomiasis (a chronic disease involving the liver) may also increase risks.

Treatment of male breast cancer

Treatment parallels that for similar forms and stages of female breast cancer and involves "local control," with surgical removal of the tumor by lumpectomy or mastectomy. When the cancer is surgically excised, some *axillary*, or underarm, lymph nodes are also taken out to test for malignancy and help stage the tumor. Positive (cancerous) lymph nodes are even more strongly associated with spreading disease than in women. Radiation is given after lumpectomy or if the lymph nodes are positive for cancer or if the surgical excision is near the chest wall. Surgery tends to be more radical in men because of the usually later stage of the disease when discovered, the smaller size of male breasts, the more frequent involvement of the chest muscles and problems with staging. Removal of testes or adrenal glands is sometimes advised. Systemic (total-body) chemotherapy is usual for men at risk of recurrence after local therapy. Hormonal therapy with tamoxifen may also be used, as in women.

The prognosis (predicted survival) is largely determined by the underarm lymph node involvement and tumor markers, as in women. If the nodes test positive for cancer chances are worse than if they are negative and show no sign of cancer. The seemingly poorer survival rates in men may be due to delays in diagnosis and lack of suspicion that cancer is present. Male breast cancer carries the same prognosis as that of a similar type and stage in females.

Producing the healthiest possible baby

Preconception preparation • Fertilization and conception • Reversing infertility • Pregnancy in the over-thirties • Modern "windows" into the womb • The course and care of pregnancy • Choice of birthplace and birth assistant • The role of midwives • Changes in the mother's body during pregnancy • Charting fetal progress • Nutrition in pregnancy • Exercise in pregnancy • Spotting high-risk pregnancies • Prenatal classes • The three stages of labor • From fetus to newborn • Cesarean birth • Newborn child-parent bonding • Breast is still best

10

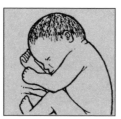

BIRTH IS A UNIVERSAL journey we've all taken —from the shelter of our mother's body out into the exterior world. But in the past few decades, attitudes to childbirth have changed dramatically. With scientific evidence being applied ever more stringently to the practice of obstetrics and childbirth methods, our ideas of how to produce the healthiest possible baby and mother have turned 180 degrees, and then turned back yet again. These changes can make it hard for women and their families to know how to make their best personal birthing choices. And choice has become the number 1 word in pregnancy and childbirth—including choice of whether and what kind of prenatal genetic testing of the fetus to have, of where and how to have the baby and who should be present to assist at the birth. The onus on the woman, her partner and family to make informed decisions is becoming greater, and the decisions more complicated and more stressful with increasing childbirth options.

As late as the mid-1700s, theorists like the French philosopher Descartes viewed the unborn child as a miniature, preformed adult, curled up inside the womb with all its tiny organs already intact. Later on unborn babies came to be regarded as tadpole-like creatures, their brains a "blank slate" upon which rearing and experience would engrave personality and other features. Today's research opposes such absolute emphasis on "nurture"—the influence of home, environment and education—proposing that biology (genes) and the environment *jointly* mold human development. The scientific literature presently suggests that babies are born with genetic "hardwiring" that, given the appropriate environmental events, stimuli and exposures during the early years of life, can reach its maximal potential.

The quest for a "superbaby"

Only in recent years have scientists recognized the many influences—such as nutrition, smoking, alcohol and medications—on fetal development. Modern obstetric care aims to produce the healthiest possible babies through prenatal care and education, good nutrition, appropriately monitored fetal progress and referral of high-risk pregnancies to specialized providers for care whenever necessary. Since time immemorial parents have always wished for a perfect baby, and the first question at birth is still an anxious "Is my baby normal?" But while everyone wants the healthiest baby possible, there's still considerable argument about how best to achieve it.

In the early part of this century, medical care for pregnancy and childbirth was minimal.

By the 1940s, physicians had become more involved in the process of childbirth and pregnancy monitoring, largely supplanting midwives in North America. Birthing began to move out of homes and into hospitals, becoming more "medicalized." The accompanying fall in infant and maternal death rates was attributed to better medical care, although better overall health and nutrition, fewer pregnancies and smaller family size likely played a significant role as well.

Studies in the 1960s and 1970s reinforced the belief in medicalized birthing, showing that women who received prenatal care from physicians and gave birth in hospital were more likely to deliver healthy babies. Not surprisingly, this led to even more medical involvement, with the introduction of obstetric specialists, prenatal tests and high-tech birthing procedures, along with authoritarian pronouncements on diet, exercise, sex and birth positions. Many a baby today has had a "medical checkup" long before emerging from the womb. Sophisticated genetic screening and high-definition ultrasound may have determined the baby's sex and diagnosed some imperfections before birth. Ultrasound screening may have shown physical defects such as a missing limb or brain and heart flaws; analysis of a little amniotic fluid surrounding the fetus or of cord blood may have revealed some genetic faults. On discovering fetal imperfections, parents may choose to terminate a pregnancy or carry it to term and prepare for a less-than-perfect child.

Nowadays, biochemical tests can also detect parents carrying certain genetic flaws before conception and assess their chances of having an affected child. For example, a simple "mouthwash" test to analyze buccal cells (from the mouth) can determine whether one or both parents carry the gene for cystic fibrosis (a serious defect affecting the lungs and digestive system), and predict the risks of bearing an affected child (1 in 4 if both parents carry the cystic-fibrosis gene). The knowledge may influence their decision to start a family. Should they decide to proceed , pre-birth tests on the fetus can determine whether it carries the faulty gene, giving them the option of terminating the pregnancy.

There is now considerable debate over the extent to which medical techniques can improve a potentially bad birth outcome—for example, in a mother who is malnourished —and how far medical interventions (such as continuous electronic monitoring of the fetal heart during labor) are desirable or can produce fewer deaths and complications.

Prenatal rubella immunization and genetic counseling are examples of how malformations can be prevented, as is persuading women not to smoke, take drugs or drink alcohol while pregnant. Detecting a fetus with specific ailments can lead to arrangements for birth in a special unit with facilities to operate on the newborn and correct or minimize the defect.

However, many medical approaches practiced in the past 20 years are being reassessed for their efficacy, their cost to the healthcare system and their possible adverse effects. For example, while earlier studies favoured the medical model hospital birth, recent scientific evidence shows that home births are as safe as hospital births for low risk women, provided that they are under the care of well-trained midwives. There is increasing support for the concept that most births are a "normal" process, with low risks, requiring little medical interference and few medical procedures. And the dogma of "once a Cesarean always a Cesarean" is also being overturned. Many women who've already had one Cesarean are encouraged to try a vaginal birth for the next baby. Until recently, physicians were also relearning how to manage breech (buttocks first) births instead of automatically doing a Cesarean, but a landmark trial completed in 2002 has shifted the pendulum back to doing Caesarian deliveries for breech births. With challengers to this evidence, future studies may again see the pendulum swing back. The practice of episiotomy (cutting tissue in the area between vagina and anus to widen the passage)—traditionally almost routine in many North American delivery rooms—has now been proven to offer no benefit in the short or long term to mothers or babies, so that allowing the tissues to tear along "natural" lines is the current practice. Use of low forceps to assist delivery of the baby's head is also now less common. (Vacuum suctioning to ease delivery is now sometimes used instead.) Also, use of forceps to "pull" a high head down is infrequently attempted. Routine continuous electronic monitoring of the fetal heartbeat during labor is now also being questioned from many quarters, as it has not been shown to improve fetal or maternal outcomes. Many centers have supplanted this practice with the use of intermittent fetal monitoring—which gives mothers more freedom of movement and more choice of positions during labor—in accordance with evidence that, for low-risk pregnancies, the maternal and fetal outcomes are equally good.

The quest to bear a "perfect" baby also raises ethical dilemmas. Some health professionals anticipate possible problems from the technology that tells parents in advance the sex of their child and some of the abnormalities it may have. In future, as more and more genes are identified and pinpointed, it may be possible to test for a wider range of defects. Some fear that genetic tests may promote eugenic or "quality" control and lead to a mentality where parents select for birth only "designer" babies—perhaps only males—and where even marginally handicapped children may be castigated or blamed for not having been "terminated." In Ontario recently, ultrasounds requested only to determine the sex of the baby have been denied across the board, even if the parents are willing to pay for the service themselves.

New emphasis on caring

Pregnancy and childbirth procedures are now moving back from high tech to lower tech, as women demand more control over their bodies. Driven by those who consider pregnancy and labor a natural, healthy life event rather than a "disease," and under increasing pressure from primary care obstetric providers such as family practitioners, nurses, midwives and women themselves, pregnancy management has moved away from the "intensive care" concept to the "family-centered" or "birthing-centered" concept. Although the basics of the medical model remain, with their emphasis on detecting and managing pregnancy risks (such as hypertension, gestational diabetes and retarded fetal growth), a supportive medical caregiver—whether physi-

cian, nurse or midwife—is emerging as the most crucial element in pregnancy care. In fact, obstetrics is now frequently termed "care in pregnancy and childbirth."

Childbirth is becoming more of a family affair

Not only is the pregnant woman receiving more care, but the well-being of the whole family, especially the father, is beginning to get greater attention. For example, a woman's relationship to her partner is seen as crucial to successful childbirth and parenting. Several new studies have shown that stress and anxiety in pregnancy are related to poor obstetric outcomes, and women with satisfying relationships have fewer adverse symptoms in pregnancy and are better adapted to parenthood 1 year after birth. In other words, happy women make happier mothers and healthier babies.

One University of Toronto family physician explains that "a family-oriented approach helps couples make room for and adjust to the new baby and give it optimal care." There are also fewer pregnancy problems—less anxiety, apprehension and denial—in couples who are well prepared for parenting and jointly supervise the pregnancy. Alerting signs of "unpreparedness for parenthood" may include: the mother's ambivalent feelings about the pregnancy, insecurity about parenting skills, no plans made for the baby, a feeling that "pregnancy interferes with my lifestyle," expectation that the newborn will "be a friend," fears of the new role alignment and a father who doesn't attend at doctor-visits or delivery. The provider should be enquiring about such issues and attitudes at prenatal visits, and may make more effort to involve the father in pregnancy care or provide extra counseling for the couple.

Support systems—the father, grandparents, siblings, friends and extended family—are seen as vitally important to the successful outcome of pregnancy. Experts in family-centered pregnancy care now include the father of baby-to-be in discussions, counseling and education, as well as in prenatal classes. "Family-centered care," explains one physician at the McMaster Medical Centre, "recognizes birth as a primal life event rather than a medical procedure, encourages the presence of fathers, siblings, even grandparents, [and does] everything possible to make it a family event, letting them share the exhaustion, exhilaration and wonder of a new baby."

Since close contact in the postbirth period may strengthen parent-child ties, maternity staff encourage parents to have some private time with their new baby. They encourage a mother to put the newborn against her body, as skin-to-skin touching makes many mothers fondle their infants more and may elicit behaviors not seen with blanket-wrapped babies. An added advantage is that putting the baby to the breast soon after delivery speeds uterine contraction, expels blood-clots, establishes the baby's sucking reflex (strong right after birth), speeds the arrival of mother's milk and gets things off to a good start. Family-centered care has now been largely accepted across North America, although some maternity caregivers say "It's more lip service than reality." (A few hospitals still don't allow partners—especially those of single mothers—to be present at the birthing.)

Fathers play a crucial role in childbirth

Fathers play an important part in helping their partners with pregnancy, birth and early motherhood, giving them confidence and establishing a family environment at the birthing scene. Yet fathers too may feel insecure and ambivalent about the pregnancy, find it hard to accept (even deny it), be reluctant to attend prenatal visits and have trouble committing to the parenting role. However, family-centered caregivers actively encourage fathers-to-be to attend doctor visits, be present at the ultrasound exam (where the baby may be seen moving), take part in discussions about labor, birth positions, breastfeeding and postpartum help, and handle the newborn in the delivery room. The evidence shows that a trained supportive partner in the delivery process, historically called a "doula," actually reduces pain for the mother and improves almost all outcomes, both maternal and newborn. Developing a personal and unique "teamwork" approach to the delivery process can make it easier for everybody.

Fathers of sick or premature babies (whose mothers may be hospitalized elsewhere) can

---

MANY ROUTINE BIRTHING PROCEDURES BEING REEVALUATED OR ABANDONED

New evidence indicates that some widely used birthing routines such as enemas, shaves, genetic tests and use of episiotomies, epidurals and fetal monitors—while sometimes needed—may do more harm than good. Studies show that episiotomy—a small cut in the vagina to reduce pain and ripping during birth (used in 70 percent of cases in some centers)—can actually increase tearing and later cause incontinence. It should not be done routinely, but can be necessary to facilitate a quicker birth if there is increased concern about the baby's safety. Giving an epidural (spinal anesthesia) to reduce labor pain often causes transient fever in the mother, and leads to increased newborn surveillance and the potential for overuse of antibiotics in babies born to mothers who had an epidural. Genetic screening, now offered to all women in some centers, may cause anxiety and should be more judiciously used (with careful genetic counseling), for those at risk. Many modern birthing procedures have not been put to the test of rigorous scientific investigation and need closer evaluation to prove their benefits.

---

help with frequent visits. A Canadian study showed that fathers of pre-term infants held them longer and took more part in their upbringing than those of full-term babies, the concern for their children overcoming any effects of separation due to initial frailty. However, the absence of the father is not necessarily a lasting or negative influence on children.

In today's changing culture many fathers are staying at home as the primary caregiver. This may be due to practical considerations (the mothers pay is more remunerative) or other reasons (the father is more suited to this activity, job flexibility, etc.).

PRECONCEPTION PREPARATION

Pregnancy should be regarded not as an illness but as a natural process or continuum that starts with conception and continues through 9 months of fetal development inside the uterus to infant life outside it. Birth is just one step—albeit a crucial one—along the way. By the time a baby is born, it has already gone through 9 critical months of development.

Ideally, pregnancy care starts before conception, by assessing fitness for childbearing. It might help if future parents find out as much as possible beforehand, so they can make informed choices on pregnancy care and birthing of their child. Testing for disorders such as hepatitis B, syphilis, gonorrhea and other conditions that could endanger the baby may be done, so that steps can be taken to lessen the risk. Preconception testing for antibodies to rubella (German measles) in the mother is *vital*, as this infection during pregnancy can seriously deform the fetus. Women without rubella antibodies should be immunized and then avoid conception for 3 months afterward.

Genetic counseling is advised for couples who know of inherited diseases in the family—such as phenylketonuria, (a protein-digesting flaw), Tay-Sachs disease (nerve degeneration, invariably fatal by age 4), cystic fibrosis (a digestive and lung disorder), hemophilia (failure of blood to clot), sickle cell anemia (with abnormal hemoglobin leading to oxygen lack), muscular dystrophy (muscle-wasting) and others. Blood tests can now detect parent-carriers of many such inherited defects.

THE FETUS IN LATE PREGNANCY

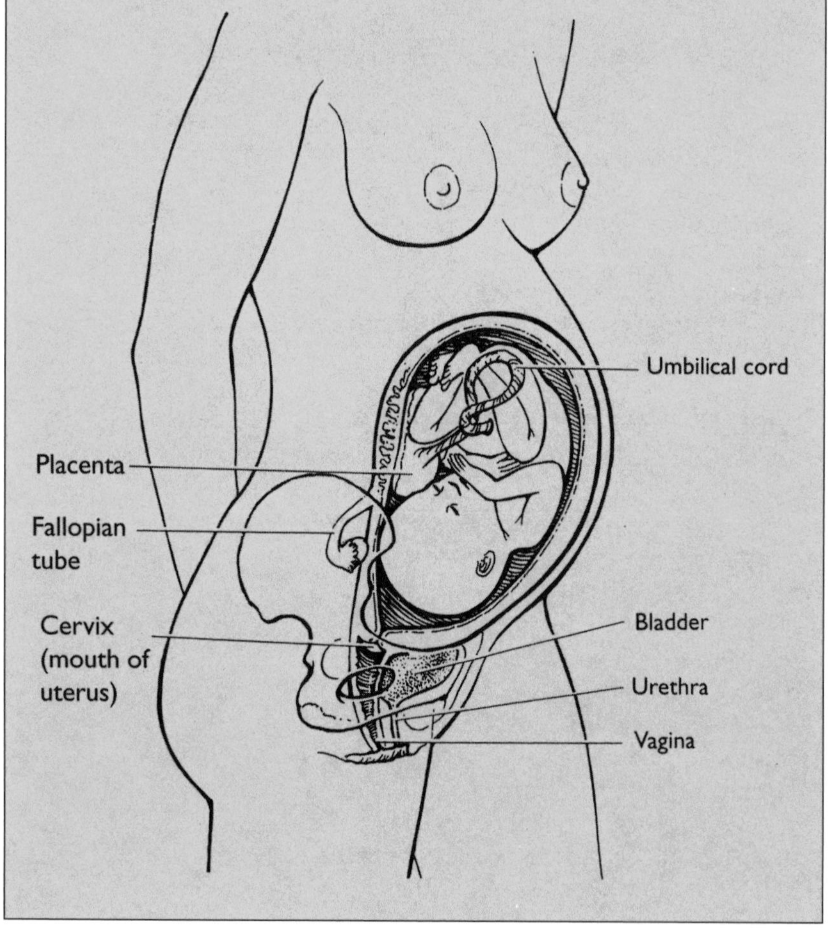

Placenta

Fallopian tube

Cervix (mouth of uterus)

Umbilical cord

Bladder

Urethra

Vagina

Sensible lifestyle habits—balanced nutrition, regular exercise, avoidance of tobacco, alcohol and drugs (unless medically advised)—should ideally begin before conception. Giving up tobacco smoking before and during pregnancy is a wise precaution. Most of the tissues destined to form vital organs are laid down during the first 12 weeks of embryonic development, when a woman may not even know she's pregnant. It is precisely during this early stage that the unborn child is most vulnerable to environmental toxins, infections, medications, alcohol and malnutrition.

Good nutritional status of mothers-to-be at or near conception, and in early pregnancy, is crucial for bearing healthy babies. One University of Toronto expert explains that "malnourishment or early nutrient deprivation is hard to make up later in pregnancy (especially after the 12th to 14th week). Mal-fed fetuses may not reach their normal growth curve, remaining underweight until birth and after." One British researcher notes that many women don't realize how nutritionally deprived their bodies are. Specific nutrient deficiencies can lead to specific infant damage. For example, a shortage of *folic acid* (one of the B vitamins) can lead to neural tube disorders—with an incomplete spine or brain. So women are now advised to make sure they have enough folic acid in their diets (or take supplements) to help avoid these congenital faults in their babies.

Ideally, women should start increasing their folic acid intake well before conception (at least 3 months beforehand), making sure they get 0.4 mg (400 micrograms) a day, preferably from a vitamin supplement. Eating plenty of folate-rich foods such as dark leafy greens, legumes (lentils, dried beans, chickpeas) and orange juice is beneficial, but most women do not get adequate amounts of folic acid through diet , hence the recommendation that all women planning conception start folic acid supplements.

FERTILIZATION AND CONCEPTION

Fertilization, the union of one egg with one sperm, is normally achieved by sexual intercourse. Chance decides which egg in which ovary is released and penetrated by which viable sperm. A woman need not reach orgasm to procreate.

Requisites for fertility

For conception, a sperm must fertilize an egg within 24 hours of ejaculation and ovulation, because both sperm and egg soon deteriorate, even though they may still be able to unite for another day or two. Although they may remain alive for as long as 4 days, sperm survival time is highly variable. Ejaculated sperm lodge at the top of the vagina, then travel to meet the egg. The path from penis to Fallopian tube (where the egg waits) is perilous. Sperm must traverse the vagina—inhospitable because it's acidic, and sperm prefer an alkaline environment—go through the uterus and up to the Fallopian tube. Millions of sperm per ejaculate are required because many perish en route to the egg and others fail to penetrate the egg's tough outer membrane. If enough sperm have survived the journey, conception generally occurs in the lower part of the Fallopian tube or upper part of the uterus. Sperm that have the slightest imperfections (being slow swimmers or short-tailed, for instance) generally fall by the wayside.

The Canadian Fertility Society estimates that sperm counts vary from 20 to 300 million sperm per ejaculate (averaging 3 to 5 ml). For unknown reasons, up to 40 percent of men on occasion have sperm counts lower than the 20 million per ejaculate usually needed for fertilization. A sperm count below 20 million per ml is unlikely to achieve fertilization. Even though they may have too low a sperm count to be classed as "fertile," there are isolated cases of men with only 2 to 5 million sperm per ejaculate siring babies. But sperm banks, which usually prefer youngish men as donors, require a minimum sperm count of 100 million sperm per ml, since the freezing process destroys some.

Once the egg is fertilized, an immediate chemical reaction on its surface prevents other sperm from entering it. Fertilization also triggers division of the egg into 2 cells, then into 4, 8 and 16 to become a zygote. Six or 7 days later having gone through many cell divisions, the hollow ball of cells becomes a blastocyst that burrows into the spongy, blood-rich wall of the uterus. This process of implantation is the start of pregnancy.

REVERSING INFERTILITY

Infertility fluctuates from place to place and decade to decade. Approximately 60 percent of couples who do not use contraception and have regular intercourse will conceive within 6 months, 80 percent within 12 months and 90 percent within 18 months. Consequently, women who have been trying to get pregnant for more than 12 to 18 months and haven't succeeded should be referred to an infertility specialist. A women's age is one of the main factors determining her fertility. Therefore, earlier referral is advisable for women who are 35 years of age or older, or for those with a history of pelvic inflammatory disease, or other infertility risk factors. Infertility is increasing in Canada, possibly due to delayed childbearing (older women being less fertile) and an increase in sexually transmitted infections (such as chlamydia and gonorrhea) that can cause sterility by scar-

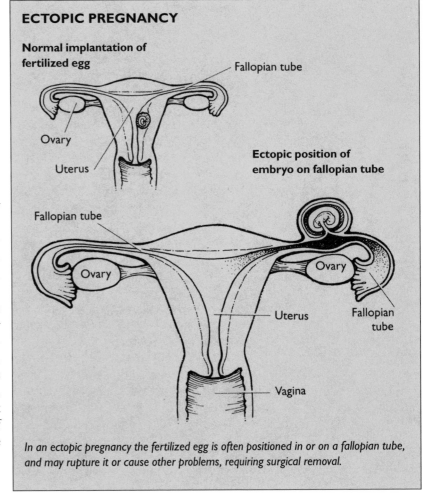

ECTOPIC PREGNANCY

Normal implantation of fertilized egg

Fallopian tube

Ovary

Uterus

Ectopic position of embryo on fallopian tube

Fallopian tube

Ovary

Ovary

Uterus

Fallopian tube

Vagina

In an ectopic pregnancy the fertilized egg is often positioned in or on a fallopian tube, and may rupture it or cause other problems, requiring surgical removal.

CAUSES OF INFERTILITY

In women:
- absence of or irregular ovulation;
- surgical or radiation treatments that destroy the ovaries;
- obstruction or damage to Fallopian tubes due to causes such as sexually transmitted diseases;
- pelvic inflammatory disease (PID) due to a sexually transmitted infection (often symptomless);
- a ruptured appendix or previous surgery;

- congenitally absent ovaries (e.g., in Turner's syndrome);
- endometriosis (where the uterine lining grows outside the uterus and blocks or damages the tubes);
- hostile cervical mucus;
- antibodies to sperm, which may explain why conception fails in the "normal infertile" couple.

In men:
- insufficient sperm or poor sperm quality;

- in men who are marginally subfertile, various factors may aggravate the infertility, such as:
  - premature ejaculation;
  - excess alcohol consumption;
  - postpubertal mumps (if there is *orchitis*—painful testicular inflammation);
  - testes that have not descended;
  - overheating of the genitals (due to tight

clothing, long spells of sitting, too many saunas or hot baths), since a cool temperature favors sperm survival;
- certain drugs that diminish sperm count (such as marijuana).

The causes of infertility in men are often harder to pinpoint than in women, and, if found, harder to treat. In about 85 percent of male infertility the reason remains unknown. Incidentally, sterility in

men—inability to fertilize an egg—should not be confused with impotence, which is the inability to sustain an erection.

Although sperm numbers are critical, sperm quality—motility, speed, vigor, size and shape—also play a vital role. It's difficult to upgrade a low sperm count—certain drugs (such as clomiphene) and hormones (which are rarely effective) may be tried.

---

ring the fallopian tubes. In Canada, 8 percent of couples experience infertility. On a global scale, unwanted fertility poses a drastic population problem; but on an individual level, when a couple cannot conceive a child, it can be a major personal challenge. Fortunately, new methods now help many infertile couples conceive, and greater options for creative adoption are also becoming available.

Officially, infertility is defined as "the inability of a couple to conceive after a year of unprotected regular coitus (without contraception)." In many couples who cannot conceive, neither partner is really infertile; with a different partner each might manage to conceive. In a small number, 10 percent or less, of such involuntarily childless couples, both partners appear normal but cannot jointly conceive a child. Such a couple is termed "normally infertile" with infertility "of no apparent cause."

About a third of all infertility is due to a female disorder, another third is caused by male problems, the remainder arising from combined incompatibility. In some cases, mistimed intercourse is the only reason for infertility. The odds of being able to conceive can sometimes be improved by explicit information, better coital mechanics (change of lovemaking position) and precise timing to the day of ovulation. About 25 percent of infertile couples become

pregnant once they seek medical help, sometimes with no treatment other than general sex and intercourse counseling. Another 30 percent respond to appropriate treatment for the man, woman or both.

The discovery of infertility, almost invariably traumatic, sets up a vicious circle of recrimination and worry. Sex life loses spontaneity and becomes joyless. The time-consuming, tedious and costly fertility tests seem demeaning; both partners feel victimized, sensing a loss of control over their bodies. All too often, infertile people suffer silently, finding their inadequacy too shameful to share with others, particularly since so many people are apt to confuse fertility with their sexual identity.

Initial fertility options

A number of solutions have become available for overcoming infertility. For many couples the first-line approach is ovulation induction with clomiphene citrate. There has been recent interest in the use of insulin-lowering agents such as metformin in women with polycystic ovarian syndrome (PCOS), a condition that affects fertility through irregular or absent ovulation. In vitro fertilization (IVF), with successful live-birth rates of 25 percent per cycle, is another option, but it's expensive, time-consuming, and complicated. If the problem is male subfertility, intrauterine insemination may be all that is required. In cases of severe deficits in men's semen quality or failed IVF, intracytoplasmic sperm injection of the ovum may be used, a procedure that is done in the lab.

Test-tube, or in vitro, fertilization (IVF)

Since the birth of the first test-tube babies, many infants have been successfully born by IVF worldwide. But the success rate remains low—around 20 percent in many centers.

In vitro fertilization (the Latin means "in glass") entails the fertilization of an egg or several eggs with ejaculated sperm in a glass dish. The eggs, artificially ripened by hormonal agents taken by the woman, are removed surgically from her ovaries.

After being incubated and fertilized, then grown in a dish for 48 to 72 hours, the tiny fertilized eggs—now embryos—are put back into the mother's uterus in the hope that at least one will develop into a full-term baby. IVF is most often successful if three fertilized eggs are inserted into the uterus; however, implanting several embryos increases the chance of twins and multiple births, should gestation of more than one proceed to term.

Before entering an IVF program women must undergo a "scout laparoscopy"—the ovaries are examined (via a viewing tube inserted through a tiny cut in the umbilicus) to make sure that eggs can easily be harvested. If for any reason the ovaries are inaccessible, the couple is refused entry into the IVF program. While some centers limit the number of tries at test-tube fertilization to 5 times per couple, others allow unlimited attempts.

Progress in laser methods to unblock Fallopian tubes may reverse female infertility, and for male-factor infertility (more common than hitherto suspected) new methods can improve sperm quality, separate healthy from defective or sluggish sperm and increase chances that one will penetrate the egg. A recently developed technology—intercytoplasmic injection, or ICSI—assists men with very low sperm counts or sperm with faulty heads (that can't penetrate the egg) by injecting a single good sperm directly into a healthy egg. The process is guided under a microscope to make sure the sperm enters the right spot in the egg to stimulate cell division and produce a 4-celled embryo, which is put back in the woman's uterus via her cervix.

Other research to improve IVF success is looking for ways to select embryos likely to implant in the uterus and to freeze spare embryos for another try. Researchers are also investigating "embryo suicide" (fragmentation), perhaps due to some chromosome flaw or an environmental agent. Freezing embryos raises thorny ethical and legal issues about unused embryos, especially their donation to another infertile couple.

PREGNANCY IN THE OVER-THIRTIES

The number of women having a first baby after age 30 has been steadily climbing in Western nations. Some studies suggest that older women are at above-average risk of problems such as miscarriage, premature birth or low-birthweight babies. Others find few extra risks in delaying pregnancy until age 30–35 or later. Some risks may be due to pre-existing disorders such as high blood pressure or a tendency to diabetes. New reports find reassuringly little evidence of increased risks of low-birthweight or premature babies in women who start a family after age 30. One study from New York's Mount Sinai School of Medicine, which followed almost 4,000 first-time pregnancies, found mothers over age 30 no likelier to deliver prematurely or have a stillbirth than younger first-time mothers. Mothers over age 35 had only slightly higher risks of producing low-birth-weight or premature babies.

Nonetheless, while mothers-to-be in their thirties are usually more ready for responsibility and more health-conscious than younger mothers, they face above-average risks of bearing babies with genetic abnormalities. The risks of bearing a baby with a chromosomal aberration (especially Down syndrome) increase dramatically after age 35. The risk of having a baby affected by Down at age 20 is 1 in 1,667 , rising at age 30 to 1 in 952, to 1 in 378 at age 35, and 1 in 106 by age 40. The risks for a woman at 40 of having a baby with any chromosomal abnormality are 1 in 66, versus 1 in 526 for the 20-year-old.

Overall, healthy women attempting a first

MODERN METHODS HELP SOME INFERTILE COUPLES

Many new centers within large hospitals specialize in treating infertility with a variety of methods:
- Ovulation may be induced by means of hormonal agents such as clomiphene, Pergonal and others.
- Tubal micro-surgery—performed under a special operating microscope, sometimes with lasers to vaporize scar tissue and adhesions—may clear or repair blocked or injured Fallopian tubes. Surgery on Fallopian tubes, which are as fine as Saran wrap, is laborious, often requiring repeat operations.
- Artificial insemina-

tion (AI) uses a syringe to insert the habitual mate's seminal fluid (or that of a donor) near to the woman's cervix at ovulation time.
- Intrauterine insemination (IUI), an offshoot of AI, uses washed, concentrated sperm—from the habitual mate or an anonymous donor—inserted right into the uterine cavity.
- Sperm-cleansing can improve sperm numbers and quality by repeated washing and centrifuging to sift out dead and defective sperm, concentrating the "best of a bad lot."
- Intercytoplasmic

sperm injection or ICSI, to insert one good sperm into a "perfect" egg by micromanipulation.
- Surrogate motherhood—rarely done through infertility clinics—involves insemination of a fertile woman other than the habitual partner with the chosen man's sperm, or transplantation of a test-tube-fertilized embryo into her womb. This surrogate (substitute) mother then carries the baby to term (a procedure fraught with ethical dilemmas and possible parenthood disputes!).

MODERN "WINDOWS" INTO THE WOMB

In the past few decades, advances such as ultrasound and fetoscopy (use of a miniature waterproof camera) have allowed scientists to peer into the uterine world to see the unborn child and check whether it has certain defects.

Ultrasound monitoring is now offered almost routinely by many pregnancy caregivers—at around 18 to 20 weeks of gestation. Ultrasound techniques bounce high-frequency sound waves off tissues in the mother's abdomen to produce an image on a TV screen that reveals the baby's shape, size and movements. Ultrasound can also detect certain abnormalities, such as retarded intrauterine growth (shown by a disproportionately small body size when growth is delayed), extra digits, missing limbs, a cleft palate, certain heart flaws, an incomplete skull (anencephaly), perhaps also other neural tube disorders such as an unfused spine (spina bifida) and new markers for Down syndrome. In fact, early first trimester ultrasound is a significant contributor to newer noninvasive methods for detecting Down syndrome. It also shows the baby's position—correctly head first (vertex), feet or buttocks first (breech) or sideways across the womb (transverse lie). Ultrasound also gives clues to fetal age, helps to estimate the due date and identifies multiple pregnancies. Combined with pregnancy genetic screening, a normal, routine 18- to 20-week ultrasound may actually reduces the previously estimated risk of genetic abnormality by a further percentage.

Besides giving the clinician some valuable information, the ultrasound exam can reassure parents (as is mostly the case) that the baby's major parts and organs are developing normally (But ultrasound doesn't pick up minor abnormalities.) Glimpsing their baby on the ultrasound screen, watching it kick and even suck its thumb, months before birth, sometimes gives parents an added sense of reality about the expected child. It can also persuade the smoking mother of a growth-retarded fetus to quit.

However, given that ultrasound is expensive and that although there are no known risks at present, fetal risks are unknown, there is disagreement about its use for routine screening of normal, low-risk pregnancies. Although tests are

pregnancy after age 30 have an excellent chance of producing a healthy baby. Although rates of successful conception declines as women age, even women in their early forties can still bear healthy babies, provided they take some simple precautions, seek professional advice and get regular pregnancy care. But it's wise to embark on pregnancy before age 40, since fertility declines quickly thereafter and the chance of fetal abnormalities increases. Childbearers of advancing years might consider being tested to see whether the fetus they are carrying has Down syndrome or other congenital problems. The tests are done by ultrasound, amniocentesis, chorionic villus (placenta blood) sampling and other methods (described below). It is salutary to remember that timing of childbirth is often not something within our control for overlapping reasons, such as lack of partner, career factors, infertility and personal issues in either partner. While the "medical" advice would be to start having children early, those who start late need to know the risks without being criticized or faulted for delaying.

typically given just once in pregnancy, they can be used more often. Any problems that arise in pregnancy (vaginal bleeding, unsure dates, etc.) usually elicit another ultrasound to reassure both caregiver and parent. Reviews of the literature indicate there is "fair evidence"—reasonable but not strong evidence—in favor of a single ultrasound test during the second trimester. Studies show that routine ultrasound at this time decreases the need for inducing post-term (late-going-to-labor) pregnancies, helps to diagnose multiple pregnancies, decreases the number of low birth weight babies and increases the number of pregnancies terminated because of chromosomal abnormalities. Whether any of this has proven to be a benefit for mother or baby remains controversial. The task force did not recommend routine, serial, repeat ultrasound examinations for all pregnant women, as the evidence of its benefits is not indisputably clear.

Amniocentesis, a test that can be done as early as 13 to 16 weeks of gestation, can detect many fetal abnormalities such as Down syndrome ("trisomy 21"), neural tube defects and many genetic (DNA) disorders such as sickle cell anemia and cystic fibrosis. If amniocentesis shows the baby has a genetic flaw, the pregnancy can be terminated, should the parents so decide. A little amniotic fluid is withdrawn from around the fetus by inserting a fine hypodermic needle into the uterus using ultrasound guidance, usually under local anesthetic. The fluid is analyzed for substances such as *alphafetoprotein* (which may indicate a baby has a neural tube defect) and the fetal cells are examined for genetic (chromosome and DNA) faults. Test results take about 3 to 4 weeks to come in. Since amniocentesis carries a 1-in-100 to 200 risk of miscarriage, it's only offered to women at above-average risk of fetal anomalies, such as those with "positive" prenatal genetic screening test, those over age 35, women who have formerly had an abnormal baby or those with known genetic defects in the family. Age 35 is chosen as the at-risk cut-off as it is the age at which the risk of detecting a genetic abnormality equals the risk of adverse outcome by amniocentesis.

Chorionic villus sampling (CVS), a newer and more specialized technique for detecting chromosomal and other fetal defects, is done at 9 to 12 weeks of gestation and offered to women over age 37. It involves taking small blood and tissue samples from the fetal side of the placenta—the *chorionic villi*—through the vagina or abdomen, via a tiny guided needle. Test results take about 21 days to come in, which allows earlier termination of pregnancy than after amniocentesis, for those who wish it. Risks of abortion due to CVS are double those for amniocentesis (i.e., about 1 per 100).

First trimester and integrated prenatal screening programs are available in some provinces. These combine the use of an early ultrasound between 11 and 14 weeks to look at the thickness of the baby's neck (the nuchal translucency) with blood markers (e.g., pregnancy-associated plasma protein). *The triple screen or maternal serum screening* test (MSS) is done on maternal blood at 15–17 weeks of gestation. Available since 1993, this blood test has replaced the previous alphafetoprotein test and screens simultaneously for alphafetoprotein (AFP), *estriol* (E3) and *human chorionic gonadotropin* (HCG), looking primarily for Down syndrome and neural tube defects. Current recommendations are that it be offered to all pregnant women. Like many genetic tests, the answers do not come back in black and white terms ("your child certainly will or will not have this disease"), but rather as an expression of risk. The risk for a condition like Down syndrome is often expressed as risk compared to other women who are the same age as the mother being tested. This can be confusing because a "positive" test, when the risk is above average for an age-matched woman, can actually present an overall risk that is still quite low. For example, the average risk for bearing a baby with Down syndrome for a woman of 37 may be 1 in 250, but her personal risk from the test may indicate a risk of 1 in 200. The test is "positive" (more than 1 in 250) but her risk is still very low. It can be calming if the woman's test is normal, or anxiety-provoking if it is "positive," —especially for people who prefer "black-and-white," "yes-or-no" answers rather than "risk-estimate" values.

Genetic screening from blood tests; either

first trimester screening, integrated prenatal screenings, or an MSS blood test can avoid the need for a woman to undergo the riskier amniocentesis; in fact, women may choose *not* to undergo amniocentesis if the triple screen test suggests a low risk of fetal abnormalities. However, this advantage is somewhat offset by the large number of false positives given by the triple screen, which may suggest defects where none exist, perhaps followed by termination of a normal pregnancy or necessitating an amniocentesis to confirm a possible fetal defect. Finally, it may be helpful for expectant parents to consider what they would do if they did have a positive test. If the answer is "nothing, but I would like to know," then it helps to put the results in perspective, especially further testing that would put the fetus at risk. If the answer is "nothing," then these people might not even bother to have the test.

Mothers-to-be can help to check fetal vigour by counting the baby's kicks in the last trimester for instance noting the usual 4–6 kicks per hour after supper. Although controversial, the method may help to monitor fetal well-being. Should the fetal activity diminish, expectant mothers can alert the physician. Pregnant women should also report any noticed changes in themselves—especially possible danger signs such as dizziness, blackouts, headaches, severe back pain, unusual swelling, early rupture of the bag of waters or bleeding.

THE COURSE AND CARE OF PREGNANCY

Normal human gestation (growth of a baby within the uterus) lasts about 266 days (9 months or 39 weeks) from conception. During the embryonic stage, spanning the first 8 weeks, most miniature organ systems are laid down, including brain, heart, liver lungs, limbs and digestive tract. In the fetal stage, which follows and lasts until birth, the development of organs is completed in preparation for life outside the mother's uterus. While birth can happen at any point during fetal life, it is safest at or near term, after 9 full months of development have made the baby ready to face the outside world and obtain oxygen by breathing air rather than absorbing it from the mother's blood supply.

While a fetus may survive if born prematurely or at below-average weight, "preemies" and low-birthweight babies do not usually thrive as well as full-term, full-weight newborns.

Pregnancy is traditionally divided into three trimesters, each roughly 3 months. The expected time of birth, or "due date," can be calculated from the last menstrual period using various formulae. It's generally estimated as 280 days from the first day of the mother's last menstrual period or 266 days from the day of fertilization (assuming normal menstrual cycles with mid-cycle ovulation). Another strategy is adding 1 year and 7 days to the date when the last menstrual period began and subtracting 3 months from the total. But due dates are notoriously misjudged. Although 90 percent of babies are born within 10 to 15 days of the estimated date, many arrive earlier or later.

A woman with a first pregnancy is called a primigravida, those with subsequent pregnancies multigravida. The risks of toxemia of pregnancy (a metabolic disturbance with symptoms such as face swelling, swollen limbs and raised blood pressure)—now often called "eclampsia"—are highest in first pregnancies and those of very young (especially teen) mothers. Bleeding problems tend to increase after three or more pregnancies, or in women over age 35. Miscarriages or spontaneous abortions may occur for no known reason among fetuses below 500 g (18 oz), and are more frequent among older women than among women aged 20 to 30. The expected rate of miscarriage is approximately 1 in 5. In fact, according to some specialists, the number may be higher as many fetuses are naturally lost because of faulty chromosomes or other flaws within the first 2 months after conception, often without a woman ever suspecting she has conceived.

Choosing "caregivers" for pregnancy and birth

Pregnant women become prey to all sorts of fears, from "Will eating tomatoes cause birthmarks?" (it won't) to other food worries, distrust of environmental chemicals, apprehension over the pain of childbirth or the use of anesthetics, ambivalence over the pregnancy, fears of being an incapable parent, apprehension about coping with the stress of pregnancy and a new baby—the list goes on and on.

Therefore, the pregnant woman is well advised to seek a really empathetic caregiver for support during pregnancy and birth—the family physician, nurse, midwife or obstetrician who can best reassure and help her and her partner cope with the changes of pregnancy, both physical and emotional. It is best to choose a caregiver who welcomes questions and encourages her to express concerns, and with whom she feels free to discuss any worries, no matter how trivial or bizarre—from heartburn to backache to fears of infanticide. Trusting relationships and good communication with the pregnancy-care team can help to achieve a safe and satisfying pregnancy and birth experience.

Prenatal care

The best present parents can give their baby is their own good health. As one expert puts it, "What women want during pregnancy, birth and lactation is not intensive care but an intensely caring situation." Woman need all the support and encouragement they can get at this time. Until a few decades ago, neither expectant mothers nor their caregivers paid much attention to the pre-birth period. The fetus was not monitored or checked and no one thought much about its development inside the uterus, all eyes being focused on the birth itself Today, care of *both* mother and developing fetus is considered crucial in anticipating and forestalling risks. "Windows into the womb" (such as ultrasound and amniotic fluid sampling) can help parents-to-be and their caregivers chart the unborn baby's progress and detect some abnormalities. But all the tests women now undergo can instill anxiety and worry while awaiting the results. All the more reason why they need reassurance and support.

A "birth plan" suits many

A "birth plan" agreed on ahead of time with the pregnancy-care team can help a couple get the conditions they want for labor and birth. "It's not a contract or a written declaration of expected rights," says a maternity care specialist at the McMaster Medical Centre, "but a flexible plan, worked out together with the support team, stating preferences for the atmosphere and conduct a couple would like for the birth of their baby. Informed decisions are the basis of good maternity care, and health professionals should share their knowledge with parents-to-be, so they can make wise choices."

Obstetricians at the McMaster Medical Centre suggest that women "interview their intended physician(s) or other caregivers, enquire tactfully about their attitudes to weight gain, childbirth education and birthing procedures (pre-birth shaves, enemas, inductions or whatever else concerns them)." They might ask how many Cesareans the physician or clinic performs, whether they encourage vaginal births after Cesareans, how much they promote breastfeeding and so on. They can also enquire about the birthing-room or ward and nursery policies and ask whether the father (or another relative or friend) can be present at delivery.

Valmai Elkins, a Montreal physiotherapist, childbirth educator and author of *The Rights of the Pregnant Parent*, suggests that women state their wishes well ahead of labor to make sure they won't be "promised one type of birth but be given another." She also advises a pre-birth tour of the hospital facilities (now routine in many centers) to become familiar with the setting and avoid being intimidated later on.

Monitoring the pregnancy

Monitoring pregnancy means regular prenatal visits to keep tabs on mother's and baby's progress. Ideally, every woman should be seen within the first 12 weeks of pregnancy to thoroughly evaluate her condition and compare it with later changes. Women with normal pregnancies are seen every 4–6 weeks, then fortnightly and weekly toward the end of gestation.

"The first prenatal visit," notes one University of Toronto obstetrician, "helps to date the baby's age, vital for correct care, and allows testing for any disorders present in the mother." At the first visit, the caregiver notes the woman's feelings and observations about her pregnancy, takes a detailed history about her background, including any illnesses and previous pregnancies. Tests are done for hemoglobin levels (to check for anemia and iron status), urinary-tract and other infections such as hepatitis B, syphilis, HIV, gonorrhea, chlamydia and others. Some infections such as rubella, syphilis, HIV, and toxoplasmosis—can seriously endanger the baby and call for protective measures or perhaps a Cesarean birth (as for women with active genital herpes). To avoid the risks of toxoplasmosis—an infection due to organisms often carried in cat feces and raw meat that can cause fetal malformation—women are advised not to change the cat litter or eat underdone meat.

At subsequent prenatal visits, the caregiver evaluates fetal growth by assessing uterus size, felt by hand and measured with a tape. At each visit, weight is checked, blood pressure taken and urine tested for protein and glucose. Besides physical evaluation of the mother and baby, the parent's emotional and psychological well-being are discussed.

Blood samples are usually examined at the first visit and again at weeks 16 and 26–28 to screen for gestational diabetes, anemia and Rh blood problems. Samples are sometimes also examined in between, for example, to check for maternal alphafetoprotein, which may suggest the presence of neural tube abnormalities. (Neural tube defects are higher in those with a previously affected child or relatives who had the disorder and in women with insulin-dependent diabetes.)

CHOICE OF BIRTHPLACE AND BIRTH ASSISTANT

The choice of birthplace in Canada is limited, but there are now proposals for free-standing birthing centers with a less clinical atmosphere than hospitals, but with all emergency procedures available in case of need. Some women still opt for a home birth attended by a midwife and physician, but most physicians prefer hospital delivery because of back-up in case of unforeseeable complications, such as sudden hemorrhaging or "failure to progress" (a sluggish labor). Nonetheless, those who opt for home birth can rest assured that midwives carry emergency equipment and will arrange transfer to hospital in case of need.

Many sites are seeking a middle ground as they make birthing centers much more "home-like." Some hospitals have set up birth units that simulate a home environment—with cosy decor soft music, even a rocking chair—and the full range of emergency technology available close by. In many hospitals, childbirth positions are now optional. The flat-on-the-back delivery position is uncomfortable—with the mother working to push the baby out uphill, against gravity. Mothers are encouraged to give birth in any position they like—sitting, squatting or lying sideways—as in many primitive societies. Walkabouts during first-stage labor—another aid to uterine contractions—are promoted in most birth units, routine pubic-hair shaves are only done in some; intravenous systems (for medication or feeding if needed) are no longer routinely set up. Mothers are given mirrors to let them view the birth.

Women are now being discharged as early as 12 to 48 hours after birth, if all goes well, from many centers. Shorter maternity stays reduce the risks of hospital infection, enhance family closeness and are also cheaper. But the downside is that women now leave the hospital without having learned enough about newborn care and breastfeeding techniques.

The debate over home vs. hospital births
Home birth remains an emotional and controversial issue, discouraged by the Canadian Medical Association, the Canadian Society of Obstetrics and Gynecology and equivalent agencies in many other countries. The argument against home birth is that it may subject mother and/or baby to avoidable risks and that even in a seemingly healthy, normal pregnancy things can go wrong at the last minute, necessitating a Cesarean section or other medical procedure. However, research shows that most emergency birthing situations can be predicted ahead and that a well-trained birth assistant can handle most emergencies at home or transfer to hospital in ample time to avoid risks to baby or mother.

Since the 1930s, home births have dwindled in most industrialized countries and "safety" has become almost synonymous with hospital birth. Statistics show that in Canada only 0.9 percent of women gave birth at home in 1989 (some unplanned), compared with virtually none in the United States, 35.5 percent in Holland and 1.7 percent in Britain. (However, in the United States there are many free-standing birth centers for women, as an alternative to hospital deliveries.) Home births in Canada were attended almost solely by midwives and a handful of physicians willing to assist. In Canada, many branches of the College of Physicians and Surgeons forbid physicians to attend home births because of "unnecessary risks to mother and infant." The success of the Dutch model, in which healthy, nonrisk mothers can opt for either home or hospital birth, depends critically on a view of birth as a normal physiological process that goes at its own pace and requires as little interference as possible. But it requires scrupulous prenatal screening and careful selection of women who are suitable for home birth.

The debate on home versus hospital births still centers on safety issues—especially as a number of women with low-risk pregnancies who opt for home birth have to be transferred to hospital because of unforeseen emergencies such as hemorrhage, unsuspected breech position, abnormal fetal heartbeat, prolonged or nonprogressing second-stage labor or a retained placenta.

One study of over 1,000 planned home births in Toronto between 1983 and 1988 found that 83 percent proceeded normally, 17 percent required transfer to hospital and 2 infants died. These figures are similar to those found in hospital births. The study found the transfer rate of planned home births to hospital 3 times higher in first-time (primipara) pregnancies than in subsequent ones. Several other studies report that home births result in fewer medical interventions—such as forceps deliveries, episiotomies, induced labor or Cesareans—than hospital births. It also appears that there are no more life-threatening emergencies than in hospital for normal, low-risk pregnancies. (More research is needed into the real risks.)

At a pregnancy-care conference in England during the late 1980s, a statistician from Nottingham University declared that "in Britain, for the 90 percent of normal, uncomplicated labors, large hospitals are the least safe places of birth, with an increased incidence of jaundice, forceps deliveries and asphyxia (from labor drugs like Demerol), and certainly less safe than small maternity units staffed by general practitioners and midwives." Another British survey concluded that the setting, environment and type of obstetric care greatly influence birth outcomes and that the "spillover of medical knowledge to the home setting may be the best situation for normal pregnancies at no anticipated risk, while hospital delivery best suits pregnancies at known risk."

The recent move to reinstate midwives in some provinces as active partners in maternity healthcare is a welcome step. In 1991, for instance, a report by the government of Alberta concluded that low-risk women may be allowed to give birth at home, accompanied by the midwife, and perhaps also the physician. There are now training centers all over Canada. With the comeback of midwives in Canada, home births may become a better-regulated and safer option, and some health authorities are considering the possibility of making arrangements for quicker transfer to hospital of home-birth babies or mothers in case of need.

THE ROLE OF MIDWIVES

Midwives have an ancient tradition of providing personalized, ongoing prenatal care through pregnancy, offering education and training for labor assisting at the birth (in former times often without a physician's help) and coming in afterward to help the mother and newborn for up to 6 weeks.

The philosophy behind midwifery is that pregnancy and childbirth are natural, healthy processes that can be facilitated by midwifery skills, and that women have a right to make choices about how and where they give birth. As defined by the World Health Organization, midwives are qualified to provide the necessary care and advice throughout pregnancy, labor and the *puerperium* (immediate post-birth period) and to conduct normal, low-risk deliveries on their own. Midwives help women and their families enjoy birth with as little intervention as possible. Their approach is client-centered and nonauthoritarian.

Part of midwives' jobs is to spot warning signs and identify women who might develop problems (such as those who are obese, have high blood pressure or have had difficult deliveries in the past), or refer those who have a troublesome labor for further consultation with a physician or at a specialized obstetric unit. Their care includes the detection of abnormal conditions in mother and child, noticing if labor fails to progress normally, getting medical assistance if needed and executing emergency measures in the absence of medical help.

Midwifery making a comeback in Canada

Despite a time-honored tradition as pregnancy and birth attendants, midwives were largely displaced by physicians during the past few decades in Canada, the United States and many other Western countries. With the medicalization of many birth procedures, midwives had no official status or legal place in the healthcare system.

Fortunately, this attitude is changing, and midwives are regaining their rightful place in

maternity care on this continent and achieving official status, so midwifery is a burgeoning profession. Prompted by the efforts of midwives themselves and by public interest, several provinces initiated legislation—amid considerable controversy—to bring midwives under formal regulation and designate them as primary caregivers in maternity care with hospital admitting privileges.

In 1993, Ontario legislation permitted the establishment of Canada's first College of Midwives to license *registered* midwives to practice autonomously and attend births in hospital (or at home) under the Canadian healthcare system. The college is a regulatory body that regulates, licenses and organizes the training of midwives (with a 4-year B.Sc. course). Currently

TRACKING FETAL GROWTH AND DEVELOPMENT

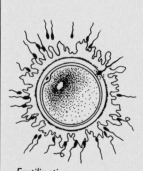
Fertilization (Conception)

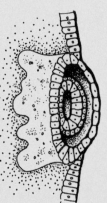

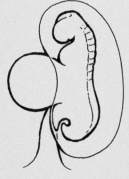

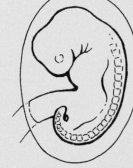

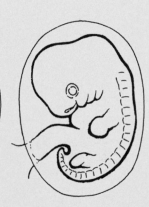

———————————————— EMBRYONIC STAGE ————————————————

WEEK 1
• fertilized egg moves along Fallopian tube toward uterus, dividing as it goes
• 46 chromosomes are copied into every new cell (except the future egg and sperm cells), giving the future child its inherited characteristics

WEEK 2
• fertilized egg attaches to uterine wall
• placenta begins to form

WEEK 3
• blood system laid down
• membranes and bag of waters begins to form around embryo

WEEK 4
• placenta formed
• heart begins beating
• backbone, spinal cord and brain forming
• digestive system forming

WEEKS 5–7
• testes form in males and start to secrete testosterone (male hormone); future sperm ("germ") cells set aside with chromosome number halved (to 23 per sperm)
• limb-buds being shaped and muscles forming by week 6
• 4 chambers formed in heart by week 7

NOTE: Normal human gestation (growth of fetus in the uterus) lasts about 266 days (39–40 weeks) from conception. The "due date" is 266 days from the day of fertilization (or 280 days from the first day of the mother's last period). About 90 percent of babies are born within 10–14 days of the estimated due date but some are "premature" (born before 36 weeks gestation), some are "postmature" (born after 42 weeks gestation).

about 20 to 30 qualify each year in Ontario. The new regulations allow registered midwives to practice and attend births in hospitals, clinics, domiciliary (home) conditions or in any other service, according to the woman's choice and risk status. Midwives provide hospital care together with other members of the healthcare team. If a woman chooses midwifery care she will be seen by her midwife for prenatal visits, and the midwife will arrange for laboratory testing and consultation with specialists if needed. Spontaneous (normal) vaginal birth can be attended by the midwife, who will examine the newborn and provide care for up to 6 weeks postpartum for baby and mother.

The British Columbia College of Midwives, established in 1998, also registers midwives to practice under the Canadian healthcare system. Manitoba has a new Midwifery Act that will license midwives as primary healthcare providers. (Other provinces are working toward full legal status for midwives.)

In the U.S., the system varies widely from state to state, some permitting only "nurse midwives" (trained nurses) to practice, others allowing midwives to practice without any standardized regulations.

For more information, contact the Association of Midwives: (416) 481-2811; the Ontario College of Midwives: (416) 327-0874; the British Columbia College of Midwives: (604) 875-3580; the American College of Nurse Midwives: (202) 728-9860; or the Midwives Alliance of North America: (316) 283-4543.

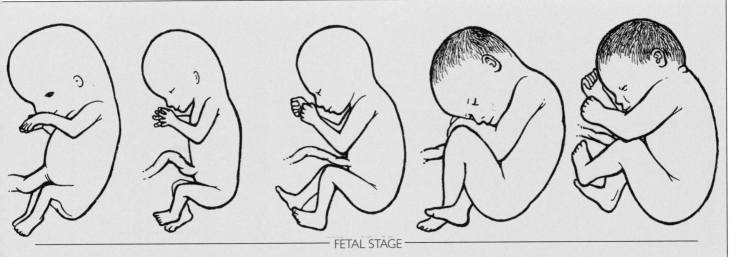

FETAL STAGE

WEEK 8
- facial features and teeth forming
- limbs taking shape
- fingers and toes forming
- long bones and internal organs developing

WEEK 12
- fetal heartbeat may be heard
- eyes almost fully developed; ears ready
- tooth buds forming
- nails present
- ovaries forming in females and future "eggs" set aside with half chromosome number (23) per egg

WEEK 16
- most bones formed
- muscles active
- facial features better defined
- external genitalia formed in males and females
- "quickening"—fetal movements—may first be noticed around week 18–20

WEEKS 20–36
- survival possible outside womb after 24–26 weeks
- baby can be clearly felt moving
- head proportions more balanced
- bones and limbs elongate
- lungs still immature, lacking surfactant

WEEKS 37–40
- baby moves down into birth position (usually head down)
- baby gains weight fast as fat deposits accumulate
- lungs mature
- hair soft and downy
- "full-term" birth is at 37 or more weeks, "premature" before 36 weeks gestation

CHANGES IN THE MOTHER'S BODY DURING PREGNANCY

Female hormones maintain the conditions needed for the developing fetus. Progesterone is first secreted by the ovary, later in large quantities by the placenta. Hormones stimulate development of the mammary glands: breasts swell, the areolae (nipple areas) increase in size and nipples protrude. Some troublesome symptoms are common at the start of pregnancy—morning sickness, heartburn, dizziness and weariness—but these tend to disappear by the fourth month. After that, many pregnant women feel amazingly energetic, often right up to the start of labor.

The cardiovascular system changes in response to the call for a larger blood supply with an increase in blood volume. Blood pressure usually decreases during the first 2 trimesters of pregnancy, returning to normal during the third. Varicose veins are quite common because of hormonal effects on blood-vessel walls, and because the expanded uterus depresses the venous blood return. As diaphragm movement is somewhat restricted, the ribcage tends to flare out, not always returning to its normal position after the birth. Late in pregnancy, breathing may become shallower and more frequent as the lungs become somewhat restricted.

The muscles of the gastrointestinal tract tend to become less contractile, with slow stomach emptying, sometimes resulting in heartburn and constipation. Urination becomes more frequent as the enlarging uterus presses on the bladder.

Other changes may include increased pigmentation on the face, known as chloasma; stretch marks on the abdomen; and changes in posture that may cause leg and back pain.

As the neck of the uterus softens—an early sign of pregnancy that may be detected by the examining physician—and as the uterus expands, it also rises, reaching the level of the navel about the middle of the fourth month. By the end of the pregnancy, the uterus has expanded to about 36 cm (15 in) above the pubis.

Fetal activity may begin as early as the 10th week of gestation, but it's not usually noticed until 18–20 weeks into pregnancy (even later with firstborns). By that time, the developing fetus is a lively little entity that moves around in its increasingly confined space and responds to loud sounds. "Quickening," the first sign of fetal movement, is usually felt around the fifth month, and often described as being like "the fluttering of a tiny bird." It's sometimes so faint that a mother wonders whether her unborn baby really moved. Unborn babies have rest periods alternating with times of vigorous action when arms flail, legs kick and the body bends and arches. The movements are more discernible when the mother is relaxed. The fetal kicks continue on and off throughout the rest of pregnancy. If they diminish markedly in late pregnancy, it may be a sign of fetal trouble, and should be reported to the caregivers.

CHARTING FETAL PROGRESS

About 4 weeks after conception, when the embryo is only 4 mm (1/6 of an inch) long, the tubelike heart begins to beat. At 5 to 6 weeks postconception, arms and legs are mere fingerless buds, becoming paws around the eighth week. By 12 weeks, the fingers can grasp objects, and the fetus can suck its toes, grimace, frown and press its lips together. By this time it's also swallowing and urinating amniotic fluid. The "hairy ape" stage of fetal development refers to a stage when the unborn's body is temporarily covered with hair. Strangely, the very first fetal hair grows in as coarse bristles, particularly on the eyebrows, lips and even the palms of the hands and soles of the feet. This primary hair is soon replaced by a soft down all over the body, called lanugo, shed just before term. Most newborns have scanty hair although some premature babies may still be downy all over. The fetal body is also covered with vernix, a thick, waxy coat—especially thick on the scalp and eyebrows—that protects the delicate skin from being chapped by the salty amniotic waters.

By the fourth to fifth month of pregnancy, the fetus wriggles within its cramped quarters, turns somersaults, and flexes and stretches its limbs—movements that feel like butterfly wings within the mother's belly. It reacts to the mother's movements and outside sounds—perhaps remaining inactive while gently rocked, or jerking sharply in response to loud bangs. Its responses to sound are measurable by changes in heartrate and body movements. A microphone inserted into the uterus shows the dominant sounds to be the mother's digestive noises and the steady beat of her heart; no doubt this is why some mothers report that holding an infant over the left breast calms it. Machines that mimic a human heartbeat (at about 60–80 beats a minute), or the tick of a grandfather clock, can also soothe fussy babies, and some hospital baby-care units use heartbeat machines to comfort preemies. But while some parents believe that reciting Blake or playing Mozart to an unborn child can shape its personality, most experts consider this a far-fetched notion.

At 22 to 26 weeks of growth the fetus is wrinkled, because the skin lacks fat under its surface layer. At this stage the genes that regulate liver function, respiration and digestion may not yet be fully "turned on," one crucial reason why babies born before 26 weeks have a tough time surviving. By 29 weeks, fat, an enormous safeguard for newborn well-being, is laid down. Fetal fat stores nourish the newborn during its critical transition from the womb to the exterior world. Brown adipose fat, a unique fetal feature, is deposited around the kidneys and in the neck. A rapid heat-producer brown fat warms the tiny newborn body, which cannot yet shiver to create heat.

Most babies are born at "term"—between 39 to 41 weeks of gestation—but some are born prematurely (before completing 37 weeks of development) and some late, after 42 weeks of gestation, as "post-term" or "postmature" babies.

NUTRITION IN PREGNANCY

While no one can choose a baby's eye or hair color eating well and gaining adequate weight can increase the chances of giving birth to a healthy, full-weight baby. An infant's birthweight is often linked to the mother's weight gain during pregnancy. In general, heavier newborns thrive better are more resistant to infection and have fewer risks of illness than small newborns (who weigh under 6 pounds at birth). Maternal weight gain in pregnancy is very variable, but should ideally be 11 to 16 kg (25 to 35 lb) to

produce a baby weighing 7.5 to 8 pounds. "Yet," comments one health consultant at Toronto's Department of Public Health, "many women still worry about gaining too much and go on diets that could harm their babies." An overweight woman should wait until after the birth to reduce, since dieting during pregnancy may release toxins that could harm the fetus. Those who are underweight at the start of pregnancy may need to put on as much as 18 kg (40 lb). Pregnant teenagers, still growing themselves, have particular nutrient needs.

Expectant mothers may gain weight steadily, but caregivers must be alert to any sudden spurts, which may herald unhealthy fluid retention or the onset of pre-eclampsia (characterized by elevated blood pressure and swelling of the face, hands and feet). The rate of gain varies from woman to woman, and is about 0.9 to 1.8 kg (2 to 4 lb) in the first 12 weeks of gestation, then roughly 0.5 kg (1 lb) a week to about 4.5 kg (10 lb) extra by the 20th week of gestation, 9 kg (20 lb) by 30 weeks, to a total of 11 to 16 kg (25 to 35 lb) by term (39 to 41 weeks). At first, the weight gain is mostly in the mother's body—putting on extra fat and breast tissue, increasing maternal blood volume, enlarging the uterus and filling it with fluid. The later weight gain is largely in the unborn child and the placenta.

A well-balanced diet of fresh foods that includes enough protein and overall calories (about 1,800 to 2,500 a day by mid-pregnancy) and adequate vitamins and minerals, with special attention to iron, salt and calcium, is advised. Protein is a crucial nutrient for healthy fetal development, and is also needed for the mother's increased blood volume. About 75 to 80 grams of protein a day is recommended, an increase of about 50 percent above average intakes, or one extra 30-gram serving of protein in the form of meat, fish, poultry, eggs, cheeses, nuts or legumes.

Iron is essential to both mother and baby for the manufacture of hemoglobin (the red pigment in blood that carries oxygen to tissues). Liver, red meat and dried beans are good natural iron sources. While most women in developed countries who eat a well-balanced diet get ample iron, many physicians recommend a daily

EATING PLENTY OF FOLIC ACID CAN PREVENT NEURAL TUBE DEFECTS

Neural tube defects (NTDs) such as spina bifida and anencephaly occur when the spinal cord fails to close properly, or part of the brain doesn't develop. These defects arise very early in fetal growth—in the third or fourth week after conception—when the woman may not even realize she's pregnant. Approximately 1 per 1,000 births involve a neural tube defect. (Anencephalic infants usually die soon after birth.) Consuming enough folate (600 micrograms per day) at least 3 months before and during pregnancy can help offset the risk of these birth defects.

iron supplement from mid-pregnancy on, especially for anemic women.

A diet that includes meat contains enough natural salt (sodium) without adding any when cooking or at the table. But salt should not be excluded from the diet except on medical advice, since sodium is vital for the growing baby and the mother's extra blood volume.

Calcium is essential for the developing baby's bones and tooth buds, and for efficient nerve and muscle function. A low-calcium diet may permit calcium to leach out of the mother's bones. Three or 4 cups of milk a day—or the equivalent in other dairy products (yogurt, cottage cheese)—should provide the needed daily 1.2 grams. Nondairy sources of calcium are broccoli, dried beans, canned salmon and some grains.

To reduce the risk of neural tube defects and certain anemias, women who might conceive or who are already pregnant need extra folic acid (Folacin)—600 micrograms a day. Experts recommend that besides the amount they get naturally from a varied diet, women who might become or are pregnant should take 400 micrograms of folic acid daily, either from fortified foods or a supplement. The new dietary guidelines also specify a safe upper limit for folate intake at 1,000 micrograms of folic acid per day. (To prevent excess, infants and young children should only get folate from natural food sources.)

Vitamin A, the rest of the Bs, C, D and F will probably be ample in a varied diet containing fresh fruits, vegetables and fortified milk products. But pregnant vegetarians are at risk of nutritional deficiencies—especially of iron, calcium and protein—because of the sheer bulk of plant foods needed to supply adequate nutrients. Vegetarian mothers-to-be may need advice on vitamin and mineral supplements.

Medications, smoking and alcohol

Medications during pregnancy may deflect normal fetal development and produce various deformities, according to the type of medication and the amount absorbed. Many substances that get into the mother's bloodstream also cross the placenta and reach the developing baby. Once regarded as a "magic barrier" the placenta was termed a "bloody sieve" by the late Virginia Apgar, the anesthesiologist who originated the

Apgar score for rating newborn well-being. For each fetal organ—eyes, lungs, heart—there's a specific critical period when its growth can be distorted by chemicals and drugs. Some medications can be safely taken in pregnancy, and for others a substitute may be available. But many seemingly innocent medications, such as anticonvulsants, antinauseants, laxatives and cold remedies, may harm unborn babies. The greatest danger of malformation for most organs occurs during their most rapid period of growth, usually in the first 12 to 14 weeks of pregnancy. If prescription drugs are essential to control a disorder such as epilepsy or diabetes, a couple should seek medical advice before conceiving.

Smoking tobacco increases the risk of placental insufficiency and premature birth, often resulting in underweight babies. About 25 to 30 percent of pregnant women still smoke throughout their pregnancies. Approximately 80 percent of women try to quit or reduce smoking during pregnancy with only 23 percent managing to maintain their cessation over the course of the pregnancy. An additional 17 percent reduce their smoking by more than 5 cigarettes per day. Overall, most smokers continue smoking during pregnancy. Nicotine is not teratogenic and does not increase the risk of congenital defects; however, smoking causes numerous adverse fetal and neonatal (near-birth) effects on the baby. Studies show that babies born to smoking mothers are shorter than those of nonsmokers, weigh less and are more susceptible to respiratory infections after birth. As well smoking increases the risk of spontaneous miscarriage in the first trimester. There is some evidence that babies born to smoking mothers may also be more prone to hyperactivity, suffer more crib deaths (Sudden Infant Death Syndrome) and be slow learners. These studies, however, have confounding factors that influenced the results, such as socioeconomic class, parental education and passive smoking (others in the family being smokers).

Alcohol consumption, now on the rise among women, is alleged by the director of the U.S. National Institute of Alcohol Abuse and Alcoholism to be "the third leading cause of mental retardation and neurological problems in infants, also causing a roster of malformations in heart, limbs…skull, head and brain," collectively termed Fetal Alcohol Syndrome (FAS). The greatest fetal dangers from alcohol occur in the first 3 months of pregnancy. Some go so far as to claim that "the only known safe limit for alcohol in pregnancy is none." Others say that, late in pregnancy, an occasional glass of wine or beer does no harm.

Saunas are considered a "no-no" during pregnancy, and hot tub soaks are also not advised (unless the belly isn't immersed), as the heat may raise the mother's "core" temperature, alter blood flow to the fetus and possibly cause fetal damage.

Genital herpes in pregnancy

Herpes simplex viruses (HSV) can cause cold sores on or near the mouth (usually type I herpes, or HSV-1), or on the genitals (generally type II, or HSV-2). However, genital herpes can also be due to cold-sore type-1 (HSV-1) viruses, often passed on through oral sex. Typically, genital herpes appears as itchy, burning sores or blisters that ooze, crust and then heal; during an active attack in women, urination can be painful. But the infection often has no or minimal symptoms, even though those infected can transmit the viruses to others. About 20 percent of North Americans carry genital herpes viruses (often unknowingly). The infection can linger in the body, with occasional "flares"—generally milder than the first episode.

Genital herpes can endanger newborn infants, especially if the mother has herpes sores at delivery (which can infect the baby as it passes through the birth canal). Neonatal herpes is a rare but life-threatening disease that attacks the infant's throat, eyes and nervous system and can be fatal, or leave lasting effects. But the condition usually only endangers newborns if the pregnant mother has active genital herpes at the time of labor, in which case Cesarean delivery is advised.

Women with genital herpes are often very worried about the possibility of passing it on to their offspring. But the risk of transmitting genital herpes to a fetus or newborn is low in those with recurrent infections, generally posing a threat only if the mother has a fresh infection

---

SOME DIETARY TIPS DURING PREGNANCY

- **Shun junk foods—they contain calories but few valuable nutrients.**
- **Avoid alcohol, known to produce fetal deformities; malformations due to alcohol absorbed from the mother arise mostly during the first trimester of pregnancy, so alcohol is best avoided in the first half of pregnancy, and restricted to an "occasional" drink for the rest.**

- **Avoid all medications before conception and during pregnancy. Check with your doctor or other caregiver about use of any over-the-counter medications, such as antihistamines, painkillers, cough medicines and so on during pregnancy, as some can harm the developing fetus.**
- **If constipated, don't take laxatives without medical advice**

(Metamucil is considered safe). Having 15 ml (1 tbsp) of wheat bran a day may overcome the problem.
- **If nauseated with "morning sickness," try some plain dry crackers and sips of water before getting out of bed. Eat smaller meals more often throughout the day, rather than a few large ones. If nausea persists, seek medical advice.**

---

picked up late in pregnancy (or a very severe flare-up). The HSV-2 infection is transmitted to about half the babies born to mothers with a *first attack* (who don't yet have antibodies that would be passed on to and protect the newborn). While Cesarean delivery can prevent transmission during labor parents must still take care not to infect the infant later on.

To reduce the risk, mothers-to-be should tell their attending physician or midwife that they have had (or may have) genital herpes and check for signs of an outbreak (vulval itching, burning or tingling). Other measures to protect the baby are to abstain from sex with a partner who has known (or suspected) oral or genital herpes—especially in the last trimester of pregnancy—even if he has no symptoms, and to avoid oral sex if he has cold sores on the mouth. Other ways to reduce the risk are to avoid early rupture of the "waters," to shun use of fetal scalp monitors (which may pass viruses to the baby), to avert a forceps delivery if possible and to take care not to infect the infant after birth (wash hands before touching the newborn). Babies can get herpes if kissed by someone with a cold sore; so don't kiss your baby if you have a cold sore, and ask others not to.

Herpes infections are treated with acyclovir tablets (preferably at the start of an attack) for 5 to 10 days, continuing until all sores have

SCREENING FOR PSYCHOSOCIAL RISK FACTORS THAT THREATEN THE BABY

Besides physical, medical and obstetric risks, social and psychological factors can endanger a baby's future health. Caregivers looking after pregnant women are alerted to watch for certain psychosocial factors that could jeopardize fetal and newborn well-being. These include lack of social support, a shaky marriage (or partnership), a pregnancy that's unwanted (after 20 weeks into it), rigid sex-role expectations, recent life stresses, substance abuse, psychiatric disturbances (such as depression), a history of child abuse or violence in the mother or her partner, low self-esteem, a poor relationship between the expectant mother and her own parents, and failure to attend prenatal classes.

crusted over. People with many recurrences may stay on acyclovir to suppress outbreaks. Two new drugs that require less pill-taking are available, but acyclovir is recommended in pregnancy as there is more experience with this medication.

For more information, contact the CDC National STD Hotline: 1-800-227-8922, or the U.S. National Herpes Hotline: (919) 361-8488.

EXERCISE IN PREGNANCY

Many women, on becoming pregnant (particularly for the first time), wonder whether they should carry on with their exercise programs or usual sports. Provided the pregnancy is progressing without complications, normal activities need not be curtailed. Women accustomed to sporting activities (used to maintaining an exercise program for 3 months or more) can continue them. Exercise regimes should be done 3 to 5 times per week with moderate intensity for 30 to 40 minutes duration. Activities such as walking, swimming and working with aerobic gym equipment are encouraged. Exercise should be done regularly to tone the muscles—including pelvic-floor or Kegel exercises—to prepare for labor. Activities such as tennis, swimming, jogging or cycling may be continued, but moderated in late pregnancy. Some caregivers might discourage the exertion of sports that have unpredictable impact, such as downhill skiing, water skiing and horse riding, and heavy lifting is best avoided. Scuba diving is *not* recommended, as the effects of underwater pressure on the fetus have not been determined. Women who exercise during pregnancy should be aware of changes in their balance due to the altered weight distribution and center of gravity. Ligaments become slacker through hormone changes in pregnancy and relaxing hormones also increase the hypermobility (excessive moveability) at some key joints such as knees and hips.

SPOTTING HIGH-RISK PREGNANCIES

"Risk scoring" is a technique used to evaluate the progress of pregnancy with parameters that help to determine whether mother or baby is in a risk bracket that necessitates referral to a spe-

cialized unit for safer birthing. A prenatal score chart is used to plot maternal changes as they appear. According to a pediatrician at the University of Western Ontario, the method can "significantly reduce risks of physical or mental handicaps in the baby. Different risks may surface as pregnancy progresses."

Overall, about 10 percent of all pregnancies pose some danger to mother; fetus or both at labor or birth, and 70 to 80 percent of these are predictable in advance. The rest happen unexpectedly, due to unanticipated problems, such as a cervix that is sluggish and won't dilate (open), baby in an awkward position, the cord wrapped around the baby's neck, maternal hemorrhage, failure to progress, the placenta blocking the baby's passage or the baby becoming distressed by oxygen shortage. Such unexpected problems underlie the modern rationale for giving birth in specialized obstetric units or hospitals, where medical help is instantly on hand. But most problems can be spotted in plenty of time to avoid mishaps, correct them or transfer to hospital if need be.

Risk factors that are obvious ahead of time include maternal obesity, narrow pelvis, incomplete cervix, drug use, poor nutrition, previous miscarriage, previous problem labors, diabetes or other medical disorders. Additional risks may surface at different times as pregnancy advances, such as eclampsia, bleeding (perhaps from a loosening placenta), retarded fetal growth, early membrane rupture ("waters breaking") and—most feared of complications—a very premature labor.

Prematurity and low birthweight bring risks

Although premature or low-birthweight babies are more vulnerable than full-term ones, and some may have to spend time in a neonatal unit (sometimes in incubators), many survive. However, prematurity is still a leading cause of infant mortality, and a number of the preemie or low-birthweight survivors have above-average risks of health and learning problems. At present, 5 to 10 percent of live births in North America are premature, and pre-term babies have less ability to withstand temperature changes, respiratory problems and infection.

"Prematurity" is defined as birth occurring before 36 weeks of gestation and "low birthweight" as newborn weight less than 2.5 kg (5.5 lb). The more premature or underweight the newborn, the greater the risks of illness and disability. Factors that predispose to prematurity are multiple births (e.g., twins), placental failure and excess amniotic fluid.

A premature or pre-term birth, whether spontaneous or engineered by induction or early Cesarean section, removes an unfinished fetus from the womb, possibly causing danger for the infant, whose body may not have enough fat stores to bridge the gap. Fat reserves are critical to survival until the mother's milk comes in, a few days after birth. Premature babies who lack brown adipose stores have more trouble regulating their body temperature than full-term babies. The digestive system is immature and the lungs may not yet be ready to breathe air. Nevertheless, perinatal units can now save smaller and smaller babies—the cut-off point for survival currently being about 24 weeks after the last menstrual period (or 22 weeks after conception). If newborns cannot feed and swallow they may have to be fed intravenously, and if unable to control body temperature will be kept in an incubator.

Many very premature infants die of infections, respiratory distress or other problems. In one Canadian study, of 260 infants born between 23 to 28 weeks of (gestational) age, one-third couldn't survive. Those that did survive had above-average risks of physical and mental disabilities. In another study on surviving preemies born at 24 to 29 weeks of gestational development, 80 percent developed normally without handicaps, about 5 percent suffered severe disabilities (such as cerebral palsy and learning problems) and 16 percent had mild disabilities. Other studies find that 14 to 15 percent of babies born earlier than 29 weeks gestation end up mildly to severely disabled. Efforts made to avert a premature birth include bedrest and certain medications. If it can't be stopped, the mother may be given medications that stimulate rapid maturation of the fetal lungs, to facilitate newborn breathing.

Low birthweight (being "small for dates" or small for a given developmental stage)—not the same as prematurity—also puts newborns at risk of health problems. Babies that weigh 2.5 kg (5.5 lb) or less at birth—even if full-term—have fewer than average reserves with which to face life outside the uterus. The World Health Organization defines low birthweight as below 2,500 g (less than 5.5 lb) at delivery; very low birthweight as less than 2,500 g (3.3 lb). Very-low-birthweight babies are at still greater risk of infection, hearing and vision problems, and possibly learning difficulties.

PRENATAL CLASSES: PREPARING FOR LABOR

Prenatal education classes, given by childbirth educators, help women make choices and prepare for labor. They include lectures and films as well as discussion and maybe physiotherapy sessions. Prenatal childbirth classes are offered in most hospitals for parents-to-be and include training in breathing, relaxation and muscle control (or pelvic-floor exercises) for an easier labor and birth.

The Lamaze system, a well-known prenatal birth-preparation system, named after Dr.

SOME PREGNANCY AND BIRTH COMPLICATIONS

- *Placenta previa*—where a fetus sits high up in the uterine wall and the growing placenta partly or completely blocks the uterine outlet—hinders safe delivery, possibly necessitating premature induction of labor or a Cesarean.
- *Abruptio placenta*—premature detachment from the uterine wall of a normal placenta—is associated with intense pain and jeopardizing fetal well-being, necessitating a Cesarean to save a distressed fetus.

- *Pre-eclampsia and eclampsia (formerly called "toxemia")*—is a still poorly understood condition, most common in young women with a first pregnancy and in those with diabetes and/or multiple pregnancies (e.g., twins). It is signalled by rising blood pressure, swelling of feet, legs, hands and face, and protein in the urine. If not halted, preeclampsia may lead to full eclampsia, which threatens mother and fetus, possibly necessitating early delivery. The

treatment is bedrest and blood-pressure medications while watching for kidney and other problems.

- *Multiple birth (e.g., twins)*, is either "identical" (with identical genes, from one egg, fertilized by one sperm) or "fraternal" (non-identical), where two separate eggs are fertilized by two separate sperm and the twins are not necessarily "same sex" or in any way similar. About two-thirds of twins are fraternal, one-third identical.

THE THREE STAGES OF LABOR

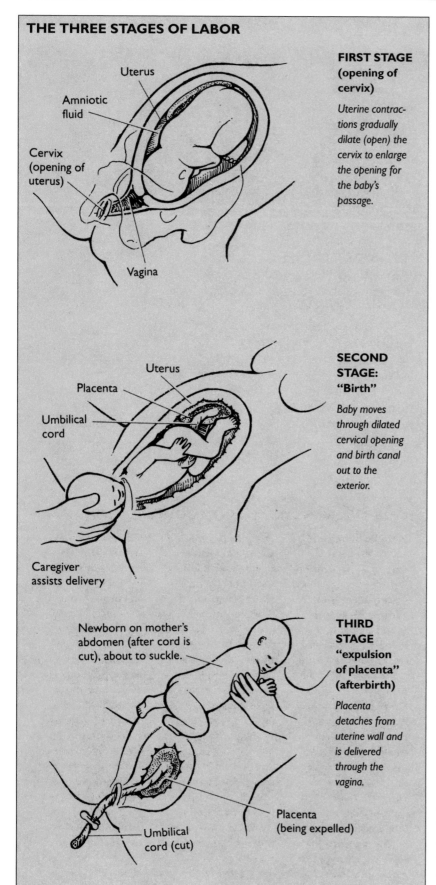

Uterus

Amniotic fluid

Cervix (opening of uterus)

Vagina

FIRST STAGE (opening of cervix)

Uterine contractions gradually dilate (open) the cervix to enlarge the opening for the baby's passage.

Uterus

Placenta

Umbilical cord

Caregiver assists delivery

SECOND STAGE: "Birth"

Baby moves through dilated cervical opening and birth canal out to the exterior.

Newborn on mother's abdomen (after cord is cut), about to suckle.

Umbilical cord (cut)

Placenta (being expelled)

THIRD STAGE "expulsion of placenta" (afterbirth)

Placenta detaches from uterine wall and is delivered through the vagina.

Fernand Lamaze, a French obstetrician, adapted Russian conditioning tactics to lessen labor discomfort. The four basic principles of Lamaze training are: replacement of the word "pain" with contraction (building an image of controllable labor); replacement of myths by detailed facts (to allay fears and build confidence): diversion of pain signals (by focusing on a known object brought into hospital): and reliance on a supportive coach (partner, relative or other helper) to time contractions, give gentle massage and encouragement. This method is not guaranteed to be painless, or to allow childbirth without anesthetic; rather; medication is regarded as a tool to use if needed. Lamaze birthing has been shown to be both pleasant and safe. Lamaze-trained childbearers tend to be relaxed, take few drugs and have fewer than usual Cesareans, forceps deliveries or episiotomies. If there is a vaginal tear; it is often less serious than with unprepared birthers.

Leboyer's "nonviolent childbirth" aims to ease newborn transit with low lights, hushed voices, delayed cord-cutting (after the blood stops pulsating—deemed dangerous by some experts because it could artificially increase newborn blood volume), gentle skin massage and placing the newborn in a warm bath at once. Some aspects of Leboyer's birthing method have now been incorporated into some obstetric units, which dim the lights, place the baby on the mother's abdomen immediately after birth (even before cord-cutting) and generally soften the birthing atmosphere.

Modern childbirth-preparation methods discuss pregnancy care and childbirth choices, support from caregivers, how to facilitate the birth, ambulation during labor; the right to privacy and rooming-in. Most amalgamate some Lamazian principles with other ideas, like those of British anthropologist and childbirth educator Sheila Kitzinger; who takes a psychosexual approach to labor. She views birth as a "keenly sensual, vaginal pleasure—especially in the final stage of labor; as the head descends—in which women trust their body, and work *with*, not against, its rhythms and see it not as a suffering vehicle, but as something over which they have control." She warns women to expect at least a half-hour of "extreme discomfort during transition" (from first to second, or pushing, stage of labor), and calls for "pain relief to be on hand when requested or needed."

Nowadays, prenatal classes also give instruction on newborn baby care—things like bathing a baby and changing diapers—which are no longer taught in hospitals because early discharge of new mothers (after 24 to 36 hours) doesn't allow enough time.

THE THREE STAGES OF LABOR

The process by which labor starts is not fully understood. The first stage begins as the cervix, or neck of the womb, begins to open and the mucus plug that fills it is dislodged. This "show," a small pinkish blob, often heralds the start of labor. There's a progressive increase in frequency, strength and duration of uterine contractions that dilate the cervix, ultimately to 10 cm (4 in)—usually wide enough to let through the baby's head.

Breathing exercises help the mother to relax and cope more easily with the discomfort. Typically, the sac that holds the water bulges in front of the baby's head and ruptures at or before full dilation of the cervix, at the end of the first stage (but it often breaks sooner; even before contractions begin). The first stage usually lasts about 12 to 16 or more hours in first-time mothers, and less—perhaps only 4 to 6 or fewer hours—in subsequent births. The baby's heartrate is checked regularly (babies at

risk may be electronically monitored throughout labor), and the mother may be occasionally examined internally to see how labor is progressing. When the cervix is fully dilated, at the end of first-stage labor; the mother often feels a tremendous pressure and an urge to "push"—in transition to the second stage.

The second stage of labor begins once the cervix is fully dilated. The mother may feel an irresistible urge to push. As the baby passes through the birth canal the mother bears down, taking deep breaths. Relaxation between contractions is usually blissfully painless, as the baby's head pushes against the cervix and anesthetizes the nerve endings!

The third stage of labor is expulsion of the placenta, or "afterbirth," which may take place in a few minutes or up to half an hour later. Sometimes it's expelled more quickly if the baby is immediately placed on the mother's abdomen, before the cord is cut, and allowed to suckle. The sucking action stimulates release of the hormone *oxytocin*, which contracts and closes up the uterus, forcing out the placenta.

Electronic fetal monitoring of the baby's heartbeat during labor is almost routine in many North American hospitals and birthing units. A belt is strapped over the mother's abdomen to record the baby's heart pattern, which is displayed on a screen. The fetal heart can also be monitored with a small electrode placed on the baby's head. As so often happens, research lags behind practice, and

BREECH BABIES

The term "presentation" refers to the position of the fetal head relative to the cervix (mouth of the uterus). As birth begins, most full-term babies present head down (in the vertex position—from the Latin for "top of the head"). In this position, the largest part of the baby, its head, pushes down and dilates the

cervix sufficiently to allow the rest of the body to slip through. But 3 percent of babies present in a breech position (from the Anglo-Saxon term for britches), where the baby's bottom or feet press down first, and may not dilate the cervix enough to allow the head through—creating an emergency situation.

Breech babies may present as:
• a frank breech, with the buttocks presenting first and fetal heels up around the ears, a position usually manageable by vaginal birth;
• a complete breech, where both buttocks and feet present with foot soles showing through (riskier but

sometimes manageable by vaginal birth);
• a footling breech, where feet appear first, a position rare at term but common with premature breech babies, which is very risky and demands a Cesarean.

The recent Canadian Consensus Report advocated vaginal delivery for fully developed frank or

complete breech babies with an estimated birth weight of 2,500 to 4,000 g (5 to 9 lb) and a pelvis considered adequate for passage of the baby's head. Both U.S. and Canadian experts require the attending physician to be experienced in doing vaginal breech births.

routine electronic monitoring is now roundly criticized by many experts. They allege that unless it's done "in conjunction with fetal scalp blood tests (for fetal oxygen levels) it does not improve fetal safety or health and is no better than regular monitoring with a stethoscope." (But often there are too few nurses to do regular stethoscope monitoring.) Many experts thus consider electronic fetal monitoring unreliable without the biochemical backup of blood-oxygen levels—taken by fetal scalp sampling to measure the blood's pH (acidity level). And even with fetal blood sampling, electronic monitoring of the fetal heart has *not* been definitely shown to improve birth outcomes. One specialist at the University of Western Ontario says, "Fetal heart patterns and reactions are often interpreted by inexperienced staff producing false alarms of fetal distress in perfectly healthy babies, resulting in much needless Cesarean surgery." Fetal distress can also be detected not only by stethoscope checks but also by a decreasing volume of amniotic fluid and other signs.

Induction of labor—inducing the uterus to start contracting with hormones such as oxytocin and prostaglandin E (to soften the cervix), or by breaking the bag of waters, or both—is done in 15 percent of Canadian births, compared to 3 to 5 percent in many European centers, where the practice is frowned upon. Usual reasons for induction include a distressed baby, a mother in trouble (e.g., with eclampsia, diabetes or a blood incompatibility) and an overdue or postmature baby. Induction of labor, however, has some disadvantages. When done by breaking the bag of waters, it allows the sterile buffering fluid to leave the uterus, which may increase risks of infection. The induction method using oxytocin may also produce overly strong contractions. And overly strong contractions may loosen the placenta. Thus caution is urged for the artificial induction of labor. The induction of labor, like other birthing practices, is being reassessed at present for its validity and usefulness.

About 10 percent of pregnancies go well beyond the due date. Those that last 2 or more weeks past the due date (or 42 weeks) are considered "post-due"—perhaps because something fails to trigger labor. Problems can then arise, such as fetal oxygen lack or a baby too big to pass through the woman's pelvis. In the past 30 years or so, post-term pregnancies have been managed either by inducing labor or by awaiting spontaneous labor while carefully monitoring fetal well-being, and inducing labor at any hint of fetal distress.

Episiotomies—making a cut in the vaginal wall to ease the baby's passage and then sewing it up again—used to be almost routine in North American deliveries, but is now done less often in most hospitals, as its usefulness is much contested. Studies show that cutting the vaginal wall may increase the tearing, cause laxity in the pelvic floor; incontinence and lead to dyspareunia (pain on intercourse), so the practice is now declining. Recent studies show a dramatic drop in episiotomy rates.

FROM FETUS TO NEWBORN: A LEAP INTO THE UNKNOWN

By the time a fetus is ready to be born, the volume of amniotic fluid (the "waters" that break when labor begins) has been reduced to about a quart. At term, the average baby is about 50 cm (20 in) long and weighs about 3,500 g (7.5 lb). Babies that weigh less than 2,500 g (5.5 lb) are labeled "low birthweight," but not all low-birthweight newborns are premature, some are just "small-for-dates" babies.

Human infants are born somewhat immature compared to most other animals, requiring a long period of parental nurturing before they become independent. In most full-term newborns, the body is plump, most biochemical systems and enzymes are ready for action, the tiny lungs are coated with surfactant (a substance vital to lung expansion) and the chest is able to take that crucial first gasp of air.

The immediate post-birth period

Baby care immediately after birth includes examination of baby and placenta (afterbirth) for signs of infection or abnormality, weight and length measurements and rating the baby's well-being on the Apgar scale at 1 and 5 minutes after delivery. The 10-point Apgar scale allots zero to 2 points each for:

• heart rate;
• skin color;

- muscle tone;
- reflexes; and
- respiration.

In Canadian hospitals, silver-nitrate drops or erythromycin ointment are routinely given to newborns to forestall possible blindness due to maternal gonorrhea. Vitamin K is usually also administered to newborns to help with blood-clotting and minimize bleeding at birth, as the immature liver doesn't yet produce this vital substance.

Caring for sick or premature babies

Health professionals now encourage parents to spend time with premature or sick newborns—even those in incubators. Neonatal units support parents in trying to feed ailing newborns, and some even encourage siblings to visit, to promote family ties. Parents can briefly hold and touch sick newborns in intensive care or neonatal units. Even putting a hand into the incubator to stroke the baby stimulates the infant and assists respiration.

Mothers are encouraged to breastfeed and express and store their breastmilk in sterile refrigerated bottles for later feedings, not only for its nutritional value, but to make breastfeeding easier when the baby arrives home. In some birth centers, parents also get psychophysiological instruction and support from the baby-care team in handling their vulnerable preemies.

A vast new field of infant psychiatry identifies communication problems and can assist parent-infant interaction and reinforce parental feelings of competence.

CESAREAN BIRTH: TIME FOR REAPPRAISAL

Once a rare and often fatal operation—previously considered an "obstetric defeat"—Cesarean surgery is currently done more often to deliver a distressed fetus and avoid damage in difficult birth situations. In fact, it is now the manner of birth for nearly 1 in 5 Canadian babies. As Cesareans have become safer, the decision to operate has likewise become easier. The dramatic rise in North American Cesareans has been paralleled by an equally sharp decline in perinatal mortality (babies

---

ASSESSING NEWBORN HEALTH

Newborn reflexes checked include:
- **The rooting reflex**— the turn of a baby's head when its cheek is touched—nature's way of ensuring that a newborn will turn to the nipple, be nourished, grow and thrive. (Right from the first moments after birth an infant will search with its mouth and turn its head to try to find the breast.)
- **The grasp reflex**— newborns hang on to an adult finger so tightly that they can often be

pulled upright.
- **The "doll's eye" reflex**—eyes pointing in a fixed direction as the head turns.
- **The startle or "Moro" reflex**—dipping of the head and stretching, then flexing of arms and legs (as if surprised, but it's not real shock, just a transient reflex!).
- **The stepping reflex**— a 1-day-old infant will "step out" as if walking when held upright on the examining table (a dramatic reflex

that disappears by a few weeks after birth).

Another system of measurement, Brazelton's Neonatal Scale, evaluates neonatal behavior with more sophisticated ratings of mental, social and temperamental capacities. The method measures infant reactions to sound, light and other stimuli, distinguishing time spent awake, semiconscious or asleep and amounts of crying, gazing, kicking or looking, assessing 26 different behaviors.

---

dying after 28 weeks of development or at 1 kg [2 lb] in weight, or up to a week after birth). But tempting though it may be to link the drop in perinatal deaths to the rise in Cesareans, studies disprove the connection. In reality, perinatal mortality dropped *before* the rise in Cesareans.

Alarmed at the escalating rates of Cesareans, many obstetricians, health officials and consumers claim that Cesareans are no longer done just for accepted medical reasons—such as a breech position, a large baby in a small pelvis or a prematurely separated placenta—but because the operation gives physicians more control and avoids the potentially serious complications of a difficult vaginal birth. But while medical advances have made Cesarean birth safer, it's still not as safe as an uncomplicated vaginal birth. Borderline cases (such as a long labor that doesn't necessarily threaten the mother or infant) raise many doubts about current practices in doing Cesareans.

What is a Cesarean section?

The origin of the term "Cesarean section" is obscure. Legend has it that Julius Caesar was born by cutting open his mother's abdomen and extracting the baby, but since Caesar's mother survived the operation (then invariably fatal for the mother) the theory is open to doubt! The procedure more probably got its name from the Latin *caedere*: "to cut." In a Cesarean operation the surgeon cuts through ("sections") the abdominal skin and muscle and lifts the baby out of the uterus. The classic vertical incision in the uterus has now been largely replaced by a horizontal incision in the uterus and also a horizontal cut in the abdomen when possible (as it's more cosmetically pleasing). In an emergency situation the surgeon may still make a vertical cut in the abdomen (because it's quicker and easier), but will still do a transverse uterine incision whenever possible, because it is stronger than the vertical, less likely to bleed profusely and far less likely to rupture in subsequent labor. General anesthesia may be employed, but the surgery is usually conducted with regional (epidural) anesthesia, which permits the mother to see her newborn immediately and avoids the slower recuperation after a general anesthetic.

Risks of the Cesarean

Newborn health can suffer from a Cesarean birth, especially if a premature baby is taken out too soon. Also, Cesarean babies tend to have a slightly greater risk of Respiratory Distress Syndrome (RDS), owing to the lack of stimulation obtained during normal vaginal birth—which squeezes the fetal lungs, or because the lungs lack the surfactant coating vital to their expansion—particularly if the Cesarean is done electively (by choice) and the baby's calculated due date is wrong, leading to premature birth.

Maternal illness or complications following Cesareans now average 11 to 18 percent, the risks being greater for those who are obese or anemic, or who have emergency surgery after a difficult labor. Infection of the wound site, uterine lining, urinary tract or pelvis is the most common complication in the mother (But infection can likewise occur after a long or difficult vaginal birth.) Fortunately, antibiotics greatly reduce the dangers of post-Cesarean infection. Complications are fewer in those who choose a repeat Cesarean than in those done as emergency operations. (The Society of Obstetricians and Gynecologists of Canada quotes a mortality figure for emergency Cesareans of 9.9 per 100,000 births, which is twice that for elective repeats and about 2 to 4 times that for modern vaginal births.)

The psychological impact of unexpected Cesarean surgery in a couple that anticipated a natural vaginal birth can be devastating if they aren't adequately prepared and made comfortable with the decision. The father's presence in the delivery room and keeping the newborn close to the mother after birth are reassuring. Some women actually welcome a Cesarean as deliverance from what they call the "painful, terrifying experience" of vaginal birth.

Vaginal birth after Cesarean (VBAC)

Well-documented studies show that, in thousands of women, trial of labor (TOL)—attempting vaginal labor after a Cesarean—is a safe, often successful, even beneficial procedure for childbirth. The risks of uterine rupture with the new lower-segment transverse Cesarean scar are minimal. In a study of 10,000 women giving birth vaginally with a transverse scar, there were no maternal deaths. Even if a transverse incision opens a little before or during an ensuing labor, there is very little risk of complications, and it usually heals easily without further attention. In fact, dangers may be lower with a VBAC than with a planned repeat Cesarean.

Many centers now promote normal labor as a safe option for women after a Cesarean birth, provided they fulfill certain criteria. Yet, despite its advantages, acceptance of VBAC has been slow and parents-to-be may have to search for a physician and center that are willing to encourage it.

The odds for succeeding in VBAC are about 70 percent. Although theoretically any woman (except someone with a classic uterine incision) can try for VBAC, some women are more likely to succeed than others. The outcome depends partly on the reason the first Cesarean was performed, since some problems tend to recur. Breech presentation, fetal distress, *abruptio placenta*, *placenta previa* and accidental cord prolapse are not likely to recur. In essence, the latest advice is that VBAC be treated like any other natural labor; except that a very long second-stage labor is discouraged in case of any uterine weakness.

NEWBORN CHILD–PARENT BONDING

Newborn–parent bonding is a concept introduced by Marshall Klaus, an Ohio pediatrician. Many maternity units now encourage parents to spend time alone with their new baby right after birth.

Immediately after birth, most normal, full-term newborns have a period of "quiet alertness," possibly due to the stimulation of birth and the release of adrenal hormones during labor. In this phase, with eyes wide open, newborns stare at faces and scan their surroundings. Seeing their infant gazing at them, parents may "bond" instantly to the new arrival. After this the babies usually doze off into a long, deep sleep.

The newborn bonding concept has recently come under fire, since the idea of a "critical period" right after birth does not hold up as a universal phenomenon. While some parents enjoy immediate contact with their newborn, others take longer to form emotional ties. Although many studies show more interaction (more face-to-face gazing, stroking, chatting and patting) after early parent–baby contact, none has found any long-term differences in closeness, or proof that the initial bonding advantages persist into later relationships. The publicity about early bonding may create a false belief that if this experience is missed, parents can never make it up. In fact, for all of those who cannot bond at once—because of medical interventions during birth (such as Cesarean section) or problems with the infant's health (such as anoxia or premature birth) or because the mother has the "baby blues" or postpartum depression—professionals stress that there are countless other bonding times. (See Chapter 14 for more on newborn bonding and postpartum depression.)

Rooming-in—babies remaining in their mothers' rooms rather than returning to the nursery between feedings—is now very common, to encourage bonding and breastfeeding. Experiments show that mothers who keep their babies rooming-in beside them exhibit greater maternal behavior—looking, soothing, cuddling, chatting and feeding—than parents of babies in a central nursery. If a mother doesn't want to keep the baby in her room all the time—perhaps after a long and difficult birth—she should be encouraged to feel comfortable with her decision, and other family members can help with baby-care at first. According to many researchers, when fathers also have extended early contact with their babies, they continue to spend more time in child care later on.

The amazing abilities of newborns

Although a newborn recognizes its mother's smell and voice, it may not feel anything special about her until several weeks later. Even the first "social smile," at around 6 weeks of age, is not uniquely directed at parents but at anyone who coos to the infant. So while parents may "bond" at once to their infant, the child may take months to become truly attached to them. But by 6 to 8 months of age, an infant generally shows a clear preference for its parents over strangers, and has separation anxiety if removed from them.

Recent research shows that the newborn possesses a perceptual apparatus that enables it to respond effectively to its new world and, more important, to shape the behavior of its parents and caregivers. Helpless as they seem, newborns come well equipped to signal their needs. Harvard pediatrician T. Berry Brazelton noted two survival mechanisms: the ability to pick out and respond appropriately to stimuli that enhance well-being, and the capacity to "tune out" disturbing stimuli (such as loud noises or bright lights), which allows the infant to avoid sensory overload. For example, a full-term newborn turns toward a rattle while a premature one turns away, not yet ready to deal with that stimulus. Newborn crying—tearless, because tear-ducts are not yet working—produces parental comforting and feeding, which causes the crying to cease, allowing caregivers to gain confidence, which encourages more nurturing.

Until recently, it was popularly believed that newborns could not see clearly. Research now shows that they not only see in three dimen-

REASONS FOR CESAREAN SECTION

- **Failure of labor to progress normally;**
- **fetal distress possibly seen on the electronic heart monitor (due to lack of oxygen);**
- **fetal malposition (such as breech—buttocks first—or a transverse lie, baby lying horizontally and unable to emerge);**
- **cephalopelvic disproportion—a woman with a pelvis too narrow for the baby's transit;**
- ***abruptio placenta*—a placenta that separates too soon and endangers the baby through lack of oxygen and the mother through hemorrhage;**
- ***placenta previa*—one that implants in an unusual position and blocks the baby's passage, with risk of hemorrhage during labor;**
- **a previous Cesarean.**

THE BENEFITS OF VBAC

- Faster post-birth recovery;
- greater parental satisfaction;
- less risk of post-birth complications such as infection in the mother;
- less risk of respiratory problems in the newborn;
- reduced healthcare costs;
- shorter hospital stay.

sions, but show distinct visual preferences. Being nearsighted, they focus best at about 8 to 10 inches, roughly the distance of a baby's mouth from its mother's face while nursing. Research also shows that even day-old babies prefer the human face and black-and-white or outlined pictures of it to abstract or blurred images. They can follow moving objects and will turn their heads to see a human face. Infants look longer at a slow-moving object than at a static one.

Newborns hear well, showing a distinct preference for the human voice, for women's voices over men's, and for high-pitched sounds to low-pitched ones. This may explain the human tendency to address infants with high-pitched baby-talk or songs. In studying the response to human voices, Brazelton and his Harvard colleagues found that about 68 percent of newborns turned toward a human voice, some actively searching for its source. Such complex, coordinated behavior involves many auditory pathways.

A baby's sense of smell is sufficiently sensitive within a few days of birth to recognize its mother's odor; even that of a pad soaked in her milk infants will ignore all other stimuli and turn to it. Touch is also sensitively developed in newborns. Skin-to-skin contact is not only soothing to parents and baby, but has various health advantages especially in colonizing the baby's system with the mother's (rather than alien) bacteria. Skin-to-skin contact often makes parents massage and stroke their babies extensively, which is less frequent with clothed contact.

New evidence about innate newborn personality may help to remove the guilt often felt by parents of extra-demanding, fussy or colicky babies, or those who fear they missed the post-birth bonding boat. Some babies are simply more "difficult" and less responsive than others—more unpredictable, irritable and easily upset. U.S. child psychologists Stella Chess and Alexander Thomas label parental anxieties over nurturing skills as the *mal de mère* syndrome ("sick mother" syndrome), typified by the fear that any innocent act, word or gesture may irreparably harm a child. This type of parent may be afraid to criticize or punish an infant for fear of lowering its self-esteem, and dare not praise it or show affection in case of "spoiling" it. Yet

parents who respond promptly to their infant's cries generate warmth and confidence; attentiveness and loving care build trust, which makes youngsters secure and less likely to demand excess attention.

There's no evidence that any one child-rearing method inevitably creates this or that type of child. For instance, domineering, authoritarian treatment may make one infant submissive, another defiant. Much depends upon the child's individual coping mechanisms. Even when parents are obviously abusive, there's no absolute or predictable outcome. Some children who grow up under horrendous conditions—with psychotic, alcoholic or violent caretakers—develop into balanced, competent human beings. Over the long haul, neglect damages children, but by the same token a day's irritation or momentary burst of anger is not disastrous, provided there's a steady undercurrent of tender affection.

BREAST IS STILL BEST

Breastmilk, specifically tailored to human development by the long process of evolution, supplies all the nutrients necessary for optimal infant development in the first few months after birth. Despite increasing public awareness and scientific validation of the enormous benefits of breastmilk for infants, many mothers who begin nursing quit too soon for lack of know-how, assistance and emotional support. While three-quarters of new mothers in Canada start off breastfeeding, a quarter give up within a month or so, usually sooner than intended, and only a third are still breastfeeding by the time their babies are 3 to 4 months old. When deciding whether or not to breastfeed their baby, new parents need accurate information in order to wend their way through the wealth of conflicting data.

For all its apparent simplicity, breastfeeding is not a reflex action or an instinct that comes naturally, but an art that must be taught and practiced. Although the sucking reflex is instinctive, women must learn how to position the newborn and latch it correctly to the breast. Good positioning is all-important. There are some infants who must learn to suck properly as well! The best way to succeed is to learn ahead about the science of lactation and watch others nursing. Successful nursing involves tenacity, confidence and freedom from emotional tension, and requires constructive help at critical moments. Given some basic information during the first weeks of lactation, and helpful support, most women have an excellent chance of success.

Although practices such as rooming-in and family-centered birth units encourage breastfeeding, shorter postpartum hospitalization is now the rule, and many mothers leave hospital within a day or two—before their milk comes in (generally on the third post-birth day). The shorter hospital stay gives little time for instruction in breastfeeding techniques. And not all hospitals have an atmosphere that encourages breastfeeding; some healthcare attendants have an inbuilt prejudice against nudity or don't regard the breast as a nurturant part of the body, valuing it mainly for its sexual appeal. While most health experts today recognize the benefits of breastfeeding, few may actually have watched a mother nurse her baby! Whether verbally or nonverbally expressed, such attitudes may subtly undermine a new mother's confidence. What nursing mothers need is plenty of practical advice and support to persevere, particularly as the inability to nurse a firstborn can be a bitter disappointment and may engender guilt feelings.

Tips for nursing mothers
Following a few simple steps and anticipating possible deterrents may help to get nursing off to a good start.
- *Obtain competent breastfeeding instruction* before the baby's birth, ideally during prenatal classes. Classes generally include details of breast anatomy, the mechanism of milk production, the stimulative effect of sucking, the benefits of demand feeding, a physical nipple examination and preparation of inverted or small nipples if necessary.
- *Have baby room in* (request it ahead) and feed on demand whenever possible, *not* by the clock. One University of Toronto expert reminds nursing mothers that "new babies with easily famished bodies need food every 2 hours or less." Newborns should be beside the mother from birth onward if possible and suckle whenever hungry. The more a

baby sucks, the more the milk comes in. Contrary to the supposition that scheduled feedings reduce demands on the hospital staff's time and attention, one British study found that babies kept beside the mother's bed (not taken away even for diaper changes) and fed on demand exerted a far smaller load on the nursing staff, gained weight faster caused fewer problems (such as nipple soreness or breast engorgement) and were easier to handle. On this basis, some hospitals have abolished scheduled feeds as a waste of nurses' time and a hindrance to successful lactation.
- *Feed the newborn immediately* after delivery. The sucking reflex is strongest in the first half-hour after birth, fading somewhat thereafter before it reappears at full force some 40 hours later. And the baby's sucking action stimulates release of the hormone oxytocin, which hastens milk secretion and also helps to expel the placenta and contract the mother's uterus, lessening the risk of hemorrhage. (Some obstetricians put a healthy, full-term baby to the breast instantly, even before the cord is cut.)
- *Remember that the pre-milk fluid, colostrum,* is a valuable first nourishment. Even the few

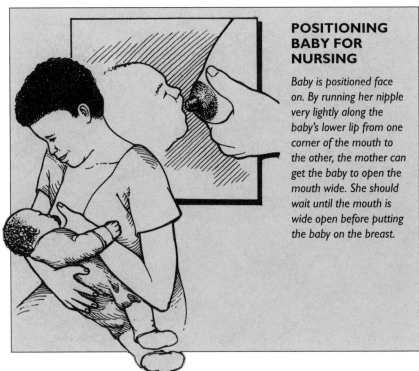

POSITIONING BABY FOR NURSING

Baby is positioned face on. By running her nipple very lightly along the baby's lower lip from one corner of the mouth to the other, the mother can get the baby to open the mouth wide. She should wait until the mouth is wide open before putting the baby on the breast.

SOME REASONS WHY WOMEN ABANDON BREASTFEEDING

- Insufficient knowledge of its benefits;
- inadequate prenatal instruction;
- failure to get off to a good start;
- too little expert help in dealing with small but common problems;
- poor positioning of the baby at the breast;
- a delay of several hours in newborn nursing (thwarting the strong post-birth sucking reflex);
- separation of newborn and mother rather than "rooming-in";
- feeding by schedule instead of on demand;
- omitting night feedings;
- early fluid supplements (which undermine the baby's breast-sucking urge);
- need or desire to go back to job after 8 to 12 weeks (but even this amount of breastfeeding is worthwhile);
- conscious or unconscious reinforcement of mother's (unwarranted) fears about inadequate milk;
- derogatory comments or attitudes about the probable difficulties or messiness of breastfeeding, which communicate a negative attitude to insecure mothers;
- exhaustion or frustration from the need to be on 24-hour call (compared to bottle feeders, who can share the load).

drops of this clear yellowish secretion obtained at an initial feeding provide some protein, minerals and vitamins, as well as maternal IgA antibodies, with concentrations many times above those found in breastmilk a few days later providing protection against infections. As an extra bonus, the laxative effect of colostrum encourages the evacuation of the sludgy meconium (which fills the newborn's bowel), making the infant hungrier and more likely to nurse vigorously, thereby bringing in the mother's milk sooner. Finally, immediate postnatal feeding and early bowel clearance reduce the absorption of bilirubin (from red-blood-cell debris), diminishing the chance of newborn jaundice.

- *Be sure to position the baby correctly.* For a good sucking position, the whole nipple and as much as is comfortable of its surrounding areola (colored part) should be well grasped in the baby's mouth

- *Avoid too-frequent post-feed weight checks.* While weekly tracking of newborn weight is essential, test-weighing after feeds to see how much milk has been swallowed creates undue anxiety. A demand-fed baby sometimes takes a snack, at other times a full meal. Some weight loss is common after birth, and it may take babies 10 to 14 days or so to regain their birthweight.

- *Assess the adequacy of the milk supply* through natural signs and infant habits. Many a woman needlessly abandons nursing for fear of scanty or poor milk. But milk adequacy can be evaluated by hearing the steady slurp of the baby swallowing, seeing a trickle of milk from its mouth, noting the many wet diapers. A mother can rest assured that she has enough milk if the infant settles down after satisfying nursings every few hours, has a steady weekly weight gain of 120 to 210 g (4 to 7 oz), 6 to 12 wet (colorless) diapers a day and frequent soft, seedy, yellow stools. A need to nurse frequently may just mean that the baby is seeking comfort or undergoing a growth spurt; frequent hunger pangs are natural, since breastmilk digests easily and leaves the stomach quickly. Leaky breasts and fussy periods are also normal and do not indicate too little milk.

Overcoming some common pitfalls in breast feeding

- *Don't skip night feedings.* Leaving a newborn unfed for several hours—perhaps to give the mother some uninterrupted sleep—may diminish the milk supply, cause breast engorgement and hinder nursing. (The mother has a right to participate in the decision-making process, and should know that around-the-clock access and more sucking increases milk production.)

- *Request or insist that hospital birthing staff avoid fluid supplements* from rubber-nippled bottles during the first few post-birth days. No studies document a regular need for water supplements in the first few days of life, and most babies do fine without a lot of fluid in the first day or two. However; many institutions still give supplemental sugared or plain water by bottle (often to allow the mother some rest, "top off" a feed, avoid dehydration, facilitate mucus-swallowing or line up hospital schedules). Some experts claim that even 1 or 2 bottles given soon after birth can subtly disrupt the complex natural sucking urge.

- *Avoid "nipple confusion" or "bottle spoiling."* The early introduction to a rubber nipple, with its different sucking style, can make newborns suck poorly at the breast. Bottle nipples give an immediate reward—different from the kind of sucking needed to extract milk from the human breast and a baby who's known the ease of a bottle nipple may fight the breast, refuse it or just fall asleep after a few token sucks. Ineffective sucking fails to stimulate milk production and, through no fault of the mother or baby, is a common cause of "failure-to-thrive" (insufficient weight gain) and a frequent reason for abandoning nursing. If the real root of the trouble (early introduction to rubber nipples) isn't spotted, the problem may be ascribed to irrelevant causes such as "a lazy baby" or "flat nipples."

• *Realize that colic or excessive crying fits are not necessarily reasons to stop nursing.* Colicky babies often do better if fed at one breast only at each feeding, for 30 minutes or so. (After the initial adjustment period, experts often advise mothers to nurse routinely at alternate breasts to empty each completely)

• *Learn how to cope with excess milk ejection.* Occasionally the milk "let-down" or ejection is so strong that the nursing infant draws back, unable to suck and unsatisfied. The problem is easily handled by a brief burping session, expressing a little milk first, and by nursing the baby at one breast only per feeding so that both the watery foremilk and richer hindmilk (last drops) are obtained. The problem fades as mother and baby adapt to each other. Lying down while feeding may ease the flow. Feeding the baby before it is fully awake, rather than waiting for a ravenous infant, may also help to avoid a sudden gush.

• *Anticipate and learn to deal with engorgement* (uncomfortably full, hard breasts). Breast engorgement, due to increased vascularity (blood supply) and milk accumulation, produces an overfull breast difficult for the baby to grasp. Severe engorgement can lead to plugged milk ducts and mastitis (inflammation of the breast), inhibiting lactation. Frequent nursing at the breasts will minimize the problem, and some milk can be expressed manually or with a pump before feedings to soften the areola so that the baby can latch on better. If engorgement occurs, hot towels or breast massage in the shower before a feeding may help. Between feedings, ice-packs can be soothing.

• *Realize that infant jaundice* is a frequently cited but usually invalid reason to abandon the breast. If a baby's eyes look yellow and its skin sallow, it may be due to a high level of bilirubin (blood-breakdown product), which peaks in the first week after birth. This was once regarded as a reason to stop nursing, but the latest research shows just the opposite. In most cases, frequent and continued breastfeeding is the best way to get rid of the bilirubin that causes newborn jaundice. (The jaundice of newborns is usually harmless and gone in a few days.)

Avoiding sore nipples

Sore nipples can often be prevented by prenatal preparation for breastfeeding, avoiding harsh soaps (which dry and harden the skin), exposing the nipples to air whenever possible and making sure the bra doesn't irritate them. To assist flat or inverted nipples, women can wear a breast shield designed to draw the nipples out during pregnancy and between nursing times. Since sore nipples are easier to prevent than to treat, it is important to remember that nipples usually become sore (and then cracked) if the baby isn't well positioned and sucking properly.

The cure for sore nipples is not less nursing but good baby positioning, nursing first on the less sore side (to satisfy the ravenous hunger) and air-drying nipples after feeds. Should soreness occur, it can be minimized by bathing with plain water (breastmilk has enough antiseptic properties) and air-drying nipples for 20 minutes after feedings whenever possible. Clothes and bra-liners that trap moisture and increase wetness should be avoided. Breast shells (shields) can be worn between feedings to help air circulate. Rubber nipple shields should *not* be worn while nursing as they reduce the baby's sucking power and drastically diminish the milk supply. Heat, ultraviolet lamps and hair-dryers may soothe the soreness. Creams and ointments only loosen the baby's grasp and make it slip off so must be rinsed off before a feed. (Most nipple creams are not recommended by experts, especially those containing steroids, antibiotics or other drugs.) With feeding position corrected, sore nipples usually improve within days. A fungal thrush infection on the breast or in the baby's mouth can be cured by gentian violet or antifungal drugs.

Mothers with breast-rejecting babies, who don't latch properly onto the breast, can be helped by temporary lactation aids. These provide extra calories from formula (without a bottle) by trickling a little through a long tube into the baby's mouth, rewarding it as it feeds at the breast, thus reviving its interest in nursing. The system, which requires patience, often manages to correct the suckle. The aid is also helpful in dealing with newborn jaundice.

Help is available

The La Leche League (LLL), founded about 30 years ago by a small volunteer band of nursing mothers, has now expanded to become an international authority on breastfeeding with branches across Canada; the telephone number is listed under La Leche League and "Breastfeeding Help." Lactation experts and breastfeeding clinics such as the one at the University of Toronto's Hospital for Sick Children can also help in breastfeeding, or ask your local health department for a public-health nurse.

THE MANY BENEFITS OF BREASTMILK

- Always ready to serve, at the right temperature; no mixing needed;
- portable and affordable;
- easily digested—its composition produces smaller, softer curds than formula;
- laxative effects help to clear bowels quickly;
- promotes good facial structure (by the breast-sucking action of the infant jaws);
- encourages interaction with mother, enhances bonding and provides lots of environmental stimulation;
- contains growth and other factors that promote infant metabolism.

Main nutritional advantages:

- Biochemical blend right for human babies (different from cow's-milk formula); calcium and zinc in particular are more readily absorbed from breastmilk than from formula;
- nutrients more "bio-available" (easily utilized) than those in formula;
- protein and salt content lower than formula, so less burden on infant kidneys;
- protein and amino-acid composition well balanced for human brain and nerve development. The proportions of whey and casein protein in breastmilk favor human metabolism, and are less allergy-provoking than cow's-milk formula;
- contains taurine—a component of neonatal bile salts—that may enhance iron absorption in breastfeds;
- contains human milk fats of the right type, with lipase enzymes that make it more digestible than formula fat;
- higher in valuable polyunsaturates;
- cholesterol content (absent in formula) may

induce enzyme action that promotes better cholesterol metabolism, possibly avoiding some health problems later in life;

- the increase in fat content at the end of a feeding (in the "hindmilk") may provide a "fullness" signal that prevents overfeeding;
- good iron absorption supplies stores sufficient for first 6 months, provided mother is not anemic and the baby's not premature (in which case iron stores may run out sooner). Formula-feds should have iron-enriched brands, but some formulas have excess iron (which may interfere with zinc absorption);
- contains more vitamin C than formula, and all other vitamins in ample amounts, except vitamin D.

Main anti-infective benefits:

- High lactoferrin content favors growth of lacto-bacilli bacteria in the infant's gut, ousting harmful microorganisms, and by binding to iron, lactoferrin impedes the growth of E. coli (diarrhea-causing) and other bacteria;
- immunological benefits from antiviral agents, white blood cells (e.g., macrophages and lymphocytes) and immunoglobulins (antibodies) that protect against infective agents—such as E. coli, salmonella, staphylococci, streptococci and microorganisms that cause giardiasis, polio, shigellosis, meningitis and pneumonia. The combined immunological properties of breastmilk help newborns resist infection, reducing the incidence of diarrhea, gastric, respiratory and other illnesses.

Note that there are two maternal conditions in which breastfeeding is not advisable: acute or chronic hepatitis B and HIV (AIDS) infection.

Helping children grow up healthy

Breastfeeding • Instilling good eating habits • Choosing the right baby formula • Toilet training • Building in self-esteem • Preventing avoidable injuries • Preventing childhood choking • Recognizing and managing childhood disorders • Understanding childhood fever • Allergies • Asthma • Autism • Birthmarks • Cerebral palsy • Chickenpox • Colic • Common colds • Croup • Juvenile, Type I or "insulin-dependent" diabetes • Diarrhea • Diphtheria • Down syndrome • Ear infections • Eczema • Enuresis (bedwetting) • Epiglottitis • Epilepsy (seizure disorder) • Fifth disease (Erythema infectiosum) • Foot disorders • Giardiasis • Haemophilus influenzae Type B infections • Hepatitis A • Hepatitis B • Impetigo • Measles • Meningitis • Mumps • Pinkeye (conjunctivitis) • Polio (poliomyelitis) • Rheumatic fever • Roseola RSV infections • Rubella (German measles) • Scabies • Sore throats • Sudden Infant Death Syndrome • Teething • Tetanus (lockjaw) • Thrush or candida (yeast) diaper rash • Tonsillitis • Whooping cough (pertussis) • Worms

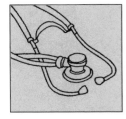

THIS CHAPTER CONSIDERS some general health topics related to children, and then describes (in alphabetical order) a number of specific ailments and conditions that may affect children.

Among the many influences on child health, pediatricians stress the need to breastfeed for the first 6 months if possible; to wean wisely in order to establish good lifelong eating habits; to refrain from smoking in the home, as cigarette smoke increases risks of pneumonia and other childhood chest infections; to ingrain self-esteem at every opportunity; to prevent needless injuries and to know the basics for recognizing and handling childhood illnesses.

BREASTFEEDING

The American Academy of Pediatrics and the World Health Organization recommend exclusive breastfeeding as the ideal nutrition during the first 6 months of life and state that no other solids or liquids are required during this period. If possible, and ideally, breastfeeding should continue for at least 1 year, but iron-enriched solids should be added in the second 6 months of life.

Despite increasing public awareness and scientific validation of the benefits of breastmilk as the only food for infants in the first few months, many mothers who begin nursing quit

11

too soon. When deciding whether to breastfeed their baby, new parents need accurate information to wend their way through the conflicting data—and they need support in persisting. Breastmilk is biologically tailored to human development. It not only supplies all the nutrients necessary for optimal infant development, but also contains antibodies and living cells (such as white blood cells) that can protect newborns against bacteria, viruses, fungi and parasites. Formula manufacturers have not yet managed to duplicate the many complex properties of human milk, a living fluid. Furthermore, breastmilk is "on tap" at the right temperature, requiring no addition of (possibly unclean) water, no mixing, no warming or night trips to the fridge. Breastfed babies seem to have stronger teeth, better facial structure and fewer dental problems than bottlefeds because of the way their tiny jaws work to get food. They are also less prone to allergies than those fed formula.

In addition to providing optimal nutrition, breastfeeding is a dynamic, personal relationship between mother and infant that may enhance emotional bonding. Since breastfed babies tend to feed more frequently than bottlefed babies, they often spend more time interacting with the world around them, and some pediatricians believe that the extra stimulation makes them livelier, with swifter eye-hand coordination—due to the interaction with the mother's body, the movement from one breast to the other and the "rooting" reflex (searching for her breast). And the mother may receive a boost in morale from the knowledge that she's providing the best possible food for her child. In addition, a nursing mother often slims down faster after delivery, because the suckling baby consumes 500 or more calories a day.

The signs of successful breast feeding in the neonate are as follows:

- 8 to 10 feedings a day
- audible swallowing
- 6 to 8 wet diapers a day
- 3 to 5 bowel movements a day
- birth weight regained by 2 weeks

While breastfeeding is the optimal nutrition in the first few postbirth months, this doesn't mean that all mothers are able to breastfeed, nor does it mean that babies fed modern, scientifically researched, meticulously produced and carefully selected formula are nutritionally deprived. However, parents should get enough information beforehand to make an informed choice about the best way to feed their infants. If, for whatever reason, a woman cannot or does not want to nurse her baby—perhaps because of job commitments or an illness (such as hepatitis B), or because she must take certain drugs—she needn't feel less competent as a mother. Better to bottlefeed than to be perpetually worried or uncomfortable about nursing. Breastfeeding can be challenging and frustrating and its success can be augmented or benefit from both personal support and help from lactation consultants, nurses, midwives, doctors and/or others. (See Chapter 10 for more on breastfeeding and ways to successful nursing.)

INSTILLING GOOD EATING HABITS

Lifelong eating patterns are often set in infancy, when a child is weaned from milk to solids. It's best to introduce a wide variety of different foods one by one, keeping a lookout for allergic reactions.

Teach children to eat only when hungry and to stop when full. Offer small servings of individual foods and remove them after 20 minutes. Try to stay calm and relaxed when feeding young children; anxious parents can make children refuse food as an attention-seeking gimmick. Accept some mess and expect day-to-

day appetite swings. Try not to coax, force-feed or insist on children "cleaning their plate"—forcing them to eat more than they want only leads to later eating disorders. If they consistently refuse to eat at mealtimes, offer water rather than juice between meals. If they keep up a "hunger strike" for days on end, remember that they rarely starve themselves.

Parents who react to all their baby's cries as though they were hunger signals and ply a youngster with tasty morsels may make the child regard food as the answer not only to hunger but to all life's discomforts—cold, wet, anxiety and stress. Similarly, it's best not to use food as a reward or bribe, which gives the impression that food equals love, attention or approval. Using food for bribes can make children (and adults) turn to favorite goodies for solace or to counter every moment of sadness.

Family and cultural attitudes to food have a tremendous impact on eating styles. Since children learn by watching other family members, parents should try to display good dietary habits themselves and avoid food faddism. For instance, if Dad refuses all vegetables or Mom turns her nose up at liver the child will likely acquire food aversions. For children who reject vegetables, caregivers can set a good example by pleasurably eating the proffered vegetable themselves before coaxing a child to eat it. Helping to prepare the vegetables may also encourage a child to eat them!

Generally, how much and how a child eats depends on his or her individual makeup. Respect true dislikes but encourage the child to sample as many different foods as possible, to instill the idea of well-varied nutrition. Children usually eat as much food as they need to keep them going, even if the amount seems too small. Childhood appetites vary with the weather illness and growth spurts.

Tips for developing good eating habits

- When weaning from breast or bottle, start with bland, nonallergenic foods: rice cereal, puréed carrots, squash, potatoes, bananas, apples and pears.
- Use sound dietary information when introducing new foods, and provide amounts required at different stages.

- Watch for signs that the child is full, such as turning the head away from the spoon, clamping the mouth shut and other obvious gestures.
- Never force or bribe a child to eat: children know when they're no longer hungry.
- Offer only small amounts of food and fluids at a time. There's always more. Children get overwhelmed by large amounts, and there is less to clean up when spills occur.
- Serve well-balanced meals that include a wide range of tastes and textures, so that your child learns about enjoyable variety.
- Watch for allergic reactions (hives, throat or tongue swelling. See "Childhood food intolerances and food allergies," below.)
- Use unbreakable dishes. Try a cup with a lid or straw for children who are first using a cup (6 to 8 months old), since both mimic sucking actions.
- Examine your own attitudes and those of other family members toward eating to determine how they might influence the child. A stress-free atmosphere promotes self-feeding skills and good lifetime food attitudes. Remember that your mood will influence the child.
- Make mealtimes enjoyable. Mealtimes are not just times to eat but also opportunities for socializing. ("The family that eats together stays together!")
- Settle your child comfortably and maintain a slow, relaxed pace.
- Don't "hurry along" meals.
- Try not to force-feed, if possible.
- With very young children, allow time for play and experimentation but stop the meal before the play and mess become too bothersome.
- Ignore food throwing or messiness at first; it's part of normal development. Children "drop" things in order to learn the "letting go" reflex, and where better to practice than dumping bits of food from a highchair? Cleanup may be made easier by putting newspaper or plastic sheeting under the highchair. Once children acquire the skill of letting go and spilling, it's just a game that shouldn't be rewarded by continually picking up the dropped food. Instead, after the third or fourth throw,

remove all food—the child is likely full.
- Encourage a child who bolts food to slow down by talking between spoonfuls. It also helps if adults eat slowly. Put small amounts of food on the plate and use gentle reminders to chew well before swallowing.
- Encourage independence. Children need time to practice eating skills. Success helps them feel good about themselves.
- Promote choice and responsibility in food selection and respect the child's decisions. For example, let the child choose between two vegetables, and once the child has chosen, express pleasure that your child is eating a vegetable. Providing limited and realistic choices encourages children to think independently and exercise some control. For example, "Would you like a few carrots or a lot of carrots?" Allowing choices makes children feel like people!
- For children who dislike vegetables, try calling them something descriptive and fun. For example, if the child likes colours, call peas "green balls" and carrots "orange circles." Let children hand-pick them from a bowl of mixed vegetables.
- Let toddlers pick food from the family serving plate, so that they feel free to decide what and how much to eat. This helps reduce frustration during the "no" stage. Offer some foods to eat with a spoon at each meal (to teach the child how to handle utensils) but allow some finger foods to make the transition easier.

BABIES NEED ENOUGH FAT FOR NORMAL GROWTH

The high percentage of fat in both human milk and formulas may come as a surprise to many adults intent on limiting fat intake. But the low-fat diets recommended for adults do not apply to infants who need a fat-rich diet to meet their high energy needs. Since there are limits to the amount of food infants can ingest and digest at any one time, the only way to get the energy density of food up to the required level is with a high fat content.

BOTTLE FEEDING TIPS

- *Follow formula preparation instructions exactly. Don't add extra powder to make a stronger feed. If it's too concentrated, the baby may become dehydrated because the mixture is too rich. Adding extra water means that the baby won't get enough essential nutrients.*
- *Never add sugar or food (e.g., cereal) to a baby's bottle.*
- *Don't put baby to bed with a bottle*, as prolonged sucking on a bottle of formula, milk or juice bathes the upper teeth in a carbohydrate-rich fluid and can produce dental decay.
- *Never prop a baby to feed alone*, in case

of choking.
- *Keep made-up bottles of formula refrigerated.*
- *Never heat bottles in the microwave; the heat can be uneven and lead to scalding from hot spots in the milk.*
- *Never reuse leftover formula*—bacteria levels could have risen.

KEY TYPES OF FORMULA

Standard	Cow's-milk-based formula for weaning from breast or for bottlefeeding full-term infants. Provides 3 mg iron/L. May contain lactose.
Iron fortified	Cow's-milk-based infant formula for use when weaning or for bottlefeeding full-term infants. Provides 7–13 mg iron/L. May contain lactose.
Lactose-free	Cow's-milk-based, lactose-free formula for infants with lactose intolerance.
Soy	Milk-free, soy-based formula, useful for infants with a milk-protein allergy. Lactose-free. May contain sucrose or be sucrose-free. Use with physician advice.
Hypoallergenic formulas	Specially designed for infants with colic, or those who cannot tolerate milk-based or soy-protein-based formulas.
"Next Step" formulas	Transitional formulas for babies over 6 months old who have started on solid foods but aren't yet ready for cow's milk (of debatable usefulness).

- Don't hover expectantly while a child eats, monitoring each mouthful, and avoid talking about food too much, as though it were the "be all and end all"! Food is for health, not for obsession.

Childhood food intolerances and food allergies

Food intolerances differ from food allergies, which are identifiable immunological reactions to a specific food ingredient, with definite symptoms such as hives, wheezing, and swelling of the tongue and throat. By contrast, a food intolerance may produce bloating, loose stools, gas or vomiting but not immune-system symptoms. Some children are lactose-intolerant, owing to the lack of an enzyme called lactase, normally present in the bowel wall, which digests lactose (milk sugar). A child with lactase deficiency develops gastric discomfort after ingesting lactose-containing foods such as milk, butter and yogurt. This food intolerance can be managed by feeding milk-free substitutes, such as soy formula, for a short time. In older children, milk intake may be limited, or they can be given special low-lactose or lactose-free milk products.

Watching for and managing cow's milk allergy

Cow's-milk allergies (to specific proteins such as whey and casein) affect an estimated 1 to 3 percent of North American children under three years old, and as many as 7 percent of those in allergy-prone families. Symptoms of milk allergy include vomiting, diarrhea, asthmatic wheezing, breathing difficulties, eczema and hives—often appearing within an hour or two of ingesting cow's milk. Those with a severe milk allergy can develop hives, swollen lips and tongue, wheezing and gastric pain within minutes of ingesting even small amounts of cow's-milk protein. Milk sensitivity often wanes around 18 months of age.

To block or mute a milk allergy, many pediatricians promote prolonged breastfeeding (for at least 9 months), avoidance of milk products by the lactating mother and use of substitute formula when weaning from the breast. In the past, infants allergic to cow's milk were switched to soy formula, but recent studies find that some infants allergic to cow's milk also develop a soy allergy. Alternatives include *casein hydrolysates* (made by heat-treating cow's milk to break down bovine proteins into less-allergy-provoking fractions)—an often well tolerated substitute, although rather bitter tasting and expensive. *Whey hydrolysates* are newer reportedly better-tasting products, although less well tolerated. Allergists stress that these substitutes may not be entirely safe for milk-allergic children—"hypoallergenic" (having little or a reduced tendency to cause an allergic reaction) does *not* mean "nonallergenic."

CHOOSING THE RIGHT BABY FORMULA

Women who wish to or must bottle feed their infants now have a wide range of formulas to choose from. Although infants don't really need

---

PREMATURE AND LOW-BIRTH-WEIGHT BABIES NEED EXTRA IRON

While experts argue about the overall need for iron-enriched formula, all agree that low-birthweight and premature infants have special requirements because of their low iron stores at birth and growth rates faster than full-term babies. The Canadian Paediatric Society recommends an iron supplement be given to them beginning at 8 weeks of age, continuing until the child turns 1 year old. Iron is given in fortified formula to bottlefeds and as commercial drops to breastfeds.

the extra iron until 6 months of age, most experts recommend iron-fortified formula from birth onward for fully bottlefeds as parents rarely like to change brands. For breastfed babies, iron-fortified formulas are recommended when weaned. Higher fat milk is generally recommended at 12 months.

Formula cannot completely mimic breast milk

Despite their best efforts, formula manufacturers have not yet managed to duplicate all the hormones, enzymes, antiviral agents (such as immunoglobins) and antibacterial factors (e.g., lactoferrin) in breast milk.

Special formulas for special baby needs

Lactose-free formulas are useful for infants with lactose intolerance—intolerance to the lactose (sugar) in cow's milk—but not for infants allergic to cow's milk. The symptoms of lactose intolerance (excessive gas, abdominal bloating and diarrhea) mimic those of milk allergy—e.g., eczema (a scaly rash), hives (red skin wheals), flushing and swollen lips.

Formulas based on soy protein are the principal alternative to cow's-milk formula but are not suitable for premature babies. They are good for infants with lactose intolerance, milk allergy and *galactosemia* (an inherited inability to metabolize the milk sugar galactose). The carbohydrates used in most soy formulas are sucrose and corn syrup, easily digestible by infants. But soy formula may not be the right choice for infants allergic to milk protein because of cross-reactivity.

Hydrolyzed-protein formulas suit babies with a cow's-milk intolerance or allergy, persistent colic, severe feeding problems and nutritional disorders. Although made from cow's milk, the milk protein is first broken into its component amino acids or "predigested," decreasing the likelihood of allergic reactions. However, hydrolyzed formulas are expensive and many physicians suggest trying others first.

Experts debate the iron needs of young infants

Iron is essential for making hemoglobin—the compound in red blood cells that carries oxygen around the body. Lack of iron can lead to anemia. Healthy, full-term babies are born with enough iron to see them through the first 4 to 6 months of life. However, within the first year an infant must triple its body weight and double its total iron content, creating a high demand. Infants aged 5 to 12 months need 7 mg of iron/day; children aged 1 to 3 years need 6 mg/day, and those aged 4 to 12 years require 8 mg daily. From the age of 6 months on, infants need extra iron—usually obtained by starting them on varied solid foods.

Experts agree that infants need extra iron after the age of 6 months; they argue about the necessity for all bottlefeds to have iron-enriched formula from birth onward. Many think it's unnecessary to start bottlefeds on iron-fortified formula until they really need the extra iron—around the age of 4 to 6 months. One key argument against iron-enrichment hinges on the fact that bacteria that thrive in the bowels of infants fed iron-fortified formula might increase risks of gastroenteritis (diarrhea) and colic. The optimal amount of iron to put in baby formula has not yet been established. North America formulas contain more iron than those in Britain and France.

TOILET TRAINING

Learning to go to the toilet is part of natural human development and should start only when the child is ready—usually between 2 and 3 years of age. But each child's physical progress differs: a child may be ready earlier or later than a sibling, other people's offspring or daycare friends. Let the child set the pace. Patience, support and understanding are essential. A child may show signs of readiness but not yet be really ready—for example, when in the "no's" stage, having temper tantrums or going through a stressful or disruptive period (perhaps because of a move to a new home or a divorce). "Accidents" will happen. From time to time even toilet-trained children may revert to diapers because of stress—perhaps a new baby in the family, a parent's absence or some illness. This is common and usually does not last long. Many find the summer—when accidents are more easily dealt with—the best time for toilet training . When the child does successfully use a "child potty," their achievement shouldreceive a warm round of approval or applause.

Children are emotionally prepared to use the toilet when:

- they tell you about the urge to urinate or have a bowel movement;
- they know what is expected when on the toilet;
- they are willing to urinate or have a bowel movement in the toilet instead of in a diaper.

Children are physically prepared to use the toilet when:

- they can control their bladders (when they can hold enough fluid in);
- they can control the sphincter (anal) muscles that hold in stool.

Tips for toilet training

- Use the same words and routines for toilet learning at home as in childcare programs. Give encouragement and verbal praise as positive support.
- Use potty chairs—they are less intimidating than toilets.
- Make toilets feel safer with a special seat, and/or secure a stool or box under the feet for children sitting on the toilet.
- Never force a child to use a potty: it only sets up a power struggle and negative feelings toward it.
- Encourage a child to sit for short periods of time, and be sure to try at key times—i.e., soon after meals, before naps and after waking up dry from a nap (once the child is comfortably awake).
- With increasing success, start leaving off diapers for a short period. Encourage the child to do this by himself or herself. Leave the potty in the same area for the child to use periodically.
- Don't reward children with food or candy (it puts the wrong connotation on food, equating it with approval).
- Try removing diapers all day once the child gets the hang of things. Most children will stay dry during the day well before they can be out of diapers at night.
- Watching older brothers and sisters or parents use the toilet provides positive role modeling.

- Praise the child for getting to the toilet on time, but don't get angry if there's an accident. Instead, reassure the child that accidents do happen, and that they're "no big deal."
- In order to teach proper personal hygiene, always wash the child's hands and your own hands after changing soiled diapers or after a child uses the toilet.

BUILDING IN SELF-ESTEEM

The critical importance to childhood health of ingraining a clear sense of self-worth is becoming ever more clear. The brain is very "plastic" during early infancy and the first years of life and although we do not know exactly the best way to influence its development, we do know that interaction and stimulation with others are crucial for optimal child development. The reactions that come naturally to parents, such as cooing, smiling and tickling a newborn can all contribute to their sense of self-worth and build confidence and trust. From day one after birth, by everything they say and do and by verbal and nonverbal actions, parents, teachers and siblings communicate approval or disapproval, likes or dislikes, which profoundly influence the way children view themselves. Displaying disapproval by a facial expression or hunched shoulders can be just as influential as open verbal criticism. For instance, a disgusted grimace while changing diapers can make a baby feel "dirty" or "ashamed" of his or her body.

To bolster childhood self-esteem, parents and caregivers should express respect, acceptance and love to children, regardless of their behavior. Children need to be unconditionally valued as worthwhile people even when their behavior is not acceptable. While expressing disapproval for bad or unacceptable behavior do not reject the child as a whole. Make children feel accepted for what they are, and emphasize the positive rather than the negative sides of their character and abilities. Make children feel loved for their own unique qualities: "I like your sturdy legs"; "You have the silkiest cheeks imaginable"; "Your drawings are great." In depressed or low times, children will remember these comments and feel better about themselves.

Always remember to acknowledge good childhood actions or progress. Relatives visiting

SIGNS OF READINESS FOR TOILET TRAINING

- **Child stays dry for longer periods;**
- **Child recognizes and mentions wet or soiled diapers;**
- **Child uses words or gestures to communicate need to urinate or defecate;**
- **Child demonstrates interest in the toilet;**
- **Child goes to the potty and sits on it;**
- **Child can pull own pants down.**

young nieces, nephews or grandchildren can help by making each child feel "special." Instead of giving a blanket greeting—"Hi kids!"—they can single out each child for separate attention. "Hello, Andrea, how is your new school?" or "Tell me, Jeremy, are you still playing the guitar? Give me a tune." For frazzled parents, the extra attention given to children by others can be a great help, while the children gain self-esteem by relating separately to other relatives, friends and teachers.

Children who don't feel accepted may think they're all bad and therefore unable to control or change their actions, instead of believing that they are okay and can change the way they behave. Child guidance should be positive, with a sympathetic but firm approach. Consider the child's viewpoint before handing out punishment. Be clear and direct in explaining what you disapprove of and why; don't just be cold or withdrawn. It's better for children to know why you are displeased than to guess they've done something far worse; better to be told that you're angry about "the lie told" or "skipping class" than to feel utterly worthless and unloved.

Showing respect for children and helping them to build self-esteem means:
- valuing the child's feelings and thoughts;
- accepting the child's ideas and contributions;
- being honest with the child;
- understanding the child's point of view;
- telling children, including infants, what to expect from you, so that any reprimand or disapproval is understood and not taken as total rejection;
- listening attentively and picking up cues from children's unique communication modes—for example, the particular way an infant coos, smiles, cries or moves; his or her preferred toys; how a toddler gestures or tries out words; the way an older child communicates ideas;
- demanding realistic rather than perfect behavior and setting realistic limits;
- offering choices to foster independence: "Would you like your medicine now or in 10 minutes?" or "It's bedtime—would you like your teddy or doggie to cuddle?";
- communicating with "I" messages or personal statements about how undesirable behavior affects you. "I" messages help children see the

LEADING CAUSES OF FATAL CHILDHOOD INJURIES

- **Motor vehicle crashes (often because of failure to wear appropriate restraints);**
- **falls—from beds, table tops, shelves, ledges, stairs or play equipment;**
- **burns (due to no smoke detectors, or carelessness with** fireplaces, matches, lighters, stoves);
- **drownings (in bathtubs, sinks, diaper pails, laundry pails, pools and ponds);**
- **suffocation, choking (on small toys, nuts, balloons, combs, candy, plastic bags of all kinds);**
- **poisoning from** medicines, cleaning products and other chemicals (very frequent);
- **being struck by heavy or sharp falling objects (bookcase, TV set, anything that can easily topple if pulled by tiny hands).**

immediate effects of their behavior; for example, "When you throw blocks, I worry that you may hurt someone or break a window even if you don't mean to." This beats saying, "Naughty boy, that's a bad thing to do!" Such scolding provides only negative, character-deprecating information, giving the child no positive direction. Allow children to make mistakes and then remain neutral so that the child learns by his or her own errors. Children need time to find their own solutions. They also learn by having to repair the consequences of their behavior—for example, wiping up spilled juice.

PREVENTING AVOIDABLE INJURIES

Injury tops the list for causes of death and permanent disability among children in Canada. Over half the deaths in people under age 24 are due to unintentional injuries. (In infants under 1 year old, however, although injury rates are high, they are the sixth cause of death, after birth problems, inherited defects, Sudden Infant Death Syndrome, infections and heart flaws.) Apart from death, accidents take an immense toll in needless injury. And Canada is a global leader in childhood injury, with rates higher than Australia, Japan and most of Western Europe. (See also Chapter 2, the section on injury-prevention.)

Knowing how injuries are likely to happen and at which ages, and planning to avoid them, can prevent much tragedy. Many needless deaths result from auto crashes (where children weren't wearing car restraints), drownings (because of unsupervised water play or baths), fires (no smoke detectors in the house) and bicycle accidents (children not wearing helmets). Other injuries, generally somewhat less serious, result from children being struck or pierced by objects, and from sports. Children have been killed or badly hurt because a TV fell on them when they pulled the cord, because they were accidentally shut in a fridge or freezer, because they roller-bladed without a helmet, drowned in a garden pond, and in countless other home and playground mishaps.

Canada has introduced laws covering child car seats, childproof packaging, flame-resistant nightwear and toy labeling, as well as fireworks and a multitude of other hazards. However, childproof packaging isn't going to work if parents don't fasten the lids properly; child car seats won't work if they aren't used. Caregivers frequently underestimate dangers to children—for instance, when crossing streets or bicycling, both common causes of childhood deaths. A recent survey found that parents were more worried about their child being kidnapped or abusing drugs than about the less dramatic but far more prevalent risk of traffic injuries. Only 6 percent of parents surveyed knew that injury is the main cause of childhood deaths.

How "accidents" happen

Injuries typically happen when caregivers relax their watchful gaze or overestimate a child's skills. They can occur with parents or other caregivers in the next room—or even in the same room. Not everyone realizes that within seconds a child can fall off a high surface (even a bed), drown or get badly burned. Anticipating how and where injuries may occur is the first step in avoiding them. The childproofing of the home, car and surroundings must be geared to each age group and the youngsters activity levels. The greatest danger arises when children's activity levels exceed their judgment.

Once babies can reach and grasp (around age 3 to 4 months), they're at risk of burns from pulling or toppling hot coffee pots, toasters or kettles, or of choking on objects reached and put in the mouth (such as beads, small parts of toys, peanuts, popcorn, candy, plastic bags).

In toddlers, the most frequent causes of injury or death are drownings, traffic accidents and poisonings. In preschoolers up to about age 5, falls, burns, choking, auto accidents and poisonings are the most frequent causes. In schoolchildren, cycling and pedestrian mishaps top the list, and in adolescents, the causes are car passenger deaths (often due to careless or drunken driving), suicide, substance abuse and homicide.

PREVENTING CHILDHOOD CHOKING

Choking is the second most common cause of death in children under age 5. It can occur from awkwardly sized bits of food, eating too fast, not chewing well, running with food in the mouth or swallowing small objects. Foods liable to cause choking and considered unsafe until chewing is mastered (around age 4) include peanuts, popcorn, hard candy, large pasta and hot dogs. (For how to handle a choking emergency, see "Choking" in Chapter 17. Do *not* slap the choker on the back. Call for emergency help *at once*, if a choking victim becomes limp, blue or unconscious.)

Tips to prevent choking in children

Practice and teach children safe eating habits:
- Take small bites, chew thoroughly and swallow *before* taking another bite.
- Don't eat while talking or laughing.
- Sit still during meals; don't run or play, or eat and drink simultaneously.
- Cut food into small enough pieces.

PROTECTING CHILDREN FROM INJURY

As primary safety measures for infants unable to protect themselves, install household smoke detectors, ensure safe cribs (remember the secondhand, older models may not conform to modern standards) and make sure any play equipment (swings, slides, seesaws, dollhouses, ladders) is in safe working order, has no sharp edges or nails sticking out, meets Canadian Standards Association (CSA) standards and bears the CSA seal of approval. Be sure to use age-appropriate, properly installed car restraints. (In one study, unrestrained children were 11 times likelier to die in auto crashes than those properly secured.)

Once children can move about and explore their surroundings, store all sharp objects, medications and household chemicals well out of reach, up and away out of sight. Drowning is a particular threat to toddlers if a child is momentarily left alone. (One child recently drowned in a small puddle of water on top of a swimming pool cover!) Burns from over-hot tap water are another hazard; keep maximum water temperature below 48°C (120°F).

TIPS FOR REDUCING CHILDHOOD INJURIES

- **Reorganize and child-proof all rooms to which young children have access.**
- **Store all sharp objects and household chemicals well out of reach of tiny explorers.**
- **Make sure play equipment (swings, slides, seesaws, dollhouses, ladders) is in good working order.**
- **Ensure that electrical cords don't dangle over counter edges. They can get caught in a cupboard door or drawer, or be pulled by a child. Unplug cords from electrical outlets when not in use.**
- **Don't carry hot foods or liquids when children are nearby.**
- **Turn pot handles toward the back of the stove.**
- **Store unopened glass pop bottles in a locked cupboard. Pressurized pop bottles easily shatter or** explode, and the shattered glass can cause serious injuries.
- **Safety-proof stairs: put handrails on both sides of the staircase and don't leave clutter on steps. Put a safety gate at the top and bottom of stairs.**
- **Keep cleaning products in their original containers or ensure that they are properly labeled, and store them safely beyond children's reach.**
- **Use special latches, locks or other safety devices to make storage areas inaccessible to children.**
- **Since plastic bags of all kinds present a suffocation hazard, don't keep them loose—instead, tie in several knots and discard, or use alternative packaging.**
- **Don't let small children play with balloons inflated or uninflated (in the last** few years, several children have perished by choking on them).
- **Don't allow children to sit on window ledges; never leave them unattended on a balcony.**
- **Never leave "crawlers" unattended on high surfaces (even a bed).**
- **Don't let children play in or around cars.**
- **Forbid playing with matches, lighters and cigarettes.**

Tips for safer childhood car travel:

- **Fasten luggage below seatback level (especially in the back of station wagons or "hatchbacks"), as a sudden stop can make it fly forward. Never put items of any weight in the back window—in a sudden stop they become dangerous projectiles.**
- **Make sure all children** are secured in car restraints approved by the Canadian Standards Association (CSA).
- **Place small infants in rear-facing child car seats that conform with the Motor Vehicle Safety Act—either portable infant carriers or convertible seats—fastening the infant well by the harness straps, and making sure the seat is securely tethered.**
- **Seat toddlers (9–18 kg or 20–40 lb) in child car seats behind the driver conforming to the Children's Car Seats and Harness Regulations (set by the Hazardous Products Act). This can be a convertible or a special child seat in a forward-facing position with a tether strap to prevent the seat from flying forward. The harness straps must be securely fastened.**
- **Teach older children to fasten seat belts at all times, before the car is started.**
- **Avoid looking at children in a rear seat—removing your attention from the road for even a few seconds can easily lead to a collision.**
- **If the child requires care, don't do it while driving—park the car first.**
- **Walk around your car before backing out of the garage or driveway to be sure it is clear of children, toys, bicycles and other obstructions.**
- **Many car-rental companies offer car seats. Check for this option and their safety when renting.**
- **Have a first-aid kit on hand for minor injuries. Even if seemingly unhurt after a car crash, have a checkup by a physician or local hospital.**

- Don't eat lying down.
- If something is difficult to swallow, spit it out!
- Don't discourage a child from coughing food up—it could save a life.
- Never force a drowsy child to eat.
- Minimize distractions while eating.
- Don't reswallow what's coughed up; spit it into a napkin instead.
- Never take off or completely push in pop can tabs, which can cause choking if swallowed.
- Babies have a strong cough reflex—encourage them to cough if choking.
- If a child begins to choke, don't pound him or her on the back; it may make the obstruction worse; don't give bread either—it causes a bigger blockage.

Be aware of items that easily cause choking in children, for instance:
- Do not give children under 5 years of age peanuts (which easily get stuck), peanut butter or soft cheese products (except spread thinly), soft bread, hard candy, popcorn, unpeeled apples, carrots, celery or grapes. (Peanuts and similar foods aren't really considered safe until around age 5 to 6.)
- To avoid trouble, grate carrots and remove pits from fruit. Note that hot dogs can cause choking because a youngster's airway is about the size of an average hot dog. To avoid trouble, skin hot dogs and either dice them or cut them lengthwise, not in coin shapes.
- Children have choked on small balls, buttons,

batteries, coins, crayon pieces, marbles, tiny toys, balloons, pieces of a plant or even bits of plastic from a disposable diaper.

- Make sure children's toys can stand up to rough play and are in good repair, with no broken or loose parts that could stick in the throat. Keep older children's toys, which may have small detachable parts, away from young children.
- Keep children's sleep and play areas free of small objects, such as marbles, that could be inhaled or swallowed.
- Note that *balloons are especially dangerous* to children. One expert tells of a child who bit a balloon on his first birthday, choked on it and died. The balloon's adhesive quality makes it very difficult to dislodge.
- Do not prop a baby under the age of 9 months with a bottle while lying down, as it may choke on the liquid.

SOME EARLY SIGNS OF ILLNESS IN CHILDREN

- **Unusual fussiness, irritability or altered behavior is a significant sign. The greater the change in a child's behavior, the greater the likelihood of serious illness. Children who remain active, hungry and playful aren't usually too ill. But those who seem unusually sleepy, dozy, irritable, lethargic or unresponsive may be harboring some serious disorder.**
- **A runny nose may signify infection. The most common causes of a runny nose in young children are viral infections—for example, the common cold. Allergies and chemical irritation are other causes. The color change of a nasal discharge is not significant, but if it persists for more than a week, the child should be medically checked.**
- **Coughing can be triggered by infection and/or irritation**

anywhere in the respiratory tract, from the nose to the lungs, or may be due to allergies, asthma, chemical irritation, cystic fibrosis, an inhaled object or a child's psychological state (anxiety). A cough often long outlasts a runny nose. If it's persistent, see a physician about it.
- **Wheezing when breathing out—due to air-passage narrowing and/or excess mucus in the airways (tubes) of the lungs— is often due to a viral infection or asthma. Rapid shallow breathing needs medical attention.**
- **Vomiting is much more frequent in children than in adults, and produces much less discomfort; it may be due to the general effects of an infection rather than a specific stomach irritation. Vomiting in itself isn't dangerous unless the child chokes on inhaled vomit, or**

vomits frequently enough to become dehydrated.
- **Diarrhea with frequent, watery or unformed stools can be a risk if the amount of water lost surpasses the amount taken in, leading to dehydration. Dehydration can be serious because it impairs the blood circulation, and occurs much more rapidly in infants than in older children or adults. If children vomit as well as having diarrhea, the danger of dehydration increases and medical attention is needed.**
- **A suddenly pale complexion, or yellowing of the whites of the eyes, may signify acute illness that needs prompt medical attention.**
- **For fever, see "Understanding childhood fever" later in this chapter.**

RECOGNIZING AND MANAGING CHILDHOOD DISORDERS

The most common childhood disorders seen by family practitioners are coughs and colds, sore throats (including tonsillitis), ear infections, roseola, chickenpox and various cuts, bruises and unintentional injuries. In the modern world, vaccination can save children from many infectious diseases that formerly killed countless youngsters.

Vaccines save young lives

Immunization against communicable diseases remains one of the most cost-effective and life-saving health measures. Widespread vaccination programs in the Western World have dramatically curtailed previously ravaging diseases such as polio and eradicated smallpox. While no vaccine is 100 percent safe, today's vaccines used for childhood immunization are very effective in preventing disease; they have *few* side effects and *extremely* low risks. They save thousands of lives each year. In fact, vaccines are so effective that many of the diseases they protect against are now rare in the Western world. Some infections now rare in Canada—such as diphtheria, tetanus and measles—still claim thousands of lives around the world. The success of immunization campaigns and antibiotic drugs has lulled many into the belief that the battle against infectious diseases is won. However, one leading Canadian expert in infectious diseases warns that "we ignore the need for vaccination at our peril."

How immunization works

The principle of immunization (or vaccination) is based on the fact that exposing the immune system to a vaccine containing weakened microbes (or parts of them) mimics an actual infection but is too weak to make the person ill. The body develops "immune memory," just as it would in response to a real bacterial or viral infection. Although artificially induced, the vaccine-triggered immune memory is then ready to spring into immediate action any time the person is exposed to these particular germs. In this way, vaccines provide long-lasting immunity without the risks of illness or death associated with the actual infection. The viruses causing some infections, such as influenza, change annually and this is why we need to get immunized with a new vaccine each year.

All children should be immunized at specified ages against diphtheria, tetanus (lockjaw), pertussis (whooping cough), polio, measles, mumps, rubella (German measles), Haemophilus influenzae B (Hib) infections such as meningitis, and hepatitis B. Health authorities are now also recommending childhood immunizations against chickenpox, pneumococcus and meningitis.

Some advances in vaccines

- *Varicella (chickenpox) vaccine* for all children in Canada. Chickenpox is caused by a virus called varicella. Since the licensure of the varicella vaccine in the U.S. in 1995, the incidence of varicella and related hospitalizations in the

VACCINES CONTAIN EITHER:
• **killed, intact bacteria (e.g., whole-cell pertussis vaccine);** • **killed, intact viruses (e.g., inactivated polio vaccine—IPV);** • **weakened or "attenuated" live virus (e.g., measles,** | **mumps, rubella vaccines and oral/live polio vaccine—OPV);** • **purified bacterial polysaccharides or sugars (e.g., Haemophilus B or Hib vaccine);** • **purified viral protein**	**(e.g., hepatitis B vaccine);** • **inactivated bacterial toxin (e.g., diphtheria and tetanus toxoids); or** • **purified bacterial proteins (e.g., acellular pertussis vaccine).**

U.S. have fallen—by 76 to 86 percent in 2001—and studies demonstrate that the vaccine provides 70 to 90 percent protection against varicella infection and 95 percent protection against severe varicella for 7 to 10 years. The routine immunization schedule is for all children to be vaccinated against chickenpox at 12 to 15 months and receive catch-up immunization up to 12 years of age. The vast majority of children get infected with chickenpox or varicella in daycare or at school. If there is a question about having had the disease, your care provider can do a blood test to check. Children under age 13 require one varicella vaccine dose, while children older than 13 and adults require 2 doses given 4 to 8 weeks apart.

- *Pneumococcus vaccine or Prevnar* protects

SOME SENSIBLE PRECAUTIONS ABOUT VACCINATION

While adverse reactions to vaccines are rare, there are certain people and some conditions that warrant caution:

- **People allergic to eggs and specific chemicals must be cautious about receiving vaccines that contain traces of egg-protein (in measles, mumps, influenza and yellow-fever vaccines), or such substances as thimerosal (a mercurial preservative in most inactivated vac**cines) and antibiotics (such as neomycin, in some polio vaccines).

- **Live viral vaccines are unsuitable for some. Measles, rubella, mumps, yellow-fever and oral polio vaccines all contain weakened but live microorganisms. While there is no solid proof that live virus vaccines can harm the fetus, it is safer to err on the side of caution and avoid them while pregnant.**

- **People who have a** moderate or severe illness should wait until they're better to be immunized (although a minor infection such as a head cold, with or without fever, need not prevent vaccination).

- **People with immune-deficiency diseases, those on immunosuppressants and children with leukemia should not receive live virus immunization, although those infected with HIV may do so.**

- **Those living with an immunosuppressed person should not take live (oral) polio vaccine, as the virus can be passed on. No problem exists with other live vaccines.**

- **The pertussis component of the DPT vaccine is generally blamed for post-vaccination discomforts: fever, redness and swelling at the injection site, and fussiness, drowsiness and appetite loss experienced in about 50 percent of inocu**lated babies. These reactions, which are usually short-lived, mild and no cause for alarm, are easily minimized by giving fretful children acetaminophen (Children's Tylenol, Tempra, Atasol, Panadol), perhaps at the time of injection and again a few hours later. A tiny proportion get further adverse reactions to the pertussis vaccine, though far less so with newer vaccines. Severe reactions are rare.

children against Streptococcus pneumoniae that causes a variety of infections in the lungs, ears and brain. In Canada each year, there are approximately 65 cases of meningitis, 700 cases of blood infection, 2,200 cases of pneumonia requiring hospitalization and 9,000 cases not requiring hospitalization, and an average of 15 deaths per year due to *S. pneumoniae* in children under 5 years of age. The conjugate pneumococcal vaccine is recommended by immunization authorities for all children 23 months and younger, although some parents may decide not to have their children vaccinated, given the cost and relative rarity of serious pneumococcal infection. The vaccine is also recommended for all children 24 to 59 months who are at risk for invasive pneumococcal infections.

- A variation on this pneumococcal vaccine that comes in one shot is now also strongly promoted for all seniors (and some other vulnerable groups), partly because antibiotic-resistance is hindering successful treatment. (See also Chapter 15.)
- *The meningitis vaccine* has been used primarily in outbreaks, especially in school, university or college settings. As authorities have found it effective, they now recommend early immunization at 2, 4 and 6 months.
- Influenza vaccine has been around for a while and has traditionally targeted elderly people. But recent evidence now favors universal vaccination, especially for and including children over 6 months of age. Immunizing children reduces the spread of influenza through families and the community. Many provinces in Canada now fund influenza vaccination for everyone aged 6 months and over.
- *An antimeningitis or Hib vaccine* to protect infants and toddlers against a certain type of meningitis due to infection by Haemophilus influenzae type b (Hib) bacteria. A new, safe and effective vaccine against Hib can protect infants as young as 2 months old and is given to children at the same time as the routine diphtheria-pertussis-tetanus (DPT) immunization—at ages 2, 4 and 6 months. The benefits of Hib immunization are already here: Hib is no longer the prime cause of

meningitis in infancy, and other forms of Hib disease, such as epiglottitis, have also become uncommon.

- *A new bio-engineered, more effective "acellular" pertussis vaccine* against whooping cough, with fewer side effects than previous forms, introduced as Pentacel in Canada.
- *New vaccines against hepatitis A*—recommended for all travelers to places where this viral disease is rampant.
- *Hepatitis B immunization* for all children and at-risk groups. Universal immunization against hepatitis B is now strongly advocated across the world. A reliable hepatitis B vaccine, made by recombinant DNA technology (from proteins in the viral coat), given in 3 doses over a 6-month period, provides immunity lasting at least 10 years. Vaccine side effects are minimal, maybe just some soreness at the injection site. Babies born to carrier mothers can be infected in the uterus or at delivery, so all pregnant women are given a blood test for hepatitis B and endangered babies are protected by immune globulin, given as soon as possible after birth, followed by vaccination. Other children are given hepatitis B vaccine in their school years.
- *Hepatitis A and B vaccines* can now be given in one injection (Twinrix).
- *A two-dose measles vaccination schedule* to replace the older 1-dose immunization, the second shot being given at school entry, around age 5 to 6 as an extra MMR (measles, mumps and rubella) vaccine. Measles is a potentially serious infection that can have lasting consequences due to complications such as pneumonia and *encephalitis* (brain inflammation). It remains a major childhood killer across the world, and adults with measles are usually very sick. Recent campaigns to revaccinate all schoolchildren against measles have dramatically reduced the number of cases.

UNDERSTANDING CHILDHOOD FEVER

Children seem to get fevers from almost everything—except, contrary to popular folklore, teething. Colds, sore throats, middle-ear, gastric and many other infections cause a child's tem-

ROUTINE IMMUNIZATION SCHEDULE FOR INFANTS AND CHILDREN

Age at Vaccination	DTaP	IPV	Hib	MMR	Td or dTap	Hep B (3 doses)	V	PC	MC
2 months	X	X	X					X	X
4 months	X	X	X			Infancy		X	X
6 months	X	(X)	X			or in		X	X
12 months				X		preadolescence	X	X	
18 months	X	X	X	(X) or		(9–13 years)			or
4–6 years	X	X		(X)					
14–16 years					X				X

DTaP   Diphtheria, tetanus, pertussis (acellular) whooping cough vaccine

IPV   Inactivated poliovirus vaccine

Hib   Haemophilus influenzae type b conjugate vaccine (against infant meningitis)

MMR   Measles, mumps and rubella vaccine

Td   Tetanus and diphtheria toxoid, adult type vaccine

dTap   Tetanus and diphtheria toxoid, acellular pertussis, adolescent/adult type vaccine

   (with reduced diphtheria and pertussis components)

Hep B   Hepatitis B vaccine (given to infants or schoolchildren)

V   Varicella (chickenpox) vaccine

PC   Pneumococcal conjugate vaccine (against pneumonia)

MC   Meningococcal C conjugate vaccine (to protect against meningitis "C").

NOTE: children with egg allergies must be cautioned against receiving mumps, measles or flu vaccines which are grown in chick eggs.

Based on *Canadian Immunization Guide*, 6th ed., 2002, published by Health Canada.

perature to climb. The degree of fever in itself generally poses no danger. The child's behavior is usually a more telling clue to the severity of an illness. But in those under 2 months of age, fevers that would be no cause for alarm in older children may signal a serious problem that requires urgent medical care.

Medication isn't always needed for feverish children. When recommended, acetaminophen, every 4 hours, is given. ASA (acetylsalicylic acid, such as Aspirin) should never be given to a feverish child or teenager because, should the fever be due to some infection such as influenza or chickenpox, taking ASA can increase the risks of Reye's syndrome—a serious disorder that often leads to severe liver and brain damage, sometimes death.

Fever in itself is no danger

Both the public at large and health professionals tend to overestimate the dangers of fever.

Saying that a child is "running a fever" or "has a temperature" means that the body temperature is elevated above the level considered "normal." Human body temperature fluctuates slightly during the day and is usually lower in the morning and higher in the afternoon and evening. When an infection or some other disease process sets in, substances may be released that elevate body temperature. Fever does *not* harm the body and may in fact assist the immune defenses. While its exact mechanism remains unclear, recent medical evidence shows that fever may actually help the body fight disease by increasing the activity of the immune system and the white-blood-cell defense activity. Thus, lowering the fever may make sufferers more comfortable, but does not necessarily assist the body in combating disease.

Children generally run higher temperatures than adults without being as ill. For instance, a 2-year-old with an ear infection can easily have a temperature of 40°C (104°F), while such high fevers are rarely seen in older children. If a child has a fever higher than 39°C (102.2°F), it's generally time to consult a physician. But fever alone isn't dangerous as long as it is not excessively high (over 41.5°C or 106.7°F), and provided fluid intake replaces the body water lost.

The definition of a "significant" temperature

NORMAL BODY TEMPERATURE

In the armpit: 36.4°C (97.5°F)–37°C (98.6°F)
In the mouth: 37°C (98.6°F)
In the rectum: 37.5°C (99.5°F)

A child has a fever if the temperature is:

In the armpit: 38°C (100.4°F) or higher (although armpit tempera-
                  tures are not very accurate and have a wide range)
In the mouth: 38°C (100.4°F) or higher
In the rectum: 38.5°C (101.4°F) or higher

CENTIGRADE–FAHRENHEIT CONVERSION CHART

37°C	=	98.6°F
37.2°C	=	99.0°F
37.5°C	=	99.5°F
37.8°C	=	100°F
38°C	=	100.4°F
38.5°C	=	101.4°F
39°C	=	102.2°F
39.5°C	=	103°F
40°C	=	104°F
40.5°C	=	105°F
41°C	=	105.8°F

N.B.: To convert Celsius readings to Fahrenheit, double the degrees C, subtract 10 percent, then add 32. (E.g., 40°C x 2 – 10% + 32 = 104°F.)

varies but is generally considered to be one that's over 38.5°C (101.4°F). A temperature higher than 40°C (104°F) is regarded as high, but even that won't cause brain damage or permanently threaten health.

Causes of childhood fever vary with age

- At all ages, viral infections are a much more common cause of fever than bacterial infections.
- In newborns (birth to 1 month), fever is often due to infection—sometimes bacterial, occasionally serious. Dehydration, overdressing or an overheated environment may also cause a mild temperature rise.
- In infants (1 month to a year), fever is primarily due to upper-respiratory viral infections, often complicated by an ear infection.
- In toddlers (aged 1 to 4) and preschoolers (aged 4 to 6), the most common fever-causing conditions are infections such as upper-respiratory viral infections, bacterial pharyngitis (sore or "strep" throat), tonsillitis, ear infections and bronchitis. Other causes are digestive- and urinary-tract infections.
- In schoolchildren (aged 6 to 12 years), respiratory infections top the list of fever-causing problems, as well as urinary-tract infections, especially in girls.

Measuring fever

Temperatures are taken by mouth or rectum, in the axilla (armpit) or in the ear. Thermometer scales are marked in degrees Celsius (centigrade), Fahrenheit or both. Commonly used fever thermometers are glass or digital and both work well. Digital thermometers are more sen-

sitive than glass ones and may be used for oral, rectal or armpit measurement. The heat-sensitive tapes or forehead strips that change color on contact with the skin are considered very inaccurate. An excellent new technique, used in some hospitals and perhaps soon to become popular for doctors' offices, employs a tiny temperature-recording instrument put into the ear which registers a very accurate reading within a few seconds. Ear measurement is easier than taking rectal temperatures in tiny babies. Rectal or armpit readings are best for home measurement in children under 5 years old, as a glass thermometer can easily break. Rectal readings are usually about .5 to 1 degree higher than those in the mouth, while underarm temperatures read lower. By age 5, most children can hold a thermometer safely in their mouths.

- When taking a rectal reading, some suggest placing the child on the stomach across your knees and cuddling him or her to keep quiet, while others prefer laying the baby face up and, lifting the legs—meanwhile smiling reassuringly! The thermometer is held about 2.5 cm (1 in) from the tip, lubricated (e.g., with Vaseline) and inserted about 2.5 cm (1 in) into the rectum—up to the point at which it's being held.
- To clean a digital thermometer, wash only the tip with soap and warm (not hot) water and wipe off with alcohol after use. Dry well. To clean a glass thermometer, wash in lukewarm soapy water and rinse with alcohol.

Fever in newborns always needs medical attention

Any fever in newborns up to about 8 weeks of age should immediately be reported to the physician. The fever itself is not the danger but the underlying cause may be serious at this young age. Fever is often the *only* sign of infection in young infants, who give fewer alerting clues than older children to illnesses they may be harboring. It is difficult to know when babies feel below par. Since very young infants cannot localize and fight infection as well as older children, they are at greater risk for bacteremia (a spreading bacterial infection) and meningitis (inflammation of the brain and spinal-cord coverings).

The challenge for doctors is to distinguish mild viral from serious bacterial infections. Because of the risk, many physicians automatically hospitalize newborns with fevers in order to observe them closely and start treatment, possibly giving them antibiotics while awaiting the results of laboratory tests. If the lab culture results are negative and the infant quickly returns to normal feeding and activity, the hospital stay will be short.

Once an infant is past the newborn period, at 2 to 3 months of age, fever is less worrisome. The illness may then be handled at home with close observation and follow-up. In infants aged 3 months to 2 years, a fever over 38.5°C (101.4°F) for 24 hours merits a call to the doctor. In children aged 3 to 6, a fever that lasts 48 hours needs medical attention, even if the child looks well and has a good appetite.

In schoolchildren, the same fever may be left for 72 hours before calling the doctor, provided the child doesn't seem ill and is lively, feeding and behaving normally. As children grow, the symptoms of illness become easier to identify because the child can explain what's wrong.

Also, parents get better at assessing the gravity of their child's condition.

Appearance and behavior are more critical indicators

Do not regard the height of the thermometer reading as the only measure of childhood illness: how a child looks and behaves are more important. A mild viral infection can cause a fever as high as 40°C (104°F), while a severely ill child with meningitis may have a lower fever, around 38.5°C (101.4°F). In general, the child's behavior tells more about the severity of the illness than does the degree of fever. When judging a child's condition and deciding whether or not to call the doctor, caregivers should be guided also by how sick the child seems.

Caregivers should assess whether the child is:

- lively and alert or droopy, apathetic and unusually listless;
- eating well or has a diminished appetite:
- playing normally or ignoring toys;
- gazing around curiously or uninterested;
- smiling at familiar caregivers or unresponsive;

TIPS FOR COOLING FEVERISH CHILDREN

Do's

- **Keep the child lightly dressed indoors, unless he or she is uncomfortable.**
- **Give plenty of cool, clear liquids to replace lost body fluid. Popsicles, ice water or carbonated beverages help to cool a feverish child.**
- **Give acetaminophen (e.g., Children's Tylenol, Atasol, Tempra or Panadol) at a dose of 15 mg/kg (7 mg per lb) every four hours, if needed to reduce discomfort, remembering that it may not bring their temperature right** down to normal. Another option is ibuprofen (Advil, Motrin) which can last longer. Since most children don't feel too uncomfortable until the temperature reaches 39.5°C (103°F), fever-reducers are unnecessary unless the child feels miserable.

- **Consider lukewarm sponge baths or sitting the child in a lukewarm bath—a strategy that, although controversial, is recommended by some physicians, especially for a high** fever. If sponging is to be done, a single oral dose of an anti-fever medication should be given first and the sponging fluid should be lukewarm (neutral to the touch). Don't use cold water as it causes shivering and raises body temperature Although some doubt its efficacy, it may be worth sponging an uncomfortably feverish child for 15 minutes—not immersing him or her completely but leaving most of the body exposed to speed evaporation. But sponge baths should be used only if medically recommended, and children should never be left alone in the bathtub (for safety reasons). If sponging makes a feverish child chilled, shivery or unhappy, forget it!

Don't's

- **Don't overdress or cover a feverish child with heavy bedding. Bundling up a child for fear of "getting a chill" is a common mistake.**
- **Don't overheat the room; keep it no warmer than 20–21°C (68–70°F).** Turn off the heat or open a window slightly, if necessary. Use a fan or an air conditioner in hot weather.

- **Don't cover the child with wet towels or wet sheets—it is uncomfortable.**
- **Don't use alcohol sponging because alcohol can be absorbed through the skin.**
- **Do not give ASA because of the link to Reye's syndrome in the presence of certain viral illnesses such as influenza and chickenpox.**

WHEN TO CALL THE DOCTOR ABOUT FEVER

Call immediately if the child:
- is under 12 weeks old;
- has fever over 40.5°C (105°F);
- acts or looks very sick;
- is crying inconsolably, hard to awaken, delirious or confused;
- has trouble breathing,
- has known medical risk factors (such as leukemia, or sickle

cell anemia) or is on immunosuppressants;
- has a stiff neck;
- has febrile convulsions (twitching or shaking) for the first time;
- has purple spots (petechiae) anywhere on the skin;
- has burning or pain with urination.

Call during office hours if:
- the temperature is over 38.5°C (101.4°F) for 24 hours or more;
- the fever runs for more than 3 days (no matter how mild, or what age the child);
- the behavior of the child is particularly fussy or cranky, or unusually quiet;
- you are anxious about the child's appearance and/or behavior.

- able to be comforted or inconsolably cranky;
- a normal pink color or pale and looks ashen:
- breathing normally or taking rapid breaths (more than 40 a minute);
- "dry" or "wet" in the mucous membranes (nose, eyes); or
- showing obvious signs of pain or discomfort, such as pulling at the ears, holding the head or indicating pain on swallowing.

Watch particularly for such signs of serious illness as a stiff neck; a pale complexion; listless behavior; *petechiae* (purple spots) on the body—all indicative of meningococcal infection (meningitis).

Seizures occasionally occur in feverish children

A few children have seizures (convulsions) at temperatures above a certain level, often when the fever starts to rise. Such seizures never cause brain damage, and the tendency usually fades as children grow, often vanishing around the time a child reaches first grade. Febrile seizures occur in 2 to 4 percent of children worldwide. Although they are scary for parents, there are typically no long term repercussions. They do however indicate a slightly increased risk for epilepsy. The background risk for epilepsy in the general population of children is 1.4 percent and among children with simple febrile seizures it is slightly higher. The doctor should be called at once the first time a child has a febrile seizure, as it could be due to an infection such as meningitis. But

once it's clear that the child is seizure-prone, and once parents know how to handle the situation, it's no longer an emergency. Fever-induced convulsions often run in families. Antipyretic (fever-reducing) medication such as acetaminophen, given every 4 hours for the duration of the fever, may prevent further seizures. (Some experts suggest calling the doctor about any seizure, even in children prone to them, for reassurance and to make sure there is no serious illness causing it.)

ALLERGIES

Allergies typically produce wheezing, coughing, shortness of breath, tongue and/or throat swelling, hives (skin redness or weals), itching and perhaps difficulty swallowing. They arise through exposure to particular substances (allergens)—such as dust mites, pollen, food ingredients, pollutants, insect stings and certain medications—which sensitize the body and cause a buildup of antibodies that set off an allergic response. Since allergic reactions can come on rapidly and in some cases may be life-threatening, people must watch for and respect them.

It usually takes more than one exposure to build up sensitivity to a particular substance. For example, the first time a child eats peanut butter, there may be no sign of an allergic reaction. But if peanut sensitivity develops, the next peanut-butter sandwich or cookie may trigger an immunological response with breathing difficulty or even anaphylactic shock.

Anaphylactic shock is an emergency, a severe allergic reaction with symptoms such as swelling of the eyes, tongue and face, hives on many parts of the body, low blood pressure, vomiting, diarrhea and possibly loss of consciousness. Once someone is "sensitized," symptoms can develop within minutes. Severe allergic reactions require prompt adrenalin (epinephrine) administration, by inhaler or injection. Allergy kits are available from pharmacies, and include full instructions. The best strategy, though, is to identify the allergy-triggering item(s) and avoid them if possible. Mild allergies are treated with antihistamines.

Managing the rising risk of childhood peanut allergies

Peanut butter and other peanut products are designated "danger foods" because so many people have developed peanut allergies. Although some peanut-allergic children have a severe reaction at the slightest taste of peanut, the condition can be well managed with common sense, vigilance and the help of recently published guidelines.

Peanut allergy is now one of the most common causes of food-induced *anaphylaxis*—a rapid, generalized, body-wide allergic response. The reaction can be amazingly swift—with red hives appearing all over the body in minutes, perhaps also swelling of tongue and throat, a flushed face, wheezy breathing and a sudden drop in blood pressure (allergic shock).

The increase in peanut allergy among North American and European children is attributed to the growing diversity of peanut products and their consumption by younger children before their immune systems are fully mature.

To protect children, parents are advised to withhold all peanut products from a child's diet until at least 3 years of age. Children diagnosed as peanut allergic must be taught to watch for and avoid all peanut-containing foods and to carry a self-injection kit containing epinephrine (adrenaline), the life-saving treatment for a severe allergic reaction.

Schools urged to adopt peanut precautions

Many physicians are calling for "peanut-safe classrooms." "It cannot be stressed enough," notes one emergency physician, "that minute amounts of peanut (often as hidden ingredients) can be life-threatening. Even a trace of peanut butter left on a knife could be fatal. The number of anaphylactic episodes in schools is increasing, emphasizing the need for greater awareness."

The Canadian Society of Allergy and Clinical Immunology (CSACI) has launched a campaign to educate schools about peanut allergies and how to manage them. Severely allergic children must have their allergy clearly stated (e.g., on a medical-alert bracelet). Identification sheets could include the child's name, photo-

WARNING SIGNS AND SYMPTOMS OF SEVERE PEANUT ALLERGY

- **itching, tingling, burning of tongue and lips;**
- **upset stomach, nausea, vomiting, diarrhea;**
- **hives (red, raised skin welts) anywhere on the body;**
- **swelling of throat, larynx and tongue;**
- **flushing;**
- **throat tightness or closing;**
- **difficulty swallowing;**
- **wheezing, troubled breathing;**
- **sudden drop in blood pressure/allergic shock;**
- **dizziness;**
- **irregular heartbeat;**
- **sense of doom, collapse;**
- **unconsciousness.**
- **N.B.: All or some symptoms can occur at the same time.**

graph, specific allergy (e.g., peanuts, bee-sting).

Schools should have on hand first-aid epinephrine kits in designated areas (e.g., lunch rooms, gymnasiums, schoolyards, swimming pools). They should be easily accessible (*not* in locked cabinets). U.S. guidelines are similar and the American Academy of Allergy is adapting the Canadian school guidelines. A total ban on peanut products is controversial as they are good sources of cheap protein, and some people feel that forbidding children to eat peanut butter at school infringes on personal liberty. Critics also say that peanut bans may make children feel ostracized, or give them a false sense of security so they're less vigilant. Allergists suggest that schools should be "peanut-safe" rather than "peanut-free," with certain classrooms (or eating areas) excluding peanut products.

For primary schoolchildren with allergic disorders, the problem should be discussed with the school staff—without overdramatizing. Informing teachers can help them understand a child's behavior, which might otherwise seem to be "attention seeking." Allergic children should not be unduly pampered or made to feel special as they could become manipulative (for instance refusing to take medication in order to attract attention).

At the secondary-school level, managing allergies requires great tact as broadcasting an allergy problem could embarrass teenage children and make them "throw caution to the winds."

Tips for preventing severe peanut allergies

- *Do not feed infants born into allergy-prone families* peanuts or peanut butter until age 3 or older.

- *If breastfeeding allergy-prone infants*, avoid eating peanuts.
- *Alert teachers, school and daycare personnel* to the presence of a peanut-allergic child.
- *If there are known peanut-allergic children in school*, try not to send peanuts, peanut butter or peanut products to school.
- *Do not share food or trade utensils* or food containers.
- *Eat only home-prepared food* whenever possible.
- *Be cautious with unlabeled foods.* Many prepared foods are exempt from labeling requirements; bakery products don't list ingredients.
- *Watch for hidden peanut*, especially hard to detect in items such as ice cream, "veggie" burgers, cakes, gravy, cookies, Chinese, Thai, Vietnamese or African food.
- *Read food labels* with scrupulous care *every time* you buy a product (products may change ingredients).
- *If you or a family member suspect a food allergy*, go to a physician or licensed allergist—don't try to self-diagnose or self-treat.
- *Wear a medical alert bracelet* if you have a severe food allergy.

- *Carry an auto-injector kit*, know how to use it, and to replace it when past the expiry date.
- *Look for the "Allergy Aware" symbol* at Canadian restaurants.
- *Speak up!* Be forthright and inform friends and colleagues about an allergy; ask about food ingredients if unsure.

(See chapter 13 for more on allergies.)

ASTHMA

Asthma is the most common childhood disease, affecting as many as 7 to 15 percent of children 3 to 6 years old, although it can start as early as 6 months of age (when it's often misdiagnosed as something else, such as croup or bronchitis). While some suffer attacks only in childhood, it often recurs during adulthood, despite the commonly held misconception that children "outgrow" asthma.

In asthma, the lung's air passages become clogged by inflammatory changes, muscle spasm and a buildup of sticky mucus. "Inflammation is the underlying pathology in asthma," emphasizes one University of Toronto respirologist. "If the inflammation is left untreated, the constriction worsens, leading to breathing troubles."

A classic asthma attack surfaces with per-

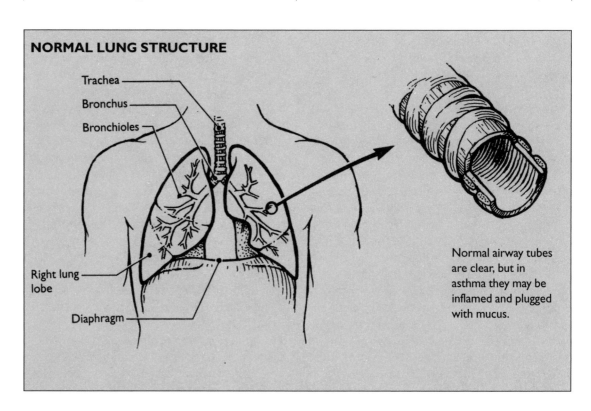

NORMAL LUNG STRUCTURE

Trachea
Bronchus
Bronchioles
Right lung lobe
Diaphragm

Normal airway tubes are clear, but in asthma they may be inflamed and plugged with mucus.

sistent coughing, chest tightness and excess phlegm (mucus). The telltale signs are labored breathing, persistent coughing and wheezing, the wheeze occurring when breathing out through clogged air passages. But not everyone with asthma wheezes—the only clue to the condition may be a persistent cough.

In children, asthma is hard to distinguish from an ordinary cold or a cough; a dry cough that drags on and on, and is especially trouble-some at night and first thing in the morning is suspect, or if a child has frequent chest colds, noticeably labored breathing and wheezing after exercise. Get specialist advice to help the child gain enough control to attend school and enjoy all the usual childhood activities. Although most (about 75 percent) of childhood asthma is mild and controllable with occasional bronchodilator puffs, it can become rapidly severe with attacks that worsen rapidly over days or hours—some-times without prior warning.

The first step is prevention, which includes reducing dust mites and cigarette smoke in the home (see the website below for specific measures). Modern treatment focuses on reliev-ing the underlying lung inflammation, with anti-inflammatory agents as the primary med-ications, plus bronchodilators to widen the airways when and as needed. The bronchodila-tors make people feel better as they work quickly. However, the "steroid" puffers are more effective at actually treating the problem (inflammation) and preventing further illness. Inhaled glucocorticosteroids (ICS) are the most effective agents in this category and are consid-ered the first-line anti-inflammatory therapy for asthma. Generally, the bronchodilators are referred to as "relievers" and the steroids are referred to as "preventers" or "controllers." The inhaler devices are colored blue and brown respectively. The steroid puffers are well toler-ated, but can cause a very slight reduction in a child's growth. Once the steroid puffer is no longer being used, however, growth usually starts up again. Newer pills called leukotriene receptor antagonists (LTRAs) have become available. The use of LTRAs as the initial anti-inflammatory treatment remains controversial, but they can certainly be used in children who will not or cannot use glucocorticosteroids or in those who show very positive responses to the LTRAs. In these cases, the kids can be weaned off steroids.

Children with moderate disease (episodes every 4 to 6 weeks) may be started on nons-teroidal puffers (perhaps inhaled cromoglycate or nedocromil), or on ketotifen (Zaditen) tablets or syrup. To facilitate inhalation of asthma medica-tion, a "spacer device" on the puffer; or an Aerochamber with a mask, can be used. There are many new types of inhaler now on the market that make it easier for children to take their drugs.

The 5 percent or so of asthmatic children who have severe problems, with troubled breathing on most days (serious enough to interfere with school and sleep), need regularly inhaled corticosteroids plus bronchodilators for "breakthrough" wheezing. Studies show few or no toxic side effects from regular, low-dose inhaled corticosteroids in children. Although there have been some concerns about steroids stunting children's growth, the low dose of the agents inhaled is only minimally absorbed into the bloodstream. Children on high steroid doses need careful monitoring.

In managing youngsters with asthma, tact and understanding are the essence, as children are often ashamed of having to use a puffer. The best advice is to treat the child as normally as possible. Using a home peak-flow meter to monitor the condition is a help in spotting wors-ening asthma. Asthmatic teenagers are notoriously tough to handle because they tend to deny the disorder and ignore breathing diffi-culties. Visit www.AsthmaActionPlan.com for a complete toolkit to help prevent asthma.

AUTISM

Autistic children can't relate normally to others, but escape into their own inner world, unable to bear too much sensory "input" or stimulation. Occasionally, the term Pervasive Development Disorder (PDD) is used to describe autism and its distorted perception, sense of reality and movement. Autistic children are not just delayed, they are very different. About 4 per 10,000 children (1 in 2,500) are autistic.

Typically, autistic children display:
• an inability to form social relationships;
• disordered speech;

SOME COMMON BIRTHMARKS

Stork bites, also popularly known as *salmon marks*, are reddish-pink marks at the nape of the neck or on the forehead, seen in 30 to 40 percent of white-skinned newborns. If the stain shows up on the neck or eyelids, it's called an *angel's kiss*. This harmless little mark is a collection of surface blood vessels that dilate and cause redness. It almost always fades during the first year, although faint signs may remain forever.

Mongolian spots, more a bluish smudge than a spot, are due to a collection of pigment-producing cells, and occur mostly on the lower back or buttocks. The name is a misnomer because the spot is by no means exclusive to (or common in) Mongols (babies with Down syndrome) or among Mongolian races, but is most frequent among blacks, Asians and Jews of Spanish or Portuguese origin.

Café-au-lait patches are light brown stains made up of pigment-producing cells, seen in about 10 percent of Caucasian newborns. These birthmarks appear mainly on the trunk and can be any size. Being inconspicuous, they rarely pose a cosmetic problem although they can last a lifetime. More than 5 café-au-lait spots on a child may signal the presence of an underlying disease, neurofibromatosis (disfiguring, sometimes progressive formation of tumors on the skin or nerves).

Spider angiomas are small, red, wispy spots on the face with networks of fine blood vessels radiating outwards, somewhat like a spider's web. Not strictly defined as birthmarks, they often don't appear until the age of 2 to 3 years and usually fade by puberty. They also sometimes develop in women during pregnancy or in older people, and are occasionally left behind after strawberry birthmarks have faded. They are generally harmless, but large numbers of them may signal liver problems or an unsuspected vitamin B deficiency. Some can now be treated with electrical therapy or lightened by tunable dye laser treatment.

Port wine stains are present at birth, affect 0.3 percent of all babies and come in many shapes and sizes, ranging from small and inconspicuous to large and obvious, on any part of the body, but mostly on the face or neck. Usually permanent, a port wine stain (*nevus flammeus*) is a malformation of blood vessels just under the skin. It usually starts off pale pink but gradually darkens, until by middle age it is a deep reddish purple, possibly with some wart-like skin changes. The chief complication of port wine stains is the psychological burden of feeling "marked."

In a minority of cases, a port wine stain affects the underlying tissues. Some children with port wine stains on the face have accompanying abnormalities of certain blood vessels in the brain, a congenital condition known as the Sturge-Weber syndrome. In its more serious manifestations, this syndrome can lead to seizures or glaucoma (increased eye pressure). When a port wine stain is large and covers both the cheek and forehead there is a 50 percent risk of glaucoma. And since about a quarter of infants with port wine stains on the face have symptomless Sturge-Weber syndrome, experts advise that all such children have a brain CT (X-ray) scan and an eye test before the age of 5 or 6 months.

Today, laser therapy has dramatically improved the treatment of port wine stains. Properly performed on adults, argon laser treatment is considered good to excellent, with effective lightening in about 70 to 80 percent of cases, although it may leave scars. In children, use of flashlamp-pulsed tunable dye lasers can give excellent results even at ages as young as 3 months. (The best time to treat port wine stains is in early childhood, to avoid the hardship of disfigurement in the school years.)

- obsessive repetition of phrases, activities and habits;
- resistance to the smallest changes in familiar surroundings;
- an impaired ability to form abstract concepts.

Children who exhibit only one or two of these characteristics for a short time are not autistic. Children with autism have the problem for many years. The causes of autism are not known, but it may stem from problems in brain function. Because many autistic children have difficult behavior, special management is a major part of the treatment. Most children with autism enter special schools, but some with good cognitive ability can be integrated into regular grade school systems.

BIRTHMARKS

Almost 1 in 3 children is born with a pink, red or brown skin spot, popularly called a birth-

HELPING CHILDREN GROW UP HEALTHY

Strawberry mark is the popular name for a bright red or pink, clearly demarcated, raised or domed, spongy, blood-filled skin tumor seen in 4 to 10 percent of babies. It purportedly arises because of the arrested embryonic development of a small part of the blood system. About 55 percent are obvious at birth; another 25 percent show up within a week and the rest up to a month after birth. The strawberry mark usually appears on the head, face or neck, sometimes on the lip, nose or eyelid, less often on the trunk. It can be tiny, but most average 2 to 5 cm (an inch or two) and a few cover a larger area. Strawberry marks affect twice as many girls as boys. They generally grow rapidly until the child is about 9 to 12 months of age and then stop expanding and gradually lighten, usually vanishing or fading to a cosmetically acceptable shade by the time a child starts school.

Most experts recommend no treatment for strawberry marks. Parents are advised to "watch and wait" for them to fade or disappear.

A small proportion of strawberry marks fail to lighten or get smaller, leaving some residual skin wrinkling or a pinkish tinge. Very rarely, complications arise from strawberry marks that become infected or ulcerated, bleed or cause irreversible facial distortion. Strawberry marks near the mouth may impede feeding, those on the eyelid may obscure vision. Large marks on the eyelid or in the ear can lead to medical problems. In such cases, steroid therapy—taking prednisone for a short time—may be the solution. But because of its potential side effects in young children (slowed growth and possible immune-system suppression) only those at serious risk are given steroid therapy. Almost all strawberry marks on the lip that don't regress on their own by age 6 or so need some form of therapy, usually surgery. Laser therapy helps some cases.

mark, the vast majority of which are small and inconspicuous. But a few birthmarks need treatment because they're disfiguring or endanger health. Although parents may despair for children born with them, most birthmarks are harmless and many fade with time, some disappearing around age 8.

A birthmark is loosely defined as any spot, stain, swelling or other mark obvious within two weeks of birth on a baby's skin, including vascular (blood-filled) lesions such as strawberry marks that show up a bit later. Most birthmarks appear on the face, neck, ears or buttocks. While the vast majority are harmless, occasionally the presence of many birthmarks, possibly along with other symptoms, may point to underlying disease.

Corrective makeups can hide birthmarks
Those with birthmark who cannot or do not wish to undergo laser therapy or other treatment can use dermatological makeups (such as Dermablend or Covermark) containing titanium dioxide, which conceals birthmark better than ordinary cosmetics. Dermablend, for example, comes in a wide range of shades, suitable for any skin. The product is waterproof and fragrance-free, and can be worn for days, even through baths or in bed.

CEREBRAL PALSY
Cerebral palsy (CP) is a disorder often acquired because of an injury to the fetal brain, which happens during pregnancy (in the uterus) or during birth, resulting in impaired movement and posture. About 1 case in 10 develops after birth as a result of, for example, a motor-vehicle crash or violent child abuse. Some, but not all, children with CP have perfectly normal intellectual abilities. However, others have hearing problems, seizures, visual difficulties and language problems, which may lead people to assume that they are mentally handicapped when they are not. The amount of brain damage doesn't increase overtime, but as children with CP grow older the movement problems may change.

The type of CP depends on the part of the brain damaged and can be:
- *spastic*—weak or jerky muscles;
- *choreoathetotic or extra pyramidal*—difficulty coordinating movement;
- *diplegic*—affecting the two lower limbs;
- *quadriplegic*—affecting all four limbs;
- *hemiplegic*—where one half of the body (left or right) is affected.

The types of CP range from merely an awkward walk or arm movements to impairment significant enough to necessitate a wheelchair. Occasionally, a teacher is the first to suspect

WHAT TO DO FOR CHICKENPOX

• If a child comes down with chickenpox, watch other children for signs of it during the next 2 to 3 weeks. If your child develops chickenpox, make sure you tell the school, and contact your physician.

• Keep children with chickenpox out of school and daycare facilities for 5 days after the rash begins or until all blisters have crusted, whichever is shorter.

• Do not give acetylsalicylic acid (ASA or Aspirin), or any products containing it, to children with chickenpox. ASA increases the risk of Reye's syndrome (a severe illness that damages the liver and brain). Instead, use acetaminophen products to control fever.

• A new medication, acyclovir, is now available to treat the complications of chickenpox. Many authorities recommend giving it if available within 24 hours of noticing the illness. This is more important for adults who get chickenpox as the disease is usually more serious at older ages. It should be given to those at high risk—for instance, children with leukemia or the immunosuppressed.

CP—for example, if a child has difficulty achieving age-appropriate learning milestones.

Treatment (for instance, regular physical therapy) aims to improve the child's skills before the problem interferes too much with function. Those who have difficulty speaking may need technical aids. Caregivers can consult the attending physician or the Canadian Cerebral Palsy Association.

CHICKENPOX

With the advent of the new vaccine, the rates of serious problems due to chickenpox (varicella) has been considerably reduced. Chickenpox is still a very common childhood infection, caused by the *varicella-zoster* virus. Usually mild in children, chickenpox begins with a fever; followed by a characteristic rash in a day or two. The rash starts as little red spots, and these turn into fluid-filled blisters that crust over in a few days. The illness is usually mild, but may be accompanied by a high fever and severe rash in some. Complications include pneumonia, secondary bacterial infection of the pox rash and encephalitis (inflammation of the brain), which is quite rare. Fortunately, provided children don't scratch, even the most awesome-looking chickenpox rash usually fades without leaving pockmarks. The usual incubation period (time since the child was exposed to the bacteria or when illness became apparent) is 10 to 21 days. The disease is infectious for 48 hours before the onset of the rash, and until the last vesicles crust over (about 1 week). When the vesicles have crusted over, the child can look diseased but is technically no longer infectious. The secondary attack rate among individuals who have not been infected previously within a family is 70 to 90 percent. It is extremely rare for an individual to get chickenpox twice; in most reported cases the original diagnosis was erroneous.

In adults, chickenpox can be dangerous. Pregnant women who get chickenpox are at increased risk of pneumonia and, in addition, the virus may infect the unborn or newborn baby, causing severe illness. Varicella infection during the first 20 weeks of pregnancy results in congenital anomalies in about 2 percent of cases. People with immune deficiencies—such as leukemia or those on steroid medication—are also at risk of severe illness if they get chickenpox.

Chickenpox viruses spread through air or via direct contact with the blisters. People remain infectious until the last blister has crusted or 5 days after the rash first appeared, whichever is shorter. The only way to stop the spread of the virus is to prevent infected people from sharing the same room or house with others—not very practical! The chickenpox virus can survive for many years in the body and may later be reactivated as shingles or zoster. (For more on shingles, see Chapter 5.) Since the same virus causes both chickenpox and shingles, someone who never had chickenpox can catch it from a person with shingles.

WHAT TO DO FOR COMMON COLDS

• Wash your own and children's hands often—especially before preparing or eating food.

• Give plenty of fluids.

• Give acetaminophen (if necessary) to bring down fever and relieve aches and pains, and decongestants (on the physician's advice) to lessen nasal stuffiness. Although these medications may make people feel better, they don't alter or shorten the course of infection.

• Contact the physician if a child with a cold has:

• earache;

• fever higher than 39°C (102°F);

• unusual sleepiness;

• excessive crankiness or fussiness;

• rapid breathing or difficulty breathing;

• persistent coughing.

(See also the section on the common cold in Chapter 16.)

COLIC

A colicky baby is one who cries often and long enough to aggravate parents and caregivers. A more practical definition is excessive crying in a healthy, thriving infant. Colic occurs as frequently in breastfed as in bottlefed babies and almost always resolves by 4 months. While most infants fuss now and then—typically for 1 to 4 hours at suppertime—colicky babies cry for hours on end, despite cuddling, feeding, burping or changing. They supposedly have some "tummy discomfort," but no one really knows what causes colic. Nothing is definitely wrong with the bowels of most colicky infants, nor is there generally excess gas or wind, or any identified food allergy. However, excessive crying makes infants swallow air, which they burp up or pass as wind. The straining and tightening of the stomach muscles during crying also forces air out of the rectum so that these babies seem "windy." Colic is best viewed as a clinical manifestation of normal emotional development and the crying does not signify harm. Organic disease accounts for less than 5 percent of colic cases but must be ruled out. Other conditions that can cause excessive crying are intussuception, testicular torsion, incarcerated hernia and child abuse.

Parents often feel stressed by the endless crying, and it may reassure them to know that this behavior during the first 3 or 4 post-birth months does not predict future irritability or health problems. While all possible efforts should be made to comfort colicky babies, their regular sleep and feeding schedule needn't be disrupted by excessive comforting attempts. The best bet is to wrap them up snugly, cradle them soothingly and handle them gently. Reducing noise and dimming lights may help. Steady, smooth vibrations such as those from a rocking chair or car ride often quiets them.

COMMON COLDS

The common cold is a viral infection that usually lasts a week, slightly longer in young children. Most children have several colds a year sometimes being quite sick (with a high fever; lack of energy and loss of appetite), at other times hardly ill at all. Occasionally, a cold can lead to complications, such as ear infections and pneumonia. Children with colds usually have runny noses, coughs and fever. Being due to viruses, colds do not improve with antibiotics, although it often seems that way. The average child has 6 to 8 colds a year.

Cold viruses spread from person to person mainly by:
• direct contact, whenever a child with a cold touches his or her saliva or runny nose and then touches another child or object; or
• indirect contact, whenever a child with a cold rubs his or her saliva or runny nose and then touches an object, such as a toy or furniture, contaminating it with the cold viruses (which are quite tough and can survive for hours on surfaces such as eating utensils, counters, towels). People catch the cold by touching the contaminated object, picking up the virus on their hands and then rubbing their eyes or nose.

CROUP

A viral infection of the throat and vocal cords (larynx), croup is a severe respiratory condition in children under age 5, called laryngitis in older children. Croup often begins as a cough with some evident breathing difficulty. The lining of the throat and larynx become red and swollen, producing a hoarse voice and a bark-like cough. The passage below the vocal cords may also be inflamed, making it difficult for the child to move air in or out. Breathing can become rapid and noisy, but croup mostly sounds worse than it is. However, children may become tired through the labored breathing and in rare, very severe cases, breathing can be obstructed. A few children are sick enough to need hospital treatment. Antibiotics do not work on croup because it's a viral infection. Short term dexamethasone, a steroid, has been shown to improve outcomes. As well, many children improve with humidity (such as a being in the shower) or in cold air. The latter explains why many children improve on the way to the emergency room on a chilly fall evening.

JUVENILE, TYPE I OR "INSULIN-DEPENDENT" DIABETES

Diabetes occurs when the pancreas does not produce enough of the hormone insulin to keep blood-sugar levels within safe limits. Insulin is a

WHAT TO DO FOR CROUP

- If a child has suspected croup, contact a physician.
- To relieve the harsh, dry cough, humidify the air well.
- Try putting the child in the bathroom and running the hot water taps to get up a good steam.
- Follow directions for any prescribed medication.
- Should any or all of the following appear, immediately take the child to see a physician or to the hospital emergency department:
  - fever higher than 39°C (102°F);
  - rapid or difficult breathing;
  - new or increased drooling;
  - severe sore throat—refusal to swallow;
  - extreme discomfort when lying down.

SIGNS AND SYMPTOMS OF UNTREATED DIABETES

- Tiredness, weakness;
- excessive, frequent urination;
- a raging thirst;
- vision blurring;
- weight loss.

hormone that helps the body store and use glucose (sugar)—the body's main fuel for energy. Without enough insulin, the body cannot survive, because the cells cannot absorb enough glucose from the blood.

One in 600 to 700 children has early-onset or type I diabetes. While the condition is largely hereditary, triggers in the environment (such as a virus or toxin) can start it off or destroy the insulin-producing pancreas cells. Children with diabetes should be encouraged to participate fully in school and suitable sports.

Juvenile diabetes is controlled by:
- insulin injections;
- carefully regulated diet;
- monitored exercise.

Those with early-onset type I diabetes need insulin injections for a lifetime—usually twice daily, to keep blood glucose at near-normal levels. The insulin doses are tailored to fluctuating blood-glucose levels, determined by testing a finger-prick drop of blood with a small portable kit. The blood droplet is put on a paper strip and its color change shows the glucose reading. New blood gloucose kits no longer reguire finger-pricking. The required insulin dose is then calculated and given by injection just under the skin, in the arm, leg, abdomen or buttocks, usually before breakfast and supper.

People with type I need a carefully regulated diet to provide sufficient calories for growth, best divided into three balanced meals and three snacks to distribute the energy evenly through the day. Youngsters must eat their entire carbohydrate (starch/sugar) content, or its equivalent, at each meal to ensure a steady sugar intake and avoid *hypo* (low) or *hyper* (high) blood-sugar swings. (See also Chapter 16).

DIARRHEA
Diarrhea is a common childhood problem that's generally harmless and brief, but occasionally severe, especially in infants. Its hallmarks are unusually frequent bowel movements with unformed, watery stools. A child with diarrhea may also vomit and have fever; loss of appetite, nausea, stomach cramps and blood and/or mucus in the stool. Diarrhea-causing microbes spread easily from person to person, especially among children who don't yet use the toilet.

Most diarrhea is due to viral infections that cannot be cured with antibiotics, although some forms are caused by food-borne bacteria.

DIPHTHERIA
Diphtheria is a very severe, contagious, bacterial throat infection, easily spread by coughs and sneezes, which can lead to heart failure and nerve damage; I in 10 cases is fatal. Symptoms include fever, rapid pulse, swollen neck glands, a thick yellow discharge from the nose and—most distinctively—a grayish membrane on the throat and tonsils. Diphtheria can totally block breathing and may cause skin or ear infections. It is now rare in Canada, because almost all children are immunized, but is still common in many parts of the world. Diphtheria vaccine, usually given in combination with pertussis and tetanus vaccines (DPT), protects most of those immunized. In some provinces/territories, DPT is also combined with polio and Hib (anti-meningitis) vaccine. Adult diphtheria vaccine boosters are required every 10 years to sustain protection. If you do suspect diphtheria, call your physician at once.

DOWN SYNDROME
Down syndrome (before known as Down's syndrome), which affects the brain, head, heart, hands and feet, was first described by Dr. Down in 1866. It was formerly called mongolism because of the slanted eyes often seen with the disorder. It afflicts I in 600 children and is now known to be associated with a specific chromosome flaw or extra number 21 chromosome (known as "trisomy 21"). The extra chromosome 21 usually arises by a quirk of nature before birth (sometimes because of faulty cell division). Occasionally the flaw is passed from parent to child. The risk of bearing children with Down syndrome increases as women get older—approaching I in 200 at age 35, and more with advancing years.

Almost all children with Down syndrome have impaired mental development. However, some, especially in preschool years, show only mildly delayed mental development. Most have impaired language skills. Children with Down syndrome tend to be more "loose" or floppy (hypotonic) than average, often with odd move-

WHAT TO DO FOR CHILDHOOD DIARRHEA

- Ignore the old adage of "starving out the diarrhea" and continue light meals—unless the child is vomiting. Contrary to the former idea of "fluids only," the modern approach is to continue eating a normal diet after the first 12 to 24 hours of diarrhea, and above all to keep on drinking enough fluid to avoid dehydration.
- Contact a physician if the child has symptoms suggesting dehydration or worsening infection:
  - has a fever higher than 39°C (102°F);
  - refuses to drink;
  - vomits repeatedly;
  - has very large, watery stools or several stools in a day;
  - has less than the usual number of daily wet diapers (or urinates less);
  - has a sunken fontanel (soft spot on top of the head in infants);
  - has sunken eyes;
  - is listless;
  - has rapid breathing;
  - has bloody stools.

As protective measures and to manage the diarrhea:

- Make sure that all household members wash their hands after changing diapers or going to the toilet, and before eating or handling food.
- Do not share toothbrushes, cups or eating utensils.
- If the child with diarrhea is on milk formula, do not boil, concentrate or thicken it, because this may worsen dehydration.
- Follow the new guidelines for feeding children with diarrhea:
  - For breastfed children under 6 months old breastfeeding can continue, but also give extra water.
  - For infants on formula, replace the formula for 12 to 24 hours with oral rehydration solution (ORS), as advised by a physician. Make up for lost fluids by offering the infant 30 to 60 ml (1 to 2 oz) of ORS every half to 1 hour when awake, or after each loose stool, more if tolerated. The ORS, marketed as Gastrolyte, Pedialyte or Riceolyte, can be bought at any pharmacy or grocery store. If juice is given, it should be diluted (half water, half juice). Avoid plain water, as it's not nourishing enough and draws out more fluid compounding the problem. Always consult the doctor if the diarrhea is severe.
- Do not give only ORS for longer than 24 hours. This could deprive the child of valuable nutrients. ORS is not given to stop diarrhea, but to replace lost fluids and electrolytes.
- Infants can also have rice cereal, bananas, potatoes and other lactose-free, carbohydrate-rich (starchy) foods. When juices are given, continue to dilute with water. Give a variety of juices.
- For older children, regular diet can continue after giving ORS for only 12 hours or so. Children over 6 months of age can eat a regular diet, although the child may not feel much like eating. However, he or she should drink as much as possible.
- After 1 day of diarrhea, feed older infants and children a light, mixed diet:
  - Jell-O;
  - frozen Popsicles;
  - noncarbonated soft drinks;
  - whole-wheat noodles;
  - cereals (especially, rice cereals);
  - light meats (fish, chicken);
  - bananas;
  - potatoes.
- Consult a physician or pediatrician if you still have any questions about feeding a child with diarrhea.
- Do not give the child medication unless medically advised. Antidiarrheal medicines are not usually recommended, as they don't cure the infection and may mask signs of illness.
- Keep the child at home until bowel movements normalize or until you are told the child can return to school or daycare.

ments known as atlantoaxial instability due to looseness of the spinal vertebrae. They are prone to respiratory-tract and middle-ear infections and tend to be nearsighted (myopic), requiring glasses at a young age. The age of the pregnant mother can be a predictor of risk for Down syndrome and prenatal testing is available to help assess risk in pregnant women.

EAR INFECTIONS

Most children will have had at least one bout of middle-ear infection—*otitis media*—by the time they reach the age of 3. Middle-ear infections are almost as frequent in children as the common cold, though far less frequent in adults.

Otitis media—from *oto* for ear; *itis* for inflammation, *media* for middle—is more common in boys than girls, most prevalent in winter and often follows a cold. When young children have a cold or other respiratory infection, or sometimes an allergy, the eustachian tube (which connects the throat to the middle ear) is likely to get blocked, allowing bacteria to flourish and reach the middle ear. If the eustachian tube becomes plugged, air cannot enter the middle ear and it fills up with fluid—either clear (serous) or infectious (purulent). The fluid presses against the eardrum, causing pain, even sometimes perforating it by creating a small hole.

Fluid replacing air in the middle ear deadens sound and can cause transient hearing loss in one or both ears. Since untreated middle-ear infections can spread to surrounding areas and cause serious complications, even mild cases need prompt medical attention.

Symptoms of middle-ear infection are pain, sometimes severe, typically starting at night, when a child awakens howling with pain, pulling at the ears. There may also be fever; appetite loss, vomiting and diarrhea. Yet some children with *otitis media* hardly seem sick at all, although the feeling of fullness in the ears (from the fluid) may make them tug at their ears.

Physicians generally diagnose *otitis media* by looking at the eardrum with an otoscope (lighted ear-examining instrument) and with a device to detect fluid in the middle ear (known as a tympanometer or reflectometer). Sometimes it's necessary to remove wax from the outer ear canal in order to see the eardrum clearly.

Antibiotics are the usual treatment and generally make children better in a few days (but to eradicate the infection, the whole antibiotic course must be completed). Middle-ear infections may also resolve spontaneously within 7 to 10 days without any treatment. The eardrum often ruptures, letting out an exudate, usually giving prompt relief.

The trouble is that many children get recurrent middle-ear infections. And even when the infection is gone, fluid may linger on in the ear for months—perhaps not suspected until some hearing loss or behavioral problem alerts parents to it. Children may adapt to the slight hearing loss without noticing it and parents may remain equally unaware, attributing the youngster's slow responses to stubbornness. A child's inexplicable crankiness—owing to the emotional toll of not hearing properly—may eventually drive parents to seek medical attention. Or the teacher may notice a lack of attention at school because of a child's inability to hear clearly or keep up with peers.

The doctor's dilemma in treating childhood

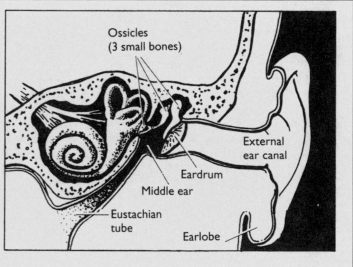

MIDDLE-EAR INFECTIONS IN CHILDREN

The middle ear contains three tiny bones or ossicles—the hammer, anvil and stirrup—that conduct sound from the eardrum to the inner ear. Normally, a little air enters the middle ear with each swallow, equalizing pressure on either side of the eardrum. But in young children the eustachian tube is narrow, short and angled so that it easily gets blocked. As children grow older, the eustachian tube lengthens and otitis media becomes less frequent.

Ossicles
(3 small bones)

External
ear canal

Eardrum

Middle ear

Eustachian
tube

Earlobe

fluid in the ear is that most cases clear up with or without antibiotics or any other treatment. Recent reviews show that only 1 in 15 children benefits from early antibiotics. By 12 weeks after a middle-ear infection, approximately 90 percent of children are better without antibiotics. Most children over 2 years of age do fine with watchful waiting and acetaminophen or ibuprofen treatment for fever and pain. Doctors make the decision to treat based on appearance, age and past history. It can be tough on parents to do "nothing," but the tincture of time is often all that is needed., Some children drag on and on with fluid in the ears, even despite antibiotic therapy that often leads to some loss of hearing. Experts stress the need for frequent checkups and hearing tests for children prone to middle-ear infections.

Myringotomy (putting a small hole in the eardrum) to drain off middle-ear fluid may be tried for persistent cases. For children old enough to cooperate, myringotomy can be done under a local anesthetic, but those under age 8 usually need general anesthesia.

Tympanostomy—insertion of ventilating tubes or "grommits" into the eardrum of the blocked ear (under general anesthesia) to let air into the middle ear—is often done to prevent or minimize hearing loss. But to tube or not to tube children's ears is a much-debated question. Some experts oppose ear tubes because their benefits are transient and time alone (about three months) makes most children better with no residual hearing loss. Tests show that with or without antibiotics, with or without tubes, 20 percent of children still have fluid in their ears and some hearing loss 1 month after a bout of *otitis media*, but by 2 months only 9 percent and by the third month only 6 percent are still not back to normal. At this point it seems that there is a benefit in giving antibiotics—for instance improved quality of life—for kids who have had more than 3 infections in 6 months, or 4 infections in a year. Some doctors prefer a trial of low-dose antibiotics for 2 to 6 months. Others may want to defer and this is also reasonable. Some oppose tubing because, although it carries no greater surgical risks than average, it is still an operation done under general anesthesia, the tubes tend to need reinsertion and there's an increased risk of scars of the eardrum after tubing. Moreover, they're a nuisance because children with tubes must not get water in the ear. Most tubes fall out after 6 to 9 months.

Those who favor tubing argue that although middle-ear infections generally heal without them, tubes help to avoid a possible developmental lag in learning due to hearing loss from fluid in the ears. Avoiding hearing loss is particularly critical between the ages of 18 months and 3 years, when language develops. But it has not been proven that the temporary hearing loss due to middle-ear infections has any long-term effects on language development or learning ability.

ECZEMA

Eczema is one of the most troublesome infant rashes—on the face, body and in any skin creases. In older children, it tends to be localized on elbows, knees, necks and behind the ears. The itchy rash may be moist and weepy or dry and scaly. The eczema rash is usually red, patchy and scaly, with flare-ups that look oozy, weeping and "angry." Most children with eczema have very itchy skin, worsened by scratching. Eczema is not dangerous unless the rash becomes infected. In some cases, eczema is an allergic reaction to cow's-milk protein in formula, citrus fruits, chocolate, eggs or other foods. While it is usually a long-term condition, 50 percent of children outgrow eczema by the age of 21. It may be linked to conditions such as asthma or other allergies. Eczema is often confused with impetigo because the rashes look alike, but eczema is not infectious. A new and effective agent called Tacrolimus is available. It contains no steroid, but is very expensive.

WHAT TO DO FOR CHILDREN WITH ECZEMA

- **Avoid known triggers, and use anti-inflammatory steroid creams, moisturizers, anti-itch medication and possibly antibiotics (if the eczema is infected). Tacrolimus (Protopic) is also helpful.**
- **Avoid anything that might irritate the skin or increase sweating.**
- **Don't overdress infants.**
- **Dress in cotton clothing.**
- **Avoid wool—particularly irritating to the skin of those prone to eczema—and also steer clear of synthetics such as nylon because they do not allow the skin to "breathe."**
- **Use bland hypoallergenic soaps for washing.**
- **Avoid bubble baths and excessive bathing, which may worsen eczema.**

WHAT PARENTS CAN DO FOR CHILDHOOD EAR INFECTIONS

- **If you suspect your child has a middle-ear infection, contact your physician, who will examine the child's ears.**
- **Call the physician if the child shows any of the following:**
- **a worsening earache despite treatment;**
- **a high fever over 39°C (102°F) in spite of treatment, or one that lasts more than 3 days;**
- **excessive sleepiness, crankiness or fussiness;**
- **a skin rash;**
- **rapid or difficult breathing;**
- **noticeable hearing loss (can't clearly hear noises, tapes or what's being said).**

WHAT TO DO FOR BEDWETTING

- Seek professional advice if:
  - the child is still wetting after age 5 or 6;
  - half the nights per week are wet;
  - the child has persistent daytime wetting after age 4 to 5 or for several months;
  - the child has been dry at night for 6 months or more and suddenly starts wetting again.
- Remember that most bedwetting eventually vanishes, given time and patience (provided there's no organic abnormality).
- Since the overwhelming majority of bedwetters do not have organic or psychological problems, refrain from scolding children for an involuntary problem.
- Try charting wet and dry nights to sharpen the child's bladder consciousness and speed up the drying-out process. Rewards can be given for dry nights, but carry the risk of creating guilt for the child. Within a year, about 25 percent of children achieve complete resolution, which is somewhat better than the spontaneous resolution rate of 15 percent. Another 70 percent of children improve.
- Some recommend getting bedwetters to help in changing and laundering soiled linen; it may do the trick.
- For the wetter's bed, plastic undersheets are essential.
- Consider alarm systems to stop the wetting. Urinary alarm systems, powered by batteries, attach to the child's pyjamas near the urine outlet (urethra); the first drops of wetness set off the alarm, and the child's bladder muscles automatically contract, squeezing off the urine flow. The slumbering child awakens, goes to the toilet and reattaches the device before going back to sleep. Alarms can take up to 16 weeks to become effective. According to learning theory, alarms change the innate signal "urinate" into its opposite, "don't urinate" (unless awake and at the toilet!). For an alarm to work, the child must be old enough, want to do something about the problem and be willing to go through the necessary steps. The most suitable candidates are older children (aged 7 or more) who are greatly bothered by wetting. The decision to use an alarm should be made only with a child's full consent. Alarm systems should be continued until the child has been consistently dry for a 3-week period.
- Ask about medications against bedwetting:
  - Imipramine (Tofranil), an antidepressant, can suppress nocturnal enuresis. Taken regularly, it makes about 50 percent of bedwetters permanently dry. But when it is stopped, bedwetting often returns. Common side effects include irritability, lethargy and mild gastrointestinal problems—symptoms that disappear once the drug is withdrawn. Since Tofranil is a dangerous drug when taken in overdose, it must be kept well out of children's reach and safely locked up, which explains why many parents prefer not to give it to children.
  - Desmopressin, an antidiuretic hormone, shows great promise for nighttime enuresis. Used as an aerosol spray (squirted into the nose), it concentrates urine, reduces flow and decreases the amount held in the bladder. This drug helps up to 40 percent or more of bedwetting children, who become completely dry as long as they're on it. Some relapse on discontinuation, and about 30 percent fail to respond. It's very useful as a short-term "fix" for children going to camp or on an overnight stay.
  - Antispasmodic drugs such as oxybutynin chloride (Ditropan) can be useful for daytime wetting by reducing the frequency of bladder contractions, delaying the urge to urinate. These drugs are especially useful for wetters for whom every tiny bladder squeeze sends them running.
- As a final ploy, buy a book called *Sammy the Elephant and Mr. Camel*, written by two psychologists (Joyce C. Mills and Richard J. Crowly). The story describes an elephant unable to carry a trunkful of water like other elephants, and who is guided by Mr. Camel to gain self-control and self-esteem. In the end the elephant puts out a fire with a trunkful of water. Children don't mind the somewhat weak plot, and the book is a "healing metaphor" whereby the child subconsciously goes through the steps with Sammy the elephant until able to hold in urine.

ENURESIS (BEDWETTING)

Parents eagerly look forward to the time when their offspring can make it through the night without wetting the bed and tiresome diapers can be discarded. Yet, although most children are dry by age 4 or 5, many go on wetting at night for several more years. About 15 percent of children are still nighttime bedwetters by the time they start school, 3 percent by age 10, and although almost all are dry by age 11 without any treatment, 1 to 2 percent go on wetting into adolescence—to their own and their parents' embarrassment. (One study even found that 2 percent of U.S. soldiers were occasional nighttime wetters.)

Enuresis or bedwetting is defined as "the involuntary voiding of urine, at least twice a month, in children aged 4 to 6 years, and once monthly (or more) in older children." It is usually due to slow maturation of the bladder's complex urine-voiding system. If there are no other symptoms or abnormalities, bedwetting is considered a variant of normal development. Male bedwetters outnumber girls by 2 to 1 up to age 11, after which the sexes even out.

Despite the popular myth that bedwetting

stems mainly from psychological reasons or bad parenting, it is not the child's fault or due to poor upbringing. Current medical wisdom advises worried parents not to scold but to let "the tincture of time" help children outgrow the annoyance. Yet although the vast majority naturally grow out of this harmless condition, children have been beaten, bled, blistered, fed nauseating concoctions, given electric shocks and otherwise tormented in efforts to make them dry.

The overall incidence of primary nocturnal enuresis is about 15 to 20 percent among 5-year-olds, 5 to 7 percent among 10-year-olds, and 2 to 4 percent among 12- to 14-year-olds. The spontaneous remission rate is 15 percent per year.

Three main types of childhood bedwetting

- *Primary nocturnal enuresis*—nighttime bedwetting in a child who's never been dry and still wets past age 4 to 5 is often hereditary, and without psychological undertones. A child with primary nocturnal enuresis requires a thorough physical examination and urine tests to rule out infection or structural causes.
- *Diurnal enuresis*—daytime as well as nighttime wetting—can stem from underlying anatomical disorders or emotional problems. Most children can stay dry during the day, with occasional lapses, by age 3 to 4. Those who consistently wet during the day after age 4 should have a full medical workup because, although it could be due to a developmental lag, diurnal incontinence is the type most likely to arise from an underlying abnormality (infection, sickle cell anemia, diabetes or structural defects). A small number of daytime wetters have psychological problems that require special counseling.
- *Secondary enuresis* (the least common form of bedwetting) starts up after children have already been persistently dry for 6 months to a year. It may be nocturnal or diurnal, and calls for a thorough medical examination. The reappearance of wetting in a previously dry child could arise from a urinary-tract infection but is often due to emotional distress—perhaps difficulties at home or school, often signaling some underlying anxiety.

BEDWETTING NOT DUE TO NAUGHTINESS, REBELLION OR POOR PARENTING

While disruptive to a family, and upsetting and uncomfortable for the child, bedwetting must be kept in perspective. For the most part, it is more a housekeeping annoyance than a medical abnormality. Nocturnal bedwetters are not misbehaving.

If undertaken at all, treatment should include reassurance, perhaps gentle attempts to increase bladder holding or possibly an alarm system. Nightly charts may encourage progress, and some drugs are worth considering. In some cases, medication helps to dry up the urine flow for special occasions (a weekend away, a holiday or going to camp).

Tracing the reasons for bedwetting

In the early 1900s, bedwetting was regarded as a childhood neurosis, even a masturbation substitute. But today it's considered a normal variation in the speed of bladder development and, except in rare cases, not a psychological disorder or a form of rebellion. Bedwetters don't do it on purpose. Enuresis does not lead to kidney failure or permanent disability.

- Organic causes include diabetes mellitus, kidney problems, epilepsy, sickle cell anemia and urinary-tract infections.
- Extra deep sleep is no longer blamed for nighttime wetting. Formerly, bedwetting was thought to occur in children who sleep so deeply that they don't respond to the bladder-emptying urge when the bladder is full. But many parents notice that even when they awaken a bedwetting child to go to the toilet, another wetting episode occurs within an hour of voiding, with a half-empty bladder. The latest research shows no link between deep slumber and bedwetting. The claim that nighttime enuresis is a dream disorder has also never been scientifically proved. Although enuretics often describe dreams of wetting the bed—after which they wake up in a puddle—it's likely that the child first passed urine and then dreamed about it.
- Some nightly wetters are deficient in an antidiuretic hormone, vasopressin, which regulates urine flow from kidney to bladder. Adults usually produce more vasopressin at night, suppressing urinary flow. Children who continue bedwetting past the usual age may be slow to produce the hormone. (Giving the

SOME DO'S AND DON'T'S FOR BEDWETTING

Do's

• Recognize that bedwetting is quite common in girls up to age 5 and in boys up to age 8, 10 or even older.
• Give reassurance: it's crucial for bedwetters and their caregivers to realize that enuresis is a normal condition and nothing to worry about, remembering that many of a child's classmates probably also suffer from it. A matter-of-fact attitude, dismissing it as "nothing out of the ordinary," is best.
• Banish feelings of guilt or shame: it's not the child's fault.
• A night light in the bathroom is useful to help children go to the toilet or change bedwear.
• Try using absorbent bed pads or a folded blanket under the bottom sheet to limit urine spread; placing absorbent pads between bottom sheet and mattress minimizes the dampness and reduces the cleanup operation.
• A reward or positive-reinforcement system can help—praising dry nights, giving the child a small reward or a star on a chart for every dry night—or bigger rewards for several dry nights in a row.
• Encouraging a child to help change and wash the wet bed sheets is a sound idea—not as a punishment but as a practical aid, to engender a sense of responsibility and the pride of "lending a hand." It should be requested in a nonjudgmental, good-humored style.
• Behaviour modification may be tried, with guidelines given by a family physician or pediatrician (or just plain common sense).
• Slow, steady training to go to the bathroom before bed can increase bladder consciousness.
• Cleanliness is essential. Be sure the bedwetter has a shower or bath before going to school; the smell of urine clings.
• For children who wet during the day, bladder retraining may work. It teaches "bladder awareness" and how to control bladder capacity by drinking fluids, then holding urine in with the sphincter muscles and releasing it at will. Regular, timed trips to the washroom, with gradually longer times between emptyings, can help.

Don't's

• Don't scold or shame a bedwetting child, even if you're angry: disapproval only compounds the problem.
• Don't curb fluids. Many parents and caregivers restrict fluids in bedwetting children after supper, in the vain hope that they'll stay dry—a strategy that sounds reasonable but rarely works. Whether or not any liquid is taken, some fluid will accumulate in the bladder, and a child with poor bladder mastery will wet the bed whether there's a little or a lot in the bladder. Since caffeine (in tea, coffee, chocolate, or some soft drinks) stimulates the bladder directly, it should not be given to wetters near bedtime.
• Don't awaken the child and take him or her to the toilet at your own bedtime. While this strategy works for some bedwetters, it isn't foolproof, and since it disturbs the child's sleep, many pediatricians consider the practice disruptive and think it may interfere with natural bladder control, stopping the child from learning to respond to the body's own signals. (Some experts dispute this, saying that if nighttime lifting works, it is unreasonable to tell parents to stop.)
• Don't put bedwetters to bed in diapers or training (padded) pants—this is strongly discouraged by most pediatricians. Despite the possible convenience to parents, continuing to wear diapers after age five may be demeaning to a growing youngster and could "infantalize" the child, encourage immature behavior and undermine security. In older children it can produce skin irritation.
• Don't be tempted by intensive "dry bed" training—"psyching" the child to get heavily involved in beating incontinence by getting up every hour at night, for example, plus other steps to persuade the child to work toward dryness. The method is controversial and advised against by most experts.

drug desmopressin acetate, which mimics the body hormone, can cut back urine production and halt bedwetting until the child's system is mature.)

• If both parents were bedwetters, there is a 77 percent chance that their offspring will also be bedwetters. If only one parent was enuretic, there is a 40 percent chance. Recognizing the inherited roots of bedwetting may deter parents from scolding or inflicting "cures" for a problem that will vanish with time. (It may also reassure bedwetting children to know that their parents also wet their beds!)

EPIGLOTTITIS

Epiglottitis is a very severe, life-threatening infection of the epiglottis, a flap of tissue at the back of the throat that closes over the vocal cords (larynx or voicebox) when a person swallows. If a child with epiglottitis isn't immediately treated, the swelling can become severe enough to block the airway within hours and lead to sudden death by suffocation. Early signs resemble croup, but with epiglottitis the child becomes rapidly ill, with high fever severe sore throat, drooling and difficulty breathing. Epiglottitis is always an emergency. It's almost always due to *Haemophilus influenzae type b* (Hib) bacteria (not related to influenza viruses). Fortunately, epiglottitis has become very uncommon through infant immunization with the new Hib vaccine.

What to do for a child with suspected epiglottitis

- Call the doctor at once.
- Keep the child upright (sitting).
- Take the child at once to an emergency room if:
  - fever is 39°C (102°F) or more;
  - breathing is rapid or difficult;
  - there's much drooling;
  - the child won't or can't swallow.

EPILEPSY (SEIZURE DISORDER)

Epilepsy (now called "seizure disorder") involves sporadic seizures (convulsions) that occur because of a temporary, unusually high level of electrical activity in the brain. During a seizure, the body loses control of its sensory systems (such as hearing), as well as breathing, body temperature and/or blood-pressure regulation. Overall, 1 to 2 percent of all children have seizure disorders, but less than 1 in 100 preschoolers. The disorder may be inherited, but the cause is largely unknown. Children with underlying brain damage such as cerebral palsy may be especially prone to seizures. For some children, certain triggers bring on the seizures.

Signs and symptoms of:

- *mild (epileptic) seizures*
  - drowsiness;
  - rolling of eyes;
  - inattention and fading awareness.
- *"Grand mal," generalized epileptic seizures*
  Grand mal or "tonic-clonic" seizures may affect just one part of the body, but more often the whole body shakes and trembles, even violently. The child may drool at the mouth and/or bite the lips, cheeks or tongue, falling down unconscious, possibly also losing control over bladder and bowel movements. Tonic-clonic seizures usually last only a few minutes. Although frightening to onlookers, they generally pass without complications for the child. A deep sleep often follows the seizure. (See also Chapter 16.)

EPILEPSY TRIGGERS MAY INCLUDE:

- infections;
- a rapidly rising fever;
- flashing or blinking lights (such as camera flashes);
- fatigue;
- a scary amusement ride (such as a roller coaster);
- certain sounds or odors.

N.B.: Seizures due to high fever are not epilepsy. (See also "Understanding childhood fever" on pg. 304 and the section on epilepsy in Chapter 16.)

- *"Petit mal" or absence seizures*
Absence seizures are usually very short in duration, often just a few seconds. The child may simply appear momentarily blank and inattentive, as though daydreaming. However, unlike daydreaming, the child cannot be aroused. Some children have many of these brief seizures during the course of a day. If you suspect a child of having seizures, consult a physician.

(For more on epilepsy, see Chapter 16.)

FIFTH DISEASE (ERYTHEMA INFECTIOSUM)

Fifth disease is an infection of the respiratory system caused by the parvovirus B_{19}, which spreads as the common cold does, i.e.,

- from the hands of someone with the infection;
- from something touched by the infected person; or
- through the air.

The infection produces a very red rash on the cheeks, as if they've been slapped. By the time the rash develops, the child is no longer infectious. One to 4 days later a lace-like rash appears on the arms and the rest of the body, lasting from 1 to 3 weeks, possibly accompanied by fever. The illness is often mild and the child may not feel at all sick. (Adults usually get a more severe case, with fever and painful joints, but at least 50 percent of adults have had fifth disease in childhood and will not get it again.) Outbreaks of the disease can occur in school-age children. There is no vaccine to prevent it and no medication to treat it. Exposure in pregnancy can be of concern, so any pregnant contacts should be informed.

FOOT DISORDERS

- *Club foot:* an inherited or congenital anomaly frequently detected in newborn infants. Children may need casts and/or corrective

---

TREATMENT OF EPILEPSY

To prevent seizures, children often need daily anticonvulsant medication such as:
- phenobarbital;
- phenytoin (Dilantin);
- valproic acid (Depakene);
- carbamazepine (Tegretol).

Side effects of anticonvulsant drugs may include: lack of coordination, behavior changes, headaches, drowsiness, dizziness, rash, increased gum size, baldness, anemia, gastrointestinal upset, liver abnormalities, double vision, blood abnormalities.

WHAT TO DO FOR FIFTH DISEASE

- Watch a child for signs of it if a school chum has it.
- Contact a physician if you are pregnant and exposed to this disease, as it can (rarely) affect the fetus.

WHAT TO DO FOR GENERALIZED (GRAND MAL) SEIZURES

- Most important, remain calm.
- If possible, place the child on the floor—on the side or stomach, not on the back—to prevent choking on saliva.
- Remove any object that could injure the child (such as toys and chairs), and move the child away from other potential dangers such as stairwells.
- Loosen tight clothing around the child's neck and remove eyeglasses.
- If possible, put something flat and soft under the head.
- Do not put anything in the mouth. Do not try to open the child's mouth (people do not swallow their tongues during epileptic seizures).
- Do not try to restrain the jerky movements: it could injure the child. Children who are having a seizure are unaware of what they are doing and their body movements are very powerful.
- Do not attempt artificial respiration unless the child fails to start breathing again once the seizure stops. If this happens, begin artificial respiration (see Chapter 17) and call an ambulance.
- Allow the seizure to stop on its own. If it lasts more than 5 minutes, or if the first seizure is followed by a second one, call for medical help. Once a seizure has started, it can be stopped only by special medication.
- When the seizure is over, place the child in the "recovery position" (see Chapter 17). This will keep the airway open and prevent the possibility of breathing vomit or saliva into the lungs.
- After a seizure, children will be sleepy for some time. Stay close by and reassure the child as soon as he or she awakens.
- Do not give food or drink until the child is fully awake.
- During a seizure, it is not uncommon for the child to urinate or have a bowel movement. Depending on the child's age, this can be very embarrassing, and should be handled discreetly when the child awakens.
- Record the seizure's duration, any injuries and how the child felt afterwards.
- If possible, prevent other children from witnessing a grand mal seizure, which can be very frightening.

WHAT TO DO FOR GIARDIASIS

- Watch the child for signs of diarrhea, if others have it.
- Contact a physician if you think your child has a *Giardia* infection. Stool samples may be taken to confirm the diagnosis. Occasionally, a sample needs to be taken from the duodenum using a special scope. Antibiotics are necessary.
- Ensure that all household members wash their hands after changing a diaper or using the toilet, and before preparing or eating food.

surgery, plus orthopedic care by a physician.
- *Flat feet:* a common childhood problem for which children must wear shoes with special arch supports to allow normal foot growth and reduce discomfort.
- *In-toeing:* an inward-pointing or "pigeon-toed" forefoot (metatarsus varus), often detected in newborns and benign. Some more severe forms require a cast. Other, rare forms of in-toeing require treatment with special shoes, braces or surgery. Most children will improve at least slightly as they grow older. •
Out-toeing: walking in a slightly out-pointing manner; this usually improves with time.
- *Limping:* a sign that something is wrong, possibly a cut, wart, infection, bone disease or just uncomfortable shoes. A child with a constant or sudden, unexplained limp should be seen by a physician.
- *Toe-walking:* usually just a bad habit, but the heel cord may be abnormally tight because of underlying cerebral palsy or spinal-cord problems. The child should be seen by a physician.

GIARDIASIS

Giardiasis is a bowel infection due to a parasite, and is quite common in daycare centers, especially where children are still in diapers. The *Giardia* parasites are often present in a child's stool without causing any illness. They spread from the hands of someone who has changed diapers or used the toilet, and their spread can be prevented by carefully washing hands after changing diapers or going to the toilet, and before preparing and eating food. Routine hand-washing is crucial to prevent the spread of the disease, even when no one has diarrhea.

Although giardiasis produces few or no symptoms, in some it may cause:
- diarrhea or mushy bowel movements (with a bad smell);
- gas, abdominal pain;
- poor appetite and weight loss.

The infection can be cleared up by medication.

HAEMOPHILUS INFLUENZAE TYPE B INFECTIONS

Haemophilus influenzae type b (Hib) bacteria frequently infect young children, but rarely adults. They can cause serious illnesses, including:
- meningitis (infection of the brain's covering membranes);
- epiglottitis (infection of the windpipe);
- cellulitis (deep skin infection);
- pneumonia;

• joint and bone infections;
• bacterial tracheitis (croupy cough).

Before widespread infant immunization with the Hib vaccine, I child in 200 came down with a serious Hib illness before age 5, children under 2 years of age being most endangered. A major consequence of Hib infection, bacterial meningitis, spreads fast among those crowded together in close quarters. Therefore parents and caregivers of an infected child should be vigilant about the possibility of transmission. The spread of Hib infections can often be prevented by immediately treating all household, childcare or school contacts with an antibiotic. Intravenous antibiotics are given to prevent complications in those with Hib illness, and to their close contacts.

Fortunately, the new and effective Hib vaccine can prevent the disease. It is given as 3 injections starting at 2 months of age, usually at the same time as the diphtheria-pertussis-tetanus shots, plus a booster at 15 to 18 months of age.

HEPATITIS A

Hepatitis A is a viral liver infection, often with few or no symptoms, but possibly accompanied by yellowing of the skin and whites of the eyes (jaundice), fever appetite loss, nausea and "feeling sick all over" It is usually a mild illness and rarely produces permanent liver damage. Many infants and children infected with hepatitis A have no sign of illness, but it can be more severe in adults. The hepatitis A virus is acquired via infected stool and through contaminated food or water and it spreads easily if people do not wash their hands after changing diapers or having a bowel movement. For those known to have been exposed, infection can be prevented by an injection of immune (gamma) globulin. There is no medication to treat the disease, but a new vaccine is very effective in preventing it, and is used mainly for travelers to infected areas and to prevent outbreaks. (See "Hepatitis A" in Chapter 16.)

HEPATITIS B

Hepatitis B is a dangerous, potentially fatal liver infection, caused by a virus different from that responsible for hepatitis A, and is transmitted

---

WHAT TO DO FOR HIB INFECTION

• **Contact your physician immediately if a sick child has:**
  • **high fever;**
  • **excessive sleepiness, or unusual crankiness or fussiness;**
  • **a stiff neck (unwillingness to move the head up and down);**
  • **vomiting;**
  • **rapid or difficult breathing;**
  • **new or increased drooling;**
  • **a sore throat;**
  • **pain on swallowing or refusal to swallow.**
• **Check your child's immunization record. A child aged 2 months to 5 years who has not been immunized should be given Hib vaccine. The vaccine is not a substitute for antibiotics in treating Hib disease or preventing it in those already exposed.**

WHAT TO DO FOR HEPATITIS A

• **Watch for signs of hepatitis A if someone else in your household has it, or a child's playmate.**
• **Be sure that all household members wash their hands after going to the toilet or changing a diaper, and before preparing or eating food.**
• **Ask whether immune globulin injections can be obtained to prevent infection.**

WHAT TO DO FOR HEPATITIS B

• **Be vaccinated if in a risk category.**
• **If pregnant, have a blood test to determine whether or not you are carrying hepatitis B, so the baby can be immunized at birth if necessary.**
• **Health authorities now urge hepatitis B immunization for everyone, before or during adolescence. (See "Hepatitis B" in Chapter 16.)**

---

via blood and body fluids. Like AIDS, it is transmitted primarily by sexual contact and via blood products or contaminated IV needles. In Canada, at least half a million people are hepatitis B carriers; they show no symptoms themselves, but can spread the infection to others. Young children are less than adults likely to have symptoms of illness. Some children develop lifelong hepatitis B infection and become permanent "carriers" of the virus. Newborns of mothers with hepatitis B are often infected.

Pregnant women can pass on hepatitis B to their developing fetus or to newborns during delivery, which can result in serious disease at a young age, even though no signs may show at birth, with a high risk of later developing liver cancer. Therefore, all pregnant women are given a simple blood test for hepatitis B. Endangered babies can be protected by hepatitis B immune

WHAT TO DO FOR IMPETIGO

- If you think your child has impetigo, contact your physician.
- Make sure that all household members wash their hands thoroughly with soap and running water after touching infected skin.
- Don't share face-cloths or hand and bath towels.
- Take all the antibiotics prescribed, even after the impetigo rash has cleared. If a topical antibiotic is prescribed, make sure lesions have resolved for at least 24 hours. (See also section on impetigo in Chapter 5.)

globulin (HBIG), given as soon as possible after birth, followed by vaccination. Older children of hepatitis B carriers should also be vaccinated. Hepatitis B vaccination is now recommended for all school-age children in Canada.

IMPETIGO

Impetigo is a common childhood skin infection caused by *Streptococcus* (strep) and *Staphylococcus* (staph) bacteria that enter via scrapes, cuts and insect bites. Some people mistakenly think that only unclean children get impetigo, however; the condition does not arise from too little washing. The impetigo skin rash is a cluster of blisters or red bumps that ooze and may form honey-colored crusts. The rash usually appears around the nose, mouth and parts of the skin not covered by clothes. It spreads when someone touches an impetigo spot, and can be prevented by washing hands after touching infected skin. Treatment of impetigo with antibiotics helps to prevent its spread.

MEASLES

Although often considered a trivial disease, "red" measles, or rubeola, is one of the most serious of common childhood illnesses. One in 10 children with measles gets an ear infection or pneumonia, and adults with measles are usually very sick.

Alerting symptoms of measles include fever (38.3°C, or 101°F, or higher), runny nose, red eyes, cough, white spots inside the mouth (hard to see, and lasting 1 to 3 days), followed by a red rash that spreads from the face to the rest of the body, lasting 3 or more days. Some children are so ill they need to be hospitalized. Measles continues to have a mortality rate of about 1 in 1,000, and encephalitis (brain inflammation) is also a complication in one per 1,000 cases, sometimes producing deafness and mental retardation. Once people have had red measles they become immune.

The measles virus spreads easily from person to person through the air and is infectious from about 3 to 5 days before the rash appears and up to 4 days after that. Almost everyone exposed to the virus who has not been immunized or already had it will get measles. In exposed children who haven't been immunized, the infection can be prevented with an immediate injection of immune (gamma) globulin. Measles vaccination within 3 days of exposure can usually prevent the illness from developing, and may even be considered for infants as young as 6 months (although they need revaccination soon after their first birthday).

The modern measles vaccine is highly effective in preventing the disease among those immunized on schedule. The standard immunization procedure is one shot of live vaccine at (or as soon as possible after) a child's first birthday. A second shot is now advised for all children at school entry, around 4 to 6 years of age. The National Advisory Committee on Immunization of Health Canada considers the elimination of measles in Canada a top priority.

Vaccination side effects are rare, other than transient swelling and redness at the injection site and fever in 15 percent of vaccine recipients.

N.B.: People hypersensitive (allergic) to eggs should not receive measles vaccine, as it contains traces of egg products.

WHAT TO DO FOR MEASLES

- Parents who suspect their child has measles should call their physician.
- Since measles is very contagious and outbreaks can be magnified by infected children passing on the virus to others in doctors' and hospital waiting rooms, special arrangements may be made to have the child examined.
- If you suspect you have measles, you should stay well away from people who may be susceptible.
- Those exposed can ask about eligibility for a protective immune (gamma) globulin shot.

MENINGITIS

Meningitis, which arises from many different causes, can be a very serious, possibly fatal illness, affecting mainly children and teenagers. Despite treatment, it may leave survivors with permanent brain damage, but fortunately antibiotics and safe vaccines can reduce the danger.

Meningitis is an umbrella term meaning inflammation of the meninges—the membranes covering the brain and spinal cord. Meningitis can arise from a variety of viral infections or bacterial *meningococci*. It can be mild and self-limiting or life-threatening, depending on the cause and the degree of inflammation. Any inflammation around or in the brain and spinal cord—no matter what the reason—can have serious consequences.

The warning signs of meningitis can come on slowly or suddenly. Since the early signs—fever irritability and headache—mimic those of less serious ailments, such as respiratory infections (e.g., flu or a feverish cold), parents or physicians may not recognize meningitis at first. It is wise to become familiar with the symptoms and potential seriousness of meningitis.

In infants, meningitis can begin with rather nonspecific symptoms—irritability and poor feeding, extreme drowsiness and lethargy.

In toddlers and young children, meningitis usually starts off with fever drowsiness and irritability—sometimes preceded by a common cold. Some children also vomit and find light disturbing. But the most telling feature of meningitis is a stiff neck that makes it painful to move the head up or down (looking at the ceiling or floor); sufferers tend to lie still with their necks straight, as the slightest neck movement hurts the inflamed nerve roots.

Older children and adults may complain first of a searing headache and, later of a stiff neck. They may also develop a strange purplish rash (petechial rash) that gives meningitis its nickname of "spotted fever."

Sorting out the different types of meningitis

Viral meningitis (the "aseptic" form) is by far the most usual and least serious variety, sometimes arising as a complication of other viral infections, such as mumps, polio, measles and chickenpox.

Viral meningitis is rarely fatal. Recovery from this form is usually complete except for rare cases (such as meningitis due to *herpes simplex*).

Bacterial meningitis, although less common, is more serious and can cause permanent neurological injury or death. The bacteria responsible include streptococci, *Haemophilus influenzae type b* or Hib (nothing to do with influenza!), *Neisseria meningitidis* and *tuberculosis*. The bacterial infection often begins in the nose and/or throat, later invading the bloodstream and spreading to the meninges and cerebrospinal fluid.

The type often called meningococcal meningitis is caused by various strains or "serogroups" of *Neisseria meningitidis* bacteria (mostly types B and C in Canada). The bacteria often inhabit the throat and nose without causing any illness, or the infection can become invasive and spread via the bloodstream throughout the body. If the meningococcal bacteria invade parts of the body that are normally sterile (free of infective agents)—such as the blood or fluid around the brain and spinal cord—they can produce a fulminant (rapid) invasive infection. Galloping or fulminating cases can progress to septic shock collapse and death in 6 to 10 hours.

While bacterial meningitis can strike at any age, three-quarters of those affected are children. Whether or not a child will come down with meningitis depends largely upon the level of natural immunity.

Meningococcal bacteria are transmitted from person to person in nasal droplets, but the infection is not highly contagious and requires close contact for transmission. It spreads most rapidly among people in confined quarters—such as schools, households and daycare centers. In North America, most of the population acquires natural immunity by early adulthood; about 80 percent of those over age 20 are immune. But even immune persons can harbor the bacteria in their noses and throats, passing it on without being ill themselves. During epidemics many people may carry and transmit the bacteria without being unwell. The incubation period for the development of bacterial meningitis is 2 to 10 days, and about half of those who develop the illness do so within a few days of contact with an infected person.

THE MAIN ALERTING SYMPTOMS OF MENINGITIS

- **fever;**
- **irritability;**
- **extreme drowsiness;**
- **intense headache;**
- **stiff neck;**
- **nausea, vomiting;**
- **confusion;**
- **a pink or purplish, pinpoint rash (in some forms);**
- **eye sensitivity or light aversion (photophobia);**
- **seizures (in later stages).**

WHAT TO DO FOR MENINGITIS

- **Watch for the main alerting symptoms: fever, unusual fussiness, irritability (in infants), extreme drowsiness, intense headache, stiff neck.**
- **Have infants vaccinated against the form due to Hib bacteria. A safe and effective vaccine against Hib-caused meningitis is now licensed to protect all children from 2 months to 5 years. (For more on Hib vaccine, see section on vaccination earlier in this chapter.) The Hib vaccine is not useful for people over age 5, since meningitis is usually due to different bacteria in older age groups.**

WHAT TO DO FOR MUMPS

- **Check your child's immunization record to see if he or she has had the mumps or MMR (measles, mumps, rubella) vaccine.**

- **If your child is in contact with mumps and has not had the vaccine, and is 1 year of age or older, contact your physician or the local public health agency to arrange vaccination as soon as possible.**

- **Contact your physician if you think your child has mumps.**

At present, Canada averages one case of meningococcal meningitis per 100,000 people of all ages—totaling 300 to 400 cases a year—with little change during the past 40 years. Meningococcal vaccines are not universally available, and none protects against all currently circulating forms. Recent outbreaks in Canada have been mostly due to *Neisseria meningitidis*, strains B and C. The vaccines available in Canada are only against strains A, C, Y and W-135, not B. Immunization against meningitis is now advised for all children (see page 305).

If detected in time, bacterial meningitis can be treated by antibiotics. Close contacts of people with Hib or meningococcal meningitis may be given the antibiotic rifampicin (rifampin) to prevent the illness. Taken within 48 hours of contact, the antibiotic can forestall illness. Rifampin may also be used during outbreaks in daycare centers or nursery schools but is not usually given as a large-scale preventive except during serious epidemics—for fear of facilitating the emergence of drug-resistant strains. Antibiotics are not effective against viral forms of meningitis, but anti-viral agents may help.

In newborns (under 3 months of age), meningitis may stem from bacterial organisms that are rarely the cause in the general population, such as *E. coli*, *streptococci* and *Listeria*. In older infants and toddlers, aged three months to 5 years, 70 percent of bacterially caused menin-

gitis was formerly due to *Haemophilus influenzae type b* bacteria. But immunization of infants with Hib vaccine has significantly reduced the frequency of this infection, and once all children have been vaccinated, Hib meningitis will become a rare disease.

MUMPS

A serious viral disease affecting mainly children aged 5 to 10, mumps can be prevented by vaccination at 1 year of age. The main symptoms of mumps are fever; headache, swollen neck glands, stiff jaw, swollen cheeks and possibly swollen testes in boys. Deafness, meningitis and sterility are rare complications. These days, mumps is usually a mild illness in children, sometimes not even producing swollen glands. The infection can be more severe in adults. A blood test confirms the diagnosis.

Mumps spreads from person to person through the air up to 7 days before the glands start to swell and as long as 9 days later. The incubation period is 2 to 3 weeks—i.e., it takes that long to come down with mumps after exposure. There is no treatment beyond time, bed rest and other comforts. Since the infection is caused by a virus, antibiotics have no effect.

PINKEYE (CONJUNCTIVITIS)

Pinkeye is an infection of the eyeball covering, usually due to a virus, but sometimes bacterial. It can also be caused by an allergy or rubbing the eyes excessively. Pinkeye turns the whites of the eyes pink or red, causes a scratchy feeling or pain in the eyes and may produce tears and pus. By morning, the pus or discharge often makes the eyelids stick together.

Pinkeye is spread when:
- an infected person touches the discharge and then touches another person or object;
- an uninfected child touches an infected child's eye discharge and then his or her own eyes;
- an adult wipes an infected child's eyes and then touches his or her own eyes, or someone else's.

POLIO (POLIOMYELITIS)

Poliomyelitis, now rare in Canada thanks to widespread immunization, remains common in many parts of the world. (Travelers to endemic

WHAT TO DO FOR PINKEYE

- **Get medical advice; it is not easy to tell whether the infection is caused by bacteria or viruses. Bacterial pinkeye can be cured with antibiotics, which also stop the** infection from spreading. There is no treatment for viral pinkeye other than hot compresses.

- **Try not to rub the eye; if you do rub it, wash your hands.**

- **Wash your hands carefully after touching infected eyes.**

- **Do not share towels or washcloths with anyone else (it spreads infection).**

areas should be sure their vaccination boosters are up to date.) Polio is caused by a virus that enters via the mouth and can produce permanent paralysis by damaging nerve cells in the spinal cord.

Although poliomyelitis is a rare disease in Canada today, some who had it in the past are now suffering post-polio syndrome, which requires special exercise therapy.

Two forms of polio vaccine are used in Canada. For details see section on vaccination, earlier in this chapter.

RHEUMATIC FEVER

Rheumatic fever now rare in Canada and the United States, is still a serious illness, and a continuing danger in many developing areas. The illness arises from strep-throat infections. Rheumatic fever is characterized by inflammation of the heart (carditis) and joints (arthritis), "St. Vitus dance" (nerve impairment producing involuntary jerky movements) and painful nodules under the skin. While most of these complications leave few or no lasting traces, the cardiac inflammation can permanently injure the heart valves. Anyone known to have rheumatic fever stays on penicillin for life (or at least up to age 18), to prevent recurrence of an illness which might further injure a heart already damaged by one bout of carditis. Despite the rarity of rheumatic fever in the Western World, concern lingers about the possibility of lasting heart defects following a strep throat.

Rheumatic fever can be prevented by antibiotics that eradicate a streptococcal throat infection before serious complications set in. (For signs of a strep throat, see "Sore throats," later in this chapter) In the developed world, antibiotics have dramatically reduced the toll of rheumatic fever a decline that, for unknown reasons, began before the widespread use of these drugs. Currently, in Canada, rheumatic fever affects only 2 to 5 people per million per year. Nonetheless, physicians warn against complacency in treating strep throats.

ROSEOLA

Roseola, a common viral infection caused by human herpes virus number 6, can produce a high fever in young children—as high as 40.5°C (105°F)—generally with no other symptoms until the third day, when a rash of small red spots appears, mainly on the face, abdomen and extremities. Typically, comments one pediatrician, "when the rash comes, the fever goes!" The telltale clue to this disorder as against more serious conditions, is that, despite high fever children with roseola do not seem particularly ill, although a few may have seizures (convulsions) caused by the fever. Roseola gets better without any treatment, and complications are rare.

But it's hard to diagnose until the rash appears, and since fever may arise from more severe illnesses, a doctor should be contacted. The infection is very common in children aged 6 to 24 months, and rare in older children.

RSV INFECTIONS

A common respiratory illness due to the *respiratory syncytial virus*, this lung infection attacks the delicate *mucosal* (inner) lining of the lower respiratory tract or lungs. It affects mainly infants aged 6 to 12 months during winter epidemics. Symptoms resemble the common cold and usually cause a mild infection from which children spontaneously recover but RSV infection can be life endangering, particularly among infants with heart or lung ailments. It is responsible for about half of all hospital admissions for childhood respiratory ailments in Canada. RSV starts off like a bout of the sniffles but can get worse, leading to pneumonia or bronchiolitis (airway inflammation). Its incubation period is 4 to 6 days, and children generally remain infectious for 3 to 8 days, or as long as they're coughing and sneezing.

Warning symptoms
- Runny nose, sore throat, cough;
- wheezing;
- rapid shallow breathing;
- periodic cessation of breathing ("apnea") in very young infants;
- respiratory failure.

Treatment for severe RSV symptoms may require hospital treatment with oxygen administration, ventilation, fluid therapy and drugs to shorten the viral illness or reduce its severity, including bronchodilators, antibiotics, steroids and ribavirin (Virazole), an antiviral agent that's given in hospital as an aerosol.

WHAT TO DO FOR POLIO

- **Remember to get booster shots every 10 years, if immunized with the inactive injected IPV form.**
- **If traveling to areas where polio is still endemic, be sure to update the polio booster shot if needed.**

WHAT TO DO FOR RUBELLA (GERMAN MEASLES)

- **Check immunization records to see if you and your child have had the MMR (measles, mumps, rubella) vaccine.**
- **If the child is not vaccinated and is aged 1 year or older, contact your physician or the local public-health agency to arrange for vaccination as soon as possible.**
- **Women of child-bearing age who aren't sure whether they've had rubella immunization should consult a doctor to get a blood test for rubella antibodies (immunity) before getting pregnant. If not immune and not pregnant, vaccination is advised. The rubella vaccine (or the MMR vaccine) should never be given to a woman who is already pregnant.**

RUBELLA (GERMAN MEASLES)

Rubella is a mild viral infection, now rare because a very good vaccine given at 1 year of age prevents most cases. Rubella causes a low-grade fever; swollen glands in the neck and behind the ears, and a rash with small red spots. The rubella virus spreads through air or by touch, and is infectious for a few days before the rash appears and up to 5 to 7 days afterwards. Children with rubella usually show few signs of illness. Antibiotics and other medicines can't cure the disease.

The infection may also be very mild in adults, but it can create serious problems for pregnant women. If a woman gets rubella in the first three months of pregnancy, there is a high chance that the unborn child will die or develop serious defects, including malformations of the brain, eyes, heart and/or other organs. Vaccination is important to prevent rubella in children and adults, so it will not spread to any pregnant women.

SCABIES

Scabies is caused by tiny insects called mites that burrow into skin and cause a very itchy rash that looks like curvy white threads, tiny red bumps or scratches. It can appear anywhere on the body, but is usually between the fingers or around wrists or elbows. On an infant, it can affect the head, face, neck and body. Scabies spreads by contact with clothing or other contaminated items. The mites can live on clothing, other objects and skin for up to 4 days, dying after that if the clothes are not worn. For items that can be put in the wash, washing clothes in hot water and putting them in a hot dryer gets rid of the mites. A child may remain itchy for weeks after treatment, because of reaction to the mites, even though the treatment has effectively got rid of the scabies.

SORE THROATS

A sore throat is one of the most common complaints seen by family physicians. Throats can become sore from prolonged overuse of the voice, swallowing a sharp object, cigarette smoke, seasonal allergies or eating spicy food. But a sore throat often heralds an oncoming illness such as measles, influenza or a common cold. Generally, as the measles, flu or cold takes hold and its identifying symptoms—such as a rash, cough or runny nose—appear; the throat becomes less sore.

The term "pharyngitis" describes an inflammation of the pharynx (throat) and surrounding tissues, including the larynx, adenoids and tonsils—if they haven't been removed. Pharyngitis is the chief symptom of unusual diseases such as infectious mononucleosis, caused by the Epstein-Barr virus. The sore throat may persist for weeks after other discomforts vanish. The ravaging sore throat due to diphtheria—which inflames the larynx—rarely occurs any more in immunized communities. However, although often associated with other illnesses, a sore throat can be a viral (less commonly a bacterial) infection in its own right, if it persists without other symptoms.

Viral pharyngitis tends to cure itself spontaneously within 5 to 7 days, generally requiring no treatment other than topical painkillers to ease the soreness, antipyretics to bring down any fever and soothing warm drinks.

Bacterial pharyngitis, less usual but more dangerous, may also vanish within a few days with or without treatment. But streptococcal pharyngitis (a strep throat) needs prompt medical attention because it may lead to a number of complications. Risk factors for strep throat include absence of cough, enlarged nodes, previous infections, pus on the tonsils and fever.

Signs and symptoms of strep throat:
- fever over 38°C (100°F);
- fiery red, inflamed tonsils;
- a painfully sore/raw throat;
- white spots at back of throat or on tonsils;
- enlarged, tender neck glands (lymph nodes);
- a yellowish fluid on the tonsils;
- a generally sick, listless state;
- occasionally, a scarlet-fever-like rash all over the body.

In the absence of complications, streptococcal pharyngitis subsides in a few days, all symptoms usually being gone within a week. The modern medical approach is to ease the symptoms and check the throat for signs of bacterial infection, especially by streptococci. The condition needs watching, as a strep throat may lead to middle-ear infections, sinusitis and more

WHAT TO DO FOR SORE THROATS

- The problem with sore throats is knowing when to consult a doctor. A mild sore throat, without fever, perhaps accompanied by a runny nose, may be no more than a common cold needing no medical help. But any sore throat accompanied by a fever merits medical attention.
- The best relief for sore throats is rest, warm fluids, gentle gargling and perhaps painkillers.
- Fever-reducers such as acetaminophen (Children's Tylenol, Tempra, Panadol, Atasol) can bring down the temperature and reduce the pain, but not reduce the risk of complications. ASA (such as Aspirin) should never be used to relieve fever in children or teens because of the risk of Reye's syndrome.
- Antibiotics are prescribed for bacterial throat infections (usually penicillin or erythromycin), but are useless against viral sore throats.
- The many over-the-counter remedies—antiseptic gargles, lozenges, sprays and throat rinses, avidly sought by sore-throat sufferers—achieve no better results than those obtained with a warm saltwater gargle, a hot cup of tea or your favorite "toddy."

serious complications such as rheumatic fever or glomerulonephritis (kidney inflammation, not prevented by antibiotics).

Physicians suspect a streptococcal throat infection when they see a feverish patient with fiery red tonsils coated by an exudate and enlarged neck nodes. But while many doctors think they can identify a strep throat on sight, studies show they may be wrong. Surveys comparing office diagnosis against throat culture (bacterial growth) laboratory tests showed that physicians can correctly spot a bacterial throat infection only 50 percent of the time. Therefore, experts recommend taking a throat swab for lab analysis.

Antibiotic (penicillin) treatment can shorten the duration of a strep throat and prevent serious consequences. But since antibiotics may be needlessly prescribed for viral pharyngitis, many experts advocate waiting out the few hours needed to get back the lab results before prescribing drugs. The brief delay does not increase risks, for studies show that even a few days after the onset of bacterial pharyngitis, antibiotics can prevent rheumatic fever.

SUDDEN INFANT DEATH SYNDROME

Also known as "crib death," Sudden Infant Death Syndrome (SIDS) is the unexpected death of a seemingly healthy infant, usually during sleep. Infants who die of SIDS show no outward signs of distress or struggle: they simply stop breathing. SIDS shatters parents and bewilders doctors. It's the leading cause of death in babies aged 2 weeks to 1 year; affecting 1 to 2 per 1,000 infants. Despite various clues and suspected triggers, the cause(s) of SIDS deaths remains unexplained.

Recent evidence suggests that, despite the outward appearance of perfectly good health before death, SIDS babies probably have "something wrong"—some as yet unidentified abnormality—that predisposes them to sudden death. The definition of SIDS has therefore been updated to discard the idea of these babies as "perfectly normal."

The new definition of SIDS excludes identifiable reasons for sudden infant death, numbering as SIDS cases only those where exhaustive investigation turns up no known

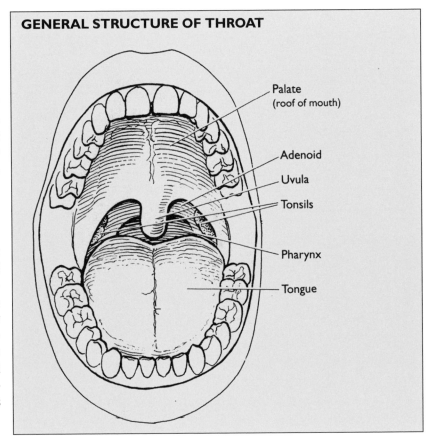

GENERAL STRUCTURE OF THROAT

Palate (roof of mouth)

Adenoid

Uvula

Tonsils

Pharynx

Tongue

reason for death. Infant deaths due to food poisoning, allergies (for instance to cow's milk or dust mites), child neglect or infanticide—formerly blamed for crib death—do not qualify as SIDS. Nor do babies who suffocate on bedding or have inborn errors of metabolism (metabolic abnormalities), or any cases not thoroughly investigated. About 10 percent of cases suspected as SIDS before autopsy later turn out to stem from other conditions, such as fulminant (galloping) meningitis, encephalitis and overlooked congenital flaws.

Most SIDS deaths occur under 6 months of age, usually in those aged 1 to 4 months and more commonly in males (about 60 percent) than females. There is also a seasonal link: two-thirds of SIDS deaths occur in winter. Some experts link the seasonality of SIDS to over-swaddling and overheating of vulnerable babies. Poor infant temperature control is believed to be one possible contributor.

The fact that SIDS babies die during sleep has prompted speculation that these infants have some flaw in the mechanism that fine-tunes breathing control. Although SIDS isn't yet traceable to any specific disorder; research indicates that they may be born with borderline breathing abnormalities that delay maturation of those parts of the nervous system which control respiratory rhythms.

There's no known way to prevent SIDS. The majority of SIDS infants don't have any noticeable breathing difficulties or warning signs of impending catastrophe. However, premature and low-birthweight babies and those with slower than normal growth rates are at above-average risk. There is no evidence that vaccination causes or increases SIDS risks. In fact, babies who die of SIDS are less likely than average to have been recently immunized.

Profiles of the mothers of SIDS infants support the notion that problems during pregnancy may predispose these babies to unexpected death. For example, women who smoke, are anemic, undernourished or prone to bladder infections, and very young mothers (especially teenagers) are at above-average risk of having SIDS babies. Such women often receive scanty prenatal health care, which could disturb fetal health. One Florida study showed a SIDS risk of 3.2 per 1,000 for mothers under age 19 compared with 1 per 1,000 for mothers aged 25 to 29. However, babies of any parents can die of SIDS.

Sleeping position recently blamed for SIDS

Recent evidence, given much media attention, suggests that some crib deaths may be related to sleeping prone (face down, on the stomach). Several studies, particularly those from Australia (Tasmania) and New Zealand, have linked this position to elevated SIDS risks. Based on the evaluation of numerous studies, the American Academy of Pediatrics and the Canadian Pediatric Society both issued 1992 recommendations that "normal infants be put to bed on their sides or backs rather than on their stomachs"—a change from the currently popular North American position.

On a cautionary note, one University of Toronto expert warns against "placing too much faith in sleeping positions until more results come in." SIDS has low prevalence rates in the United States, where so many babies sleep on their stomachs. And some argue that the sleep-position studies done in Australia and New

---

WHAT TO DO TO HELP PREVENT SIDS

- **Have good medical care and adequate nutrition during pregnancy.**
- **Keep baby in smoke-free surroundings (smoking by either parent, as well as secondhand smoke, is clearly linked to SIDS).**
- **Put baby to sleep on a firm mattress.**
- **Breastfeed if possible.**
- **If apnea, breathing stoppage or "blue spells" are noticed in the infant, get prompt medical advice.**

- **If a breathing lapse is noticed, awaken the infant with a small jolt or stimulus—a flick of the finger on the feet—which may set the baby breathing again. If that doesn't do the trick, the next step is vigorous stimulation—perhaps a hard pinch. If that doesn't work, the parent should begin mouth-to-mouth resuscitation. (See "The ABCs of AR and CPR" in Chapter 17.) (Never shake the baby hard, as it could** cause a head injury, even death.)
- **Try not to let the baby get too hot (don't overswaddle).**
- **Never have the infant's face covered by bedclothes.**
- **Avoid thick blankets, pillows or bumpers in the crib.**
- **Try not to let the infant sleep on his or her stomach. Put the baby to sleep on his or her side or back (a rolled-up towel along the back will help to keep the baby on his or her side).**

Zealand didn't allow for the popular Antipodean habit of putting babies to sleep on sheepskin bedding to keep them warm in the absence of central heating; the high SIDS rate may have gone down when infants slept on their backs because they no longer breathed in bits of sheepskin.

Apnea, a momentary halt in breathing, has also been blamed as a possible forerunner of SIDS. Tiny infants often stop breathing for a few seconds, especially after a deep sigh. Breathing stoppage lasting less than 20 seconds is not considered hazardous, but if the lapses last more than 20 seconds they may signal danger. Such Apparent Life-Threatening Episodes (ALTEs)— to give them their scientific name—often happen in the same age range as SIDS, also more commonly in males than females, and 1 to 2 per cent of infants who suffer ALTEs eventually die.

The mysterious death of a seemingly healthy infant can cause immense grief, self-blame and anxiety. Parents and other caregivers may mull endlessly over the events leading up to the death. Guilt may worsen the usual anger denial and intense sense of bereavement, even though no known measures could have prevented the infant death. Counseling for families after crib death aims to reassure them that nobody was to blame. Medical experts explain the importance of autopsy results. The police investigation of sudden infant deaths—while initially distressing—ultimately serves to lighten the burden. Parents also need reassurance that SIDS wasn't the doctor's fault. Marriages can become strained and siblings understandably distressed after a SIDS death; the siblings must be encouraged to express their sadness, self-doubts and confusion. Some may not show their grief directly but "act it out" by renewed bed-wetting, naughtiness or poor schoolwork. Expert counseling and sharing experiences with others who've been through similar situations can be a help.

TEETHING

In the vast majority of healthy children, the incisor teeth (the front four on the top and the front four on the bottom) come through painlessly. Discomfort is sometimes experienced with the molars and canine teeth, which erupt at between 12 and 36 months of age. However, teething, like growing, is mostly painless. Occasionally, when a tooth is about to break through, the gum may become tender and look obviously swollen, with a purplish bulge over the site of the new tooth, and the area may be painful when touched. The discomfort is usually short-lived. Medications are rarely necessary and should be avoided as much as possible.

If a fever cold or diarrhea develops, it is probably due to an infection, not teething. It is a mistake, and can even be dangerous, to assume that teething is the cause of any change in the infant's behavior. Teething does not cause fever. The fact that infants want to suck their hands does not mean they are teething but simply that infants find sucking pleasurable. Teething goes on continuously throughout the first 2 years of life, and the hand-sucking is a coincidence, not the result.

TETANUS (LOCKJAW)

Tetanus is a disease that results if bacteria from soil, rust, manure or animal dirt enter cuts, scratches, wounds or grazes in people who have not been immunized. The infection kills 6 out of every 10 people who get it, but vaccination effectively prevents this lethal infection. Tetanus is rare in Canada today because most people are vaccinated, but they must remember to get their vaccination boosters every 10 years. (Each year, about 20 to 30 people are hospitalized with tetanus in Canada, and there are a few deaths from it.) Tetanus remains very common in parts of the world where the vaccine is not used. Tetanus vaccine—usually given in combination with diphtheria toxoid and pertussis vaccine (DPT) during childhood—protects almost everyone immunized with the recommended 3 shots.

THRUSH OR CANDIDA (YEAST) DIAPER RASH

Candida is a fungus or yeast that infects the skin, mouth or throat. If it's in the throat or mouth, it's called thrush. The candida fungus is present in the intestines of many people without causing any illness and is common among youngsters still in diapers. It may also occur after prolonged treatment with antibiotics for

---

WHAT TO DO FOR TEETHING

- **Give painkillers (acetaminophen, not ASA) to relieve discomfort, but only if really necessary.**
- **Be patient—it's all over by about age 3, once the canines are through.**
- **If there's any fever, lethargy or diarrhea, don't automatically dismiss it as "just teething"; it is more likely due to an infection that needs medical attention. (Teething doesn't cause fever or stomach upsets.)**

WHAT TO DO ABOUT TETANUS

- **For any cut or puncture or animal bite, wash thoroughly and disinfect.**
- **Make sure that tetanus immunization is up to date. Booster shots are needed every 10 years to ensure continuing protection. (Many adults, especially the elderly, neglect to get their required booster shots. But provided tetanus boosters have been given, the vaccine isn't necessary for every little cut or injury.)**

WHAT TO DO FOR A CANDIDA (YEAST) INFECTION

- If you suspect your child has a yeast infection, contact your physician.
- Make sure you follow directions for any prescribed anti-thrush medication.
- For babies with mouth thrush: regularly sanitize the bottle nipples and soothers by boiling them for 10 minutes.
- For babies with diaper rash: when changing diapers, wash the child's buttocks and genitals with mild soap and warm water. Rinse, dry and apply prescribed ointment. Wash your own and your child's hands carefully after changing diapers.

WHAT TO DO FOR WHOOPING COUGH (PERTUSSIS)

- Check your child's immunization record to see if he or she has been vaccinated against pertussis. (Note that the vaccine is given together with diphtheria and tetanus shots.)
- See a physician at the earliest hint of possible whooping cough.

other infections. Thrush appears as a tough, whitish-gray coating on the tongue and insides of the cheeks and gums that's hard to wipe off. Over-vigorous attempts to remove it may leave a bleeding, raw surface. In severe cases, the mouth may be so sore that the infant finds it painful to suck. Most infants do not get complications from thrush.

Candida diaper rash tends to settle in the creases of groin and buttocks as a rash that can be very red, with a clearly defined border and small red spots close to larger patches. Candida infections can be cured with prescribed antifungals, such as pills, lotions or ointment.

TONSILLITIS

Throat infections that affect the tonsils—known as tonsillitis—were a serious threat before the advent of antibiotics. Infected tonsils were routinely removed to prevent complications such as middle-ear infections, glomerulonephritis (kidney inflammation) and rheumatic fever Tonsillectomy (tonsil removal) usually was, and often still is, done in combination with adenoid removal.

However; once antibiotics became available in the 1950s, physicians took a more conservative "wait-and-see" approach, resorting to surgery only in extreme cases. The pendulum is now swinging back as it's becoming clear that a few children benefit from tonsil and/or adenoid removal, especially if sleep and breathing problems result from the enlarged tonsils or adenoids. Currently, about 15 percent of children have their tonsils and/or adenoids removed, with about two adenoidectomies for every 10 tonsillectomies plus adenoid removals.

The first step with tonsillar infections is antibiotic therapy (penicillin being the drug of first choice). The antibiotic must be taken for the full period prescribed, even if the person feels well sooner, in order to completely eradicate the infective organisms. A throat swab is usually sent to a lab in order to identify the microorganism responsible for tonsillitis. While awaiting the lab results (which may take 24 to 48 hours), nonallergic patients are often put on penicillin. The current policy is to treat bacterial sore throats and inflamed tonsils or adenoids with antibiotic therapy to prevent spread to the ears or other organs.

Reasons for tonsil removal include:

- "kissing tonsils"—enlarged tonsils that meet in the middle and cause breathing problems, particularly at night. It's generally accepted that any child who is a persistent mouth breather (in the absence of a cold or respiratory infection) should have the tonsils out;
- Obstructive Sleep Syndrome, or sleep apnea, a serious condition due to obstructed airways that cause heavy snoring, daytime sleepiness and night sweats. Owing to poor nighttime rest, youngsters may be tired and lazy throughout the day. Adults too sometimes have disturbed sleep patterns due to tonsil enlargement, a newly recognized problem. Enlarged tonsils that cause sleep or breathing difficulties must come out at any age;
- quinsy (abscess)—an unusual but serious infection in and around the tonsils which makes it difficult to swallow; tonsil removal is done once the abscess heals;
- recurrent middle-ear infections accompanied by tonsillitis—3 to 4 times yearly;
- an "adenoidal" or elongated face associated with mouth breathing due to swollen tonsils and/or adenoids.

Less common indicators for tonsil removal include:

- increasing unilateral (one-sided) tonsil enlargement;
- recurrent bleeding from an infected ulcer on the tonsil;
- diphtheria (now rare in Canada);
- halitosis (bad breath) in teenagers or adults, due to decaying food caught on the tonsils.

WHOOPING COUGH (PERTUSSIS)

Whooping cough (pertussis) is a very contagious bacterial infection that affects all ages and is preventable by an effective vaccine. Most usual in children under age 7 (and very dangerous in youngsters under age 2), whooping cough usually begins with a runny nose and racking cough, which gets more frequent and severe, with a prolonged spasm ("whoop") when breathing in. During attacks, the child may become blue in the face, perhaps vomit, have convulsions and appear very weak. The temporary bouts of oxygen shortage can damage the brain. It takes children a long time to recover from whooping cough.

The disease is most severe in infants under 1 year old, many of whom are so ill they must be cared for in hospital. The illness can be fatal in young children. If an unvaccinated child catches the infection, antibiotics can treat it—but vaccination is far safer. The risk of dangerous complications from the disease in infants is much greater than the vaccine risks.

Whooping cough spreads easily, through the air or by touch, until up to 3 weeks after the coughing attacks start. It takes from 7 to 10 days to come down with whooping cough after exposure to the pertussis microbes. Although complications are rare beyond the age of 2, whooping cough is still quite common among adolescents and adults. About 20 to 25 percent of adults with a cough lasting longer than 7 to 10 days have whooping cough—even though they may not know it and rarely whoop!

A new, more effective acellular pertussis vaccine, containing only the disease-causing components, not the whole bacterium, has recently been developed that stimulates a stronger immune response against whooping cough and has fewer troublesome side effects than previous forms. This vaccine also protects against mild pertussis—an added advantage as the mild form plays a key role in spreading the illness (and is often mistaken for a less serious cough).

Key advantages of the new pertussis vaccine

- *Greater efficacy*, giving more of those immunized lasting immunity;
- *fewer "vaccine failures"* (common with previous forms), where those not adequately protected by immunization spread the disease;
- *fewer side effects* such as soreness at the injection site, fever inconsolable crying and seizures;
- *protection against mild disease*—which might not be recognized as whooping cough, but would help cut down spread.

WORMS

Pinworms are tiny, white thread-like worms that live in the intestines; they crawl out of the anus at night and lay their eggs on nearby skin. Most children with pinworms have no symptoms, although some get very itchy around the anus and vagina. Pinworms are a nuisance rather than a disease. They are very common and spread easily among children and staff in childcare facilities, especially when those infected scratch the itchy area and get pinworm eggs on the fingers or under the fingernails and then touch someone or something else. Uninfected people can

WHAT TO DO ABOUT PINWORMS

- **To halt the spread, stop children from scratching.**
- **Ensure that all household members wash their hands carefully after going** to the toilet or changing diapers, and before preparing or eating food.
- **Ask your physician whether all household members** should also be treated with medication.
- **Inform school or daycare staff that the child has pinworms.**

WHAT TO DO ABOUT RINGWORM

- **To prevent the spread, check your child for signs of a typical "circular rash" on the head, skin or feet.**
- **Call the doctor if you think your child has ringworm.**
- **Ensure that the hands are washed after touching the infected skin.**
- **If a child has ringworm on the scalp, make sure that no one else uses the same comb, hair-** brush, facecloths or towels.
- **Don't let children with ringworm return to school or daycare until after treatment has started.**

WHAT TO DO ABOUT ROUNDWORMS

- **Contact your physician if you notice that a child is scratching the anal** area, or if you see a worm emerge.
- **Inform the school or daycare authorities.**
- **Give the prescribed medication as instructed.**

pick up pinworm eggs from infected clothes, pyjamas, sheets or surroundings. (The eggs can survive for several weeks outside the body.)

Ringworm is a fungal skin infection—not a worm at all—which causes a ring-shaped rash, with a raised edge, that is usually quite itchy and flaky. When the scalp is infected, there is often a bald patch: ringworm on the feet is usually very itchy, with cracking between the toes. Ringworm spreads from person to person by touch. When someone with ringworm touches or scratches the rash, the fungus sticks to the fingers or gets under the fingernails. Ringworm on the scalp can spread via combs and hairbrushes.

It can be cured with medication, taken by mouth or as ointments or creams put on infected areas.

Roundworms (Ascaris) are a common but harmless affliction in young children, with large worms (up to 20 cm or 8 inches long) that may emerge from the anus or even the nostrils. The sign of infestation is itching in the anal area. Mostly innocuous, the worms may occasionally cause a mild form of pneumonia. Treatment is with suitable medication for a few days. (A different form of roundworm, much smaller in size, can be picked up from the feces of infected cats and other pets. It also requires special medication.)

Puberty and adolescent changes

The stages of adolescence • The physical changes of puberty • Body-image concerns • The tragic pursuit of thinness • Psychosocial development in adolescence • Helping adolescents through the transition • Medical checkups for adolescents • School problems • Adolescent sexuality • Risk-taking behavior • The heavy toll of adolescent suicide • Teenage and student drug use

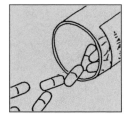

DURING THE LONG plateau of childhood, girls and boys look and behave much alike, but from ages 10 and 11 and onward, each gender develops different sex-specific changes as hormonal triggers initiate puberty and the development of secondary sex characteristics—changes that signify the transition from boy or girl into man or woman.

Adolescence is a biopsychosocial process that involves intense physical, emotional and psychological changes, with a huge variation of what's considered "normal." Each teenager reacts somewhat differently to the demands of growing up. Rather than being a sudden event, adolescence is a gradual transition with many social and emotional demands both on teenagers and on their parents. But while it has been described as a period of "extreme instability," or "normal psychosis," most adolescents remain relatively unruffled by the process, cope well with the transition and survive with no lasting difficulties. "In reality," says one University of Toronto pediatrician, "about 30 percent have an easy growth process, 40 percent have periods of calm intermingled with turbulent times and 30 percent have a tumultuous adolescence marked by storm and stress."

Adolescents eagerly seek greater control of their lives, but although no longer children, they're not yet fully equipped—or allowed—to take on adult roles or responsibilities. Despite the outward trappings of bravado, many feel deeply unsure about their changing looks and ability to cope with things ahead. It is normal for adolescents to feel uncertain—young and unsure one minute, mature and confident the next.

The primary tasks of adolescence are separation from parents and the establishment of a new personal identity. In achieving them, adolescents must accept their new body image, adopt peer codes, establish a sexual ego, plan vocational goals and formulate their own opinions—no mean feat! Some feel overwhelmed by the sudden body changes and the pressure to look after appearance, worry about weight, keep up with schoolwork and conform to peer values. During this period, psychological conflicts from early childhood may resurface and cause additional turmoil as adolescents work through and resolve them.

The emergence of a new physical, cognitive and social self may result in a person with values different from (and sometimes contradictory to) parental expectations. Parents and other caring adults can ease children through the process by knowing what to expect, being tolerant and explaining to teenagers what's ahead—for example, the many emotional, cognitive and relationship changes, as well as physical maturation, such as developing breasts and menstruation in daughters, "breaking" voice and nocturnal emissions in sons.

12

THE STAGES OF ADOLESCENCE

Some experts divide the period into early adolescence (the junior-high years); middle adolescence (the high-school years); and late adolescence (the university years or early employment years). These three stages overlap, but by the time they're completed most adolescents have gained autonomy, attained a psychosexual identity and begun to support themselves emotionally and financially.

Early adolescence (approximately ages 12 to 14)

This phase is marked by rapid physical growth, the emergence of secondary sexual characteristics, a focus on the changing body and a wish to "belong" to peer groups.

- Rapid physical changes lead to intense "self-centeredness"—concerns about being normal, preoccupation with body image, uncertainty about appearance, interest in sexual anatomy, anxieties about breasts and periods in girls, about wet dreams and penis size in boys.
- The tendency to "size themselves up" leads adolescents to compare themselves (often with despair) against their peers.
- Along with the rapid, somewhat discomfiting physical changes comes a testing of new strength in sex-appeal and opinion-forming skills.
- In forming close, intense (possibly idealized) friendships with same-sex chums, boys may swear "eternal comradeship" and girls may develop a "crush" on another (sometimes older) female.
- The social world appears to early adolescents as a place in which to explore their burgeoning potential and practice adult-like behavior—even though they are still far from having a stable identity.
- An independence struggle may begin, with a shift from reliance on parents to greater peer-group involvement—turning to friends as a source of advice and comfort.
- Cognitive abilities rapidly develop, with increased capacities for abstract reasoning.
- A tendency to daydream and build a fantasy world is a normal component of identity development (not a "waste of time").

- A sense of being constantly "on stage," scrutinized and evaluated by others, is accompanied by a tendency to magnify and dramatize personal problems or events.
- Testing authority is commonplace as teens try to define themselves and their powers— behavior that may create friction within the family.
- Journal writing is common; feelings, emotions and thoughts are expressed.
- The inability to control impulses may lead to dangerous risk taking.

Middle adolescence (approximately ages 15 to 17)

This stage is typified by still more rapid growth of cognitive skills, the ability to conceptualize and operate according to abstract thought, increased intensity of feelings, further separation from parents and greater reliance on peer groups. Peer relationships play a key role in the development of personal identity, their support and advice replacing that of parents.

- Body-image concerns wane as most start to feel more comfortable in their new body, spending more time on making it look attractive.
- With the distancing of family ties, peers set the going standards, helping to compensate for the frustrations of everyday life or "not being understood" by adults.
- Middle adolescents live almost entirely in the present, swaying with whatever peers decide to do, annoyingly unable to state or stick to plans, never knowing what they're going to do the same evening, let alone the next day.
- They avidly seek more privacy and many complain about the lack of personal space and a place of their own to meet in, preferably devoid of adults.
- Family conflicts may become more frequent with the adolescent's declining interest in parental wishes; new "power lines" are forged.
- In addition to peer attachments, middle adolescents often ally themselves emotionally with adults *outside* the home, perhaps as idols, mentors or "hero" figures—attachments that can profoundly influence ideas, career and the future course in life.

- Many start dating, testing their new-found sex roles.
- Some claim to be "stressed out" by the concurrent demands of school, extracurricular activities, home duties and maintaining same-sex as well as "dating" relationships.
- Identity development bounds ahead, with an enhanced ability to express feelings and explore those of others.
- A sense of omnipotence frequently increases risk-taking behavior (leading to accidents, alcohol use and other dangers).
- The still-limited economic independence of middle adolescents curbs their activities— many don't have the money or opportunity to explore as fully as they would like.

Late adolescence (approximately ages 18 to 21)

In this last phase of the quest for independence, if all has gone well, the young person will be well on the way to handling the tasks and responsibilities of adulthood. Having successfully separated from the family, the late adolescent often comes to reappreciate parental values and support.

- Parental advice may once more be sought and a new, positive relationship with the family often emerges. (However, some late adolescents are still struggling with independence issues.)
- The perfected adult body of late adolescence has acquired a self-image to go with it and a clear sexual identity.
- Peer-group attachments become less important as the adolescent becomes secure in his or her own values.
- Late adolescents develop more of a "conscience," a sense of perspective, the ability to delay gratification and to compromise, with a refinement of religious, moral and sexual values.
- Relationships become less exploitative and more reciprocal, the focus being on enjoyable companionship rather than peer adherence.

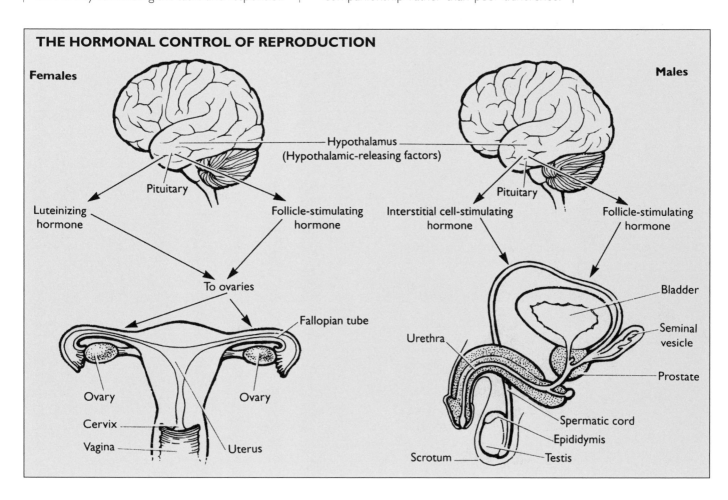

THE HORMONAL CONTROL OF REPRODUCTION

Females — Males

Hypothalamus (Hypothalamic-releasing factors)

Pituitary — Pituitary

Luteinizing hormone — Follicle-stimulating hormone

Interstitial cell-stimulating hormone — Follicle-stimulating hormone

To ovaries

Fallopian tube

Ovary — Ovary

Cervix

Vagina — Uterus

Bladder

Seminal vesicle

Prostate

Urethra

Spermatic cord

Epididymis

Scrotum — Testis

THE ENDOCRINE (HORMONE-PRODUCING) GLANDS

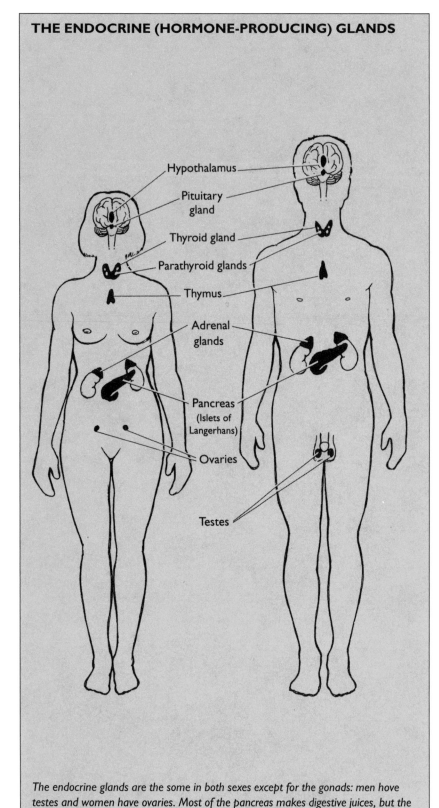

Hypothalamus

Pituitary
gland

Thyroid gland

Parathyroid glands

Thymus

Adrenal
glands

Pancreas
(Islets of
Langerhans)

Ovaries

Testes

The endocrine glands are the some in both sexes except for the gonads: men hove testes and women have ovaries. Most of the pancreas makes digestive juices, but the specialized islets of Langerhans make the hormone insulin. The brain, stomach and intestines also make and release hormones.

More sustained friendships are forged, involving tenderness and responsibility.

- The late adolescent thinks in more concrete terms about career, job and plans for the future, and can organize time better and plan a productive lifestyle.

THE PHYSICAL CHANGES OF PUBERTY

Girls usually begin puberty between ages 9 and 12, boys 2 to 3 years later. The changes in height, weight and sexual development encompass a wide range of normal. The fastest growth in height occurs around ages 12 or 13 in girls and 14 to 16 in boys. Growth tends to be greatest in spring and summer. Muscle strength in girls increases up to ages 15 or 16, then tapers off, but increases steadily in boys up to ages 16 to 18 or beyond.

The secondary sexual changes of puberty are triggered by hormones from the *hypothalamus* and *pituitary* glands in the brain. The hypothalamus produces gonadotropin-releasing hormones (GRH), which cause the pea-sized pituitary gland at the base of the brain (just behind the eyes), to produce two hormones: follicle-stimulating hormone (FSH) and luteinizing hormone (LH), which in turn trigger production of sex hormones by the male testes and female ovaries.

- FSH stimulates sperm maturation in males, ovarian follicle development in females;
- LH stimulates testosterone output in males, ovulation and progesterone production in females;
- estradiol increases bone growth in boys, and in girls it triggers the development of breasts, labia, vagina and uterus;
- testosterone accelerates growth and stimulates in boys development of penis, scrotum, muscle mass, pubic and underarm hair, larynx size (and voice-deepening), and in girls the development of pubic and underarm hair.

The onset of menstruation

Menarche, the first menstrual period, is a memorable—sometimes unexpected, occasionally unnerving—event. The normal age of menarche ranges from 9 to 16 years, averaging 12.4 years in North America today.

Once menstrual periods begin, a girl can get pregnant any time, even at her very first sexual encounter. Some mothers do not bother to tell their daughters much about menstruation, assuming they will learn about it in school. But schools do not always do a thorough job of sex education, often failing to explain adequately the meaning of menstruation and also giving too little information about birth control and sexually transmitted diseases. Yet if parents prepare a daughter well ahead for her first menstrual period, the event can be celebrated in a positive manner. It can also be used as an opportunity to discuss birth control, sexuality and parenthood.

Body fat plays a key role in the onset of periods

For menstrual periods to begin, a girl's body must have about 22 to 24 percent of body fat. (At maturity, the average girl's body has 24 to 28 percent body fat, compared to about 14 percent fat in boys.) Results from many countries confirm that menstrual periods become irregular or cease when body fat dwindles below 22 percent in women of average height. Halted ovulation may be a protective biological mechanism that prevents pregnancy when a woman has insufficient energy stores to nourish a developing fetus or breastfeed a newborn.

Changes of puberty in boys

For most boys, the first hint of imminent manhood is growth of the testicles and penis, and the development of pubic hair which gradually becomes darker and more abundant, with hair also appearing under the arms and on the legs and perhaps on the chest and back. Later usually between ages 13 and 18, the beard starts to appear and the voice deepens. Although boys generally start growing later than girls, they go on growing for several years after most girls have stopped, often reaching full height between ages 16 and 18.

Wet dreams and penis fantasies

Wet dreams—nocturnal emissions or the ejaculation of semen while asleep—are common during puberty. But the first nocturnal emission can be very upsetting, even though it's an involuntary response to erotic thoughts or dreams.

Nocturnal emissions are a normal part of adolescence, and parents usually understand better than boys think they will! Some boys also have involuntary erections at awkward times during the day. There is not much that can be done about such erections, but it may help to remember that this happens to most boys and diminishes with maturity. Boys naturally tend to compare penis size and some hold contests to see who can ejaculate or urinate the farthest. Penis size has nothing to do with potency, sex drive or fertility, nor does it make any difference to the ability to conceive children. Similarly, it has nothing to do with the capacity to give sexual pleasure. An erect penis of even 7 to 10 cm (3 to 4 in) can stimulate the vaginal nerves and give ample pleasure. (While the vagina's entire length is erotically sensitive, the outer third is most sensitive, especially to tactile stimulation.) Yet macho myths often lead men to equate masculinity with penis size—just as women can be led to believe that sex appeal has to do with the size of their breasts. Such unfounded notions only exacerbate natural adolescent uncertainties.

BODY-IMAGE CONCERNS

Dissatisfaction with body shape and size is almost a rite of passage for teens, and in one survey 54 percent of adolescent girls and 33 percent of boys reported "dissatisfaction" with their bodies. Other surveys reveal that 90 percent of young women and a growing number of young men in Western societies dislike their bodies and are preoccupied with weight and shape, sometimes for life.

The wish to acquire a fashionably thin body makes many adolescents resort to unhealthy practices such as dieting, fluid deprivation, or overuse of saunas or weight-lifting equipment. Dieting, fasting, "binge and purge" behavior and abuse of laxatives and diuretics (water-loss pills) are widespread among adolescents—especially females—sometimes leading to malnutrition. "Since weight concerns are almost universal," notes one U.S. nutrition expert, "we should no longer consider them pathological but an adaptive response to growing up in a society obsessed with thinness." Given that the media and fashion industry portray successful women as thin and asexual, adolescent girls tend to regard a naturally soft or buxom female shape as undesirable.

Basing self-esteem more on outward appearance and body shape than on other assets—such as musical, artistic, creative, scholastic, nurturing or other abilities—many of today's adolescent girls have an appallingly low sense of self-worth, poor views of their value to society and often less confidence than boys of similar age. One Canadian survey found that while 60 percent of girls aged 8 to 9 report they are "happy with the way they are," by the time they reach 16, only 29 percent of girls are content and confident about themselves, compared to 48 percent of similarly aged boys.

Dieting and nutritional deficiencies

In trying to conform to the media portrayal of a desirably thin body, many adolescents—girls in particular—adopt unhealthy practices such as smoking (to curb appetite) and very restricted diets. Efforts to acquire a lean, svelte shape lead many of today's young women to consume too few (and/or the wrong) calories. They may select "lite" foods for the wrong reason—not as part of a healthy eating regimen, but because they don't like themselves the way they are.

Believing that "mind over matter" should allow them to achieve a skinny look—despite today's biological tendency to be larger and heavier—many young women feel guilty for being even slightly overweight or less slender than TV or magazine models. And if they fail to adhere to the self-proclaimed diet, they feel ashamed, further lowering self-esteem.

One reason for the dieting mania is the current view of female beauty found in most media, which equates a slim body with success and desirability. As one specialist puts it, "today's images tell women that thinness equals power and confidence, leading to an unhealthy preoccupation with weight, shape and dieting." Struggling to reduce or maintain their weight, many young women restrict their food choices and limit calories to 1,000 or less a day—generally too little to supply the needed nutrients. Yet most women can never achieve the idealized slim shape—no matter how rigorously they diet—because of the body's biological tendency to maintain a "set-point" and to put back the

weight lost as soon as a diet ends. (For more on the pitfalls of dieting, see Chapter 2.)

According to some experts, "weight preoccupation has become a way in which people, especially women, express control, and for some weight control is a substitute for gaining mastery over other aspects of their lives." Focusing on weight may be a coping strategy to avoid dealing with painful emotions or experiences such as sex abuse. Those with low self-esteem may hope to gain approval through being thin, precariously relying on body-image as tangible proof of worthiness rather than on more substantial qualities, achievements and attributes. Becoming or staying thin may become a primary goal in life, overshadowing attention to family, career and friendships. Weight preoccupation and eating disorders are basically an expression of "dissatisfaction with oneself." They fall on a continuum with inveterate dieters at one end and those diagnosed with anorexia nervosa and bulimia at the other.

The massive preoccupation with dieting, which often starts in the primary grades, gives adolescent females the nutritional challenge of obtaining enough nutrients while restricting calories to avoid weight gain. Surveys reveal that the challenge is often unmet and that many women aged 15 to 24 are malnourished and consume less than the recommended daily intakes of key nutrients such as calcium, iron, zinc, magnesium, some B vitamins and vitamin D. Health problems arising from the nutrient lack include fatigue, an inability to learn properly, disturbed (or halted) menstrual cycles, anemia (from lack of iron), depleted bone density (from shortage of calcium), and—in extreme cases—dangerous illnesses such as anorexia nervosa and bulimia. The disordered eating habits may last a lifetime and the tragedy is that the yo-yo dieting spiral that starts in the teenage years may lead to obesity later on.

Society needs to set new values to help young people get out of the dieting trap, overcome the idolization of thinness, and base their self-worth on assets other than appearance, a good figure or body shape. An Australian study found that 8 percent of 15-year-old girls dieted at a "severe level" and 60 percent at a "moderate level." The risk for an eating disorder was increased eighteenfold in severe dieters and five fold in moderate-level dieters compared with nondieters. The study's authors recommend exercise rather than dieting as the optimal strategy for weight control in adolescents.

THE TRAGIC PURSUIT OF THINNESS: ANOREXIA NERVOSA AND BULIMIA

Western society's idealization of thinness is producing an alarming increase in eating disorders, especially among young women. The never-ending efforts to lose weight and conform to the media image of an "ideal" shape are leading more and more young people to diet at the cost of health. Weight preoccupation is now widespread in our society, affecting people of all ages, classes, occupations and ethnic backgrounds.

There's a steadily rising incidence of eating disorders such as anorexia nervosa and bulimia nervosa, which can cause devastating health problems, even death. The incidence of these eating disorders is especially high in adolescent girls. Crude mortality rates as high as 18 percent after 30 years have been reported with some of these deaths due to suicide. Over 300,000 Canadians suffer from these eating disorders, which may coexist, overlap or occur separately. Men are also becoming increasingly prone to eating disorders, however the relative rates of anorexia nervosa in women compared to men are 10 to 1 for women, 20 to 1 for men. Anorexia nervosa involves the pursuit of thinness to the point of starvation, seriously endangering health. Bulimia nervosa also involves food and weight-obsession, but with frequent binge eating—the compulsive consumption of vast amounts of food—followed by vomiting and purging sessions to counteract the possibility of weight gain through overeating.

Besides those actually diagnosed with anorexia nervosa and bulimia, countless others—an estimated 10 to 20 percent of all North American women—are weight-obsessed and engage in many of the self-harming behaviors associated with these eating disorders. Many who are not strictly anorexic or bulimic nonetheless share some characteristics of these illnesses, such as an obsessive desire to be fashionably thin, relentless dieting and an intense fear of weight gain. Girls and women make up about 95 percent of those struggling with severe eating problems, boys and men the rest. Studies find a high rate of depression, anxiety and other psychiatric disturbances (including the psychological results of sex abuse) among those diagnosed with serious eating problems.

Anorexia nervosa

Anorexia nervosa (AN) affects about 1 percent of young females aged 14 to 25 (and some males), of whom 15 to 18 percent are in danger of dying from the disorder. The disorder afflicts primarily adolescents and young women, who starve themselves in the relentless quest for a slender figure. The term "anorexia nervosa," barely heard of 30 years ago, has now become a familiar household word. But "anorexia nervosa," meaning a nervous loss of appetite, is a misnomer since appetite loss usually appears, if at all, late in the disease. While the disorder was previously confined mainly to girls from affluent

CHARACTERISTICS OF ANOREXIA NERVOSA

- **Increasingly desperate pursuit of thinness.**
- **Terror of becoming fat or "losing control."**
- **Misperception of inner sensations such as fatigue, anger.**
- **Low sense of self-worth—dependence on external looks.**
- **Feelings of helplessness (lack of initiative, failure to gain autonomy, being overly tied to family or peers).**
- **Denial of illness, refusal to acknowledge "anything wrong."**
- **Stubborn insistence on "being too fat" despite extreme thinness and weight loss.**
- **Fear of growing up.**
- **Lack of trust in self and others.**
- **Preoccupation with cooking the family dinner (even high calorie items) but eating very little of it themselves**
- **Perfectionist tendencies—excessive desire to perform well.**
- **Withdrawal from social or sexual contacts, increasing isolation; avoidance of social occasions that involve eating.**
- **Endless weighing and measuring of body size and weight, all activities being regulated by "what the scales say."**
- **Compulsive exercise (even standing all day to hasten weight loss).**
- **Intense preoccupation with food—collection of menus, recipes, cookbooks, utensils.**
- **Subterfuges to avoid eating (giving food to dog, throwing it in garbage); peculiar patterns of handling food (e.g., hoarding but not eating it; preparing meals for others but not eating themselves).**
- **Undivided attention to meals—hours taken to consume even tiny amounts.**
- **Reproductive changes: amenorrhea in women, impotence in men.**
- **Osteoporosis (bone loss).**

families, it has now spread to all social classes and ethnic groups.

An English doctor first described a case of anorexia nervosa in the 1800s as a "skeleton clad only in skin"—a woman who stubbornly refused to eat, "giving no reason for her obstinacy." Typically, people with anorexia nervosa have an unshakable preoccupation with dieting and are at least 15 percent below their normal weight. Many feel fat despite their emaciated appearance and are socially withdrawn. Some subsist on as little as 300 calories a day. They refuse to acknowledge normal hunger pangs, seeing resistance as a sign of self-discipline. AN can result in many metabolic, hormonal and physical disturbances. Sufferers may finally seek medical advice because of fatigue, slow heart rate, low blood pressure, bloating, brittle nails, fine or "lanugo" hair development on the body, a yellowing skin and other characteristic signs of starvation.

The causes of AN are multifactorial and include biological, family, psychological and societal influences, including a history of sex abuse. Some blame its prevalence on our society's excessive weight-consciousness. Scientists are debating whether chronic dieters and compulsive exercisers differ from those with full-blown anorexia nervosa only in degree—with AN representing an extreme consequence of dieting—or also qualitatively. (Mild anorectic symptoms occur in many compulsive exercisers and obsessive dieters.)

Most medical specialists regard anorexia nervosa as a psychiatric illness. As defined by the American Psychiatric Association's Diagnostic and Statistical Manual of Mental Disorders, its hallmarks are: a relentless pursuit of thinness; body weight 15 percent or more below desirable weight; intense fear of being fat or putting on a gram or ounce; misperception about inner sensations (such as anger, disappointment); absence of at least three consecutive menstrual cycles and a distorted image of body size and shape (viewing an emaciated body as fat). The outwardly defiant and stubborn demeanor of those with AN often hides an extreme vulnerability and lack of self-esteem.

The disorder may delay sexual development if it starts young. Female anorexics typically become amenorrheic (menstrual periods cease), their breasts diminish, their fat dwindles, their feminine curves vanish, osteoporosis (bone loss) occurs, their body may become covered with fine hair (lanugo) and many medical disorders appear—such as pancreatitis, anemia, low blood pressure, cold-intolerance (blue extremities), heart irregularities and liver ailments. Weight-loss is pursued to the exclusion of all else. Many anorexics also exercise compulsively—perhaps walking or swimming great distances each day—to the point of utter exhaustion, in order to "burn calories" rather than for fun or good health.

The symptoms of AN may start imperceptibly, with a narrowing of food choices, making remarks about "being too fat," increasing preference for diet foods, counting calories, omitting meats, eating primarily fiber-rich foods, a refusal to dine with the family, excuses of "eating later" and withdrawal from social occasions.

Self-starvation may be a drive for control

While the bizarre eating patterns may seem to come out of the blue, they often result from childhood experiences, overly strict upbringing, excess emphasis on high grades, excellent performance or perfect behavior, neglect or abuse, all of which produce an extremely low sense of self-worth. Recent research reveals that 65 percent of those with anorexia and other severe eating disorders have experienced some form of abuse, whether physical, sexual, verbal or emotional, or have witnessed violence between parents. The abuse can leave children with feelings of revulsion, shame, guilt and powerlessness, leading them to think that they can't control their bodies or anything else in their lives. These feelings of helplessness may translate into an extreme need to control or "punish" the body through self-starvation. The focus on weight and the maintenance of a thin, childlike form may help women to avoid growing up and thinking about victimization or unpleasant experiences.

The family of someone with AN is often restrictive and overprotective. The child's needs may be denied, communication may be restrained and family members may avoid conflict only by suppressing emotions and feelings. While outwardly harmonious, the family may discourage independent opinions or actions, expecting total obedience. Although AN is called an eating disorder, many believe it might more aptly be called a disorder of control, since most anorexics have a profound feeling of inadequacy in directing their lives. The weight preoccupation may deflect their thoughts and stop them from dwelling on an intolerable situation.

The underpinnings of AN are apprehension about maturing and an overwhelming sense of ineffectiveness. Some experts view the disorder as a push for autonomy and a way to escape or rebel against stifling domination. The relentless drive for thinness and its attainment prove mastery over *at least one area*—their own bodies. Typically, but not always, anorexics base their self-worth entirely on external appearance and the approval of others, especially their peers.

The pre-illness personality of anorexics is often described by parents, teachers and peers as being that of a "perfect little girl," someone who has always complied with the wishes of others. Such children tend to be obliging, industrious and academically bright, with a desperate wish to succeed but no clear self-identity. Long before the illness manifests itself, these children are obedient and reluctant to test their own capacities. Anorexia nervosa is now spreading to a broader range of adolescents who are less compliant, industrious and achievement-oriented.

Precipitating events

The triggering events that may start someone on the anorectic dieting spiral often seem no different from those facing many women in our slimness-obsessed society. The dieting may be set off by a teasing remark about being chubby, a dieting parent or friend or some stressful circumstance such as going to camp, starting university or doubts about dating.

Alerting signs may be excessive weight concern, a diet with repeatedly lowered weight goals, avoidance of foods considered "fattening," eating smaller and smaller portions, leaving meals to go to the bathroom, worries about imagined flabbiness, loss of hair, complaints of feeling cold,

expressions of self-loathing, wearing oversized clothes and withdrawal from social life.

By the time anorexics come to medical attention there are usually clear signs of starvation. A typical case might be a quiet, studious girl who continues a more and more restricted diet until she consumes a daily ration of one grapefruit, two slices of melba toast, a morsel of cheese and plain tea. The reduced food intake may create great distress among family and friends, who urge her to eat normally, but denial of sickness is typical. Anorexics may consider their bodies obese no matter how thin, failing to recognize that the emaciated body is neither beautiful nor healthy.

Family background may set the stage

Although no single home scenario predetermines anorexia nervosa, there are recognizable family dynamics and risk factors, particularly authoritarian rules, overprotection, an emphasis on appearance and scholastic grades rather than on other attributes, and "over-enmeshment"—where actions and achievements are valued in terms of the family, not the individual. Predisposing influences include parents who discourage independence and expect the child to subordinate her wishes to those of the family. These are generalizations and describe features found in many families of anorexics. Living with someone who has AN is very difficult for all parents and loved ones as there is no "secret pathway" that avoids, prevents or cures AN. It may help if parents take stock of their parenting styles and see whether they are too controlling or are adequately helping their teenager grow up by clearing the way to independence while setting limits, but at the same time making sure they show enough love, approval and affection.. Coping with a child who has an eating disorder can be very challenging. Many parents find it helpful to talk with other parents who are, or have, gone through the experience of dealing with an eating disorder, or discussing it with a knowledgeable health professional.

A stifling, overprotective attitude may retard the development of a child's identity in families that try at all costs to keep up appearances, never allowing any argument or disagreement to surface. One expert describes

USUAL EFFECTS SEEN IN STARVING PEOPLE (PRESENT BUT NOT UNIQUE TO ANOREXIA)

- **Sleep disturbances—insomnia, restlessness;**
- **hair loss (on head) but growth of downy hair (lanugo) on body;**
- **dry skin, brittle nails;**
- **cold extremities—bluish hands and feet;**
- **altered cardiovascular function—lowered or irregular heartbeat;**
- **potassium depletion (which can cause cardiac arrest);**
- **bloating—even if fasting;**
- **unabated ravenous sensation on eating;**
- **mood swings: irritability, poor concentration, apathy;**
- **nail-biting and gum-chewing (food substitutes).**

a typical anorexic's family as "too involved with each other—unwittingly preventing the teenager from gaining independence or coping skills." When all activities are dictated by the parents' concept of what is right, the child grows up with a deficient sense of self and poor decision-making skills. Some have deep fears of maturity and the responsibilities of growing up—sometimes labeled "phobic avoidance" of the demands of adolescence. By bringing back an immature, unthreatening body contour and stopping menstruation, weight loss delays the need to face adult womanhood.

Treatment of anorexia nervosa

Although food avoidance is the overt feature of anorexia nervosa, any other underlying psychiatric problems or mental illnesses—such as depression, anxiety and obsessive-compulsive disorders—must also be assessed and tackled.

Support and guidance can come from a trusted friend, relative, co-worker teacher or counselor. In helping anorexics it is crucial to maintain a nonjudgmental attitude, to listen without trying to exert control and to guide them to professional therapy. Therapy may take the form of individual or group sessions, sometimes best in a hospital setting—on an outpatient or inpatient basis—and may involve medication as well as psychotherapy. Hospital admission is mandatory for some anorexics, because of severe starvation and accompanying health hazards. Bed rest and a reasonable goal for weight-gain reinforce the idea of anorexia as an illness that needs nursing, and close monitoring of mealtimes. Antidepressants may be tried, as well as zinc supplements—said to help some cases but still under debate.

Since anorexia is such a complex problem, recovery too is complex and may take several years. About 30 to 50 percent of anorexics recover fully within a few years, either spontaneously (on their own) or with correct therapy. Those in whom the eating disorder continues untreated face complications such as osteoporosis, metabolic disorders, cardiovascular and other illnesses. The outlook is best if treatment starts before weight loss is too extreme and if the family dynamics are not too distorted.

The top priority is to reverse the weight loss,

mitigate any damages of starvation, and support a desperately unhappy, ill person. For successful treatment, a good psychiatric assessment is essential, with cognitive and behavioral therapy. Hospitalization and controlled refeeding are also essential for children who are critically ill with anorexia. Most individuals whose weight is 75 percent or less of expected body weight require medical attention and treatment. The major therapeutic modality for long-term management is cognitive-behavioral psychotherapy that tries to replace negative thinking styles with a more reality-based and positive approach to improve everyday coping skills. A recent randomized trial found that both behavioral family system therapy and ego-oriented individual therapy (plus collateral sessions with the parents) were effective, but that more rapid improvement occurred with the behavioral family therapy. Most treatments also include re-educating the family, to improve relationships and to correct the anorexic's eating habits, with clear information about the hazards of starvation, including its effects on thinking and behavior. In the past, some experts recommended that the topic of eating be avoided, focusing on psychological factors. Today this is not considered useful; issues of weight and food must be addressed. The goal is not control of the anorexic, but relief of suffering and cognitive therapy to reverse the individual's poor self-image.

The family is advised to participate in therapy—especially if the anorexic is still living at home—even though many resist involvement, regarding the illness as the "child's problem" or denying it to save face. Some blame the adolescent for not eating, saying, "If only she'd eat properly we'd all be happy again." The physician's insistence on family involvement may arouse strong parental feelings of guilt or recrimination that must be faced for treatment to succeed. Some parents of anorexics ignore their offspring's plight, feel ashamed or won't devote time to their ailing teenager, preferring to leave treatment to medical experts—an attitude not likely to help the anorexic, as the problem is aggravated by the family dynamics. The family members must be taught to see themselves as helpers, not "scapegoats," and as an integral part of the treatment plan.

The most basic elements in refeeding

anorexics are getting them to trust the medical caregivers and to stick to a meal plan with enough calories. Clinicians try to establish an empathetic relationship by discussing the anorexic's feelings, going beyond weight gain to deeper worries. Anorexics generally respond well to frank information about the cultural, familial and biological roots of their condition and how their behavior arose. Sufferers often express amazement at their misconceptions about nutrition and family influences.

Bulimia nervosa

Once considered just a subclass of anorexia nervosa, bulimia nervosa is now recognized as a bingeing disorder in its own right, occurring mainly in females aged 16 to 25, especially prevalent among high school and college students. Bulimia nervosa afflicts an estimated 2 to 4 percent of Canadian females aged 12 to 25 (and some adolescent males). Like anorexia nervosa, it too involves extreme weight-preoccupation and fears of losing control, but alternate bouts of bingeing and fasting, vomiting and purging are its distinguishing hallmarks. A "binge" may be one cupcake or an entire apple pie, depending on personal perceptions. Predisposing factors include a family history of alcoholism and depression.

There's been a dramatic upsurge in the number of cases of bulimia in recent years, and again, this is blamed on society's worship of thinness in the face of increasing average body weights for women. Adolescent anorexics may later become bulimics. Sadly, many remain eating-disordered and dissatisfied with themselves for life. Bulimics share the anorexic's fear of losing control, are similarly obsessed with weight loss, and also have a high incidence of depression and other psychiatric disorders. Like those with anorexia, bulimics embark upon restricted diets but can't stick to them, and engage in cycles of restricted eating, bingeing and self-inflicted vomiting and purging—with excessive use of laxatives, diuretics and perhaps ipecac syrup (to induce vomiting). When their dietary restraint breaks down, bulimics binge on vast amounts of food—cakes, desserts, hot dogs, whatever—then vomit it all up to avoid weight-gain. Since hunger returns after vomiting, bulimics are constantly tempted to binge again, and face dangerous medical consequences. The binge-and-purge pattern allows many bulimics to keep a normal or slightly below normal weight so that their disordered eating may remain hidden from all but close family members. Bulimia, however, can occur with any body weight. Bulimic individuals are more likely than nonbulimic women and children to have had mothers who were obese during their childhood, to have been exposed to family members who were dieting, and to have experienced negative remarks about their eating habits, appearance, size or weight.

Bulimics often use laxatives in vast quantities, on the false premise that they reduce calorie absorption, when in fact they only cause dehydration. The purging doesn't rid the body of unwanted calories, as laxatives work on the large intestine after the calories have been absorbed (higher up, in the small intestine). Self-imposed vomiting, which may take hours per session, gets rid of only a few calories and is extremely hard on the digestive system, throat and heart. Diuretics or water pills rid the body of some water as well as valuable minerals. Loss of potassium can seriously disturb the heart rhythm.

The diagnostic criteria for bulimia nervosa are: persistent over-concern about body weight, a morbid fear of being fat, recurrent episodes of binge eating (rapid consumption of vast amounts of food in a short period)—averaging at least two binge-and-purge sessions per week for 3 or more months—and behavior that aims to offset the overeating, such as regular self-induced vomiting, overuse of laxatives and diuretics, together with feelings of shame and "loss of control." Alerting signs may be a chipmunk-like face—with swollen cheeks (from enlarged parotid or salivary glands)—and dental problems from teeth enamel eroded by the acidity of frequent vomiting. Many bulimics seek medical advice because of constipation, fatigue, rectal bleeding and Russel's sign—callused hands, rubbed by being stuck down the throat to induce vomiting. Laxative abuse may produce alternating diarrhea and constipation or rebound water retention. Diuretics, used to eliminate body water compound the health risks. Other complications of bulimia nervosa include stomach bleeds, kidney disorders and electrolyte imbalance—possibly producing serious, sometimes fatal, heartbeat irregularities.

Bulimics may need hospitalization, but less often than anorexics. Treatment means understanding and accepting the diagnosis, and offering cognitive and behavioral therapy—to modify the disturbed body-image, overcome feelings of shame, perhaps to deal with previous sexual abuse and improve social and family interaction. Group therapy may be particularly successful. Antidepressants (such as imipramine, fluoxetine and others) may also help to reduce binge eating or stabilize a depressed mood. Recovery takes a variable time and relapse rates average 30 to 40 percent.

TIPS FOR BUILDING SELF-ESTEEM AND IMPROVING BODY IMAGE

For the person with low self-esteem:

• Think about how you treat your body and the way it works for you—by carrying you around, bending and stretching, housing your thoughts—and focus on parts you like or consider okay. Enjoy being in your own body.

• List the things you do well and the things you like about yourself—ask friends and school or workmates what they appreciate most about you.

• Ask whether you are good to yourself and your body or always depriving it. Reward yourself for things well done—a drawing, helping a friend, writing an essay. Give yourself non-food

treats, whether taking a bubble bath, going to a movie or renting a favorite video.

• Find ways to express painful feelings or memories—write them down, draw or paint them, share the feelings with a friend or even with a pet.

For family and friends:

• Avoid making comments about weight or looks—they'll only perpetuate the obsession with body image and weight.

• Do not try to tempt with or engage in a power struggle around food—those with eating disorders have deep psychological reasons for the behavior and need to be in control of their eating.

• Be available to give support, advice and to listen, to provide information and suggest treatment choices for the anorexic, while leaving the decision to her.

• If close to or trying to help someone with disordered eating, examine *your own* attitudes to dieting, size and appearance so that you don't convey any prejudices or exacerbate the weight preoccupation. Don't unwittingly reinforce or pass on society's harmful idolization of thinness.

For more information, contact the National Eating Disorders Information Centre: (416) 340-4156.

PSYCHOSOCIAL DEVELOPMENT IN ADOLESCENCE

The teenager's world, filled with new experiences and the acquisition of new skills, may produce a jumble of emotions, which many find hard to articulate. What seems important to the adolescent may seem trivial to the adult. Parents may deplore the adolescent's erratic schedule or tendency to daydream, not realizing that these are normal aspects of development.

Adolescence also provides a "window" or an interval of time when psychological difficulties or struggles of early childhood—for example, separation anxiety, desolation over a divorce, fears of going to daycare, sibling rivalries—may be reworked, sometimes with "acting out" behavior and rebellious conduct. Parents who are perturbed by what seem to be exaggeratedly emotional or hostile attitudes might note that the teenager is likely working through deep-rooted psychological problems from earlier years. They may be encouraged to bear in mind that it's only a transient stage in growing up.

In the teenage years, the values and mores of peers begin to supersede those of parents. Suddenly the parents—who previously seemed all-knowing—are revealed as ordinary people with normal human flaws, which sometimes come as a revelation to adolescents. In developing independence and their own opinions, teens may discover a gulf between their views and those of their parents, which can engender conflicts. It takes a deft parental touch to set limits that permit teenagers the freedom and exploration needed to foster self-esteem, while protecting them from danger. Adolescents need rules and guidance, though they may stridently oppose them.

HELPING ADOLESCENTS THROUGH THE TRANSITION

Parents, confronted by their children's emergent, sometimes flamboyant, independence, also face major adjustments as their offspring pass through puberty. Some parents find it hard to accept teens as sexual persons and shun casual or dinner-time chats on the subject, perhaps limiting discussion of sex to occasional advice about birth control and sexually transmitted diseases. Mother–daughter discussions about sex are far more frequent and wide-ranging than mother–son discussions. Few boys receive (or seek) sex education from parents. Fathers often don't fill the communication gap. Yet parents can help adolescents formulate their ideas by using TV shows, news headlines or magazine articles as an opening to discuss sex, relationships, violence and other issues.

Some parents become reticent about physically showing affection to adolescents, just when these young people need reassurance about still being wanted. Parents who frequently cuddled their children when young may be uncomfortable about hugging a teenager or fathers and sons may avoid physical contact because it seems "unmanly." Sometimes barriers to parent–child affection are raised by adolescents themselves because of stories heard about sex abuse or molestation by family members. Yet adolescent boys and girls need reassurance more than ever. Although they may appear offhand and independent, most teens desperately need positive feedback. If physical affection is withdrawn, this may be taken as rejection and breed resentment and feelings of no longer being desirable.

It's salutary to remember that most teenagers have deep concerns about their self-worth and sometimes feel uncomfortable with themselves. They may have ambivalent feelings about the roles of family and friendship, about school performance, employment possibilities, their future. Such feelings of inadequacy are compounded if parents unconsciously reinforce

THE CHIEF DEVELOPMENTAL TASKS OF ADOLESCENCE

- **Developing an identity distinct from that within the family;**
- **overcoming worry about body changes and physical appearance; accepting a new body image and forging fresh self-esteem to match it;**
- **forming intimate relationships with same-sex and opposite-sex peers outside the home;**
- **understanding and gaining control over sexual urges;**
- **developing an adult role that fits (or**

doesn't) **the sex-specific behavior patterns expected by society;**
- **gaining a sense of "self," believing in personal opinions, knowing who one is;**
- **perfecting a personal value system and vocational ambitions—developing a world view—and sorting out which values will form a guiding principle for one's life and behavior;**
- **creating a perspective of the**

future—**setting goals that seem worthwhile, realistic and attainable;**
- **making study/employment decisions: deciding what one wants to accomplish or must learn;**
- **developing marriage thoughts or plans: ideas of what one's partner might be like;**
- **assuming responsibility for personal decisions and actions—learning to run one's own life.**

a teenager's self-doubts by avoiding the closeness of physical touch. Withholding expressions of affection can impede intimacy and create relationship problems later in life.

One 16-year-old girl beset by self-doubts described how her mother stopped stroking or kissing her once she entered puberty, making her feel totally rejected. The feeling was luckily offset by her aunt, who boosted her self-esteem and—sometimes to the girl's embarrassment—continued to hug her repeatedly telling her how attractive, creative and intelligent she was.

As adolescents strive to consolidate personal values it's worth remembering the hurdles they face, especially when one is exasperated by

COMPARING PARENTAL AND ADOLESCENT CONCERNS

Typical concerns of parents include:
- **rebellion—common in early and middle adolescence (severe rebellion needs professional attention);**
- **daydreaming—a normal part of adolescent development;**
- **excessive risk-taking— best handled by family discussions, limit-set-**

ting, evaluation of unmet adolescent needs or wishes;
- **rudeness and hostility;**
- **reluctance to adhere to the limits set;**
- **violent mood swings—which require assessment to check for depression, bipolar disorder (manic-depression)**

or other psychiatric disorders;
- **school problems— which call for evaluation of type and frequency;**
- **sexual interests— possibly intercourse, risks of pregnancy and STDs (especially AIDS). Sexuality needs frank discussion and information**

about birth control and STD avoidance.

Typical teenager concerns include:
- **family conflicts, limits, arguments over curfew, friends, privacy;**
- **peer relationships, dating;**
- **school—academic record, popularity,**

teachers, changing schools;
- **identity: who am I? body image, shyness, loneliness;**
- **medical/health worries—am I normal? too short? too fat? acne; psychosomatic problems (such as headaches, stomach aches, insomnia);**
- **mild depression.**

COMPARING ADOLESCENT AND PARENTAL DEVELOPMENT TASKS

Adolescent task	Parental task
Accept physical changes of puberty	• Accept that adolescent is no longer a child, and treat as an emerging adult; • recognize that behavior and mood are affected by hormonal changes of puberty.
Develop new self-image.	• Be content with less intimacy: • allow privacy but maintain enough contact to affirm love and concern.
Build independence from family	• Determine what behavior is desirable or unacceptable (set clear rules); • determine, communicate and negotiate limits (boundaries), and penalties for exceeding them or transgressing agreed limits; • adapt to changing needs of adolescent; • teach adolescent how to make decisions by role-modeling.
Develop stable role identity	• Encourage self-esteem-enhancing activities to boost adolescent's sense of self-worth; • recognize parental influence in identity problems; • maintain long-term view of process rather than arguing over minor infringements.
Develop adult thinking skills.	• Differentiate between egocentrism, self-evolution and selfishness; • recognize adolescence as a transitional and developmental stage.

their untidiness, erratic mealtimes or other provocations. The best bet for parents is to keep open the lines of communication, make sure that their teenager stays in touch, avoid a judgmental attitude and see that the teenager still feels wanted and valued.

By the same token, parents have a right to expect a modicum of responsibility and should negotiate "fines" or removal of privileges if the agreed rules are transgressed or duties left undone. Teenagers still need firm guidelines and empathy even though their behavior may be annoying. It may help to remember that other parents probably face similarly erratic behavior. However hard it may be to accept, detachment from parents and family is an inevitable part of growing up. Adolescents must be encouraged to develop their own opinions, values and friends. It happens in each generation!

MEDICAL CHECKUPS FOR ADOLESCENTS

Teenagers should be medically assessed in early and middle adolescence. Physicians generally prefer to see the adolescent alone, chat informally, listen to concerns and treat comments seriously. They try to build confidence, establish rapport and ideally act as the teenager's advocate. Establishing rapport can be challenging as many adolescents are uncomfortable with authority and find the medical system too rigid and authoritarian, mistrusting physicians.

The doctor takes a full medical and psychosocial history, asks about home, family relationships, friends, hobbies, drug and alcohol use, dating and sexual activity. The medical evaluation will also screen for psychological/mental health and assess risk behaviors, giving physicians a chance to spot adolescent anxieties about physical maturation, allowing discussion of breast and penis size, acne, skin and hair care, exercise and diet. It also offers an excellent opportunity to check on school pressures and discuss family conflicts, social isolation, loneliness, and anxiety or depression. Physicians may counsel on accident prevention and are often the first to spot substance abuse. Physicians often assume that the young person is sexually active or using drugs, or at least contemplating these activities, and counsel accordingly to be on the safe side.

A skilled physician listens for any "hidden agenda" that may reveal inner worries. For instance, a teenager who visits a physician about stomach pains or a headache may really be worried about family conflicts or becoming pregnant. Open-ended questions—for example, "Tell me more about it"—often bring out the adolescent's true concerns. Providing the youngsters with the doctor's telephone number allows them to go for advice on their own if they wish.

The checkup generally includes measurements of height, weight, blood pressure and pulse rate; and evaluation of vision, hearing, teeth and gums, neck (thyroid), abdomen and pelvis, as well as immunization status—with booster shots being given if needed. Since myopia (shortsightedness) tends to worsen in puberty, this may be the time to suggest glasses or contact lenses (usually soft, replaceable types that need minimal cleaning and care). Pubertal progress is evaluated by examining the external genitals—testes and pubic hair in boys, breast development, pubic hair and menstrual regularity in girls.

The physician will likely inquire about sexual activity, knowledge of STDs and how to prevent them. It is a good opportunity to provide counseling on birth control and to instruct teenagers in contraceptive choices and their correct use. Nutritional status is assessed, with discussion of diet, weight-maintenance and any eating disorders possibly present. Some teenagers may feel awkward and worry about confidentiality if discussing worries with a doctor who has seen them through childhood and who may also look after the rest of the family. Sensing this, a physician may recommend a colleague. Finally, a physician might try to get a sense of the "burden" that a clinical problem places on the adolescent. For example, a mild case of acne may seem like a minor health concern to older individuals but can be devastating for teenagers.

SCHOOL PROBLEMS

Scholastic problems frequently appear in adolescence, partly because of the many competing demands, hormonal changes and new friendships. School grades may fall short of parental expectations, and the expressed "disappointment" can engender a sense of failure, perhaps depression—even if the teenager is really doing fine. Academic failure, particularly in high-achieving families, is a recognized factor in teen suicides. Parents should avoid creating needless stress at this sensitive age and remember that an academic shortfall is often made up later on. It may help if concerned adults outside the family give teens a chance to air their anxieties. If concerned, contact the teacher school principal, guidance counselor or the physical education staff.

ADOLESCENT SEXUALITY

Making the decision to have or not have sexual intercourse is serious business for teenagers. And the fact that adolescents now attain reproductive capacity at an earlier age has widened the gap between physical maturity and economic independence. Caught between peer and parental values and media images of sexuality, adolescents often have hazy notions of realistic sexual relationships. Current North American culture gives young people conflicting messages about sex, sometimes showing it as a "sign of maturity," and other times disapproving of teenage sexuality. Parents may say one thing, friends or favorite TV programs the opposite. On the one hand, young people are told to

TIPS ON COMMUNICATING BETTER WITH TEENS

- **Listen attentively.**
- **Be sensitive to teenage feelings and a "hidden agenda" of worries.**
- **Treat problems seriously, do not scoff at or minimize them.**
- **Avoid power struggles.**
- **Show interest and concern, but express trust.**
- **Acknowledge the adolescent's maturity by offering choices and exploring them.**
- **Be open and honest—adolescents quickly pick up on deceit.**
- **Use an interactive rather than an interrogative style, progress from neutral to more sensitive topics and try a third-person, objective approach to delicate subjects.**
- **Maintain nonjudgmental frankness.**
- **Assure confidentiality. Be mindful that intimate teen disclosures are delicate matters. Having promised confidentiality, stick to it!**
- **Use and explain the proper terms, avoiding slang. "Do you know exactly what's meant by sexual intercourse?" "Do you know what STDs are and what they can lead to?" "Do you know why it's dangerous to drink and drive and what to do about it?"**
- **Don't lecture, moralize or be self-righteous: instead try to stand back and gently help in the decision-making.**
- **Be firm and don't condone risky behavior.**
- **Avoid barriers to communication such as:**
  - comparison with other teens;
  - minimizing a problem;
  - excessive talking;
  - "taking over" an adolescent's problem;
  - using phrases such as, "The trouble with you is...," "How could you do this to me?", "In my day...," "Is that all?", "You're all wrong...," "How can you think like that?", "That's a dumb thing to say," "I'm busy right now..."
- **Make resources, advice and expert help easily available.**
- **Let the adolescent know that if he or she indicates an intention to pursue illegal activities, you may need to inform the authorities.**

FOR HEALTHIER, SAFER SEX, ADOLESCENTS MUST:

- clearly understand male and female reproductive roles and functions;
- be well informed about sexuality and intercourse, its pleasures, risks and health consequences;
- feel proud and comfortable about their bodies;
- have a strong sense of self;

- be aware of sexual feelings;
- realize that sexuality is natural and normal;
- be able to share and discuss sexual wishes or aversions;
- know about birth control and how to avoid unwanted pregnancy;
- know about the different sexually trans-

mitted diseases, how they're contracted, what the signs and effects are and what to do about them;
- know where to get information, advice and help (e.g., from family physicians, school nurses, guidance counselors, planned parenthood organizations or STD clinics).

refrain, and on the other they are bombarded by TV shows that implicitly encourage them to be sexually active. Adolescents are understandably confused about what's right or wrong, and some claim to be formidably pressured to have sex before they feel ready for it.

Since many high school students spend a lot of time glued to the TV, it should come as no surprise that many get much of their sex education from what sociologists call "alternative sources." In one year of prime-time TV viewing, a typical teen will see an estimated 20,000 scenes of sexual behavior or innuendo. But what the media show about sexuality is often exploitive, with too little emphasis on tenderness and responsibility, too much on violence.

Sexual violence is a distinct risk among young people. One study found that more than 10 percent of students had been involved in one or more abusive relationship, beginning around age 15. Acquaintance-assault is common. Because of their immaturity, vulnerable teenagers may feel compelled to act as though they can handle any situation. Their inexperience in sexual situations makes them easy victims, and they may minimize or even deny an assault, blaming themselves or fearing that no one will believe them.

Many young females allegedly also feel "put down" by males and may put up with exploitive, even violent, behavior in the belief that they somehow provoked the undesirable action, whether date rape or other abusive behavior.

In one survey, over 90 percent of teenagers cited TV shows that pressured them toward early sex. Four out of 5 teens mentioned at least one popular TV program that portrays casual sex, depicting it as "power not love." A 1986 poll conducted for the U.S. Parenthood Federation ranked peer pressure first as the incentive to have sex, curiosity second, the idea that "everyone does it" third, sexually excited boys pressuring girls fourth, and the wish for sexual gratification last.

Although sexual activity is rare in Canada before age 13, statistics show that, by Grade 11, 41 percent of girls and 49 percent of boys have had intercourse at least once. By the time they leave high school, over half have tried intercourse. However, despite the prevailing myth that "everyone does it," these statistics reveal that only *half* of all Canadians actually have had sex before ages 18 to 20. Surveys also reveal that the first sexual encounter(s) in adolescents are unexpected and frequently unprotected by birth control or measures to reduce risks of sexually transmitted infections. Adolescents frequently act on impulse, and are completely unprepared at first intercourse—despite the seeming plethora of information and the push for safer sex.

Studies show that 1 in 3 Canadian teenagers currently uses no birth control at the first sexual encounter. The teenage sense of immortality may make them disregard the risks. Some teens say they consider condoms unaesthetic or too open an admission of the intention to "do it." They thus start their sex lives in a manner that's quite likely to give them a sexually transmitted infection (including AIDS) and/or an unwanted pregnancy. Many teenagers commonly wait over a year after first intercourse before receiving reliable contraceptives or infection-prevention advice. Main reasons given for the delay are fear that parents will find out, aversion to a pelvic exam and mistaken beliefs about the side effects of contraception.

Adolescents need much guidance in coping with sexuality and strong support for the decision to postpone sexual involvement until they feel ready for it. They need reinforcement in believing that their body is their own private possession and that no one—including relatives and friends—has the right to touch it sexually if not wanted. Saying no to sex is every person's option, no matter who they are or what someone else says, and teenagers need to know that it's perfectly normal to do so.

Sex education is still far too scanty

Parents and educators need to candidly discuss sexuality well before youngsters reach adolescence, with explicit information on both pregnancy avoidance and prevention of sexually transmitted infections. Adolescents should recognize the similarities and differences between male and female roles, how values affect decisions, the importance of self-confidence in one's own choice, the need to respect the choices of others and that prompt treatment of an STD can prevent serious health impairment. And they need to know how to say no to sex and feel comfortable with the decision.

Yet many teenagers don't know where to get precise advice on sexuality and ways to avoid unwanted pregnancy or protect themselves against STDs. School sex-education courses tend to be short and factual, emphasizing reproductive function rather than sexual choices, emotions or decision-making skills. While many parents relegate sex education to health professionals and educators, studies suggest that that is hardly enough. And parents don't fill the gap. Surveys show that high school students would like to receive sex-related information from parents but perceive parental knowledge as "inadequate." Numerous studies report that two-thirds or more of adolescents can't communicate with their parents about sex, and many parents wrongly assume that their children don't wish to, even though in fact they'd like to talk to parents about it.

Contrary to popular opinion, sex education is not part of everyday schooling. According to one Planned Parenthood Association, while Canadian national guidelines for sex education are underway, at present education given in schools is haphazard and hampered by controversy and lack of trained leadership. "In fact," states one counselor, "between Grades 8 and 13, most teens may encounter one non-mandatory unit on sexuality in one required physical health and safety course (if they are not off

---

TEENS CARELESS ABOUT CONTRACEPTION: TEENAGE PREGNANCIES ON THE RISE

Canada's teen pregnancy rate rose alarmingly in the late 1990s to 49 per 1,000 women aged 14 to 19—levels not seen since the 1970s, (with over 20,000 teen abortions in 1996). Although still only half that of the U.S., the high rate of teen pregnancy shows that Canadian sex education isn't working, and it poses a huge burden in healthcare costs (as babies of teen mothers are often sickly) and lost years of education and employment for the young mothers.

The only way to reach teens better is to provide open and explicit sex and contraceptive information, and for physicians to be easily accessible to young people, give them clear (non-judgmental) advice, assuring them of complete confidentiality. Only about 20 percent of sexually active teens use any birth control (usually condoms or the Pill), but they use it inconsistently and often wrongly. For example, many women forget to take the contraceptive

pills regularly, may "share them with friends," or think they "go on working" even if some are missed. The newly approved Depo-Provera (3-monthly progesterone) injections are becoming popular. And physicians remind teens that the "morning-after Pill"—which stops pregnancy if taken within 24 to 48 hours of intercourse—is freely available on request from hospital emergency departments and physicians.

---

doing an alternative project or team practice or skipping class). Sexual health is just not a number-one priority for harassed educators."

In talking to teenagers about sexuality it's wise to be matter-of-fact and nonjudgmental, steering away from joking about a matter they take very seriously. Parents can admit to embarrassment or discomfort (if that's the case)—teenagers respect honesty. It's essential to honor the adolescent's privacy and not to pry about things they don't want to talk about. And it's useful to provide detailed, practical, up-to-date pamphlets, books and other materials answering questions about sex, and to suggest easily accessible, neutral sources for reliable advice—such as family-planning units, STD clinics, pediatricians, family doctors and local health units.

Physicians can play a major role in helping to prevent unwanted adolescent pregnancy and STDs by encouraging questions, giving explicit information and making it clear that adolescents are responsible for their own sexual health but that adults can and will arm them with knowledge. Although teens ultimately decide for themselves when, how and with whom to have sex, it may help to suggest that they talk to each other about the use of condoms and other safer ways to have sex.

Adolescents need to know that they are not alone in having to practise safer sex in the age of AIDS. Although not a long-term option for most young people, abstinence from intercourse is increasingly considered an acceptable choice. (And it's still all right to say no even if you're not a virgin.) "Calls for abstinence are probably less effective," says one University of Toronto pediatrician, "than suggesting postponement of sexual intercourse until ready." Abstinence can be defined as refraining from intercourse rather than restraint from all sexual activity. Teenagers can be encouraged to choose nonpenetrative yet pleasurable intimacy (or "outercourse") rather than intercourse—in short, "everything but." Kissing and mutual massage are safer, noninsertive ways to enjoy sexual contact, provided there is no exchange of body fluids. Giving valid scientific reasons can strengthen the argument: the sexual health of teenage girls is enhanced by postponing intercourse because the immature cervix is easily invaded by the human papilloma virus, chlamydia, gonorrhea and other infective organisms.

RISK-TAKING BEHAVIOR

Embarking on the road to emancipation and self-determination, adolescents may participate in potentially destructive activities. Experimenting with a vast variety of new experiences, many take inordinate risks—sometimes unaware of or stridently denying the possible consequences.

Parents may be dumbfounded by the adolescent's urge to practise dangerous behavior often with an air of invincibility that belies the uncertainty beneath. The gap between the teenager's abilities and the adult view of them frequently leads to arguments. The failure of adults to appreciate and encourage developing teenage capacities can increase reliance upon peer groups, which may encourage further risk-taking, where teenagers participate for the badge of "belonging."

Risk behaviors are usually exacerbated by alcohol or drug use and early sexual activity. Although most adolescents don't lie when questioned about their actions, they are unlikely to volunteer such information. Often, knowledge of friends and a glance around the teenager's room—which typically contains the adolescent's entire worldly belongings—may reveal risk-taking tendencies. Discarded games and stuffed animals are jumbled together with objects portraying new interests—posters, books, audio, video and computer equipment. Parents may be alerted to sexual activity or drug use by the discovery of injection and other paraphernalia left lying around, or by the types of books and magazines.

Runaway behavior

Defined as "unauthorized absence from home," the behavior is tried by many adolescents, typically those aged 15 to 17, mostly from white, suburban families. The average stay away from home is less than 3 days (72 percent of runaways), with about 15 percent staying away up to 2 weeks and only 13 percent leaving home for longer. The return home is a personal decision in over half the adolescent runaways, and prompted by parental or peer influence in the rest. About 6 percent never return home.

Reasons given for running away range from school failure or lack of communication with parents to revenge for some disciplinary action or peer imitation. Family rows may trigger the action. It's often a declaration that things at home have become unbearable due to excessive "tightening of the reins"—or a statement of autonomy perhaps because of a lack of trust, or the family's refusal to grant independence. One out of 4 runaways is labeled a "throwaway"— forced to go or excluded from the family rather than running by choice. In some parts of the United States, an estimated 1 in 8 teenagers runs away at least once. Sometimes the adolescent's strengthening peer relationships and shifting loyalties lead the family either to try to bind closer ("enmesh") or to unwittingly "expel" the youngster. Family dynamics that may predispose adolescent runaways include emotional arguments, overly strict rules, lack of interest or adult alcohol and drug use.

Peers can play a strong role in runaway behavior. As one psychiatrist puts it, "Having a friend who's not liked or sanctioned by the parents might force a choice between family and friend. With disrupted family ties or frequent conflicts at home, the teen will likely opt for the disfavored friend or peer group (which promises acceptance and support)." But running away may endanger the teen, who gives up a caring, concerned environment for uncertain shelter and security. The result can be a disastrous chain reaction with reduced opportunities, inadequate nutrition, poor hygiene, lack of support, loss of the sense of "belonging" and increasing isolation. Separating from the family before they have forged a clear identity of their own puts runaway adolescents at high risk.

THE HEAVY TOLL OF ADOLESCENT SUICIDE

The intentional self-destruction of a life is an almost incomprehensible tragedy. Yet suicide is now a leading cause of death among Canadian males aged 15 to 24, the rate having tripled in the last 30 years, especially among teenagers. With about 3,500 completed suicides a year, Canada supposedly has one of the world's highest suicide rates, males greatly outnumbering females as suicide "completers," although females outnumber males as "attempters."

Statistics for 1990–91 show a suicide rate in Canada of 13 per 100,000, with 4 times more men than women completing the act but more women attempting it. For children under age 14, the suicide rate is very low, rising at ages 14 to 19 to 11 to 13 per 100,000 for males and 1 to 3 per 100,000 for females. (The rate is highest between ages 20 and 29.) Of those who try to kill themselves, 1 in 50 to 1 in 100 succeeds, and there are repeat tries in 6 to 16 percent of suicide attempters. Of methods used in Canada, firearms top the list for males, followed by suffocation (hanging, drowning), piercing with a sharp instrument and poisonings. In females, poisonings are the most frequent method, followed by hanging, jumping from heights and suffocation, only a few trying firearms.

Suicides are especially common among Aboriginal populations. Death by suicide among Canada's Aboriginal populations is almost 4 times higher than for the rest of Canada, half the suicides being in the 15-to-24 age range, often occurring in clusters. One suicide often sets the stage for more—perhaps by making it

appear to be "permissible" behavior. Contributing factors are the loss of traditional values, religion and culture, alcoholism, dysfunctional families, poor adult role models and media publicity about suicides.

Adolescence is an especially vulnerable period

Adolescence is a particular danger time for suicide, as it's a period of change and challenge. One U.S. study found that 10 to 20 percent of 15- to 19-year-olds had "some suicidal thoughts and intentions"; a French study of 13- to 16-year-olds living outside Paris found that 1 in 20 boys and 1 in 10 girls frequently "thought about suicide." In an Ontario survey, the prevalence of suicidal behavior or thoughts was 5 to 10 percent in boys, 10 to 20 percent among girls. A suicide attempt may be a call for help or may represent a final gesture of hopelessness. For the family, suicide imposes grief at the loss, rage at the act, a sense of waste and guilt for having failed as parents.

Factors commonly linked to suicide

Conditions thought to play a role in suicide include: unemployment, broken homes, low morale, social chaos and mental illness. Suicides are especially prevalent among the mentally disordered. Retrospective studies show that up to 80 to 90 percent of suicides had definable psychiatric problems, such as major depression (not just sadness), bipolar disorder (manic-depression), anxiety disorders or schizophrenia. Someone may also be predisposed to suicide if there's a family history of depres-

THOSE MOST AT RISK FOR COMMITTING SUICIDE

- **Aboriginal populations, such as Indians, Métis and the Inuit (with suicide rates 4 times that in the rest of Canada);**
- **the bereaved—those who have suffered the recent loss of a loved one;**
- **alcohol abusers— alcohol impairs**

judgment and may induce someone to "finish the job";
- **people from dysfunctional homes with a disrupted family life or hostile family relationships;**
- **persons with a history of previous suicide attempts;**
- **people with relatives**

who committed suicide;
- **isolated individuals, with no social support network (family, friends, church group);**
- **people with a major depressive episode;**
- **those who've experienced a recent relationship breakup.**

FACTORS AND EVENTS THAT MAY TRIGGER SUICIDE

- loss or death of a "significant" person;
- break-up of an intimate relationship with a friend, relative, girlfriend or boyfriend;
- alienation from family and friends;
- low self-esteem;
- feelings of failure;
- divorce or separation of parents;
- too few rules or guidelines within the family;
- overly high parental expectations;
- obsessive perfectionism and teenage

- anxiety about falling short of expectations (their own or those of parents or peers);
- reduced school performance—an inability to achieve or maintain a valued position in school or to get good grades;
- truancy, running away, theft;
- inability to cope with stress;
- disciplinary incidents at school or at home;
- a family history of major depression or alcoholism;
- family turmoil, quar-

- rels or disputes;
- physical or sexual abuse/assault;
- publicity about suicide in others—inducing a chain reaction (especially common in Native peoples);
- a chronic or debilitating physical illness;
- mental illnesses (e.g., anxiety disorders, schizophrenia, major depressive illness, manic-depression, obsessive-compulsive disorder);
- a previous suicide attempt.

sion or manic-depression. Substance abuse, especially of alcohol, may contribute by undermining personal functioning and social relationships and by encouraging impulsive, self-destructive acts.

Social factors also count. Isolated individuals without a network of supportive friends are at higher risk. Among adolescents, low self-esteem and anxiety arising from the changes they experience often lead to thoughts of self-destruction. Given their inexperience, young people may not realize that disappointments and setbacks are part of everyday life and can be overcome. Poor job prospects, marriage breakdown, moving house, family violence and sexual abuse are also known to fuel a sense of hopelessness and increase suicide risks. Besides stressful life events and emotional fluctuations, having the means of self-destruction—such as firearms or dangerous medications—close at hand increases suicide rates.

Repeated or sensationalized media stories of suicide have a greater impact in precipitating more suicides than a single report about the incident. Media publicity about suicide is often followed by a "rash" or cluster of teen suicides—maybe because this seems to condone the behavior, persuading vulnerable youngsters to mimic it. Schools and communities need to be aware of the dangers and implement preventive strategies.

Depression may play a role in suicide

Depression is more common during adolescence than hitherto recognized and a frequent reason for suicide attempts. Although its extent is unknown, most specialists believe that childhood depression can be as severe as in adults, but identifying it can be difficult. It may be hard to recognize the depth of despondency felt by some young people because their apparent "coolness" or air of invincibility hides the inner despair. Tragically, parents and other adults may overlook it because they expect adolescence to be a time of turmoil.

Depression in adolescents is still poorly understood and may vary from mood swings or short-lived episodes to chronic recurrent feelings of worthlessness, helplessness and hopelessness. Depressed adolescents often "act out" their despondency with out-of-control behavior and a rebellious attitude that hides the underlying dejection. The alerting signs of adolescent depression include withdrawal from the family, noncommunication, loss of interest or pleasure in usual activities and changes in sleep and eating patterns.

Treatment of adolescent depression is psychotherapy or antidepressant medications such as the selective serotonin reuptake inhibitors (SSRIs) or the newer serotonin-norepinephrine reuptake inhibitors (SNRIs). However, authorities such as the FDA have issued strong warnings about the need for extreme care in prescribing antidepressants to adolescents because these medications can sometimes increase suicide risks. (For example, the use of Paxil in the U.K. is contraindicated for adolescents.) Youngsters on antidepressant medications need careful surveillance and the medications must never be suddenly discontinued: use must always be tapered off slowly. Psychotherapy, in particular cognitive behavioural therapy (CBT), may help to relieve teenage depression by overcoming negative, self-denigrating thought patterns.

Warning signs or markers for suicide

Talk of suicide is often a plea for help and should never be taken lightly. Studies reveal that two-thirds of successful suicides had hinted at their intention before carrying it out. Yet parents often remain oblivious to their youngster's suicidal thoughts, far less aware of their dejected feelings than peers. Physicians, families and teachers should be on the alert for possible signs of suicidal intent—sadness, hopelessness, emptiness, lack of energy, loss of interest in friends, school or hobbies, irritability, conduct disorders (such as truancy), emotional disturbances and mood swings.

Some experts call suicide a "deficiency disease"—a lack of close friendships and social connections. There is a growing recognition that even children aged 5 to 6 can already harbor suicidal ideas. In many teens who attempt suicide, a vulnerability already present in childhood is exacerbated by the demands of adolescence and by family conflicts (if the parents fail to deal adequately with the teenager's developmental process). However, many suicide attempters (and completers) are not "social misfits," but ordinary, anxious teenagers. They may feel increasingly distanced from their family, friends and society, becoming outsiders or loners. The final triggering event may be a failed exam, loss of a boyfriend or girlfriend, pregnancy or a family quarrel. Family cohesion appears to be a protective influence.

Any expressed wish to end life must be taken seriously and never dismissed as an idle threat. Far from being impulsive or "spur-of-the-moment" actions, most suicides are carefully planned. It's crucial to be available to comfort the distressed person and get him or her into treatment promptly if possible. Be particularly suspicious when someone's previously gloomy mood suddenly changes to cheerfulness without sufficient reason. This is often a sign that the person has finally resolved to commit suicide and is relieved that the decision is made.

FACTORS IN AND SIGNS OF ADOLESCENT DEPRESSION

- decreased sense of self-worth; achievements falling short of aspirations;
- significant loss— death of a loved relative or boyfriend/girlfriend;
- separation or divorce of parents;
- loss of boundaries and guidelines within the family;
- inability to cope with developmental tasks of adolescence;
- parental substance abuse;
- family conflicts or poor communication;
- problems with peer relationships; real or imaginary rejection by peers, which can tip an insecure adolescent into depression;
- a perpetually sad or worried expression;
- loss of interest or pleasure in all previously enjoyed activities;
- refusal to go to school, participate in peer activities;
- poor concentration;
- low energy all day long, every day;
- declining schoolwork;
- glum outlook, bleak view of future and own relationship to it;
- excessive self-criticism;
- poor stress-coping skills—which may make the slightest challenge seem overwhelming;
- rapid mood swings, irritability, angry outbursts;
- "acting-out behavior"—truancy, running away, sexual promiscuity;
- substance abuse;
- a wish to be "left alone."

Physiological changes (psychosomatic clues):
- constant fatigue;
- "somatization"— unexplained physical complaints (e.g., abdominal pain, muscle aches);
- insomnia or excessive need for sleep;
- anorexia and weight loss, or significant weight gain or loss even if not dieting;
- menstrual irregularities;
- headaches.

POSSIBLE HINTS OF SUICIDAL INTENTION

- mention of death wishes, or "being a burden," which may remain unvoiced unless someone inquires;
- suicidal letters, quotes, poems, allusions;
- references to death or suicide, even in jest;
- sense of hopelessness;
- a bleak view of the future;
- aggressive or antisocial conduct;
- irritability, angry outbursts, hostility directed at self or others;
- "acting out"— conduct disorders, truancy, running away;
- boredom, loss of interest in usual activities;
- understated or vague allusions to suicide or of "being better off dead," possibly revealed in letters, diaries, notes or essays;
- excessive guilt and expressions of unworthiness;
- expressed fears of becoming insane, losing control, hurting others;
- giving away cherished possessions for no apparent reason;
- sending people unexplained "goodbye" notes;
- inappropriate preoccupation with making a will;
- a sudden tranquillity or cheery mood in the formerly depressed—indicating that death has been accepted as inevitable.

ASSESSMENT AND ACTION FOR SUICIDAL IDEATION (OBSERVED THOUGHTS OR IDEAS OF SUICIDE)

If:
Suicidal thoughts, expressions seem to be frequent and/or overwhelming,
   OR
The teenager seems to have a plan
   OR
The adolescent has no reliable support,
Emergency psychiatric referral is necessary.

If:
The thoughts are fleeting,
AND
There is no plan,
AND
There is reliable support and people to help care for the person,
Emergency psychiatric referral is not necessary, **but referral to a family doctor or mental health professional is warranted. Follow-up is essential to ensure that symptoms do not worsen.**

The easiest way to ferret out suicidal thoughts is to ask whether the teenager has ever thought of "ending it all" or that "things are unbearable," or "the world is a horrible place." Don't be afraid to raise questions for fear of putting ideas into the person's head. Teenagers may come right out and confess suicidal intent, and most will talk about other forms of distress, or leave obvious clues to their desperation. Allow adolescents to open up and speak about what's troubling them. Try questions such as:

• Have you ever felt that life is not worth living?
• Is the feeling urgent?
• How long has the feeling been there?
• Is it increasing in intensity?
• Have you formed any specific plans for killing yourself?

Although each suicide try is different, many adolescent cases have a pattern that falls into three stages. First, there's a deficiency of close social connections—few family ties, frequent quarrels and no intimate friendships, creating an underlying vulnerability. The background scenario may include alcoholic or abusive parents, unwanted step-parents, divorce or death of a cherished person, being abandoned by a friend. In the second or "escalation phase," insecurity is magnified because of family conflict, isolation and again, lack or loss of close friendships. The final event that caps the despair and precipitates the suicide may be the loss of a girlfriend or boyfriend, a broken relationship , an inability to surmount hurdles, fear of impending exams, a family quarrel, peer rejection, school failure or some other disappointment.

Access to firearms greatly increases suicide risks

Access to means of suicide, especially firearms, will endanger those at risk and can help them to succeed in killing themselves. Owners of firearms should weigh their reasons for keeping a gun at home against the possibility that it might some day be used for the suicide of their children. Attempts at suicide are a warning sign of future tries—the risk being higher with someone who attempted suicide in a remote site with little chance of discovery. For such instances, family and school should be especially vigilant and try to restrict means of self-destruction.

Suicide-proofing: preventive measures

The best preventive strategy is to promote the mental health and self-esteem of adolescents, to try and identify troubled youngsters at home or in school and to make counseling and mental-health care available to them via teen clinics and mental-healthcare providers. There's a crying need for more suicide-proofing. "Rather than taking a blunderbuss approach to all school-children," says one educationalist, "we must make efforts to screen for and identify vulnerable adolescents, specifically counseling those at risk. This means training parents and high school educators to identify mentally ill youngsters who are at particular risk, such as those suffering from depression, anxiety disorders, schizophrenia and other psychiatric problems."

It's also vital to curb excessive publicity about teen suicides. In order to forestall a copy-cat rash of suicides, the press might be persuaded to act responsibly and restrict themselves to single, rather than multiple and sensationalized, statements about suicide, preferably not putting them on the front page or at prime viewing time—and refraining from casting the suicide in a heroic or flattering light.

Schools and communities might have a preventive contingency plan in case of a suicide cluster rather than taking a "wait-and-see"

ARE YOUR KIDS ON ILLICIT SUBSTANCES?

Signs of excess alcohol/drug use in teenagers:
- suddenly become less affectionate, more irritable, secretive, hostile, depressed, apathetic, withdrawn, unable to sleep or sleeping too much;
- behave less responsibly, neglect chores, don't keep curfew, forget family birthdays or occasions, don't do homework, cut classes;
- drop old friends and adopt new ones, acquiring the habits and language of the new friends, lose interest in school and hobbies;
- become uncommunicative or aggressive, defensive when drugs are mentioned, and voice approval of or concern for friends who use drugs;
- complain of parents "hassling" or "trampling their rights";
- disordered thinking, memory lapses, difficulty with concentration; increased or decreased appetite, heightened sensitivity to taste, touch or smell.

Tips for dealing with drug-taking adolescents:
- Don't jump to unwarranted conclusions.
- Respect the adolescent's privacy—searching through belongings will only erode mutual trust and respect.
- Talk with another trusted adult to put things into proper perspective before going to the adolescent.
- When you confront your son or daughter, don't assume he or she is immature, or a drug addict. The first time you discuss drugs (or alcohol) is very important—how parents react can put an end to the whole matter, or make it worse and drive it underground.
- Handle the problem objectively; face the reality of drug use.
- Avoid moralizing, saying things like, "How could you do this?" or, "Think of your dismal future."
- Dwell on the person's positive attributes and avoid showing resentment.
- Be honest, empathetic, firm, even-tempered and avoid personal attacks on the adolescent's character.
- Express concern about health; explain that you feel worried, hurt.
- Try to stay calm. Reaffirm your continuing love while expressing disapproval of drug use.
- Say what action you intend to take, then follow through.
- If professional help is needed, don't be afraid to seek it.

approach. Families can help by showing concern, interest and empathy. There's often a tendency by parents and teachers to brush aside the possible danger of suicide, a reluctance to intervene or say anything in case of worsening the problem. Anyone who is worried about a youngster's suicidal intent should face the possibility and take or guide the adolescent to professional assistance.

Many people find parents' support groups invaluable. For example, Parents Against Drugs, an Ontario nonprofit organization, has several chapters across the province, operates a phone-in support line and holds regular seminars for parents, teenagers and teachers, helping kids to say no to drugs. The Centre for Addiction and Mental Health (CAMH) in Toronto and other units across the country can also furnish help and information.

If an adolescent talks or even hints of suicide or shows other warning signs, it's imperative to seek professional help at once so that the risks can be assessed and real intent separated from fleeting thoughts. A thorough examination by a child psychiatrist, psychologist or mental health team can determine if an adolescent is truly depressed and suicidal. Handling suicidal people deftly depends on familiarity with the person, a good psychiatric assessment and supportive therapy. People who admit that they have definite plans to commit suicide should *not* be left alone and, in many cases, are best admitted to a psychiatric unit. Follow-up of suicide attempts is essential—with counseling and attention to improving school and family relationships. Help for despondent teens is available via pediatricians, psychiatrists, school counselors and telephone hotlines. Make sure the numbers are posted and accessible.

Aboriginal or First Nations populations—among whom suicide rates are particularly high—are in special need of suicide-prevention strategies. Because of poverty, poor education and unemployment, many have a low sense of self-worth and try to escape via alcohol use and/or suicide tries. They need Aboriginal-run crisis centers, special training schemes and education in traditional practices that can promote self-esteem, enhance self-awareness and help redefine an individual's "purpose in life."

Suicide-prevention strategies might also include efforts to make lethal methods—such as firearms, poisonous gases and medications—less available by stricter gun laws, detoxification of car exhaust and restricted access to subway lines.

Boosting adolescent self-esteem is crucial

Boosting self-esteem is the key to preventing suicide. Every decision made by young people is influenced by the way they feel about themselves. To prevent suicide, we must promote self-confidence among adolescents so they can better avail themselves of openings and opportunities. Instead of the common tendency to dismiss youth as "callow," "superficial," "self-indulgent" or "lazy," we should value their abundant energy and creative potential, explore their thought styles and try to understand the current teen culture. We must do all we can to make youth feel respected—listening to their opinions and treating them as valued members of society. Young people can be encouraged to participate in the decision making at home, in school, at work and in the community. A positive step is to signal to teens that their innovative and questioning attitudes offer an invaluable counterpoint to adult perspectives.

Communities should provide recreational facilities and gathering places where young people can meet, enjoy and define themselves freely, without adults present. Many teenagers complain of a lack of privacy, no place to be on their own, away from the ever-watchful gaze of adults. Teenagers typically say they feel as though they're constantly under scrutiny, being observed, and not trusted or allowed to develop autonomy. We should tap young people's amazing energy, originality and enthusiasm to run their own peer counseling and support groups. Every positive action or contribution by adolescents should be recognized and praised by relatives, teachers, workmates and health professionals.

TEENAGE AND STUDENT SUBTANCE USE

Drug use increased rapidly among high school and college students during the 1960s when many experimented with alternative lifestyles. It peaked in the late 1970s and has declined dramatically since then. The good news is that among both Canadian and American students, drug use is less fashionable than in past decades, perhaps because of rising health concerns.

Experimenting with a various substances doesn't inevitably lead to addiction. Many young people sample drugs at school or college, for fun or to go along with their peer group, trying whatever is the "in" thing. Alcohol, tobacco and marijuana remain the most popular teen substances and, being an illicit substance, marijuana may act as a "gateway" to use of other illicit drugs. If drug use begins in adolescence, it's more likely to occur in adult life, although most young people who do drugs try them out of curiosity once or twice and then abandon them.

The teenagers most likely to try illicit substances are those with companions who can procure them. Those who do use drugs may use several. Adolescents who use drugs just to go along with the group are less likely to continue beyond their twenties than those who take them up for personal enjoyment or because of underlying psychological factors. Teenage use of alcohol is also a matter of concern. Having experimented with many illegal substances, young people today seem to prefer legal, easily obtainable alcohol.

If illicit drug use does continue, however, new associations and new companions may be woven into everyday life, making the pattern hard to break. The story of a young Montreal art student is typical. As a shy teenager low in self-esteem, she smoked marijuana at school to please her peers, gradually becoming a regular user. Later she tried heroin too, mainly to alleviate depression after her boyfriend left her. After that, she took marijuana daily and heroin several times a week, neglecting her studies. Her finances were depleted by her drug habit, which finally led her to a therapist for help. Explaining the powerful grip of heroin on her life, she told a therapy group that "at first I only took a little at weekend parties, but then I bought my own supplies, because even if my body didn't physically desire the drug, inside my head I was terrified I'd run out when I needed it. Now I haven't had 'smack' [heroin] or marijuana for over six weeks, and I think I'm going to kick it." (See also Chapter 2, the section on drug and alcohol use.)

Modern environmental health hazards

Allergies • Hay fever • Insect allergies • Food allergies • "Total allergy syndrome" • Tight-building syndrome • How safe is our drinking water? • Getting the lead out • Coping with temperature extremes • Staying fit on the job • Toward healthier global travel

13

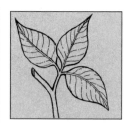

ENVIRONMENTAL pollution is an unavoidable by-product of modern industrialized society. Our consumer-driven culture provides us with a high standard of living but also exposes us to ever-increasing contaminants in the air we breathe, the water we drink, the food we eat and our workplaces. We know that certain substances (such as PCBs and dioxins) cause cancer that workplace chemicals (such as cereal dusts and soldering fumes) worsen asthma and that heavy metals (such as lead) can cause learning problems. While we can't protect ourselves from all environmental risks, being aware of them and minimizing our exposure to some of them can help us to reduce their health-harming effects. For example:

- Running the water in older homes (mostly those built before 1950) with lead pipes for 3 minutes each morning before drinking it can reduce risks of lead poisoning.
- Avoiding the midday sun and consistently using sunscreens can reduce skin-cancer risks.
- Breastfeeding an infant born to allergy-prone parents can delay the onset and possibly reduce the likelihood of allergic reactions (such as hay fever or asthma) in that child.
- Wearing protective clothing (long sleeves and long pants) and using insect repellents can

lessen the danger of insect bites and the disorders they spread—such as West Nile Virus (from mosquitoes) and Lyme disease (from ticks).
- Keeping the house dust-free can reduce asthmatic attacks in those sensitive to dust mites.
- Regularly cleaning air conditioners and humidifiers can minimize the risk of infections from the microorganisms they harbor.
- Not smoking in the home reduces risks of childhood respiratory illnesses.

ALLERGIES

Physicians have long wondered why some individuals develop serious symptoms, and a few even die, from innocuous agents that don't trouble most people. Allergies are non-contagious reactions: itching, sneezing, wheezing, swelling up, breaking out in hives, having difficulty breathing or occasionally collapsing. People prone to allergies are said to be hypersensitive or *atopic*—meaning "strange or unusual"—having abnormal responses to certain triggers.

An estimated 15 to 20 percent of North Americans have allergies, and they tend to run in families. A child with one allergic parent has a 1 in 4 chance of developing allergies. If both parents are allergy-prone, there's a 2 in 3 chance.

The tendency to regard all pollutants as allergy-provokers is a false generalization, as some merely cause irritation—such as a cough, sore throat or skin irritation—rather than a true allergic reaction.

Allergies are definite immunological reactions

A true allergic reaction is an inflammatory or immune-system response, with observable skin, breathing and/or other changes, brought on in certain people by repeated exposure to specific substances.

The allergy-provoking agents—known as allergens—include biologicals (such as pollens or other plant components), pharmaceuticals (such as sulfa drugs or penicillin), foods (such as components in eggs or nuts) and synthetics (such as toluene dyes or isocyanates in furnishings). The most common and annoying allergens include inhalants—such as animal dander, pollens and molds. More dangerous allergens include insect venoms and specific foods such as peanuts (which are not really nuts but legumes), nuts (for example, walnuts) and shellfish (such as lobster, crab and shrimp).

An allergic response results from the body's remarkable ability to distinguish "self" from "nonself" or "foreign" substances, and its attempt to fend off those that are "nonself." In sensitive individuals, the offending substance or allergen, which is harmless to most people, causes overreaction of the body's immune system. Whether inhaled, ingested, injected or absorbed through the skin, the allergen provokes the manufacture of specific antibodies known as IgE (immunoglobin type E) antibodies. The IgE antibodies bind to special mast cells or are carried around the body by the bloodstream.

The reaction between the allergen and IgE antibodies on the mast cells triggers the release of a powerful cocktail of vasoactive (from the Latin *vas*, meaning "vessel") mediators. These substances, such as leukotrienes, histamines and others, make blood vessels leak and cause swelling and congestion, producing a sometimes violent inflammation.

Scientists speculate that the allergic response arose as a protective evolutionary strategy to ward off parasites. Nonallergic people also produce some antibodies to common allergens, but their central control mechanism suppresses an unnecessarily large immune response.

Specificity is the hallmark of the allergic response: it's a specific immunological reaction. For example, someone allergic to plicatic acid, found in western red cedar dust, will form IgE antibodies on inhaling this chemical, reacting with throat swelling, wheezing and other symptoms. Those sensitive to the allergen (protein) in cat dander form IgE antibodies and react with wheezing, hives, skin itching and other symptoms. Thus, while the "foreign" substances that cause allergies vary widely, the reactions they set off are specific, identifiable and predictable.

A rare but severe *generalized* allergic response that affects the whole body can put it into anaphylaxis shock—a life-endangering condition with such reactions as flushing, swelling of the eyelids, mouth and throat (which threatens breathing), confusion and perhaps a sense of impending doom. Blood pressure may drop precipitously, depriving the heart and brain of oxygen—leading to blue lips (cyanosis) and unconsciousness, and possibly death within minutes unless immediate medical relief and an injection of adrenaline is available. (See "Allergic shock" in Chapter 17 for emergency treatment.)

Delayed allergic reactions are less common but may occur in some instances, starting 4, 6 or more hours after exposure to the allergen, peaking at around 48 hours. Delayed reactions, which may be a result of IgE or other types of antibodies, are also very distressing and the major factor in allergic asthma.

It takes more than one exposure to sensitize someone to a particular allergen. As a rule, on the first encounter nothing happens. It may even take several exposures to get the manufacture of IgE antibodies going. But once the body is fully sensitized to a specific allergen, the IgE antibodies are produced quickly whenever it enters the body, setting off the reactions.

A typical case is a 40-year-old man, sensitized to penicillin (which he'd received for an infected leg wound in his teens), who went into allergic shock when he was again injected with the drug after a car accident. The emergency crew recognized the reaction, guessed he was allergic to penicillin and immediately administered a life-saving epinephrine (adrenaline) shot. Sometimes allergic shock goes unrecognized,

DIAGNOSING ALLERGIES

Allergists try their best to pinpoint the offending allergen(s) so that people can avoid them, but that's not always easy. Sometimes the culprit is obvious—a family pet or eating eggs—but often it's hard to discover exactly what sets off the allergic reaction. Accurate diagnosis depends on detailed history-taking and sometimes a series of tests.

Skin or "prick" tests, although not very specific, are commonly used as a cheap, easy way to identify allergens. Tiny amounts of suspected allergens are inserted into a series of shallow punctures (scratches) in the skin of the arm or back. An allergic person responds within about 15 minutes with histamine release and the development of a local red weal and flare where the allergen was inserted.

The RAST (radio-allergosorbent test) analyzes a small sample of blood for the presence of specific IgE (immunoglobin type F) antibodies. It is more complex, less reliable, less sensitive, more expensive and more time-consuming than skin testing.

SORTING OUT THE ANTIHISTAMINES—OLD AND NEW

Today's number 1 anti-allergy medication, antihistamines come in a bewildering variety—including "old" and "new," "short" and "long-acting," "sedating" and "non-drowsy" forms. Antihistamines are H1 or H2 histamine blockers, depending on their action.

Most of those used today are H1 blockers, classed as first generation (more sedating) or second generation (less sedating), both available mainly as nonprescription drugs.

Choosing the right antihistamine is very individual; some people try many types before finding the most effective. One common mistake is to take them as "rescue" medications, when symptoms worsen—

perhaps when the pollen season hits or a cat sets them sneezing. Yet antihistamines are most effective if started before symptoms start—for example, at least half an hour before visiting a friend with a cat.

First-generation antihistamines are still popular, and their sedative side effects often lessen within the first week. They come as tablets, emulsions and drops in many forms, under numerous brand names, including *diphenhydramine* (e.g., Benadryl), *clemastine* (Tavist), *chlorpheniramine* (e.g., Chlor-Tripolon), *hydroxyzine* (Atarax) and others. However, first-generation antihistamines depress brain and CNS (central

nervous system) function, reducing alertness and reaction time and the ability to concentrate. They must be used with caution, as they diminish performance and can seriously impair coordination. First-generation antihistamines also cause *anticholinergic* effects, producing a dry mouth, blurred vision, urinary retention and sometimes impotence. Side effects worsen in combination with alcohol, another brain depressant. They should be used with caution (and medical advice) by the elderly and children under 12 years old, and are not advised for people with asthma, glaucoma, breathing problems or prostate trouble, or for pregnant women.

Second-generation antihistamines—generally less sedating, with fewer side effects (although some can cause insomnia and hair thinning)—include *ketotifen* (Zaditen), *loratidine* (Claritin), *levocobastine* (Livostin), *cetirizine* (Reactine), *fexofenadine* (Allegra) and others. Although many individuals swear by one brand, it is likely that they are all equally effective. Combined with certain antibiotics such as *clarithromycin* and *erythromycin*, some antihistamines can produce serious heartbeat irregularities. In addition, anyone taking antifungal drugs such as *ketoconazole* (Nizoral) and *fluconazole* (Diflucan), should not take terfenadine or astemizole, as the antifungals inhibit the

liver's metabolism of these antihistamines, allowing concentrations to reach toxic levels. As well, the elderly, people taking the anti-ulcer drug, *cimetidine* or *disulfiram* (Antabuse)—for alcohol problems—and those on antidepressants are cautioned against these two antihistamines. They are not safe for use during pregnancy or lactation.

Antihistamines should *never* be used by people who:
• have a heart or liver ailment;
• are taking *ketoconazole* or other antifungals;
• are taking the antibiotics *erythromycin* or *clarithromycin* (Biaxin).

and a sudden death may be mistakenly attributed to a heart attack or some other disorder.

People who know they are susceptible to acute allergic reactions should wear a medical identification bracelet mentioning their particular allergy and carry a pocket emergency kit—such as the EpiPen, a spring-loaded syringe containing adrenaline that's very easy to use and available by prescription. When needed for an allergic attack, EpiPens should be used immediately, without delay—on the way to the hospital emergency department, for instance.

Managing allergies: a three-pronged strategy

The three key steps in treating and managing allergies are avoidance, pharmacotherapy (appropriate medications) and immunotherapy (allergy injections).

Avoidance or "environmental control"—strat-

egy number one—means keeping away from whatever allergen(s) trigger the allergic symptoms: specific foods, pollens, molds, animals or allergy-provoking medications. Sometimes people with severe allergies must change jobs to avoid an allergy-causing substance (such as latex or a hair dye) or must get rid of a much-loved pet.

Pharmacotherapy, the second line of allergy treatment, now offers a wide variety of medications. Antihistamines are the mainstay—they block histamine receptors and reduce or stop the effects of histamine, responsible for the itching, swelling, etc. The newer second-generation antihistamines are less sedating and some are longer acting than the older types.

Steroid nasal sprays are also weapons in the allergy-relieving drug arsenal. For asthma, corticosteroid inhalers are now extensively prescribed as first-line drugs, and asthma med-

MEDICAL HAY FEVER (ALLERGIC RHINITIS) REMEDIES

- **Topical corticosteroids such as *beclomethasone* (Beconase), *flunisolide* (Rhinolon), Fluticasone propionate (Flonase) and *budenoside* (Rhinocort)—the mainstay of allergy treatments—are the agents of choice for hay fever. Used as a nasal spray and inhaled daily during the hay fever season, they are about 90 percent effective in relieving nasal symptoms with no major side effects.**
- **Antihistamines— whatever type suits you best—can help to control symptoms. However, antihistamines can have side effects—especially drowsiness and fatigue—that may interfere with driving, work and other activities. (They should not be taken with alcohol, as the two make a dangerous mix.) The new, nondrowsy varieties suit some hay fever sufferers.**
- **Topical (local) nasal decongestants can be used very occasionally, but never regularly, or they may cause "rebound" congestion. In the long run, decongestant nose sprays exacerbate rather than halt hay fever symptoms and are best reserved for situations of extreme nasal stuffiness such as at night when sleep is hampered.**

  A number of antihistamine-vasoconstrictor ophthalmic drops can be used as adjuncts to nasal steroids or antihistamines to ease eye discomfort in dealing with allergic rhinitis. These eye drops include antazoline-naphazoline (Vasocon-A), pheniramine-naphazoline (Naphcon-A) and pheniramine-phenylephrine (Vernacon).

  For people who do not respond to the above medications, some may improve with the antileukotriene drugs such as zafirlukast (Accolate) in doses of 20 mg or montelukast (Singulair) in doses of 10 mg once daily.

ications also include bronchodilators (airway wideners) for occasional symptom relief, and other anti-inflammatory medications. Still other medications act on other aspects of the immune reaction—for example, *cromoglycate*, which suppresses the mast-cell response and stops symptoms from surfacing. For anaphylaxis, injected epinephrine is the right treatment.

Immunotherapy or "desensitizing" allergy shots, the third weapon in treating allergies, is considered suitable for selected people with certain allergies. Immunotherapy, if used properly, is the one form of therapy that alters immune system activity and offers a chance of cure for IgE-dependent allergies. It involves a lengthy course (up to 5 years) of regular injections using specific allergen extracts to decrease immunological sensitivity and prevent or reduce the allergic response. Immunotherapy is used primarily for cases where avoidance and medication fail to control symptoms, being especially helpful for those allergic to insect venom, dust mites, specific pollens and a very few with allergic asthma.

The treatment of life-threatening anaphylaxis or a severe allergic reaction requires the immediate injection of epinephrine—either a self-administered shot of adrenaline from a pocket auto-injector, or from a medical physician or hospital staff.

People who know they have a severe allergy should always wear a medical identification bracelet naming their particular allergy and carry a pocket-sized epinephrine injection kit—such as the spring-loaded EpiPen, which is easy to use and available by prescription. After self-injecting epinephrine, people with anaphylaxis or a generalized allergic reaction should always get to hospital as soon as possible, as they may require other life-support assistance. There can also be a "late" reaction (up to several hours afterward) requiring further medical aid. Always seek advice from an allergist after experiencing a severe allergic reaction.

The ultimate goal of allergy treatment is to find some way to "down-regulate" the immune system's overly aggressive reaction. Although "cure" isn't yet possible, well-tailored therapy can control most allergy symptoms, except for the most severe or unusual.

HAY FEVER CAN RUIN LIFE'S PLEASURES

Hay fever is a popular misnomer for allergic rhinitis—it's *not* usually due to hay. Afflicting 15 percent of Canadians, it's a seasonal irritation of the nose, eyes, throat and lungs in response to lightweight, wind-carried pollens. Said to be a modern epidemic, this condition now affects millions around the world.

In Canada, the pollens that cause hay fever come from trees during early spring; in June and July the villains are grass pollens; and in late summer and fall, weeds, particularly ragweed, are the culprits. (Heavier, sticky pollens of plants such as goldenrod, dandelion and most garden flowers do not trigger this type of allergy.) Allergies provoked by other allergens typically occur at different times. House-dust allergies, for example, are usually worst in fall when windows are closed and the furnace starts up.

The all-too-familiar symptoms of hay fever

The first sign of hay fever is often a smarting, burning sensation in the nose and eyes. The nose becomes red from constant blowing. Children often develop an "allergic salute"—an upward nose-rubbing action to alleviate the allergic itch. As the nasal passages get swollen and obstructed, sneezing fits ensue and the nose discharges a clear, thin fluid unlike the thick, colored drip of a typical cold. The eyes get watery—eyelashes of hay fever sufferers are typically wet and silky, the eyes often encircled with dark "allergic shiners" caused by the engorged blood vessels around them. The voice becomes husky as the irritation spreads to throat and lungs. Hay fever can start up within 10 minutes of pollen grains entering the body, and tissues become more responsive with con-

tinued aggravation, giving almost constant misery. Once the triggering pollens have left the scene, usually after the first fall frost, the symptoms vanish.

Much seasonal discomfort can be prevented if hay-fever sufferers take a few simple measures:
• Avoid treks through woods and fields.
• Air-condition the home or at least the bedroom, and keep the windows shut; keep the vent on the air conditioner closed to prevent the inflow of pollens.
• Use bedding made of synthetic fibers, as it's easily washed. Consider covering mattresses with plastic or other impervious covers, sealed with a zipper. Wash bed sheets weekly, and blankets regularly, on the hot-water cycle.
• Allow no pets in the bedroom and remove all carpets from the bedroom.
• Try lingering in the morning shower, while breathing deeply, to clear the sinuses.
• Take exercise indoors in pollen season.
• Discard mildewed or damp objects, which may harbor molds.
• Keep the basement clean and dry.
• Steer clear of nonspecific irritants that may aggravate hay fever—cigarette smoke, dust, drafts, alcohol (which is a histamine-releaser) and even contact lenses (which may aggravate the eye irritation).

A FEW CAUTIONARY TIPS ABOUT INSECT STINGS OR BITES

• Avoid insect attractants such as cooking smells, outdoor picnics, messy garbage, pet food, perfumes and cosmetics.
• Don't wear bright or shiny objects or clothes, as these attract most daytime insects, especially stingers (although mosquitoes like dark colors). White, light green and khaki seem least attractive to insects.

• If you know you're severely allergic to insects, try not to be alone outdoors, so that others are around in case of need.
• Behave calmly around insects. Sudden movements and flailing arms frighten them into self-defensive action.
• Be especially vigilant when it's humid, as some insects are

angrier in wet weather.
• Garden cautiously. Take care not to disturb a nest or a bunch of wasps feeding on garbage; avoid use of clippers on hanging plants or places that may conceal insects or their nests.
• Be on the lookout for hidden nests—often under eaves, decks, fallen logs, compost heaps, hanging vines.

• Should a hazardous insect enter your vehicle, don't attempt to drive. Pull off the road and swish it out carefully.
• Try using insect repellent containing diethyl-m-toluamide (DEET), for instance, Muskol. Products containing citronella oil, ethyl hexanediol and dimethyl phthalate may also repel some insects. Put repellents on the skin

(avoiding the eyes) or spray on clothes.
• Immunotherapy or desensitizing shots are recommended for those allergic to honeybees, yellow jackets, hornets and certain wasps. Appropriate skin testing with very dilute amounts of pure venom can pinpoint the allergy and indicate who's a suitable candidate for immunotherapy.

INSECT ALLERGIES: WHAT BIT OR STUNG YOU?

Insect secretions can produce reactions ranging from a barely perceptible itch to a life-threatening allergic response.

Specific insect venoms can cause an immediate response or a delayed reaction—hours or even days after an encounter. The faster the allergic response, the more serious it usually is. In some allergy-prone individuals, insect venoms can not only trigger production of IgE antibodies, but sometimes cause a massive histamine release that rapidly affects the entire body.

Insect allergens can penetrate the body via a piercing bite or a sting from the insect's rear, or by inhalation of wind-blown hairs, spines or other insect parts. Most of these insects either bite or sting, but a few, such as some ants, are both biters and stingers. Bites normally cause milder symptoms than stings because less venom is injected.

Biting insects—such as blackflies, horseflies and deerflies, bedbugs, lice, fleas, mosquitoes and ants attack humans mainly in search of blood. In order to obtain the blood, biters release enzymes that soften the skin and dilate the blood vessels. These salivary secretions can trigger an immediate or delayed allergic response.

Stinging insects—such as the honeybee and other bees, hornets, yellow jackets and wasps—attack either in self-defense or to subdue prey. Their stingers inject venom, a potent substance that can cause severe allergies, even sudden death. Insect venom is a remarkably powerful toxic substance—mostly protein—in some instances able to totally paralyze prey by a neuromuscular block. Although some experts reserve the term "venom" exclusively for insect-sting chemicals, the scientific definition is "any poisonous matter that animals secrete and insert into other animals by biting or stinging."

Those allergic to insects are usually sensitive to just one species, although there can be cross-reactivity: for example, people allergic to hornets may also react to yellow-jacket stings. The most frequent insect allergies arise from yellow-jacket stings, followed by wasps, hornets and bees. Children tend to grow out of their insect allergies. By contrast, those never previ-

ALLERGIC REACTIONS TO INSECT STINGS OR BITES MAY BE:

- **a moderate local reaction with swelling and itchy redness appearing within about 20 minutes, lasting a few hours and fading without serious consequences;**
- **an extensive local reaction with a huge, hot swelling—reaching maybe from wrist to shoulder, or ankle to thigh—that is very bothersome but still more or less around the attack site;**
- **a generalized systemic reaction, occurring within minutes or (rarely) seconds, involving many other areas of the body, with itchy hands and feet, widespread hives, chest tightness, wheezing, abdominal cramps, diarrhea and faintness. These symptoms may occur without much local discomfort at the actual sting or bite site and require prompt medical assistance. (See above and in Chapter 17, under "Allergic shock.")**

ously allergic to insects may become so in later life. If someone has had a generalized body reaction to insects, even a mild one, skin tests should be done to determine the type and extent of the allergy, and preventive steps should be taken. Removing the stinger (which can often be done by scraping a credit or bank card along the skin) can reduce the reaction.

What to do about insect attacks

If stung or bitten, gently flick off the offending insect. Don't run but walk (overheating increases toxin absorption); a dip in cold water or a nearby lake may minimize the reaction by constricting blood vessels and by stimulating a natural adrenaline release through the shock of hitting cold water.

If stung by a bee, which leaves its stinger in its victim, flick or scrape off the stinger. Never squeeze the stinger as it only injects more venom.

For mild local symptoms such as redness, swelling and itching, wash the attack site, perhaps swabbing with antiseptic. Use an ice pack or cold compress and elevate the stung part, if possible. Try antihistamines to reduce itchiness. Apply a steroid or combined steroid-antibiotic cream to reduce inflammation and prevent

POISON IVY

The poison-ivy plant, toxicodendron, is a common weed of the cashew family that grows from coast to coast in North America. (There are several related plants, and names vary from place to place—"poison ivy," "poison oak," "poison sumac"—but the term "poison ivy" will be used here to cover all of them.) Contact with the leaves or oil of poison ivy causes a nasty skin eruption or allergic contact dermatitis in about 70 percent of people. All parts of this plant—leaves, roots and stem—contain the chemical urushiol, responsible for the skin reaction, which ranges from mild to severe.

Poison ivy causes a delayed hypersensitivity reaction which, in contrast to hay fever and most food allergies, involves not IgE antibodies but sensitized T-cells. An initial exposure is necessary to "sensitize" the person, after which subsequent exposures result in the typical poison-ivy rash—a red, itchy, weepy eruption with fluid-filled blisters. The rash may occur in streaks where the plant or its oil touched the skin, usually develops within 24 to 48 hours of contact and may last for days or weeks.

Washing immediately may prevent the itchy rash from developing, but unfortunately many people are unaware that they have encountered this noxious plant or its oils until the streaky, red, itchy rash appears.

Poison ivy or its oil can cause a rash even if someone touches the dead plant in winter, or if it gets onto a sensitive person's clothes from the smoke of burning plants or if the oil is touched on the fur of pets. Most commonly, though, the oil is released onto the skin when the plant is trodden on or broken, and it is spread by touch. People can suffer a repeat outbreak if they later don contaminated clothing. The rash itself is not contagious and doesn't spread from person to person once the oil is washed off the skin. However, it is not unusual to be exposed to poison ivy by touching the fur of a household pet , such as a dog or cat, that has been exposed to the plant.

The problem is usually worst in those with other skin problems, such as psoriasis or acne. If someone is very sensitive or allergic to the urushiol, a severe reaction can occur that requires immediate medical attention.

The best remedy is prevention—learning to recognize the plant and avoid touching it. If it grows in your neighborhood, post a color photo of the plant where children (and guests) will see it. Next best is to remove the oil from the skin as soon as possible. If the oil has been on the skin for less than 2 to 6 hours, thorough washing with ordinary soap (not forgetting to clean under the fingernails) will often prevent or lessen the reaction. If the oil is removed within 5 to 10 minutes of contact, a rash may be avoided. Alcohol-based cleansing tissues, available in pre-packaged form (such as Alco-wipe), are effective. Rubbing alcohol on a washcloth is even better. Clothing should be washed separately in hot water and detergent. Also wash a pet suspected of contact.

The best treatment for mild local cases is a topical corticosteroid cream (such as Cortone, Cortaid or *betamethasone valerate*), and for severe cases or generalized rashes a 7- to 10-day course of oral corticosteroids (such as *prednisone*). Antihistamines such as Benadryl may help to reduce the itching. Always see a physician for a severe poison-ivy rash.

Once the rash appears, keep the blisters clean and dry. Cool compresses, ice packs or aluminum acetate (Burow's) solution applied for 20 to 30 minutes every few hours helps to dry out the blisters and soothe the itching. Bathing in tepid water with colloidal oatmeal (Aveeno) may also help. Soothing calamine lotion may be applied to the affected skin. Beware of other over-the-counter preparations that could worsen the condition—especially those containing benzocaine.

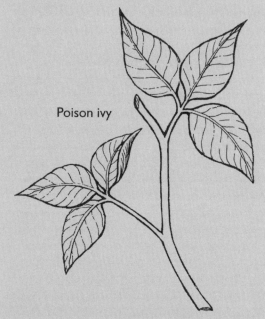

Poison ivy

The identifying features of poison ivy are its three (and sometimes more) shiny, toothed or lobed leaves, the middle leaf being larger than the two side ones. It grows as o droopy vine or shrub, and its flowers and berries are greenish to white.

infection. The absorption can be enhanced by rubbing the cream in and covering the area with plastic wrap secured with cellulose tape.

For a severe local response, seek medical attention. As first aid for a sting on a limb, put a tourniquet between the attack site and the heart, to prevent the spread of venom—releasing after 60 seconds. The physician may prescribe steroid tablets (such as prednisone).

For an ensuing infection at the bite site consult a physician.

Be alert to the possibility of spread to the rest of the body, and get to hospital quickly at the first hint of anaphylactic shock (see above and Chapter 17, "Allergic shock" and "Bites and stings.")

Beware of insects that carry diseases

Blackflies, common day-biters in northern U.S. and Canadian cottage country (particularly in May and June), are tiny, stout-bodied insects, sometimes visible in swarms. Their razor-sharp mouth parts can bore a hole in you silently and swiftly, producing a large, red weal 3 to 4 centimeters (an inch or more) across. Although blackflies are more a nuisance than a danger in Canada, in West Africa and some parts of South America they carry small nematode worms responsible for river blindness.

Sand flies, known as gnats or "no-see-ums" because of their tiny size, get through some screens and can cause extensive local allergies, but while one person itches madly, another remains untouched!

Mosquitoes, known as the "king of disease-carriers," are the most medically devastating of insects, owing to the various disease organisms they carry—the protozoa responsible for malaria, tiny nematode worms that cause elephantiasis and, in Canada, West Nile virus and western equine encephalitis. This viral illness—a sporadic problem in the western provinces, especially in a heavy mosquito year—attacks the nervous system, hitting more children than adults (about 5 to 15 cases a year) and sometimes inflicting permanent paralysis, deafness and mental disability. West Nile virus is a classic example of a mosquito-borne illness. Most people don't even know when they have contracted this virus, but approximately 1 in 150 of those

with the illness can get quite ill, especially as the virus can affect fluid surrounding the brain.

Fleas are blood-eaters that carry no diseases in Canada, but are renowned elsewhere for spreading bubonic plague. Fleas prefer other animals (especially rodents) and only jump onto humans when pets die or go away.

Fire ants, named after their fiery bite, are not a hazard in Canada but are a fearsome pest in many parts of the United States, particularly Florida. Residual scarring and severe allergic reactions can occur from fire-ant venom.

Spiders, universally feared owing to the superstitions surrounding them, are usually harmless, but some, such as the tarantula and black widow, can inflict lethal injury on humans. Another type common in North America, the brown recluse spider, causes considerable aggravation, with nasty, spreading blisters that can leave unsightly scars.

FOOD ALLERGIES: ONE PERSON'S MEAT IS ANOTHER'S POISON

Although virtually any food can trigger an allergy in a susceptible person, some of the most common allergens are in eggs, cow's milk, peanuts, nuts, seafood (especially shrimp, oysters and lobster), wheat, celery and certain seeds. People can be allergic not only to natural food ingredients but also occasionally to preservatives and "fresheners" (such as sulfiting agents).

Someone who reacts to one food may also have an allergic response to other similar foods. For example, those sensitive to peanuts may also react to soy products. (For details on peanut allergy, see Chapter 11.) Those allergic to tree pollens may react with an itchy mouth to certain fruits (such as apples, plums, pears, cherries). Some foods are less allergenic if cooked. A few specific allergens have been isolated from the foods that contain them, such as those from codfish (antigen "m"), shrimp (antigen II), milk (betaglobulin), soybeans (trypsin-inhibitor) and peanuts (antigen I). But many others aren't yet identified.

Sometimes, exercise aggravates a food allergy. In one instance, a young man always became nauseated and broke out in hives when he exercised within 2 hours of eating celery—to which he was slightly allergic—but had no reaction if he ate it without exercising.

TIPS FOR SAFER FOOD HANDLING AND PREPARATION

- *Buy perishables and frozen foods last at the supermarket;* get them home and into the refrigerator promptly. Check "best before" dates on perishable items. If expired, report to the store manager.
- *To avoid botulism, take great care in home bottling,* don't buy foods in cracked jars, swollen or dented cans and don't eat canned goods that have a milky instead of the usually clear liquid around them. Never taste suspect goods—discard, well-wrapped in plastic. ("When in doubt, throw it out!")
- *Freeze meat, fish and poultry* as soon as possible after purchasing. Freeze in freezer bags to prevent "freezer burn," which makes meat tough when cooked. Date the frozen packages. In general, fresh meats can be kept safely frozen for 6 to 12 months, hamburgers for 3 to 4 months, ham for 2 months, bacon for only 1. Fish shouldn't be kept frozen for more than 4 months.
- *Refrigerate raw poultry, fish, ground meat and liver* for no longer than 2 days and other uncooked meats no more than 5 days. Keep cooked meat dishes refrigerated for at most 3 to 4 days.
- *Refrigerate cooked leftovers* promptly, dividing into small portions for fast chilling. Make sure that the warm food doesn't touch cold, already refrigerated products.
- *Defrost or thaw foods inside* the refrigerator or in a microwave oven rather than on the kitchen counter. Cook soon after thawing.
- *Carefully follow package instructions* for store-bought frozen foods (e.g., frozen dinners that state "do not thaw before cooking").
- *Eat hot foods hot, cold foods really cold,* not lukewarm.
- *Keep food at safe temperatures*—at 0°–5°C (32°–40°F) for cold foods, over 60°C (140°F) for hot foods.
- *Do not keep prepared dishes at room temperature for longer* than 1 hour before cooking and 2 hours afterward.
- *Consider all raw meat and poultry contaminated.* Rinse well before cutting or cooking. Never let other foods touch them because microorganisms can "jump ship." Also rinse the sink well after washing poultry and meats. Never serve cooked meats or poultry on the same plate that held the raw meat or chicken.
- *Marinate meats inside the fridge* and never use the marinade for gravy without boiling for several minutes.
- *Cook meat, poultry and fish really well;* hamburger and poultry in particular must never be pinkish in the middle.
- *Use a meat thermometer.* Beef, veal, pork, poultry and lamb should be well cooked, to temperatures of at least 74°C (165°F).

As with other allergies, the reaction results because the body mistakes a harmless nutrient for a dangerous substance and reacts with IgE antibody production. Also as with other allergies, a reaction doesn't usually appear until a second or subsequent exposure to the food allergen. Once the allergy-prone person is sensitized, future exposure can elicit symptoms within minutes or hours of eating the offending morsel.

Some food allergies cause delayed symptoms that come on hours later. About 40 percent of those known to have a food allergy suffer nausea, cramps, vomiting and diarrhea. Many also have hives or, in children, eczema (on the face in infants; behind the ears and on arms, neck and legs in older children). Occasionally the allergic reaction spreads to the entire body, causing life-threatening anaphylactic shock (see earlier in chapter).

Someone sensitive to a certain food component may react from merely inhaling or touching the ingredient. One woman allergic to oysters collapsed at an oyster-shucking party after just inhaling the sensitizing ingredient; she had neither eaten nor touched them! (An adrenaline shot revived her.) A boy allergic to peanuts collapsed and died within minutes of eating a sandwich prepared with a knife previously contaminated with a tiny amount of peanut butter. For this reason it's vital to take allergies seriously. *Never* assume that someone just "doesn't like" a food, and won't notice a small amount—the results could be tragic.

Young children are particularly vulnerable to food allergies, especially if the first solids given on weaning are cow's milk or meat proteins. Breastfeeding for as long as possible may help to delay and possibly reduce the risk of food allergies and is encouraged for offspring of allergy-prone parents. Starting solid foods one by one at intervals of 2 or 3 weeks, and watching for adverse reactions, can also help to detect and minimize childhood allergies. (See Chapter 11 for more on childhood allergies.)

Warning signs of food allergies
- Swelling of tongue and throat;
- stomach and intestinal upsets;
- eczema on the hands or cheeks;

- When *barbecuing* a whole chicken or roast, preferably precook or pre-microwave it. After barbecuing, meat often stays raw on the inside.
- *If stuffing poultry*, insert cooled stuffing immediately before roasting or preferably cook separately and then insert.
- When *buying and cooking fish*, choose one with the head still on; nonsunken, glossy eyes; shiny, tight scales and pink gills.
- *To increase egg safety*, buy government-inspected, grade A eggs (washed before marketing), throw out obviously cracked eggs, cook eggs well and do not cool hard-boiled eggs by plunging into cold water (which may create air pockets where bacteria can grow).
- *Drink only pasteurized milk*; if buying from farms, shun unpasteurized milk (not legally sold in Canada).
- *Wash fresh fruit and vegetables carefully* to remove dirt, soil and bacteria; also wash the tops of cans and jars before opening.
- *Wash all utensils, dishes, sponges, cloths, cutting boards* and counters with hot soapy water (not just rinse water) after use, perhaps also rinsing with bleach. Remember that cutting boards may harbour harmful bacteria in crevices.
- *Cut foods to be eaten raw* (such as salad) on a clean board with a clean knife. If using the same board for both meat and other

foods, maximize safety by shredding other items before cutting meat.
- *When packing lunches*, allow time to chill items containing meat. Tell children to keep lunches as cool as possible. At work, refrigerate your lunch.
- *Chill picnic perishables* well before packing and carry in a cooler. Use insulated containers to keep hot foods hot and cold foods cold. Preheat or precool them for extra safety.
- *When microwaving*, rotate foods for even heating. (Although microwaving heats food fast, it heats unevenly.) Cover foods with plastic to create steam that heats the food surface.
- *When eating out*, make sure that food is served well cooked and hot—if not, send it back.
- *Note that; contrary to popular belief, commercial mayonnaise does not usually cause food poisoning.* The lemon juice or other acid in mayonnaise usually thwarts bacterial growth.
- *Wash hands and clean fingernails*, using soap, before and after handling food, especially raw meat, poultry, fish and shellfish.
- *When on kitchen duty*, wear clean clothing and don't touch the face or hair while preparing food.
- *Never prepare food if you have boils, sores or other skin infections*: if no alternative, use extra precautions.

- hives (weal or rash) anywhere on the body; or
- a sudden drop in blood pressure with weakness, perhaps oncoming unconsciousness—requiring emergency medical aid.

Treatment of food allergies is simple: avoid any foods known to bring on the distress, and exclude all foods containing even traces of the identified allergen. Allergy-prone people must become careful label readers and food watchers. When dinner invitations are accepted, the host can be tactfully advised that a certain food is a problem. People going to a party where unknown foods may be served can take an antihistamine an hour or so beforehand to moderate the allergy (although it won't block it). Those known to have severe food allergies can carry an emergency EpiPen.

Distinguishing food allergies from food intolerance

General surveys report that 25 to 30 percent of adults claim to have a food allergy, but when samples of these individuals were investigated, the actual number turned out to be 0.5 to 2.5 percent. Many people can't distinguish an aller-

gic reaction from a food intolerance or toxicity—such as lactose intolerance or food poisoning (e.g., due to bacteria in chicken or fish). While the symptoms of a food intolerance may resemble an allergy, the causes, mechanism and treatment are very different. A food intolerance does not involve the immune system or IgE (allergy) antibodies.

Unlike food allergies, which are immunological responses that can occur suddenly in minutes or seconds in response to a certain ingredient, an intolerance usually requires large amounts of food and takes longer (often hours) to appear. A person who develops a headache, gets diarrhea or feels nauseated after consuming a certain food does not usually have an allergy. Someone who feels faint or develops migraine after eating overripe cheese is reacting to the tyramine in it, but not with an allergic response. Red wine also contains *tyramine*, which dilates blood vessels and may produce a headache, but that's not an allergic reaction.

Chocolate—often accused of causing allergies—rarely causes allergic reactions. The phenylethylamine in chocolate may make people "hyper" (edgy and restless) but doesn't usually trigger an allergic response. Strawberries and tomatoes are rich in histamine, and eating a large amount may cause histamine-induced symptoms—not a true allergic reaction. Bacteria in underdone beef may cause "hamburger disease" with vomiting, diarrhea and fever—but that's also not an allergic disorder. Non-immunological food reactions are *not* allergies.

A true food allergy is a distinct and observable immune system response to a specific food allergen (protein). It involves the production of IgE antibodies and release of mediators (such as histamine) from mast cells, producing identifiable symptoms. Although most food allergies are immediate IgE-antibody reactions that appear within 15 minutes at most, a few are delayed forms (involving a different immune mechanism) that surface 12 to 48 hours after ingesting a food allergen.

It's surprising how many people are eager to blame what ails them on what they eat, and especially on a suspected food allergy, without any scientific back up for it. Although up to 40 percent of people *think* they are allergic to food, only 3 percent suffer true immunological food reactions.

Here are some common nonallergic food reactions:

Lactose intolerance is an inherited lack of the enzyme lactase, required to break down lactose (milk sugar). The disorder may mimic a milk allergy and is prevalent in groups whose ancestors weren't exposed to milk from domesticated cattle (most common in Aborigines, American blacks and Indians, Bantus, Chinese and Finns). Symptoms include vomiting, diarrhea and bloating. This is a very common problem, especially as people age. The incidence and prevalence of lactose intolerance is 3 out of 10 in non-Caucasians and 1 in 10 Caucasians. Frequencies observed between males and females are essentially the same. Racial statistics show that 5 to 12 percent of American Caucasians; 60 to 75 percent of African-Americans, Mexican-Americans and American Jews; 90 percent of Asian-Americans and 75 to 100 percent of Native Americans are lactose intolerant .

Celiac disease, which affects 1 in 3,000 peo-ple, is a chronic diarrheal condition characterized by malabsorption of nutrients and precipitated by the ingestion of gluten commonly found in foods with wheat, rye and barley. In children, symptoms may be serious diarrhea, bloating and cramps.

Hemolysis (red-blood-cell destruction)—or favism—is a reaction to broad (fava) beans in those deficient in a particular enzyme, leading to fever, headache, anemia and coma.

Tyramine, an amino acid commonly found in red wine, aged cheeses, canned fish and yeast fermentation products, may cause headaches, nausea and other symptoms.

Monosodium glutamate (MSG), a flavoring used in Asian cooking and some prepared foods and seasonings, can cause headaches, palpitations, weakness and numbness.

Metabisulfite, a preservative used in red wine and on many foods such as potatoes, apples, restaurant salads, dips and beer, may trigger asthma and hives.

Food poisoning—not a food allergy

An estimated 1 in 6 Canadians suffers at least one bout of food poisoning in any given year, usually contracted from cafeteria meals or goodies eaten at a catered gathering. Foods likely to harbor health-harming microorganisms include undercooked meat and poultry, rice dishes, custards, cream, unpasteurized milk, shellfish and commercially prepared foods. Food poisoning in North America has been traced to such unsuspected sources as Belgian chocolates, low-calorie ice cream, commercially prepared garlic in oil, grilled onions and baked potatoes.

The alerting signs of food poisoning are primarily diarrhea, nausea, perhaps also chills, fever and vomiting. But often the only indication of a food-borne infection is diarrhea. The discomfort may begin within a few hours of consuming the contaminated food or only appear days later, when it no longer seems linked to a particular food and may be self-diagnosed as stomach flu. Food poisoning usually causes no more discomfort than a stomachache and transient diarrhea, but it can be severe, even fatal—especially in the elderly, children, pregnant women, diabetics, alcoholics and the immune-deficient.

What to do about food poisoning

- Never let your dinner or sandwich become a "microclimate" for bacteria. Remember that bacteria do best in warm, moist, protein-rich surroundings such as meaty broths, gravies, soups, mayonnaise mixtures and custards, where they can multiply by the million.

- To reduce risks of food poisoning, keep hot foods really hot and cold foods really cold; reheat leftovers thoroughly. Heat food to 74°–100°C (165°–212°F), or cool it to 0°–5°C (32°–41°F). Never leave spoilable food like meat, fish or eggs at room temperature for more than 2 to 3 hours.

- Don't let raw meat and poultry or their juices contaminate other foods, especially those that will not have further cooking—for example, don't let raw meat touch delicatessen meat or salads.

- When barbecuing meat, cook it well and place cooked barbecued food on a clean plate, not the one that held the raw meat.

- Avoid stuffing a raw bird with a warm cooked dressing; cool the dressing well first.

- Always wash the hands well with soap before and after handling food. Cross-contamination via dirty fingers and unclean cooking utensils is frequent.

- In a case of food poisoning, give plenty of clear fluids, preferably water, flat ginger ale, or oral rehydration solution (ORS).

- If a food-borne infection is suspected, report it to the family physician (it's a reportable disease in some provinces).

- See a physician if symptoms are severe, there's persistent diarrhea and/or vomiting, and/or there is a high or persistent fever.

- Don't take antidiarrheals without medical advice.

- If the sufferer is an infant, continue breast-feeding.

- If you believe the food was already tainted when you bought it from a store or restaurant, advise your local public-health department.

LATEX ALLERGY: A BURGEONING ENVIRONMENTAL PROBLEM

Latex is causing concern because of increasing reactions to latex gloves (and other medical devices), as well as to condoms, erasers and even balloons. Nowadays latex is found almost anywhere, including bicycle hand grips, escalator handrails, hot-water bottles, shoe soles, goggles, rubber bands, sports equipment, bandages and numerous dental devices. Most likely to cause sensitization and allergy are thin, dipped products (such as rubber gloves, balloons and condoms).

Among the general public the risk of an allergic reaction to latex remains below 1 percent, and serious reactions are rare. But the incidence is climbing in healthcare workers, and currently 25 percent of dental workers and 17 percent of other healthcare professionals report latex reactions of varying severity.

Latex allergy arises through sensitization to residual proteins from the rubber tree that produces it, or to the additives used for vulcanization. The most common form is a delayed reaction that peaks 24 to 48 hours after contact, and is not usually severe—producing a rash or eczema at the point of contact. (Women may develop vaginal irritation and itching if their partner wears latex condoms.) The more serious form of latex allergy arises through inhaling airborne particles, especially from the powder used inside surgical gloves. In operating rooms and dental offices, where pre-powdered gloves are removed and donned many times, breathing in latex proteins can produce a sudden and severe reaction.

Although it has long been known that latex can cause contact rashes, allergic shock and death from this product were almost unknown before reports trickled in during the late 1980s. Physicians and nurses with this allergy may have to stop doing activities that require them to wear latex gloves or work in latex-laden environments.

Use of non-powdered, "low-protein" gloves are a possible solution. (In one case, a switch by all co-workers to powder-free latex gloves allowed an allergic employee to keep her job.) But finding alternatives for latex is a problem, as other materials are less flexible, crack, split more easily and cost more. Moreover, gloves made of alternative products such as vinyl may provide an inferior barrier and are more permeable to blood and water with a risk of allowing infectious agents through—less likely

---

TRACKING DOWN THE ELUSIVE CAUSES OF TIGHT-BUILDING SYNDROME

- Physical and mechanical ventilation problems (blamed for 50 to 70 percent of discomforts) include temperature and humidity imbalances, a lack of fresh air with adequate oxygen, and poor maintenance.
- Chemical irritants (blamed for roughly 15 percent of TBS symptoms), include:
  - outdoor contaminants—such as carbon monoxide, nitrogen oxide and other compounds drawn in from parking garages, storage sites or loading docks (which account for about 10 percent of cases);
  - chemicals emitted indoors—such as tobacco smoke, and emissions from office furniture, equipment, carpets, drapes, cleaning materials and other sources (responsible for about 5 percent of cases);
  - biological (microbial) contaminants that accumulate in the moist slime of uncleaned HVAC systems.
- "People-pollutants"—such as perfumes, aerosol sprays and personal odors—may also add to the problem.
- Mass hysteria and group suggestibility are sometimes cited as contributors to TBS, but this is widely considered implausible by experts, particularly as hysteria tends to appear and disappear suddenly, while TBS symptoms are remarkably consistent and persistent.
- Job stress and work demands may be a factor. A British study suggests that stress owing to lack of control over the indoor environment underlies some tight-building problems—especially among clerical workers "stuck in one place" all day long. This study found more than twice as many cases of nasal stuffiness, headaches and other symptoms among people in mechanically ventilated offices as among workers in naturally ventilated buildings where fresh air could be let in through windows.

N.B.: These factors may act, in combination, to produce cumulative effects.

SYMPTOMS TYPICAL OF TIGHT-BUILDING SYNDROME

- Extreme fatigue and lethargy (especially in the afternoons);
- mucous membrane (throat and nose) irritation;
- eye soreness;
- dry, itchy skin (redness and irritation);
- decreased performance and concentration;
- headaches;
- respiratory infections and wheezing;
- allergic reactions with no allergen pinpointed;
- exacerbation of asthmatic symptoms;
- nausea and dizziness;
- flu-like chills, fever;
- mental confusion.

with gloves manufactured from other non-latex but more expensive materials such as neoprene. Becoming aware of the problem, manufacturers are now trying to make latex products lower in rubber-tree proteins.

People with latex allergy may cross-react to certain foods and develop an itchy mouth when they eat bananas, avocados, kiwi or chestnuts, which contain proteins resembling those of the rubber tree. *Ficus benjamina* (weeping fig) is a houseplant with aerosolized sap that is a latex product able to trigger allergic reactions in latex-sensitive people.

TIGHT-BUILDING SYNDROME

The health complaints designated as "tight-building syndrome" first surfaced during the energy crunch of the 1970s, when many buildings were tightly sealed and heavily insulated in an effort to cut energy consumption and fuel costs. (The syndrome is also dubbed "stuffy-building," "sick-building" and "sealed-building" syndrome.) As well, new "off-gassing" synthetic products were increasingly being used indoors, causing malaise.

Tight-building syndrome (TBS) is generally defined as a set of nonspecific, environmentally caused discomforts reported among a significant number (at least 20 percent, sometimes up to 40 or 50 percent) of occupants in buildings such as schools, offices, retail and residential structures and is sometimes confused with a syndrome called Multiple Chemical Sensitivity (MCS). (Synonyms for multiple chemical sensitivities include environmental illness, 20th-century disease [see below], total allergy syndrome, sick building syndrome, and immune dysregulation.) Sufferers generally feel dramatically better when they leave the building, even on a lunch break, but worse again on re-entry. Health complaints are most frequent after the ventilation system has been shut down over a weekend, the malaise typically appearing at the start of the work week and gradually worsening during the working day.

Experts use the term "tight-building syndrome" to describe vague discomforts—such as fatigue and mild nasal irritation—reported when there are no physical or medical findings to support the complaint. They reserve the name "building-related illness" for the less common allergic reactions and fevers (such as humidifier fever) identifiable by laboratory tests.

Sometimes, TBS complaints are restricted to people in certain parts of a building. Very often, the sickness is too vague to warrant sick leave.

SOME SUSPECTED INDOOR AIR CONTAMINANTS AND THEIR EFFECT ON HEALTH

Substance/irritant	Some major sources and entry paths	Possible health effects	Suggested control measures
Volatile organic compounds (VOCs)—organic chemicals that easily evaporate into indoor air at room temperature—e.g., solvents, benzene products, adhesives, plastic polymers, combustion products. Paints, plastics, tiles, pesticides, sealants, wood substitutes, synthetic furnishings, liquid-process photocopiers, foam fillings, insulation, upholstery.	NB.: indoor concentrations may be 5 to 10 times above those outdoors.	Eye, mucous-membrane or skin irritation, dizziness, nausea, respiratory impairment, depressed brain function. Benzene products may increase cancer risks.	"Bake off" gases before occupying a new building: substitute less volatile compounds: use charcoal filters; ventilate well. Although U.S. and Canadian guidelines set upper limits for permissible amounts of certain chemicals in indoor air, none are yet established for VOCs.
Formaldehyde, a VOC (an aldehyde) with a potent smell, has been a much-publicized TBS problem in modern buildings.	Building materials; urea-foam insulation; pressed-wood products (plywood, particle board): carpets, upholstery foams and fabrics; adhesives, household waxes, wallboard, dyes, plastics, combustion products, preservatives.	Eye, nose, throat irritation; skin rashes: headaches; memory lapses; allergy-provoking (sensitization). May increase cancer risks (not proven).	Select materials carefully when furnishing home or office, avoiding synthetics and glued products whenever possible.
Phenols—organic compounds, antiseptics, also called carbolic acid.	Disinfectants, plastic resins, wood preservatives, tobacco smoke, household cleaners, air fresheners, polishes, glues.	Skin sensitization, nausea, breathing difficulties in those who are susceptible.	If sensitive, select phenol-free household products (look at labels).
Nitrogen dioxide—strong-smelling toxic gas (the brown haze in city smog).	Combustion byproducts, furnaces, wood stoves. cigarette smoke, car exhaust; portable kerosene heaters and gas ranges.	Eye-burning and watering, throat irritation, lightheadedness. Lung damage at high exposures.	Ventilate combustion appliances well. Supply enough outside air; minimize back-drafting of flues.
Carbon monoxide (CO)—a toxic, odorless. odorless gas.	Incomplete combustion from indoor heat sources, automobile exhaust.	Headaches; combines with blood-hemoglobin, displacing oxygen, reducing its supply to body tissues. Fatal in large amounts. Symptoms of CO poisoning include dizziness, vision blurring, nausea, loss of consciousness.	Watch for exposure to car exhaust or other incomplete-combustion products.
Ozone (O_3)—a colorless, unstable gas, irritating even in tiny amounts to those with respiratory problems. Traces in "natural" air are usually higher outside than indoors.	High electrical discharges, action of sunlight on "smog," photocopiers, dirty electronic air cleaners. (Concentrations of 0.001 parts per million are normal indoors; levels 40 times higher may cause symptoms.)	Nose, throat, sinus, lung irritation (perhaps burning sensation), eye watering, blurred vision.	Ventilate well if ozone sources are present. Change or clean electrostatic filters regularly; run only with fan on.
Airborne or aerosolized microorganisms—bacteria, viruses, fungi, protozoa and other microbes that grow in dark, damp conditions, e.g., inside air conditioners, vaporizers, humidifiers.	Live on dirt; thrive in damp conditions and poorly maintained HVAC systems.	Can cause allergic reactions or flu-like illnesses such as Humidifier fever; Pontiac fever; Legionnaires disease.	Reduce humidity below 50 percent. Discard damp furnishings. Check that HVAC systems work as designed. Clean well, maintain properly to prevent sludge (microbial buildup). Use humidistat control of ventilation fans.

But among any group of employees, there will be a few hypersensitive individuals who are severely affected by even small changes in temperature and airflow, or tiny concentrations of chemicals, far below the amounts that would bother most.

Microorganisms can cause serious problems

Stagnant water and moisture in humidifiers, filters, condensers, drip pans, cooling towers, ducts, coils and pumps provide the damp, dark, warm conditions ideal for breeding microorganisms such as bacteria, fungi, algae, amoebae and mites. If dispersed within contaminated droplets and inhaled by people and pets, these microbes can cause illness. Microbial contamination of indoor air arises from poor maintenance and infrequent or nonexistent cleaning of air-conditioning and humidifying systems, not only due to negligence but also because design flaws may hinder access.

TBS health problems due to microorganisms include:

- *Allergic rhinitis*, a sinus and nose irritation that strikes susceptible people soon after they enter a contaminated building.
- *Asthma*, which may be triggered or exacerbated by microorganisms, especially fungal spores.

- *Hypersensitivity pneumonitis*, also known as allergic alveolitis, a lung impairment due to allergic sensitization to organic dusts, aerosols or fungal spores disseminated through dirty HVAC systems. One of the more serious tight-building sicknesses, its symptoms include chills, coughing, breathing difficulties and diminished lung function.
- *Humidifier fever*, a noncontagious, mild, flu-like infection that results from microorganisms dispersed in fine airborne droplets from contaminated HVAC systems. Although the specific microbes responsible remain obscure, certain bacteria and protozoan amoebae (or their components) are under suspicion. The infection typically develops a few hours into a workshift, following a weekend or vacation. This illness, which primarily affects industrial workers (particularly in grain and cotton works), is signaled by fever, chills and coughing (normally without lung involvement). Attacks may last a day or two, be few or frequent, and mild or severe enough to necessitate sick leave. Recovery is usually rapid.
- *Pontiac* fever, named for an outbreak in Pontiac, Michigan, when 95 of 100 hospital employees were struck by chills, fever, headache and muscle pains due to bacterial contamination of air conditioners. This mild,

SOME TIPS AND SOLUTIONS FOR TIGHT-BUILDING SYNDROME

- **Ensure that building managers meet air-quality guidelines and introduce sufficient outside "makeup" air.**
- **Check that temperatures remain at 20–23°C (68–73°F) in winter, and 23–27°C (73–81°F) in summer.**
- **Maintain humidity around 30 to 60 percent for optimal comfort and minimal microbial growth.**
- **Change air-conditioning filters as often as recommended, and**

make sure filters fit properly.
- **Ensure that HVAC systems are adequately maintained, cleaned and periodically checked (metal ducts and fans are easier to keep clean than fiberglass, which attracts moisture).**
- **Adopt a nonsmoking policy, or at least arrange separately ventilated areas for smokers.**
- **Do not partition space in a way that impedes airflow.**

- **Avoid cool-mist and ultrasonic humidifiers or vaporizers; if not well cleaned, they breed microorganisms (the steam type is preferable).**
- **Discard or remove for cleaning water-damaged items—e.g., porous materials, carpets, drapes, upholstery, moldy ceiling tiles. Promptly repair all internal leaks.**
- **Wash smooth surfaces well with bleach to keep down**

microbe levels.
- **Make the indoor climate as health-promoting as possible by substituting nonirritating, natural materials for synthetics when feasible (especially at home)—e.g., use cotton instead of synthetics; wood instead of vinyl; avoid particle-board (which emits VOCs); avoid carpet and other glues or use no carpets; cut down on solvents when possible.**
- **"Bake out" new**

buildings (freshly laid carpet and furnishings emit volatile organics) by turning up the heat and then the ventilation, to vaporize and flush out volatile fumes before people move in.
- **Restart ventilating systems in work premises before the work week begins.**
- **Urge building owners to attend promptly to occupant health complaints by calling in experts to examine HVAC systems.**

self-limiting, flu-like condition is sometimes called "Monday fever" It typically starts on return to work, lasts 3 to 5 days, and carries no risk of pneumonia.

- *Legionnaire's disease*, a life-threatening bacterial pneumonia, usually spreads through air-conditioning systems.

Home humidifiers can be a health hazard

Home humidifiers can also cause ill health and symptoms similar to those discussed above if not kept clean. Steam or evaporative humidifiers are less likely to contaminate the air with microorganisms than cool-mist types. Whatever you choose, keep it scrupulously clean. Wash the tank thoroughly according to the manufacturer's instructions. Any standing water (even a pan on the radiator) can quickly become contaminated by molds and bacteria. Vinegar or hydrogen peroxide will kill molds; chlorine bleach kills bacteria.

"TOTAL ALLERGY SYNDROME": TWENTIETH-CENTURY DISEASE OR MULTIPLE CHEMICAL SENSITIVITY

The concept of "total allergy syndrome"—first dubbed "twentieth-century disease," but now called "multiple chemical sensitivity" (MCS), also known as environmental illness or indiopathic environmental intolerance—has led to many so-called allergy treatments for a syndrome not yet proven to be either allergic or total. Those hit by this incapacitating syndrome typically report multi-organ symptoms that are triggered by exposure to one or more chemicals. People with MCS are diagnosed with so-called "somatization syndrome" (where psychological ills are translated into physical complaints), and they have an irrational fear of all chemicals and suffer panic attacks triggered by non-noxious agents or stimuli. They often attribute their reactions to being "allergic" to a vast range of products and stimuli, from electromagnetic fields and automobile exhaust to paint, perfume, adhesives, furnishings, carpet glue, detergents, numerous plants, cigarette smoke and any items with distinct odors. People afflicted by MCS experience profound distress from minute amounts of the incriminated chemicals—well below threshold levels that bother most people.

Failing to obtain satisfactory medical treatment, MCS sufferers often seek help from clinical ecologists and self-proclaimed specialists in environmental medicine—sometimes traveling to distant clinics and undergoing costly therapies of unproven usefulness. Some are advised to drink only triply distilled water administer sublingual "neutralizing drops" at the onset of symptoms and isolate themselves in "environmentally safe" havens within their homes. In many cases, they entirely withdraw from society, spend most of the time at home, permitting only a few select visitors "free of all scents and pollutants."

Although people with MCS frequently see themselves as "victims" of multiple chemical allergies, their complaints—headaches, poor concentration, bloating, gastric upsets, throat tightness (although the throat looks normal) and an inability to get air into the chest (but no wheezing)—lack the hallmarks of real immunological reactions. "The majority of people with multiple chemical sensitivity," says one allergist, "have no evidence of allergy—no elevation in IgE levels, no sign of increased mast cell mediators (histamine, cytokines or leukotrienes)."

Some researchers have theorized that MCS could arise in certain people through an inability to detoxify chemicals or because of the proximity of the brain's limbic (emotional) center to the olfactory (smell) lobe, with no blood-brain barrier between to keep out large molecules. The limbic system, or so-called primitive brain, is the seat of human emotions and urges—anger love, sadness, sexual drive, self-preservation and survival. Whether there is any truth to this surmised connection remains to be seen. In any case, MCS sufferers need to reduce exposure to irritating volatile odors and organic solvents, and many benefit from counseling, nonjudgmental psychotherapy, support and stress management advice.

Very recent (2004) findings from a University of Toronto study suggest that people suffering from MCS might have a genetic predisposition to the condition because of alterations in the genes that control certain monoxygenase enzymes responsible for the body's biotransformation or detoxification of various drugs and environmental chemicals. (Some of the altered

METALS IN DRINKING WATER THAT COULD INJURE HEALTH

- Aluminum—a component of a material used in purifying water—is not easily absorbed by the body. Suspected of being linked to Alzheimer's disease, aluminum is a nerve toxin and endangers those with kidney failure. In countries such as Canada, Norway and Sweden, with a big acid-rain problem—i.e., where large amounts of aluminum are released into the water—authorities set strict limits on concentrations.
- Arsenic—widely found in the earth's crust, and present in trace amounts in food—is a poison that may damage bone marrow, and also a human carcinogen; the ideal level is zero.
- Barium can harm the heart, circulation and nerves, so authorities recommend strict controls.
- Cadmium—a metal highly toxic even at low concentrations—occurs naturally and leaches into soil and water from vehicular exhaust and industrial wastes.
- Mercury—known to damage human nerves—may be present at danger levels in large fish such as lake trout, whitefish and swordfish. Eating them may pose a health risk far greater than mercury absorption from drinking water!
- Lead can damage the developing brains, blood systems and bones of unborn and young children. Currently, both U.S. and Canadian health agencies strictly limit lead levels in household water, calling for still lower allowable levels. Household tap water is likely to contain lead if it is carried by lead, lead-soldered or brass pipes. U.S. regulations ban the use of lead pipes, lead solder or flux in the installation or repair of public water systems, and Canada is doing likewise.

genes possibly linked to MCS are also thought to be involved in Gulf War Syndrome.) However, this theory awaits further confirmation and replication of the research results.

Anyone considering unconventional tests or cures should try to distinguish fact from fiction, remembering that allergies arise from definable, distinct immune system activity with a recognizable set of blood chemistry changes and defined symptoms. Many allergists and immunologists warn people to beware of self-styled "ecologists" claiming they can identify allergic triggers by unvalidated tests such as hair analysis, feeling the pulse, self-urine injection or "cytotoxic" tests. The result of misguided trust could be a long course of unproven (perhaps expensive) therapy, false hopes and failure to get correct diagnosis and suitable treatment. Alongside medical therapy, many unconventional therapies work well, but anyone considering their use should discuss the pros and cons with a medical caregiver.

For more information on dealing with allergies consult your family physician, an immunologist or allergist, or a local Allergy Information Association; and read *The Complete Allergy Book* by June Engel.

HOW SAFE IS OUR DRINKING WATER?

Given today's sophisticated water-purification methods, Canadians can rest assured that their municipal supplies are relatively free of disease-causing organisms.

While wide-scale outbreaks of waterborne infections have become a rarity here, there's still a need for vigilance. A recent U.S. outbreak of cryptosporidosis—a severe diarrheal illness due to protozoan organisms—is a dramatic reminder of the need to be on the lookout for waterborne microbes. (The probable cause of the U.S. outbreak was a sewage spill containing the protozoa or their eggs, which came from infected cattle feces.)

The U.S. Centers for Disease Control (CDC) still report sporadic cases of illness from waterborne pathogens such as *Giardia* and *Campylobacter* from public or private water supplies. While Canada is spared the worst of such microbial illnesses by virtue of location—because the main pathogens thrive in hotter climates—giardiasis ("Beaver fever") is still common in the lakes and rivers of northern Canada. Campers, hikers and travelers who drink unboiled and untreated stream or lake water can get serious diarrheal infections from these microorganisms.

Increasing worries about chemical contamination

Canadians have now shifted their concerns about drinking water to chemical pollutants. Such fears have made increasing numbers turn to bottled water.

THE CHIEF POSSIBLE CONTAMINANTS IN DRINKING WATER

Metals

Water naturally contains dissolved metals and their ions (charged forms), some of which, such as zinc, copper, cobalt, magnesium, molybdenum and manganese, are essential in trace amounts to human life. Current research indicates that the health risks of exposure to other metals in drinking water are generally low, and that in the small amounts present most do not harm human health, although some have potentially injurious effects.

Asbestos

Asbestos fibers can get into drinking water from naturally occurring rock deposits and industrial uses. Although we may inadvertently consume a little asbestos through drinking water, studies to date find no link between asbestos absorbed from tap water and cancer or any other diseases.

Nitrates

Nitrates occur naturally and also seep into drinking water from sewage, fertilizer and septic tank runoffs, as well as from feedlot wastes. Although the health risks of current intakes from tap water remain unclear, there are concerns that quite low nitrate levels may increase risks of stomach cancer. High concentrations (more than 10 mg/l of water) can cause a rare blood disease in young children—infantile methemoglobinemia—in which nitrates (reduced to nitrites in the stomach) disrupt the blood's oxygen-carrying ability. Authorities remind us that nitrates abound even in natural foods such as fiber-rich vegetables, and if eaten in great excess could endanger the health of those who are vulnerable.

Organic chemicals

Organic chemicals comprise a vast array of substances both natural and synthetic—pesticides, herbicides and petroleum products. Some synthetic organics, which in high doses promote cancer, can pose a health risk by accumulating in meat, poultry, milk or fish. Animal studies show that in high doses, these substances produce sterility, impair the nervous system and damage the heart Drinking-water levels of synthetic organics—such as dioxins, aldrin, chlordane, DDT, PCBs and furan—are therefore kept as low as possible. While their trace-level danger is hard to evaluate, tiny daily doses of such organic contaminants could have cumulative health effects.

Salt

In areas where salt (sodium chloride) is used as a de-icing agent, sodium can seep into water supplies, and high sodium levels may threaten the health of people with high blood pressure. Commercial water softeners, which replace calcium with sodium salts, may also exacerbate high blood pressure and increase the risk of heart problems. However, for most people, the amount of sodium obtained in drinking water is negligible compared to the quantity ingested in food.

Dissolved radon gas

Radon, a radioactive gas (a decay product of uranium), can dissolve in water from uranium ore, granite, shale, phosphate and pitchblende or, more infrequently, through uranium-contaminated buildings. Radon is one of several naturally occurring radioactive elements in drinking water. It can enter household air from basements and, along with radon from other sources, contribute to lung-cancer risks. Water from lakes, rivers and reservoirs generally contains very little (one picocurie or less per liter), but underground water may contain more. Public utilities usually monitor the total radioactivity of their water, but not radon levels specifically. Even drinking water from high-radon sources often remains in reservoirs long enough for the dissolved gas to dissipate. But if radon-rich water is drawn from wells and goes straight into the home, it may later emit radioactivity in a bathtub or teakettle.

Fluoride

An ever-increasing number of countries and cities around the globe fluoridate their water to prevent tooth decay in children, a practice that may also diminish osteoporosis risks in later life. Many experts believe that adding fluoride to drinking water is a wise health measure.

N.B.: On balance, drinking water provides more benefits than health hazards.

Since World War II, through improper waste disposal, global waters have become contaminated by a steady buildup of chemicals, including:
- industrial and synthetic chemicals;
- chlorinated and other compounds formed during water-chlorination and -treatment processes;
- naturally occurring chemicals, such as arsenic;
- natural and industrial radioactive materials, such as radon;
- substances such as lead that leach in from water-conducting pipes.

Among the most potentially health-harming contaminants in Canadian drinking water are the chlorinated compounds—formed by water disinfection with chlorine and coming from chlorinated industrial byproducts such as PCBs (polychlorinated biphenyls), dioxins, cyclodiene pesticides (e.g., aldrin, chlordane, lindane, heptachlor), trichloroethylene and carbon tetrachloride. Being fat-soluble, these chlorinated hydrocarbons endanger fish and other marine life by being absorbed into their fatty tissues, and are then perhaps consumed by humans and other animals.

Industrial, agricultural and household chemicals enter ground and surface waters via a few main routes, namely:
- sewage-treatment plants;
- direct industrial discharge or industrial spills;
- surface runoff of pesticides, herbicides and fertilizers;
- improper disposal of hazardous chemicals (some of them from households);

- storage-tank leaks;
- garbage- and dump-site seepage.

The "dirty dozen" water contaminants

About 400 chemicals, 360 of them synthetics, have already been identified in the Great Lakes, which provide drinking water for millions of people. The number is hardly surprising, since there are 164 toxic-waste sites along the U.S. side of the Niagara River alone. Twelve of these chemicals, popularly called the "dirty dozen"— among them the dioxins, toxophenes, PCBs, DDT benzo (alpha) pyrene and hexachloroben-zene—are known to endanger health. Some of them cause birth defects; others are cell deformers.

To the best of their ability, health officials keep tabs on the levels of these compounds in drinking water and their long-term effects. Most chemical contaminants are present in such tiny amounts that the health hazard, if any, will creep up slowly, becoming noticeable only after years or decades of exposure. In our search for clean water we may forget that the possible dangers from food contaminants far outweigh those from drinking water. It is estimated that eating a single fish contaminated with PCBs, or filling up just once at a leaky gas pump and breathing in benzene, could endanger health more than a lifetime of drinking municipal tap water in most parts of Canada.

Is our tap water safe?

The answer is that, while there is good reason for concern, there's no cause for alarm. Experts assure us that the trace levels of most chemicals currently present in drinking water are not a health risk.

The good news for now is that Canadian drinking water provides a safe beverage that poses a far lesser danger than smoking tobacco or eating too much animal fat. The bad news is that there may be as-yet-unrecognized health risks from daily exposure to trace contaminants that will endanger future generations.

Are bottled waters any safer?

Annual sales doubled to 5 L (1.1 gallons) per capita in Canada from 1982 to 1990. Some people prefer the taste of bottled water (and there's no disputing tastes), but it's not necessarily safer than tap water. Bottled water simply comes out of some alternative water source—like an artesian well or a natural spring—but can contain contaminants in amounts that are well above the guidelines set for tap water. The label "natural" means only that its mineral content hasn't been altered, not that it is healthy.

Although tap-water quality may be open to question, it is at least rigorously tested for 100 or more substances. Only three contaminant levels must be checked in bottled waters: bacteria and coliform organisms; fluoride levels; and TDS (Total Dissolved Solids such as magnesium, iron and sodium). Labels need only identify the source of the bottled water and state the amount of fluoride and TDS. (Quebec has tighter bottled-water regulations calling for the analysis and listing of eleven substances—requirements not necessarily observed!)

In Canada, bottled spring water must, by law, come from underground springs, but there is no law dictating that it must be pure. Even waters advertised as "impeccably purified" may be less pure than consumers expect. American consumer studies have detected several contaminants in commercially bottled water including acetaldehyde and toluene (possibly carcinogenic), arsenic (toxic), high sodium, a range of industrial solvents and traces of plastics. One Canadian consumer study found that some bottled water contained arsenic in amounts well above those allowable in tap water, and lead in quantities above proposed guidelines. Other bottled waters were unacceptably high in sodium. Some bottled waters have more fluoride than allowed for tap water (one brand contained 4 times the maximum allowable concentration), but most bottled waters contain none. A child who drinks only bottled water without taking fluoride supplements, may therefore be at risk of tooth decay and osteoporosis.

Being ozonized but not chlorinated, bottled water doesn't smell of chlorine or contain any of the potentially health-harming chlorinated chemicals. More critical from a health standpoint, however, unchlorinated water may be contaminated at the bottling plant by bacteria and other microbes. Once the bottles are opened, any microorganism present begins to

WATER-TREATMENT DEVICES

• **Activated carbon filters are the most popular type: water from the tap is flushed through or stays in contact with a carbon filter that traps impurities. Large below-sink units containing granular activated charcoal are the most efficient of these devices. They remove bad tastes and smells caused by impurities and in addition, when new, filter out many organic chemicals (such as chloroform and pesticides). The activated carbon** binds some, but not necessarily all, organic compounds. However, once the filter becomes saturated, it may actually release impurities into the water rather than removing them. Users must be aware that:
  • **carbon filters should be used only with water disinfected according to microbiological limits;**
  • **filters need to be changed regularly— at least every 3 to 6 months;**
  • **taps should run for** 30 seconds before the water is used, to flush out the filter.
• **Reverse-osmosis devices—originally used to convert salt water to fresh— attach under the sink. The tap water goes through a semipermeable membrane that traps impurities. These appliances can remove inorganics but are not very good at eliminating organics, particularly chloroform. The membrane requires changing every 2 to 4 years, and it can rupture, allowing** concentrated chemicals and bacteria to pass into the water. Users must be aware that:
  • **high water pressure is needed with reverse-osmosis devices;**
  • **devices should only be used with disinfected water that meets present guidelines.**
• **Distillation devices distill water by boiling, steaming and then condensing it into a holding tank, a method that disinfects the water and precipitates out some** metal salts and organic chemicals. Since distillation may concentrate volatile organics that evaporate with the distilled water, most distilling units incorporate some other method, such as a vent, to discard the first distillate collected. Users must be aware that:
  • **maintenance and thorough cleaning are essential;**
  • **distillation uses a fair amount of electricity;**
  • **the water tastes flat!**

proliferate. In one study, researchers analyzed the microbiological content of bottled water sold in stores across Canada; of 114 lots, both domestic and imported, 46 percent were bacterially contaminated and 12 lots were "grossly contaminated"—to the point of threatening health. Another study found 25 percent of bottled water to be ordinary tap water! Whatever concerns there may be about drinking water bottled water has not proved to be the answer.

Checking out home drinking-water quality
Your local branch of Environment Canada should be able to answer general queries about water safety, but questions about specific drinking-water sources should be directed to local water suppliers and/or local departments of public health.

People can have their private well water tested (free of charge in some cases) for nitrate, fluoride, sodium and hardness levels, and for bacterial content. What's needed, according to one University of Toronto expert, "is a program enabling private well-owners and tap water drinkers with justified concerns to request additional tests for contaminants such as lead and PCBs, for a minimal fee, by local environment or health departments." At present, it can cost several hundred dollars to check for 20 or more chemicals.

• Turbid drinking water is usually a sign that excess particulate impurities are present, which may encourage the growth of bacteria and other microorganisms. Turbidity-causing material also interferes with chlorine disinfection. Home owners should consult local health authorities.
• If radon levels are known to be high in the neighborhood, householders can ask to have an atmospheric test done by local Environment Canada or health-department officials, and if airborne radon is high and the house depends on well water it should be checked for radioactivity.
• Ask to have lead levels in tap water checked in houses built before World War II (when lead pipes were commonly used), particularly if there are small children in the household.
• People drinking water from private or shared wells should—as a rule of thumb—have a once-only test for lead, petrochemicals (if a gas tank is located nearby), and specific

pesticides or herbicides used in the area. In some areas testing of wells is advised 2 to 3 times a year during spring runoff and periods of drought/dry spells thereafter which can be done by local Environment Canada officials if health concerns are legitimate.

Two simple measures to improve drinking-water quality

• Before using water for drinking or food preparation, first thing in the morning or if the water has been unused for several hours, run the cold tap until the water is as cold as possible, to get rid of metals such as lead. Never consume water from the hot tap (hot water dissolves lead and other metals more easily than cold).

• Let water sit overnight in the fridge in an uncapped container to get rid of the chlorine smell.

NB.: Water Analysis and Evaluation Kits that test for 92 substances are available from The Consumers' Association of Canada, tel.: (613) 723–0187, Box 9300, Ottawa, ON K1G 3T9.

GETTING THE LEAD OUT

Lead is everywhere—the metal occurs naturally in rocks, and industry transfers it into the air snow and rain, whence it is deposited back onto land and into rivers, lakes and seas. And it can seriously damage health. Severe lead poisoning leads to coma and death; smaller amounts have subtler effects, and may damage learning ability in children and bone strength in adults.

One legendary theory attributes the downfall of Ancient Rome partly to mental deterioration and infertility caused by absorption of this toxic metal from plumbing, water cisterns, lead-glazed dishes and, above all, wine sweetened with lead acetate ("sugar of lead"). A recent archeological find in Canada uncovered three members of Sir John Franklin's 1845 expedition to the North Pole who reportedly died of lead poisoning—perhaps from defective tin cans—judging by the large amounts discovered in their bones.

Getting the lead out of our lives is no easy matter. A global increase in lead pollution took place during the Industrial Revolution, and

another when tetraethyl lead was added to gasoline as an antiknock agent. Even in the mid-Atlantic, lead levels are now 40 times above presumed prehistoric levels. Lead enters the body from food, as small particles inhaled from the air via the ingestion of lead-laden dirt, and to a small extent from drinking water and other beverages. Most of the lead in our bodies comes from lead-contaminated food. Plants pick up lead from the soil and are consumed by animals, and human beings—at the top of the food chain—eat the contaminated livestock as well as plants. Thus our entire food supply is contaminated, but since lead concentration diminishes on its way up the food chain, animal products contain less than plants.

Drinking water poses a minimal lead hazard in most cases, and any lead in tap water can be largely eliminated by flushing the pipes for a few minutes before taking a drink or using water for cooking. Schools in some areas have been advised to let their drinking taps and fountains run for a minimum of 5 minutes before permitting children to drink.

Over the past couple of decades, "safe" levels of lead in the blood have progressively gone down. The U.S. Centers for Disease Control in Atlanta pronounced 30 µg/dL (micrograms per deciliter) as the upper limit for health safety in 1978, but lowered this figure to 25 µg/dL in 1985 and to 10 µg/dL in 1991. This is the "action" level that should trigger active steps to find the source of exposure and reduce or avoid it. Canadian public-health authorities have set similar but slightly higher action levels, varying slightly from province to province.

However, many health authorities consider today's "safe" level of lead not safe enough. Recent studies show childhood brain and neurological impairment can occur at lead levels well below those previously accepted as safe. Below the "action" level of blood lead, there is a "concern" level that may adversely affect health and behavior (especially in children), but is not considered bad enough to warrant active steps for lead removal.

According to one Health Canada official, the real level at which health damage could occur is 5 to 10 µg/dL, or even lower in groups at particular risk—such as young children and the fetus. Many experts also argue that, for the sake of reproductive safety, permissible lead levels for women in the childbearing years should be set as low as for young children—although this could bar them from certain types of employment.

Aided by the phase-down of lead in gasoline, average blood-lead levels in Canadians have declined, but worries remain about people living in lead-polluted residential areas and those who live close to industrial lead-emitters.

Tracing the lead in household sources

- *Paint*—in many countries, including Canada, lead-containing paint is forbidden for use indoors or on children's toys, pencils and other items. Canadian children living in older homes (pre-1940s) still face a possible but rare risk of lead poisoning even from indoor paint, if bits from old layers of lead-based paint are inhaled or swallowed. Lead-containing paint for outdoor use must bear warning labels on the can.
- The use of vinyl mini-blinds, a newly discovered source of lead poisoning, remains an issue. Until relatively recently, lead was used as a stabilizing agent in the manufacturing process of these blinds, and as they aged, lead dust accumulated on the surface of the blinds.
- *Food cans soldered with lead*—recognizable by their dark inner seams—are a known source of lead contamination; in the past, heavy consumers of canned goods often spooned lead into their bodies along with the food. Modern welded cans and molded plastic ones (recognizable by their rounded bottoms) are gradually replacing older leaded types.
- *Dishes, ceramics, lead-glazed earthenware, crystal decanters and pottery* can leach lead into their contents, especially if the contents are acidic. Lead-glazed ceramics pose a greater health danger if the coating is cracked or when in contact with acidic liquids—for instance, citrus juices, wine or vinegar—that attack the lead-containing glaze or glass, leaching the metal into food or drink. One Montrealer who regularly used a cracked ceramic jug for his morning orange juice suffered acute lead poisoning. Imported earthenware (and imported paints) may

sometimes slip through Canadian regulations. Recently, U.S. researchers reported that wine kept for 4 or more months in crystal decanters contained up to 200 times the level of lead deemed hazardous.
- *People who work with ceramics* run the risk of lead poisoning from lead-containing glazes and paints, whether the craft is pursued as a job or a hobby. Arts councils strongly advise against the use of lead glazes.
- *Antiques* such as old pewter mugs (pewter being a mixture of lead and tin) and *lead seals* on wine bottles (now being phased out) are other possible sources of lead poisoning.
- *Colored comics*—which may contain lead-containing pigments—are occasionally chewed by children.
- *Firearms ammunition*—many cases of lead poisoning have been reported among gun-club members using poorly ventilated indoor firing ranges. Ducks and other waterfowl with drooping necks have been found to have lead poisoning from eating lead shot and nibbling fishing weights!
- *Renovations and home construction*—although dozens of countries banned the interior use of lead paint in the early 1900s, North America did so only in the late 1970s. Many homes still have lead-based paint on their walls. Home renovators may thus inhale lead dust while sanding off old paint or tearing down painted wood and steel structures. Oxyacetylene torches used for cutting and burning lead paint can create dangerous lead fumes. Proper ven-

---

HOW LEAD ENDANGERS HEALTH

- **Raises blood pressure (perhaps even at currently permissible blood-lead levels), with possibly increased risk of strokes and heart attacks;**
- **impairs the nervous system—which may cause learning problems and stunted growth in children;**
- **is linked to gastroin-**
- **testinal problems;**
- **may trigger gout;**
- **causes kidney damage (usually at high toxic levels);**
- **disrupts red-blood-cell function and interferes with the action of enzymes needed for hemoglobin formation, possibly causing anemia;**
- **possibly impairs**
- **male sperm;**
- **may damage the fetus, as lead in the mother's blood is transferred across the placenta to the developing baby; miscarriage is a risk if the maternal blood lead is high;**
- **possibly damages bone, leading to osteoporosis and other problems.**

tilation and cleanliness are essential when renovating, and special care must be taken not to contaminate young children.

- *Soil near a metal refinery,* smelter or heavily traveled highway may be far higher in lead than in most urban areas. Above the 500 ppm (parts per million) mark, residents of some provinces can ask to have their soil retested by local authorities, to see whether replacement should be considered. There is, however, no strong scientific evidence that soil replacement is the solution in all situations. On a cautionary note, environmentalists remind us that the discarded lead-rich soil would create a disposal problem.
- *Vegetables grown* in soil containing over 500 ppm should probably be regarded as toxic. Turnips, potatoes and onions are those most likely to absorb lead. As a safeguard, people are advised to wash hands well before preparing food, discard the outer leaves of leafy vegetables (such as cabbages and lettuces) and peel root vegetables grown in lead-rich areas.

Treatment to rid the body of lead

In most cases, all that's required to lower blood-lead levels is to get away from the lead contaminator(s). Chelation therapy (using substances that bind to lead so that it can be extracted) may be used in severe cases to get rid of lead already in the body. But chelation carries the disadvantage of pulling lead in the bone out into the bloodstream, producing transiently high levels that may endanger the kidneys. Chelation therapy has been touted to reduce heart disease, but has not proven to be of any use in well-designed trials.

COPING WITH TEMPERATURE EXTREMES

Many animals—like fish and reptiles—have to function at the temperatures they find themselves in, adapting their behavior to whatever their bodies are capable of in the warm or the cold. But humans (like other mammals) are warm-blooded our bodies expect to be maintained within a very narrow temperature range (at least for the body's core) and cannot work for long outside that range. We have developed complex mechanisms—such as shivering, sweating, and constriction and dilation of blood vessels—to protect our bodies from losing or gaining too much heat. When these mechanisms are overwhelmed by excessive or prolonged heat or cold, our body functions can be severely affected. Thus, anticipating climatic changes, and being prepared for them, can easily become a matter of survival.

Avoiding heat illness (hyperthermia)

Heat stress, or heat-related illness, ranges from mild to severe. The start of heat stress often goes unnoticed—perhaps producing only irritability and somewhat slowed reaction times. But a severe rise in the core body temperature impairs coordination and hinders the ability to focus or think clearly. Hot, confused people may further endanger themselves by failing to don hats, losing sunglasses, forgetting to take off excess clothes or not drinking enough fluids.

HOW TO GET THE LEAD OUT OF YOUR LIFE

- **Never drink water that's been standing overnight in household lead plumbing.**
- **Run water from the cold tap for a few minutes—until it runs very cold—before drawing water for drinking or cooking.**
- **Never use water from the hot water tap in food or drink, and especially not for baby's formula, because hot water may dissolve more lead than cold water does.**
- **Practice good hygiene—wash hands before eating or snacking, and after playing outside or handling pets.**
- **Wash children's hands well after they've played out-** side; discourage them from swallowing soil, dirt or paint chips.
- **Avoid burning colored newsprint, comics, magazines or wrapping paper in the barbecue pit or fireplace—they may give off lead-laden fumes.**
- **Wash leafy vegetables well and discard outer leaves.**
- **Peel root vegetables, especially if grown in lead-rich areas.**
- **Keep home as dust-free as possible.**
- **Avoid food from lead-soldered cans.**
- **Have any paint chips from old buildings checked for lead by local health authorities.**
- **If renovating, avoid using a heat gun on leaded paint; wear a** mask and coveralls; wash work clothes separately from the family wash.
- **Eat well away from any renovating area.**
- **If using an old electric kettle (which may contain lead solder), empty stale water and replace with fresh before boiling.**
- **Grow vegetables as far as possible from roads and highways.**
- **Don't preserve foods in glazed pots that may contain lead.**
- **Don't store acidic food or drink in lead crystal or lead-glazed containers.**
- **If your home has lead pipes, consider having the water tested by the local board of Environment Canada.**

If heat buildup outstrips the body's ability to lose it by sweating and evaporation from the skin, the body's normal heat-regulating mechanism can fail, leading to the cessation of sweating—a dangerous situation where the brain's hypothalamic temperature-regulating center loses control. Huge swings in blood volume and pressure may produce sudden collapse, even death.

Anyone who succumbs to heat stress must be rapidly cooled off to avoid damaging the brain and other organs. Since there's all too often a lack of water, ice and medical expertise on hand to treat those affected by heat, prevention is definitely best. (See Chapter 17 for first aid measures against heat illness.)

Avoiding cold injury (hypothermia)

Hypothermia—dangerous body cooling—can occur if normal body temperature falls by even two degrees. Mild hypothermia occurs if body temperature drops to 33 to 35°C (91 to 95°F); below 30°C (86°F), hypothermia is life-threatening.

As the body loses heat, metabolism and heartrate slow down. With mild to moderate hypothermia, shivering—the body's way of building heat by muscular activity—remains violent but the person may stagger as if intoxicated and speech may be slurred. Hypothermic people become quiet, may refuse food and drink and become sluggish, fatigued and drowsy. The skin may be deceptively pink even though icy cold. The pulse is slow and weak, and breathing is shallow. As body cooling progresses, shivering lessens; the person appears weary, withdrawn, confused and irritable and may act strangely—perhaps undressing despite the cold—due to a deceptively warm sensation. With severe hypothermia, shivering stops; people hallucinate, stare with fixed pupils and may lose consciousness. The pulse, heartbeat and breathing may seem imperceptible—as if the person is already dead.

The treatment for mild hypothermia—for someone still shivering and coherent—is to prevent further heat loss, find shelter and rewarm the casualty by adding extra clothes (preferably woolen), covering with blankets, cuddling against others or sharing a sleeping bag. Contrary to popular folklore, alcohol does *not* warm people up. On the contrary, it dilates blood vessels and gives them a false sense of warmth.

If hypothermia is more severe—if the person is no longer shivering—get medical help as soon as possible. Severe hypothermia is a medical emergency; the casualty needs expert rewarming to prevent further damage and avoid endangering the heart. (See Chapter 17 for details of emergency first aid for hypothermia.)

STAYING FIT ON THE JOB

A healthy employee has fewer accidents, takes fewer sick days, uses less health-insurance benefits, is more productive and costs less than an ailing worker. Accordingly, many companies are now introducing fitness and lifestyle programs to decrease absenteeism, reduce staff turnover,

---

TIPS TO BEAT THE HEAT

- **Minimize physical activities and outdoor exposure during the hottest parts of the day (11:00 a.m. to 3:00 p.m.).**
- **Drink plenty of liquids (preferably a gallon a day!); thirst is quenched long before lost fluids are really replenished. Vigorous exercisers are advised to drink at least 15 to 20 ounces (t2wo cups, or .5 liter) of water before working out or starting a race.**
- **If running a long race or exercising vigorously, replace fluids with plain water. While some people favor *iso-molar* solutions (balanced electrolyte drinks) like Gatorade, plain water is the best drink in hot weather**

and immediately before and during vigorous exercise, because it dilutes and counteracts the rise in plasma (blood) potassium that can occur in these circumstances.
- **Limit alcoholic beverages and caffeinated drinks (such as tea, coffee and colas) as they are diuretics and increase fluid loss.**
- **Wear a hat (wide-brimmed if possible) or use an umbrella or sunshade, and wear loose, lightweight, light-colored garments (preferably cotton).**
- **Acclimatize the body gradually by increasing heat exposure slowly.**
- **Walk on the shady side of the street.**
- **Spend as much time**

as possible in air-conditioned rooms or buildings, set air-conditioners at 24°C (75°F) or place large fans in windows to draw heat outdoors.
- **Park vehicles in the shade and open car windows and doors before entering a parked vehicle.**
- **Take frequent cool showers or baths.**
- **Slightly increase dietary salt intake during hot summers or if regularly exercising hard—by adding a little to cooked food or salads. (Do not take salt tablets unless medically advised to do so.)**
- **Omit heavy, fatty foods, desserts, gravies and sauces.**
- **Cook during the cooler part of the day.**

improve productivity and boost morale. Classes range from regular aerobics to lifestyle-improvement workshops in nutrition, smoking cessation, and so on.

Fit employees feel and work better and are cheaper to maintain. One study, conducted by the University of Toronto together with two life-insurance companies, showed the cost-effectiveness of a worker-fitness program. Over 1,000 employees participated. Half of the test-employees at the Canada Life Assurance Company exercised regularly, and they were compared to a control group of nonexercisers in another insurance company. The Canada Life classes included graded exercise routines as well as seminars on nutrition and weight control. A monthly newsletter gave practical tips on diet, hypertension, smoking and other health matters.

The results were gratifying. The fitness programs attracted 35 percent of all employees (as many clerical as managerial staff), and after 6 months participants were doing regular 17-minute aerobic sessions, compared to no workplace exercise in the control group. Employee turnover during the 10-month study went down from 15 percent to 1.5 percent among exercising employees. Absenteeism in this group declined by 22 percent, and they used the medical system less often than the sedentary group. The life-insurance company calculated a potential overall saving of $150,000 annually if just 28 percent of employees participated in the health-promotion program—a saving of 1 percent of the payroll. Needless to say, even after the study ended, the company retained the health program.

In general, about 30 percent of employees will take up a regular workplace fitness and lifestyle program, but half are likely to defect over the first 6 to 18 months. Dropout rates are greatest among older people; the unpunctual; the obese; smokers; blue-collar workers; those with high blood pressure, angina, heart pain or arthritis; people with unsupportive partners; and those who consider the instructor "uncaring" or "inattentive."

A recent University of Toronto study found that those adhering to fitness programs perceived them as fun, worthwhile, healthy or "tension-relieving." Noncompliers, on the other hand, saw no link between exercise and good health, and many reported that they got enough exercise anyway—a false conviction common among nonexercisers.

The ABCs of a worksite fitness and lifestyle programs

Programs range from simple exercise classes to full-scale health clubs with gymnasiums, swimming pools, running tracks and badminton or squash courts. To achieve its aims, a fitness program must be lively, safe, enjoyable, conveniently located, effectively led and attractively packaged. As a minimum effort, a company could offer a running track or an exercise room.

- *Creative planning* should include collaboration with employees. A fitness committee, with a director, proposes a budget, obtains funds, discusses how and where classes should be held.
- *A preliminary questionnaire* measures employee eagerness, exercise preferences (aerobics, swimming, jogging) and willingness to pay

---

TIPS TO BEAT THE COLD

- Dress appropriately, in layers (for details, see section on winter sport tips in Chapter 2).
- If stranded or very cold, find or build any kind of shelter (under a tree, in a hollow or cave) and stay out of the wind.
- Try to remain dry. Dampness against the skin increases heat loss. However, it's not always advantageous to change damp or wet garments. In very cold air, changing clothes may produce extra heat loss, so use your discretion. It may be better simply to cover up the damp clothes with more clothes on top.
- Avoid exercise that makes you sweat. Although movement creates body heat, the resulting perspiration may wet clothes and enhance heat loss. Move slowly and methodically rather than quickly.
- Put on extra clothes or blankets if possible, or wrap up in plastic.
- Keep head, neck and hands covered. As much as 40 percent of the body's heat loss occurs through the neck and head, and up to 20 percent via the hands. Covering the head, mouth and nose lightly with a cap or scarf creates a heat flow that allows you to breathe warmer air.
- Stay awake at all costs. The body's metabolism and heat production diminish even more during sleep.
- Don't sit or lie directly on the cold ground. Insulate yourself with objects such as branches, leaves, dry, loose soil, backpacks or shoes.
- Huddle close to others in a group.
- Remain with others; do not wander off alone.
- Don't eat snow. It doesn't satisfy thirst and wastes precious body heat.

minimum fees to defray costs and maintain participation.

- *Involving upper management* is a key to success; if superiors take part in exercise classes, workers are encouraged to join in.
- *No universal blueprint* works for all; the program must be geared to target participants, whether clerical or sales staff, executives or laborers.
- *A preliminary fitness test* for participants is wise, and is best done in conjunction with the company's health department, to assess safe limits for exercising.
- *Showers* are an absolute requirement.
- *The program should attract 20 to 30 percent of employees* as regular adherents. It may also draw in the unfit and nonexercisers, not just the already converted. In Canadian companies, less than 5 percent of employees are usually committed to vigorous physical activity; hence, a fitness program that attracts even 20 percent is enhancing the health of at least 15 percent more.
- *Limiting initial enrollment*, far from deterring participation, often creates interest.
- *Set realistic goals* that don't raise false hopes for a magic route to guaranteed health.
- *Broad-based, varied programs* work best—with graded exercise classes and varied activities (as seasons permit), including lifestyle-improvement seminars.
- *Skilled, well-trained, enthusiastic leadership* is crucial. An invigorating, creative and credible fitness instructor who can explain things clearly and individualize exercise prescriptions, is a top priority, and well worth the cost entailed.
- *The fitness instructor should be qualified in first aid* and CPR; if not, other employees with these skills should be on call.
- *Classes should be convenient and accessible*, preferably conducted at the worksite.
- *Good facilities* improve adherence and are more important than expensive equipment in making classes a success.
- *Flextime is best*, allowing various exercise times.
- *The approach should be lighthearted*, nonjudgmental and sociable. Participants will broadcast the success of an enjoyable program.

TOWARD HEALTHIER GLOBAL TRAVEL

As tourists increasingly venture off the beaten track, they become more susceptible to infections such as traveler's diarrhea and rare diseases such as Lassa and Dengue fever. It's wise to obtain health advice from reliable sources such as travel clinics before you leave home. If you get sick during or after your travels, be sure to tell the doctor where you have been and ask whether the problem could be travel-related.

Travel to most parts of North America and Europe (including the former Soviet Union) and the Caribbean requires fewer precautions than going to Asia, Africa or South America. Staying in clean, air-conditioned hotels poses fewer health risks than camping, going to less traveled places or renting a local room. The well-nourished are less apt to become ill than the poorly fed. Remaining in disease-ridden areas for lengthy stays obviously brings greater risks than a short vacation.

Tips to keep adventurous trippers healthier:

- *Travel tip #1*

  See your physician before departure, especially to exotic places. Get advice on sensible precautions, what to take in a medicine kit and where and when to get any needed immunizations. Take a medical kit containing bandages, adhesive plaster, antiseptic and antibiotic creams, antinauseants, antimalarial tablets (if needed), antihistamines, painkillers, antidiarrheal agents, tablets for purifying water, insect repellents, antibiotic pills (to treat traveler's diarrhea), any special prescription medications and needles plus syringes in a commercial kit (with a physician's letter explaining why you're carrying them, i.e., to have a clean, non-AIDS-contaminated set in case of need). Keep records of any drugs used. Take spare eyeglasses. One University of Toronto travel expert suggests including condoms because, as he rhymes it, "a tisket, a tasket, a condom or a casket." If appropriate, wear a Medic-Alert bracelet documenting allergies and special individual health problems. Consider visiting the Center for Disease Control's travel website (http://www.cdc.gov/

BENEFITS OF A SUCCESSFUL WORKPLACE FITNESS PROGRAM

- **Convenient and easy to attend;**
- **no need to commute or find parking space;**
- **better morale and productivity due to less illness and less staff turnover, and greater concentration on tasks;**
- **boosted self-esteem, owing to fitter self-image and the feeling that the employer cares about employee wellbeing;**
- **solidarity and group spirit, from the shared camaraderie;**
- **reduced healthcare costs;**
- **lowered life-insurance costs—some insurance companies offer reduced premiums to individuals who practice healthy lifestyles;**
- **better public image of organization; a health-promotion program improves corporate image at local and national levels.**

SHIFT WORK AND CIRCADIAN RHYTHMS

Companies can improve productivity and employee health by careful scheduling of shift work. Since many jobs are now done around the clock, some workers are exposed to "occupational jet lag." Many shift-work schemes are arranged for convenience and economic expediency and ignore the body's natural circadian rhythm (biological clock), possibly wreaking havoc with worker health and efficiency.

While about a third of shift workers say they enjoy the changing schedules, citing the advantages of more free time, and days off that give them a chance to shop, bank and share family activities, others dislike it and feel unwell. Individuals vary in their susceptibility to health problems from shift work (gastrointestinal upsets, fatigue from lack of sleep). Those who are "owls" and adapt to changing sleep times may be more suited to shift work than "larks" who like set sleep and wake-up times. As their biological clocks struggle to adapt at the start of a shift change, most workers complain of discomforts such as headaches, mood swings and stress. An accumulated sleep debt may cause lapses in concentration and vigilance. Also the inner biological clock may keep body temperature and hormone levels low just when they should be high for optimal efficiency. Well-documented studies from many countries indicate a performance dip, with diminished attention, between 2:00 and 4:00 a.m.—with a parallel increase in errors, performance failures and mishaps among train drivers, truckers, pilots, healthcare workers and others.

There is much debate about the best way to overcome these problems. One-week shifts are considered the most disrupting to physical, social and psychological health. It takes about a week for sleep-wake rhythms to adapt, and they're no sooner adjusted than a new shift begins and circadian rhythms must change afresh.

Although it's not always feasible, many experts suggest that shift-work rotations should be every 3 weeks instead of every week, to give the biological clock more time to adjust. While many North American companies now favor 21-day shifts, Europeans prefer shifts that change every 2 or 3 days, which don't disturb the circadian sleep-wake rhythm as much and avoid forcing the biological clock to adapt. This system also proves less disturbing to family and social life, as workers return to normal every third day.

---

travel/) or the Canadian Travel Medicine Program (http://www.phac-aspc.gc.ca/tmp-pmv/pub_e.html) to educate yourself about any current travel risks.

- *Travel tip #2*
Review your inoculation status and seek advice about any immunization boosters needed against diphtheria, polio, tetanus, measles, rubella and mumps. Get your required shots in good time. Immunization requirements vary from country to country (See "Immunization schedule" in Chapter 10.) Some of these vaccinations need time to take effect so try and get in to see the doctor at least 6 weeks before you leave. Inoculations against some diseases rare in North America, such as yellow fever and cholera, are regulated by the World Health Organization (WHO). Since vaccination requirements and travel risks change, travelers should check with a travel clinic, officer of health or Health Canada to see what is advised for the areas you plan to visit. *Tetanus vaccination* is essential for all non-immunized travelers. Tetanus is caused by a bacterium that exists in the soil, and is found throughout the world but is more prevalent in damp, warm climates. Tetanus vaccine gives effective protection, but booster shots are needed every 10 years. Check your tetanus antibody status.

- *Diphtheria reimmunization* may be needed (every 10 years) because, although diphtheria is uncommon in Canada, it's still widespread elsewhere.

- *Rubella* (German measles) is a relatively mild and innocuous infection in adults, but can drastically malform unborn babies; all women of childbearing age should ensure they have the necessary booster shots.

Travelers may also need vaccination for the following, less common diseases:

- *Yellow fever*, a viral disease transmitted by mosquitoes. The WHO requires inoculation (which lasts 10 years) at designated yellow-fever centers for anyone entering or passing through an infected zone. Some countries demand yellow-fever vaccination for all entering visitors, others only for those from certain areas.

- *Cholera*, a bacterial illness transmitted through

water is still rampant in Asia, Africa and the Middle East and has recently broken out in South America. Cholera is not much of a danger to travelers provided they drink safe water and don't eat unpeeled fruit or uncooked shellfish. Since existing vaccines give little protection, cholera inoculation is no longer recommended. For countries that still require vaccination certificates, some Canadian doctors issue exemption certificates or give one dose of cholera vaccine to satisfy foreign authorities.

- *Typhoid fever*, a worldwide febrile disease transmitted via food and water is prevalent wherever there's poor sanitation and hygiene. The currently available typhoid vaccines (including the new oral Vivotif Berna and the injectable Typhin-V) offer partial—about 75 percent—protection.

- *Meningococcal disease* (meningitis) can occur in epidemic proportions. Vaccines are available against strains A, C, Y and W-135 and are advised for those staying 2 weeks or more in areas where the disease is a major problem for instance, in Central Africa, Egypt, Chad, Ethiopia, Morocco and parts of India.

- *Hepatitis*, a viral liver infection, is acquired from fecally contaminated food and water or the blood and secretions of carriers. The various forms of viral hepatitis (A, B, C, D and E) are caused by different viruses. There are now effective vaccines against hepatitis B (which is especially prevalent in South East Asia and Africa) and against hepatitis A. Those traveling to areas where hepatitis B is epidemic should be immunized against it, as it has a 1 percent mortality rate and leads to liver cancer. Although less dangerous than hepatitis B, the A form is more frequently encountered by travelers. Hepatitis A can be prevented by a new hepatitis-A vaccine. There is now a dual or combined vaccine against both hepatitis A and B given in one shot. (For more on hepatitis, see Chapters 11 and 16.)

- *Japanese B encephalitis* vaccine is suggested for travelers to rural Southeast Asia, especially in summer and fall. This mosquito-borne disease is prevalent in rice-growing areas of China, Nepal, Thailand, Vietnam, Taiwan, Korea and the Philippines. Three doses of the Biken vaccine, one week apart, are recommended—if it's available.

- *Rabies* is a worldwide viral disease spread by wild and domestic animals such as foxes, raccoons and dogs. Those likely to come into intimate contact with wildlife and those staying for a long time in rabies-ridden areas of the developing world should be immunized.

- *Travel tip #3*
Protect yourself from malaria if traversing mosquito-infested areas. Malaria is still one of the greatest health threats to travelers abroad. It's a protozoal infection spread by mosquitoes that feed on human blood, usually biting between dusk and dawn. The main risk areas are: tropical parts of Africa, Asia, Mexico, South and Central America, Haiti, South East Asia and some Pacific islands. At present, malaria is on the upswing, partly owing to the cutback of insecticide spraying for environmental and other reasons. Although malaria can be transmitted from mother to unborn baby, and (rarely) via a contaminated blood transfusion, it is usually acquired from the bite of an infected female *anopheles* mosquito. The incubation period is 10 to 60 days but can be longer. The parasites enter the liver where they multiply, then break out, reenter the bloodstream and cause fever, chills, headache, muscle aches, fatigue, perhaps also vomiting and a cough. The illness can be fatal.

Even though malaria infects over 300 million people a year, and causes about 2 million deaths annually, it is still regarded by some as a rare and exotic affliction. Yet not so long ago malaria was quite common in Canada. Canada still reports about 250 cases a year, mainly among immigrants and those returning from trips to South America, Asia and Africa.

A drug-resistant killer strain of malaria, not treatable by the main antimalarial drug, chloroquine phosphate, has now emerged in many tropical areas. Of the four types of malarial infection in humans, *Plasmodium falciparum* is the most lethal, and those going to risk areas need special preventive drugs. None of the drugs currently available guarantees complete protection, but mefloquine is now the drug of choice for travel to areas with chloroquine-resistant malaria.

As a preventive, get and take antimalarials, cover yourself well, sleep under mosquito nets and use DEET insect repellent. New, light, portable mosquito nets with bamboo frames are a good idea. (Bear in mind that the mosquitoes that carry Dengue fever may even bite during the day.)

Treatment of malaria must be swift and appropriate, to prevent respiratory failure and even death. A fever in any traveler coming from a malarial area should be considered a medical emergency. Since some forms of malaria linger in the body (even in those who have been conscientiously taking antimalarials), people who have visited a danger zone and develop a fever or chills within two years of their travels—especially within the first few months—should suspect malaria and seek prompt treatment.

To protect yourself from malaria:

- Reduce time spent outdoors from dusk to dawn, and wear protective clothing, covering legs and arms.
- Apply a nonaerosol insect repellent to all exposed skin, the most effective being 30-percent or higher-strength *diethyl-m-toluamide* or DEET (a chemical found in Muskol, Off, Deep Woods and other preparations). The strength of the DEET indicates how long it will be protective. Lower strength is recommended for kids (under 10 percent) but it needs to be applied more often, never near the eyes.Sleep in screened lodgings or under mosquito nets.
- Mefloquine needs to be taken 1 week before entering a malarial setting. Other anti-malarials have variable starting times. These drugs need to be continued regularly throughout your stay and for 4 weeks after returning.
- Watch for and report any adverse side effects from antimalarial drugs—such as itchiness, swelling, nausea or a skin rash. Mefloquine can, rarely, cause depression and psychosis. Although antimalarial drugs do not prevent the mosquito from infecting you, they usually stop the symptoms from appearing. See the CDC site for more information (http://www. cdc.gov/travel/) .
- *Travel tip #4*
Avoid or learn to treat "traveler's diarrhea,"

also known as turista, Montezuma's Revenge, the Hong Kong dog, Delhi belly, Casablanca crud, the Rangoon runs and the Aztec two-step. Traveler's diarrhea, due to bacterial organisms, affects up to 80 percent of unwary vacationers to areas such as Mexico, Southern Asia and the Caribbean. Typically, it causes one or more short episodes of watery stools, often starting 1 to 5 days after arrival or 5 days after leaving an endemic area. It is due to bacterial contamination of food or water. The diarrhea may be accompanied by abdominal cramps, vomiting, chills, fever and appetite loss. Blood and mucus are not usually present in the diarrheal stool; if they are, get immediate medical advice. Self-remedies are fine for mild to moderate diarrhea but severe bouts need medical attention—because of the risk of more serious problems.

Drink clear fluids such as broth, bottled carbonated drinks and clear tea (no milk) until the diarrhea stops. Use oral rehydration solutions to replace lost fluids (rather than just plain water). Stick to rice, noodles, puréed cooked foods (carrots, apples, potatoes) until better and resume full diet gradually. Add milk products last. Don't take medications such as Enterovioform or those containing chloramphenicol (a bone-marrow depressant). Use medications that slow diarrhea, such as Lomotil, Imodium or paregorics, sparingly (Imodium and Lomotil can also be used in children: they work by slowing the bowel spasms.) These medications are useful when you are traveling and access to a washroom is limited, but it is important to understand that the diarrhea is your body's way of getting rid of the infection (viruses or bacteria). When this elimination pathway is blocked, the infection may last longer. Do not use even these drugs when there is high fever chills or persistent (bloody) diarrhea. In such cases, consult a doctor.

To clear up traveler's diarrhea, take 28g (2 tbsp) or 2 tablets of Pepto-Bismol every half-hour. Eight doses often clear up traveler's diarrhea. Some travel advisors suggest carrying self-treatment antibiotics such as norfloxacin, ciprofloxacin or trimethoprim sulfamethoxazole, to be taken when the diarrhea starts; the dose for moderate to severe diarrhea is 1 tablet twice daily for 3 days. These same antibiotics, or Pepto-Bismol, can be taken as preventives for traveler's diarrhea, but are usually so advised only for high-risk travelers (with health problems). Antibiotics should not be used lightly. If they are used, the antibiotic regimen most likely to be effective is ciprofloxacin (500 mg) taken twice a day.

- *Travel tip #5*
Drink only "safe" water or purify it. Water (including ice cubes) in most tropical countries is contaminated because of poor sewage disposal and improperly treated water supplies. Animals and humans may defecate in the water supply. Filtration alone isn't enough. Even staying at first-class hotels doesn't guarantee pure water.

Safe drinks include:
- beverages (such as tea and coffee) made with boiled water;
- canned or commercially bottled carbonated beverages, including bottled water soft drinks, beer and wine. Wipe obviously dirty bottles or cans before drinking;
- coconut juice directly from the shell;
- water you have purified yourself.

To purify water add chlorine bleach (2 drops per liter or quart) until the chlorine smell is just detectable after mixing, or add 2 percent tincture of iodine (5 drops per liter or quart), or boil the water—bringing it to a boil is usually sufficient. The Water-Tech portable purifiers are lightweight and ideal for short-term trips, work well and last a long time. They can purify more than 455 liters (100 gal) of water.

To make water safe for tooth brushing, collect the hottest water possible from the tap in a clean glass and let it cool.

- *Travel tip #6*
Do not wander barefoot in unknown places. Protect the feet against cuts, abrasions, snakebites, insects (sand fleas and ticks) and parasites such as hookworms and threadworms. Several parasites and worms can burrow through the foot's unbroken skin. (See also below, tip #9.)

- *Travel tip #7*
Be aware of a few rare but potentially deadly infections that may afflict travelers to exotic places:

- *Lassa fever* first described in Nigeria in 1969, is one of the most dangerous viral illnesses. It is transmitted by an arenavirus found in the urine of rodents in rural areas of West Africa, producing high fever and prostration.
- *Dengue fever*, generally mild and short-lived, is transmitted by day-biting mosquitoes and is common in the Caribbean, Southeast Asia, Central America, the South Pacific and Africa. It comes in various forms and characteristically produces a sudden high fever, sore throat, severe joint and muscle aches and a rash on the torso and face—rather like measles.
- *Encephalitis*, a viral infection of the nervous system spread by mosquitoes and ticks, occurs in rural areas of Europe, the former Soviet Union and the Orient, especially during summer months. General anti-insect precautions should be taken—wear long-sleeved shirts and long pants, use DEET insecticide.
- *Sleeping* sickness (*trypanosomiasis*) is a rare, insect-borne disease that causes acute fever and can strike visitors to African game reserves. The African variety is carried by tsetse flies. South American trypanosomiasis (also called Chagas' disease) is transmitted by bugs that live in the mud cracks of adobe huts and in thatched roofs.
- *Leishmaniasis*, transmitted by sand flies, has an incubation period of months to years and results in skin sores and a rarely serious febrile illness. It occurs mainly in India, Asia and some Mediterranean areas.

- *Travel tip #8*
Acclimatize yourself and combat "jet lag." Maintain adequate fluids and get enough rest to avoid stress, heatstroke and immune-system problems. Wear loose-fitting clothes in hot climates, bathe often and dry well afterwards. If you have high blood pressure and go to a hot climate, minimize blood-pressure problems due to the heat by seeking air-conditioned rest places.

In adapting to a warm climate, your body must adjust to sweating without undue loss of salt, and to working in the heat. Pretravel preparation, suitable clothing, sunglasses, sun lotions and adequate fluid intake assist acclimatization, which is especially tough for the old, the obese and those who are in poor health or have chronic ailments such as diabetes.

Reduce stress on the body by taking two suitcases instead of one massive, heavy one. Take an inflatable neck pillow for comfort while traveling. Since acclimatization takes several days, travelers should rest after arrival, particularly if their flight has taken them through several time zones. Take along a few candy bars, dried fruit or other energy foods in case altered schedules lead to long delays without food. (Diabetics in particular should prepare for this contingency.)

Avoid jet lag by paying attention to your biological clock, which automatically regulates temperature, hormone secretion and many other body functions in a 24-hour rhythm. For a westward time shift, the biological (circadian) system requires about 2 days to readjust the sleep-wake cycle, 5 for body temperature, and 8 days or more for other rhythms. Jet lag lasts longer and is more troublesome going east than west. Diabetics and heart patients must keep accurate track of time to take their medication as needed. People with angina or other heart trouble should beware of high altitudes and bring plenty of their prescribed medication. (Bring twice the usual amount in case the stay is extended.)

- *Travel tip #9*

Do not swim, wade or even dabble in unknown, untreated fresh waters (chlorinated swimming pools are fine). Many water-dwelling parasites in hot climates can enter the skin, including schistosomiasis. Schistosomas are blood flukes that go from snails to humans and then back again from human feces to snails. The schistosome parasites are released by snails into the water (river stream or pond) and infect people by penetrating the skin. Once inside the body, they travel through the bloodstream and damage the large intestine, bladder liver and lungs. Schistosomiasis, also known as bilharzia, is prevalent in all African fresh waters, the Middle East, the Caribbean, parts of South America and Southeast Asia. Ask about contamination before wading, swimming or plunging into foreign waters. If accidentally wet, dry off as fast as possible.

- *Travel tip #10*

Be wary of your means of transportation in foreign places. Next to heart disease and cancer the next major cause of death among vacationers is motor vehicle accidents. Travelers should avoid overcrowded public vehicles and especially motorcycles (the number-one killer abroad). Rural travel should never be attempted at night. Taxi drivers who are reckless or drive too fast should be cautioned. Always buckle up—if there's a seatbelt! Know your blood type. If you need a transfusion and have time, locate blood that's been tested and shown free of HIV (AIDS) and hepatitis B viruses, and call your embassy (or other official representation).

HINTS FOR AVOIDING TRAVELER'S DIARRHEA

- Avoid salads and raw vegetables (often contaminated by night-soil—excrement used as fertilizer) and dressings such as mayonnaise. Eat only freshly cooked, hot vegetables.
- Wash all fruit and vegetables with previously boiled or bottled water.
- Tomatoes should also be washed, and should be unbruised.
- Eat no leftovers.
- Don't use food from bent or dented cans.
- Avoid buffets or a "chef's special table," particularly if food is outdoors and exposed to flies. Cold meats provide an excellent milieu for infective organisms, particularly in tropical heat and humidity. Stick to well-cooked meats, served hot. (Even in Canada, eaters of raw sushi risk infection.)
- Stay away from unpasteurized ice-cream and other dairy foods. Tuberculosis and brucellosis may be passed on from infected cow's milk, and contaminated water may be added to milk to make it go farther! Consume only dairy products labeled as "pasteurized."
- Avoid ice cubes. Freezing water does not kill organisms, nor does the alcohol in a drink (although strong liquor does reduce bacterial numbers).
- Don't swim, wade or wash in unfamiliar fresh or sea water, only in chlorinated pools. Swimming in the ocean is safe only if the beach is far from the mouth of a river or sewage outlet.
- Remember that besides traveler's diarrhea, which is usually mild and self-limiting, other diseases with diarrhea as a symptom—such as typhoid, cholera, hepatitis and parasitic infections—can be acquired from contaminated food and drink producing bloody stool, fever and other symptoms besides diarrhea.

MELATONIN UPDATE: CAN IT RELIEVE JET LAG?

In recent years, melatonin has been touted as a "wonder drug," but researchers and government officials warn that claims for its therapeutic benefits are vastly overrated and unproven. The only evidence-based benefits of melatonin in humans are its ability to combat sleep disorders, reset the biological clock and perhaps overcome jet lag. Despite no scientific confirmation of its benefits, melatonin sells well across the United States, where it is classed as a "food supplement." In Canada, it is classified as a drug. Until proper large-scale random studies have been done, its efficacy, benefits and safety remain to be proven. Researchers caution that the tablets sold in health stores (usually in 1 to 5 mg doses) produce blood concentrations 10 to 100 times higher than the usual night-time peak, with long-term effects, safety and efficacy still to be determined.

What is melatonin?

Melatonin is a hormone secreted by the brain's tiny pea-sized pineal gland during the hours of darkness, in tune with a natural circadian or 24-hour rhythm. Only in the 1950s did scientists find that the gland produces melatonin, its output stimulated by the dark and suppressed by light. In humans, melatonin secretion starts in the evening, promoting drowsiness, a drop in body temperature and reduced secretion of some hormones such as corticosteroids. Any bright light above a certain intensity—whether from natural daylight, fluorescent or ordinary indoor lighting—inhibits its secretion. Researchers are studying how the substance could be used to help those with sleep-wake disorders and to reset the body's biological clock in shift workers and travelers.

Melatonin, jet lag and shift work

Melatonin may help globe-trotters who cross several time zones recover more quickly from jet lag—disturbed sleep, daytime drowsiness, irritability and diminished concentration—by helping to reset the circadian rhythm or body's biological clock.

Modern jet travel disrupts that rhythm, putting the body out of kilter with activities at the arrival zone—rising time, work schedule, mealtimes, bedtime. Melatonin can accelerate "entrainment" of the biological clock. In one experiment 28 travelers flying between New Zealand and England were given 5 mg of melatonin at bedtime 3 days before and 3 days after their flights. The hormone reduced the severity of jet lag and its duration by a couple of days. However, a trial following 257 Norwegian physicians who had visited New York City for 5 days were randomized to either placebo or 1 of 3 doses of melatonin (5.0 mg at bedtime, 0.5 mg at bedtime, and 0.5 mg taken on a shifting schedule, showed no benefit to melatonin. Although scientists are optimistic that large-scale studies may establish melatonin as a useful sleep aid, they are skeptical of claims for other benefits that come from poorly designed studies.

No serious side effects have been reported from the occasional use of melatonin. The U.S. Food and Drug Administration has had only four reports of side effects, none serious. Informal surveys suggest that some who take melatonin experience nightmares, headaches, depression and morning drowsiness. But the hormone's physiological effects—lowered body temperature, increased drowsiness, decreased alertness and possible effects on reproductive function—need to be evaluated. The effects of high doses of melatonin are unknown; they could interfere with the body's own production of the hormone or with the production of other hormones such as estrogen or testosterone. Studies must also determine how melatonin interacts with other drugs, such as antidepressants, and its effects in the elderly. The U.S. National Institute of Aging is launching a major clinical trial to test melatonin's efficacy and safety as a sleep aid for the elderly.

Despite the fact that its sale remains illegal in many countries, people flock to buy the hormone. For them, the experts have a few cautionary tips:

• Consult a physician before using the drug, especially if you are also taking other medications.
• If using it for occasional (not chronic) insomnia, take a *very low dose*—0.1 to 0.3 mg—about half an hour before bed.
• Don't take melatonin if you:

- are pregnant or breastfeeding (its effects on the fetus or breastfed babies are unknown);
- are depressed or taking drugs for depression (it may worsen depression);
- are trying to get pregnant (melatonin has been found to have contraceptive effects in large doses):
- have a severe allergy or autoimmune disease, such as arthritis or diabetes (it may affect the immune system).
- Children, who produce high levels of melatonin naturally, should not take the hormone.

In conclusion

Usually sold in a synthetic rather than natural form, the melatonin product currently available may be adulterated or unsafe. Laboratory analysis of some showed no trace of the hormone; others contained various contaminants. The wise course at present is to refrain from taking it until we have more evidence about its benefits and risks.

Home again—what to do on your return

Since infections can remain latent in your body for a long time before erupting, it's a good idea to be on the lookout for their signs and symptoms during and after distant travels. See your physician if you feel at all unwell, feverish or overly tired, or if you have persistent diarrhea. Report any unusual swelling, skin rash, sore or itch. Tell your physician where you have been,

and about any medical complaints or treatments while you were away. And be sure to keep on taking your antimalarial drugs for the full 4 weeks after you are back.

For more travel health information, contact public-health units or travel clinics (where they exist) in hospitals—such as those in Toronto at the Toronto Hospital, tel.: (416) 595-3670, or St. Michael's Hospital, tel.: (416) 360–4000; your family physician; Health and Welfare Canada offices; CATMAT (The Committee to Advise on Tropical Medicine and Travel)—established by Health Canada and its websites. Or consult Missionary Health Institute International Travel Services, tel.: (416) 494–7512, 4000 Leslie Street, Willowdale, ON M2K 2R9. Consult MMWR (Morbidity and Mortality Weekly Report from the U.S. Centers for Disease Control), which has a supplement called "Health Advice for International Travel" providing updates on current recommendations and infectious-disease outbreaks around the world—the travel expert's "bible," at www.cdc.gov.travel. Read "Don't Drink the Water," published by the Canadian Society for International Health and the Canadian Public Health Association. See the Canadian "Recommendations for Preventing and Treating Malaria among International Travellers," published by CATMAT, or contact the International Association for Medical Assistance to Travelers (IAMAT); in Ontario, call (416) 652–0137.

Coping with mental and emotional problems

Where does stress come from? • Coping with stress • Depression • Modern treatments • Depressive variants • Holiday blues • Manic depression • Chronic fatigue syndrome • The disabling effects of anxiety disorders • Schizophrenia • Finding therapy for mental and emotional problems

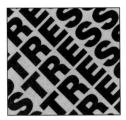 HEALTH SURVEYS consistently reveal that 15 percent or more of North Americans have emotional or mental disturbances severe enough to require professional help. Mental health problems range from stress-related discomforts to anxiety disorders and phobias—and at the far end of the scale—mental illnesses such as schizophrenia. Since anxiety, depression and other mental disorders may express themselves in physical terms, it's not always easy for physicians to discern the underlying problem.

According to one University of Toronto professor of psychiatry, mental and emotional disorders often masquerade or "somatize" as physical ailments. In fact, more than 50 percent of people with psychosocial distress first present to doctors with physical complaints, such as muscle aches, headache, back pain, dizziness, nervousness, digestive upsets, sleeplessness and fatigue. Somatization is defined as "a tendency to express emotional or mental disturbances in physical terms, especially common in those with anxiety disorders or depression." The psychiatrist explains that "Somatizers typically find it difficult to acknowledge emotional upsets, personal feelings, losses or conflict. They may view mental or emotional disturbances as a weakness, preferring to assume the sick role because of organic ailments—such as allergy or fatigue

syndromes—which are regarded as beyond control and not one's fault." In other words, somatization helps people unconsciously disguise the reasons for the distress and so avoid the stigma of mental illness. According to psychiatrists, some chronic somatizers will embrace each "newly discovered, poorly defined, fashionable ailment," such as candidiasis (bodily yeast invasion), "Yuppie flu" or twentieth-century allergy disease, to explain undiagnosed complaints of unwellness.

WHERE DOES STRESS COME FROM?

Stress, which is the demand placed upon the body's physical and mental reserves, is essential to human productivity. Without it we become passive and wither—as sometimes happens when people are bored or unoccupied, or retire without planning ahead. A little stress acts as a human motivator and mobilizer making us more alert and "on the ball." Students, for example, often do best with the pressure of exams: athletes may excel under the tension of a race: actors deliver their best lines before an audience rather than during rehearsal.

While stress can improve performance, too much is counterproductive. Everyone is exposed to some everyday stress, but how much is too much? In one evaluation, the stress levels of various events were rated comparatively. Ranked in order of highest to lowest stress-producers were: death of a spouse or other loved one, divorce, jail term,

14

SOME SIGNS OF MENTAL OR EMOTIONAL DISTURBANCE

- **A pervasive sense of helplessness;**
- **inability to function normally;**
- **unexplained anxiety;**
- **irrational fears;**
- **worry or anxiety out of proportion to the actual stressors experienced**
- **incapacitating fatigue;**
- **sleep disturbances— unusual difficulty falling asleep, frequent nighttime awakening;**

- **diminished concentration powers, wandering attention;**
- **nervous restlessness;**
- **unmerited guilt feelings;**
- **obsessional behavior (e.g., checking endlessly to see if the stove's turned off or the toothpaste cap is in place);**
- **unshakable thought preoccupation (overriding usual interests and social interaction);**

- **lack of interest in family, friends; neglect of usual companions;**
- **dismal outlook, negative thoughts, crumbling defense mechanisms—a feeling of nothing working out "as it should";**
- **diminished sense of self-worth (a frequent sign of depression).**

robberies/hold-ups, personal injury, being fired, getting married, retirement, illness of a relative, moving house, changing schools, children leaving home, trouble with in-laws, mortgage foreclosure, workplace conflicts, holidays (especially Christmas).

What is stress?

There is no universally accepted definition of stress. Some psychologists define it as "a reaction to an observable event (stressor) that influences the person in a harmful way." Others call stress "a situation where the internal or external demands exceed the person's coping skills." Stress is harmful only if the events or situations causing it are *perceived* as burdensome, and if the body cannot adapt to the demands made upon it. Failure to adapt to stress may cause hormone changes that ultimately damage health.

Scientifically, stress is a "state of arousal" in which psychological, physiological and biochemical changes are provoked by specific stressors. A stressor is any force, change or event that calls upon a person's coping skills and inner resources. Stressors may be positive or negative. For instance, a job promotion or marriage, although a welcome event, nonetheless produces stress by necessitating change. A negative stressor such as a loved one's death or losing a job, brings disturbing stress.

Stressors may be acute (such as nuclear accidents, divorce, bereavement), developmental (such as marriage, adolescence, a job promotion), or ongoing (such as poverty or an alcoholic parent). Workplace stressors include job overload or underload, time pressures, role ambiguity (uncertainty about lines of responsibility), role conflict (simultaneously trying to please those above and under oneself), fear of making mistakes, thwarted career plans, underused skills, lack of control, lack of promotion, shift work, an aggravating work environment (noise pollution, cigarette smoke, inadequate safety precautions).

Certain workplace stressors may be an integral part of the job. Telephone operators, for example, undergo stress from being constantly monitored for their voice and client approach, while also being bombarded with consumer questions they can't answer—about weather conditions, road reports, hospitals, restaurants and movies. Bus drivers too are plagued by job stress, pressured by the simultaneous need to meet schedules, be polite to passengers and deal with traffic. Worldwide, bus drivers suffer more than most employees from stress-related gastrointestinal disorders and hypertension (high blood pressure).

Tracing the stress pathway

Evolution marvelously prepared human beings to react to danger through the "fight-or-flight" response. In the immediate, alarm stage of this reaction, the adrenal glands release stimulatory hormones, the heart races to send oxygen faster around the body, extra glucose is supplied for energy, the hair "stands on end" (a throwback to the days when our heavy body-hair made us look larger), blood is diverted from the gut to the working muscles, and other changes make the body stronger and swifter. But this fight-or-flight response—very apt for fighting or fleeing tigers—hardly equips us to face most stressors of modern life. Imagine a car alarm that's occasionally very useful, but loses its utility if it goes off all the time.

Continued or frequent stress results in profound physical, emotional and psychological

STRESS PATHWAY

| Stressor | → | Perception | → | Response | → | Outcomes |

Stressor

A change, event or situation that calls upon inner resources to adapt to or neutralize it.

Perception

How the stressor—event situation or change—is perceived; e.g., as a threat or as a challenge that might promote growth.

Response

Short-term
Alarm/light-or-flight reaction.
Rise in adrenal medulla hormones, increased heartrate, blood sugar.

Long-term

		Outcomes
Physical:	Increased corticoid hormones	Changes in blood lipids (fats)
	Exhaustion	Peptic ulcers
	Elevated blood pressure	Reduced immune defenses
	Gastrointestinal upsets	
	Appetite changes	
Emotional:	Shock	Depression
	Denial	Burnout
	Anxiety	
Cognitive and Behavioral:	Self-medication	Chronic alcoholism/drug addiction
	Refusal to face situation	Hide and give up
	or	or
	Rational problem solving	Rise to challenge and develop more coping skills

N.B.: At each arrow, many individual factors influence the reaction.

---

changes. Skyrocketing levels of corticoid (adrenal gland) hormones and other biochemical changes can lead to extreme exhaustion; physical ailments such as chronic muscle aches, headaches and back pain; anxiety disorders; poor concentration; insomnia; social isolation; depression; burnout; high blood pressure; heart disease; weakened immune defenses (with increased risks of infection); and escape into alcohol and/or other drug abuse.

One person's challenge is another's threat

The amount of stress people can handle depends on genetic makeup, upbringing, coping mechanisms and social support. Reactions to a stressor also vary depending on the way we perceive it. While the outcome of stress can be very damaging, what one person finds devastating may stimulate another. In some people a stressful challenge even leads to personal growth and better coping mechanisms. Compare one widow who, unable to face her loss, never ventured out and became clinically depressed, to another who, after mourning her

husband's death, took up a career and found satisfaction in new relationships.

These individual differences explain why—faced with events such as war hijacking, job demotion or relocation—people react differently. The same situation can seem challenging ("the spice of life") or terrifying ("the kiss of death"), depending on how it's interpreted. Thus, a new supervisor added duties or office computerization may present an intriguing challenge to some, while in others it provokes terror. Or a noon-hour fitness class may relieve tension in some but prove stressful to others who, perhaps, dislike group activities or hate wearing shorts. Jumping out of an airplane would daunt most of us, but is exhilarating to those who choose it as a personal challenge.

It's a fallacy to think that only high-level occupations or positions induce stress. Although executives, bureau chiefs and medical officers do bear heavy burdens—for looking after money, human beings and resources—they also possess the authority to carry through their aims. Bosses who "run the ship" tend to be less

THE OUTCOME OF STRESS IS INFLUENCED BY:

- family background—for instance, whether there is a predisposition to depression, heart ailments or alcoholism;
- learned behavior and upbringing—someone who was taught problem-solving skills and acquired self-esteem at a parent's knee is likely to cope better with stress than a child of more punitive or authoritarian parents;
- mindset—individual cognitive (thinking) styles. A flexible, constructive, "problem-solving" mode in the face of difficulties, rather than panic, improves stress management;
- social support—having close relatives and friends to share problems with;
- a sense of "belonging" to a religious, national, ethnic or other group;
- solidarity with compatible colleagues and fellow workers who can give practical advice and "cover" when asked. A study of air-traffic controllers showed that those with close confidantes suffered fewer headaches, sleep disturbances, anxiety and other signs of stress.

stressed than subordinates who shoulder responsibility but have little overall control. Assistants, secretaries and nurses, who often bear front-line responsibility for making things run smoothly but lack the authority to make decisions, are highly prone to stress. Traditionally, middle managers suffer the most stress. Consider three key aspects of a job: the amount of control you have over it, the degree of responsibility it entails, and the reward you receive for doing it. The person working on an assembly line, who has a fair amount of responsibility, but has no control over the speed at which the line moves and receives little pay, can certainly experience more stress than the manager who has greater responsibility, but far more control over the job situation.

People who allow others to make all their decisions can also suffer great stress, particularly if suddenly forced by circumstances (perhaps a death or separation from a spouse) to abandon the dependent role and take on responsibility. The ability to make decisions about your life is called "locus of control." Although some things are certainly beyond one's control, it is healthier to feel that most aspects of your life are within your internal control.

The three Cs that lessen stress

People who feel in control of their own actions and on top of circumstances tend to deal more effectively with stress than those who see themselves as helpless victims buffeted by adverse circumstances. A recent study of executives showed that under prolonged stress some (but not others) developed hypertension and heart disease. Those who successfully withstood long-term stress not only felt "in command" but also had a so-called hardy personality, exemplified by the three Cs: Control, Commitment and Challenge.

Effective stress-copers were *confidently* in control—with faith in their own abilities; were *committed* to any task in hand; and welcomed *challenge*. They tended to be involved in many activities—whether work, family or social—and viewed change, even if stressful, as part of life, not something aimed personally at them. Being curious and confident, they sought new ways to overcome setbacks and surmount hurdles. Lack of control combined with high pressure is a deadly stress combination.

COPING WITH STRESS

Stress-managing skills include the ability to communicate and share feelings, thoughts and problems—dialoguing with others at work or at home—and to put expectations in line with reality. Gaining control and learning to take charge of one's life is another powerful stress-coping strategy. Regular exercise helps to reduce tension. However, experts warn against regarding exercise, jogging or other sports as a panacea for stress reduction, since overachievers often take the same compulsive attitude to exercise programs as to the rest of life, and may become stressed by activities undertaken for relaxation!

General stress-management programs

Stress-management courses and programs help people change the way they perceive and respond to stress. The biggest predictor of stress is one's own interpretation of it. For some people stress is a welcome challenge or interesting exercise in problem-solving. For others, coping with stress is difficult and requires self-therapy such as using relaxation techniques, deep-breathing routines, music therapy, power naps, mind-focusing techniques, meditation, exercise and biofeedback. Most people try to

PRACTICAL TIPS FOR COPING WITH STRESS

- Ferret out your particular set of stressors and assess which are avoidable, which not; avoid the avoidable.
- Try to alter or remove stress-provoking situations.
- Do frequent reality checks.
- Take stock of priorities—decide what's a "must" and what can be deferred or delegated.
- Assess expectations and their achievability, admitting that no one can always be perfect.
- Get rid of unrealistic expectations of yourself and others.
- Adopt a flexible "problem-solving"

mode in the face of difficulties.
- Confide in others, share emotions and worries.
- Don't condemn yourself for failure or occasional lapses.
- Neutralize or silence the inner "self-critic"—try to be kinder to yourself and more self-accepting (no one's perfect).
- Check your mindset from time to time: are there too many "shoulds," "oughts" or "must do's" in your head? (If so, try to eliminate some of them.)
- Restructure thinking patterns—downplay the negative and emphasize strengths and positive assets

rather than weaknesses.
- Adopt a philosophy of uncertainty to replace rigid anticipation.
- Dissect and analyze your work situation—its demands and benefits.
- Improve time-management; space and pace work better. Parcel tasks into smaller portions.
- Diversify interests, cultivate hobbies, cherish relationships.
- Practise "detached concern" rather than overinvolvement.
- Try to turn stress into a positive challenge whenever possible.
- Learn relaxation techniques such as "power napping"

visualization (imagining a soothing activity to attain tranquillity).
- Use mind-focusing strategies, repetition of personally meaningful words or phrases to help you calm down.
- Experiment with music therapy. sound tapes and soothing imagery.
- Incorporate rest periods into daily schedule; make time to be good to yourself at least once a day. (For mothers, that's often after midnight when everyone else's needs have been met—try to change that routine!)
- Find time to exercise whenever possible—

try yoga, Tai-chi, walking, swimming (whatever works for you).
- Get advice on managing leisure time and vacations—perhaps take several small holidays rather than one long one (which can bring its own stresses).
- Consider what you can "control" and what you cannot. Focus on solving the problems you can control or manage to deal with. Try to evaluate and cope with problems you can't control by putting them into perspective so they don't become all-encompassing or overwhelming.

improve their sense of personal control. Therapists who can help with this range from medically trained psychiatrists to social workers, psychologists, relaxation therapists, massage therapists and employee assistance counselors.

Occupational burnout

"Burnout"—a popular but misapplied catchword—is often used to mean "stressed out" or exhausted by job-related activities. The term has become part of our modern vocabulary, loosely used for anyone who devotes too much time and energy to specific activities. There is considerable debate about the validity of this label applied to the complex, psychobiological outcomes of stress.

The term "burnout" was coined during the 1970s as street slang for excessive drug use, and later adopted to denote stress among healthcare personnel such as nurses, social workers and physicians, especially those working in pedi-

atric wards, intensive-care and psychiatric units. Nurses caring for sick infants frequently became emotionally attached to their tiny patients, suffering stress for those who later died. In these situations, health professionals complained of irritability, anxiety, apathy, exhaustion and an inability to carry on. Psychologists attributed the syndrome to the relentless stress of daily exposure to conditions that were physically and emotionally taxing, and often worsened by budget cuts and staff shortages.

The concept of occupational burnout has since spread to people in many occupations, such as teachers, homemakers, air-traffic controllers, transit workers, administrators, dentists and lawyers (particularly those dealing with low-income clients). Experts emphasize, however, that burnout is a complex interaction between the job and people who tend to overinvest in their work.

A classic example of burnout is that of an

STAGES AND SIGNS OF BURNOUT

Stage 1: *The "eager beaver"*
- Overly high expectations of self and job.
- Feeling of omnipotence, perfectionism: "I can do anything"; "I will conquer all"; "I will never make mistakes."
- Idealistic, single-minded attitude.
- Unrealistic concept that job should be 100 percent satisfying.
- Expectation of continual praise and approval.
- Inability to detach from work situation.

Stage 2: *Disillusionment*
- Job not measuring up to expectations or fulfilling hopes.
- Guilt if any time taken off for self.
- Trying even harder; striving and pushing more.
- Dissatisfaction with own performance.
- Progressive loss of self-confidence.
- Reduced enthusiasm and creativity; disenchantment.
- Disappointment in coworkers.
- Sense of being unappreciated.
- Becoming impatient and argumentative.

Stage 3: Frustration
- Increasing fatigue, irritability, angry outbursts.
- Lowered job performance and morale; inappropriate reactions to people or situations, bitter remarks.
- Repetitive accidents, unfinished tasks.
- Spending more time achieving less.

- Finding fault with everyone and everything.
- Callous, detached attitude.
- Hostility toward formerly revered supervisors or well-liked colleagues.
- Denial of emotions, feelings; not sharing or discussing thoughts.
- Restless search for risky diversions (e.g., parachuting, deep-sea diving).
- Boredom, bouts of absenteeism.

Stage 4: Despair and apathy
- Negative self-image; sense of failure.
- Apathy, loss of energy, resignation.
- Helplessness, sense of drowning.
- Alienation, emptiness, refusal to see friends.
- Conflict-laden dreams.
- Neglected personal appearance.
- Extreme cynicism: the former workaholic, having lost all devotion to the cause, becomes increasingly bitter.
- Forgetting appointments, deadlines.
- Losing possessions.
- Rash of minor physical ailments—headaches, stomach upsets, bowel problems, colds, backaches.
- Morbid fear of death.
- Mental, physical and emotional exhaustion—spiritual malaise
- The endpoint of burnout—inability to continue daily activities.

intensive-care nurse who, having entered her career with idealistic hopes, found that, despite her dedication and best efforts, many patients—

IT'S NOT JUST THE INDIVIDUAL'S PROBLEM

Since the reasons for job stress stem jointly from the organization and the individual, minimizing it should also be a shared venture. Healthy organizational approaches could include the following:
- Allowing workers to participate in decisions that affect their jobs.

- Job rotation to give periodic relief from front-line positions—perhaps by temporary transfer to an administrative, training or research position.
- Organizational attempts to foster peer support networks, either through team-building or by allotting

time to discussion of staff stress.
- Feedback about performance; praise for tasks well done.
- Flexible schedules.
- Fitness programs to enhance well-being.
- Helping people channel stress, which is an integral part of existence, toward enhanced productivity.

including tiny children—failed to recover. Case loads were excessive, overtime was frequent and too little time was provided to comfort patients or relatives. Few thanks were given. Disappointed at her inability to save everyone, the lack of gratitude and the frustrations of the job the nurse would come home angry and "dump" on her husband, with uncontrollable crying fits. She finally lost all interest in both her patients and her household. The only solution was a complete break from nursing and a new career (She went back to school, with the financial support of her spouse, and became a librarian!)

Job-person mismatch is usually to blame

The job environment alone is rarely responsible for occupational burnout; there's no such thing as a job that's equally taxing for all. Job stress arises not just from the specific task but from the *interaction* of the person and the job. If the demands of a position exceed someone's abilities, or if an employee lacks the mental agility needed, that position will prove stressful for that individual. For example, a job that requires typing at 80 words per minute will pressure someone who can do only 40 words per minute. A job that requires knowledge of math will prove stressful to someone who dropped it in Grade 9. Working in an air-traffic control tower may seem extremely stressful, but given the necessary expertise, together with a personality that thrives on a hectic pace, it may in fact be exciting.

Occupational stress is likely to produce burnout in people with unrealistic notions about their own capacities and what the job can offer. It is common in those who devote their "all" to work and little to outside interests. Burnout is often seen in "type-A" overachievers. The type-A personality is said to have free-floating hostility and overaggressive competitiveness, typified by a confrontational approach, a tendency to shout, abuse and blame others and "hurry-sickness"—an exaggerated sense of urgency, and a compulsion to do everything in a rush rather than ponder actions. Others who fall prey to job stress may have striven too hard to reach their goal, or may have exaggerated expectations.

Experts warn against jumping to the conclusion that someone is "burned out" when the symptoms may stem from another disorder. Burnout must be differentiated from depression and other mental illnesses before diagnosis is made. Signs of depression often mimic those of burnout—namely, changes in sleep patterns (typically early awakening), diminished appetite, diurnal mood swings (feeling low in the morning, more cheerful as the day progresses), muscular fatigue (as if "walking through molasses"), a dry mouth.

DEPRESSION: MORE THAN JUST TRANSIENT BLUES

Occasionally feeling glum and discouraged is a normal response to the strains and stresses of everyday life; sporadic bouts of the blues may arise because of some loss or disappointment or for no obvious reason. But although such spells are colloquially described as "depression," the term really refers to a clinical mood or "affective" disorder or disturbance that needs professional help. Effective treatment is now available and in most cases can do much to alleviate the misery of true depression, even though, to those in its grip, recovery often seems impossible.

Health professionals subdivide depressive illnesses into unipolar and bipolar forms. If depression is the only mood (affective) disturbance, the disorder has one "pole" and is called *unipolar depressive disorder*. If there are alternating phases of depression and mania (exaggerated elation or "highs"), with mood swings at two extreme poles, the condition is termed *bipolar disorder*—also known as manic-depressive disorder or "la folie circulaire" (circular insanity).

Clinical depression (unipolar disorder)

True *clinical depression* is a definite psychiatric illness accompanied by changes in brain chemistry. It is an affective or mood disorder with emotional, cognitive (thinking), behavioral and physical changes that require medical treatment. Truly depressed people may lose touch with reality and barely summon up the will to eat, speak or move. Depression may occur reactively—in reaction to some negative life event, loss or tragedy—or it can hit like a bolt from the blue. In the past, depression was viewed as a weakness or personality flaw to be overcome by greater resolve or strength of character. Today, it's regarded as a serious illness with biological, social, emotional and psychological aspects that can be treated with antidepressant medications and psychotherapy.

The tendency to clinical depression may be inherited and the mood change may be precipitated by a crisis or loss such as the death of someone close, a relationship breakup, divorce, move or career disappointment. Sexual or other abuse may be an underlying trigger. Stress due to working conditions, role conflicts, financial worries, interpersonal problems or other stressors can lead to a major depression. Certain drugs (such as tranquilizers, blood pressure medications, codeine and indomethacin) can also trigger it.

A HISTORIC, UNIVERSAL AND RAVAGING AFFLICTION

Depression respects no boundaries, affecting people of all races, religions and cultures. One early account of depression is the Biblical story of King Saul, whose episodes of despair were relieved only when David, the Bethlehem shepherd boy, played his harp. As his illness progressed, the king's black moods became less and less affected by the shepherd's music, and ultimately Saul killed himself. The list of historic figures who suffered from depression includes George Washington, Charles Darwin, Lord Byron, Abraham Lincoln and Winston Churchill—who named depression his "black dog." Shakespeare called depression that "sad companion, dull-eyed melancholy," and Sigmund Freud, who wrote extensively about it as "separation loss," self-treated his depressive episodes with opium. In our era, those who have admitted to battling the affliction include media mogul Ted Turner, writer Sylvia Plath (who committed suicide), actress Margot Kidder and poet Leonard Cohen.

Too few of the depressed seek or get proper help

Depression is far more prevalent than many realize. Overall, depressive illness affects 10 to 15 percent of North American men and 25 percent of women at least once in a lifetime. Employers notice increasing problems due to its debilitating effects, with a rising toll of absenteeism, lost productivity, re-staffing and financial costs. Prescriptions for antidepressants are soaring. But although safe, effective treatment is available, depression remains a much misunderstood, underdiagnosed and hugely undertreated condition. Despite long-standing recognition of the affliction and effective new treatments, good counseling services, mood disorder clinics and self-help groups, too few depressed people seek or get appropriate therapy.

Studies show that fewer than one-quarter of depressives seek medical therapy. Many depressed people are reluctant to admit to their distress or disclose emotional problems for fear of being condemned or labeled as "weak," and because of the continuing stigma of mental illness. The biggest hurdle in obtaining proper treatment is failure of both patients and doctors to recognize its symptoms and severity. Many of the depressed think they're just tired or "under the weather" (Pervasive fatigue is a telltale clue.) Those caught in its dark grip often believe recovery is impossible or not worth the effort, or that they do not deserve help. Some don't go for treatment because they're ashamed of having a mental disorder or think depression isn't a real sickness.

The increasing recognition of depression as an illness involving an imbalance in the brain's neurotransmitters has removed some of the stigma, misconception and mystery surrounding it. Once people realize that depression is not their fault, that it is not due to a character flaw but involves biochemical changes, many find it easier to accept and manage. People are urged to learn and watch for symptoms of depression, to know when and where to get professional advice. If one treatment doesn't work, another likely will, or combination therapy may do the trick. It is well worth seeking expert help from the family physician, a psychiatrist, employee assistance unit or one of the new mood disorder clinics.

Women are more prone to depression than men

In all cultures, many more women than men suffer from depression. "Overwhelmingly," says the head of a women's health program, "women list social factors as key sources of stress, fatigue and depression." They are stressed by role conflicts, and by being "torn in different directions" through a combination of home duties and outside work, child care, sleep deprivation, financial burdens, relationship worries, lack of emotional support, "too little control over their lives" and insufficient exercise. Harassment, victimization, violence, abuse and poverty can all play a part. Young, unemployed women, especially single mothers living alone with dependent children, are particularly prone to depression.

How to recognize clinical depression

Major depression is considered a serious illness that requires professional treatment. It is diagnosed in North America by criteria defined in *the Diagnostic and Statistical Manual of Mental Disorders* (4th edition) or DSM-IV (published in 1994 by the American Psychiatric Association). In severe depression, the mood becomes joyless and thought patterns negative; actions often slow down as though the person is heavily burdened. The key alerting symptoms of serious depression are *anhedonia* (a persistently low mood, loss of interest or pleasure in activities

SIGNS AND SYMPTOMS OF CLINICAL DEPRESSION

Criteria that identify a major depressive episode:

A major depressive syndrome is characterized by a deeply despondent or sad mood and pervasive loss of pleasure lasting a minimum of 2 weeks along with at least four of the following symptoms:

- poor appetite and weight loss (or increased appetite and weight gain)
- energy diminution
- fatigue and weakness
- sleeping poorly or oversleeping (altered sleep rhythm)
- sluggishness, slowed movements or restless agitation and jumpiness
- anxiety, helplessness, despair
- loss of interest in usual activities
- reduced sex drive
- slowed, confused thinking, inability to concentrate
- unusual indecisiveness
- self-reproach, feelings of worthlessness
- inappropriate guilts
- crying spells, recurrent brooding, suicidal thoughts

N.B.: Symptoms must be present almost every day for 2 or more weeks, be severe enough to impair everyday functioning, occur without other medical conditions (such as diabetes, anemia, thyroid dysfunction) and not be preceded by other psychiatric disorders (such as schizophrenia). In children under 6, at least three of the first four symptoms should be present for at least 2 weeks, nearly every day (with a constantly sad expression and inability to cry).

N.B.: Depression often accompanies certain diseases as lung, pancreatic and other cancers, hypothyroidism and drug/alcohol abuse; it can be induced by certain medications, such as anti-hypertensives (blood pressure drugs) and steroids.

In fact, depression may be the first indicator of certain physical diseases, requiring treatment both for depressive and disease symptoms.

Common signs and symptoms by which to recognize clinical depression:

1. PHYSICAL (VEGETATIVE) CHANGES:
- *Appetite and weight disturbances.* Waning appetite and weight loss, a bad taste or a dry mouth and altered bowel habits may signal depression; the depressed person may become thin and haggard. Paradoxically, a few depressives overeat and rapidly gain weight.
- *Sleep and circadian rhythm alterations.* Many depressives have distorted circadian rhythms (biological clocks), with disturbed sleep patterns. Typically, depressives awaken early in the morning and lie awake brooding. Trouble falling asleep and night-insomnia can occur but are more characteristic of anxiety. Many depressed people sleep less than usual, awaken in the middle of the night, perhaps weeping inconsolably. Hypersomnia (oversleeping), where the

depressed sleep as much as 12 to 14 hours nightly, can occur, but is less common. Rapid eye movement (REM) sleep (with dreaming) tends to be more frequent, the dream state coming on more abruptly and vividly than normal, although the total amount of dream-time may be below normal.
- *Slowed movement.* The depressed seem to droop, sag and walk slowly—as though laboring under a great weight. But psychomotor agitation can also occur, with twitchy restlessness. Depressives may find it hard to sit still; they may pace up and down, wring their hands, pull at their hair or twist objects interminably in their hands.
- *Waning sex drive.*
- *Loss of energy, weakness and extreme fatigue.* No "get up and go," a reluctance to dress, go to work or do tiny chores (which appear as monumental tasks).

2. EMOTIONAL FACTORS:
- *Lack of interest, feelings, pleasure, merriment and inability to have fun.* The most universal sign of depression is an absence of pleasure in activities which normally give satisfaction. An expressionless, blank face, emptiness, numbness, reduced eye-scanning, a downcast look or a slow, monotonous voice can signal the mood change. Severely depressed patients may become unable to move, eat or talk, all willpower seemingly gone.
- *Anxiety.* Some 60–70 percent of depressives feel anxious with impaired autonomic (involuntary) nervous system control (resulting in increased heart rate, blood pressure and respiration).
- *Irritability and unusual hostility.* The depressed may appear abnormally upset by minor unpleasant events that increase their sense of guilt and worthlessness, with sudden outbursts.

3. COGNITIVE (THINKING) DISTORTIONS:
- *Loss of concentration and decision-making ability.* Impeded performance can magnify feelings of self-doubt and failure, especially in perfectionists who recognize their reduced mental prowess; the simplest decisions—such as writing a letter or beginning a meal—may take hours.
- *A sense of worthlessness.* Rumination about faults and failures, either real or imaginary, is common. Plagued by remorse, depressives blame themselves for their illness, insisting they have let others down—a disturbed judgment about which it is usually impossible to reason.
- *A hopelessly bleak outlook.* All goals—including recovery—seem unattainable.
- *Hypochondriacal preoccupation about health.* Exaggerated, unfounded fears of nonexistent madness or impending death are common.
- *Suicidal thoughts and death wishes.* The unendurable prospect of continued misery often involves amazingly well-constructed plans that may be hinted at and, unless picked up and dealt with, may lead to a successful suicide or repeated attempts to terminate life.

that usually give pleasure), a pervasive sense of sadness or emptiness, and deep feelings of inadequacy or worthlessness. In diagnosing major depression, the loss of pleasure and despondent feelings beyond the bounds of normal behavior must last at least two weeks. For a confirmed diagnosis of major depression, the person must have exhibited either the continually despondent mood or loss of pleasure in usual activities (anhedonia) for a minimum of 2 weeks, along with four other symptoms from a specified list (see box). People with anhedonia and fewer than four other symptoms may have just moderate to minor depression.

Sleep disturbances are a common sign of depression and the very first sign of depression is often extreme fatigue and disturbed sleep patterns (especially awakening early). Typically, depressed people feel worst in the morning, with a gradual mood lift as the day wears on. Other warning signs include sluggishness and slowed movements or psychomotor agitation (restless fidgeting) and excessive feelings of worthlessness. Accompanying features may include anxiety, chest tightness, loss of appetite, weight changes, decreased concentration, slowed thinking, difficulty making decisions and a waning sex drive. The classic depressive is a self-critical brooder, interminably mulling over shortcomings. Many have a very low sense of self-worth, guilt feelings over minor incidents, thinking they're "no good." Many are obsessed with thoughts of death and suicide. We all have occasional "blue" days, but when a person's low mood and lack of pleasure are overwhelming, affecting every aspect of life at home and at work, it is time to seek professional help.

Depression in children is often hard to recognize. In young children it frequently reveals itself by a constant woefulness despite a reluctance to cry, or in school by behavioral or learning problems, withdrawal, antisocial actions, slow speech, reading difficulties and refusal to attend class.

During adolescence, depression may produce antisocial or aggressive behavior, perhaps accompanied by grouchiness, withdrawal from the family, irritability and inexplicably worsening school grades. It can lead to suicide attempts, and parents who notice such changes should keep a sharp and vigilant eye on their teenager and have the behavior investigated by a professional caregiver or counselor, perhaps with referral to a psychiatrist.

Among the elderly its signs—appetite loss, sleep problems, delusional thoughts—are often mistaken for signs of aging and not given proper attention. (About 3 percent of the elderly have clinical depression, but many more of those who live in institutions are affected.) Failure to treat depression correctly, especially in the "healthy elderly," leads to needless despair and suffering. It's often treated with tranquilizers rather than appropriate antidepressants, perhaps without taking into account drug interactions with other medications being taken. Correct treatment of depression in seniors can bring remarkable improvement in outlook and function, and may help avoid the suicide attempts so common among elderly men.

Many influences contribute to depression

Most experts believe there is no single cause of depression, that it is multifactorial and stems from a variety of biopsychosocial factors that include physical, biochemical, social, psychological and emotional influences. In adults, a tendency to depression may arise from a biological vulnerability coupled with such early predisposing factors as childhood abuse, deprivation or the loss of a loved companion or caregiver. An episode of depression may be triggered by adverse life events such as a relationship breakup, death of a cherished person, job loss or being forced to move. According to one University of Toronto expert, "Neither a biological, genetic or biochemical predisposition alone, nor environmental events, nor purely psychological reasons explain clinical depression." Depression often follows or accompanies a physical illness such as arthritis, hypothyroidism, Parkinson's disease or heart attacks.

The biological roots of depression

Modern evidence shows definite changes or an imbalance in neurotransmitters (chemical messengers) in the brains of many people with depression, mainly involving "amine type" transmitters such as serotonin and norepinephrine. Researchers believe that one or both of these transmitters may malfunction, be depleted or ineffective, during depressive episodes. This theory gains validity from the effectiveness of antidepressant medications that increase the transmitters' availability. Despite the biochemical abnormalities linked to depression, no clear cause-and-effect link has been defined. Nonetheless, antidepressant medications often help to redress the neurotransmitter imbalance.

The psychological roots of depression

Parental death or absence, feelings of abandonment, a disapproving or withdrawn parent or guardian, and a lack of intimacy, friendship and unconditional love during childhood, feelings of rejection and lengthy hospitalizations—before about age 6—can predispose someone to depression in later life. But the depression may also be triggered by some stressful experience—a career failure, relationship breakup, job loss or house move. Without other contributing reasons, childhood losses alone are unlikely to produce depressive illness.

Depression-prone individuals are sometimes described as dependent, insecure and introverted—perfectionists with obsessional traits and low stress tolerance. And although the theory is controversial, some experts say depressives tend to depend on the external approval of others for self-esteem rather than relying upon innate or inner qualities.

The genetic connection

Clinical depression tends to run in families. Those with siblings, parents or other relatives who are or have been depressed are at above-average risk. Although a genetic influence may predispose someone to depression, several twin studies show that biological reasons alone do not necessarily produce the condition, but do so only in combination with other forces or events.

Depression may lurk beneath physical complaints

Clinical depression often hides behind physical symptoms such as stomach upsets, neckache, backache or loss of sex drive. This "somatization" can make it hard for unwary physicians to detect the underlying problem. Misled by the vehemence of physical complaints, they may prescribe remedies that can't relieve symptoms because the depression hasn't been diagnosed. The depressed often "doctor shop," visiting one physician after another for relief of physical complaints such as stomach or backaches that mask the depression. Somatization helps them disguise the reasons for distress and avoid the stigma of mental illness.

MODERN TREATMENTS CAN HELP: IT'S WORTH "STICKING WITH IT"

Today's therapies—more humane and effective—include:

- *Pharmacotherapy*, with various antidepressant medications, alone or in combination, to rebalance brain chemistry.
- *Psychotherapy* (usually with a psychiatrist) to help reverse the depressed person's negative and self-blaming thought patterns. Two of today's most proven psychological therapies for depression are cognitive-behavioral therapy (CBT)—which tries to reframe or replace negative thinking patterns with more reality-based and positive interpretations—and interpersonal therapy (IPT), which aims to help the person improve the dynamics of key relationships.
- *Exercise* now turning out to be as effective for mild depression as many other therapies.
- Electro-Convulsive Therapy (ECT), which applies a brief electric current to the brain while the person is anesthetized, is still used occasionally when other therapies do not work or in people who don't want to take antidepressant drugs. Despite its negative image, ECT gives good results for severe depression.

Sadly, in the midst of their debilitating torment, depressives often feel too down—physically, mentally and emotionally drained—to bother with medical advice, imagining their suffering is justified, and that treatment is useless. Yet even those who believe they're not ill enough to need medical attention or who think it "won't help" can benefit from treatment. "It's essential," notes one psychiatrist, "that the depressed—and their friends, partners, family, employers and workmates—realize that *help is available*. No need to tough it out alone or try to handle it themselves."

Family, friends and colleagues can assist by persuading the depressed person to get professional help, pointing out that therapy is worth a try. The best idea is to express compassion, empathy, interest and a steadfast willingness to listen attentively (without being judgmental), to show understanding, never accusing the depressed person of faking it or telling them to snap out of it.

Anyone whose depressed mood lasts over 2 weeks needs expert assistance. The family physician is usually the first person to consult, and will, if necessary, refer the depressive to a psychiatrist or mood disorder clinic. Employee assistance programs may also be available for confidential professional help. For suicidal people, the emergency department of any large hospital usually offers assistance around the clock. Anyone expressing suicidal thoughts, especially with a concrete plan, needs immediate emergency or psychiatric referral.

Antidepressant medications central to modern therapy

Pharmacotherapy is today's mainstay for treating depression, with medications that act on specific neurotransmitters. Antidepressants are nonaddictive drugs that don't remove life's problems but allow people to feel better so they can work at solving them. For example, after a few months on *sertraline* (Zoloft), one severely depressed woman, frustrated in her job, vexed with her husband and disappointed with her new house, changed her viewpoint and reported that her job was "quite challenging," her husband "okay" and the house "really quite nice."

Since full-blown depression is a serious illness it requires medical attention. Being partly due to a biochemical imbalance of brain transmitters, depression is often best managed by pharmacological (drug) treatment, perhaps with several combined antidepressants, often along with psychotherapy. With so many new medications now available, most people can find help for their depression; if one antidepressant doesn't work, another may. If we imagine our brains as having lots of neurochemicals driving around and parking slots for them to slide into, medications such as the serotonin re-uptake inhibitors simply fill the parking slots so the chemicals can remain in action, elevating the mood. The medications generally work best in conjunction with counseling and psychotherapy. Antidepressants usually take at least 2 to 6 weeks to work at full dosage, so people need to persevere during that time. Different medications suit different depressives, but they must be continued for long enough (usually 6 to 12 months) to work. If side effects are severe, or if the medication fails to bring relief after several weeks, or if the dose is wrong, it can be corrected or another drug substituted. For a first episode, antidepressant therapy usually continues for 6 months after the person feels better, and should be continued for several months after apparent recovery. (Continuing for at least 4 months after symptoms abate lessens chances of relapse.) Once treatment ends, the medication must be *gradually* tapered off under physician guidance, not suddenly stopped. Going off antidepressant medication abruptly can precipitate severe reactions such as dizziness, nausea and nightmares.

Mood stabilizers such as Epival, Tegretal and lithium carbonate (used mostly in manic depressives) can also improve mood, especially in people with bipolar disorder. But lithium carbonate requires several weeks to work and must be carefully regulated to reach the therapeutic range without toxicity. As well, there is emerging evidence that multiple therapies seem to work a bit better, so now depressed people can benefit from two different types of antidepressants, such as Wellbutrin and an SSRI. Sometimes addition of a low dose "anti-psychotic," or a tranquilizer, seems to help sufferers.

Rundown of main antidepressant medications

The antidepressant medications most frequently prescribed for major depression are the *selective serotonin reuptake inhibitors* (SSRIs), and the newer *serotonin-norepinephrine reuptake inhibitors* (SNRIs), as well as the older tricyclic class of drugs, which, although they are often less well tolerated and can produce more severe side effects, are still useful for some people. Common side effects of these medications include dry mouth, diarrhea (or constipation), weight gain (with some), headaches and decreased libido, but these effects are usually transient and not too bothersome.

- *Selective serotonin reuptake inhibitors* (SSRIs)—which prevent or slow reabsorption of the brain transmitter serotonin by inhibiting certain breakdown enzymes—are now the mainstay and first-line drugs for depression.
- **The SSRIs include:**
  fluoxetine (Prozac)
  sertraline (Zoloft)
  paroxetine (Paxil)
  citalopram (Celexa)
  fluvoxamine (Luvox)
- Nefazadone (Serzone) was recently removed from the market because of rare liver problems. Mirtazapine (Remeron) is a newer medication that is quite sedating, which can be a useful side-effect for patients struggling with both depression and insomnia. Some types (e.g., Prozac) are longer acting; others (e.g., Luvox) stay in the body for less time. Side effects vary and may include irritability, fuzzy thinking, nausea, appetite loss, loose stools and sexual dysfunction as well as stimulant effects (such as nervousness, insomnia, tremors and anxiety) and headache.Sexual dysfunction as a side effect can be hard to delineate because diminished libido or decreased sex drive can themselves be one aspect of depression. However, a specific effect of SSRIs is delayed orgasm, and some clinicians in fact treat men with early ejaculation issues with SSRIs. SSRI side effects tend to be dose-related and transient. These drugs also work for anxiety and other mental health conditions. People who can't tolerate one SSRI may do well on another, and older people may need smaller doses.
- *Serotonin and norepinephrine reuptake inhibitors* (SNRIs) are effective (new and still being investigated) products that also work well for anxiety. Chief side effects are nausea, dry mouth, constipation and drowsiness (which tend to wear off) and some sexual dysfunction.
- **The SNRIs include:**
  venlafaxine (Effexor)
  duloxetine (Cymbalta)
- *Tricyclic* and other older antidepressant medications are still sometimes prescribed. The

tricyclics affect various neurotransmitters and are just as effective as some newer types, although side effects (which include vision blurring, dry mouth, urinary hesitancy, and dizziness) tend to be more bothersome than with the SSRIs or SNRIs. These tricyclic drugs are not safe for use in people with heart problems. They should not be prescribed to anyone who may try to overdose on them because they are extremely dangerous in these situations.

- **The tricyclic antidepressants include:**
  amitriptyline (Elavil)
  desipramine (Norpramin)
  doxepin (Sinequan)
  imipramine (Tofranil)
  nortriptyline (Aventyl)
  chlomipramine (Anafranil)
  trimipramine (Surmontil)
- *Atypical antidepressants*, another class of antidepressants (so-called because they don't fit neatly into other drug classes), are also becoming more widely used. Mirtazapine (Remeron) is quite sedating, which can be useful in depressed people who are anxious or agitated. Wellbutrin (bupropion) has a different mechanism and affects dopamine regulation. It resembles the molecule in Zyban, the anti-smoking medication, so these two drugs should not be taken at the same time. Because of its different mechanism Wellbutrin can be quite useful in combination with other medications or when other antidepressants have failed. It causes less sexual interference than some other antidepressants.
- **The atypical antidepressants include:**
  mirtazapine (Remeron)
  bupropion (Wellbutrin)
  moclobemide (Manerix)
- *Monoamine oxidase inhibitors* (MAOIs) such as *phenelzine* (Nardil), still used for depression, especially if accompanied by much anxiety, have become less popular mainly owing to side effects (such as a dry mouth, tremors and constipation) and the dietary restrictions (owing to a possible high-blood-pressure crisis if MAOIs are taken with foods containing tyramine, such as red wine, ripe cheeses and smoked meat). These medications are now

rarely used as they can interact adversely with other anti-depressants.

Psychotherapy may help boost the mood lift and is a useful adjunct to medication

Various forms of psychotherapy, used in combination with antidepressant drugs, can enhance recovery and are especially useful for mild to moderate depression. However, psychotherapy is usually done by trained practitioners who may be hard to find or access.

Psychodynamic therapy—an analytical approach that may involve quite brief therapy (partly adapted from the older psychoanalysis methods)—tries to uncover the precipitating event(s) or reason(s) for depression and decipher any unconscious meaning that may not be evident, thereby helping to dispel the bleak outlook.

Interpersonal therapy (IPT) analyzes changing roles and the way someone relates to others, trying to improve relationship dynamics, communication skills and self-image. It focuses on the here and now, creating ways to work out immediate problems and strengthen the ability to build personal relationships. IPT often helps resolve personal and marital conflicts. Depending on the nature of the problem, the therapy may be quite brief and do well for anxiety disorders, moderate depression and borderline personality disorders.

Brief therapy encompasses several recent forms of psychotherapy—such as behavior and rational-emotive therapy—replacing the older time-consuming analytical methods, with specific objectives and a shorter time-frame. The goals (a more positive outlook, and better functioning) may be achieved in 10 to 65 sessions rather than the previous 500-plus sessions.

Cognitive-behavioral therapy (CBT) is increasingly used for depression with good results. CBT tries to correct the depressed cognitive ("thinking") mode by exerting "mind over mood" efforts that enhance coping skills. Rather than reversing the actual mood, it relies on correcting faulty thought patterns and beliefs, based on the premise that the maladaptive behavior and emotional distress of depression stem primarily from distorted thoughts, low self-worth and false appraisal of situations. Cognitive therapy helps depressed people think through their situ-

ation and correct self-blaming and negative thought patterns, constructing a more self-forgiving outlook. Even if the despondency doesn't lift entirely, cognitive therapy can help depressives carry on with everyday life.

How about electroconvulsive shock therapy (ECT)?

Despite its bad press (much of it due to misinformation), electroconvulsive therapy (ECT) remains the most effective remedy for severe depressives who are suicidal or don't respond to other treatments. ECT is done using premedication with muscle relaxants and short-acting general anesthesia. Electrodes on the head painlessly apply an electric current for half a second. Treatments are usually given 2 or 3 times weekly, for 6 to 12 sessions. The main side effect is temporary memory loss, usually only with successive treatments. The psychiatric associations of Canada, the United States and Britain advocate selective, judicious use of ECT for severe depression, where it is often 80 to 88 percent effective.

DEPRESSIVE VARIANTS
Dysthymia

Dysthymia is an increasingly diagnosed, longer-lasting but milder form of depression, with similar but less severe symptoms. However, the negative outlook, fatigue, social withdrawal, helplessness and discontent of dysthymia may continue for years, and may never lift completely. In contrast to major depression, dysthymia tends to come on gradually, is less intense and waxes and wanes. Few sufferers suspect they have dysthymia, and physicians often don't detect it. One recent study found that 3 percent of the U.S. population has dysthymia, the rate being highest in older people. The causes of dysthymia are unclear, but antidepressants that potentiate serotonin—the SSRIs such as Prozac and Zoloft are the drugs of choice for treating it. Cognitive-behavioral therapy is also effective.

Seasonal affective disorder (SAD)

Seasonal affective disorder or SAD is a type of depression in which symptoms vary with the amount of daylight—worsening in fall or winter, perhaps relieved by a trip south! It typically comes on in October or November and fades in April or May and is often accompanied by carbohydrate craving, significant fatigue and oversleeping. This type of depression may be related to levels of melatonin (a hormone secreted by the pineal gland). Daily phototherapy with a special light box can bring a significant mood lift.

Postpartum depression

Postpartum depression (PPD) is a depressive episode that occurs within a year of childbirth. It is the most common complication of childbearing, affecting 13 percent of new mothers. Studies show that women are at increased risk of developing mood disorders in the first 4 to 6 weeks after delivering a baby, with a greater need for psychiatric care in that period than at any other time in life. Apart from the fact that it happens soon after childbirth, postpartum depression does not differ from depression that occurs at any other time in a woman's life. It must meet the same DSM-IV diagnostic criteria (see above). However, with PPD, the sense of worthlessness typical of depression may revolve around concern for the baby's wellbeing and the woman's negative feelings about her value as a parent. She may express fears of failure or anxiety about not being a "good mother."

Aside from this, the symptoms of PPD are the same as for any other major depression, namely, a pervasive sense of sadness (*anhedonia*) or inability to feel pleasure, sleep disturbance, extreme fatigue, sluggishness (or agitation), inability to concentrate, excessive feelings of worthlessness and recurrent ideas of suicide. Symptoms of PPD usually begin within the first few weeks of the baby's birth, although they can surface up to 12 months later. A bout of PPD may last anywhere from a number of weeks to several months. or even up to a year. It may remit and resurface. Once women have had PPD, they have a 40 percent chance of experiencing another episode with subsequent births, and a 25 percent chance of developing depression at other times.

One key problem in detecting PPD, however, is that the fatigue, sleep disturbance and appetite changes may be taken as normal for a mother caring for a new infant. It may help to ask the woman whether she is able to sleep when the baby is resting peacefully or when someone else is caring for the child. Because the feelings of inadequacy, low self-esteem and guilt typical of depression tend, with PPD, to center on the infant and anxiety about parenting abilities, the depressed woman may express thoughts of being a "bad mother," a "useless parent" or "unable to cope." Since motherhood is expected to be a happy experience, many mothers with PPD are reluctant to reveal their feelings of despair and lack of pleasure in their infants. They may avoid talking about their sadness for fear of being labeled as inept or stigmatized for having a mental illness. Given the reluctance of new mothers to disclose despondent feelings at what should be a joyous time, PPD often goes undetected and undertreated. Women with PPD tend not to recognize it as a serious illness, and their health care providers may fail to diagnose it because they are unfamiliar with its symptoms and neglect to ask mothers about their feelings and emotions. (Deeper questioning often reveals that the depressive symptoms started well before PPD was diagnosed.)

Identified risk factors or possible warning signs that a woman is at risk of developing PPD include:
- a previous bout of major depression
- depression or anxiety during pregnancy
- family history of psychiatric illness
- recently experienced stressful or negative life events
- poor support networks (lack of emotional and practical support from partner, friends, relatives)
- relationship conflicts or marital discord.

Fortunately, PPD can be effectively treated and most (85 percent) of sufferers recover fully. As with depression at other times, treatment of PPD includes psychotherapy, antidepressant medication, counseling and support groups. Receiving plenty of support during pregnancy and after the birth (especially from an attentive partner) can protect women from PPD or mitigate its effects. Psychotherapy includes interpersonal therapy (IPT) and cognitive-behavioral therapy (CBT), which can be most effective (see above).

The antidepressants most frequently prescribed for PPD are the SSRIs (*selective serotonin reuptake inhibitors*) and newer SNRIs (serotonin-norepinephrine reuptake inhibitors), although the older tricyclic medications and other antidepressants are also sometimes used. Side effects are the same as those described above for antidepressants, but as women who have just given birth may be extra sensitive to drugs, lower starting doses may be advised. As with treatment for general depression, the medication may take several weeks to bring relief. Doctors suggest antidepressants be continued for several months after recovery and *never* stopped abruptly, in order to avoid withdrawal problems.

The use of antidepressants while breastfeeding remains controversial. Mothers may refuse the drugs for fear of adverse effects on the baby of exposure to small amounts transmitted through breast milk. However, current evidence suggests that commonly prescribed antidepressants—such as sertraline (Zoloft), paroxetine (Paxil) and nortriptyline (Aventyl)—are probably safe for mothers to use while breastfeeding full-term, healthy babies. Nonetheless, the mother's decision about taking antidepressants while breastfeeding needs careful evaluation. The mother, her partner and caregivers must weigh the harmful impact of the mother's depression on the baby against possible risks of exposing the infant to antidepressant medication via breast-milk. They must jointly decide which feeding method is the best for mother and baby. The main goal is prompt treatment of PPD. Severe, long-term or chronic, untreated maternal depression may hamper mother-infant attachment and could hinder the baby's behavioral, social and cognitive development. Current evidence suggests that a prolonged bout of depression in the mother may undermine the child's development of language skills and IQ, more so in boys than girls. At the same time, it is important to stress that any impairment of child development stems from *prolonged* depression, not from a single, short-term postpartum episode.

Support from a partner, family and friends are invaluable in countering postpartum depression. Support is especially helpful when partner, relatives and friends act as sympathetic, attentive, non-judgmental listeners, reassuring the mother of continuing love, making her feel val-

ued and taking on as much of the baby care and household chores as possible while she's down and despondent. Partners who notice the mother's low mood can be helpful in alerting health care providers to the possibility of PPD.

Postpartum depression must be distinguished from other mood disorders that are common after childbirth. In particular, PPD must be differentiated from the "baby blues" (also called "maternity" or "postnatal" blues), which is a transient mood change affecting 50 to 80 percent of women after childbirth, and from puerperal psychosis, which is a rare but very serious psychotic illness (affecting about 0.1 to 0.2 percent of new mothers). Puerperal psychosis requires immediate emergency care and, usually, hospitalization.

The baby or maternal blues are mild and self-limited mood swings generally appearing 2 to 4 days after delivery and lasting just a week or so. The blues typically show up as rapid changes from smiling joyousness to tearfulness, with the woman seeming irritable and anxious, and having inexplicable crying spells. Some researchers ascribe these rapid swings to postnatal hormone changes after delivery. The blues usually require no treatment other than support and reassurance, and vanish on their own within 2 weeks. However, some women with the blues go on to develop depression within the first year of having a baby. In some cases the blues worsen to become true depression, or they may lift, later to be followed by a bout of PPD.

Puerperal or postpartum psychosis complicates 1 to 2 deliveries per 1,000. In contrast to the blues and PPD, psychosis is an extremely severe illness with sudden onset, requiring emergency attention. It can surface within 48 to 72 hours of birth, usually becoming evident within 2 weeks of delivery. Studies suggest that postpartum psychosis has a biological, possibly genetic basis, being most common in women who have relatives with psychiatric disorders. Its warning symptoms are rapid alternation of depressed and elated moods or "highs," with bizarre, confused or disorganized behavior. However, as postpuerperal psychosis usually comes on rapidly and unpredictably, it can be hard to discern and health professionals often miss it.

The warning signs of psychosis include an

empty, numbed or emotionless expression, delusions (fixed, false beliefs about happenings that have no basis in reality) and hallucinations (seeing things or actions not visible to anyone else, or hearing voices telling them to do certain things). Any woman exhibiting such behavior needs immediate psychiatric attention. Infanticide and/or suicide are distinct risks in women with postpartum psychosis. Possible clues to suicidal intentions may be the mother's incessant preoccupation with the infant's safety, or remarks such as "the world's such an awful place, we'd both be better out of it."

The trouble is that when a mother's home alone with her new baby, no one may notice that she's in dire need of professional help. Women with new babies are exhausted anyway—getting little sleep—and the fatigue may not be recognized as due to depression, so the illness may not get needed treatment. Hospitalization may be necessary, the baby being admitted along with the mother or taken in for visits. The good news is that this kind of depression has a high recovery rate. About 80 percent of women with postpartum depression improve within 2 to 3 months, although a few have persisting depression.

For help or information about depression, contact your family physician, a local branch of any psychiatric association or, in some centers, self-help groups: Depression Information Resource & Information Centre (DIRECT): 1-888-557-5051); Depression Information Line of McMaster University: 1-888-557-5051, extension 8000; Parent Help Line: 1-888-603-9100; www.parenthelpline.ca; Centre for Suicide Prevention: www.suicideinfo.ca; Mood Disorders Society of Canada: www.moodisorderscanada.ca/depression/ppd.htm; in Toronto, the Centre for Addiction and Mental Health at www.camh.net, the Manic-Depressive Association: (416) 486-8045 or Motherisk Home Line: (416) 813-6780 or www. motherrisk.org/; in Montreal, Depressives Anonymous: (514) 842-7557 or the Quebec Association of Depression: (514) 529-7552; the Winnipeg-based Depression and Manic-Depression Association of Canada: (204) 786-0987; the Mood Disorders Association of British Columbia: (604) 873-0103, the Depression and Manic-Depression Association of Alberta: 1-888-757-7007.

ST. JOHN'S WORT—A NATURAL ANTIDEPRESSION REMEDY?

Herbal therapies for depression are becoming increasingly popular—in particular St. John's Wort, derived from the hypericum perforatum flower. In Germany, St. John's Wort (SJW) outsells Prozac (America's third biggest-selling prescription drug), and the herb is fast gaining popularity in North America as a natural antidepressant. Initial studies showed that SJW, typically at 300 mg three times a day, was an effective therapy for depression. More rigorous studies have narrowed this niche to mild to moderate depression. SJW should not be used as a first-line agent for patients with major depression. Side effects include some gastric upsets, dizziness, possible allergic reactions and increased sun sensitivity. It does interact with some medications, so inform your doctor if you do take SJW. It is unclear how this herbal remedy might work. Some speculate that—like the monoamine oxidase inhibitors and SSRIs—St. John's Wort may increase levels of the brain's "mood-lifting" neurotransmitters (serotonin and epinephrine).

"Natural isn't necessarily better," warns one U.S. expert, "and it can be risky, if the belief leads people to abandon effective medical therapy, or self-treat a condition that needs professional help." People should not take this herb alongside other medications without first consulting their physician, as the combination could be dangerous. Although results seem promising, more research is needed to determine whether, how and to what extent St. John's Wort works as an antidepressant. It's not recommended for use during pregnancy.

HOLIDAY BLUES

Holidays—especially the yuletide season—are traditionally a time of generosity, love and fulfillment, yet few survive the festive period without some disappointment and conflict. As our society has come to observe them, holiday times promise fun and enjoyment. Christmas in particular dangles the lure of boundless warmth and material wishes magically granted by sugarplum fairies. Western society goes berserk at this time, exaggerating the occasion beyond its original meaning with media hype and an orgy of commercialization, and the season intensifies the contrast between fantasy and reality, the difference between the way we wish our lives to be and the way they really are.

Most people manage to have a satisfying time at Christmas, family rifts being glossed over and assuaged by the pleasures of eating, drinking, togetherness, hearing from old friends, phoning distant relatives, visiting the elderly and generally taking stock before another year begins. However, because of the high expectations, the time for reflection and the comparison with others, disappointments are inevitable. The term "holiday blues syndrome" has been coined by psychiatrists to describe the downside, which brings fatigue, irritability, bitter nostalgia for lost youth, awareness of mortality, regrets about failed ambitions and relationships, coupled with a strong hope for magical solutions. As many of us struggle with unspoken anxieties or conflicts, stress starts to take its toll—shown by the higher rates of people seeking psychiatric advice at Christmas time.

Everyone goes to such lengths to have a merry Christmas that the failure to enjoy the holiday can create unbearable stress. People who usually manage to maintain their equilibrium may break down because of inner loneliness, boredom, removal of the usual routine and the image of everyone else apparently having a great time.

Holiday times are especially hard on those who feel abandoned. The lonely, isolated, sick and recently bereaved often feel private despair in the face of holiday activities. For people who cope with isolation year round, feelings of loss are exaggerated. By no means are feelings of loneliness confined to those who are truly alone. Even in the midst of their families, some feel desperately lonely, surrounded by people they don't really care for who fail to live up to their expectations. To those with incipient psychiatric problems, holidays can prove stressful enough to precipitate a breakdown.

People who are troubled by the holiday season can take solace in the fact that Christmas is but 1 week out of 52, and try to make the annual event as pleasant as possible. Coping strategies may include setting realistic goals, not expecting too much of yourself or others, examining your expectations, planning ahead, assigning and parceling out specific tasks to others willing to help, and sharing responsibilities.

MANIC DEPRESSION

Manic depression (bipolar disorder), a mood disorder with alternating episodes of depression and mania, is a serious illness with sometimes devastating effects on the sufferer and his or her family. A manic depressive's mood swings from one emotional pole to its opposite—bouts of mania or "highs" alternating with glum depression. However, in many cases the depressive episodes greatly outnumber the manic ones. The depression in bipolar disorder is identical to that of major clinical depressions, and the *manic* episodes identify the condition.

Although we often envision the "manic" side of bipolar illness as its defining feature, most of the time people with this disorder just experience the depressed phase of a bipolar cycle. Mania seldom occurs on its own, without depression. Bipolar patients often mainly experience depression, with only a few bouts of mild mania—"hypomania"—rather than full mania. Bipolar disorder is divided into two subtypes. A diagnosis of bipolar I disorder requires that the person has had at least one manic episode with or without a previous depressive episode. The diagnosis of bipolar II disorder implies that the patient has had one or more major depressive episodes, as well as one or more hypomanic episodes (during which the person needs less sleep and is functional but not psychotic), without evidence of prior mania. The cycles of depression and mania may not be predictable or regular. In certain cases, known as "rapid cycling," the manic and depressive stages may alternate rapidly—a condition that can be hard to control or treat.

As in clinical depression, suicide is a serious danger in manic depressives. About 15 percent of bipolar patients commit suicide during the depressed phase. (For more on suicide, see earlier in this chapter and the section on adolescent suicide risks in Chapter 12.)

The manic phase identifies bipolar disorder

Usually, the mania appears quite suddenly—within days to weeks—often, but not always, emerging from a period of deep depression. At first, before they have had the experience of living with a manic person, family and friends may be delighted at the mood elevation, welcoming the increased energy, cheerfulness and sociability. However, it soon becomes apparent that the "hyper" mood and the person's actions are odd, with rapid speech, disconnected, racing thoughts, decreased sleep needs, exaggerated self-praise, grandiose notions and irritability.

Sometimes extreme irritability is the most prominent mood alteration in the manic stage.

Mania tends to distort thinking and judgment. About 60 percent of manic people have omnipotent thoughts in their "up" mood, perhaps thinking they're God, the queen or a rock star. Some have hallucinations, and hear voices or see visions. Fueled by their mania, some bipolar patients behave dangerously and foolishly. For example, while in a manic state they may spend money recklessly and embark on crazy schemes that bankrupt themselves and their families, or they may become angry, sometimes paranoid and even violent. Some become hypersexual, with openly promiscuous behavior "Young manic males are among the most difficult patients we encounter," says one University of Toronto psychiatrist. "They may exhibit an extraordinary increase in muscle strength, which combined with a lack of judgment and sense of invincibility, can be a formidable challenge." The manic episodes can last for months, long enough for sufferers to wreck their lives, lose their jobs or break up their marriages—good reasons why mania should be treated as soon as it's discovered. A few manic depressives exhibit bursts of productivity or creativity during their elated phase.

Diagnosing manic depression

The diagnosis of bipolar disorder can be confirmed only after identifying a manic episode, which ranges from mild to severe and typically first appears in adolescence or between ages 20 and 30—although the disorder is increasingly seen in people over age 50. In contrast to clinical depression—which affects more women than men—manic depression afflicts both sexes equally.

Treatment of manic depression

Persuading those in a manic state to get treatment can be difficult, as they often not only don't feel sick, but in fact may say they feel great—although most manics find the experience is distressing and show signs of irritability. Since it is hard to reason with manic people, most receive treatment in hospital, usually with drugs and perhaps also with psychotherapy. Before treatment, tests are done to rule out kid-

CRITERIA FOR DIAGNOSIS OF MANIC EPISODES

A. A distinct period of abnormally and persistently elevated, expansive or irritable mood.

B. During the mood disturbance, at least three of the following symptoms (four if the mood disturbance was mainly irritable):
- **inflated self-esteem, grandiosity;**
- **decreased need for sleep, e.g., awake after only three hours of sleep;**
- **more talkative than usual;**
- **flight of ideas or "racing" thoughts;**
- **distractibility, e.g., attention too easily drawn to unimportant or irrelevant stimuli;**
- **increase in goal-directed activity either socially, at work, at school or sexually;**
- **excessive involvement in risky activities—e.g., unrestrained buying sprees, sexual indiscretions or foolish business investments.**

C. A mood disturbance severe enough to damage job or social functioning or relationships with others, or requiring hospitalization to prevent harm to others or self.

D. Hallucinations or delusions.

E. Not superimposed by other psychiatric illness, such as schizophrenia.

F. Not caused by an organic disturbance or drug.

ney ailments, thyroid abnormalities (especially important for those with frequent rapid cycles) and other possible causes. Routine tests include electrolyte measures, blood counts and electro-cardiograms.

Lithium salts are the backbone of therapy for manic depression. How lithium manages to modify both manic and depressive mood swings isn't known, but it is an effective mood stabilizer in 50 to 60 percent of manic depressives. Lithium may be combined with an anti-psychotic drug such as haloperidol or, increasingly, with antiepileptic drugs such as carbamazepine or valproic acid. Combined medication using lithium plus haloperidol is frequently prescribed at first, because lithium takes about 14 days to work and several weeks to become fully effective.

Since there is a narrow range between the therapeutic and toxic levels of lithium, periodic monitoring of blood levels is essential. Symptoms of lithium toxicity include hand tremors, nausea and decreased coordination. Annoying but usually tolerable side effects include frequent urination, thirst, mild nausea, diarrhea and weight gain—a very troublesome side effect that often leads to noncompliance and relapses.

RECOGNIZING THE HALLMARKS OF THE MANIC PHASE

In differing degrees, the following symptoms define mania:
- indefatigable restlessness—always on the go;
- increasingly less sleep—sometimes only a few hours nightly;
- cheerfulness and optimism, verging on euphoria—as if perpetually "high";
- lack of judgment;
- loud, rapid, pressured speech, full of jokes and puns, that's hard to interrupt;
- jumping from idea to idea—completely unintelligible in the severely manic;

- irritable, suspicious outbursts.

In diagnosing manic depression, doctors must rule out other possible causes of mania such as:
- *endocrine and metabolic disorders*—for instance, adrenal diseases (such as Addison's disease or Cushing's syndrome), liver ailments, hyperthyroidism (excess thyroid function), porphyria (a metabolic disorder) and vitamin B_{12} deficiency;
- *hemodialysis* (kidney failure);
- *neurological problems*—for

instance, Huntington's disease, brain tumors, encephalitis, multiple sclerosis, Wilson's disease, consequences of AIDS, temporal-lobe lesions;
- *certain medications*—e.g., the antianxiety drug alprazolam, cimetidine and ranitidine (stomach-ulcer drugs), corticoids, levodopa (for Parkinson's disease), some psychostimulants (such as amphetamine) and antidepressants;
- *drug abuse*—of alcohol, cocaine, phencyclidine.

Long-term lithium therapy makes it possible for many manic depressives to live productive, normal lives. The therapy may have to be lifelong, as stopping it is a major reason for relapses. The burden is therefore on sufferers to understand why they need the medication. A trusted physician who is sensitive to individual problems can help in minimizing side effects and persuading the sufferer to stick with the therapy. Earlier fears that lithium can damage the kidneys have not been realized, and today, after 40 years of lithium use, renal failure is not considered a danger. But those on lithium must be aware of fluctuations in its level (with fluid intake) and of interaction with other drugs. Fevers, excessive dieting, diarrhea, non-steroidal anti-inflammatory drugs (including ASA) and chlorothiazide may increase blood lithium levels.

Alternative medications for those who don't respond well to lithium—for example, rapid cyclers—include anticonvulsants alone, or antidepressants together with lithium for episodes of severe depression. In addition, newer antipsychotics have proven useful as well as an anti-seizure drug called lamotrigine. The evidence is more powerfully in favor of

starting treatment with lithium, but some patients prefer to start with lamotrigine as it has fewer side effects.

BORDERLINE PERSONALITY DISORDER

Borderline personality disorder is an increasingly recognized mental illness, affecting an estimated 1 percent of the North American population, twice as many women as men. This psychiatric problem usually manifests itself in late adolescence or during the early twenties, but it occasionally appears during childhood. Borderline personality disorder (BPD) shows up as a pervasive pattern of instability and emotional turbulence, with an inability to control mood, impulses and aggression, deep-seated self-image problems, trouble with personal relationships and frequent suicidal thoughts. (Suicide rates are high among those with BPD.) The impulsive behavior may include spending sprees, verbal outbursts and reckless driving. Eating disorders (especially bingeing) and depression are also common.

Typically, people with this disorder feel "good" one minute, and "bad" or "ashamed" the next. Their emotional swings are extreme and unpredictable. Within a few minutes they may exhibit tenderness, rage, sorrow and panic. The person with BPD can, for example, be pleasantly agreeable one moment, vehemently angry the next with no apparent reason for the emotional switch or flare-up, except possibly being hypersensitive to some imagined slight or insult. Many have paranoid tendencies and suspicions about the intentions and actions of those around them. People with BPD tend to form unusually intense, often tumultuous personal relationships, marked by repeated arguments, temper tantrums, breakups and a profound fear of losing the primary "attachment figure." The fear of abandonment and poor distress tolerance may show up as excessive "clinging" and constant demands or frantic phone calls for reassurance. Understandably, the maladaptive behavior of people with BPD can frighten others, drive them away and exacerbate relationship problems.

Clinical signs of the disorder include the extreme emotional swings, excessively low self-worth, repeated self-mutilation or "slashings," depression and suicidal tendencies, making sufferers frequent users of psychiatric services. Many have several hospitalizations and require ongoing care from various therapists.

The causes of BPD are complex and remain largely unknown, but may include genetic factors (a family history of mental illness) and adverse childhood experiences such as parental violence, poor attachments or sexual abuse. Some researchers view the disorder as a continuing form of post-traumatic stress disorder (PTSD), stemming from childhood experiences. Recent neuroimaging techniques show that certain brain regions (particularly the amygdala and limbic system) are disturbed in those with BPD, suggesting "hyperarousal" and weakening of the inhibitory controls that normally regulate emotional responses. However, whether these changes are due to genetic factors or arise as a consequence of the disorder remains unclear.

Prompt treatment can help people with BPD continue to function and prevent the dire consequences of self-harm. Strong support networks are also essential. Medication may include tranquilizers and antidepressants to calm the emotional turbulence and get the person to "think before acting." However, the key to treating this illness is ongoing psychotherapy. Various forms of cognitive-behavioral therapy, in particular dialectical behavior therapy and group therapy, seem to be most helpful. Therapy for BPD aims to increase the person's coping skills and tolerance for emotional distress, improve reality assessment and problem-solving, enhance self-esteem, build behavioral skills for everyday living, resolve interpersonal conflicts and get the person functioning and productive. Suicidal intentions must be carefully monitored, with constant and easy access to therapeutic or emergency care if needed. Accompanying problems such as distorted self-image and eating disorders must also be tackled.

Recovery rates for BPD are good and this disorder has a better prognosis (chance of remission) than many other psychiatric illnesses such as bipolar disorder. Studies show that 75 to 80 percent of people with BPD achieve remission after a few years of therapy. Outcomes are best in those with a high IQ, cases where there's

no evidence of parental brutality and in those who seek care in late adolescence or adulthood (rather than during childhood). Nonetheless, people with borderline personality disorder must consider it a lifelong problem.

CHRONIC FATIGUE SYNDROME

Known by many popular names, chronic fatigue syndrome (CFS) hits mainly achievement-oriented, well-educated young adults, primarily those from middle and professional classes. For over a century, reports from many countries have described a perplexing ailment typified by prolonged fatigue, feverishness, sore throat, tender neck nodes and decreased concentration powers. Unrelieved by normal rest, the persistent tiredness is enough to stop people from working, exercising and having fun.

During the past century, fashionable complaints involving overpowering lassitude bore exotic names such as chlorosis ("the green sickness," attributed to iron-deficiency anemia), epidemic neuromyasthenia (nerve-and-muscle weakness) and neurasthenia (described by one famous U.S. physician as "a lightheaded nervous exhaustion, inability to concentrate, and exquisite intolerance to coffee and alcohol").

Similar symptoms have been ascribed to other poorly defined diseases, such as twentieth-century disease (total allergy syndrome), hypoglycemia (low blood sugar), severe vitamin-mineral deficiencies and the "Royal Free disease" (a cluster of unmitigated fatigue cases among nurses at Britain's Royal Free Hospital in 1955— ascribed by some to mass hysteria). Outbreaks in Britain were labeled myalgic encephalomyelitis (muscle and brain inflammation.

Prevailing chronic fatigue problems were attributed to Epstein-Barr virus (the virus responsible for mononucleosis), which is accompanied by pervasive fatigue. But the link to the Epstein-Barr virus (EBV) remains unproven. One nickname for the inexplicable fatigue is "Yuppie flu," the name deriving from the flu-like symptoms and the prevalence of the condition among ambitious high-achievers and young professionals. (Epidemics of so-called "fashionable" illnesses are rare in underdeveloped areas.) Hallmarks of the condition are constant, lingering exhaustion—sometimes debilitating enough

WHAT IS CHRONIC FATIGUE SYNDROME?

Chronic fatigue syndrome is now seen as a nonspecific, complex syndrome with persistent fatigue that lasts at least 6 months (or longer) and is not attributable to an existing medical condition (e.g., hypothyroidism, sleep apnea, obesity), psychiatric disorder (e.g., major depression, dementia, anorexia nervosa), or alcohol or substance abuse. The origins of CFS are unknown, although theories about its possible causes range from organic causes—such as a viral infection or immune system dysfunction—to psychological disturbances. CFS by definition includes new-onset, persistent or recurring mental and physical fatigue that substantially impairs a person's ability to function, causes post-exertional malaise or fatigue with slow recovery lasting over 24 hours, sleep problems, pain in muscles and joints and various other challenges such as memory problems or enlarged lymph nodes. For a diagnosis of CFS, the symptoms need to persist for more than 6 months in adults and 3 months or more in children.

to ruin a career and family life. Many people today blame it for their low energy and "lack of wellness." Publicity about the ailment, frequently inaccurate, has encouraged many to think they have it, often with a remarkable absence of abnormal findings and no medical foundation. Although CFS was originally suspected of being a viral infection, recent evidence finds no consistent link to infectious agents, and experts suggest this syndrome may be the physical expression of underlying psychological dissatisfaction, depression or a need to "opt out."

Fatigue syndrome is commonest among hard-driving young adults

Prime candidates for chronic fatigue syndrome are career-oriented professionals, especially unmarried, well-educated overachievers aged 25 to 40. About one-quarter of sufferers are healthcare workers (doctors, nurses, therapists), and it affects twice as many women as men. Those afflicted tend to be perfectionists who strive to excel in all areas—job, sports, appearance—and many are ardent exercisers, working out strenuously several times a week. The syndrome's impact on these overscheduled sufferers can be devastating, especially if pervasive fatigue forces them to give up part or all of their activities. They may then adopt the "victim" role and, despite their fatigue, display inexhaustible energy in fighting for the validity and recognition of their illness.

Frequently cited complaints

The fatigue syndrome typically produces unmitigated exhaustion, a niggling sore throat, muscular weakness and a general malaise sufficient to prevent usual activities. Sufferers frequently report peculiar headaches, tender, swollen lymph nodes, joint pains, disrupted sleep, chills, night sweats and feverishness. Some also experience light aversion, an inability to abide the slightest noise, nausea, appetite changes and bladder problems. Many report a shortened attention span and a decline in normally sharp thinking processes. There may be some memory loss, confusion and slurred speech. Often severe enough to diminish the mental acuity needed for job performance, the illness leads to lengthy sick leave and numerous disability claims. The least exertion greatly exaggerates the weariness. Symptoms may be severe enough to halt all activity, with sufferers spending hours each day in bed. The average duration of the disorder is 2 years, but many improve in a few weeks to months. The disorder tends to return at times of emotional and/or physical stress.

The good news is that, despite the distressing impact of the disorder most sufferers gradually recover at least 80 percent of their former capacities when it wanes. Perhaps guided in part by the "wisdom of their bodies," once they recover, many don't resume their previously unrealistic, overextended, action-packed lives, instead reevaluating their priorities and choosing a slower pace.

There is considerable overlap between CFS and fibromyalgia, as well as with multiple chemical sensitivities and irritable bowel syndrome, all of which have a considerable psychological component and are dubbed so-called "fashionable" ailments. Given current lack of knowledge about the etiologic (causative) and mechanistic, factors, it may be useful to view these conditions as multifactorial disorders, involving an inability or unwillingness to adapt to surroundings and environment. Consequently, the person's tolerance for combined stressors, no matter what their source, is exceeded, producing a complex of symptoms. Many people with CFS feel their malady is not taken seriously by healthcare providers, and physicians are urged not to dismiss their suffering as trivial or as a "pseudo-illness." In a large population-based sample of 28,000 adults, the prevalence of CFS was found to be 0.5 percent among women and 0.3 percent among men. These people are ill and need appropriate care. The distress of people with CFS is real, and like any chronic disease, sufferers need to accentuate the positive. The current medical approach to CFS is to foster self-awareness and a sense of personal limits. Exercises that are gradually increased have proven to be very therapeutic. A randomized controlled trial of graded aerobic exercises versus flexibility exercises and relaxation therapy found a marked improvement with aerobic exercises. Management also includes reassurance about the condition and the likelihood that it will improve, discussion with family and friends about its impact, good nutrition, and cognitive or behavioral therapy.

No consistent infection found in CFS

Reliable medical and laboratory tests have failed to reveal a consistent link between CFS and any infection. Most patients who "felt feverish" actually had normal temperatures. The CDC (Center for Disease Control) cautions that in this illness, with its "wide-ranging, nonspecific symptoms, the connection to Epstein-Barr is tenuous and unproven." Well-controlled studies also found no correlation between CFS and a high antibody level, or evidence of any consistent immune-system flaw. Many of the chronically fatigued actually had *less* suppressed immune systems than healthy, nonfatigued control subjects. None of the reported immune-system abnormalities correlates with the severity of CFS or the improvement noted during therapy.

Psychological factors usually play a major role in CFS

Since researchers find no credibility for a consistent organic cause in CFS, they look to mental disturbance as an explanation—the more so because the severity of symptoms seems to ebb and flow in harmony with mood and emotional states. According to recent research, a high proportion of the ceaselessly fatigued (over 60 percent in some studies) have had one or more past episodes of psychiatric disturbance, such as

---

BASIS FOR DIAGNOSING CHRONIC FATIGUE SYNDROME (CFS)
(recognizing that there may be several joint causes)

Common signs and symptoms of chronic fatigue syndrome (a designated number must be present to confirm the diagnosis):

To be confirmed as having CFS a person must have:

- new onset of persistent or recurrent fatigue lasting over 6 months (not resolved by rest), severe enough to reduce average daily activities by 50 percent
- reliable, thorough medical and laboratory tests to exclude other, treatable, clinical diseases and conditions that could cause the fatigue. such as:
- psychiatric diseases (e.g., depression, anxiety, somatization disorders);
- diabetes;
- endocrine/hormonal disturbances (e.g., Thyroid or adrenal disorders);
- heart kidney, blood diseases,
- anemia;
- cancer;
- infection by bacteria (e.g., TB);
- parasitic diseases (e.g., toxoplasmosis);
- fungal invasions (e.g., histoplasmosis);
- chronic hepatitis;
- street-drug or medication side effects.

Subjective symptoms experienced:

- extreme prolonged fatigue (lasting over 6 months);
- chills, feverishness;
- nighttime sweats;
- sore throat;
- tender swollen lymph nodes in neck and/or armpits;
- headaches;
- unexplained muscle weakness;
- muscle aches;
- joint pains that come and go;
- sleep disturbances;
- difficulty concentrating;
- memory loss;
- mood changes;
- visual changes;
- stomach (abdominal) cramps;
- appetite change;
- weight loss or gain;
- irritable bladder;
- dizziness;
- lightheadedness;
- "blue" spells, crying fits;
- rapid pulse.

Laboratory and medical or physical findings*:

- low-grade fever (37.6°–38.6°C, or 99.7°–101.5°F)
- pharyngitis (red, inflamed throat);
- swollen lymph nodes;
- minor immune-system changes (in 30% of sufferers), such as:
- elevated antibodies to some viruses, e.g., Epstein-Barr virus, measles, Coxsackie, herpes;
- low gamma globulin;
- increased synthetase enzymes:
- decreased "killer cell" activity (lowered immune defenses).

Other syndromes/illnesses sometimes mistaken for CFS:

- depression, anxiety;
- infections, e.g., AIDS, Coxsackie virus, Epstein-Barr; brucellosis;
- fibrositis (arthritic syndrome/fibromyalgia);

- sleep apnea;
- diabetes;
- hypothyroidism (underactive thyroid);

- anemia;
- cancer;
- Addison's disease.

* to be documented by a physician

depression, panic attacks or phobias. In addition, many CFS sufferers admit to having blamed other well-publicized "diseases of the year" (which they heard about through the media) for their malaise. Experts speculate that in those prone to mental disturbances, CFS represents a maladaptive response to physical and mental pressure. A stressful event—moving house, changing jobs, marriage, divorce—often precipitates it.

Many psychiatrists believe that CFS emanates largely from a propensity to mental and emotional disturbances, which express themselves in the guise of fatigue and other physical symptoms. One University of Toronto specialist found that 67 percent of CFS sufferers in her practice "had episodes of depression and other psychiatric disorders, several years before the onset of their debilitating fatigue." One U.S. study from the National Institutes of Health (NIH) in Maryland found that 75 percent of CFS sufferers "warranted a psychiatric diagnosis of anxiety disorder, affective [mood] disorder, substance abuse or antisocial personality problems."

The combined evidence shows that two-thirds of those with CFS meet the criteria for psychiatric illness, usually depression. Depression bears distinct similarities to the syndrome, being also accompanied by extreme fatigue, headaches, muscle pain, weakness, dizziness, dysuria (bladder dysfunction) and gastrointestinal upsets—all cardinal symptoms of CFS.

However, many CFS sufferers object to being labeled as "psychiatrically ill" and deny psychological problems (for which they might feel guilty), preferring to pin their discomfort on an organic condition. But whether its roots are organic or psychological, the syndrome is equally distressing. The dearth of medical evidence for anything organically wrong does not diminish the very real pain and frustration of those with CFS.

Treatment: life must go on

Key points in handling CFS are a thorough medical evaluation, investigation of lifestyle issues, laboratory tests and psychiatric assessment to exclude treatable physical or mental disorders.

Since psychiatric disturbances may underlie the disorder, they must be considered in recommending treatment. The best therapy is rest, supportive counseling, a graduated program of physical activity, avoidance of a "catastrophic" attitude and symptomatic drug therapy with painkillers, antihistamines, and antidepressants. Accurate scientific information helps to dispel misconceptions and lessen the frustration felt by CFS sufferers. They are not malingering—they really feel ill—but they can be encouraged to feel better. The key is to help them accept some discomfort as a normal part of life. On the one hand, CFS is like any other chronic disease that requires self-management, on the other hand it is unique in that sufferers may not get the empathy or understanding that most diseases generate.

As for medications, anti-inflammatories, antibiotics and tranquilizers don't offer a cure or even much relief for CFS, but many sufferers do improve on one or other of the newer antidepressant drugs, especially types that act as both mood-lifters and pain-relievers if they can be persuaded to take them. Low doses of doxepin (Sinequan), nortriptyline, desipramine and fluoxetine (Prozac) may help. However, trials have not shown large benefits to date. Some patients have responded to low-dose cortisone. But close monitoring is crucial.

Activity, modeled on rehabilitation programs, with gradually increasing energy levels, is strongly encouraged. It helps to reduce anxiety, affirms the ability to move and avoids anticipation of prolonged bed rest and disability. Since many people feel most energetic in the morning, wearying as the day progresses, exercise is best planned for the early hours. Rewards are given for increased activity.

Treatment may also include cognitive behavioral therapy to stop CFS sufferers from "catastrophizing"—believing they will never again be fully active—giving reassurance that the illness isn't lethal and will likely diminish and vanish with time. Sufferers are taught to attribute the symptoms to real reasons—perhaps just "work overload," a bad day or staying up late. They are encouraged to take it easy, but *not* to stay in bed—to "continue with their lives" while awaiting recovery. Psychotherapy can help if anxiety, depression or a somatization disorder is present.

THE DISABLING EFFECTS OF ANXIETY DISORDERS

Anxiety disorders are a group of different conditions with anxiety as their common core. Recent studies have exposed the surprising prevalence of anxiety disorders in modern society, a hidden epidemic now known to affect over 10 percent of North Americans at some point in their lives. The word "anxiety" comes from the Greek "to strangle," capturing the strong physical sensations of tightness or choking prominent in these disorders. The key symptoms of anxiety are worry and fear. Agoraphobia, where the person has a difficult time leaving home and translates it to, literally "fear of the marketplace," is a marker for the severity of the anxiety.

Distinguishing normal anxiety from true anxiety syndromes

There is a profound difference between normal anxiety, which is a protective human response, and anxiety as a debilitating psychiatric disorder. Fear is a biologically adaptive reaction to real danger. By contrast, unfounded or unrealistic anxiety—a vague fear of hostility, of "danger at every turn" (even when there's no real threat), is destructive. Fear arouses the body's autonomic (involuntary) nervous system, evoking the fight-or-flight response and triggering production of the hormone norepinephrine (adrenaline), which puts all senses on the alert, speeds the heartbeat, dilates the pupils and diverts blood to the working muscles. Anxiety is a very "physical" illness.

In anxiety disorders, a similar but uncalled-for fight-or-flight response releases norepinephrine when there's nothing to fight or flee. Human beings cannot endure intense anxiety for long without feeling ill or developing a "phobic" avoidance of the fear-arousing situation(s). Unresolved anxiety problems may lead to clinical depression, alcoholism and suicidal tendencies. If anxiety destroys the ability to function normally, it requires professional help.

Anxiety disorders are more disabling than hitherto recognized

Since all of us fret to some extent about everyday problems, anxiety disorders tend to be trivialized; they often go undiagnosed, and are considered less troublesome than other psychiatric conditions. A recent University of Toronto study showed that many who suffer from anxiety syndromes are misdiagnosed, and get extensive cardiac, neurological and other medical workups and perhaps even faulty treatment, because an anxiety disorder that might have responded to simple therapy has gone unrecognized. Yet true anxiety disorders are far from trivial. They can destroy careers, families and friendships. The life of someone with post-traumatic stress disorder (following a life-threatening assault) or of an obsessive-compulsive may be almost as disrupted as that of a schizophrenic.

A 1988 National Institute of Mental Health survey of more than 18,000 people in five U.S. cities astonished the psychiatric community by revealing that anxiety disorders are now the most prevalent psychiatric illness in North America. The largest survey of psychiatric problems ever undertaken, it found the rate of anxiety disorders among the population over a period of 6 months to be 7.3 percent, with 14 percent of respondents reporting transient anxiety problems at some time in their lives. (By contrast, the level of alcohol and drug abuse was 3.8 percent, schizophrenia 0.6 percent and depression 2.2 percent.)

Anxiety symptoms mimic those of medical conditions, such as shortness of breath (as in asthma), chest pain (as in heart disease), diarrhea (as in bowel disorders)—an added reason

ANXIETY DISORDERS INCLUDE:

- simple phobia;
- social phobia;
- panic disorder;
- agoraphobia;
- generalized anxiety disorder (GAD);
- post-traumatic stress disorder (PTSD);
- obsessive-compulsive disorder (OCD).

Although each anxiety disorder is distinct, with its own set of symptoms, different forms can coexist.

UNDERSTANDING HOW ANXIETY BUILDS

Anxiety disorders usually first appear in adolescence or early adulthood, and often persist for life. They were once ascribed to "separation anxiety" (being separated from parents), castration anxiety, punitive parenting or conflict. Nowadays, experts believe that biochemical plus psychological, cognitive, behavioral, social and cultural factors jointly produce these disorders. Many researchers lean toward a biological explanation for anxiety disorders, with an overactive nervous system and specific abnormalities or imbalances in the brain's neurotransmitters.

Finding the trigger(s) for anxiety problems is not easy, but in about half the cases therapists can piece together a scenario that at least partly accounts for the disorder. Many sufferers can point to stressors such as a family loss or conflict with an "important other" that precipitated the problem.

for incorrect diagnosis. Also, anxiety may accompany other illnesses, such as thyroid disease, asthma, heart ailments and gastric problems. Some drugs, licit and illicit—for instance, caffeine, cocaine, bronchodilators and amphetamines—provoke anxiety-like symptoms. Surveys show that many patients in family-practice units (one-quarter of patients, according to some studies) have transient panic attacks in certain situations or due to drugs such as marijuana or cocaine. Occasional panic attacks or those linked to drug use are not true anxiety disorders.

General treatment for anxiety disorders

Whatever the cause(s) of anxiety disorders, treatment usually entails psychological counseling, behavior or cognitive therapy and sometimes medication. A good therapist assesses the reasons for the anxiety, traces events that might have triggered it and evaluates its impact on everyday activities. The link between the underlying anxiety and physical symptoms such as chest pain and gastrointestinal upsets is pointed out to the anxious person.

For many, the most frightening part is the dread that some terrible disease is causing these symptoms. Many people seem to cope once they get a clear explanation of the condition, and know there's no incipient heart failure or other illness about to strike. Those whose anxiety is related to only a few situations can often get by without much professional aid. For example, someone who is afraid of public speaking faces no anxiety problem unless forced to address large groups; a woman who's afraid of dogs will be fine unless she is a veterinarian or marries someone who adores dogs. However, obsessive hand-washers who peel off their skin, or agoraphobics too afraid to leave the house, need intensive therapy. Fortunately, specific behavior therapy is often very effective.

Exposure therapy, which is becoming increasingly popular will quickly relieve some anxiety disorders, especially phobias. It helps people to confront the fear-evoking situation(s) in a controlled and graded way, enabling them to develop coping mechanisms. For example, an arachnophobic may be asked first to look at pictures of spiders, then to keep a spider in a cage at home,

then in the bedroom, until the discomfort subsides. An individual fearful of the subway is first taught relaxation exercises (deep breathing, visualizations, etc.) and then starts by going to the ticket counter or turnstile, then the following week goes down to the platform, possibly with a friend. At each stage, the anxiety comes on and is accepted and dealt with by the individual. Slowly the person becomes "immunized". This can be scary and counterintuitive for the anxious patient, especially the concept of "if it feels good that's bad, and if it feels bad, that's good."

Cognitive therapy means helping sufferers to understand the reason(s) for anxiety and to rationally reappraise the beliefs that make them feel defenseless and "forced to flee." The fearful thought mode—expectation of dreadful things that might happen—is replaced by logical patterns to break the cycle.

Pharmacotherapy employs anxiety-relieving medications (anxiolytics), for instance, the benzodiazepines, such as alprazolam, clonazepam or lorazepam. A major change has been the use of antidepressants for anxiety. Antidepressants have become first-line therapy, with benzodiazepines sometimes used at the beginning as it takes some time for the antidepressants to take effect. Some anxiety sufferers require benzodiazepines long term, others on an occasional basis. Many anxious people are reluctant to take such drugs for fear of dependence or addiction, but addiction is very unusual in those taking benzodiazepines for anxiety. Withdrawal symptoms of rebound anxiety, insomnia and tremors can be a problem when discontinuing benzodiazepines, so it's best to taper down dosages gradually.

Panic disorder in particular

The word "panic" comes from the Greek god Pan, who used to jump at passersby as a practical joke. But panic disorder is no laughing matter. Panic attacks often begin in the teens or early adulthood, and may come out of the blue, as episodes of terror that hit for no discernible reason. Previously mislabeled "housewives' disease" or "soldier's heart," panic attacks can immobilize people from all walks of life. Panic-ridden people may think they're having a heart attack or some other crisis; the typical symptoms—chest pain, shortness of breath and a sense of choking—

send many rushing to the hospital emergency department with the first few episodes. But the chest tightness is due to the anxiety, and is not a cardiac problem. Other symptoms include palpitations, flushing, chills, sweating, difficulty swallowing, dizziness, unsteadiness, feelings of unreality and a sense of incapacity. During an attack, many people feel strangely disconnected from their surroundings. Some think they are going to die or go mad. If the attacks continue, they begin to wonder whether they're crazy. Comments one University of Toronto specialist, "They may imagine it's due to something they did or that there is something about the situation during which the attacks happen that somehow triggered them. In trying to come up with answers, many misattribute the cause of panic attacks to the context in which they arose." For example, someone who had an attack while driving a car may believe there is something about driving or the destination that caused the panic. Panickers who link attacks with the situations in which they occur may avoid more and more places, developing an increasingly constricted lifestyle and sometimes becoming completely housebound. Yet those beset by panic attacks may not seem outwardly agitated. A U.S. National Institutes of Health report notes that many anxious patients see 10 or more doctors before their condition is accurately pinpointed and properly treated.

Panic attacks may start during major life changes, and in some cases therapists can piece together a psychosocial picture of what triggered the attacks—such as a divorce, a death in the family, stress or excess work. Some people function all right during the stressful event(s) and then panic when things calm down. Some have panic attacks mostly at night, others more in the daytime. Some experience several attacks a day—very unnerving. A typical panic attack lasts for 2 to 10 minutes, sometimes up to an hour. Even when the attack is over, anxiety can linger on for hours or days.

The diagnostic manual of the American Psychiatric Association defines panic disorder as "one or more panic attacks per week for four weeks or one or more, followed by persistent fears of panic." To qualify as panic disorder some attacks must be spontaneous and unexpected,

AGORAPHOBIA—OFTEN LINKED TO PANIC ATTACKS

Agoraphobia is the terror of being away from a safe place, or being somewhere from which escape is difficult. Agoraphobics typically develop a fear of driving, tunnels, bridges, shopping malls and subways. "What underlies the fear," says one expert, "is being in a place or situation where they can't get immediate help in case of a sudden panic attack. At its most extreme, agoraphobics won't even leave the house because of the terror expected."

Agoraphobia is often linked to or follows panic attacks, but it may also arise independently. The agoraphobic fear may relate to specific places: if a woman was in the laundromat when she first experienced panic, she may be reluctant to go into any laundromat. Treatment for agoraphobia is similar to that for panic disorder—psychotherapy, reassurance and antidepressants, as well as anxiolytic drugs, e.g., clonazepam (Rivotril).

not triggered by a definite event such as an exam or sighting a snake. Since alcohol may relieve the panic, it's not surprising that some panickers (about a third) become alcoholics. Panic disorders may also result in depression and suicide.

Treatment for panic attacks is the same as for most anxiety problems—behavior therapy, knowledge of what's going on in the person's life and reassurance that disease or death isn't imminent. Many panickers calm down once they know that the condition likely stems from a biochemical transmitter imbalance in the brain. Cognitive-behavioral therapy has proven effective, as well as pharmacotherapy with antidepressants. General education regarding the mechanisms of panic is almost always helpful.

Simple phobia

Simple phobias, among the commonest of anxiety disorders, entail persistent, irrational fears (sometimes amounting to panic) of circumscribed events or situations. Among the countless specific phobias, the most frequent fears are of animals (such as dogs, snakes, mice), heights, blood, crowds, enclosed spaces, lightning or air travel. More unusual phobias include arachnophobia (fear of spiders), photophobia (fear of light), sarcophagophobia (fear of being buried alive) and apiphobia (fear of bees). Phobias are more common in women than in men. They often begin around ages 7 to 9, but may persist through life. Many phobic people prefer to hide their phobias, just avoiding the triggers, but if circumstances force them to be in repeated contact with the feared situation—as with politicians afraid of air travel—therapy may be sought.

Treatment is with exposure therapy (see above), which often works well; sometimes a single session lasting a few hours eradicates the phobia. For example, one woman terrified of cats was confronted with a small cat in her therapy session, stood trembling by the door for 40 minutes, gradually came nearer touched the cat on the therapist's lap and, at the end of a 4-hour session, ended up with the cat on her lap, the phobia gone.

Social phobia

More common in men than women, social phobia is the fear of performing, of being scrutinized by peers or by the public, of "not being liked." Fearing evaluation, the social phobic blushes, trembles, feels faint and may be totally unable to perform. Social phobias typically revolve around speaking in public, going to restaurants, using public washrooms or signing one's name in front of a bank teller (for fear of a trembling hand and wobbly signature!). Most people experience these symptoms to some degree, but people with social phobia experience significant functional impact. Often beginning in adolescence, social phobias affect about 2 percent of the population. The inhibition or shyness can cripple social and professional life, possibly resulting in alcoholism and depression. For example, an 8-year-old who can't speak up in class may skip school; a lawyer unable to address the jury without trembling may change careers; an advertising creator afraid to present ideas, may turn to writing copy for others; or someone asked to join the head table at a banquet may refuse for fear others will see his or her inability to swallow.

Therapy may include antidepressants, education, and CBT. Beta blockers have not been examined for use in treating social phobia, but are used by many professionals to improve performance.

Generalized anxiety disorder (GAD)

Although less debilitating than panic disorder, generalized anxiety disorder (GAD) is a dis-

tressing complaint, with free-floating anxiety and jitteriness that are not usually crystallized into discrete panic episodes. General anxiety often manifests itself as physical symptoms with no anatomical or identifiable basis—such as tension (trembling, twitching, restlessness), gastric upsets, urinary problems, chest pain, headaches, autonomic system overactivity (dizziness, sweating, palpitations) and hypervigilance (being perpetually keyed up). GAD sufferers often report pervasive fatigue, insomnia and an inability to fall asleep. To qualify as GAD, symptoms must be prominent for 6 months or longer. GAD affects 2 to 5 percent of the population, striking more women than men. There is significant overlap with depression. The disorder resembles panic, but people with GAD get worried about far less severe symptoms than true panickers, often consulting physicians not only about physical ailments, but to discuss unrealistic worries such as fussing over a perfectly well child's health, anxiety about money when there are no financial problems or fear of losing a job when there is no cause for concern.

Treatment for generalized anxiety disorder is psychotherapy and medication, plus reassurance that it's not a deadly disease. GAD sufferers often recover once they realize that the physical manifestations stem from underlying anxiety and that lifestyle changes may solve the problem—for example, more rest periods, exercise and holidays.

Post-traumatic stress disorder (PTSD)

This anxiety condition arises after some overwhelming trauma such as rape, assault, car accidents, plane crashes, war, torture, imprisonment or natural disasters such as earthquakes or floods. Its prevalence and severity are often underestimated. "Shell shock" was the expression used for the World War I veterans in whom post-traumatic stress disorder was first documented. It is frequent among U.S. Vietnam combat veterans, as many as 50 percent of those who engaged in heavy combat apparently suffering from it. A University of Toronto study showed that 50 years later many World War II concentration camp survivors, especially those from Auschwitz, still suffer severe PTSD. Its striking features are recurrent nightmares, flashbacks of the traumatic event and intense anxiety on exposure to any reminders—such as helicopters for Vietnam veterans, and news bulletins or anti-Israeli propaganda for Nazi concentration-camp survivors. Those with PTSD may have numbing emotional detachment, recurrent insomnia, an exaggerated startle response (jumpiness) and profound guilt over having survived when others perished. The prevalence of post-traumatic disorder in the overall North American population is 1 percent.

Treatment for PTSD is psychotherapy to dispel the terrifying flashbacks, plus tricyclic antidepressants (such as imipramine) or MAOI antidepressants. But despite treatment, many with PTSD continue to suffer great distress.

Obsessive-compulsive disorder

Once regarded as a psychiatric curiosity, obsessive-compulsive disorder, or OCD, is now proving to be very common, affecting as many as 1 in 50 North Americans. After a flurry of media interest, evoked by 1980s television talk shows publicizing the usefulness of the drug buspirone for treating OCD, many people revealed their strange, sometimes bizarre, often secret behaviors. Obsessive-compulsives whose problem had nearly wrecked their lives told fellow sufferers how therapy had helped them. When columnist Ann Landers wrote about OCD, she was deluged with 8,000 letters in 1 week.

Many people with OCD try to hide their behavior even from family and close friends. Sigmund Freud noted that obsessives were adept at concealment because, having devoted several hours to their "secret doings," they functioned well for the rest of the day. The secret doings that Freud referred to were rituals performed to relieve the anxiety caused by obsessive thoughts. These obsessive thoughts are often "taboo" and so the rituals are the only outlet. A person who touches every lamppost, chews every mouthful hundreds of times, must brush his or her hair 200 times, spends hours opening and closing cupboards or is afraid to use the toilet for fear of germs may resemble a schizophrenic. But unlike psychotics, who believe their thoughts come from outside sources—from aliens or devils—obsessives know that their thoughts are their own. Nor are they neurotics; they know their actions are pointless, struggle to resist them, describe their behavior as "dumb," but are convinced that if they don't continue the rituals something bad will befall them or others. A well-known journalist feels compelled to check 10 times that her front door is closed every morning before going to work. An internist calls the lab a dozen times to make sure the test results are right, noting that his compulsion seems senseless, but still feels obliged to call. Some OCD sufferers stretch a routine activity like dressing from minutes to hours. Some feel compelled to go from the car to the front door in a certain way four steps forward, two back, or singing "Yankee Doodle Dandy" (to the despair of their families and the possible amusement of neighbors).

It should be noted that mild "obsessions" can simply be rigid ways of doing things. For example, some ultra-neat people can't sleep until every dinner dish has been cleared, all ashtrays emptied or crooked paintings straightened. Such eccentrics do *not* necessarily have OCD.

The American Psychiatric Association describes OCD as an illness with recurrent obsessions or compulsions, or both, severe enough to cause marked distress, be time-consuming (over 1 hour a day) or interfere significantly with normal routine. The obsessive thoughts are deeply disturbing, not pleasurable. In severe cases, the thoughts become so tormenting that the person sacrifices relationships, work, school and basic comfort to escape them. In some instances obsessives do nothing all day except attend to their rituals.

OCD tends to emerge in adolescence through to the mid-thirties, although it can start in childhood. It often remains hidden for many years. Fear of contamination is a common theme, many obsessives being afraid to shake hands or touch doorknobs because of possible dirt, or to eat for fear of poisoning. Others fear loss of control—they are afraid of strangling their children or killing a dog. Some have disturbing sexual thoughts, tormenting fantasies, blasphemous images, pathological doubts or concerns about sin or hell. Families often worry that the person with OCD may act out hostile obsessions, but obsessives want to avoid their thoughts, not derive pleasure from them. OCD patients very rarely put violent thoughts into action.

Common types of obsessives

- *Cleaners* (85 percent of those with OCD) have a fear of contagion that compels many to spend hours in the shower, or to wash their hands 50 or 60 times a day, often with harsh soaps, until their hands are raw. Although the obsessive knows that the dread of filth is irrational, the thoughts create such psychic distress that they must be relieved by constant cleansing. Washing eases the tension, but the distress soon builds up again until the cleaning must start over.

- *Checkers* (doubters) are compelled to continually recheck their actions—for instance, to make sure they have turned off the stove or locked the door. Some repeatedly visit the scene of an imagined accident to be certain they haven't run over a child on the way home. "They are reassurance addicts," comments one therapist, "constantly checking to make sure nothing's amiss."

- *Hoarders* may save every piece of mail they've ever received, every scrap of paper, even Christmas trees from past years—for fear that they'll throw out something valuable. Common obsessions are:

- fear of contamination: "Everything I touch is full of germs";

- doubt: "Did I hit that dog with my car?";

- orderliness: "I can't attend class until everything in my room is in perfect order";

- fear of aggression toward oneself or others— "If I had a knife, I might lose control and stab my mother"—necessitating compulsive acts to make sure the violence cannot happen (e.g., throwing out all sharp objects).

OCD was traditionally viewed as a psychological disorder attributed to restrictive parenting, early toilet training (causing an unhealthy obsession with cleanliness) or anxiety over sexual urges. But modern scientists believe it to be caused by a biological abnormality, probably an imbalance in one or more neurotransmitters (chemicals that act as messengers between nerve cells)—particularly serotonin, which modulates repetitive actions, sleep, aggression and grooming behavior. There may be too little serotonin in some areas of OCD brains, causing grooming behavior to go out of control. The fact that one-third of OCD cases improve with serotoninergic drugs (which raise serotonin levels) supports this possibility.

Treatment for obsessive-compulsive disorder is with psychotherapy, antidepressants, buspirone and serotonin-activating drugs, often in high doses, such as clomipramine (Anafranil), fluoxetine (Prozac), paroxetine (Paxil), sertraline (Zoloft), citalopram (Celexa) and fluvoxamine (Luvox). Even after several decades, only 20 percent of patients have made a complete recovery and 28 percent have "recovered" but continue to have symptoms that do not cause distress or interfere with daily activities. Since the medications suppress symptoms rather than curing the illness, the disorder may reemerge if the drugs are discontinued. In serious cases, several drugs may be needed. However, OCD is a complex disorder and therapy is not a matter of handing out a few pills and expecting lifelong horrors to vanish overnight. Many OCD sufferers have devoted hours each day to their obsessions for years, and it takes a great deal of psychotherapy to eradicate such deep-rooted behavior.

Behavior therapy employs "exposure" and "response prevention," exposing patients to the feared situations to reduce the rituals. In some studies, these methods are as effective as medication. Behavioral techniques provide relief for about 50 to 70 percent of patients. The therapist guides sufferers to confront the situation being avoided, such as touching door handles, shaking hands or eating certain foods, helping them to refrain from the ritualistic practices. Someone who detests dirt, for instance, will be asked to rub dirt on the hands and abstain from handwashing for a while. Alternatively, the person might be encouraged to visualize the anticipated catastrophe, such as running over a cat, become accustomed to the thought and extinguish the anxiety. In the most severe cases, when OCD makes life unlivable, brain surgery may be a last resort.

For further information, contact anxiety-disorder clinics or the Centre for Addiction and Mental Health (CAMH) at www.camh.net.

SCHIZOPHRENIA

Schizophrenia is a serious, often lifelong psychiatric illness that usually starts in young adulthood. Among historic figures thought to be schizophrenics, Louis Riel and the painter Hieronymus Bosch are two of the better known. Schizophrenia affects .5 to 1 percent of the population in all races and cultures. Many of us probably know someone who is a schizophrenic. The tragedy of schizophrenia is that it often comes as a bitter and unexpected blow, during or soon after the difficult teenage years, just when a youngster seems about to fulfill the promise of his or her childhood.

There is a genetic element—not yet fully understood—to schizophrenia. If one or other parent is a schizophrenic, the chance of a child having the illness rises to 10 percent. Should both parents be afflicted, the risk for their offspring is 40 percent. Although males and females are equally at risk, schizophrenia tends to show up earlier in males—in the late teens and early twenties—while in females the first schizophrenic crisis usually hits 10 years later between age 25 and 30. Traditionally, schizophrenics have been feared as violent criminal types—a myth to be dispelled, since the rate of violence among schizophrenics is no higher than among the rest of the population. However, their behavior often seems odd, owing to their distorted perception and thought patterns.

Defining schizophrenia

Still imperfectly understood, schizophrenia is a brain disorder now controllable by various drugs. The term "schizophrenia" originates from the Greek *schizo* and *phren*, meaning split mind, a term formerly used to describe the disorder's more common symptoms such as disconnected ideas, the hearing of voices and an inability to comprehend reality. Until recently, much confusion surrounded the definition of this and other mental illnesses, which were often indiscriminately lumped together.

A new diagnostic rigor has clarified the definition of schizophrenia as a "thought disorder." By the currently accepted definition, schizophrenia is an illness with psychotic episodes, heralded by an initial, acute (active) phase occurring before age 45, often in adolescence,

with continuous, intense symptoms (such as delusions and disordered thoughts) lasting at least 6 months. Its minor features may creep up slowly (before the onset of an obvious breakdown) and seem little different from the ordinary ups and downs of adolescence. In others, the illness hits like a bolt from the blue, with a full-blown, acute psychotic attack. Before schizophrenia is diagnosed, other possible causes of the symptoms—such as drug abuse, epilepsy, a brain tumor or metabolic disturbances—must be ruled out, and the condition must be clearly differentiated from affective (mood) disorders. The use of standardized, well-structured interviews has made the diagnosis of schizophrenia more accurate.

The natural course of schizophrenia is deterioration, which is usually greatest in the first few years following diagnosis. Rates of deterioration or symptom worsening vary markedly from one individual to another. The prognosis is better for women than men, for those who have a later onset of disease, for those who respond well to an initial course of medication, and for those who live in a relatively serene family environment. The prognosis is considerably worse if negative symptoms are prominent, if the patient also has a substance abuse disorder, and if social and cognitive functioning were poor before the onset of illness. The longer the duration of untreated psychosis, the worse the prognosis.

Some schizoid symptoms are hard to handle

The illness is signaled by a number of features, none of which is unique, but which together confirm and characterize schizophrenia. The most usual signs of an acute phase are the so-called "positive" (although detrimental) behavior changes:

- distorted thought processes—incoherent and illogical reasoning—shown by fragmented speech, jumbled or "nonsense" talk and use of idiosyncratic, sometimes unusually concrete phrases, often with a fixation on body parts;
- perceptual problems, in which schizophrenics think their thoughts are being deciphered or broadcast aloud, or that they can read the thoughts of others;
- auditory hallucinations—typical of the

illness—in which those affected hear voices inside their heads telling them what to do, or behave strangely in response to such instructions;

- delusions—false convictions of grandeur power or persecution, during the psychotic stage. Classic examples are a schizophrenic who imagines that he is Jesus or that an accidental bump in the subway is an assassination plot. Such convictions are tenaciously held against all reason;

- paranoid suspicions—where an innocent smile, remark or joke is misconstrued as being directed solely against the schizophrenic, perhaps with malicious intent;

- intense and prolonged spiritual and other preoccupation; schizophrenics may become lost in ideas that, if communicated, seem bizarre to others.

- inability to distinguish fantasy from fact; a belief that daydreams are true.

The reappearance of some of these symptoms during a quiescent phase of the illness should alert the schizophrenic, caregivers and family to the possibility of a repeat breakdown.

Apathetic inactivity awaits many with schizophrenia

Alternating with psychotic interludes in schizophrenia are calmer intervals when the person is not really back to normal, but exhibits "negative" aspects of the condition—not easily amenable to drugs or psychiatric treatment. These include extreme lassitude (often mistaken for laziness), passivity or a tendency to shun social contact, slow and impoverished thinking, sluggish movement, incongruous emotions (such as laughing at a sad event), ritualistic behavior and isolation. There may be an inability to complete even small jobs or to organize and plan daily living. Poor hygiene, sloppy dressing and social withdrawal make it difficult for the schizophrenic to cope with jobs, friendships and dating.

The apathetic state continues—sometimes for a lifetime—with occasional psychotic flare-ups, which can be triggered by stress or excitement. Some people with schizophrenia find the quiescent stage of their illness dull, empty and harder to bear than its hallucinatory highs. A few may try—by quitting medication or

seeking tense situations—to reawaken the acute phase and lose themselves in delusions of grandeur rather than face the reality of an unsatisfying existence.

Research probes the causes of schizophrenia

Although the exact nature of the malfunction is unknown, neurochemists believe that schizophrenia probably involves an imbalance in dopamine, a brain transmitter and that the disorder may stem from an abnormal reactivity to dopamine. In certain areas of some schizophrenic brains, an excess of dopamine-sensitive receptors has been found. The drugs used for the illness work by suppressing dopamine action. Some studies suggest alternative causes of schizophrenia, such as early viral infection, birth injuries that deprive brain cells of oxygen, and anatomical brain abnormalities—shown by CAT scans (special brain X-rays).

The knowledge that schizophrenia arises from some organic or biochemical dysfunction, rather than from faulty upbringing or psychological influences, comforts many parents who might otherwise feel responsible for bringing about their child's disorder.

Treatment with drugs can usually control symptoms

Thanks to psychotherapy, a broad range of neuroleptic (antipsychotic) medications and a more tolerant public attitude toward mental illness, those with schizophrenia are no longer shamefully shunted off to psychiatric institutions. Some now live and work within the community (about 25 percent have full-time employment). Brief admissions to hospital may be necessary for relapses when symptoms flare, but hospital treatment, although a crucial element, is no longer the only therapy. Like diabetes, schizophrenia is a chronic lifetime disorder that needs regular attention, though some suffer only one attack and recover fully. Regular use of antipsychotic drugs can help prevent attacks.

The standard (older) antipsychotic medications used for schizophrenia include *chlorpromazine* (Largactil, Thorazine), *haloperidol* (Haldol) and *trifluoperazine* (Apotex, Stelazine). These drugs bind to and block dopamine recep-

A FEW GUIDELINES FOR FAMILY AND FRIENDS OF THOSE WITH SCHIZOPHRENIA

- Above all, persuade sufferers to stay on their prescribed medication regime and keep doctors' appointments.
- Provide a calm, supportive, unstressful atmosphere.
- Explain clearly at all times what you're doing and why; speak precisely.
- Be realistic in your expectations.
- Avoid being too inquisitive or probing thoughts too deeply, while still inviting schizophrenics to share ideas and experiences.
- Arguing or calling schizoid delusions irrational only leads to mistrust and anger. A better response to a sufferer's belief that he or she is Jesus would be "I guess you feel special and different today. Let's try a low-key routine for the next few days."
- Encourage a structured lifestyle with a regular routine and small tasks, praised if well done; include sanctions and rewards as suitable.
- Remember that motor actions—such as cooking, carpentry, drawing and other mechanical tasks—may be easier than verbal efforts (although this varies according to former ability); most will attempt whatever activities they did before becoming ill.
- Enlist help in volunteer jobs, such as making cookies or helping the blind, provided it's within the abilities of the individual patient.
- Remember that, depending on the severity of the illness and previous abilities, each person with schizophrenia can tackle different challenges.
- Coax the sufferer to engage in gentle social interaction, but avoid large parties or big family gatherings.
- Since schizophrenics are shy people and find intimate and sexual relationships difficult, don't push them unduly.
- If in doubt about what to do, consult the patient's therapist, and consider joining a friends' and relatives' discussion group.

tors at nerve endings in the brain, cutting down the excess dopamine action. Long-acting injections are sometimes better than tablets, which many forget or neglect to take. The older antipsychotics control the so-called positive symptoms of schizophrenia (the distortions, hallucinations and delusions) in many who take them, but are less effective against its negative aspects (the lassitude, emotional numbness, thought limitation and withdrawal).

The older antipsychotic drugs have some troublesome side effects, which include agitation (a restless desire to pace about), vision disturbances, some weight gain, muscle tremors (like those in Parkinson's disease), a mask-like expression and drowsiness. Late-onset side effects include extrapyramidal (jerky) movements and tardive dyskinesia—involuntary, restless movements of fingers, head, jaws and tongue, which produce strange gestures and grimaces that schizophrenics are largely unaware of but that can disconcert others. Side effects may seem worse than the disease itself although some can be reduced by counteractive medication.

The newer "atypical" antipsychotics, available since the late 1980s, have greatly improved the treatment of schizophrenia, helping many who previously resisted treatment to function better. Atypical antipsychotics include *clozapine* (Clozaril), *risperidone* (Risperdal, Risperdone), *olanzapine* (Zyprexa) and most recently, *quetiapine* (Seroquel). These atypical antipsychotics combat both the positive and the negative aspects. As added advantages they have fewer side effects than other agents, with less (or no) extrapyramidal tremors, tics and twitches. (Side effects of the atypicals include dizziness, drowsiness, dry mouth and weight gain.) Rather than targeting just the dopamine neurotransmitter pathway, newer drugs also block some serotonin transmitter action, rebalancing the brain's chemistry. While still not a cure, the new antipsychotics allow many schizophrenics to reintegrate into the community and workforce.

In general, schizophrenics are maintained on a steady low dose of medication to suppress the most distressing symptoms of their illness, with temporarily higher doses when a breakdown or flare seems imminent. Full recovery, relatively uncommon, depends on the severity of the illness. If it happens, recovery usually comes within the first 2 years: it's rare after 5 years of the disease. However, a degree of social recovery—the ability to function outside hospital—occurs in many of those afflicted. With time, each schizophrenic learns his or her limits and realizes the usefulness of the medication. After a person reaches 40, life with

THE CHOICE OF THERAPISTS FOR EMOTIONAL AND PSYCHIATRIC PROBLEMS INCLUDES:

- medically trained psychiatrists (fees covered by health-care plans);
- psychologists, who practice various forms of psychotherapy and may be research-oriented or clinical (giving practical advice);
- psychoanalysts, who usually have no medical degree but have themselves undergone some kind of rigorous analysis (Jungian, Freudian, Adlerian, Reichian, Gestalt, whatever)

and now administer similarly oriented psychotherapy to others;
- social workers, who may provide individual or group psychological and lifestyle counseling, or do mainly community or organizational social work. Clinical social workers generally provide therapy in the context of family, marital, work, lifestyle and other problems;
- pastoral counselors

(perhaps for those with religious affiliations);
- relaxation therapists;
- various types of relationship and sex-counseling services;
- child- and family-service associations for marital and child-care counseling;
- workplace employee-assistance programs, often an excellent place to get advice and therapy;
- group therapists;
- self-help agencies.

schizophrenia often becomes less distressing—psychotic episodes diminish, maintenance drugs can be minimal and the quality of life improves.

Skipping medication is a big problem

Often, those with schizophrenia feel so well on the antipsychotic medication that they go off their drugs, risking relapse. Many patients quit because of the false illusion that they're cured, in denial of their illness or because of discomfort from side effects. They miss medical appointments and often move—even out of town—to avoid supervision. Some heap abuse on their caretakers, venting the frustration of their illness on others. Quitting or skipping medication usually produces a slow deterioration, a return of acute symptoms and rehospitalization, so people looking after schizophrenics should aim to be viewed as aides rather than adversaries. Treatment programs should be flexible and nonjudgmental and help patients remain in treatment.

Rehabilitation is an uphill battle

Since this illness strikes the young, their lives are often interrupted during the formative years by repeated hospital stays. They therefore have

little schooling or job skills. Owing to unemployment, apathy and neglect, many schizophrenics are malnourished and poor forced to live in hardship and deprivation. A few rehabilitation programs are available to help them learn new job skills, and to teach them to look after themselves, manage their illness and avoid relapses. For lack of alternatives, many schizophrenics use emergency departments of hospitals as primary care (medical help) facilities.

Some schizophrenics ultimately manage to live alone and hold a job—a situation that not only lessens the burden on the family but also helps raise self-esteem. Others live in group homes, which provide a range of supervision from round the clock to once a week or so. Families can join support groups and share their worries with other families of schizophrenics. Various organizations have sprung up to help schizophrenics and their families and helpers, such as The Canadian Friends of Schizophrenics, 95 Barber Greene Road, Suite 309, Don Mills, Ont. M3C 3E9, tel.: (416) 445-8204.

FINDING THERAPY FOR MENTAL AND EMOTIONAL PROBLEMS

In deciding where to find help for mental, emotional and psychological disorders, people are often confused by the multitude of different therapists out there—ranging from psychiatrists and psychologists to social workers, marital counselors and behaviorists. It's wise to find out what's what in the world of psychosocial counseling, and distinguish between "stress-related distress" (which may stem from work or lifestyle habits), remedied by simple relaxation therapy, and deeper problems that need the attention of a psychologist or psychiatrist. Mentally troubled or disturbed people have to decide whether they need advice from a psychiatrist (who has a medical degree, with fees usually covered by provincial healthcare plans) or nonmedical therapy from a clinical psychologist, social worker or other counselor. It is difficult to generalize about effectiveness as much of it depends on the nature of the relationship with the therapist.

In general, psychiatrists are best equipped to handle mental illnesses such as schizophrenia, OCD, PTSD, or severe depression. For emotional or stress-related issues talking to a nonmedical therapist about worries and feelings may be as good as or better than psychiatric treatment.

The way to start is by discussing the problem with your family physician, who can help in advising you where to turn and give you an appropriate referral. Most family physicians have considerable expertise in managing depression and anxiety. Some also have a special interest in mental health, have received advanced training, and spend some or all of their clinic time conducting psychotherapy. They are also often "connected" with experts in the more complex mental health illnesses. Psychologists have received special training in talk therapy and can be an excellent resource. Often the choice comes down to finances as psychiatrists and family doctors are covered by provincial funding. Social workers, psychologists and others can be covered when associated with a hospital or special program, but often are not. Friends and colleagues at work are also good people to ask for advice on where to get help. The plethora of different therapists can be confusing, as it's diffi-cult to know who does what! There is no licensing body for psychotherapists, and so anyone can hang up a sign as a "therapist." To distinguish one therapist from another ask for credentials and inquire about the therapist's training and background. Does he or she belong to a licensed body or association? Does he or she have a special license to practice?

Overcoming the stigma of mental illness

Discrimination against those with psychiatric illnesses has a long, dark history. Even today the stigma remains, and people with manic depressive disorder depression or other psychiatric illnesses often hesitate to seek help because of it. Millions who suffer from psychiatric disorders, which respond well to modern treatment, do not obtain professional care and suffer needlessly. In recent years, efforts have been made to heighten the awareness of mental illness as a major health problem. Many employers have developed employee-assistance programs (EAPs) through which people can get confidential help for mental or emotional problems.

Keeping up the quality of life with advancing years

The aging brain • Caring for well elderly relatives • Incontinence • Parkinson's disease • Osteoporosis • Alzheimer's disease

15

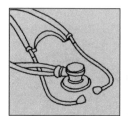

AGING IS NOT A disease. Mental ability and intelligence do not inevitably dwindle as we age. While there's some loss of brain cells and non-disease-related loss of memory as people age, other mental functions such as wisdom, knowledge and judgment often improve with advancing years. Seniors vary widely in their retention of mental capacities.

The vast majority of older people are the "well" elderly, who remain healthy into their later years, often needing little or no help. Given safe household organization, social involvement and an active lifestyle, many can go on living at home to a ripe old age.

THE AGING BRAIN

Contrary to earlier beliefs, the brain remains open to learning even in the very old, provided it's not diseased. Crystalline intelligence, which uses past experience and verbal ability, may actually increase with advancing years, provided there are no serious health problems and the person continues to use the brain by reading, socializing, game playing and taking on new interests. Cognitive decline in aging humans may increase with boredom, depression or loss of interest. The popular saying "Use it or lose it" may be trite but is likely quite apt.

The exact nature of the brain's cognitive (thinking) changes with increasing age remains controversial. While some experts argue that functions such as memory and reasoning tend to diminish, others suggest that such apparent changes may be a matter of prejudice and per-

LAYING TO REST SOME COMMON MYTHS ABOUT AGING

• *Myth:* The elderly are all alike.
Fact: People over age 65 are more unlike one another than members of any other age group. Immune-system function and mental agility differ more widely in the elderly than at other ages,

and personality too seems to differentiate more with advancing years. As the saying goes, "People remain themselves, only more so."
• *Myth:* Aging means degenerative diseases and disorders.
Fact: Few diseases are directly due to aging.

While conditions such as atherosclerosis (artery blockage) and arthritis (joint stiffness) are more common in old age, they are not just a consequence of advancing years. Similarly, many disorders such as cataracts, hearing loss, depres-

sion and incontinence are not a normal or inevitable part of aging. Old age is not a disease!
• *Myth:* Younger people don't really think about old age.
Fact: Modern society has an obsessive fear of both growing old and the ultimate,

common destiny of death.
• *Myth:* It's too late to start healthy habits in old age.
Fact: The elderly benefit as much as other age groups from good nutrition, regular exercise and other health-promoting activities.

ception, or may stem from a lack of stimulation or too little motivation to do well on mental function tests. In many of those who do poorly on such tests, the failure stems from physical illness, depression or medications taken, rather than old age.

Modern research shows the brain to be far more adaptable than hitherto imagined. Scientists have recently discovered that one type of neuron (nerve cell) abundant in adulthood is preserved in the healthy elderly, perhaps contributing to their wisdom. Recent research also suggests that while many brain cells do die off and cannot be replaced, the decay of synapses (nerve connections) is not necessarily irreversible. The growth of new nerve connections is the brains way of sculpting quicker pathways. Many experts now think that the brain possesses more neuroplasticity and restructuring ability than formerly believed, and that new nerve pathways replace old ones after injury or cell death.

Normal versus abnormal mental changes

There is generally some slowing of reaction times with advancing years, but recent studies show that the healthy elderly are only fractionally slower than younger people. For example, a 70-year-old may take one quarter of a second more time to identify a familiar object or read a speedometer than a 30-year-old. In practical terms, reaction times slowed by even a fraction of a second can be dangerous when quick reflexes are essential—as in crossing the street or driving a car; however; the greater experience and caution of older people may compensate for their slightly slower reactions.

Memory declines with advancing years, but memory problems are complex, related to both storing and retrieving facts. The retrieval of recent knowledge when wanted, at a particular moment in time, is often difficult for the elderly, but the information frequently surfaces later—not really amounting to memory loss. If asked to associate a memory with a familiar reminder, the memory degradation over time is often found to be minimal. So-called memory-pills such as Gerovital, Ribaminol, lecithin and various vitamin and dietary supplements have *not* been shown to be efficacious, and experimental drugs

---

USUAL CHANGES OF THE NERVOUS SYSTEM WITH AGE

The average brain of a 75-year-old man weighs 45 percent less than that of a 30-year-old man. Cerebral blood flow, oxygen and glucose metabolism decline with age. These changes produce various sensory, perceptual and behaviour alterations, but the effects of these changes can be minimized or accommodated.

- *Diminished heat and cold regulation* Elderly people are less adaptable to temperature extremes and feel the heat and cold more than the young. A reduction in sweating makes them more susceptible to heat exhaustion, and an impaired ability to increase the core body temperature makes them more vulnerable to the cold.
- *Dulled taste and smell* Starting in middle age, many people experience dimin-

ished taste sensitivity due to a loss of taste buds. A combined loss of taste and smell may make older people more vulnerable to appetite disorders and malnutrition.

- *Hearing changes* Hearing may begin to deteriorate starting at age 30, and it becomes progressively harder to hear high frequencies. Speech processing too becomes more difficult, and many elderly people can't distinguish among certain sounds (in particular c, t, s). Speaking clearly when addressing the elderly and facilitating lip-reading by keeping one's face in the light can ease communication.
- *Eye and vision alterations* Changes in both the structure and the function of the eyes mean that many people come to need reading glasses. With

advancing age, they find it harder to adapt from a bright environment to a darker one, and they need brighter lights for reading. Most of these changes (as opposed to disease-related disorders) can be accommodated—for example, using sunglasses in bright light, night lights in the dark or large-print books. Peripheral vision (being able to see at the edges of the visual field) may also become impaired. The elderly may have difficulty focusing on near objects (such as the speedometer) after looking at distant objects, and many find glare a problem—which can increase the hazards of driving a car or crossing the street. (Seniors must beware of driving at night, especially in vehicles with tinted windows.)

---

such as cognitive and metabolic enhancers—ergoloid mesylates (Hydergine), phystigimine and tetrahydroaminoacridine—which target certain neurotransmitter systems, have only limited (if any) benefits. At present, there are no effective memory drugs.

Although old age is commonly equated with senility and dementia (a decline in intellectual abilities such as language and abstract thought), less than 30 percent of the population ever suffers from any form of dementia, including Alzheimer's disease. However, such disorders cannot at present be prevented, even with early detection.

CARING WELL FOR ELDERLY RELATIVES

One of contemporary society's challenges is care of an increasing elderly population. In Canada, as elsewhere, family members—mostly women—are the primary caregivers of aging relatives. Their support is critical in keeping older people out of institutions. Yet, with growing numbers of women in the workforce, these added responsibilities may cause considerable strain. The goal is to give enough help while not "taking over," letting elders retain as much independence as possible for as long as possible, while at the same time ensuring that caregivers don't abandon or neglect their own interests. While the population of the "frail elderly" (over age 85) grows, the number of children aged 14 and under is steadily declining. Even at present, the elderly use more healthcare services than any other segment of the population.

According to experts from the University of Toronto's Centre for Studies on Aging, the job of keeping "frail older people out of institutions rests mainly on the backs of informal caregivers—relatives and friends—who provide about 80 percent of needed assistance to the elderly." Those looking after the unwell or fragile elderly can enlist varied services—home-support agencies, visiting nurses, aides, physiotherapists, social workers, homemakers, social clubs and Meals on Wheels—which help to maintain a senior's independence.

Maintain elderly independence as long as possible

Surveys show that seniors fear the loss of independence and admission into long-term care facilities above all else. The specter of reliance on others is upsetting; even losses such as no longer driving a car can be hard to accept, and may be resisted long after it is unsafe for the driver to be on the road. Anyone looking after older people must recognize this intense anxiety and respect their wish for continued independence. The average age of entry into geriatric institutions in Canada is 82, but we tend to overinstitutionalize our old people.

Geriatricians see an urgent need for more varied living arrangements that suit seniors, especially since premature institutionalization may accelerate a decline in functions such as memory and walking ability. Supported housing (with centralized care available), retirement homes or innovative boarding arrangements (e.g., a live-in student who gives assistance in return for a room) can help seniors to remain independent. Accessory apartments, garden suites or other residential options may help families care for aging relatives. High- and low-tech devices can prolong the ability of frail seniors to stay at home—for instance, vital-function monitors, surveillance devices for wanderers or emergency alarm systems—but they are not publicized enough, readily available or easily affordable.

When the condition of an older person deteriorates to the point that home caregivers can no longer cope, full investigation of all possible institutional options and a thorough discussion of the choices are advised. This will help to reduce and possibly eliminate resistance from the elderly relative, and relieve the caregivers inevitable feelings of guilt and doubt.

Moving in with family members

While most older people prefer to go on living in their own homes, there are several other choices—for example, housing plans or "continuing-care" retirement communities that offer residential and healthcare facilities under one roof.

People who decide to live with their children should plan the transition thoughtfully, express feelings openly, anticipate how the arrangement might work and ask themselves a few key questions:
- Do I really want to live with this child?
- Can I adapt to my offspring's lifestyle?
- How good a relationship do I have with my children?
- Would I feel like a "constant visitor"?
- Could I still pursue my personal interests?
- How much space and privacy would there be?
- Are there stairs to climb? How convenient are the toilet and bathroom?
- How about the financial arrangements; would I share household expenses?

Use all available support and community services

Caregivers should investigate and use all the supplemental support services they need or can afford from community, government, nonprofit and private home-support services. It's wise to enlist simultaneous help from several organizations, such as seniors' health centers, day hospitals, outpatient and in-patient medical and psychiatric services, hospital-based home care, geriatric day centers, community and social clubs (e.g., Second Mile or Senior Link in Toronto).

- *For housekeeping help:* visiting homemakers will clean the house, prepare meals, shop and do laundry. Cost is usually geared to income, and provinces and municipalities may subsidize services.
- *For personal hygiene:* a private or nonprofit trained helper, suggested by a physician or other healthcare professional, may come in to assist an elderly person with bathing, dressing, eating and some homemaking activities.
- *For safety:* to alleviate anxiety and summon emergency help if needed, telephone security checks may be organized. A volunteer; friend or neighbor may telephone seniors each day and, if there's no answer initiate emergency procedures. Many hospitals and private organizations supply electronic devices such as beepers that alert emergency medical units if seniors need help.
- *For social needs:* many clubs and senior day programs offer companionship and rehabilitative activities. Studies show that social support benefits health—even support as simple as someone to chat with, to share the occasional meal with, to provide companionship or to facilitate attendance at religious services.
- *For food:* Meals on Wheels (or other agencies) may deliver hot meals several times a week.
- *For medical disorders:* some healthcare services provide multidisciplinary assessment teams (of nurses, social workers, physical and occupational therapists, recreation experts, physicians, dentists, audiologists, dietitians, respirologists, speech therapists and others) to offer advice and help. Therapeutic, educational, social and recreation programs may be provided, with costs sometimes covered by provincial healthcare plans. Home-care visits may be arranged for those who qualify under Ministry of Health guidelines. Geriatric day-care or home-care programs (sometimes funded by provincial agencies) have many advantages over hospital stays. Pioneering efforts include New Brunswick's Extra-Mural Hospital or "Hospital without Walls," which provides hospital care at home, British Columbia's Quick Response Team (in Victoria) and the Regional Geriatric Program of Metro Toronto (affiliated with the University of Toronto).
- *For relieving caregivers:* some nursing homes provide temporary (vacation or respite) admittance for a day or week, or a relief caregiver may come into the house for a few hours weekly. Geriatric daycare, short stays in an institutional setting and even round-the-clock in-home services for a limited time can ease the caregiver's burden.

Encourage exercise: it can make people act and feel younger

Reduced cardiovascular function, muscle wasting and bone loss are no longer considered a natural part of aging, but a result of inactivity. Yet only about one-fifth of the current elderly population is physically active at a level that upgrades heart health. Studies confirm that the elderly can greatly improve their quality of life, and perhaps ward off osteoporosis, by regular weight-bearing exercise. A brisk walk gives a good workout, provided it's done at the right pace and for at least 20 to 30 minutes, 3 times a week. (Getting a dog often gives seniors an extra incentive to walk!) For those who can't walk, swimming and stationary bicycles give a good workout. One University of Toronto expert says that "even in their seventies, some people can push their functional ages back by as much as 20 years by regular exercise, the gains showing up as more efficient cardiovascular function (heart able to pump blood with less effort). Exercise also enhances the ability to cope with stress, offsets depression, facilitates sleep and enhances appetite." Recent studies show that exercise may even help to keep the brain in shape.

CARE OF THE ELDERLY SHOULD:

- **provide support while preserving independence and the best possible quality of life;**
- **identify and ameliorate physical and psychiatric disorders;**
- **ensure that seniors get all needed immunizations (e.g., tetanus boosters, yearly influenza shots and a one-only pneumonia vaccine.**
- **help organize living arrangements to promote independence—especially by preventing possible falls, monitoring medications taken, ensuring adequate nutrition and encouraging activity;**
- **find supported housing when needed;**
- **counsel those facing serious or terminal illnesses;**
- **ease the burden on caregivers—giving them periodic respite as well as physical and psychological support.**

Promote good nutrition

Nutritional requirements in old age roughly parallel those for other adults, although after age 50 fewer and fewer calories are required. But some of the elderly are malnourished because of poverty, physical disabilities, multiple medications, social isolation and a natural decline in smell and taste which reduces appetite. Widowed or single people often lose interest in preparing meals for themselves, and their food choices may be restricted by poverty. Difficulties in mobility, seeing and chewing may make it hard to prepare and eat food. Also, many illnesses of the elderly (such as stroke) can profoundly alter mood, which in turn can have a strong effect on nutritional intake. In particular, older people must remember to eat high-quality, easily digestible protein such as fish, chicken and eggs. Getting enough calcium is also essential, to reduce the risks of osteoporosis. Besides milk, good sources of calcium are canned salmon (eaten with mashed bones), milk products such as yogurt and cottage cheese and other soft cheeses and some green vegetables such as broccoli. Since chewing can be difficult for some, especially those with ill-fitting dentures, they may prefer soft foods and puréed fruit or vegetables. But they should choose meat, vegetables and fruit rather than pre-prepared combination dinners or soups.

Avoiding falls is a top priority

Bone and soft-tissue injuries from falls are the sixth major cause of death among people over 65. For those who are 80 years old and over who suffer hip fractures, the 6-month mortality rate exceeds 20 percent because of postoperative complications. The chance of falling in a given year increases from 25 percent at age 70 to 40 percent after age 75, and half of those who fall do so repeatedly—acquiring a fear of falling and severely curtailing their activities. Until age 75 women outdo men in falls, but after that the sexes even out. Besides broken bones, other injuries (bleeding, sprains, joint dislocations) contribute to the toll of falls. Repeated falls are a major reason for institutionalizing the elderly, and for the reduction in activity that can cause further deterioration.

Thorough medical checkups are advisable

Successful care of the elderly means distinguishing the so-called normal changes of aging from those due to underlying diseases that can be treated. Besides ongoing therapy for chronic, long-term conditions (such as diabetes and arthritis), medical exams permit early detection of newly developing conditions (such as low thyroid function or vision loss). During medical visits, the elderly shouldn't remain passive but should discuss any worries about their health or treatment. Make a list beforehand and report any abnormal

WAYS TO AVOID INSTITUTIONALIZATION

- **Granny flats (zoning requirements permitting) are self-contained, portable units temporarily installed on the property of relatives with single-family homes. (They are not very successful—nobody seems to want them and the elderly won't stay in them.) One expert says, "Either take them into your home as 24-hour members of the family or find** another solution."
- **Accessory apartments are part of a family member's home, or an added room converted to create a small, self-contained unit.**
- **In group homes people share the expenses, staff and management of a property and communal rooms such as the kitchen and living room, while retaining their own bedrooms and possibly bath-** rooms. Jointly hired staff can help with or provide cooking and maintenance. (Consult local health departments for contacts.)
- **Foster care suits elderly people who cannot live alone; they move in with an unrelated family that provides meals and personal care for an arranged fee.**
- **In home-sharing, elderly home owners with extra space take** in tenants who give housekeeping help in exchange for reduced rent.
- **Supported housing refers to residences within a neighborhood or a section of an apartment building, or specially designed multiple-unit buildings, which provide elderly people with self-contained units connected to a central administration area by a call system.** Residents usually come together for some meals and social activities.

 To find help, consult the local Ministry of Health, Ministry of Community and Social Services, provincial offices for seniors affairs (some of which have a toll-free 800 line) and municipal health departments, which provide information on local homes for the aged, seniors apartments and social clubs.

occurrences, pain or discomfort. Even a seemingly small or meaningless symptom may give clues to some underlying disorder. Caregivers can act as affirmers or advocates, helping to overcome language difficulties and explain things, but should never assume the role of "parent" or exclude the elder from the discussion. The elderly person and caregivers should disclose any and all symptoms and bring along all medications being taken, inquire about the medications prescribed—what they do, how they act, whether they have side effects—and about possible non-drug alternatives. Those worried about an aged person's ability to live alone or the extent and appropriateness of medication can ask the physician how best to manage the situation. Referral for specialized geriatric evaluation helps to reveal the overall picture. Geriatricians stress the need for house calls by family physicians, particularly for the frail elderly, to permit assessment in the home surroundings. A home visit may reveal hazards such as an unsafe bathroom, a poorly lit staircase, unopened pill containers (suggesting failure to take prescribed medication), a hidden whisky bottle or the inability of a seemingly competent 80-year-old to use the telephone (perhaps revealing memory loss due to Alzheimer's disease).

For further information on care of the elderly, contact the National Advisory Council on Aging (NACA); senior-care services; regional geriatric programs; makers of special alert devices; the Parkinson Foundation of Canada in Toronto, tel.: (416) 964–1155; the Alzheimer Society of Canada, tel.: (416) 925–3552; Meals on Wheels; visiting homemaker associations; local Ministry of Community and Social Services; in Ontario: the Baycrest Centre for Geriatric Care, tel.: (416) 789–5131, 3560 Bathurst St., North York, Ont. M6A 2E1; Senior Care, tel.: (416) 635–9492; the Regional Geriatric Program of Metropolitan Toronto, tel.: (416) 785–2488. Read *Planning Your Retirement* by Blossom Wigdor; *Old Enough to Feel Better* and *An Ounce of Prevention: The Canadian Guide to Healthy and Successful Retirement* by Michael Gordon.

INCONTINENCE
Previously considered an unmentionable subject, the elderly and not-so-elderly leaky bladder

---

KEEP TABS ON ALL MEDICATIONS

Overmedication, inappropriate prescribing (doses not properly geared to the elderly) and harmfully interacting drug combinations can compound the disabilities of aging. Most drugs are tested in young and middle-aged adults and standard drug doses may endanger older people, who metabolize the same drugs differently. The World Health Organization (WHO) and other agencies have issued guidelines for prescribing drugs to the elderly.

WHO drug guidelines for the elderly:
- **No drug should be used if there is an effective and reasonable nonpharmaceutical alternative (e.g., exercise, physiotherapy or behavior therapy).**
- **A medication should not be prescribed if it is only marginally useful and has possible adverse effects.**
- **Pharmacists should be consulted to avoid drug interactions between substances prescribed for different conditions. (Fill prescriptions at the same pharmacy to aid monitoring.)**
- **Prescribing practices that contradict these principles should be questioned.**

---

is now taken more seriously. Incontinence is the involuntary loss of urine to a degree that causes social and/or health problems. It plagues many people, old and young, and is often the final event that puts the elderly into chronic-care institutions when the family can no longer cope. Recent studies reveal not only that incontinence is amazingly common, but that it can often be completely cured or dramatically relieved.

REGULAR MEDICAL CHECKUPS FOR SENIORS MAY INCLUDE:

- **An eye examination and history to check for glaucoma, cataracts, retinal degeneration and other problems;**
- **a yearly dental examination;**
- **ear and hearing tests;**
- **monitoring of ongoing conditions such as diabetes, arthritis, high blood cholesterol or hypertension, and disorders prone to complications;**
- **breast examination;**
- **encouragement to get recommended immunizations— yearly flu shots, a once-only anti-pneumonia shot, tetanus boosters.**

Other examinations, if warranted, are:
- **mobility checks (joint flexibility, range of motion, strength);**
- **a full review of all medications being taken;**
- **evaluation of the ability to perform the activities of daily living (dressing, bathing, toilet use, cooking, cleaning, shopping);**
- **mental status assessment for mood, memory, cognition and depression;**
- **review of the use of aids and support services such as wheelchairs, canes, visiting healthcare helpers and homemakers.**

SENSIBLE TIPS FOR THE ELDERLY AND THOSE LOOKING AFTER THEM

Ensure adequate nutrition

- *Watch for signs of malnutrition* such as weight loss, low energy, mental confusion. Act early to correct poor eating habits.
- *Eat enough high-quality protein* (e.g., fish, chicken, eggs).
- *Prepare and freeze small portions*—for reheating in boiling water or a microwave oven.
- *If chewing is a problem*, choose nourishing puréed foods.
- *Avoid sudden or drastic weight-reduction programs*; there is always a trade-off between the fun of eating and diets that undermine health.
- *Caregivers can provide transportation to the supermarket*, do the shopping, carry heavy parcels or ask volunteers from a home support service to help.
- *Consider Meals on Wheels.*

Get enough exercise/activity

- *Activity should continue* within personal limits.
- *Promote weight-bearing activity*, which helps to ward off osteo-porosis—especially walking, which can build bone strength. Wear nonslip shoes with good support. Try balance exercises.
- *Check Out the YMCA/YWCA and other community organizations* for seniors' exercise programs.

Monitor medications

- *Assist the elderly person to check* on the drugs being taken from time to time.
- *Discuss whether medications are taken correctly*; use clocks, notes and phone calls as reminders.
- *Label containers* VERY clearly.
- *Check expiry dates*, throw out and appropriately replace expired items.
- *Ask the physician and/or pharmacist about adverse side effects* and possible complications of prescribed medications; try to use the same pharmacist for all prescriptions to establish a personal relationship and systematic file.
- *Ask the physician if there are nondrug alternatives* to prescribed medicines (especially if falling is frequent).

Prevent falls and accidents (a top priority)

- *Watch for causes and risks of falls* such as: waning muscle strength; weak hand grip; acute illnesses (e.g., influenza, food poisoning); vision disturbances (cataracts, glaucoma, macular degeneration); arthritis (stiffened joints); previous strokes; gait disturbances and multiple medications (especially sedating, tranquilizing and blood-pressure drugs).
- *Periodically review all drugs taken*, making sure instructions are followed. Inquire about medication side effects. Some drug combinations, such as tranquilizers, antihistamines, sedatives and antidepressants, increase the risk of falls. Decreasing doses can reduce the danger.
- *Encourage the elderly person to get vision checks* and obtain proper eyeglasses.
- *Get the right walking aids*, ensure good footwear (with enough support and nonslip soles).
- *Eliminate obvious* home hazards: e.g., loose rugs, high-pile carpeting, slippery or polished floors, obstacles, stairs without rails.

- *Put handrails on each side of stairs*; identify the edge of each step with paint or tape in a contrasting color. Carpet the stairs with low-pile material.
- *Simplify the furniture layout.* Use contrasting colors on floors, stairs and walls to clearly demarcate stairs and obstacles.
- *Improve lighting* and minimize glare.
- *Use nonslip mats in the bath*, install grab bars for bathtubs, showers.
- *Keep a night-light on* in the hall and bathroom.
- *Have snow and ice removed from walkways.*
- *Check safety aids* such as canes for wear and tear (the rubber tip on a cane can become slippery when worn thin).
- *Consider a personal "emergency response system"* (worn at home around the neck or wrist) that summons help at the push of a button.
- *In the kitchen*, use safety devices such as kettles with an automatic turnoff when boiling.
- *Remember to turn off the stove.* A microwave might be a safer alternative.
- *Use smoke detectors to warn of fire*, and carbon-monoxide detectors to signal gas dangers.

Promote good personal hygiene

- *Help to maintain cleanliness* and an attractive appearance, even if the elderly person has lost interest.
- *Keep up oral hygiene* and get regular dental care.

Combat loneliness, anxiety and depression

- *Discuss grief at loss* of friends and family.
- *Watch for signs of depression.* Frequent signs include appetite or weight loss, agitated behavior, fitful sleep, early morning awakening, reduced energy, lack of pleasure in things previously enjoyed.
- *Watch for evidence of alcoholism* or excess drug use.

Encourage social interaction and stimulation

- *Investigate community programs* that augment the support provided by family and friends. Explore church and other group activities, daycare for seniors, community-care organizations, geriatric or seniors' centers, the "Y" and so on.
- *Consider a pet* for those fond of animals. A cat, dog or bird can help to keep up or rekindle an elderly person's interest in life.
- *Promote as much mental and social stimulation as possible*—integrate into family activities; take on outings; visit often; try to keep seniors involved, wanted and useful.

Investigate aids for the disabled

- *Look into aids for independent living*, e.g., Velcro closings on clothing, nonskid dishes, special utensils to overcome arthritic stiffness.
- *Bell Canada has a "Special Needs Centre"* to serve visually and hearing impaired customers. See your phone book for the toll-free number.
- *Use memory aids*, routines, clocks, notes, oral and written reminders about medications, appointments and mealtimes.

Too much needless suffering

Untreated incontinence can lead to poor hygiene, urinary-tract infections, rashes and other skin disorders. In rushing to the washroom the incontinent often suffer falls and fractures. Fears of being far from a restroom and of unpleasant odors can cause sufferers to avoid outings, friends and family gatherings, leading to isolation and depression. Many give up their sex lives for fear of leaking. A recent consensus conference of the National Institutes of Health (NIH) in the United States concluded that millions suffer in silence due to embarrassment, failure to seek advice and lack of proper treatment. The shroud of secrecy and the myth of inevitability are perpetuated by adult diaper manufacturers, many of whom wrongly imply that urinary incontinence is a normal result of aging and that diapers are the best remedy. Believing incontinence to be incurable, only a fraction of sufferers seek medical help, turning prematurely to pads without ever having a proper diagnosis. Yet incontinence can almost always be relieved once its cause is pinpointed. It requires a thorough medical examination and laboratory workup, and specific treatment, not diapers.

According to the NIH and other studies, only 1 in 5 of the incontinent gets properly evaluated for this much-neglected health problem, and only about 1 in 3 physicians treats it properly.

About 5 to 10 percent of the population is incontinent at some time or other (some during childhood), increasing to 15 to 20 percent in older people—more in women than in men, although after age 70 the two sexes even out. An astonishing 37 percent of women over age 65 and 50 percent of nursing-home residents suffer from incontinence, partly explaining why the condition costs billions. (In 1989, the United States spent 15 billion dollars on incontinence—far outstripping the amounts spent on AIDS, heart surgery or kidney dialysis.)

More common in women than in men

Although getting older does not in itself cause incontinence, normal changes in the genitourinary tract make the condition more common in the elderly, and far more prevalent in women than in men. With advancing age most people void more frequently than when young—especially at night, as the kidneys produce more nighttime urine. The elderly are also more likely to have detrusor instability (bladder spasms or uninhibited bladder contractions), producing a sudden, uncontrollable urge to urinate. As people age, their bladder capacity declines, the urethra (urine-conducting tube) becomes less elastic and the bladder base may sag. Childbirth in women and an enlarged prostate or prostate surgery in men can damage the urinogenital muscles and lead to incontinence. The common ailments that afflict the elderly (such as arthritis, failing eyesight, strokes, Parkinsonism) and the many medications they take, compounded with difficulties in reaching the toilet, can increase bladder problems and tip a borderline case into full incontinence.

Identifying the cause of incontinence is a top priority

Finding the cause of incontinence often suggests the cure. A good medical workup will establish whether it's nocturnal (only at night) or diurnal (both during the day and at night); whether it's continuous, intermittent, severe or mild; how much urine is lost and what triggers it. A list of medications taken (both prescription and over-the-counter), assessment of the person's mental state plus instructions for keeping a micturition or voiding diary (recording fluid intake and urine output) help to establish the reason(s) for the incontinence. Testing for leakage on coughing or bending may indicate stress incontinence. Measuring how well the bladder empties may pinpoint an overflow problem. Occasionally, more extensive bladder testing may be required. Once the pattern of incontinence is determined, appropriate therapy can be started.

Treatment for incontinence

For the most part, incontinence can be successfully relieved. Clearly, if some medication or disease is behind the problem, the disease should be treated or the drugs discontinued if possible. If the cause is basically irreversible, as with Alzheimer's disease or dementia, the patient can be made more comfortable with absorbent undergarments, by use of bedpans, or intermittent use of catheters (flexible voiding tubes)—a last resort, since catheterized patients

TYPES AND CAUSES OF INCONTINENCE

Transient, reversible or acute forms

Reversible incontinence accounts for as much as one-third of all cases and can be triggered by other disorders. A sudden bout of incontinence calls for prompt medical attention. Common reasons for transient incontinence include urinary-tract infections, medications (especially sleeping pills, tranquilizers and antidepressants), illnesses that limit movement or cause confusion, such as hip fractures or high fever.

One physician has proposed the acronym DIAP-PERS to list the reasons for transient incontinence (mainly in the elderly):

- D for delirium. Someone who's confused may be unaware that the bladder is emptying without control.
- I for infection. Urinary-tract infections often cause urgency, but are treatable with antibiotics.
- A for atrophic urethritis or vaginitis. Thinning of pelvic and urinary-tract tissues in women after the menopause (when estrogen levels drop) can produce symptoms similar to urinary-tract infections, treatable with hormones or other medication.
- P for pharmacologic—over-the-counter and prescription medications that contribute to incontinence include:
  - diuretics (which increase urine output);
  - sedative hypnotics or sleep-aids (which relax the bladder muscle);
  - anticholinergics (e.g., anti-Parkinson drugs), which cause urine retention;
  - antipsychotics and antidepressants (sedating and accident-causing);
  - blood-pressure medications (e.g., beta-blockers such as propranolol) or other drugs (e.g., prazosin, clonidine, methyldopa, reserpine) that induce urine retention;
  - antihistamines and anti-inflammatories (e.g., nonsteroidal anti-inflammatory drugs), decongestants and cold remedies (e.g., ephedrine, chlorpheniramine).
- P for psychological problems such as depression or anxiety;
- E for endocrine or hormonal reasons, such as diabetes and hypercalcemia;
- R for restricted mobility, which makes it hard for people to get to the toilet;
- S for stool impaction, where constipation allows the bowel to press on the bladder.

Chronic, persistent or long-term incontinence

- *Genuine stress incontinence*—the most common type—arises from a sudden increase in abdominal pressure, for example, when coughing, lifting, sneezing or laughing. If severe, just standing up may release a dribble. It's thought to arise from weakened urethral muscles, which control bladder outflow. Smoking, obesity, constipation and respiratory problems can precipitate stress incontinence. It can occur at any age but is most often seen in middle-aged and older women, sometimes following childbirth. It is less common in men, except when the urination muscles are damaged by prostate surgery. Pelvic exercises and medications often cure it. If due to postmenopausal tissue thinning in the urinary or genital tract, estrogens may help by building up the lining tissues.
- *Urge incontinence*—the second-most common type—is due to uncontrollable bladder spasms, called *detrusor instability*. Most frequent in older adults, urge incontinence may produce a sudden need to pass urine before a toilet can be reached. Accidents occur while hurrying to the bathroom or on rising from a chair. The condition can appear spontaneously or may stem from a urinary-tract infection or problems such as strokes and spinal-cord disorders. In *reflex urge incontinence* (common with some spinal-cord disorders), accidents happen without any warning—the unsuppressed voiding occurs without any sense of urgency.
- *Overflow incontinence*—which involves frequent, almost constant urinary leakage—occurs when a full bladder doesn't empty properly and becomes permanently overdistended. Overflow incontinence accounts for only 5 to 10 percent of cases of urinary incontinence. Although there may be no identifiable cause, this form is more common in men and may be related to prostate problems. The ureter (a tube that extends from the bladder and out the penis) runs through the prostate. Over time, the prostate commonly enlarges (developing benign prostate hyperplasia) and this enlargement may obstruct the ureter, so that when the older man urinates he doesn't completely clear the bladder, which eventually leads to overflow problems. Incontinence can also arise because of anatomical obstructions such as a tumor, diseases that impair the bladder's normal contractions, certain back problems (e.g., spinal stenosis), strokes and other neurological disorders, or from medications.
- *Functional incontinence* develops when someone becomes unable or unwilling to use the bathroom, perhaps because of an illness that restricts movement or some psychiatric condition.

N.B.: Different types of incontinence may occur together.

are prone to infection. The idea is to start with the least invasive strategies, such as behavior therapy and toilet habit improvement. If that doesn't work, the physician may move on to drugs or surgery. Treating incontinence also depends on the personality of the sufferer—for instance, a confused older person with severe, long-standing incontinence is less likely to manage pelvic-floor exercises than a younger person with mild stress incontinence. Overflow incontinence is often treated surgically—for example, by reducing an enlarged prostate or with intermittent catheter voiding. Surgery doesn't help urge incontinence due to detrusor instability—it's generally best managed with medication.

- Exercises often help. Many experts suggest Kegel (pelvic-floor) exercises as the first remedy for stress and urge incontinence. Some will benefit, some will not. Exercises are now recommended not only for women with moderate stress incontinence, but also increasingly for men. Contracting the pelvic floor muscles also tightens the loop of muscle around the urethra (which holds back gas or bowel movements) and strengthens the muscles that support the bladder. To benefit from Kegel exercises, it is vital to first identify the right muscle; a physician or nurse can demonstrate how to squeeze the muscle around a gloved finger inserted into the vagina (or rectum in men). Alternatively, many clinicians describe the maneuver as being as if you were holding back flatus (gas). Once people figure out which muscles to exercise, the usual regime is to squeeze the muscles for 5 seconds, release for 5 seconds, and repeat this cycle for 5 minutes at least 3 to 4 times a day. Doing the exercises at specific times or accompanying certain activities can help the patient to remember them. Kegel exercises must be done *regularly and consistently*. Properly done, they can be highly successful in strengthening the bladder outlet, although noticeable improvement takes weeks to months. (Kegel exercises should not be done while sitting on the toilet trying to void, as this only promotes incomplete emptying.)
- Bladder or behavior training, using breathing and relaxation to suppress the urge to urinate, is another effective therapy for those with urge or stress incontinence. People are taught to "hold on" for increasing times and learn to void at regular, scheduled intervals, the interval being gradually extended over the weeks and months of training to the normal 3- to 4-hour lapse between voidings. The retraining scheme teaches people to resist urgency, postpone voiding and urinate by the clock rather than because of the urge. The cure rate is around 10 to 15 percent, with marked improvement in 75 percent of cases. Patience is key as it may take up to 6 weeks to notice any improvement.
- Combined bladder training, Kegel exercises and variations on these strategies help many to overcome incontinence. These remedies are sometimes also combined with hypnosis, biofeedback and other behavioral therapies. But the training requires a high level of commitment and is generally best for younger or middle-aged groups.
- Medications include muscle calmants for urge incontinence and estrogens for the stress type—estrogens help to build up the urogenital tract's lining tissues. Some drugs work by dampening bladder contractions or increasing bladder capacity. Self-medicating with over-the-counter products is strongly discouraged. Estrogen can be applied topically or taken orally.
- For detrusor instability or urge incontinence the best medication is oxybutynin chloride (Ditropan)—an antispasmodic, helpful even for the very old, that increases bladder storage and dampens bladder spasms, delaying the urge to void. (One side effect is a dry, bad-tasting mouth.) Flavoxate (Urispas) and dicyclomine (Bentylol) are similar drugs.
- Calcium channel blockers, which are widely used heart drugs, the tricyclic antidepressant imipramine or the drug desmopressin can be useful for drying out a leaky bladder, but may cause undesirable urinary retention, and are therefore not yet widely used.
- For nocturnal enuresis (nighttime bedwetting) a small dose of desmopressin may resolve the problem.
- Bladder surgery can be 90 percent successful in women with severe stress incontinence. The "vaginal sling" operation creates a

TIPS FOR MANAGING INCONTINENCE

- Take steps to avoid increasing intra-abdominal pressure (e.g., weight reduction, avoiding coughing if possible).
- Don't consume foods that increase urination or irritate the bladder (e.g., parsley, coffee, tea, alcohol), and avoid smoking.
- If constipation is troublesome, increase fiber and fluid intake.
- If urinating too frequently, try bladder training—consciously extending the interval between voidings by 15 to 30 minutes, aiming for 3- to 4-hour gaps.
- Quench the urgent need to void by remaining still, relaxing and then moving slowly to the toilet.
- When urinating, empty the bladder completely, and after it seems totally empty, always give an extra push to get out the last drops of urine—"double voiding."
- Drink plenty of fluids during the day but nothing for 2 to 3 hours before going to bed.
- Use absorbent pads, inserts, belts or adult diapers as a last resort. They are not generally encouraged because people who use them tend not to get correct treatment. However, those who must use these garments can find a wider variety at a health-supply house than in a pharmacy. Search the Yellow Pages under "Hospital Equipment and Supplies." (Delivery is often available.)

"hammock" under the urethra to give support; several other operations can also be used. More complicated surgical procedures include implantation of an artificial sphincter—a cuff that can be inflated to squeeze the urethra, impeding urine flow.

- Contigen injection, using a type of collagen injected into the urethral lining, is a promising new treatment for stress incontinence. Types of Teflon have also been tried. The advantage of contigen injections is that they can be done as a rapid office procedure under local rather than general anesthetic. Preliminary results are encouraging: studies show a success rate of 60 percent in men and 96 percent in women. The procedure is already offered in certain specialist centers across Canada.

Incontinent patients must be their own advocates

Often, physicians don't know what to do about their incontinent patients. If your doctor doesn't understand or is unsympathetic to the problem, demand referral to a urologist, gynecologist or incontinence expert. There's no reason to live with untreated incontinence.

For further information write to the Simon Foundation, P.O. Box 264, Station F, Toronto, Ont. M6H 4E2.

PARKINSON'S DISEASE

Parkinson's disease is a neurological disorder, clinically defined as a "movement disorder," usually of unknown origin, while "parkinsonism" refers to similar symptoms that mimic those of Parkinson's disease, resulting from other brain disorders or injuries. Parkinson's disease occurs mostly in middle and old age, and can be ameliorated (but not cured) by various drugs used alone or in combination. Named for the British physician Dr. James Parkinson, who first described it in his 1817 essay "The Shaking Palsy," the disease affects about 1 percent of Canadians over age 60 and 2 percent over age 70. It occurs slightly more often in men than in women, and in whites more often than in blacks. Although about three-quarters of those afflicted develop the disease between ages 50 and 65, it occasionally strikes younger people. No genetic predisposition to the disease has been found for those who acquire it after 50 years of age, but when it develops before 50, those affected generally have a strong familial history. The cardinal symptoms include tremor, rigidity, akinesia (difficulty moving) and gait disturbance.

After a global pandemic of *encephalitis lethargica*, or sleeping sickness, following World War I, many people developed parkinsonism up to 30 years later—attributed by some experts to the high fever, by others to contaminants in the rubbing alcohol used to cool feverish brows. Current research is uncovering the mechanism that causes parkinsonism and may ultimately lead to ways to prevent it.

What happens in Parkinson's disease?

Parkinson's disease is a central nervous system disorder involving a lack of the neurotransmitter dopamine, caused by the accelerated death of a group of dopamine-producing brain cells deep within a cerebral region known as the substantia nigra. The brain needs dopamine to send correct signals to the muscles. Symptoms of Parkinson's disease appear when 60 to 80 percent of these dopamine-producing cells are gone, no matter how they are destroyed. As people age, some dopamine-producing cells die off naturally, but it's not clear whether or not normal aging processes contribute to Parkinson's disease or parkinsonism. There's some evidence that age-related cell loss in the *substantia nigra* differs from the changes found in parkinsonism. In any case, the shortage of dopamine leads to neurotransmission failure in pathways that normally regulate muscular skills such as standing, sitting and walking, gradually producing movement disorders including an involuntary tremor and a stooped shuffle.

Although scientists now know which areas of parkinsonian brains die off and which neurotransmitter is lacking, they do not yet know what leads to the dopamine depletion. While many cases of Parkinson's have no known cause, studies reveal that certain environmental agents can destroy dopamine-producing brain cells. Together the normal neuronal losses of aging plus possible environmental brain damage will cause parkinsonism when 60 to 80 percent of the brain's dopamine-producing cells have gone.

Clues to the mechanism of Parkinson's disease came from the observation that the substance known as *methylphenyltetrahydropyridine* (MPTP) causes parkinsonian effects. The link between MPTP and parkinsonism surfaced when a young drug-user who was trying illegally to make a kitchen-brewed version of the narcotic meperidine (a morphine substitute known as Demerol) accidentally produced and took MPTP Within days he developed a "frozen" parkinsonian pose. (He was subsequently "unfrozen" by the drug L-dopa, commonly used to treat Parkinson's.)

Scientists at the U.S. National Institutes of Health showed that MPTP, a chemical similar to some herbicides (such as paraquat), can kill dopamine-producing brain cells in the *substantia nigra*. Since then, experiments with monkeys have demonstrated that MPTP induces permanent parkinsonism similar to that in humans, a discovery that gave scientists an animal model in which to investigate Parkinson's disease.

Exposure to other toxins may also produce parkinsonian disabilities. Parkinsonism has appeared among some inhabitants of Guam who, in times of famine, make flour from sago palm seeds, which contain a toxin (cycasin) that produces extensive nerve degeneration decades later (But the role of the cycad plant is still somewhat controversial.)

Neuroleptics (antipsychotic drugs) such as haloperidol and phenothiazines and a few antinauseants can also produce parkinsonism by temporarily blocking the action of dopamine at receptor sites in the brain.

Scientists think that environmental toxins, such as MPTP, that easily enter the brain may damage glial (binding) and other cells by blocking the action of their mitochondria (energy-producing particles), thereby damaging brain cells and causing them to die. In addition, there may be some link to excess iron, as the nerve cells that die seem to have accumulated iron.

Treatment benefits many with Parkinson's disease

The big breakthrough in managing parkinsonism came when a Canadian researcher developed the drug *levodopa* (L-dopa) in 1967 to help restore the brain's flagging dopamine production. Although this and other antiparkinsonian medications can partly replenish or compensate for the lost dopamine, most drugs are disappointing because they work only for a while, and can't reverse or arrest the disease. After about 5 to 10 years, problems arise with L-dopa therapy. But adding other drugs can prolong its usefulness.

Medications to alleviate parkinsonism

- Anticholinergic drugs (e.g., Artane, Cogentin and Kemadrin) inhibit the activity of acetylcholine, a neurotransmitter relatively plentiful in the brain. These drugs may reduce some parkinsonian symptoms, particularly tremors and drooling in the early stages.
- Antiviral agents (e.g., amantadine or Symmetrel) may help to increase dopamine release in the brain.

- Antidepressants can relieve depression.
- Levodopa (L-dopa), now the mainstay of treatment, is taken by mouth several times a day. Once inside the brain, L-dopa is converted to dopamine, replenishing neurotransmitter supplies and giving temporary relief of symptoms. About 80 to 90 percent of Parkinsonians respond well to L-dopa therapy, but a small percentage cannot tolerate the side effects, such as hypotension (low blood pressure), cardiac irregularity, insomnia, nausea, weakness, sweating, confusion, hallucinations and emotional changes. Some experts believe L-dopa should be delayed as long as possible; others advise giving it as soon as the diagnosis is made.
- Decarboxylase inhibitors, such as carbidopa and benserazide, prevent L-dopa breakdown in peripheral tissues, and are usually added to L-dopa so it won't disintegrate before reaching the brain. (L-dopa with carbidopa is Sinemet; with benserazide it's Prolopa).
- Dopamine agonists such as bromocriptine, pramiprexole, pergolide and ropinirole result in fewer motor (movement) fluctuations and dyskinesias (uncontrollable muscle twitches) compared to L-dopa. They are also associated with significant side effects (such as nausea, dizziness, drowsiness) and are not as efficacious as L-dopa in the long term. Dopamine agonists are, however, recommended as adjunctive treatment to L-dopa or as first line therapy in younger patients with mild-to-moderate disease who can deal with their side effects better. They can complement L-dopa's effectiveness by direct stimulation of the brain receptors where dopamine acts.
- Selegiline, or Eldepryl (also known as deprenyl)—a drug similar to MAOI antidepressants usually given early in the disease, often delays the onset of disabling parkinsonian symptoms by 13 to 24 months and puts off the need for L-dopa. The recently completed DATATOP (Deprenyl and Tocopherol Antioxidant Therapy of Parkinsonism) study—combining research at 28 medical centers, including the University of Toronto—showed a marked slowing of cell death and a delay in disabling symptoms among those with early Parkinson's disease. The tocopherol (vitamin E) had no beneficial effect. How deprenyl retards the progress of the disease isn't clear, but one University of Toronto researcher believes deprenyl "rescues" damaged brain cells rather than protecting the cells from harm.
- Amantadine, an antiviral drug, may help reduce the tremor in early Parkinson's.
- In animals, transplantation of adrenal medulla cells (which produce dopamine) from the adrenal gland into the brain can reverse some parkinsonian symptoms. Transplanted adrenal tissue may replace damaged neurons, or in some way partly restore dopamine secretion. The results of adrenal medullary grafts in humans have so far been disappointing.
- Experimental implantation of fetal embryonic tissues (which manufacture dopamine) into the brain—tried in Sweden and other centers—restored some dopamine-producing capacity in animal experiments. Preliminary studies in humans show promising results.
- New approaches use posteroventral pallidotomy—microsurgery on specific brain areas—to try to alleviate stiff parkinsonian movements, and deep brain electrical stimulation of the thalamus to relieve the tremor.
- Insertion of neurotrophic nerve growth factors (NGF) may someday help to promote the recovery of dopamine-producing brain cells. Experiments are underway with genetically engineered NGF in animals.
- Physiotherapy and exercise (especially swim-

SOME POSSIBLE CAUSES OF PARKINSON'S DISEASE

- *Previous encephalitis infection;*
- *damage by toxins or environmental poisons:* e.g., manganese dust, carbon monoxide; MPTP (a "designer" street drug that resembles Demerol);
- *certain medications;* such as neuroleptics or antipsychotics, that are dopamine depleters (e.g., reserpine, haloperidol), phenothiazines such as fluphenazine, chlorpromazine (Largactil), trifluoperazine (Stelazine) and some antiemetic drugs (such as benzamides—Maxeran or metoclopramide);
- *trauma/injury to head;*
- *other neurodegenerative disease:* e.g., Wilson's disease; Huntington's chorea (juvenile representations); Creutzfeldt-Jakob disease; Steele-Richardson-Olszewski disease (progressive supranuclear palsy), which mimics Parkinson's but involves degeneration of different brain regions and rarely includes tremor.

THE HALLMARKS OF PARKINSON'S DISEASE

Parkinson's, or the "shaking palsy," produces progressive rigidity, tremor and slowed movement. As Dr. Parkinson himself put it, "the disorder may first show itself by an involuntary tremulous motion, with lessened muscular power, in parts not in action and even when unsupported, with a propensity to bend the trunk forward, and to pass from a walking to a running pace." Parkinson's typically starts with some muscle stiffness, an altered gait and limb shaking in repose. The very first signs may seem insignificant—slightly clumsy fingers, a little trouble placing one foot before the other, a bit of a shuffle, the hint of a stoop, an almost imperceptible hand-trembling. A few sufferers deteriorate quickly, but many can carry on their usual lives with mild symptoms for years. Some never become significantly disabled.

The various parkinsonian symptoms appear at different rates, in any order, with varying intensity. They include vague symptoms that often go undiagnosed for months or years and may be shrugged off as mere aging, namely:
- a slow, heavy feeling
- unusually easy tiring;
- a hand that trembles ever so slightly.

Later signs include:
- stiffness of the limbs;
- involuntary trembling;
- walking with a shuffling, stooped gait;
- reduced facial animation;
- soft, monotone voice;
- the parkinsonian tremor—not necessarily the first but often the clearest sign of Parkinson's, and one of its more annoying signs. At first an intermittent "tapping" of the hand (when hands are resting or supported on the lap), the shaking usually subsides when hands are moved or during sleep, but increases with stress. Later—often years later—the tremor may spread to legs and lips;
- bradykinesia—acute difficulty in movements such as rising from the table, reaching for objects or getting out of bed;
- akinesia—loss of automatic initiation of movement; loss of spontaneous movement, which diminishes ability to carry out movements such as arm-swinging while walking; reduced emotional expressiveness (it may create a somewhat stony stare with infrequent blinking);
- a shuffling gait—"festination"—the inability to walk slowly and a tendency to take increasingly tiny, fast steps;
- rigidity (often disabling), muscle stiffness which in advanced stages "freezes" patients in place;
- depression, which may need treatment as urgently as the physical problems;
- intellectual impairment, which can include reduced problem-solving ability, visuospatial abnormalities and slow thought;
- parkinsonian dementia in later stages;
- diminutive handwriting (micrographia);
- increased body secretions (saliva, perspiration and skin oil); muscle cramps; leg swelling;
- susceptibility to bladder and chest infections (partly due to immobility).

ming and walking) can help maintain fitness and muscle tone in parkinsonian patients, helping them to stay mobile.
- As depression frequently accompanies Parkinson's disease, antidepressant therapy may also be advocated.

Some complications of long-term drug treatment

People with Parkinson's can continue on a levodopa drug regime for 5 or more years without bad effects, but, unfortunately, after extended therapy, involuntary movements and rigidity become increasingly troublesome. Drug side effects may become worse than the symptoms they're meant to suppress.
- *Dyskinesia*, which involves bizarre, involuntary, jerky movements of head, tongue and extremities, is a particularly troublesome side effect of L-dopa. The abnormal movements can gradually become incapacitating unless the dosage is reduced.

- *"Freezing"* episodes, especially when starting to walk, turn or change direction, are frequent as the drug wears off.
- *End-of-dose deterioration* means that, as each dose of medication wears off, symptoms may return, with varying "good" and "bad" times through the day. More frequent L-dopa doses, sometimes together with bromocriptine, may help.
- The *"on-off" phenomenon* refers to sudden spells of immobility, apparently unrelated to drug doses, which may occur several times a day and last from minutes to hours. Drugs do not help this type of parkinsonian immobility, but lowering L-dopa dosage (and perhaps adding bromocriptine) may be useful.
- *Psychiatric side effects* may occur especially in elderly patients or those with underlying cognitive decline. Often the dose of medication has to be lowered, with the result that parkinsonian symptoms increase.

For further information, consult your family

physician, a neurologist or the neurology unit at your local hospital, or the local chapter of the Parkinson Foundation of Canada.

OSTEOPOROSIS

Osteoporosis is a common and disabling ailment in which both the amount and the quality of bone tissue diminishes, leading to a weakened skeleton that easily fractures. It afflicts men and women of all ages. Approximately one in four North American women past menopause suffers fractures of bones made fragile by osteoporosis, breaks of the spine, wrist and hip being most typical. Women lose bone faster than men of the same age for about 5 to 8 years after the onset of menopause. Between ages 70 and 75, male and female bone loss evens out. Since osteoporotic bone loss can't be restored, prevention is by far the best bet by ensuring adequate calcium and vitamin D intake, doing enough weight-bearing exercise and not smoking.

What is osteoporosis?

Basically, osteoporosis stems from an imbalance in the body's bone-building mechanism, whereby bone loss exceeds the amount of bone re-formed. In some cases there is also an initial bone deficit (perhaps because of a long-term lack of calcium in the diet).

There are two main types of osteoporosis:
- *primary osteoporosis*—of which type I, seen mainly in postmenopausal women aged 55 to 65, affects the trabecular (spongy) part of bone, and type II (previously called "senile osteoporosis"), which is age-related and affects both sexes over age 75 equally, involves cortical (compact) bone;
- *secondary osteoporosis*—affecting young and middle-aged persons—which is often of unknown cause but is sometimes due to an inflammatory condition, anorexia nervosa (extreme dieting and malnourishment) or excessive exercise in women (which disturbs menstrual function, halts periods and diminishes estrogen output).

Bone consists primarily of minerals (largely calcium phosphate), together with collagen, proteins and other components. It undergoes a continual, dynamic turnover with a process that repairs minor damage and brittle areas, replac-ing them with new bone. The process of "resorption" chews up the damaged parts of bone, allowing it to be "remodeled" by the laying down of fresh tissue. The remodeling cycle takes about 100 days and is influenced by hormone output (for example, levels of insulin, estrogen and parathyroid hormones) and by calcium and vitamin D intake. After a certain age, around 30 to 35 years, there is normally a gradual decline in bone density—attributed to an imbalance in the remodeling process whereby bone resorption outpaces its buildup. However, bone strength and fracture resistance depend not only on bone mass, but also on its architecture and the distribution of minerals within it.

Fractures are the chief health problem in osteoporosis

Health problems from osteoporosis arise not so much from the bone loss, which in itself poses no real difficulties, but from multiple fractures. All bones will snap under enough force, but with bones made brittle by osteoporosis, fractures can occur with hardly any impact at all. In severe cases, breaks can occur from the mere wear and tear of daily life—even while resting in bed. In advanced stages, osteoporotic bones become so fragile that a mere hug, a stumble or the slightest pressure can cause a fracture. But until bones break, many remain unaware that they have the disease.

The main sites for osteoporotic fractures are the hip, wrist, arm and spinal vertebrae, less often the ribs. While broken wrists are common for postmenopausal women in their fifties and sixties, they are only nuisance fractures, as most heal well without surgery. But hip fractures—which are more frequent after age 75, in men as well as women—often require surgery. And although the operation is usually successful, the elderly do not always tolerate major surgery well, and may require lengthy convalescence. Many never regain their former agility, finding their daily activities seriously handicapped.

Spinal "crush" fractures—where the vertebrae collapse or become greatly compressed—are a particularly painful result of osteoporosis. A single vertebral fracture that's just a hairline crack hardly visible by X-ray may not be noticed and may cause little or no pain.

BONE STRUCTURE

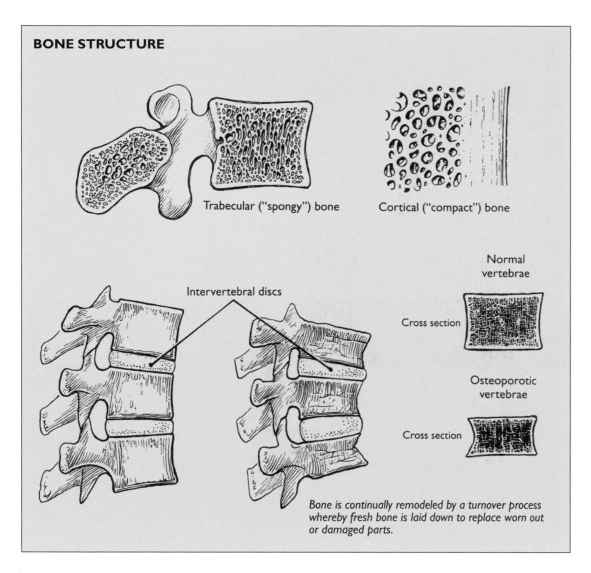

Trabecular ("spongy") bone

Cortical ("compact") bone

Intervertebral discs

Normal vertebrae

Cross section

Osteoporotic vertebrae

Cross section

Bone is continually remodeled by a turnover process whereby fresh bone is laid down to replace worn out or damaged parts.

However, several vertebral crush fractures can be extremely disabling. If every movement hurts, as it may in those with severely osteoporotic backs, daily activities can be burdensome. Successive vertebral fractures—more a crumbling of bone than a clear break—can be very painful and lead to years of deformed posture and restricted activity, although some produce no pain at all, the person only becoming aware of them through lost height and a bent back. If several back vertebrae are injured by crush fractures, the spinal compression noticeably diminishes height—sometimes by 10 to 20 cm (4 to 8 in)—giving the humped look. With the reduced height, the abdominal cavity becomes compressed, making those afflicted feel bloated after eating even small meals.

Estrogen drop at menopause is a key cause

In women, bone loss is greatly accelerated at and for a few years after the menopause. Whereas in premenstrual women the annual bone loss averages 0.25 to 1 percent, it rises to 2 to 3 percent during the first 3 to 7 years after menopause begins. The accelerated bone loss stems from estrogen deficiency, as the ovaries stop producing this hormone and the gap between bone resorption and bone remodeling increases. Changes in the output of parathyroid hormone and in vitamin D metabolism may also aggravate the bone loss.

Female athletes, especially distance runners, and young women with anorexia nervosa (self-inflicted starvation) may experi-

HIP FRACTURES A COMMON PROBLEM IN THE ELDERLY

Hip fractures are now often repaired with the help of metal screws which allow an earlier return of mobility.

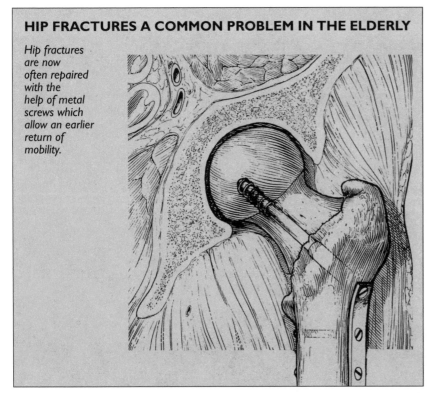

Lack of weight-bearing exercise is a major cause

Skeletal strength and health depend on the mechanical stresses and daily forces exerted on the bones by physical activity. Regular weight-bearing exercise such as walking, jogging or dancing (but not swimming) can help to offset osteoporosis. The few studies done to date on the relationship between exercise and osteoporosis show that people who stay active, such as athletes and dancers, have denser bones than sedentary types. One study showed that women enrolled in a regular exercise program lost less bone than a similar group of nonexercisers.

The inevitable reduction in activity as we age contributes to osteoporotic bone loss. Any further immobility, through fear of injury or actual confinement to bed, compounds the problem. It is well known that anyone immobilized for an extended period—as with a limb cast, paralysis or a prolonged illness—quickly loses bone mass, as much as 30 to 40 percent disappearing after 6 months of immobility. The lost bone may or may not come back. Curiously, astronauts floating weightlessly in space lost bone despite vigorous exercise routines. Metabolic studies on one Skylab crew revealed a bone diminution analogous to that seen with prolonged confinement in bed.

One cautionary note: osteoporotics who have already had fractures, or have weakened backs, should take great care about the type of exercise they do so they don't cause further injury, but they should still do recommended exercises.

Nutrition also plays a key role

People of all ages, including children and adolescents, need to eat enough calcium as an investment to prevent or minimize later bone loss. A lack of dietary calcium contributes to osteoporosis even if it occurs at an early age. Most Canadians consume enough calcium for daily needs but not necessarily enough to prevent bone loss later in life.

The recommended daily dietary intake of calcium is 800 mg, but some researchers suggest a need for yet more—about 1 gram a day premenopausally (the amount in a liter or quart of 2 percent milk). After the menopause, as much

ence early-onset osteoporosis because of disturbed menstrual cycles. The drop in estrogens sometimes causes a loss of bone mass even greater than that usually seen in postmenopausal women.

Who's at greatest risk of osteoporosis?

Most at risk for osteoporosis are thin, small, Caucasian people, those with relatives who have had multiple senile fractures, people on certain medications or with diseases known to exacerbate bone loss, and some under-exercised, inadequately fed individuals.

The risk of osteoporosis is increased by certain lifestyle habits, such as smoking, excessive alcohol intake and lack of exercise, and some disorders, such as diabetes mellitus, hyperthyroidism (overproduction of thyroid hormone), parathyroid hormone disturbances, excess corticosteroid output (from the adrenal gland), anorexia nervosa and some sex-hormone deficiencies. Medications such as cortisone derivatives (e.g., prednisone), tranquilizers, heparin (a blood thinner), some anticancer medications and antacids (which affect calcium absorption), as well as radiation, can increase risks.

as a gram and a half (1,500 mg) of calcium a day may be necessary to preserve bone strength in women. Yet studies show that the middle-aged and elderly, as well as many adolescents (especially girls watching their weight), fall short of the recommended intake. Some of the elderly consume no more than 400 mg calcium a day.

Both vitamins D and C are also essential to a healthy skeleton, but megadoses should be avoided—particularly of vitamin D, which can be toxic in excess. The skin can synthesize vitamin D, but only if it receives adequate sunlight; in a country like Canada, which has limited sunlight for many months of the year people may be short of vitamin D, especially if their diet is low in the vitamin-D-supplemented foods, such as milk products. In age-related osteoporosis type II, there are also changes in vitamin D metabolism, so the elderly should be extra sure to get enough vitamin D. Up to an extra 800 units a day of vitamin D may be advised if sun exposure

RISK FACTORS FOR OSTEOPOROSIS

- Advancing age;
- being female (twice as many women as men have osteoporosis at age 60, although risks equalize later on);
- lack of weight-bearing exercise;
- Caucasian (white) or Asian ancestry;
- having a thin, lean, small-boned body frame;
- family history of osteoporosis;
- smoking tobacco;
- excess alcohol consumption;
- high caffeine intake (from coffee, tea, colas);
- very high protein consumption;
- lack of dietary calcium (especially during adolescence and early adulthood) and/or lack of vitamin D;
- medical disorders (e.g., diabetes, hyperthyroidism, anorexia nervosa), and using certain medications (e.g., aluminum-containing antacids, some diuretics, steroid-type drugs).

is low and dietary sources are insufficient. Generally, menopausal and post-menopausal women over age 50 are advised to take a vitamin D supplement of 400 units per day, sometimes combined with their calcium supplement. Foods rich in vitamin D include fortified milk, eggs, canned sardines (in oil), canned

OSTEOPOROTIC SPINAL "CRUSH" FRACTURES SHORTEN BACKS

Successive crush fractures of the vertebrae may deform the back and cause loss of height and a severely bent posture.

Crush fractures

Severely bent osteoporotic spine

M. B. MACKAY 82 ©

salmon and eels. (See Chapter 4 for recommended vitamin and mineral intakes.)

The obese are somewhat protected against osteoporosis, possibly because adrenal hormones convert to estrogen in fat tissues.

Diagnosing osteoporosis

Early warning signs may include a stab of pain in the back while doing routine chores, coughing, sneezing, laughing or even standing still! But all too often the disease creeps up with few premonitory signs, and is discovered only after multiple fractures have occurred.

The first step in diagnosing it is a thorough medical investigation to rule out causes such as the diseases and drugs known to increase bone loss. Examination may include blood and urine tests for hormone function, assessment of calcium and vitamin D intake and perhaps X-rays. New bone density tests make it simple to determine bone mass and detect osteoporosis or its precursors (low bone density). Bone densitometry methods include computerized tomography (CT) scans, photon absorptiometry, neutron activation (to measure body calcium), and dual-energy X-ray absorption. Modern bone densitometry is a good and inexpensive tool for measuring bone mineral density and assessing the risk of osteoporosis. It's done by scanning parts of the skeleton— usually the spine and femoral neck (hip)—while the person lies beneath a slowly moving X-ray machine. The radiation dose is very low and the test takes only a few minutes (20 minutes at most). If the bone density measurement suggests decreased bone mass and a risk of fracture, other scans may be done to confirm diagnosis. Many physicians suggest a bone density test for women at possible risk of osteoporosis (for instance, those with a family history of the disorder; anorexics, people taking corticosteroids), to determine the need for treatment, and to follow its success in increasing bone strength. Bone density tests are usually not repeated until at least 18 months after initiation of treatment to improve bone mass as it takes that long to be effective. People who have a normal BMD (bone density) and are low risk do not need to be re-tested for 2 to 3 years.

Consuming enough calcium critical for bone strength

Eating a calcium-rich diet from childhood onward helps build the strongest bones possible and retains bone strength in later life, reducing fracture risks. If food does not provide enough calcium, the body will take what it needs from the skeleton.

Bones stop growing in length around the late teens in girls and early twenties in boys, but bone mass continues to increase until about age 35, when bones reach peak density. The greater the "peak bone mass," the slower the later bone loss and the less the risk of fractures. Women reach the fracture threshold at an earlier age than men because they have less bone to start with, and because they lose it faster during and after menopause. Men also lose bone mass with advancing years.

To build and retain strong bones, average adult men and menstruating women (with normal estrogen outputs) need about 1 gram (1,000 mg) of calcium a day. Postmenopausal women need more. The U.S. National Institutes of Health and the Osteoporosis Society of Canada recommend 1,000 to 1,500 mg a day for teenage girls and postmenopausal women. Although a calcium-rich diet is essential to optimal bone strength, all too many North Americans consume far too little, leaving them with fragile bones. Adolescent girls, especially those who shun milk products (perhaps in an effort to stay thin), often have serious calcium deficits, setting themselves up for later osteoporosis. (See Chapter 4 for more on dietary calcium.)

There is an ongoing debate about exact the role of calcium in preventing, arresting or reversing age-related bone loss. The U.S. National Institutes of Health has recommended the following daily allowances of calcium:

Children aged 1–10 years	800–1,200 mg/day
Adolescents and young adults aged 11–24	1,200–1,500 mg/day
Pregnant and lactating women	1,200–1,500 mg/day

Adult men
    aged 25–65   1,000 mg/day
Adult women
    aged 25–50   1,000 mg/day
Postmenopausal
    women 51–65   1,500 mg/day
Everyone over
    the age of 65   1,500 mg/day

Most experts suggest that all postmenopausal women (and men over age 65) get *at least* 1,500 mg calcium a day—either through diet alone or with added supplements. The basic North American diet without dairy products provides a daily intake of 300 to 400 mg of calcium. One 8-ounce (250–ml) glass of 1 to 2 percent milk contains 300 mg of calcium. Other good sources of calcium, supplying about 300 mg per serving, are firm cheeses (45 g or 1 1/2 ounces), canned salmon (125 ml or 1/2 cup) and canned sardines (7 medium-sized) if the bones are eaten. In addition, 125 ml (1/2 cup) of tofu has about 150 mg, 250 ml (1 cup) of cooked soy beans about 200 mg, and 125 ml (1/2 cup) of dry-roasted almonds about 200 mg. "However," stresses one bone specialist, "calcium supplements are not a treatment for osteoporosis. Women who have or are at high risk of osteoporosis should consider one of the medications now available for preserving or rebuilding bone."

Calcium supplements come in a bewildering array of preparations, matched by an equal variety of opinions about the best formulation. In general, chewy or effervescent preparations that dissolve easily are best absorbed. Since reactions to the different preparations vary, people can try various brands and formats, selecting the one that suits their taste, digestive system and pocketbook.

Calcium supplements are best absorbed when taken with meals, in divided doses. For example, two 500 mg tablets (each containing 500 mg elemental calcium) taken at different meals are better than one 1,000 mg calcium tablet. Those that contain bone meal, fossil shell and dolomite also contain lead and should be avoided. People who also take iron supplements should take them at a different time, as calcium hinders the body's iron absorption (and vice versa).

Vitamin D is also crucial for bone building. Even 20 minutes of ultraviolet (UV) exposure a day from sunlight on a small patch of skin can produce enough vitamin D for bone health. However, our winters do not provide sufficient UV rays for vitamin D formation, and few foods—except for fatty fish and fish oils, eggs, fortified milk and cereals—are rich in this vitamin. Certain food items (such as milk and some cereals) are fortified with vitamin D, and people who are housebound or don't get enough sunlight should eat D-fortified items. Older people may need a supplement of 400 to 800 IU of vitamin D per day.

Treatments for osteoporosis

Current therapy to halt or prevent osteoporosis includes weight-bearing exercise and medications that either decrease bone resorption (e.g., estrogen, calcitonin and biphosphonates) or stimulate bone formation (e.g., parathyroid hormone, fluorides and anabolic steroids). Most therapies also call for a high calcium intake and adequate vitamin D consumption.

Present treatments include:
- *Biphosphonates*, which rank high in the fight against osteoporosis. They slow resorptive bone loss, increase bone mass and can be given alongside other medications. By inhibiting bone resorption, biphosphonates shift the balance toward bone formation, reducing fracture rates (although very high doses can distort bone modeling). *Etidronate* (Didrocal), which is taken for 14 days and then followed by calcium for 76 days, has been shown to be effective. Newer biphosphonates, such as *alendronate* (Fosamax) and *risedronate* (Actonel)—the latest to come on the market—restore bone strength (by 6 to 9 percent) and reduce fracture rates in hip and spine. These newest forms can be taken on a daily or weekly basis, usually before breakfast after getting out of bed, on an empty stomach with no food eaten for half an hour after taking it (not even juice or coffee). Calcium and vitamin D supplements may also be advised. Biphosphonates are well tolerated, apart from some gastric discomfort in a few who take them.

- *Estrogen-replacement* with conjugated estrogens, called "hormone replacement therapy" (HRT) with the addition of another female hormone (progestin), to reduce the risk of endometrial (uterine lining) cancer caused by "unopposed" estrogen. (Women who have had their uterus removed can take estrogen alone). Recent trials have indicated that HRT is not as effective or as safe as once thought, but estrogen is still protective for bones. (See section on HRT in Chapter 8.)

- *Designer estrogens*, also known as *selective estrogen-receptor modulators* (SERMs), are a family of compounds developed to replace the use of estrogen—shunned by many women because of side effects (such as breast tenderness, menstrual bleeding, weight gain) and for fear of breast cancer. The SERMs are being designed to retain the benefits of estrogen—such as its bone-preserving and heart-protecting features—without undesirable effects on the uterus and breast. *Raloxifene* (Evista), the first of the designer estrogens to be approved for preventing osteoporosis, maintains bone density and improves the cardiovascular profile (by lowering LDL-cholesterol), with no ill effects on breast or uterine tissue, thereby bypassing some key risks of estrogen therapy. Main side effects of raloxifene are hot flashes and leg cramps in some women taking it, and since it can affect the fetus it should not be taken by anyone who is pregnant or planning to conceive. Trials are currently delineating whether raloxifene delays onset of the diseases or actually has a protective effect in preventing breast cancer. At present, Raloxifene is generally used as a second-line medication.

- *Calcitonin*, a hormone made by the thyroid gland, can—in large doses—inhibit bone resorption and may help preserve bone mass, although its anti-fracture efficacy has yet to be demonstrated. It is given by injection or, more recently, as a nasal spray, which is easier to use. A daily dose of 200 IU per day plus a 500 mg calcium supplement has been shown to increase spinal density. It is often used to reduce pain in people who have osteoporotic fractures.

- *Synthetic parathyroid hormone (PTH)* is a calcium-regulating agent that can stabilize bone mineral for as long as it's taken; it is believed to stimulate bone remodeling. This is effective but is still being examined for safety.

- *Sodium fluoride treatment*, first tried in 1961 for osteoporosis, can stimulate new bone growth in up to 80 percent of those who take it. But although fluoride can stimulate the regrowth of *trabecular* bone, found in the vertebrae and ends of the long bones, it has no demonstrable fracture-reducing effect in *cortical* bone—the compact long bones in the arms and legs.

Given at the correct, individualized dose, with supplemental calcium, fluoride can put back some bone lost through osteoporosis. Within 2 years, fluoride-treated patients generally have significantly fewer spinal crush fractures than those not treated. However, fluoride therapy is controversial and only hesitantly accepted by the medical profession. The new bone is not as strong as hoped for; there's a narrow line between the therapeutic and toxic dose and excess fluoride can pose a health threat. Fluoride toxicity, or *fluorosis*, is known in regions of India, China and South Africa, where water is naturally high in fluoride, and occupational exposure is a recognized health problem in industries such as smelting, ceramics, battery manufacture, brick production and metalworks; fluorine emissions can produce skeletal deformities. It was the observation that people exposed to high levels of fluoride developed dense bone that sparked the idea of using it to replace bone lost through osteoporosis.

The optimal length of fluoride treatment depends on the amount of bone already lost, but should not be less than 2 or longer than 5 years. Those likely to benefit most are people with spinal osteoporosis and many fractures, regardless of age. It is especially useful for those who don't respond to other therapies. Additional calcium intake (to total intakes of about 1,500 mg a day) is essential during fluoride treatment, and enough vitamin D (400 IU/day) is also needed. Side effects of fluoride therapy include digestive upsets (such as nausea and vomiting) in about 10 to 40 percent of patients—mostly mild and diminished by taking the fluoride with, or right after, meals. Joint and limb pain—like "growing pains"—in the ankles, feet and knees is also felt by 10 to 50 percent of those treated, due to active bone reformation. Fluoride treatment is not advised for people with kidney disorders, osteomalacia (a bone mineralization disorder), peptic ulcers or previous hip or wrist fractures.

- *Strengthening weight-bearing exercise* is highly recommended to prevent or diminish osteoporosis—suitable even for the elderly, who can walk, dance and participate in special classes. Many 70-year-olds and even 80-year-olds are surprised at their agility once they get going under expert guidance. The aim of exercises is not only to stop bone loss but to improve posture and balance, prevent falls, reduce fracture rates and impart a sense of well-being. Even a short-term (9 to 12 months) regimen of weight-bearing exercise may enhance bone strength in older people and relieve back pain. Regular walking can reduce the risk of falls and hip fractures. Recommended exercise routines include:
  - muscle strengthening, with weights on the limbs;
  - low-impact aerobics, e.g., walking, slow dancing;
  - *preventing falls* is another top priority in managing osteoporosis, as falls are a prime reason for hip fractures in the elderly, with a risk of permanent disability, or even death from complications following the injury.

Raising awareness a must

While the announcement of new drugs to strengthen bones made fragile by osteoporosis is welcome, raising awareness about the disease and how to prevent it are equally or more urgent. At present, too many remain unaware of osteoporosis, fail to assess their risks or get the simple tests that can detect it.

As always, prevention is best

The main strategies in preventing osteoporosis are to maintain bone strength by consuming adequate calcium throughout life, doing regular weight-bearing exercise and avoiding smoking and alcohol abuse. At menopause, women can consider taking estrogen supplements for a short time (a few years only) to retard bone loss. The elderly should do all they can to avoid falls by

---

> ### THE STAGES OF ALZHEIMER'S DISEASE
>
> - **The first stage is a slow, subtle loss of short-term memory—an inability to remember what happened an hour or a week ago—irritability and an aversion to new situations.**
> - **The second stage is increasing forgetfulness—perhaps an inability to remember grandchildren's** names—neurological and spatial distortion, impaired speech and loss of coordination. Alterations in personality—from a previously trusting person to one who is constantly suspicious, easily upset, even hostile—are typical.
> - **The third or terminal stage is profound deterioration in** motor and mental function, sometimes with seizures, limb twitches and loss of bladder and bowel control, necessitating around-the-clock nursing. There may be an almost total absence of response to people or activities.

---

checking for loose steps or tiles, installing good lighting, wearing nonslip footwear, making sure eyesight is corrected, limiting use of balance-disturbing drugs, removing scatter rugs and installing safety rails on the stairs and in the bathroom.

For more information, contact the Osteoporosis Society of Canada at (800) 463–6842 or (416) 696–2817.

ALZHEIMER'S DISEASE

Senile dementia, including that due to Alzheimer's disease, is already of great concern and is likely to be the greatest public health problem of coming decades.

Alzheimer's disease (AD) accounts for about 20 percent of severe elderly dementia and affects 5 percent of the over-65s. Its prevalence rises steeply with advancing years, and it affects 20 to 25 percent of those over age 80. The disease is marked by a decline in judgment, memory and thought processes, usually ending in death 5 to 10 years after its onset. First-degree relatives of an affected person have a 2 to 4 times increased risk of developing Alzheimer's disease. It exacts a devastating toll on human emotions, family relationships and the healthcare system.

What exactly is Alzheimer's disease?

Alzheimer's disease (AD), the commonest type of dementia, is a progressive degenerative disease of the central nervous system that can be definitively diagnosed only after death, by an autopsy examination of the brain. Named after the German psychiatrist Alois Alzheimer who

CHARACTERISTIC SIGNS OF AD REVEALED AT AUTOPSY

- Shrinkage of brain mass, due to loss of neurons (nerve cells) in regions crucial to learning, memory and thinking;
- death of brain cells at above-average rates in specific brain regions;
- twisted neurofibrillary tangles within the neurons of the brain's cerebral cor-

tex. While most aging brains have some tangles and plaques within brain cells, they occur in vastly greater amounts in AD brains;
- abnormal "senile plaques" (clusters);
- enlargement of the brain's ventricles or cavities;
- lack of the neuro-

transmitter acetyl-choline, due to reduced amounts of choline acetyl trans-ferase, the enzyme needed to make this neurotransmitter (essential for learning and memory);
- clumps of abnormal beta-amyloid protein in and around brain cells and within senile plaques.

first described the condition as a "disease entity" in 1907, it involves a gradual loss of motor ability and a general decline in intellect. Originally, Alzheimer's disease was defined as presenile dementia, or "intellectual decline starting before age 65," but today—despite some disagreement—most experts believe AD is the same disease at whatever age it strikes. Unlike other dementing conditions, such as vascular dementia or dementia due to strokes, AD has nothing directly to do with faulty arteries or poor circulation. It results from massive brain-cell death involving abnormal tangles, plaques and a buildup of amyloid protein within nerve cells.

Its slow, insidious onset allows those affected to adopt compensating strategies that may mask its early stages. Sometimes a sudden stress, such as a move, an illness or the loss of spouse, can precipitate signs of the illness, such as carelessness about one's appearance, forgetfulness of time, mental confusion and wanderings. Knowledge acquired from learning and memories of past experiences are gradually destroyed, until the AD sufferer has no real exis-tence in the past or present.

There are stable periods or plateaus when AD's destructive path seems to slow down or improve. But despite these "good" times, which may last a few hours, days or weeks, intellectual deterioration inevitably sets in again.

Diagnosis of Alzheimer's disease

So far; the only sure way to confirm diagnosis of Alzheimer's disease is to examine the brain after

death for signs of the telltale tangles and amyloid protein plaques. Since testing a sample of brain tissue from living people can be risky, clinical diagnosis at present rests primarily on a good medical history obtained from a reliable infor-mant (not from the patient, who may minimize symptoms), and excluding other possible reasons for the symptoms such as depression, infections, drug reactions, thyroid problems, cerebral blood vessel disease or a brain injury or tumor.

There are now a few markers—such as the ApoE4 gene mutation, and a high level of beta amyloid protein in spinal fluid—that can help to predict the likelihood of having Alzheimer's. In addition, brain imaging techniques known as positron-emission tomography (PET) scans may reveal Alzheimer-like brain changes.

Descriptions by friends and relatives in situ-ations where they can talk freely without embarrassing the sufferer are key elements in diagnosing Alzheimer's disease—especially in its early stages, when sufferers tend to deny their memory loss and gloss over deficits with excuses about absentmindedness, fatigue or anxiety. The accounts given by a relative or friend often con-tradict those of the patient, revealing the inability to continue usual tasks such as shopping, going to work or getting clothes cleaned. To the casual observer; someone moderately affected by Alzheimer's disease may appear totally normal—well groomed, polite, pleasant and competent—whereas a more penetrating analy-sis reveals conspicuous errors of reasoning. The chief hints of oncoming AD are repeated lapses of memory and an inability to do usual tasks, last-ing at least one year.

Recently, researchers have found a sub-stance known as glutamine synthetase that's elevated in the spinal fluid of those identified with AD and may provide a marker for the dis-ease. Others have found antibodies to the beta-amyloid protein found in Alzheimer's suf-ferers' plaques that may some day provide a diagnostic tool.

Strong evidence for a genetic link in AD

Amid conflicting data, studies show that one in 10 cases has some family or genetic connection. Genes related to Alzheimer's disease have already been located on chromosomes 21, 14

GUIDELINES FOR FAMILY AND FRIENDS OF PEOPLE WITH ALZHEIMER'S DISEASE

Symptom, behavior or personality change	*Suggested coping strategy*
• Memory loss and repetitious behavior; inability to remember things said minutes earlier; names of friends and object forgotten; inability to find possessions; lost interest in personal hygiene.	Tell friends to expect less responsiveness; place items in visible accessible places; ignore repetitious actions or questions; supervise daily dressing and washing routines.
• Missed appointments and skipped meals.	Give constant reminders with calendars, schedules, clocks, notes, lists, diagrams and repeated instructions.
• Depression, frustration, anger and despondency.	Be understanding, give reassurance with messages of continued affection; discussion of illness may or may not help.
• Loss of judgment and sensory feedback about climate, time of day and behavior; with inappropriate dressing, wandering about inadequately clothed and spilling of food, etc.	Provide nighttime supervision; give patient assistance in dressing; try to be a cheery "cleaner-upper."
• Sudden mood swings—from sadness (with crying) to laughing euphoria (a passing phase).	Reassure, support and avoid disapproval or rejection.
• Spatial disorientation—inability to find own room, familiar places; attempts to board bus on wrong side; getting lost risk of injury.	Avoid radical changes of surroundings, moving furniture; accompany on outings; beware of scatter rugs, sharp-edged furniture, loose objects.
• Pacing and aimless wandering, especially at night.	Get a hard-to-open door lock to restrict excursions; supply an ID bracelet.
• Sleep problems and insomnia, nighttime fears.	Encourage sufficient daily exercise (within individual limits) to facilitate sleep; use a night-light to reduce anxiety; arouse slowly if asleep.
• Increasing apprehension and anxiety in line with increasing inability to do simple tasks.	Provide greater reassurance with a touch, a hug, a smile and a calm attitude.
• Irritability and aggression—with temper outbursts.	Try to stay cool, avoid arguments or attempts at logic; if possible, don't raise the voice but be soothing.
• Decreased social skills with diminished responses and avoidance of eye contact.	Maintain eye contact, talk facing the person; when possible, continue social and group activities as usual, helping others to realize that avoidance doesn't mean rejection; help with telephoning and letter writing.
• Slowed motion and coordination.	Employ only for sheltered tasks; allow daytime rests, flexible routines.
• Speech and language deterioration with diminished comprehension.	Continue to communicate; repeat questions phrased for yes or no answers; don't talk down or condescend but speak clearly, expressing one idea at a time; lower voice pitch rather than talking loudly.
• Increased safety hazards due to disabilities.	Prevent driving, cooking, smoking, use of appliances and other risk situations; adjust hot water heater to a safe temperature, store medicines out of reach.
• Loss of bladder control.	Discreetly remind about toileting; help clean up; curtail evening liquids; use pads and protective bedding.
• Inability to move or feed self.	Need attending team to move from bed to chair and assist in feeding, bathing and other functions.
• Increasing isolation.	Try to keep up efforts to encourage visitors, remembering that seeming unresponsiveness may not mean total lack of interest.
• More physical dysfunction with seizures, loss of sphincter control, weight loss, increased susceptibility to infection.	Adopt medical treatment with doctor and nurse in team; discuss possibility of death openly, allowing for honest discussion. Make sure caregivers get adequate respite and time off so they don't get sick. Inform doctors of any noticeable changes.

and 19, and a dozen families have surfaced around the world with a dominant genetic mutation linked to the beta-amyloid protein buildup—a hallmark of the disease. Those carrying the dominant gene all develop AD in their forties or fifties, with abnormal deposition of beta-amyloid protein. The genetic model gains support from the fact that nearly all people with Down syndrome, or trisomy-21 (where individuals have an extra chromosome 21 in their cells) develop Alzheimer's disease if they reach age 40 or over.

Besides the genes for early-onset Alzheimer's, people with late-onset disease often carry a faulty gene for the production of apoliprotein E (Apo E)—hindering neuronal repair in certain brain regions. Recent research shows that Apo F is essential for repairing injured brain cells. While a normally aging brain loses neurons at a steady rate by cell death and shrinkage, an Alzheimer brain undergoes far greater structural damage, especially in the temporal lobe and hippocampal regions needed for memory.

Precise risk factors remain elusive

Of some 40 possible causes and risk factors explored since Alzheimer's disease was first defined, only two are relatively uncontroversial: old age and family history. Risks of Alzheimer's disease definitely increase with age. After age 65, the risks double every 5 years, until by age 85, 20 percent of people suffer Alzheimer's dementia. But neuroscientists are mystified by the triggers that set it off.

Suspected triggers of AD include:

- an unusual or slow-acting transmissible agent, perhaps a slow virus akin to those responsible for kuru (a disease transmitted in cannibals who eat human brains) and Creutzfeldt-Jakob disease (a rare transmissible dementia)—but evidence for a viral cause remains scanty. AD is not currently considered to be transmissible.
- environmental agents leading to the degenerative brain changes—aluminum, in particular; is strongly under suspicion. Many studies find elevated amounts of aluminum in Alzheimer brains, at levels known to be lethal in animals. Researchers are investigating whether aluminum (a known neurotoxin or nerve poison), widespread in the earth's crust and in

many foods, medicines and drinking water; could be a participating factor.

Treatment: no cure, but some helpful strategies

A central dilemma in coping with Alzheimer's disease is that it creeps up in such a gradual fashion that it's hard for the afflicted person and family to acknowledge that anything is wrong. Support and understanding can be slow in coming. Sharing knowledge may help caregivers to cope with patients, who are often the last to recognize their illness. The frustration of trying to help someone who often seems bent on defeating every effort may drive caregivers to the limits of self-control and beyond.

The newest treatment for Alzheimer's is the use of drugs called cholinesterase inhibitors. They enhance the action of the brain's neurotransmitter, acetylcholine, by blocking its enzymatic breakdown; but it may take some months to obtain any improvement. These drugs include Aricept (Donepezil), Exelon (Rivastigmine) and Reminyl (Galantamine). For some people these can turn back the clock somewhat (typically by 6 months), but for others with Alzheimer's there is not much obvious benefit.

Treatment of Alzheimer's disease also means managing the declining memory and gradually worsening behavioral symptoms with medications such as anticonvulsants, tranquilizers, antidepressants, mood stabilizers, sleep-aids, antianxiety drugs and psychiatric counseling (for both patient and caregivers).

The key to caregiving and helping people with Alzheimer's is to focus on things the person can still do and reduce the impact of waning abilities. Suggested tactics include:

- Use of memory-joggers: lists of things to do—giving times, places and phone numbers—to help the person complete tasks.
- Providing structure and stability—minimizing undue noise, disturbances, rush, hustle and bustle—to help stabilize schedules and reduce anxiety, also speaking slowly and calmly.
- To reduce the risks of wandering and getting lost, provide a pocket card with the person's name, address and phone number.
- Making the home environment as safe as pos-

sible by keeping furniture in the same place, removing clutter; using soft (soothing) carpeting (not throw rugs), installing locks on medicine cabinets and setting the water heater at a low (non-scalding) temperature.

- Enhancing communication by speaking clearly and from a spot where you can be seen, presenting one thought or instruction at a time—using gestures and cues, such as pointing to objects—and showing friendly affection.
- Absolutely forbid driving—control access to car keys.

Although there's no cure, better management of early Alzheimer's can help postpone its debilitating end. For example, preventing strokes can reduce the impact of Alzheimer's; recent evidence shows that stroke contributes sizably to the ravages of AD. (See the section on stroke in Chapter 16.)

So far; no drug can halt or reverse the brain destruction in AD. Finding a medication that can even transiently relieve symptoms involves painstaking trial and error.

Coping with Alzheimer's disease is an agonizing challenge

For many patients and caregivers this fatal aging disease brings untold turmoil, guilt and almost insurmountable challenges. Aggressive behavior, night wandering, obstinacy, paranoia and an inability to understand what's happening make the disease especially difficult. Yet despite the great emotional toll, many families try to care for afflicted relatives at home. In handling someone who was once a source of support but is now a totally dependent, mentally impaired and, eventually, immobile person, caregivers must tread a fine line between assisting sufferers in doing what they can still do and recognizing what's impossible. Home visits by health professionals can greatly ease the burden.

For more information, contact the Alzheimer Society in your community or write to the Alzheimer Society of Canada, tel.: (416) 789–0503, 491 Lawrence Ave. West, Suite 501, Toronto, ON M5M 1C7; the McGill Centre for Studies in Aging, 6825 blvd. LaSalle, Verdun, PQ, H4H 1R3; the Alzheimer Association, tel.: (800) 272–3900, at 919 North Michigan Ave., Suite 1000, Chicago, Ill. 60611–1676: the National Council on Aging, tel.: (202) 479–1200; the National Association for Home Care, tel.: (202) 547–7424.

CAREGIVERS ALSO NEED RESPITE AND SUPPORT

Amid the "save and rescue" stance expected of those looking after the elderly and frail, today's caregivers—90 percent of whom are women—must not forget to nurture themselves. Becoming a caregiver to elderly or ill parents, spouses or partners carries many implications, both physical and emotional. While to the receiver care means security and protection, for the caregiver it may entail endless juggling of conflicting demands and tasks, creating undue stress and worry.

Recent Canadian surveys show that 46 percent of working Canadians provide some eldercare, half of them also caring for dependent children. One U.S. estimate finds that women spend about 17 years of their lives in childcare and another 18 years caring for elderly parents (or other relatives).

Compared to non-caregivers, informal caregivers are more economically disadvantaged, less likely to be gainfully employed, and more likely to report physical health problems and mental disturbances. Studies also show that family legacies and tradition tend to designate one member as the "caregiver," others remaining relatively unencumbered and perhaps offering no or little help. This can pose an enormous burden on the caregiver, as well as losses—perhaps giving up a job or career foregoing leisure, recreational and social activities. Yet despite the stress, women caregivers are less likely than their male counterparts to ask for help. Instead, they may cut back on leisure activities with no time for self-replenishment.

Health professionals say it's high time to change these patterns—to place more value on informal caregiving, to provide more easily-available support networks and resources and to set boundaries and limits on what's possible. Above all, it's crucial to remember that not only the old, disabled and ill but also their caregivers need support and nurturance.

Some specific diseases and disorders

AIDS • ALS • Anemia • Arthritis • Asthma • Athlete's foot • ADHD • Back problems • Bovine encephalopathy and Creutzfeldt-Jakob Disease • Bowel problems • Bronchitis • Carpal tunnel syndrome • Common cold • Cystic fibrosis • Diabetes • Dizziness • Dry eye • Emerging infectious diseases • Epilepsy • Fibromyalgia • Gallbladder problems • Halitosis • Headaches • Heart disease • Heart murmurs • Heartburn • Hemorrhoids • Hepatitis • Hernias • Hypertension • Influenza • Itching • Kidney failure • Kidney stones • Leukemia • Liver cirrhosis • Lung cancer • Lupus • Lyme disease • Peptic ulcers • Strokes • Stuttering • Thyroid disorders • Tuberculosis • Urinary tract infections • Varicose veins • Does your work environment make you sick? • Workplace health • Zoonoses: diseases from pets

16

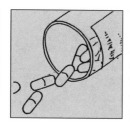

THIS CHAPTER DOES not attempt to catalogue all human diseases in an encyclopedic manner; but deals with conditions of special concern in North America today, and a few newly emergent disorders of particular interest. The topics are arranged in alphabetical order. Some of the subjects are also discussed, in other contexts, in other chapters.

AIDS

The discovery of a new, fatal and non-treatable infection known as AIDS, or acquired immunodeficiency syndrome, in 1981 shattered the complacent illusion that infectious diseases had been vanquished or are curable. Since its discovery, this infection—spread by sex, blood and injection drug use—has become a pandemic, with millions around the world already carrying the virus responsible for AIDS.

AIDS is thought to be caused by the human immunodeficiency virus (HIV), which gradually undermines the body's defenses by destroying the immune system's *CD4 + T-lymphocytes* (white blood cells) also known as T-4 helper cells. When the CD4 T-lymphocyte count drops below a certain level, the body can no longer fight off the many infections that produce the syndrome called AIDS.

HIV is a retrovirus in which the genes are packaged as RNA molecules (similar to DNA)

within a protein capsule or coat. As a retrovirus, HIV has the rare capacity to incorporate its genetic material right into the human cell's DNA. Once inside a human cell, the retrovirus uses its own enzyme, reverse transcriptase, to copy and incorporate its genes into the host cell. Thus HIV becomes an integral part of the human body, where it lies hidden, perhaps for years. There are two known forms of HIV—HIV-1 and HIV-2—producing identical forms of illness. HIV-1 is the predominant type, and HIV-2 (less easily transmitted) is found mainly in West Africa, with some cases in France and Portugal.

Even when there are no signs of infection, HIV-positive carriers can pass the virus to others. During the long incubation period, the HIV viruses quietly undermine the human immune system—destroying more and more CD4 T-lymphocytes—with no outward hint that the body's defences are being sabotaged. When the CD4 count drops below 200 cells per microliter, the body succumbs to the multiple infections that signal AIDS. The latent (incubation) period from initial HIV infection to the appearance of AIDS averages 10 to 15 years—half of those infected develop AIDS within 10 years, and three-quarters within 13 years.

HIV does not kill, it merely renders the body defenseless against opportunistic infections such as thrush or oral yeast (candidiasis) infection—often the alerting sign of AIDS—toxoplasmosis, cytomegalovirus infections, tuberculosis, cancers such as Kaposi's sarcoma (a skin cancer), invasive cervical cancer and a deadly form of pneumonia (*Pneumocystis carinii*), the killer in half of all AIDS cases. As the body's immune defenses crumble, there's an ever-greater chance of developing AIDS. Between bouts of infection, people with HIV may remain well, especially with the help of modern antiretroviral drugs. But even with currently available treatments, once someone develops AIDS, survival only averages 2 to 3 years; risks of death increase when CD4 counts fall below 50 cells/mml.

Transmission modes: how HIV spreads

The HIV virus has been isolated from blood, tears, semen, cervical secretions, saliva, urine and breastmilk. There's no evidence that AIDS can be spread through saliva or tears, or by casual domestic contact—by sharing household items—or by mosquitoes or bedbugs. HIV is less contagious than measles, hepatitis or herpes. There is no evidence that kissing has infected anyone with HIV, although cuts in the mouth or bleeding gums can expose people to infected blood.

AIDS is predominantly sexually transmitted (especially by anal sex and in those with genital sores). Female HIV carriers can infect male sex partners and vice versa. Heterosexually acquired AIDS has occurred from a single unprotected act of vaginal intercourse. Transmission risks increase if a woman is menstruating. Using latex condoms plus spermicide greatly reduces the risk. HIV also spreads via shared injection equipment, as well as from mother to baby in the uterus or at delivery. There are known cases where mother's breastmilk infected her infant.

Infection through blood products has dropped since testing began, but there are still cases acquired through artificial insemination and organ transplants. Occupational exposure among healthcare workers—for instance by a needlestick injury or splash of contaminated body fluids—can cause infection, but to date there have been very few deaths from occupationally acquired HIV.

Tests for HIV

Tests for HIV include blood tests to detect antibodies to HIV proteins, detection of viral antigens and culturing the virus itself. Most people seroconvert—develop detectable antibodies to HIV—within 3 to 12 weeks of infection. But there's a window period during which people can transmit the disease before they have developed detectable antibodies. Since about 5 percent of those infected have no signs of antibody production for up to 6 months, a negative test result can be falsely reassuring. (A second test some months later is advised for those who think they may be at risk.) The key message here is that if someone engages in high risk activities such as unprotected sexual intercourse or injected substance use, it will take 3 to 6 months for the antibodies that are being tested for to become apparent, so it takes that long before you can be fully reassured that you have no HIV infection.

The primary test for HIV is the ELISA (Enzyme-Linked Immunoabsorbent Assay), which tests the person's serum (blood) for HIV antibodies. If the ELISA is positive, a confirmatory Western Blot test will be done. Additional tests include the viral antigen assay, which may be used to screen blood donors as it shows infection during the window period when HIV antibodies may not yet have been formed. Recently, rapid (3-minute) screening lab kits have become available, as well as home diagnostic kits (using a modified ELISA method) to test for HIV antibodies in urine (not too reliable) or oral (mouth) samples (more trustworthy). Positive home test results must be confirmed with a Western Blot follow-up.

The global picture

The good news is that in developed countries AIDS has become more like a chronic disease, albeit one that depends on a complicated cocktail of medications to prolong survival and one that nonetheless remains a potentially fatal disorder. The bad news is that the World Health Organization (WHO) and UNAIDS report that by the end of 2004 there were globally already 39.8 million HIV-infected people, half of them women (and that in sub-Saharan Africa 60 percent of those infected are women who can pass the disease to their offspring). By the year 2000, the WHO had estimated that there would be 40 million HIV-infected men, women and

COMMON EARLY SYMPTOMS OF HIV DISEASE

- **Weight loss and "wasting"—an increasingly gaunt look;**
- **fevers, night sweats;**
- **diarrhea;**
- **oral candidiasis ("thrush");**
- **skin infections with herpes or varicella zoster (shingles);**
- **tuberculosis (TB): in West Africa, one-third of AIDS patients are dying of TB.**

children around the world, and sadly that prediction has come true. In some African cities, 1 in 3 adults tests positive for HIV infection. Worldwide, WHO estimates that 1 per 100 sexually active people aged 14 to 49 carries HIV infection, of whom 10 percent don't know it. AIDS is also spreading at an alarming rate in Latin America, the Caribbean, Eastern Europe and Central and Eastern Asia—especially through injection drug use and failure to use condoms. In the U.S., AIDS is the leading cause of death in men aged 24 to 44 years. However, the good news is that in the U.S. and particularly in New York City (which has many AIDS cases) fewer babies are being born HIV-infected largely because of campaigns urging pregnant women to be HIV-tested and take the necessary drugs to prevent their infants from being infected and dying of the disease.

The groups at greatest risk vary from place to place. For instance in North America, even though homosexuals had the highest HIV infection rates at first, heterosexual AIDS is becoming more common. Globally, 90 percent of AIDS is now heterosexually acquired or transmitted from mother to baby.

In Canada, by the end of 1997 there were 15,101 cumulative AIDS cases reported since the epidemic began (158 of them children), over half having already died. An estimated 54,000 Canadians are now living with HIV infection, about 5,000 of them women. Increasing numbers of women are getting and dying of AIDS; currently about 13 percent of those newly HIV-infected in Canada are women. (Estimates include adjustments for underreporting and/or delayed reporting.)

Stephen Lewis, UN Special Envoy for HIV/AIDS in Africa, made the following comment in a keynote speech in San Francisco regarding the pandemic in 2004: "On the continent of Africa, it is estimated that 4.1 million people need treatment now…i.e., their CD4 counts are below 200…and approximately 70,000 to 100,000 are actually in treatment, or roughly 2 per cent. It's important for everyone here to recognize that you're part of the most significant battle against a disease that has ever been waged in human history…and when you're consumed in your laboratories, or wrestling with the esoterica of science, at the end of that long exploratory road there lies the whole fabric of the human family fighting for survival, searching, desperately, for hope. The grieving villages, the funerals, the hospital wards, the orphans, the women at the clinics; it's an hallucinatory nightmare; it should never have come to this."

Amidst the global scene, the annual number of Canadian AIDS deaths is falling—due to the success of combination drug treatments. But while fewer are dying of AIDS, the number living with the disease is rising and there is a surge in new HIV infections, especially among young people: the average age when AIDS strikes is now 25 (compared with 35 a decade ago). Given the idea that AIDS can be treated with a slew of new drugs, people are being lulled into a false sense of security about contracting the disease, so that fewer and fewer young people are using condoms, heeding "safe sex" advice and taking precautions to prevent themselves from HIV-infection. Ottawa's Laboratory Centre for Disease Control estimates there are now at least 5,000 new HIV infections per year. "In a way, it's one step forward, two back," notes one expert. "The falloff in AIDS deaths has led to fewer warnings, and more and more people forgetting to practise safer sex."

AIDS incidence is even rising once again among young men who have sex with men, after having declined. Many of those who are HIV-positive fail to tell sex partners they are infected—increasing the danger. Only 40 percent of sexually active young people in Canada use condoms, even when having sex with unknown partners. "We need to repeat the unvarnished facts about AIDS," stresses one expert, "and the sober truth about treatment; it's no cure, but just buys time. While AIDS drugs cost about $40 a day, condoms cost only 40 cents, or are provided free in many instances."

Since AIDS is increasing among needle-sharing injection drug users, Canada as well as the U.K. and Netherlands have set up programs for free needle and syringe exchange—also handing out condoms—in efforts to curb HIV spread.

Treatment strategies and management

Because it's a retrovirus that amalgamates itself into human DNA, reaching or killing HIV is difficult. The main strategies tried are stopping virus multiplication, interrupting its growth cycle or boosting the body's immune system (e.g., with lymphokines and thymus gland hormones or by adding antibodies). Anti-HIV agents include

- *neutralizing antibodies* (to stop HIV action);
- *deoxynucleoside reverse transcriptase inhibitors* (NRTIs) such as *abacavir* (Ziagen), *zidovudine* or *AZT, stavudine (Zerit), lamivudine* (Epivir) *didanosine* or *ddl*, and *zalcitabine* (Hivid), which arrest the enzyme action of HIV's reverse transcriptase and stops or decreases HIV viral replication. These drugs are usually taken in 2 to 3 doses daily, but can cause side effects such as lactic acidosis and liver problems;
- *protease inhibitors* (such as *amprevanir, saquinavir, ritonavir, nevirapine, nelfinavir* and *indinavir*)—potent drugs that block the protease enzyme that finalizes the assembly of HIV virus particles, preventing viral replication;
- *non-nucleoside reverse transcriptase inhibitors (NNRTIs), which, like the NRTIs inhibit reverse transcriptase, but in a different manner.* Together the NRTIs and NNRTIs seem most effective in inhibiting HIV replication within infected cells. They include *efavirenz, delavirdine* and *nevirapine*. However, resistance to NNRTIs often develops quite quickly so they are of limited usefulness if used alone.
- *integrase inhibitors* that prevent viral material from being integrated into the host DNA; and
- *interferons* that stop the release of new HIV viruses produced within human cells.

Common side effects are: dizziness, rash, hallucinations, insomnia nausea and headache, damage to blood cells and liver toxicity, depending on the drugs used and their dosages.

The NRTIs such as zidovudine (AZT), among the most widely used anti-HIV agents, prolong survival in many cases, and since they can cross the "blood-brain barrier," their use also helps suppress the cerebrally damaging effects of HIV (e.g., dementia). Side effects of zidovudine include nausea, insomnia and possible bone marrow or liver damage, so people on it need careful and continuous monitoring.

One problem with drug therapy for HIV is the development of drug resistance and loss of efficacy as the HIV viruses mutate to different forms that no longer respond to or are killed by the medications. So, combination therapy with several agents—for example NRTIs plus protease inhibitors and also other viral suppressors—is often tried, with some success, although it's very costly, and adverse drug interactions may develop from simultaneous use of several medications. Toxicity of each of the drugs also limits their usefulness and the duration for which each can be given. Meanwhile, treatment is improving for each of the opportunistic infections of AIDS, for instance pneumocystis carinii pneumonia, herpes, cytomegalovirus and others.

Use of anti-HIV drugs in pregnancy, especially zidovudine (AZT) alone or in combination with protease inhibitors, beginning at 14 to 34 weeks of gestation, and continued in the newborn for the first six weeks of life, can substantially reduce the chance of transmitting HIV to the baby and possibly save its life. Taking AZT on its own (or together with lamivudine) even just for 3 to 4 weeks before delivery and during labor can also reduce the risk of infecting the baby by as much as 50 percent. More recent evidence shows that for HIV-infected women who have never taken antiretrovirals, giving them anti-HIV drugs at the start of labor and then also to the newborn can lessen the risk of prenatal infection. Such practices can reduce the huge and tragic toll of infant deaths among babies born to HIV-infected mothers.

Owing to concerns about drug toxicity and the development of viral resistance, antiretroviral treatment guidelines for combating HIV/AIDS are constantly being updated, e.g., by the WHO and U.S. Department of Health and Human Services (www.hivatis.org). An effective vaccine against AIDS may be decades away, partly because of the extreme variability of the viral agent, which quickly mutates, producing slightly different strains. A vaccine effective against one strain may not protect against another. Currently, researchers are working on both weakened whole-virus vaccines and those containing subunits of the viral envelope or its core.

As a preventive strategy, everyone should practise safer sex and use a latex condom for each and every sex act. Since HIV can stay dormant in the body for so long, to be certain a sex partner doesn't carry AIDS, one must either insist on a test, or know that he or she has not been exposed for at least 15, maybe 18, years! And who can be absolutely sure on so delicate a matter? Therein lies the dilemma of our times—how to choose a "safe" sex partner in the age of AIDS.

Treatment regimens for AIDS are constantly evolving.

For more information or help regarding AIDS, call local AIDS committees or public-health departments: AIDS hotlines (e.g., 1-800-392-2437); local STD clinics; the Bureau of HIV/AIDS at Health Canada's Laboratory Centre for Disease Control, Ottawa. Health Canada's HIV/AIDS website: http://www.hc-sc.gc.ca/english/diseases/aids.html is good for general information from a Canadian perspective; also try www.iac.org; or www.unaids.org/wad2004/report.html.

ALS OR AMYOTROPHIC LATERAL SCLEROSIS

First described in 1869 by Jean-Martin Charcot, a French neurologist, ALS or *amyotrophic lateral* sclerosis, also known as Lou Gehrig's disease, is a gradually progressing muscle-wasting disorder that destroys motor neurons (nerve cells) in the brain and spinal cord that control voluntary movement. As neurons die off, muscles throughout the body weaken and lose the ability to move. The average duration from diagnosis and noticeable symptoms of ALS to death is 3 years, although some survive much longer.

The reasons for the massive neuronal loss in ALS remain unknown, but about 5 to 10 percent of cases have a genetic link. Researchers at Montreal's McGill University have recently located one gene responsible for ALS. Scientists also suspect a slow-acting or latent virus, trauma/injury or environmental triggers—perhaps metals (such as lead, mercury, manganese or aluminium) or other toxins. However, about 95 percent of ALS is sporadic and of unknown cause.

ALS affects about 2 per 100,000 people around the world, twice as many men as women. Although its age of onset peaks in the mid-50s, younger people can also develop it. The earliest symptoms are vague, and elderly people may take them for normal changes of aging. The first hint of ALS is often hand weakness—trouble opening a jam jar, fastening a button or manipulating car keys—or it may first show itself by difficulty swallowing. By the time someone with ALS seeks medical advice, there may already be considerable muscle wasting. As the disease continues, disabilities increase—lips weaken and saliva drools, speech slurs, chewing and swallowing become troublesome. (The ocular or eye muscles are generally spared.) People with ALS may lose the ability to talk or gesture and find breathing difficult, although they're seldom in pain. Eventually sufferers are confined to a wheelchair, then bed. But since the disease attacks mostly motor neurons, it leaves intelligence, memory, reasoning and other mental capacities untouched. Those with ALS remain lucid and in full possession of their senses—sight, hearing, taste and smell—to the end, distressingly aware of their progressive decline.

At present, there is no known treatment, drug, cure or means of preventing ALS. Special exercises can help maintain muscle function, drugs can alleviate the cramps and swallowing difficulties are overcome by use of high-calorie, non-gagging foods. Suction devices help with excess saliva. Given a supportive home environment, many with ALS can continue fairly comfortable lives with help from assistive devices. Death usually occurs from respiratory failure.

For more information, contact the ALS Society of America, (818) 990–2151; the National ALS Foundation, (212) 679–4016; or the Canadian ALS Society, (800) 267–4257.

ANEMIA

Anemia is a condition in which the concentration of the oxygen-carrying hemoglobin molecule within red blood cells falls below normal, consequently depleting the body's oxygen supply. Hemoglobin is the iron-containing pigment in red blood cells which binds and transports oxygen throughout the body, delivering it to cells as needed. The body's production of red blood cells in the bone marrow depends on an adequate supply of nutrients, particularly iron and certain B vitamins such as folic acid and vitamin B 12. If for any reason hemoglobin levels drop or the number of red blood cells decreases, the body's tissues may become short of oxygen causing symptoms of anemia such as pallor (pale complexion), fatigue and shortness of breath.

There are many different forms and causes of anemia but by far the most common is iron deficiency anemia (IDA) due to lack of dietary iron, the essential component of hemoglobin in red blood cells. With this type of anemia, the body cannot manufacture sufficient oxygen-carrying hemoglobin for its needs. Short-changed of oxygen, people with IDA become weak and non-functional. In fact, iron deficiency anemia is the world's most common nutritional deficiency disorder affecting millions, especially in developing countries. Many women die during pregnancy and in childbirth because of iron deficiency anemia. And over 750 million children in the developing world suffer from anemia due to lack of nutritional iron, undermining their health, impairing mental development and producing learning disabilities.

In developed Western countries, 2 to 5 percent of individuals experience some form of anemia. Symptoms of all types of anemia, which arise from the blood's diminished oxygen-carrying capacity, typically include: paleness, unusual tiredness, lethargy, headaches, dizziness (due to lack of oxygen to the brain), shortness of breath on exertion and palpitations. Severity of symptoms depends on how low the blood's hemoglobin level drops and the extent of oxygen depletion. Normal hemoglobin levels range from 130 to 180 grams per litre for men, and 115 to 160 g/L in women. Levels below 130 g/L in men and under 120g/L in women are categorized as anemia; hemoglobin levels below 100 g/L can cause noticeable symptoms and at under 80 g/L they may be severe.

Anemia is not really a discrete disease but a feature of many different disorders. The different types of anemia belong to several major categories some caused by defects in the bone marrow's red blood cell production. Red blood cells are manufactured in bone marrow from specialized *stem cells*, becoming young red cells (reticulocytes) before maturing into adult red cells which circulate in the bloodstream, deliver-

ing oxygen for about 120 days before they die and are destroyed in the spleen. Forms of anemia due to reduced or defective bone marrow production of red cells include:

- *aplastic anemia* (failed maturation of red blood cells) a rare condition involving depletion of both red and white blood cells in which the bone marrow fails to produce the stem cells from which blood cells evolve. It can be triggered by autoimmune processes, anti-cancer treatments (such as chemotherapy), viral infections or possibly long-term exposure to nuclear radiation or certain pesticides.

- *megaloblastic anemia* due to vitamin deficiencies (mostly lack of vitamin B 12 or of folic acid), leads to the production of large but faulty red cells low in hemoglobin. Although this form of anemia is hard to detect, it can cause numbness, burning or tingling in the feet, fatigue and irritability. Vitamin B 12 deficiency can occur for dietary reasons, especially among strict vegetarians as this vitamin is found only in animal products such as fish, poultry, red meats, eggs and dairy produce. Pernicious anemia arises through the body's inability to absorb vitamin B 12 owing to autoimmune or other disorders. (It is detected by Schilling's test which measures vitamin B 12 absorption.) Another similar megaloblastic anemia, common among alcoholics and those with Crohn's disease, is due to lack of dietary folic acid. Pregnant women are especially prone to this anemia, as folate requirements are high in pregnancy and a lack can cause fetal deformities (such as neural tube defects). Therefore, experts now recommend supplements of this vitamin for all women of child-bearing age (to provide 400 micrograms daily) and some cereals are also folate-fortified. (Good sources of folic acid are liver, dark green vegetables and lentils, beans or other legumes.)

- *iron-deficiency anemia* due to lack of dietary iron necessary for hemoglobin manufacture (see below).

Other anemias (for instance hemolytic anemia) arise from premature or excessive destruction (hemolysis) of red blood cells or their decreased survival, possibly accompanying malaria or other disorders.

Still other forms of anemia are inherited as genetic mutations that result in deformed hemoglobin molecules with reduced oxygen-transporting capacity, or red blood cells that are fragile and easily ruptured. Inherited anemias include *thalassemia,* common among people of Mediterranean, Middle Eastern, African and Southeast Asian descent, and *sickle cell anemia,* common among West African and West Indian peoples (and, to a lesser extent, in Mediterranean populations), and the rare *Franconi's syndrome.* Thalassemia and sickle cell anemia are caused by recessive genes, so it takes two flawed genes (one inherited from the mother, one from the father) to produce the disease.

Anemia can also occur through blood losses, for example, in women with heavy menstrual periods, following a serious injury or through bleeding due to chronic conditions such as peptic ulcers, various cancers (such as leukemia or lymphoma), irritable bowel syndrome, Crohn's disease or other gastrointestinal tract disorders, bone or kidney diseases, frequent use of certain medications (such as ASA/Aspirin or other NSAIDs) and because of parasitic infestations (e.g., hookworm). Anemia can also accompany conditions that impair nutrition such as alcoholism, poor processing of vitamin B12 or because of nutrient-poor diets.

Diagnosis of anemia depends on measuring hemoglobin levels, doing a red cell count, observing the size, shape and color intensity of red blood cells by examining a sample (smear) of the person's blood under the microscope, and through serum ferritin tests to detect an iron-depleted state. Measuring blood levels of folate, vitamin B 12 and homocysteine may also help to identify anemia. However, all too often anemia goes undetected because it is masked by symptoms of the diseases that cause it or with which it is associated.

Treatment of anemia, tailored to its type and severity, may include use of iron or vitamin supplements, vitamin B 12 injections, blood transfusions, erythropoietin (to stimulate red blood cell production) and bone marrow transplants.

Iron Deficiency Anemia

The most common form of anemia, iron deficiency anemia is due a shortage of iron needed to produce the oxygen-carrying hemoglobin in red blood cells. Iron is an essential part of the hemoglobin molecule, and without sufficient hemoglobin. anemia develops because the body is shortchanged of its required oxygen delivery. The body is very efficient at storing iron, recycling amounts freed when red cells die, storing it as a protein called *ferritin.* Iron deficiency anemia usually starts slowly, with gradual depletion of the body's iron stores, either through continuing iron loss or because of inadequate intake. As iron stores dwindle, absorption from food increases, and anemia develops only after the body has been short of iron for a lengthy time. As hemoglobin production falls, red blood cells become smaller and oxygen in short supply. In those with anemia, the heart must compensate and work harder to provide the body with its needed oxygen.

People at particular risk of iron deficiency anemia include pregnant women and those with heavy periods, young children and the elderly with poor eating habits, people with peptic ulcers, hemorrhoids, gastrointestinal and other cancers. Children are at greatest risk of iron deficiency and its consequences, especially between the ages of 6 to 24 months. At birth, full-term healthy babies get enough iron to see them through the first few months, but after the age of 4 to 6 months they often need fortified infant foods. In Canada and many other developed countries, iron is added to all baby foods to offset impaired mental development and learning disabilities due to iron deficiency. At the University of Toronto's Hospital for Sick Children, researchers have recently developed a cheap, easy-to-use iron supplement as a nice-tasting powder to be sprinkled on baby foods or mixed with children's drinks. Already tested in eight countries, this iron-rich product can significantly reduce the prevalence of iron deficiency anemia. (See Chapter 4 for more on children's nutritional iron needs.)

Treatment of iron deficiency anemia often requires use of iron supplements taken in three daily doses. For the treatment of iron deficiency anemia, adults usually require 100 to 200 mg/day of elemental iron in divided doses, and children 3 mg/kg/day in divided doses. But it can take several months to correct the problem, depending on the severity of the depletion and how long it takes to restore the body's iron stores. Numerous formulations of ferrous iron preparations are available for treating iron deficiency anemia, the most popular being oral ferrous sulfate tablets, ferrous fumarate and ferrous gluconate. The amount of elemental iron varies among these products. In general, elemental iron makes up 20 to 30 percent of ferrous sulfate, 30 percent of ferrous fumarate, and 11 percent of ferrous gluconate.

The most frequent adverse effects of iron therapy are upper gastrointestinal tract discomfort, constipation and sometimes diarrhea, their severity depending on the dose of elemental iron. To minimize side effects, people can take the medication with meals, increase the dose gradually, and try to keep the total daily iron dose as low as possible. For those with a very low hemoglobin level, blood transfusions might be necessary.

ARTHRITIS

Arthritis is an umbrella term encompassing 116 different disorders formerly called rheumatic complaints. One of the most common chronic disorders, it afflicts 1 in 7 Canadians, half in the prime of life (aged 30 to 50). Arthritic disorders may be inflammatory in nature, such as rheumatoid arthritis; metabolic, as with gout and pseudogout; or degenerative, like osteoarthritis. Osteoarthritis is by far the most common form of arthritis. Some affect primarily the joints; others are associated with inflammation and damage to other body organs. For instance, *lupus erythematosus* may present with a facial rash but often spreads to other organs including the joints, kidneys and lungs; scleroderma not only produces skin thickening but also harms many parts of the body such as the kidneys and lungs.

Although the roots of many arthritic diseases remain unknown, scientists believe that inflammatory forms may be triggered by bacterial or viral infections along with a flaw in the body's immune system, setting the stage for an abnormal immune response that turns against

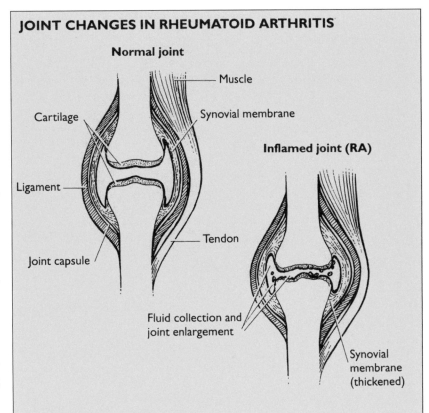

JOINT CHANGES IN RHEUMATOID ARTHRITIS

Normal joint

Muscle

Cartilage

Synovial membrane

Inflamed joint (RA)

Ligament

Tendon

Joint capsule

Fluid collection and joint enlargement

Synovial membrane (thickened)

Joints, which are hinges that enable the skeleton to bend and move, are subjected to a great deal of pressure, particularly weight-bearing joints like the knees and hips. They require lubrication and mechanisms to absorb the shock of movement or they would wear away. Cartilage, a tough elastic coating covering the ends of bones, performs both of these functions. The high water content of cartilage gives it a cushioning effect. When weight is put on a joint, the water is squeezed out and the cartilage flattens like a sponge being squeezed; when the weight is removed, the water moves back in and the cartilage expands. Every joint is encapsulated in a sac-like structure, which stops the water from escaping. Lining the sac is a membrane called the synovium, which supplies nourishment to the cartilage. Each type of arthritis affects the joints in different ways: the cartilage can be worn away; the cartilage and synovium can be inflamed; or gritty substances floating free in the joint sac can get in between the layers of cartilage.

and destroys the sufferer's own tissues. Heredity plays a part in some forms of arthritis. An example is *ankylosing spondylitis*, for which many people carry a specific genetic marker.

Symptoms and warning signs of the more severe forms of arthritis may include persistent unexplained soreness; pain; redness; early-morning stiffness; swelling and loss of movement in the fingers and toes, wrists, knees and hips; and lower back pain.

Among the myriad forms, five main types

account for more than half of all arthritic diseases diagnosed in North America.

- *Osteoarthritis (OA)*, the commonest form, affects more than 1 million Canadians, particularly people over age 60. In this degenerative condition the joint cartilage wears away, leaving bone ends to rub painfully together; but giving little discomfort until its more advanced stages. OA may be primary, developing spontaneously for no apparent reason, or secondary, where the joint damage or degeneration results from trauma, surgery or injury to the weight-bearing surfaces, or is caused by other forms of arthritis (such as rheumatoid arthritis). OA may follow bone fractures that damage the cartilaginous joint surfaces, explaining why many ex-athletes suffer from it. Overall, OA occurs equally in both sexes, but under age 45 it is more prevalent in men.

In OA's earliest stages, the cartilage covering bone ends begins to degenerate, producing irregularities and loss of shock absorption. With time, larger sections of cartilage wear away, leaving the bone totally unprotected. In severe cases, fragments of bone and cartilage can float freely in the joint capsule, producing inflammation. Cartilage has no nerve endings, so the osteoarthritic pain sensation arises from other parts of the joint—bone, muscle, ligament or tendon—due to distension or inflammation, typically after activity. Joint pain from OA is relieved by rest. As the disease progresses, the soreness becomes more frequent, continuing at night, often with a few minutes of morning stiffness. OA sufferers often try to stop using the afflicted joint because of the pain, but inaction can weaken the muscles, worsening the condition. Numerous studies have shown that activity, especially low-impact exercise for the large bones (legs, arms), reduces arthritis pain.

Treatment is more aggressive than in the past, with vigorous exercise programs to maintain muscle tone and a battery of pain-relieving and anti-inflammatory medications. Acetaminophen is the first-choice medication for long-term use, with others added as needed such as anti-inflammatory medications like ibuprofen. When these fail, other options that could be added are Capsaicin (a

hot pepper cream), another anti-inflammatory cream, stronger painkillers such as codeine, and local steroid injections into the affected joint(s). In those severely disabled by OA, surgery may help to clean out the joint sac or replace the joint with a substitute. Although it is only considered as a "last line" treatment, many report a significant improvement in quality of life with joint replacement. Glucosamine and chondroitin, both herbal preparations, have become very popular for arthritis and the evidence shows that they are effective. The trials typically used the dose of 500 mg 3 times a day and often took 1 month to work. There are, however, two caveats: the review showed that only "positive" trials were published and the product, available over the counter, is not regulated in North America for purity and concentrations.

- *Rheumatoid arthritis (RA)*, better known but less common than osteoarthritis, strikes 1 to 2 per 100 persons, more women than men. It typically starts in the fingers and toes on both sides of the body, progressing to other joints (including knuckles, wrists, elbows and knee joints). The disease usually strikes between ages 30 and 50, but can start at any time, even in young children aged 2 to 5. It may begin suddenly with a severe attack or come on gradually. Symptoms generally linger on, although there are extended times of remission without pain. The pain is caused by an inflamed and thickened *synovium*, or joint lining. Fluid also builds up in the joint cavity, causing swelling and more pain. Surrounding tissues, such as the ligaments or muscles, can also swell, making the whole joint and the area around it painful to touch and move. If pain becomes severe, muscles contract in spasm and become stiff from inactivity. Over time, the muscles weaken and the joint becomes increasingly difficult to move. Rheumatoid arthritis sufferers may be constantly fatigued by the pain.

Therapy for rheumatoid arthritis includes specially tailored exercises and several types of medication—anti-inflammatory drugs (e.g., ASA and other nonsteroidal anti-inflammatories) and, more recently, a range of disease-modifying anti-rheumatic drugs (DMARDs), which take time to work. DMARDs are an important advance because although medications such as anti-inflammatories do help with pain, unlike DMARDs, they do not alter or halt the progress of RA. Formerly reserved for severe cases, these drugs have been shown to be less toxic than imagined and are now prescribed early to prevent joint destruction. The disease modifiers include *methotrexate* (Rheumatrex), *hydroxychloroquine* (Plaquenil), gold salts, *sulfasalazine* (Azulfidine), low-dose corticosteroids (Prednisone) and immuno-modulators such as Imuran and cyclosporine. In addition, self-help devices like long-handled combs and brushes help sufferers perform everyday tasks. Replacement of severely damaged joints, once the inflammation has subsided, is now an option.

- *Gout and pseudogout*, classified as crystal-associated arthritis, involve crystal deposits within the joints. The symptoms of both are acute joint inflammation, swelling, heat, redness and pain, but the causes differ.

Gout occurs from the accumulation of uric acid, a waste product from the breakdown of food and drink. The excess uric acid forms sodium urate crystals that collect in many tissues, including the joint linings, producing inflammation. A gout attack is extremely painful, generally lasting 5 to 7 days, infrequently up to 3 weeks. The first attack often starts in the big toe, but the ankles, knees, elbows and fingers can all be affected. Over 80 percent of gout sufferers are men; women hardly ever suffer gout before menopause. Evidence suggests that primary gout is genetic, but it can also be precipitated by excessive alcohol consumption, obesity and conditions where large amounts of tissue are suddenly broken down. Renal (kidney) failure may also be linked to high uric-acid levels. Sufferers have a tendency to high blood pressure and elevated blood-lipid (fat) levels. Since the buildup of uric acid is due to metabolic causes, the popular image of the gout-ridden person as one who overindulges in food and drink seems exaggerated.

Treatment for a first attack of gout includes nonsteroidal anti-inflammatories (NSAIDs)

GENERAL MANAGEMENT OF ARTHRITIS

There's no cure for most forms of arthritis, so the goal of treatment is to reduce the inflammation and pain by lifestyle changes and exercise regimes tailored to the disease. Early diagnosis is crucial for good control; attention to the warning signs can help to prevent disability, frustration and disfigurement. Many types of arthritis are managed by the family physician in consultation with rheumatologists, orthopedists, and physiatrists—as needed.

Treatment includes ice (for acute inflammation), heat (for relief, once inflammation subsides), specific medications, physiotherapy and psychological and occupational counseling with attention to social life and family dynamics. New creams such as Capsaicin (from hot peppers) or Pensaid (an anti-inflammatory cream) may relieve the local pain and hotness of arthritic joints if applied directly to the skin.

Medications for arthritis, either local or systemic, are generally used in a "stepped" manner. ASA is the first line of defense and one of the most powerful anti-inflammatory agents known, but only if its concentration in the blood remains high enough (at a level prescribed by the healthcare provider). NSAIDs, which include over 20 modern medications, are used when ASA fails, followed by disease-retarding, second-line anti-arthritic agents. For rheumatoid arthritis specifically, the second-line drugs (such as gold salts, hydroxychloroquine and other agents) are given earlier in the course of disease, as the anti-inflammatories don't prevent deformity and joint destruction. The failure of NSAIDs to achieve improvement in 2 to 4 months calls for the introduction of second-line drugs, often first trying hydroxychloroquine, followed by gold salts or methotrexate if needed. Use of second-line drugs must be medically monitored.

other than ASA and—if possible—local steroid injections to control inflammation. (ASA is not advisable, as it affects the manner in which the kidneys handle uric acid and may lead to kidney stones.) Depending on the frequency of attacks, and if blood uric acid levels stay high, patients may be put on a lifetime regimen of *allopurinol*, a uric-acid-synthesis inhibitor. For those allergic to allopurinol, an alternative (but less effective) medication is *sulfinpyrazone*.

Pseudogout involves excess calcium pyrophosphate crystals in the joints. The attacks come on suddenly, with acute pain and inflammation lasting from days to weeks—often indistinguishable from gout. The acute form most commonly affects the knees, while chronic forms attack several joints, such as wrists and knees. Those who develop pseudogout are generally 65 or over, equal numbers of men and women being affected. There is a possible link between pseudogout crystals and diseases such as hyperparathyroidism and diabetes. People with pseudogout often have gouty associates—high blood pressure, kidney stones, arteriosclerosis (artery hardening) and hyperlipidemia (high blood fats). Pseudogout is best treated with NSAIDs, if possible, or local steroid injections.

- *Seronegative arthritis* (in which the blood test for rheumatoid factor is negative) is a related group of rheumatic disorders characterized by asymmetric (one-sided) arthritis, often in the lower limbs (possibly including the shin bone), perhaps with accompanying inflammation of the spine, eyes, genitourinary tract and bowel (colitis and Crohn's disease). The causes of this arthritis-like condition aren't known, but there may be an inherited susceptibility or an abnormal immune response directed at the body's own organs. Treatment is aggressive anti-inflammatory therapy with NSAIDs and disease-modifying agents.

- *Ankylosing spondylitis*, which affects 1 in 400 persons, attacks the spinal joints, causing inflammation and eventual stiffening as bony overgrowths fuse the vertebrae. Until recently, scientists believed the disorder affected only men; however it is now clear that both sexes can suffer from it, although it is often less severe in women. Its first symptoms are a dull ache in the buttocks, possibly extending down to the knees, and/or mid-spine. It strikes mainly young people aged 18 to 30. The pain can be noticed when turning over in bed, and may waken sufferers, who often dismiss it as stiffness. Later symptoms include morning stiffness in the mid and lower back, which is often relieved by hot showers and activity. But eventually the pain can move all the way up the spine, affecting the chest and neck, as well as larger joints such as hips and shoulders.

SOME ARTHRITIS REMEDIES

- **Acetaminophen (e.g., Tylenol).**
- **Anti-inflammatory medications, which include ASA (e.g., Aspirin) and other nonsteroidal anti-inflammatories (NSAIDs). Recent studies indicate that although the medication may stop further joint degeneration, half of all rheumatoid arthritis sufferers don't take their medications as prescribed. Yet long-term pain relief depends on keeping medications at the correct concentration.**
- **Diet. Despite some people's faith in its healing properties, diet doesn't usually alleviate or cure arthritis, but well-balanced nutrition will help keep the body at its strongest. Research shows no link between dietary changes and the progress of arthritis, except for gout, where eliminating foods such as liver, kidneys and other organ meats (which produce uric acid) may help to forestall attacks.**
- **Methotrexate, a mild immunosuppressant and anticancer drug, increasingly tried early in arthritis therapy; its effect is seen within six to eight weeks of treatment. It is usually well tolerated and an effective antiarthritic drug, although it can cause stomach upsets, abdominal cramps and coughing when first taken. Its use must be carefully monitored to avoid liver problems.**
- **Solozopyrine, a recent addition to the therapeutic arsenal—like chloroquine, best used early in the disease to prevent or reduce joint deformity.**
- **Gold salts, an old standby for arthritis, given by injection or as tablets are potent drugs used to combat rheumatoid arthritis. How and why they work is unclear. They somehow reduce the progress of the disease, but efficacy varies from person to person and it can take months before benefits are noticed. Side effects of gold salts include a skin rash, nausea and (rarely) anemia.**
- **Chloroquine and hydroxychloroquine (antimalarial drugs), which may alleviate rheumatoid arthritis but must be taken for at least 2 months before any improvement appears. Serious side effects are rare, but may include skin and bone-marrow problems.**
- **Disease-modifying anti-rheumatic drugs (DMARDs) such as low-dose corticosteroids (Prednisone) and immunomodulators (such as Imuran, cyclosporine) given to arthritics who fail to respond to other treatments or have serious complications. These drugs weaken the body's natural defenses, leaving it open to infection. Regular blood tests are required to ensure that bone-marrow cells are not damaged.**
- **Sulfasalazine, a drug long used for bowel disease, may also alleviate rheumatoid arthritis, and gout, with few adverse effects, although some patients are allergic to it.**

Treatment for ankylosing spondylitis is mainly exercise and postural training. NSAIDs are given to reduce inflammation and help improve exercise therapy. Surgery is recommended only when hips or knees are badly damaged.

Caution is required with NSAIDs

The need for care in those taking NSAIDs cannot be overstated. These anti-inflammatory medications can have serious side effects such as dizziness, drowsiness, tinnitus (ringing in the ears), kidney problems and *in particular* gastrointestinal bleeding, which may damage the stomach lining and cause serious peptic (stomach) ulcers, which can lead to fatal bleeding. Some may tolerate other NSAIDs better than ASA (e.g., Aspirin), but all of them may cause problems. NSAIDs are particularly dangerous in the elderly and people with impaired liver and/or kidney function, or in those with previous or current stomach ulcers. (See also "Peptic ulcers" later in this chapter.) Some NSAIDs are now marketed in combination with agents that protect against peptic ulcers—such as *misoprostol* (Cytotec), *ranitidine* (Zantac) or *omeprazole* (Losec). All people taking NSAIDs need careful medical supervision. Protection by antacid medication and agents that coat the stomach is recommended for high-risk patients. New anti-inflammatory medications called COX-2 Inhibitors, such as mobicox or Celebrex, have been touted as more effective and possibly safer in high-risk patients, although their safety and optimal dosages are now under intensive investigation. They are convenient medications as their effects tend to last all day. However, *rofecoxib* (Vioxx) has recently been taken off the market in some countries due to increased rates of heart problems among people taking this medication, and there are similar and escalating safety concerns about heart problems developing from use of Celebrex (especially long term, for more than 3 or 4 years), which are also currently being investigated.

For more information about arthritis, contact the Arthritis Society of Canada, 920 Yonge St., Suite 420, Toronto, Ont. M4W 3J7, (416) 967-1414. (www.arthritis.ca).

ASTHMA

Asthma, which means "gasping for breath," is an obstructive lung disease characterized by shortness of breath, wheeze and cough, in which inflammatory changes block the lung's breathing tubes or airways, hindering the movement of air in and out. The *bronchi* (lung's airways) become inflamed and overly sensitive or "twitchy," with diminished air flow. The airways may also hyperreact and contract—developing *bronchospasm*—which narrows them further, making it hard to exhale. The telltale asthmatic wheeze occurs as air is forced out through clogged airways; but not everyone with asthma wheezes. The only clue may be a persistent cough, especially at night and first thing in the morning.

Asthma affects about 5 to 10 percent of North Americans, causing about 5,000 deaths annually in Canada, and 5,000 in the U.S. Despite the commonly held misconception that children outgrow asthma, it often recurs in adulthood. There is great concern about this disorder because, as one expert from the International Asthma Council puts it, "Asthma is one of the few treatable diseases with a climbing death rate, especially among children and young adults." Asthma specialists blame the heavy toll partly on a failure to get the message out and not teaching asthmatics about their disorder, its potential severity and how to avoid its dangers.

Several processes contribute to the breathing difficulty

- The airway's mucosal lining swells in response to some trigger or irritant, releasing potent mediators (such as histamine and leukotrienes).
- Excess eosinophils (white blood cells) accumulate in the airways.
- Bronchospasm (contraction) of the muscles encircling the bronchi narrows their lumen (passageway).
- Excess mucus is produced by irritated bronchial tissue.
- Damaged cells shed from the inflamed tissues increase the blockage.

Allergies may set off attacks

Asthma may be triggered by intrinsic (internal) factors, such as an inherited predisposition to

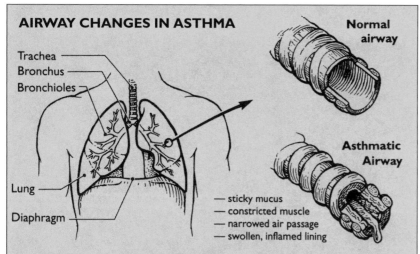

AIRWAY CHANGES IN ASTHMA

Normal airway

Trachea
Bronchus
Bronchioles

Asthmatic Airway

Lung

Diaphragm

— sticky mucus
— constricted muscle
— narrowed air passage
— swollen, inflamed lining

Bronchial (airway) narrowing in asthma follows a complex chain of events that may occur spontaneously or be provoked by certain triggers. It involves contraction of the muscles encircling the air passages, inflammation and thickening of the airway linings (walls) and increased mucus secretion. With obstructed breathing tubes, asthmatics find it hard to move air in and out of their lungs, which makes them feel short of breath. Breathing through clogged airways leads to the characteristic wheezing sound sometimes made by asthmatics on exhaling. Think of your lungs as essential filters that occasionally go overboard and start overreacting to substances in the air (smoke, viruses, mold, etc.), causing the lungs to inflame, which in turn causes mucus and swelling.

twitchy breathing tubes, or by external (environmental) factors, such as indoor air pollutants, pollens, animal fur, tobacco smoke, food or food additives, even exercise or cold air. In those prone to asthma, a viral infection such as a cold, influenza or bronchitis often sets off an attack. An estimated 40 to 60 percent of people with asthma are allergic to dust mites, pollens, molds

(fungi), animal dander or other substances. But the rest have no known allergies, and asthma often has no identifiable trigger.

Asthma best managed by patient–doctor partnerships

Treatment usually works best when physician and asthmatic together create an action plan to manage the disease and prevent severe attacks. Pharmacotherapy with a battery of asthma medications allows good control for most asthmatics. Anti-asthma drugs are chiefly inhaled forms that come in a variety of convenient pocket-sized puffers. Inhaled drugs can be taken at lower doses than pills or syrups, as they are absorbed directly into the lungs. New inhaler systems such as spacers and breath-activated "powder puffers" make asthma drugs easier to use. But people must learn how to use their puffers correctly, and choose the type that best suits them.

To avoid severe attacks, it's essential to take medications as prescribed. If asthma interferes with usual activities or keeps sufferers awake at night, the treatment is inadequate and needs to be reviewed. Those whose asthma remains troublesome despite adherence to doctor's orders should request a second opinion from a respirologist or other specialist, or a local asthma center or clinic. Simply tossing back more pills or taking more inhaler puffs without medical advice is *not* a sensible way to handle this disease.

Asthma must be treated as an inflammatory condition

While asthma was formerly viewed as a disorder of airway narrowing—calling for bronchodilator or airway-widening drugs—it's now regarded as an inflammatory condition requiring anti-inflammatories. "Inflammation is the underlying problem in asthma," explains one respirologist. "The airway narrowing and breathing difficulties are the end result. If the inflammation is left untreated, the bronchi become still more hyperreactive [twitchy], increasing the constriction, leading to a possibly life-endangering attack."

Anti-inflammatory agents (inhaled corticosteroids) are now considered first-line agents for

WAYS TO IMPROVE ASTHMA CONTROL

- **Heed warning signs of increasing severity (e.g., interrupted sleep, increasing cough or need for more bronchodilator puffs).**
- **Avoid overreliance on bronchodilators.**
- **Know when to call the physician and what to do if a physician is unavailable (e.g., take steroid pills or go to the nearest emergency); never delay seeking**

medical help.
- **As changing airflow rates reveal increasing severity, invest in a cheap, portable, home-measuring flow meter.**
- **On holidays, know where to go for help if needed.**
- **Watch for nocturnal asthma (increasing nighttime or early morning symptoms), which signal worsening asthma. Nocturnal asthma is**

a signal to get in touch with your physician.
- **Remember that viral respiratory infections increase the risk of serious asthma attacks—take precautions.**
- **Get an annual flu shot—recommended for all asthmatic adults not allergic to eggs.**
- **Have regular follow-up medical visits.**

controlling asthma, with bronchodilators (air-way-wideners) used as backup, if and when needed, for the shortest time possible, at the lowest possible dose. Bronchodilators swiftly widen narrowed airways but do nothing to reduce the lung inflammation that leaves people open to fresh attacks. "Bronchodilators are best reserved for blunting flares," notes one specialist, "not for regular use. Asthmatics who need bronchodilating drugs more than twice (or a maximum of 4 times) a day should seek further medical advice."

Many asthmatics need reassurance about the safety of inhaled corticosteroids, and experts stress that these inhaled drugs act locally on the airway tubes and little is absorbed into the bloodstream. In low to moderate doses, inhaled corticosteroids cause few side effects. With higher doses, side effects may increase, but using nonsteroidal agents (such as cromolyn or nedocromil) at the same time lessens side effects. (To reduce possible effects on the eyes, they can be closed while using the puffers.)

Learning to use the new inhaler devices

The best way to deliver asthma drugs is by inhalation through the mouth because it puts the drugs directly into the lungs, achieving an effect similar to oral medications at far lower doses. There is now a wide range of inhalers to choose from, including *metered-dose inhalers* (MDIs)—some of which are pressurized (pMDIs) or deliver the drug as a dry powder. MDIs require coordinating each puff of medication with breathing in, and need time to recharge between puffs. The addition of spacers (aerosol-holding chambers) to MDIs improves drug delivery to the lungs and makes the devices easier to use. Trial and error can show which inhaler works best for each asthmatic. (Ask your physician or a pharmacist for a lesson.)

Dry powder inhalers use dry-powder aerosols, requiring just a small click to release the drug before it's inhaled. The amount can be accurately controlled, and the inhalers are easy to use and carry. The Rotahaler and Diskhaler deliver *salbutamol* (Ventolin) or *beclomethasone* (Beclovent); the Spinhaler is used for *cromolyn* (Intal), and the Turbuhaler for *terbutaline* (Bricanyl) or *budesonide* (Pulmicort). One disad-

vantage is that during a bad attack it can be hard to suck enough powdered drug into the lungs.

Nebulizers deliver a fine mist of drug droplets inhaled through a mask. They are useful for those unable to manipulate an MDI, such as young children and the elderly, but are bulky to carry and require a power source to activate them.

Home measurement of air-flow rates aids self-management

Using a peak-flow meter—a small, easy-to-use portable device to measure *peak expiratory flow rates* (PEFR) helps to determine how well air is expelled from the lungs. It assesses lung blockage independently of the actual symptoms—which may not portray the worsening situation—so asthmatics know better when to increase medication. If airway blockage worsens, flow rates fall below expected levels, even though the symptoms may not have noticeably worsened. Trials have shown that the objective measurement of breathing ability with a peak-flow meter is more accurate than subjective measurement.

Individual action plan helps achieve control

Individually tailored to the person's symptoms by a physician and the asthmatic, and usually simple and short enough to fit on a small index card, an action plan precisely defines the doses and types of medications to use, when to step up the frequency or dose, when to add or change medications and when to call the doctor or go to an emergency unit.

OVERUSE OF BRONCHODILATORS CAN SPELL TROUBLE

Ironically, the easy availability of bronchodilating drugs may be dangerous because they give a sense that all is well, even in the face of relentlessly progressing lung blockage. Overreliance on bronchodilators may even worsen asthma, because they open up the airways and allow in more irritating triggers. Even though the troubled breathing and shortness of breath may subside within minutes of taking a bronchodilator puff, the airway inflammation remains—leaving the risk of a severe attack. Indeed, bronchodilators may mask worsening lung inflammation, so that people are unaware of its severity—or deny it—waiting too long before seeking medical aid, finding themselves in a crisis. If more bronchodilator puffs are needed than usual, it's time to seek medical advice.

OXYGEN SHORTAGE IS THE MAIN DANGER

The asthmatic inflammation and airway narrowing vary, but the net effect is a diminished oxygen supply for the body. An accumulation of stale, unoxygenated air in the lungs means that the lungs cannot effectively push out stale air with its carbon dioxide load. This prevents new, oxygen-rich air from entering, leading to oxygen shortage and possible *acidosis* (carbon dioxide buildup in the blood).

A FRESH LOOK AT ANTI-ASTHMA MEDICATIONS

Anti-inflammatory agents

These medications reduce airway inflammation and decrease mucus production but take time to work—perhaps weeks—before their effects peak. Corticosteroids come as low- and high-concentration products, as inhalers or tablets. More and more commonly t corticosteroid medications are being used for individuals with longer-lasting coughs, some of whom might have a mild form of asthma.

Steroidal anti-inflammatory drugs

• Inhaled corticosteroids include *beclomethasone* (Beclovent, Becloforte), *budesonide* (Pulmicort) and *fluticasone* (Flovent), *flunisolide* (Bronalide), among others. They are the mainstay of asthma therapy. People may start out on 8 to 12 puffs a day to bring their asthma under control, later tapering to 2 to 4 puffs daily following an attack. Side effects from inhaled corticosteroids are minor at usual doses and may include *dysphonia* (voice hoarseness) and perhaps a mild fungal (yeast) mouth infection (thrush or candidiasis), preventable by inhaling before a meal, using a spacer device, rinsing the mouth with water or gargling after inhaling the medication. Some newer puffers combine long-acting beta agonists with corticosteroids (such as Adavir, which combines Salmeterol + Fluticasone). They are chiefly used for preventive purposes as they are not effective in acute situations nor for asthma flare-ups. Consult a physician if symptoms worsen or change.

• *Oral steroids* (such as *prednisone, prednisolone*) are required for severe asthma and emergency situations. Asthmatics at risk of severe episodes often keep steroid tablets on hand as part of their action plan. The tablets are usually taken at breakfast time to mimic the body's own natural rhythm of corticosteroid release.

Nonsteroidal anti-inflammatories

• *Cromoglycate* or *cromolyn* (Intal, Nedcrom), one of the safest anti-asthma drugs, comes as a metered-dose inhaler or in powder form, and is used as a preventive for regular control rather than for swift relief. It's especially useful in children with mild asthma (given from a nebulizer) and for exercise-related asthma (before a workout).

• *Inhaled nedocromil sodium* (Tilade), more powerful than cromolyn; effectively reduces an asthmatic cough, although not as well as the new high-dose steroids. It doesn't work in all asthmatics.

• *Oral ketotifen* (Zaditen) is a mild, user-friendly anti-inflammatory, often more useful in children than in adults.

Bronchodilator (quick-fix) medications

Bronchodilators rapidly open up the airways by relaxing the smooth muscles encircling them, giving relief within minutes. Short-acting forms are used mainly as rescue medications to ease troubled breathing, taken alongside regular anti-inflammatories. Longer-acting forms may be used for more severe episodes as "add-on" drugs to be taken as well as anti-inflammatories.

Beta-2 agonists

• *Short-acting inhaled beta-2 agonists*, such as *salbutamol* (Ventolin), *terbutaline* (Bricanyl), *fenoterol* (Berotec) and *procaterol* (Pro-Air), relieve breathing within minutes.

• *Lang-acting beta-2 agonist* include *salmeterol* (Serevent) and *formoterol* (Oxeze), with bronchodilating effects that last up to 12 hours. They are used as add-on drugs, alongside anti-inflammatories for hard-to-control cases. They should *not* replace fast-acting forms for acute relief of symptoms as they take time to work and require careful monitoring.

NB: *Side effects* include tremors and a rapid or irregular pulse.

Anti-cholinergic bronchodilators

• *Ipratropium bromide* and *oxytropium* are inhaled drugs that are not recommended as first-line asthma drugs, but are a suitable alternate for people who are unable to take or tolerate short-acting beta-agonists. They have a slower onset but their bronchodilator effect lasts longer so they are useful as an adjunct to the short-acting bronchodilators These medications may also be more beneficial in people with emphysema or COPD and for elderly patients. Side effects are rare but may include mouth dryness and vision blurring.

Xanthine (caffeine-like) compounds

• *Theophylline* and *aminophylline bronchodilators* (e.g., Uniphyl, Theolair, Theo-Dur), taken as pills or syrups, are second-line airway dilators, now used less often. Theophylline interacts with some drugs and various illnesses that distort its effects—for instance, viral infections, heart and liver diseases, antibiotics and ulcer medications (e.g., *cimetidine*). These interactions, as well as side effects (e.g., nausea, diarrhea, headache, insomnia, tremors), are a frequent problem, and theophylline use must be carefully monitored.

Mediator-blockers (e.g., leukotriene-blockers)

These drugs antagonize the mediator chemicals that cause inflammatory changes They are different from most other asthma medications in that they are taken as tablets. Although promising, the potential of medications such as zafirlukast (Accolate) and montelukast (Singulair) for modifying the natural course of the disease and their long-term toxicity and safety have yet to be confirmed. Their current role is as an adjunct treatment along with moderate to high doses of inhaled corticosteroids to control more persistent asthma symptoms. When taken regularly, they reduce exercise-induced bronchospasm and are also useful in patients with aspirin intolerant asthma. Although generally not recommended as first-line therapy, leukotriene blockers are considered drugs of choice in people who are unable or unwilling to take or tolerate inhaled steroids. Montelukast may be used in children over age 6, while zafirlukast should not be used in anyone under 12 years old.

The action plan aims to help people lead a normal life with no (or minimal) wheezing, coughing and shortness of breath and no nighttime flare-ups, with only occasional use of bronchodilators.

Mild deterioration (perhaps a slight increase in breathlessness or sleep disturbed by coughing) may call for a higher dose of inhaled anti-inflammatory. If symptoms don't abate in a day or two, the next step may be to add another medication—perhaps a long-acting bronchodilator or a brief course of oral corticosteroids. Telling caregivers about worsening symptoms and communicating worries are crucial to good management.

Risk factors for potentially severe attacks

- More than two previous emergency-room visits for an attack;
- having been admitted to hospital for a severe attack;
- a near-fatal episode;
- steroid-dependent asthma (requiring oral steroids);
- recent withdrawal of oral steroids;
- noncompliance with prescribed therapy;
- failure of physician and asthmatic to recognize a severe attack.

Why the baffling rise in asthma severity and deaths?

Not only are more young people being diagnosed with asthma, but there are more emergency-room visits and deaths from this disease—with mortality rates almost doubled in the past 14 years in many industrialized countries. Yet those who die from asthma often had prior warning—previous life-threatening episodes, recent hospitalization for a severe attack or poorly controlled symptoms.

Exactly why more people are dying of asthma remains a mystery. One possible reason is that the condition is more accurately and more frequently diagnosed, and more often cited as the cause of death. Urban air pollution—increasing levels of ozone, sulfur dioxide, free radicals and other pollutants—is another suspected cause. Others are the increase in allergies, modern sealed buildings that expose people to high levels of indoor

---

SEEK IMMEDIATE EMERGENCY HELP IF YOU:

- **have symptoms not relieved by usual medication;**
- **need bronchodilators more than 6 times in 24 hours;**
- **can't carry on usual** **daytime activities because of asthma;**
- **are kept awake or wakened by symptoms for several consecutive nights;**
- **notice worsening air-** **flow readings (on home flow meter);**
- **can't say a complete sentence without gasping for air.**

---

pollutants and aeroallergens such as dust mites.

One British expert lists the "two absolute requirements for treating emergency asthma as: measuring the extent of air-flow diminution (to check the extent of lung blockage) and immediate use of high-dose corticosteroids." Guidelines for emergency management of asthma stress the need to measure air-flow rates because the wheezing and shortness of breath may not accurately portray the severity of an attack. Hospital stays range from hours to days, and treatment may include high doses of airway dilators (given through a mask), supplemental oxygen and oral or injected corticosteroids. "Any asthmatic sick enough to need emergency department treatment," states the specialist, "needs a course of oral steroids."

For more information, contact your local branch of the Canadian Lung Association; the Allergy, Asthma and Immunology Society of Ontario, (416) 633-2215; or the Allergy Asthma Information Association (AAIA), (905) 712-2242.

ATHLETE'S FOOT

With its scaling, spongy, sometimes itchy skin between the toes, athlete's foot—*dermatophytosis* of the foot or *tinea pedis* ("foot fungus")—is the most common fungal skin infection, affecting 1 in 10 North Americans at any one time, more men than women, adults more than children. In about half of those plagued by athlete's foot, the condition recurs time and again because the hardy fungal spores survive in skin cracks between the toes. Modern medications can clear up most cases, and Mother was certainly right in telling children to dry well between the toes.

The fungi that infect human feet live on the skin protein, keratin. They flourish in tropical climates and are relatively recent imports to Europe and North America, brought in by travelers and by soldiers returning from duty abroad. Athlete's foot has now become a world-wide problem—aggravated by the fashion for tight (non-breathing) running shoes.

Athlete's foot usually occurs between the fourth and fifth or third and fourth toes, producing white, soggy toe webs and scaling, fissured grooves (cracks), sometimes intensely itchy. The infection can spread to the soles of the feet, and it's aggravated by foot sweatiness and tight socks or shoes that keep in moisture. Bacterial invasion of the area may worsen the fungal infection, making it into a macerated, oozy, burning, malodorous condition.

Various types of athlete's foot

- *Moccasin-type athlete's foot* on the sole is generally a non-itchy, non-inflamed but very troublesome form that's hard to eradicate. The entire sole, possibly including the heel, becomes dry and flaky with loose, white scales in a moccasin-like pattern. The toenails may also be involved and it can be notoriously difficult to eradicate athlete's foot from them. But recently developed antifungals such as *ketaconazole* (Sporonox) and Lamisil can help. This type of fungus may also affect one hand—but curiously not both.
- *Vesicular (blistered) athlete's foot* is thought to be an allergic reaction to fungal organisms causing it (usually *T. mentagrophytes*)—a reaction somewhat like contact dermatitis. People with vesicular athlete's foot suffer from sore, fluid-filled blisters not only between the toes but also on the arch, instep and sides of the foot.

- *Ulcerative tinea pedis* tends to occur when there is a secondary bacterial infection on top of the fungal foot invasion, producing a severe condition with painful, purulent ulcers between the toes that can be very disabling and may take a long time to clear up.

Diagnosis: how to tell if you've got athlete's foot

The telltale signs of athlete's foot are scaling between the toe webs or on the soles, possibly some itching, perhaps a strong foot odor, and (if there are fissures), a painful stinging, burning sensation. Tinea pedis most often starts between the little and fourth toes; if it invades a toenail, the nail may become thick and discolored. In diagnosing athlete's foot, physicians must exclude other skin conditions such as eczema, psoriasis and ringworm, which produce similar skin scaling. The condition must also be distinguished from contact dermatitis which could be an allergic reaction to shoe materials.

Treatment of athlete's foot

Good hygiene, especially keeping the feet as cool and dry as possible—*drying well between the toes*—is a must, with special creams for troublesome areas. Uncomplicated cases often respond well to a hydrocortisone cream plus an antifungal. Many cases clear with a course of over-the-counter antifungal products, or with prescription creams such as *clotrimazole* or *terbinafine*. If topical medications don't work, an oral antifungal such as *terbinafine oral* or *itraconazole* may be suggested.

Commonly used antifungals include *miconazole, nystatin, clioquinol, tolnaftate, clotrimazole* and *terbinafine*. Some modern creams and pills used to treat athlete's foot contain both antifungals and antibacterials. Paradoxically, use of certain soaps—for example, germicidal soaps such as pHisoHex, Dial and Safeguard—may worsen rather than relieve the condition.

A foot problem that doesn't clear may not be a fungal or bacterial infection but some other skin disorder. Many people who immediately self-treat a foot rash with antifungal drugs may not only be in for useless therapy but also waste money, unless what they're treating is really a fungal infection. It is best to seek medical advice

HOW ATHLETE'S FOOT SPREADS

The organisms that cause athlete's foot can be transmitted from person to person by walking barefoot in locker rooms, fitness clubs, prisons, army barracks, swimming pools, on hotel rugs and bathroom mats, and in other moist places where many potentially infected feet shed their fungus-laden scales. However, it takes more than casual exposure to contract athlete's foot. Damp sweaty skin covered by nonporous footwear favors fungal growth. Ill-fitting footwear that causes sores or blisters increases susceptibility. A slight cut, blister or trauma to the foot helps the organisms gain access. People with diabetes mellitus and the immune-compromised are especially prone to athlete's foot.

from a family physician or dermatologist before self-medicating. Athlete's foot that's soggy, oozing, inflamed and foul-smelling requires prompt medical attention. If the foot is inflamed, or if a bacterial infection is identified, the inflammation and infection must be cleared before starting on antifungals. If the toenail is affected, consult a physician or podiatrist.

Common-sense tips for treating athlete's foot

- *Keep the feet clean, dry* and as cool as possible.
- *Take off the shoes* whenever possible to "air out" the feet.
- *Wear open footwear* or sandals whenever possible.
- *Bathe feet daily* with soap and water.
- *Dry really well* between the toes—maybe with a hairdryer!
- *Apply an absorbent powder* such as talcum powder, aluminum chloride powder or Burow's solution (aluminum acetate).
- *Wear absorbent socks* (e.g., made from cotton) and change socks daily or more often.
- *Avoid tight occlusive footwear*—sweaty feet provide an ideal microclimate for fungi.
- *To prevent relapses*, keep feet dry, change socks often, perhaps try ongoing antifungal creams. For example, following several weeks of local medication that has cleared the initial infection, tolnaftate cream may be applied once a week or so to prevent the fungus from taking hold again.

ATTENTION-DEFICIT HYPERACTIVITY DISORDER

Previously called hyperactivity, minimal brain dysfunction, hyperkinesis or attention-deficit disorder, but now named attention-deficit hyperactivity disorder (ADHD), this childhood problem is increasingly recognized. It usually shows up before age 7, typified by restlessness, inattention and impulsive behavior bad enough to undermine school and family relationships. Between 3 to 7 percent of children in North America are diagnosed as having attention-deficit hyperactivity disorder (and boys are more often affected than girls). The actual number of affected girls is probably higher than is generally reported because fewer girls than

boys with ADHD have oppositional or conduct disorders so that fewer are brought to medical attention. Even when girls are seen by physicians, the diagnosis of ADHD may be missed because it is often overshadowed by other concurrent conditions such as anxiety disorders, mood disorders or substance abuse. A family history of ADHD is common; 30 percent of first-degree relatives of children with ADHD

CAUSES ELUSIVE: BORN TO BE HYPERACTIVE?

The cause of ADHD is unknown, but since it runs in families, a predisposition may be inherited. One in four children diagnosed with ADHD has a biological parent who is similarly affected, and researchers believe genetic factors play a part in at least one-third of ADHD cases. Scientists also theorize that parts of the brain are underaroused in **ADHD**, perhaps owing to an imbalance in neurotransmitters (the brain's chemical messengers), especially an imbalance in *dopamine* and *norepinephrine*. New imaging studies with **PET** (Positron Emission Tomography) scans show that specific parts of the brain may be affected, particularly prefrontal regions, the corpus callosum and caudate nucleus. Others blame poor family dynamics or abuse as possible causes, but while stress, abuse, poor parenting and neglect may worsen the condition, family dysfunction is not considered the root cause.

MULTIMODAL THERAPY MAY INCLUDE:

- *Parent training* to learn how to deal in the best possible manner with the problem—especially ways to avoid exacerbating situations. To improve management, parents might consider joining one of the many groups available, and getting some of the excellent literature on the market—both for their own use and that of the child's teachers.
- *Behavior modification* and positive reinforcement rather than punishment—giving the child rewards for good behavior and any tasks completed, however small.
- *Adjusting school or classroom environment* in ways that help the child succeed—individualizing it to make assignments manageable, so they can be completed and provide a sense of achievement.
- *Social skills training*—to help curb aggressive behavior.
- *Individual counseling*—which may help alleviate the sense of failure and boost self-esteem.
- *Psychostimulant medications.* About 70 to 80 percent of children with ADHD benefit from stimulant drugs, but medication should be part of a total treatment plan, *not* a replacement for other therapies.
- *Support groups*, provided by some specialty clinics and organizations such as Children and Adults with Attention-Deficit Disorder (CHADD), can be invaluable.

KEY DRUGS USED TO TREAT ADHD

• *Methylphenidate* (Ritalin), the most commonly prescribed stimulant for ADHD, peaks 1 to 2 hours after being taken, its effects lasting about 4 hours It's generally taken 3 times a day, 7 days a week—in order to improve home as well as school performance and socializing. Although the afternoon dose eases home relationships, it may exacerbate side effects such as poor appetite and insomnia. (One slow-release capsule taken in the morning may last the day.) A few develop drug tolerance and need increasing doses of Ritalin to suppress symptoms, but large amounts can have some growth-retarding effect, requiring a drug change. It must be used with great caution in anyone with tics (such as Tourette's syndrome) or in very anxious children.

Side effects of Ritalin can be troublesome. They include headaches, insomnia, reduced appetite, weight loss, occasional tics (grimaces, nail biting), a zombie-like stare, obsessive overfocusing (becoming overengrossed) and emotional constriction (for instance, shown in drawings where everything is minuscule or shoved tightly into a corner). The drug is fast-acting and leaves the body quickly, producing a "wearing off" effect 4 to 6 hours after the drug is taken. Omitting the 4 p.m. dose might overcome sleep problems, but at the cost of a disrupted home life.

Some children object to the roller-coaster feeling while on the drug, and want to feel normal again, leading to a drop-off in drug-taking. Some hate the idea of having their behavior controlled, and some parents oppose the idea of mind-altering drugs for their kids. If giving a noon dose at school is difficult, slow release formulations of *methylphenidate* (Concerta, Metadate CD, Ritalin LA) or mixed *methylphenidate/D-amphetimine* (Adderal) can be administered instead. (Note: as of 2005, Health Canada has suspended use of Adderral owing to safety concerns.) *Dextroamphetamine* (Dexedrine, Dextrostat) is as effective as *methylphenidate*. Some children respond only to *methylphenidate,* and others only to *dextroamphetamine.* Treatment with stimulants has been shown not only to offset the abnormal behaviors of ADHD, but also to improve self-esteem and cognitive, social and family function, supporting the importance of treating children or adults with ADHD beyond school or work hours to include evenings, weekends and vacations. Evidence does not support the notion that children will abuse their medications, given proper diagnosis and monitoring. However, the medications come at a cost as the most common side effects of stimulant medications are sleep disturbances and decreased appetite leading to insomnia and poor weight gain or weight loss.

Evidence suggests that at least 30 percent of individuals with ADHD will not respond to stimulant medication. Other drugs that have been used for the treatment of ADHD are: *pemoline* (Cylert), *tricyclic antidepressants* (Tofranil, Norpramin), *clonidine* (Catapres), and *guanfacine* (Tenex). *Pemoline* can cause toxic hepatitis, and deaths have been reported from the use of *tricyclic antidepressants, clonidine* and *guanfacine* in children. *Bupropion* (Wellbutrin) has a safer side-effect profile, and has been used in adults, but its efficacy in children is not as well-documented.

---

also have the condition. The increased risk for siblings of a child diagnosed with ADHD is 5-fold for boys and 3-fold for girls. The condition is managed by education, changing family dynamics and the use of stimulant drugs such as Ritalin.

The hallmarks of ADHD are excessive restlessness, inattention and impulsivity. The nonstop activity disrupts family, school and social relationships and may be disruptive enough to put children with ADHD academically behind their peers. One specialist at Toronto's Hospital for Sick Children explains that "the problem is pervasive and severe enough to qualify as ADHD in about 1 percent of all children, in all societies and all countries." Not all children "outgrow" ADHD; about half continue to experience symptoms into adulthood. Recognizing the disorder may be particularly difficult in adults if it was not identified in childhood. Presenting problems in adults usually involve difficulties at work or with studies, inattention or hyperactivity which often manifests itself as "restlessness," particularly with increasing age. The diagnostic criteria for adult ADHD require that the symptoms start by age 7 and are persistently present thereafter.

Are too many being tagged with ADHD?

Although its causes remain unclear, more and more children are being diagnosed with ADHD. In the U.S., 5 to 9 percent of schoolchildren have been diagnosed with ADHD and are taking stimulant drugs such as *methylphenidate* (Ritalin). As many as half a million Canadian children are also on medication to dampen their impulsive behavior. (By contrast, in the U.K., where diagnostic criteria are stricter, only 0.3 percent are said to be hyperactive or suffering from ADHD.)

There are rising concerns about the seeming ease with which families, teachers and medical caregivers label children—especially energetic, high-spirited boys—as hyperactive, relying on drugs to calm them down. Critics question the tendency to regard any unusually rambunctious, fidgety or restless child as hyperactive and in need of special education or attention-focusing medication.

Spotting the telltale signs

Children with ADHD generally have boundless energy, ceaselessly fidget or tap their fingers and seem unable to finish any game or task—always moving on to something else. They are easily distracted, don't seem to pay attention and cannot play peacefully for long with siblings or interact sociably with schoolmates. They may become excessively angry on slight provocation. Unable to control their impulses, or wait their turn, these children often frustrate playmates who get fed up and shun them. The social isolation creates low self-esteem and a deep sense of failure.

One specialist explains that a large part of the difficulty is "disinhibition" or the inability of children with ADHD to put on the brakes. For example, most 5-year-olds swear, but not in front of the school principal, whereas children with ADHD can't stop themselves in the presence of authority. ADHD shows itself somewhat differently in girls than boys: girls may be less obviously disruptive, especially at home, and less likely to be identified with ADHD at a young age.

Typically, children with ADHD have trouble learning to read and write at the usual age; some are dyslexic and some have more deep-seated learning disabilities. Symptoms are often first pointed out by schoolteachers, usually because of academic failing rather than just the behavior problems.

The triad that defines ADHD

To qualify as ADHD, three behavior patterns must be pervasive and persistent, present for 6 or more months—before age 7—cause observable impairment and occur in more than one setting (e.g., both at school and at home). About 1 to 2 percent of children have all 3 behaviors, while in others the chief sign of ADHD may be inattention or impulsivity. The three key symptoms are:

- *inattention*—easy distractibility and an inability to focus for long on any game, task or chore;
- *restlessness* (*hyperactivity*)—endless fidgeting, being always "on the go," unable to sit still;
- *impulsiveness*—inability to stop the impulse to interrupt, be aggressive or rush on to new things.

Before ADHD is identified, a thorough medical workup is needed to find out whether it is the primary problem or tied to a child's learning disability, depression, an anxiety or conduct disorder. Symptoms of ADHD often accompany or are part of syndromes such as conduct disorders, Tourette's (tic) syndrome and autism.

Confirming diagnosis can be tricky

Since ADHD can be mistaken for other disorders, the condition is diagnosed by careful history taking, gathering information from parents and teachers and building a detailed picture of home and family dynamics. A complete medical and psychological exam rules out neurological or psychiatric problems (such as schizophrenia), those resulting from hearing problems and those due to dysfunctional family life.

Experts caution that it is critical "to interview the child alone, without the parents, to pick up on abuse or other causative factors." The condition must also be differentiated from lookalike syndromes such as depression, anxiety, learning disabilities, mental retardation and oppositional (rebellion/defiance) or conduct disorders. For example, depressed children often exhibit some symptoms of ADHD (e.g., restlessness), although it's not the primary problem.

Clinicians must also distinguish between the impulsive behavior of ADHD and frank rebellion, malice or aggression. Parents may be asked about discipline, the child's response to reprimands and whether he (it's usually a boy) gets into trouble because he acts without thinking, or because he plans to misbehave or wants to oppose. Does the child refuse to do what's asked, or just seem unable to do so?

ADULTS WITH ADHD CAN ALSO BENEFIT FROM TREATMENT

Formerly, children with ADHD were thought to outgrow the problem—usually around puberty. However, it's now clear that the function-impairing symptoms can and do persist into adult life, in at least one-third of cases. The telltale signs may be difficulty concentrating, trouble being organized and sometimes also social and emotional problems (such as mood and anxiety disorders). Many (but not all) adults with ADHD benefit from stimulant medication, to help them function. There is always some possibility of drug abuse with stimulants, but taking the medication by mouth at standard doses (commonly the same as childhood doses) has so far not been linked to dependence.

There are no neurological or lab tests to confirm ADHD. Diagnosis based on a trial of medication—giving the child some Ritalin or other drug to see if attention improves—is discouraged.

Making classroom environments fit the child

The goal is to teach the child to think of solutions—i.e., how can I fix this problem?—rather than always being told what to do. "The teacher is pivotal," comments one specialist. "Assignments can be made shorter and easier so the child gains the satisfaction of completing them, leading to a sense of achievement that may improve the motivation to stick with it and lift some of the frustration generated by constant failure."

Medications a key part of ADHD therapy

Stimulant medications used for ADHD are thought to work by adjusting the brain's chemical balance and reversing the underarousal. They decrease restlessness and aggressive outbursts, prolong the attention span and facilitate social interaction. About 75 percent of children with ADHD respond well to stimulant drugs such as Ritalin or Dexedrine, with improved behavior and better scholastic success.

Treatment works, but not by drugs alone

While most who take them benefit from stimulant drugs, medication alone is not enough to overcome ADHD. Parenting tactics, teacher attitudes, self-understanding and insight, psychosocial interventions, group therapy and other ways of achieving control are equally important. As one specialist puts it, the medications provide a "window of opportunity" for hyperactive children to "pay attention, learn to read, finish assignments, gain confidence, make friends and get an education."

For more information, consult CHADD (Children and Adults with Attention Deficit Disorders): 66 Rykert Crescent, Toronto, Ont. M4G 259, tel.: (416) 813-6858; or Child Development Clinics.

BACK PROBLEMS

Almost 90 percent of Canadians aged 29 to 65 have back pain at some time. In fact, sore backs follow the common cold as the most frequent reason for doctor visits. Ordinary backache varies from mild and gradual to the sudden, excruciating pain (*hexenschuss* or "witch's blow") brought on by a single acute stress. Fortunately, even without medical aid, 90 percent of back pain improves or is gone within 4 to 8 weeks. But as backache tends to recur, early diagnosis, prompt treatment and education to prevent recurrence are essential. Backache commonly is not a disease but stems from a combination of aging, wear and tear and poor posture, much of it preventable. Holding objects

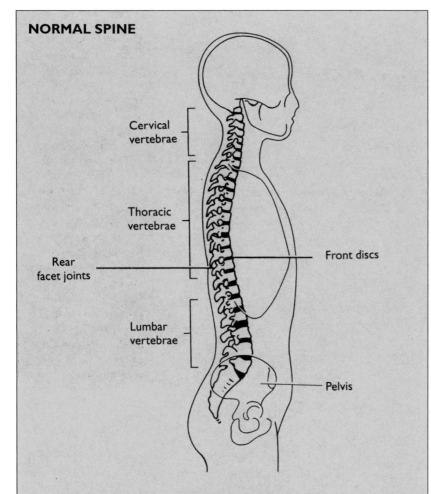

NORMAL SPINE

Cervical vertebrae

Thoracic vertebrae

Rear facet joints

Front discs

Lumbar vertebrae

Pelvis

Viewed from the side, the spine is a column with three gentle "curves"—the cervical, thoracic and lumbar regions. The back's bony elements are 33 flat-surfaced, circular bones (the vertebrae), stacked on top of each other, separated by discs (little oval pads made of fibrous tissue) that act as shock absorbers. The vertebrae articulate with each other by means of knuckle-sized facet joint at the rear, and connect via the cushioning discs in front The discs allow smooth motion without bone rubbing abrasively on bone. Somewhat like truck tires, the discs have a tough, fibrous outer coating (the annulus) and a soft, inner, jelly-like portion, the nucleus pulposus.

COMMON REASONS FOR BACKACHE

- *Muscle spasm* from irritation or damage to the spinal nerves. Back muscles go into spasm to immobilize the back and protect it from injury. Since pain from a muscle spasm in the back may travel down to the buttocks and legs, it's often difficult to pinpoint the exact location of the problem.

- *Worn facet (spinal) joints* can cause a stab of pain after some minor exertion or twisting motion such as picking up a golf ball. Pain may be immediate or worsen a day or two later. Leaning backward accentuates facet joint pain, while bending forward usually eases it. Common symptoms are: an inability to roll over or get out of bed easily; difficulty getting out of a chair or car; trouble walking erect. While felt mainly in the lower back, facet-joint pain may radiate into the buttocks and down the back of one or both thighs, typically with one hurting more than the other (possibly mimicking sciatic pain—radiating down the leg). With rest, facet-joint pain usually recedes within 4 to 14 days. It may return a few times a year, or never recur.

- *Disc trouble* (discogenic back pain) is due to bulging discs that irritate spinal nerves. With advancing age, discs lose water and elasticity wanes. They may then develop thin spots through which the soft inner material protrudes and presses on a nerve, producing back pain. Disc pain often escalates from mild to severe over a couple of days, and although it usually recedes in a week or two, it can linger on as a nagging ache. When a disc's inner portion bulges but doesn't actually protrude through the outer shell, it causes a dullish ache rather than a sharp pain. Disc pain usually worsens on bending forward; hence, disc sufferers prefer to stand erect and avoid bending.

  Those with short, acute attacks alternating with longer bouts of backache, and pain on bending both forward and backward, could have *both* worn facet joints and thinning discs. Thinning discs can throw the facet joints out of kilter, making them more prone to strain; reduce the back's suppleness, lessening its range of motion; bulge and pinch a nerve sufficiently to cause sciatic leg pain.

- *A herniated, prolapsed or ruptured* disc occurs when part of the inner pulp bursts through the tough, outer coat and irritates the spinal nerve(s) to produce persisting back and leg pain. Herniated discs tend to be a problem in younger age-groups (in the thirties and forties), most often in those who spend more than half their time sitting, such as truckers, and those who make repeated twisting movements. The sign of a truly herniated disc is intense sciatic pain down the leg, reaching the foot (in contrast to other disc problems that generally don't cause pain below the knee). Pain from a ruptured disc often worsens on coughing, sneezing and certain movements; it may be accompanied by muscle weakness, numbness and, if serious, bowel and bladder problems. Disc rupture is confirmed by CAT scans, a myelogram (X-ray pictures taken after dye injection) and other tests. If diagnosis is reasonably certain and conservative management (rest, heat and painkillers) fails, surgery or chymopapain (enzyme) dissolution may be advised.

- *Sciatica* (leg pain), which arises from a pinched spinal nerve compressed by a protruding disc or bone spur, usually builds up over a day or two and may last for 2 to 6 weeks. It tends to worsen with movement, especially bending forward, and frequently runs past the knees to the feet, sometimes accompanied by tingling or numbness. Sciatic leg pain may exceed the backache and shouldn't be ignored, since, with sufficient nerve pressure, muscular weakness and even bowel and bladder dysfunction may result. If not relieved by conservative treatment, sciatica may call for surgery to remove the nerve-pinching part.

- *Bone spurs* (osteophytes) may jut out from vertebrae and compress nerves. Fortunately they're sometimes self-limiting and tend to fuse spontaneously after about age 60. Once the bones are immobilized ("rusted stiff"), they no longer cause pain, although the trade-off is diminished suppleness.

- Spinal stenosis arises when the canal that houses the spinal cord becomes narrowed— usually by encroaching bone spurs—causing a diminished nutrient and oxygen supply to the nerves. If minor, spinal stenosis poses little threat; but in the few cases where it is severe and accompanied by symptoms such as numbness and reduced mobility, a CAT scan or MRI may be used to assess the need for surgery.

TREATING LOW BACK PAIN

• Treat the whole body, not just the spine. Most back pain tends to diminish or disappear on its own within 6 weeks.

• Relieve the initial, acute pain with anti-inflammatories, painkillers (such as ASA or aceta-minophen) and a cold pack.

• After the initial phase (about 1 week), try heat (perhaps a hot bath twice a day) as well as painkillers and muscle relaxants. (Heat should not be used in the initial phase as it may aggravate inflamed tissue.)

• Rest and immobi-lization should last only a few days (5 days max-imum) followed by a gradual return to mobility.

• Learn back-strength-ening exercises and do them regularly, plus 15 minutes daily of slow, static stretch exercises.

• Regular walking, cycling or swimming strengthens the back without strain.

• Consult a physio-therapist about back care and self-manage-ment, including how to move, stand, work and lift.

• Try TENS (transcu-taneous electrical stimulation).

• Massage helps some, provided it's done by a registered practitioner.

• Consider back manipulation by a physician or chiroprac-tor. Manipulation of the spinal vertebrae often brings speedier improvement than standard medical approaches alone; it's not a cure, but it pro-vides relief for certain types of low back pain such as facet-joint problems and sacroil-iac irritation.

• Surgery is a last resort for back condi-tions that result in nerve deterioration severe enough to weaken the legs, or produce long-lasting sciatica or loss of bowel or bladder function. Spinal-bone fusion is still occasionally rec-ommended for discogenic problems that remain incapaci-tating despite several months of nonsurgical treatment.

HOW ABOUT "FAILED BACK" PROBLEMS?

The term "failed back syndrome" is used for backs that have under-gone repeated surgery or been subjected to multiple interventions such as manipulation and injections. "Failed back" problems follow-ing surgery usually result from one or more of three possible "wrongs": the wrong (i.e., intractable) back problem, the wrong diagnosis or the wrong surgeon. One Univer-sity of Toronto specialist points out that "about 15 to 20 years ago there was an epidemic of back oper-ations when surgeons operated on almost any kind of back prob-lem. Pain clinics are now dealing with the aftermath." The pain may persist because, in a back stabilized by surgical fusion, other parts of the spine become burdened by the extra load, which may make *them* degen-erate faster. Another problem is that repeated back surgery may lead to scarring of the epidural nerve roots. The new credo is "Avoid back surgery if possible!"

near the body rather than at arm's length and making legs do the work eases spinal stress. Learning to stand, sit, lift and bend correctly, plus a few daily exercises to strengthen the abdominal muscles, can relieve or eliminate a vast amount of back pain. Less than 5 percent of back sufferers need surgery.

SOME POPULAR MISCONCEPTIONS ABOUT BACKACHE

• Discs don't "slip," "disintegrate" or "turn to dust," although they may bulge, touch a nerve and cause pain.

• Backs don't "go out," but spinal joints can be strained in the same way as other joints if overextended.

• Sitting is far harder on backs than stand-ing, and much unnecessary backache occurs because of poor body posture when seated, as well as faulty lifting and bending techniques.

• Backs aren't ultra-sensitive. Although they get a bit worn from daily wear and tear, they are quite strong.

• Back pain isn't usu-ally due to disease; it hurts but rarely harms. In less than 1 percent of cases does back pain stem from a serious underlying dis-ease.

Diagnostic findings may not match pain felt

Paradoxically, the intensity of back pain, which is highly individual, correlates poorly with X-rays, which may show seemingly serious back damage when the patient reports little or no pain. Nonetheless, X-rays and maybe also an MRI must be taken for severe back pain to rule out serious conditions such as a tumor, infection or nerve injury. Many experts claim that using a battery of tests, some of which (like the myelo-gram) are invasive, may lead to further, often needless, tests, and is only warranted when the pain is disabling, is felt right down the leg or lasts long enough for surgery to be contemplated.

Mobility is better than inactivity

Although many people suffering from low back pain want to lie in bed, this has been convinc-ingly shown to worsen the back pain. If possible, it is important to get moving. Most back problems are manageable by simple corrective measures, posture improvement and daily exercise routines. It is now recognized that surgery, bed rest and other traditional methods have failed to help the vast majority of people with low back pain. Surgery benefits only about 1 percent of sufferers—for example, those with proven spinal instability, *spondylolisthesis* (misaligned vertebrae) or persistent nerve compression. Countless studies confirm that prolonged inactivity harmfully debilitates the muscles, leads to bone loss, increases risks of a blood clot, induces depression and delays the return to normal activities. Therefore, physicians now prescribe only a short rest period, painkillers and anti-inflammatories while the back pain is acute, followed by exercise geared to the specific disorder and efforts to improve fitness. Provided it's done correctly, movement does not aggravate back pain, and brisk walking, cycling and swimming are particularly good forms of exercise for those with bad backs.

BOVINE ENCEPHALOPATHY AND CREUTZFELDT-JAKOB DISEASE

British studies suggest possible ties between mad-cow disease or *bovine spongiform encephalopathy* (BSE) and its human equivalent, *Creutzfeldt-Jakob disease* (CJD). Mad-cow disease or BSE belongs to the same group of diseases as *scrapie* in sheep and is thought to have been transmitted to cows from sheep offal feeds. These spongiform brain diseases are known to spread from one species to another—e.g., from humans to monkeys or from sheep to cows. Transformable, gene-like proteins called *prions* are thought to be responsible.

A newly discovered variant of CJD is suspected of having spread to humans from infected cattle. Although research has found no definite link between BSE in cattle and CJD in humans, the suspicion arose because the new variant of CJD, which strikes at an unusually young age, has affected several people in Britain and France. Transmission from BSE-infected cattle could possibly have occurred before control measures were implemented in 1989. However, feeding monkeys with contaminated meat and milk from BSE-infected cows has so far not transmitted the disease to these primates.

Creutzfeldt-Jakob disease has a very long incubation period—up to 30 years or more—with no overt signs of its silent presence. Worldwide, between 0.5 and 1 case of CJD per million population occurs annually, with peak onset around age 60. Once symptoms such as disturbed balance, muscular deterioration, myoclonus (leg twitching) and speech problems appear, dementia and death invariably follow within a year. Postmortem examination of CJD brains reveals a spongy look—somewhat like Swiss cheese—full of holes and riddled with amyloid plaque (protein clumps). There is no known way to screen for CJD during its long incubation period, nor is there any treatment or cure.

Most CJD in humans arises sporadically, by chance, but about 5–10 percent is genetic (inherited) due to a mutation in chromosome number 20. A small proportion (about 1 percent) is iatrogenic or due to medical treatment—for instance, transmitted via transplanting material from infected persons. Person-to-person transmission has occurred through infected growth hormone, transplanted dura mater, one transplanted cornea and use of contaminated silver electrodes for EEG (brain) recordings. (Around the world, there are 80 cases of CJD due to tainted growth hormone.)

Health professionals worry about the possibility of CJD transmission through the blood supply. One hematologist testifying before the Krever Commission of Inquiry on the Blood System in Canada warned that "CJD could become a major problem for the blood system." Most studies show no evidence of CJD transmission through blood, but one Health Canada official notes that "a few studies suggest it might be possible." One investigator from the U.S. Food and Drug Administration adds that "some of the experimental results suggesting possible blood transmission cannot simply be shrugged off." (See also p. 490.)

BOWEL PROBLEMS

The undigested remains of food enter the bowel from the intestines, which, in an adult, measure up to 6 m (20 ft), about half of that making up the small intestine, the rest the large intestine or colon. The intestines extract essential nutrients,

STRUCTURE OF THE BOWEL OR LARGE INTESTINE

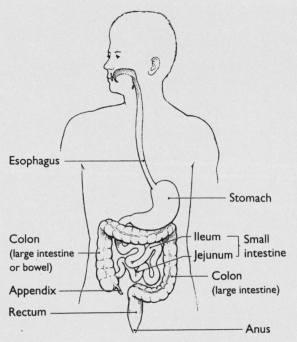

Esophagus

Stomach

Colon
(large intestine
or bowel)

Ileum ⎤ Small
Jejunum ⎦ intestine

Colon
(large intestine)

Appendix

Rectum

Anus

The medical name for the large intestine or "large bowel" is "colon"—describing the looped part of the large intestine extending from the end of the small intestine, the cecum (near the appendix), to the anus (exit point). The lower portions of the colon or bowel are called the sigmoid colon and rectum.

tions. The bowel contents are gradually moved along by wave-like muscular movements. The unabsorbed food is evacuated as a semisolid called feces or stool by a bowel movement.

Constipation

Most healthy adults have a bowel movement 3 times daily to 3 times weekly with soft, watery (but not too watery) stools. Provided bowel habits don't alter drastically, and given well-formed stool eliminated almost daily, people needn't worry much about bowel function. Constipation, however is a frequent North American complaint more common in women than men, especially frequent in the elderly. There are two main types of constipation: one due to delayed movement of stool through the colon (large intestine), the other involving a blockage at the colon outlet, perhaps with faulty defecation. Drinking more fluid and eating more dietary fiber (for example, from bran, cereals, vegetables) often relieves constipation. Overuse of laxatives is strongly discouraged. Over three million North Americans regularly use laxatives, often overstimulating their bowels into sluggish inactivity.

Constipation can be defined as the passage of hard stools fewer than 3 times a week, possibly accompanied by gas and discomfort. It may result from poor diet (low in fiber), bowel disorders and/or the use of certain drugs (such as aluminum-containing antacids and medicines containing codeine) that prolong stool transit time or alter the amount of water absorbed.

fluid and electrolytes (such as sodium and potassium) from food and dispose of undigested waste. Undigested food may remain in the descending colon for days, while fluids and electrolytes (salts) are reabsorbed into the bloodstream. One to two liters (quarts) of fluid pass through the colon every day, much of it absorbed in its ascending and transverse sec-

Diverticulitis

Outpouchings of the colon, affecting almost one-third of the Western population over age 50, produce the condition known as diverticulosis. It usually causes no discomfort, but in about 15 percent of cases the outpouchings become inflamed—producing diverticular disease, or *diverticulitis*—signaled by crampy pain, abdominal tenderness on the left side, fever, low appetite, nausea and perhaps vomiting.

While most attacks of diverticulitis are mild and need no treatment, severe forms (possibly accompanied by infection and an abscess or diverticular rupture) may require surgery. Occasionally the condition causes painless

HOW TO PREVENT CONSTIPATION

- **Eat plenty of fiber (about 20–26 g/7–9 oz a day) from fruit, vegetables, wheat bran, high-fiber cereals and breads.**
- **Drink enough fluids—6 to 10 glasses daily (including soups, juices, water, tea and other drinks), remembering that alcohol and coffee and other caf-** feinated products are diuretics that increase the body's fluid losses. It is important to drink plenty when consuming fiber-rich foods as fiber absorbs fluid in the digestive tract.
- **Develop regular bowel habits—don't delay emptying.**
- **don't strain or push at stool.**

- **don't read on the toilet.**
- **don't overuse laxatives.**
- **If stool evacuation is infrequent and fiber intake is low, try other bulk-formers or stool softeners (e.g., Surfak, Colace, Metamucil), along with enough fluids.**

bleeding (which usually stops on its own), but heavy bleeding an uncommon occurrence—may require surgical management. A new treatment is to inject remedial materials right into the bleeding bowel vessel through a hollow tube, under X-ray guidance.

As with other bowel trouble, eating more fiber may help to prevent the condition.

Irritable bowel syndrome

Irritable bowel syndrome, or IBS—also known as spastic colon, nervous bowel, mucous colitis or functional bowel disorder—is an annoying malady characterized by bloating, gas, abdominal cramps and erratic bowel habits. About 10 to 15 percent of North Americans have IBS, with a 2 to 1 female predominance. The decision to investigate and treat should be based on the severity of symptoms and the degree to which they affect the person's quality of life. Sufferers experience episodes of constipation interspersed with explosive diarrhea, sometimes many times a day. Some only experience one of these problems. Although a source of much embarrassment and annoyance, IBS is not a disease or a forerunner of serious disorders. It's an aggravation that many ignore or learn to live with, few considering it distressing enough to merit medical attention. The problem is often relieved by eating more fiber.

The hallmarks of IBS are pain-relief after bowel movements, and loose stools when the pain occurs. IBS is diagnosed "negatively," by excluding other bowel diseases as the cause of the discomfort. Symptoms that do *not* usually signify IBS and *do* require medical attention include rectal bleeding, continuous (non-crampy) pain, weight loss and nighttime discomfort. IBS symptoms generally fade at night, not disturbing sleep, whereas serious conditions (such as colitis) continue or worsen at night. A new medication called *tegaserod* (Zelnorm) has proved somewhat successful in women with constipation-dominant IBS. Safety and efficacy is still being examined. Another similar medication called *alosetron* (Lotronex), a 5-HT3 antagonist, is helpful in patients with diarrhea-predominant IBS. However, the drug was withdrawn from the market after causing the deaths of five women. (There has been some lobbying to bring it back.) Finally, cognitive-behavioral therapy has been proven to be useful, as sufferers often cite the importance of stress management in dealing with chronic IBS symptoms.

The elusive reasons for IBS

What is frequently found—or at least suspected—in IBS is an unusual pattern of intestinal movement, where the colon's normal wave-like activity is particularly sensitive and the muscles of the colon undergo abnormal contractions that sometimes show up on a routine bowel exam (with X-rays or sigmoidoscopy—looking up the colon with a special instrument). The exaggerated movements may produce bowel spasms that accelerate or delay the movement of the bowel contents, causing diarrhea or constipation. Delayed stool passage may prolong the mucosal contact with the intestinal wall, which allows further absorption of water and aggravates the problem.

Many experts think IBS is closely linked to feelings of uncertainty, tension, anxiety and/or depression. Since the colon is controlled by cerebral nerve pathways (influenced by emotions), stress can stimulate abnormal colonic movements. Many sufferers first notice their bowel problem after some distressing or upsetting event. And although recent studies on IBS have focused on colon motility rather than psychological factors, many people with the disorder have underlying psychiatric disturbances that may show up as intestinal symptoms. Two U.S. studies found that approximately 50 percent of those reporting IBS suffered from psychiatric illnesses such as anxiety disorders. By comparison, only one-fifth of people with organic gastrointestinal diseases (such as colitis) have accompanying anxiety syndromes. While not all IBS sufferers are psychologically disturbed, they share certain characteristics:
- a tendency to be hypochondriacal;
- frequent doctor visits;
- a history of being pampered as children, given treats when sick and allowed to stay home from school more often than others;
- other family members with IBS—suggesting "learned illness behavior".

TREATMENTS FOR IRRITABLE BOWEL SYNDROME

- Reassurance about its harmless nature, alleviating fears of colitis, cancer or other serious disorders. Counseling and perhaps psychotherapy. Recognition of the link between anxiety and an irritable bowel helps to overcome the problem. Brief use of tranquilizers may be suggested.
- Stress-reduction classes.
- Hypnosis and relaxation techniques.
- Dietary changes, especially the addition of fiber—much promoted. Many IBS sufferers do well just by adding 60 ml (2 tbsp) of bran a day to their food—the less refined the bran the better, wheat bran being best—adding fiber to the diet up to a level of about 26 g (9 oz) a day (more could increase symptoms). The added bulk keeps the colon mildly distended, preventing pockets of high pressure that may cause pain. (Abdominal cramping and gas may worsen for a short while after adding bulk but usually subside after a month or so.)
- Small, non-fatty meals.

For more severe cases of constipation-predominant IBS in women, a trial of *tegaserod* (Zelnorm) could be contemplated.

MEDICATIONS FOR SHORT-TERM MANAGEMEMNT OF IBS SYMPTOMS

- *Antispasmodics* (such as Buscopan and Levsin) may reduce colonic spasms and may be advised for short-term use. (Side effects include mouth dryness, a hesitant or sluggish bladder, vision blurring and slow bowel function.)
- *Carminatives* (such as peppermint oil)—smooth-muscle relaxants—are sometimes recommended.
- *Trimebutine* (Modulon) may alter stool transit time and relieve IBS. especially in those with both diarrhea and constipation.
- *Stool softeners* such as *docusate sodium* (e.g., Colace) are useful for excessively hard stools that are uncomfortable to pass, although more fluid intake and bulking agents do much the same and are preferable.
- *Cholestyramine* (Questran)—a resin that binds bile salts—may be worth a try for those with continuous diarrhea.
- *Loperamide* (Imodium) may lessen crampy pain and prevent severe, explosive diarrhea, but can also worsen constipation in the long run.
- *Maxeran, Motilium* and other drugs that alter gut motility may accelerate transit time and help sufferers whose symptoms arise from slow stomach emptying.
- Periodic use of tranquilizers such as *benzodiazepines* for stressful times can calm the gut, but should not be taken for more than 1 or 2 months.
- *Antidepressants* may help IBS sufferers with underlying depression. Besides elevating mood, they also have antispasmodic properties that reduce bowel spasms.

Inflammatory bowel disease (IBD)

Although lumped together under the umbrella term "inflammatory bowel disease" (IBD), ulcerative colitis and Crohn's disease are two distinct disorders: Crohn's disease can attack any part of the digestive tract from mouth to anus, but most often affects the small intestine. Ulcerative colitis is confined to the colon (large intestine). Inflammatory bowel disease can arise at any age, even during infancy, but usually appears between the ages of 5 and 25, affecting males and females equally.

Symptoms of both include severe diarrhea, abdominal cramps, waning appetite, weight loss. Of the many possible complications of IBD, the most serious are weight loss, weakness and fatigue, anemia, kidney stones, arthritic complaints, rash, eye disorders, and growth retardation and delayed sexual maturation (in children). Some of these conditions arise directly from the disease itself (nutrient deprivation); others, such as arthritis, are related to mechanisms not yet fully understood. Neither surgery nor drugs can cure Crohn's, but removal of the colon will permanently eliminate ulcerative colitis.

THE VARIABLE SYMPTOMS OF IRRITABLE BOWEL SYNDROME

- Constipation alternating with diarrhea (changing from day to day or week to week), lasting many months;
- abdominal bloating (gas), seemingly relieved only by defecation;
- constant urge to defecate;
- mucus in the stool;
- cramping pain beginning about one hour after eating, usually in the lower left abdomen (above the sigmoid colon), perhaps radiating to other abdominal regions;
- pain eased after bowel movement;
- possibly abnormal intestinal motility (contractions);
- spasm of the colon (may "feel hard");
- occasional pain around the anus at defecation;
- emotional or psychological stress/instability—frequently present.

RECENT STRIDES IN IBD MANAGEMENT

- *Corticosteroid drugs* reduce bowel inflammation in moderate to severe ulcerative colitis and Crohn's flare-ups. Besides relieving symptoms, corticosteroids increase appetite and help people to regain lost weight. Unfortunately they have undesirable side effects—headaches, face flushing, facial puffiness, increased body fat especially around the trunk and fluid retention (particularly around the ankles)—and also more serious side effects such as osteoporosis, blood-pressure elevation and reduced immune resistance.

New corticosteroid preparations, now in clinical trials, promise fewer side effects.
- *Sulfasalazine*—a mixture of *sulfapyridine* (an antibacterial) and *5-amino-salicylate* (5-ASA), a relative of ASA—is widely used to prevent flare-ups and alleviate mild to moderate ulcerative colitis, and also for Crohn's disease confined to the colon. Side effects are common in the first few weeks of use (headaches, nausea, loss of appetite) but minimized by taking the medication on a full stomach or as coated pills. Some people are allergic to sulfasalazine, devel-

oping a rash or hives.
- Use of 5-ASA in a variety of forms is a big advance in managing ulcerative colitis. Since most side effects of sulfasalazine stem from the sulfa component, use of 5-ASA on its own, without sulfapyridine, as daily enemas, suppositories or by mouth, may avoid problems. Various coated tablets can deliver the medication right to the affected part of the intestine. Enemas of 5-ASA now achieve remission in 80 to 90 percent of ulcerative colitis (confined to the left side of the colon), although, to maintain remission,

sufferers may also need oral drugs (e.g., Asacol, Pentasa, Salofalk, Mesasal, Dipentum) or need to continue thrice-weekly enemas.
- *Metronidazole*, an antibiotic, is increasingly used for Crohn's sufferers, especially to alleviate anal complications.
- *Immunosuppressants* (*6-mercaptopurine* and *azathioprine*) may be helpful in Crohn's disease by reducing the required dosage of corticosteroids and healing fistulas, or for cases that don't respond to corticosteroids. Cyclosporine—an immunosuppressant widely used for trans-

plants—is also being tried for IBD.
- The new pelvic pouch surgery—used for ulcerative colitis (not Crohn's)—avoids the need for an external stool-collecting bag. The operation removes the colon and rectum, leaving intact the muscles of the anus, connecting the small intestine to them. A "pouch" made out of the small intestine serves as a surrogate colon. Although it doesn't permit completely normal bowel movements, the operation reduces the inconvenience of frequent defecation without disturbing daily life.

Possible causes of inflammatory bowel disease

- *Infections*—bacterial or viral triggers.
- *Altered immunological responses.* An immune response mounted against the body's own cells is now considered largely responsible.
- *Diet.* Studies implicating such foods as sugar and cornflakes in IBD have been largely discredited. There is some evidence that lack of fiber is a cause, but the jury is still out.

- *Genetic makeup.* Between 20 and 40 percent of people with IBD have one or more relatives with the disease.

It is no longer believed that psychological problems trigger IBD, although IBD can certainly cause psychological problems. People ill from IBD may experience a sense of hopelessness, which may lead to depression as a consequence rather than a cause of IBD.

SCREENING FOR BOWEL CANCER

The current Canadian guidelines suggest that individuals aged 50 to 74 with average risks be screened every 2 years with the fecal occult blood test. This test means examining the person's stool sample in a lab for traces of blood. The occult

blood test however often comes out "positive" when there is actually no bowel cancer present. In turn, a positive fecal blood test may lead to needless further investigations, such as a colonoscopy (examination of the colon with a

long fiberoptic tube) for a cancer that's not there. The current indications are that people should have a colonoscopy every 10 years when there are no known or observed bowel problems. Occasionally, a colonoscopy reveals the presence of

small polyps in the bowel/colon that can be removed during the examination procedure. Further visits may be arranged as frequently as necessary to remove polyps on a regular basis as they can be "pre-cancerous." Individuals known

to be at high risk—people who have already had bowel polyps or cancers, those with ulcerative colitis or other predisposing conditions and people with a family history of bowel disease—are screened more frequently.

A COMPARISON CHART OF ULCERATIVE COLITIS AND CROHN'S DISEASE

Ulcerative colitis

- First described in 1875, ulcerative colitis is an inflammation of the colon's inner lining, sometimes extending to the rectum. Once thought to be restricted to North America and Europe, ulcerative colitis is now increasingly reported in Japan, India, Thailand and many other parts of the world. It afflicts young adults, three-quarters of the cases developing before age 30, although it occasionally affects children and older people. It's especially common among Jewish people.
- Ulcerative colitis may be restricted to one side of the colon (often the left) or spread to the whole large intestine (pancolitis).
- Symptoms are severe bloody diarrhea, weight loss, poor appetite, mild fever, anemia and loss of body fluids.
- Attacks vary in frequency and severity. Ulcerative colitis is mild in 60 percent of cases, moderate in 25 percent, severe in 15 percent. Some people have one attack, then none for years; others suffer frequent relapses. The disease is unpredictable. Mild disease may suddenly erupt into a severe form or go into remission for years. Flare-ups can occur for no identifiable reason.
- Complications include blood loss or, rarely, toxic megacolon (dilation of the colon) or colonic perforation—a medical emergency.
- The risks of colon cancer increase with ulcerative colitis, especially if it lasts 10 or more years and if most of the colon is affected.
- Treatment must correct malnutrition, restore disturbed fluid and electrolyte imbalance (resulting from diarrhea), control inflammation and reduce the risk of ulcers.
- Medications include sulfasalazine, 5-amino ASA products (e.g., Asacol), used as enemas, suppositories or tablets, steroids (hydrocortisone, prednisone or new forms) and cyclosporine (experimental).
- Some must stay on maintenance medication to prevent flareups.
- Surgery, reserved for those who don't improve with other treatment, entails removal of the colon and rectum and perhaps an ileostomy (artificial opening to which the small intestine is attached, allowing feces to empty into a small, disposable bag). The removal of the (entire) colon cures ulcerative colitis, since, unlike Crohn's, the disease affects only this part of the digestive tract. Such surgery may seem drastic, but many colitis sufferers prefer it to a debilitating illness.
- The new pelvic pouch operation or ileo-anal anastomosis—connecting the ileum to the anal canal—avoids an ileostomy (external bag), and makes bowel surgery easier for those who need it. More people with ulcerative colitis now opt for surgery earlier in the course of the disease, based on an informed decision taken jointly by patient and physician.
- Regular follow-up and checkups are advisable. After 10 years or so, people with ulcerative colitis should undergo yearly colonoscopy (fiber-optic visualization of the colon) to detect incipient cancers.

Crohn's disease

- Named after the physician who first described it, Crohn's disease has increased dramatically since World War II in Europe and North America but remains rare in the developing world. It is most frequent among Europeans, especially Jews. The reason for the sudden rise in Crohn's disease in the Western world remains a mystery. It's not traceable to any specific features of modern urban life, such as stress, diet, infant-feeding practices, toxins or infectious agents.
- Crohn's disease can attack any part of the digestive tract but typically affects the lower portion of the small intestine and the colon, with thickening and inflammation of the intestinal wall.
- Symptoms, depending on the areas affected, are usually diarrhea, abdominal pain, diminished appetite, weight loss, weakness and fatigue. By the time it's diagnosed, people with Crohn's may be quite ill, partly due to malnutrition from inadequate food intake. Symptoms may also include, nausea and vomiting (stomach affected), mouth ulcers, heartburn (esophageal involvement), hemorrhoids (anal disease) and infection. In some, mild symptoms drag on for years. Others have single attacks followed by long remissions.
- Major complications are bowel obstruction, fistulas (abnormal channels between intestinal loops) and mild bleeding.
- Although the risk of colon cancer in those with long-standing Crohn's is marginally increased, it is not clear how much likelier than average they are to develop colon cancer.
- Treatment aims to restore good nutrition, control inflammation and delay relapses. Since many Crohn's sufferers are malnourished by the time of diagnosis, the first step is to restore nutritional well-being with fluid, electrolyte and vitamin replacement. Many new feeding methods can help.
- Medications include: corticosteroids, sulfasalazine (for disease confined to the colon) and antibiotics such as metronidazole.
- New steroids with fewer side effects are bringing relief to some (e.g., budesonide)—still experimental.
- Intravenous feeding or *total parenteral nutrition* (TPN) often achieves remission, obviating the need for surgery. At first it was thought that TPN gave the bowels a rest. However, recent research suggests that "resting" the bowel may not be the main benefit. Merely restoring nutritional status, whether by intravenous or normal feeding (together with appropriate medication), produces great improvement in many Crohn's sufferers. An "elemental" diet of basic nutrients helps some.
- Strictureplasty, a new procedure, shows promise in alleviating the obstruction due to bowel scarring by a technique that widens the bowel and relieves the stricture. The great advantage is that strictureplasty can be done without removing any bowel sections—especially useful for those with widespread disease.
- Surgery cannot permanently cure Crohn's disease, as it may recur in other parts of the digestive tract and call for repeat surgery.

POSSIBLE SIGNS OF BOWEL CANCER

About 10 percent of persons with bowel cancer have no warning symptoms at all. However, most observe some signs:

- Visible red blood in or on the stool (perhaps as a red streak), which occurs if the polyp bleeds. The color of the blood may be bright or dark red according to the polyp's position in the colon. However, most rectal bleeding arises from hemorrhoids, and is characteristically not mixed into the stool but on top of it or just on the toilet paper.
- Occult (hidden) blood in the stool, which may be present at an early stage and is detectable by a simple test, which, although not entirely reliable, is a useful marker of bowel cancer.
- A change in bowel habits persisting more than two weeks.
- Abdominal pain.
- If the growth is large enough, bowel obstruction and severe abdominal pain, perhaps nausea and vomiting (uncommon) and a sense of incomplete defecation.
- Iron-deficiency anemia (from intestinal bleeding).

Anyone who notices these changes should see a physician at once, for investigation and treatment if necessary. Experts stress that although the vast majority of rectal bleeding is due to hemorrhoids, the possibility of colon cancer warrants medical investigation when rectal blood is noticed.

TESTS FOR COLON (BOWEL) CANCER INCLUDE:

- a digital palpation (with a gloved finger Inserted up the rectum), which allows clinicians to feel growths in the rectal area and assess their size but not whether they are malignant. A thorough digital exam detects roughly 10 percent or less of all bowel tumors;
- sigmoidoscopy—with a flexible sigmoidoscope (illuminated, metal, fiberoptic tube) inserted through the rectum that allows visualization about 35–40 cm (14–15 in) up the colon, revealing growths in the rectum, sigmoid, even lower descending colon;
- colonoscopy—direct fiberoptic visualization using a colonoscope, a 1.8-m (6-ft), flexible tube that allows clinicians to peer into every nook and cranny of the intestine and at the same time to snip off small growths for biopsy (cell sampling). During colonoscopy all but the smallest of polyps are usually removed, however innocent they appear, and tested for cancer. Colonoscopy is done without anesthetic, but Valium and other drugs are given to mute pain. Virtual colonoscopy has yet to be proven as a reliable method of detection;
- an air-contrast barium enema X-ray is still a key diagnostic tool for bowel growths. After liquid barium solution is instilled in the rectum, X-rays detect unusual lumps, bumps, elevations, polyps or tumors along the colon. But X-ray pictures do not reveal whether growths are malignant, and may miss subtle changes that show up better with colonoscopy.

Dietary treatment of IBD

Nutrition is crucial in IBD, but the exact role of diet is controversial. Experts have tried low-sugar, high-carbohydrate diets, exclusion diets and low-fiber diets with inconclusive results. The response of IBD sufferers to food varies widely. Ulcerative colitis sufferers are often lactose intolerant and must avoid milk products. Some with bowel stricture (narrowing) do best by avoiding bulky high-fiber foods. One study on Crohn's patients who had undergone surgery found that the most troublesome foods were corn, nuts, fizzy drinks, raw fruits, shellfish, lettuce, pickles, alcohol and tomatoes. Least likely to cause problems were chicken, white bread, rice and potatoes. Each IBD sufferer must identify the foods that aggravate symptoms and avoid them, remembering that regular, well-balanced meals are essential for good nutrition. One recent approach being investigated by a University of Toronto team is an "elemental diet" of nutrients in their basic format, fed through a tube, used without any medications or surgery, which helps many Crohn's sufferers. Pioneered as a diet for space travelers, it contains premixed amino acids, fats, carbohydrates and other essential nutrients, producing minimal digestive activity and little stool formation.

Bowel cancer

Bowel cancer follows lung cancer as the commonest form of malignancy in men, ranking third in women after breast and lung cancer. The incidence of bowel cancer among Canadians is about 45 per 100,000 males per year slightly less for women. People with close relatives who have had

WHEN TO CALL THE DOCTOR OR GET MEDICAL ADVICE ABOUT A COUGH

It's wise to get medical advice for a cough if you:
• are a tobacco smoker;
• are elderly;
• have heart or lung disease;
• have a fever above 38°C (101°F);
• are having chest pains or shortness of breath;
• have earache;
• notice blood in the phlegm coughed up;
• find the cough gets suddenly worse;
• feel very ill with it.

bowel cancer have a greater than average risk of getting the disease. Certain families with an uncommon condition known as familial polyposis have a propensity to develop many—even thousands of—bowel polyps before age 30, with a high risk of developing cancer if the entire bowel isn't removed. Individuals with long-standing ulcerative colitis involving the left side of the colon, are also more at risk than the general population. (See preceding section, "Inflammatory bowel disease.")

Benign bowel polyps may become malignant

There is increasing evidence that people who develop bowel (colorectal) cancer have previously had harmless growths (polyps) in the bowel wall. Opinions differ, but many believe that certain bowel polyps can become malignant—especially adenomatous polyps, with finger-like fronds. With bowel polyps smaller than one cm (less than half an inch) in diameter cancer is rare; from 1 to 2 cm (0.4 to 0.8 in), risk increases to 1 in 10, and with polyps over 2 cm (0.8 in) there is almost a 50 percent chance of malignancy. Why some polyps become malignant while others don't remains a mystery. In Canada and the United States, the majority of bowel polyps and cancers arise in the lower (sigmoid) part of the colon and the rectal area.

Treatment of bowel cancer

Fortunately, many bowel growths can now be removed via colonoscopy, obviating the need for major surgery. If the cancer has invaded the bowel's inner lining, surgical excision (resection) with lymph node removal is still advised, depending on the person's overall well-being. These days, surgical excision of a piece of bowel requires less drastic techniques than formerly, with rapid recovery for most people. Only infrequently is a *colostomy* (removal of the rectum, requiring an external feces-collection bag) necessary.

BRONCHITIS

Every fall and winter the organisms responsible for influenza and the common cold descend on us, causing sniffles and sneezing, sore throats, coughs and all-round misery, sometimes lingering as a persistent and sputum-laden cough known as bronchitis.

Key symptoms of bronchitis
• Lung congestion;
• wheezing;
• loose chesty cough, with phlegm;
• possibly chest pain when coughing.

Bronchitis can be brief and acute or persistent and chronic

Typically, the cough that heralds bronchitis surfaces a few days after the worst of a cold's runny nose stage. The term "bronchitis" covers two distinct disorders—acute bronchitis, with a cough lasting a few weeks, and chronic bronchitis, which can persist for months, year after year. Bronchitis occurs when invading micro-organisms attack the lung's mucous membranes (inner linings), irritating and inflaming them. The passages become clogged, leading to prolonged coughing, increased mucus production and sometimes bronchial spasm (contraction of the bronchial muscles).

Acute bronchitis is a mucus-producing cough that lasts 2 to 3 weeks in people with no underlying lung problems (such as asthma or emphysema), and is mostly viral, although it can be due to bacteria. The condition tends to be worst at night when copious amounts of phlegm, often yellow or greenish in color, may be coughed up. In diagnosing acute bronchitis, physicians must distinguish it from other (possibly more serious) conditions—such as pneumonia, tuberculosis, another bacterial infection or an allergy. In particular, they must make sure the symptoms aren't due to pneumonia, which is often accompanied by fever, wheezing and a crackling sound in the lungs, heard through a stethoscope. Pulmonary function tests—an office procedure—may be done to measure the volume of exhaled air before and after taking a bronchodilator.

Chronic bronchitis is a deep, mucus-producing cough that lasts for at least 3 months, for more than 2 consecutive years. The cough may become almost continuous and breathing can be difficult—especially in smokers. Chronic obstructive lung disease (COPD) may develop. (About 90 percent of those who suffer from chronic bronchitis are smokers.)

Some bronchitis may be whooping cough!

Adults who come down with bronchitis may in fact be infected with *Borderella pertussis* (the bacteria that cause whooping cough). Although children with pertussis have violent coughing fits with a characteristic whoop, many adults with the infection don't whoop—or the sound goes unrecognized. Pertussis is becoming more common among adults in whom childhood immunization has worn off. Although *natural* pertussis infection confers lifelong immunity against whooping cough, the vaccines used in childhood only provide immunity for a few years, waning by about age 12. Thus, despite childhood pertussis vaccination, increasing numbers of adults are susceptible to the disease.

The doctor's dilemma: Choosing the right treatment

The challenge for family physicians is to weigh up the evidence and decide how best to treat bronchitis, especially given new guidelines that call for less antibiotic use. Acute bronchitis was formerly treated with rest, increased fluid intake (to keep the lungs hydrated and secretions thin), cough suppressants, expectorants and antibiotics. The role of expectorants is now questioned and use of antibiotics for simple bronchitis is discouraged as several randomized studies have shown that antibiotics do not shorten the course of acute, uncomplicated viral bronchitis. New guidelines suggest treating bronchitis just by suppressing symptoms and letting it clear up without antibiotics. Bronchodilators—airway-widening medications (such as beta-agonists)—may help.

Although few physicians suggest antibiotics for everyone with bronchitis, "the doctor's dilemma," explains one family physician, "is knowing who might benefit from antibiotics." Those most likely to benefit are older people (over age 55), smokers, those who feel very ill and cough incessantly, people whose cough lasts longer than two weeks and those with asthma, emphysema or other lung problems.

Recommended therapy for bronchitis
- Bed rest;
- drinking lots of fluids to thin the secretions and lessen congestion;

MOST BRONCHITIS IS DUE TO VIRAL INFECTION

Acute bronchitis usually occurs when a virus invades the lung's air passages as the aftermath of an upper respiratory infection. Particularly to blame are influenza and common cold viruses (coronaviruses and rhinoviruses); bronchitis can also follow measles, adenovirus and herpes simplex infections. The viruses stimulate an immune response that inflames the bronchial lining.

Depending on the agents responsible, there may or may not be fever—influenza, adenovirus and pneumonia infections usually cause fever; common colds normally don't. Since most cases of simple, acute bronchitis are due to viruses, they do not respond to or need antibiotic therapy. Most episodes clear in 2 to 3 weeks with rest, increased fluid intake and over-the-counter medicines. However, occasionally a bacterial invasion may follow a viral infection, in which case antibiotic therapy may be advised. Bacterial infection is suspected when the cough persists for longer than 2 weeks, if it worsens considerably, if there is fever above 38°C (101°F), chest pain, shortness of breath and if the person feels really ill.

- not smoking cigarettes while ill (preferably quitting for good);
- limited use of cough suppressants, such as dextromethorphan or codeine, in those who cough incessantly or are unable to sleep; consult your physician before using these drugs, which are narcotics;
- ASA (Aspirin) or acetaminophen (Tylenol) to reduce fever or flu-like aches and pains;
- bronchodilators, such as *albuterol* or *fenoterol*, which may shorten the course of bronchitis and ease breathing;
- for cases complicated by bacterial infection antibiotics may be required, first trying older narrow-spectrum forms such as *erythromycin* or *tetracycline*, and for more serious cases, perhaps *doxycycline*, *clarithromycin* or one of the other new broad-spectrum drugs.

CARPAL TUNNEL SYNDROME

Carpal tunnel syndrome (CTS) is an easily treatable wrist and hand disorder, more frequent in women than in men. The problem arises through compression of the median (arm) nerve in its narrow passageway through the wrist, often starts up in mid-life to old age and generally affects both hands, the dominant (most-used) one more severely CTS can arise from certain jobs or hobbies where repeated movements or vibrations inflame the wrist tissues—for instance, knitting, computer keyboard work, driving or operating certain hand-held power tools such as drills, hammers, chain saws. The disorder is frequently seen among miners, roadmenders and others whose jobs involve use of hand-held tools that vibrate.

The first hint of CTS is a sensation of numbness or pain, usually on first awakening—as if parts of the hand had "gone to sleep"—typically felt in the thumb and index finger but sometimes all the fingers tingle. The tingling sensation worsens on flexing or extension of the wrist, subsiding when the hand is bent inwards or at rest (in a "neutral" position).

Numbness from carpal tunnel syndrome may appear after any movement that keeps the wrist overextended for long periods: stitching, keyboarding, doing manicures or giving a massage. Besides being annoying, the sensory loss may lead to burns (due to lessened sensation of heat, pain, pressure), and the muscle-wasting can make wrist movements clumsy. As CTS progresses, wrist and thumb strength may seriously decline. The reduced grip may make it difficult to grasp even light objects.

The tingling can be set off or worsened by anything that makes the wrist tissues swell and compress the median nerve. Fluid accumulation during pregnancy or before a menstrual period, a Colles' (wrist-bone) fracture, gout, rheumatic (arthritic) swelling, and adrenal or thyroid diseases are typical causes.

Diagnosis of CTS is relatively easy by the typical nighttime or early-morning hand tingling, use of Phalen's test (flexing the hands at a 90-degree angle to see if and when tingling occurs) and Tinel's test (tapping the median nerve at the wrist to see if and how strongly it produces tingling). The sooner the tingling appears, the more

serious the condition. Confirmation is with a nerve-conduction study and electromyogram (EMG), in which small electric shocks are applied at different spots along the median nerve and the muscle twitch is charted to show whether and to what extent, the hand muscle has retained or lost its nerve supply.

Treatment for carpal tunnel syndrome can be conservative: wearing a light plastic wrist-splint at night, taking anti-inflammatory medications by mouth or injected into the wrist, altering sleep positions and avoiding movements that worsen the disorder. With correct therapy, time and patience, the loss of nerve conduction can often be reversed.

If other methods fail to correct CTS, surgery to decompress the nerve may be suggested—a simple procedure done under general or local anesthetic that frees the trapped nerve and usually provides rapid relief. After a few days, stitches are removed, but splinting may be needed until the wound heals.

COMMON COLD

The common cold is an upper-respiratory-tract viral infection, which, being due to viruses, cannot be cured by antibiotics. Colds are self-limiting infections generally fought off by the body's immune defenses within a week. The first sign of a cold—usually a sore throat—appears after an incubation period of 2 to 3 days, and symptoms usually peak on the third day. The sore throat is followed by swelling of the nasal membranes and a discharge that starts out clear but later becomes turbid. To date, no one has improved upon Sir William Osler's classic description of the common cold as "an acute inflammation of the upper air passages, whereby the patient sneezes frequently, feels indisposed, perhaps chilly, with a slight headache—rarely (adults) having a fever more than a degree above normal." If the virus invades the larynx (voice box) and inflames the vocal cords, laryngitis may also occur, with a husky, muted or silenced voice for a few days.

Colds afflict young children more than adults, and schoolchildren often bring colds into the home. The average preschooler has 5 to 10 colds annually and spends almost 3 months of the year with a runny nose. Fortunately, the

COLD REMEDIES: MAY HELP WITH SYMPTOMS BUT TRY TO USE SINGLE-DRUG, NOT COMBINED, PRODUCTS

- *Topical decongestants* (such as Otrivin, Privine or Afrin) come as drops or sprays—sprays being somewhat superior to drops. Their effects last from 4 to 10 hours, depending on the type. Topical decongestants should be used only for a *maximum of four days*, strictly as directed, to prevent rebound congestion (increased stuffiness)—which can surface even after short use. Topical sprays are best reserved for "must clear" occasions (e.g., air travel).

- *Oral decongestants* (such as pseudoephedrine) come as short-acting or sustained-release products that act more slowly than sprays, but are not habit-forming or likely to cause rebound stuffiness. Hypertensives should use oral decongestants cautiously as most raise blood pressure.

- *Antihistamines* have only a marginal impact on colds, but are useful for allergy-related nasal stuffiness. Most cold remedies contain too much and too many antihistamines. Largely sedative in their effect, antihistamines may be helpful at night.

- *Cough suppressants (antitussives)* often contain codeine (as in Tylenol No. 1), *dextromethorphan* or DM (as in Benadryl DM, Triaminic DM or Robitussin DM) or *hydrocodone*, a stronger cough suppressant. Available without prescription, dextromethorphan is almost as good a cough suppressant as codeine, with fewer side effects. These agents suppress coughing by acting on the brain's cough center, *not* on the throat, and are just as, if not more, effectively absorbed from pills than syrups. Some physicians advise caution in using cough suppressants, as it is not always desirable to suppress a cough, the protective mechanism that clears the respiratory tract of mucus (phlegm). However, a dry, hacking cough that hampers work or sleep may call for control with cough medicines, which generally do no harm.

- *Expectorants* (e.g., *guaifenesin*), said to loosen and help expel secretions and enhance a productive cough, are considered useless by most experts. (Pure steam is better.)

- *Vitamin C*, widely promoted in small doses (about 250 mg daily) to prevent colds, and in massive doses (up to 10 g) to stop a cold at the first hint of symptoms, has not lived up to its promise. No anticold claims for vitamin C have been scientifically validated.

- *Zinc gluconate lozenges*, which have an unpleasant taste, have recently been shown capable of shortening some colds by a day or two, because zinc ions may reduce rhinovirus replication. However, they cause stomach pain and nausea. A new zinc gel for the nose is being evaluated.

- *Echinacea*, an herbal remedy, is very popular. It is meant to boost the immune system but to date trials testing its efficacy have shown no consistent benefit.

- *Analgesics and fever reducers* such as ASA (Aspirin), Ibuprofen (Advil, Motrin) or acetaminophen (Tylenol) are useless against most common-cold symptoms, but can combat headaches, reduce muscle aches or fever—typical of flu but rare with mere colds.

NOTE: Children with fever from an apparent cold should not be given ASA (Aspirin) because the symptoms may resemble a mild case of flu. Together with ASA, influenza viruses can produce Reye's syndrome (a dangerous liver and brain complication). To avoid the risks of Reye's syndrome, fever in young sufferers can be reduced with acetaminophen products (e.g., Tylenol or Tempra).

---

number of yearly colds dwindles to about 3 to 6 by age 10 to 14, and decreases with advancing age. Children with colds may have a fever and an upset stomach, but no runny nose.

Catching a cold is a contact sport

Cold viruses are transmitted by direct contact with infected nasal secretions, typically picked up from the hands or from some other object, transferred to the virus-permeable membranes of eyes or nose. Cold viruses can survive for hours on hard surfaces (dishes, counters) but not as long on porous items such as disposable tissues. When fingers contaminated with cold viruses touch or rub the eyes or nose, the viruses enter and multiply in the nasal passages. The mucous membranes of the mouth are quite resistant to cold viruses, so it may be easier to catch a cold from a handshake than a kiss!

No scientific data support the notion that a cold, despite its name, is actually caused by chilly conditions, scanty clothes or damp weather, but being cold can lessen the body's defenses. Arctic explorers, continually cold and damp, are less rather than more likely to catch colds, because they are isolated. Volunteers infected with cold viruses who spent days sitting in damp, chilly rooms clad only in their underwear did not develop more colds than warmly dressed controls. Nonetheless, in northern climates, colds occur with higher frequency in fall and winter because of more time spent indoors, with people herded close together.

Despite the popular belief that colds settle in the chest and cause pneumonia, this doesn't usually happen, although they are sometimes followed by bacterial infections of the sinuses or, especially in children, of the middle ear. Staying indoors doesn't necessarily help. Some people, especially children, feel better outdoors.

Are there ways to prevent a cold?

Scrupulous handwashing and avoiding crowded places may help to reduce the spread of cold viruses. Hopes for a preventive vaccine have dimmed with the isolation of over 100 subtypes of the common cold rhinovirus. But researchers are experimenting with virus-destroying solutions, "killer Kleenex" (saturated with chemicals that destroy the viruses) and antiviral drugs. New antiviral agents such as interferon (produced naturally by human cells) and *enviroxine* (a synthetic drug) offer some hope of prevention.

Beware of multi-ingredient cold remedies

Cold remedies typically clutter our medicine cabinets, but experts warn against *combination* remedies that contain multiple ingredients—for example, remedies containing antihistamines, caffeine (to counteract sedating effects), decongestants, painkillers, cough suppressants, vitamin C, and sometimes even antacids. Combined cold-relief products, especially those overloaded with antihistamines and short on decongestants, do nothing for most colds. Decongestants alone are best to clear a stuffy nose. The U.S. Food and Drug Administration finds "no justification for the large number of combined ingredients in a single blunderbuss anti-cold product." Some ingredients, such as cough stimulants or laxatives, are frankly irrational; some act against each other; some (e.g., phenylpropanolamine) are toxic in excess. Single-ingredient products are best: analgesics for pain; antipyretics to combat fever; antihistamines for some nasal drying; decongestants against nasal or sinus stuffiness; cough suppressants to reduce a tiring cough. There is no point in treating symptoms that you *don't* have!

CREUTZFELDT-JAKOB DISEASE (AND LINKS TO "MAD-COW" DISEASE OR BSE)

The discovery of a possible connection between mad-cow disease or *bovine spongiform encephalopathy* (BSE) and its human equivalent—*Creutzfeldt-Jakob disease* (CJD), a spongiform brain disease—led researchers around the world to investigate the dangers of eating beef from BSE-infected cows. Human CJD is a slow virus disease due to tiny, gene-like infective particles called prions that are similar to the agents responsible for causing *scrapie* in sheep and BSE in cattle. Mad-cow disease or BSE, which belongs to the same group of diseases as *scrapie* in sheep, is thought to have been transmitted to cows from sheep offal put into cattle feeds. These spongiform brain diseases are known to spread from one species to another—e.g., from humans to monkeys or from sheep to cows.

In its traditional form, human CJD is a rare condition, affecting about 1 per million people worldwide, with a very long incubation period (up to 30 or more years) during which there are no signs of its "silent presence." CJD generally appears in older persons (over age 65 or so), with symptoms such as disturbed balance, muscular degeneration, limb twitches, rigidity, blindness, speech problems and eventually confusion, dementia and death. While most CJD is sporadic, and of no known origin, about 5 to 10 percent is a genetic or hereditary form that affects specific families (due to gene changes or mutations in chromosome number 20).

Occasionally, CJD occurs in younger age groups, usually through transplants of corneas, *dura mater* (brain matter) or other organs from infected people, or from administering human growth hormone prepared from a CJD-infected person. Unfortunately, there's no way to screen for the disease during its long incubation period. Post-mortem examination of CJD brains (or brains from "mad cows" afflicted with BSE) reveals a spongy look, with the cerebral matter riddled with holes—somewhat like certain Swiss cheeses—scattered with grainy amyloid protein plaques.

In 1996, a new variant of CJD (named "variant CJD"), with brain changes very like those seen in BSE-infected cattle, that attacked young people (in their teens or 20s) was identified in Britain and France. By 1997, 20 new cases had been identified among young people. Researchers concluded the new cases were due to eating beef from BSE-infected cows, and since then more cases of variant CJD have surfaced among young people in various countries. To date, 150 people are known to have died from new variant Creutzfeldt-Jakob disease in the UK, and France has recorded nine cases, Ireland two cases and Canada, the U.S. and Italy have each recorded one death from variant CJD. (The Canadian case is thought to have contracted the disease from eating beef while residing in Britain.) In Canada, so far five mad cows with BSE have been officially identified since 1993, none apparently having entered the Canadian food chain. To curb the possibility of acquiring CJD from beef, and to eliminate BSE from cattle herds, authorities in most countries now ban the use of ruminant feed (containing cattle parts such as eyes, spinal cord or brain) for cows.

There are however emerging concerns about the possibility of CJD transmission via transfusion of contaminated blood or blood products. Therefore, to avoid infection through tainted blood, Canadian Red Cross policy now excludes blood donations from any known or possible CJD carriers such as those with a family history of the disease or people who have received pituitary-derived growth hormone, cornea or dura mater transplants. (This position may change as additional data come in.)

CYSTIC FIBROSIS

Cystic fibrosis (CF) is the most common potentially fatal inherited disease among Caucasians, especially those of North European descent. Until about 10 years ago, all that was known of CF was the fact that it causes chronic lung and digestive problems linked to abnormal salt transport, and its classic inheritance pattern as a single-gene, recessive disorder. (If both parents carry the CF gene, each child they bear has a 1 in 4 chance of being born with the disease.)

About 1 in 25 persons in North America and Europe carries the flawed gene, usually without knowing it and without any signs of the illness. Hence, the parents of an affected child may be unable to understand why their baby has the disease. They need to understand that CF is *not* due to diet, stress or any problems during pregnancy, nor can it be passed from one child to another; it's entirely due to genes inherited from both parents.

While the exact mechanism behind cystic fibrosis remains unknown, the good news is that the recent discovery and cloning of the CF gene has enabled scientists to identify and analyze the structure of the abnormal protein involved in the disease, and locate its site in affected cells— knowledge that will ultimately lead to more effective treatment of this devastating disease.

What is cystic fibrosis?

Cystic fibrosis involves an inability to move salt (sodium chloride, particularly the chloride part) and water through the channels in the cells that line certain organs. The flawed chloride transport and consequent dryness of cell surfaces produces abnormally thick secretions that hamper the normal function of organs such as the lungs, sweat glands, intestines and pancreas.

The first detailed report of the disease, in 1936, described it as "cystic fibrosis of the pancreas" because of the thick mucus that blocks the flow of secretions and causes fibrosis (scarring) of the pancreas. However, the pancreatic problem isn't usually the most dangerous aspect of CF, nor is the pancreas always seriously affected. It's the thick, sticky mucus in the lungs that usually poses the greatest danger and leads to frequent respiratory infections.

Digestion may also be impeded, because thick secretions slow the flow and deplete the supply of pancreatic enzymes, hindering food absorption, perhaps leading to malnutrition. In afflicted males, reproductive-tract blockages often lead to sterility. The sweat of CF sufferers is unusually salty. The "sweat test" which detects the elevated salt content, has become the standard diagnostic tool for CF.

Treatment has gradually improved, prolonging survival so that some CF sufferers now live well into their forties. However, most need lifelong medication to combat lung infections and assist digestion.

SIGNS OF CYSTIC FIBROSIS

- **Intestinal (bowel) blockage in infancy, which causes abdominal swelling, vomiting and dehydration, often requiring surgery;**
- **unusually salty taste of baby's skin when kissed;**
- **inability of the pancreas to deliver necessary digestive enzymes, and failure to gain weight despite a normal or unusually large appetite;**
- **fatty stools (greasy, flecked with fat);**
- **frequent respiratory infections;**
- **finger clubbing (abnormal fingernail growth)—also seen in other chronic illnesses;**
- **sinusitis or nasal polyps;**
- **delayed puberty, possible reproductive abnormalities—especially male sterility (over 90 percent of males with CF are infertile).**

The inheritance pattern in cystic fibrosis

Cystic fibrosis is a single-gene recessive disorder so a child must receive a flawed gene from each parent to have the disease. Someone with one faulty and one normal gene will be a carrier but will not have CF A child with one carrier parent and one non-carrier parent may or may not be a carrier (depending on which genes are transmitted) but will not have CF. However, if *both* mother and father are CF carriers, there's a 1 in 4 chance that a child will receive the defective gene from *both* sides, and therefore have the disease. It's purely a matter of chance. The risk remains one in four for each further child conceived.

Managing a devastating disease

Since there's no cure at present, therapy must usually be continued throughout life—a demanding regime for CF sufferers, parents and doctors alike. Besides medical care, patients generally require psychological, occupational, social and genetic counseling.

Medical care for CF means primarily managing the lung and digestive problems. Treatment for lung congestion includes exercises to drain fluid, methods to assist in clearing mucus and antibiotics to combat recurrent bacterial infections. While not all CF sufferers have pancreatic insufficiency, most have some degree of abnormality in the production and supply of pancreatic enzymes and many need pills to make up the deficit. Children with CF may improve so markedly with supplements, achieving excellent school records and participation in sports, that parents wonder whether their youngster really has CF. A child's response depends largely on the severity of the illness when first detected.

Gene discovery brings fresh hope of cure

A stunning piece of collaborative research done by scientists at the universities of Toronto and Michigan has located the gene responsible for CF, worked out its genetic code and defined many of the mutations that produce the disorder. Knowing the gene's chemical (base) sequence, scientists deduced the structure of the protein controlled by the gene a protein now named CFTR (TR stands for "transmembrane conductance regulator"). This gene-product, CFTR, resides in the cell membrane and seemingly assists in regulating the transport of chloride (and perhaps other substances) through cell surfaces.

Until the precise flaw (exactly how salt regulating goes wrong) is known, treatment can slow down but cannot halt the disease. However, the discovery of the CF-causing gene and its protein-product opens up the chance of developing drugs to correct the abnormal salt movement.

Gene therapy may soon provide a cure for this disease. Inserting a normal gene into CF cells to replace the defective one could overcome cystic fibrosis. The first step has already been achieved—transferring a normal version of the gene into defective pancreatic cells in a culture dish, thereby regularizing chloride/water transport.

Carrier screening and prenatal diagnosis are now possible

The discovery of the CF gene has set the stage for carrier tests. Before the discovery, parents were alerted to the possibility of having a child with CF only if they'd already had an affected child. Now, carriers can be detected with reasonable accuracy before they bear children. And genetic tests on unborn babies (examining cells removed from the amniotic fluid around the fetus) permit prenatal diagnosis as early as 2 months after conception. If the flawed gene is found, the fetus has CF and the parents can decide whether to terminate the pregnancy.

There is, however, a vigorous debate as to whether widespread, universal screening for CF should be performed before all existing mutations are known. Since the mutations reported to date add up to only 85 percent of the possible gene errors, mass screening done now would miss some carriers. And while the benefit of identifying carriers is clear most experts oppose widescale screening until at least 95 percent of the possible CF mutations are in.

For more information contact the Canadian Cystic Fibrosis Foundation.

DIABETES

Currently, in North America, diabetes is becoming a killer among all age groups, its increasing toll blamed on poor eating habits, obesity, and our couch-potato lifestyles. Diabetes is a health threat because it can damage so many parts of the body: blood vessels, eyes, feet, kidneys and heart. Over the past couple of decades, much has been learned about the causes and complications of diabetes, but there's no cure for this widespread disease. It still ranks as a major killer because it damages the circulation through coronary artery disease, the leading cause of death in North America. Diabetes affects about 5 percent of people living in the Western world, including at least 1.5 million Canadians, both adults and children. Yet many who have the disease remain unaware of it until major complications appear. *Diabetes mellitus*, to use its clinical name, is a disorder in which the body fails to keep blood sugar (glucose) at normal levels because of either a lack of the hormone insulin or failure to use it correctly. Made by beta cells in the *islets of Langerhans* within the pancreas, insulin is normally released into the blood stream as needed to help cells absorb and use glucose, keeping blood-sugar levels steady. But in those with diabetes, insulin fails to keep blood sugar within safe limits. Almost a quarter of those with diabetes require daily insulin injections.

There are three major types of diabetes

- Type 1 diabetes, also known as IDDM or insulin-dependent diabetes mellitus, in which the body makes too little or no insulin, with symptoms typically starting up during childhood, and requiring regular, daily insulin injections;
- Type 2 diabetes, also known as NIDDM or non-insulin-dependent diabetes mellitus, in which the body cannot regulate or use insulin properly, accounts for the vast majority of people with diabetes, typically appearing in adults, especially those who are obese or overweight. This group tends to be treated initially with dietary changes and weight loss, and may later require medications. Type 2 diabetes is also becoming more common among younger people, even teenagers, owing to the rise in obesity;
- Gestational Diabetes, which appears during pregnancy, affects 2 to 4 percent of all preg-

nancies, possibly predicting a tendency to develop the disease down the road.

Understanding the basics of diabetes

Diabetes is a disease where the body's cells cannot use glucose (sugar) properly for lack of or resistance to the hormone insulin, produced by the pancreas. In severe, untreated diabetes the body's cells are starved of the "fuel" needed for energy, and the tissues may "melt away" in a state resembling severe malnutrition.

Normally, insulin keeps blood levels of glucose within safe limits, ranging from 4–7 mmol/L. But in people with type 1 diabetes who have too little or no insulin, blood glucose may reach dangerously high levels, and if left untreated the high blood sugar can lead to dehydration, coma and possible brain damage. Some of the excess blood sugar may spill out into the urine—"sweet urine" is a telltale sign of the disease.

The most immediate danger in diabetes is *hyperglycemia* or high blood sugar, which can lead to ketoacidosis, with a buildup of ketone bodies in the blood and possible diabetic coma, even death. Persistently raised levels of blood sugar may lead to long-term circulatory complications such as blindness, kidney failure, nerve degeneration, stroke and heart disease.

The modern management of diabetes emphasizes good nutrition, adherence to diet, regular exercise and medications to keep blood sugar in the desirable range and offset the worst consequences. Experts advise those with diabetes to eat at regular times and exercise at the same time each day if possible.

Probing the insulin connection

The body normally regulates the absorption of glucose into cells and controls its level in blood with the help of insulin, a hormone produced by an area of the pancreas known as the *islets of Langerhans*. The pancreatic beta cells secrete insulin into the blood as needed—especially after meals.

Glucose is vital to life, but it cannot get into cells without insulin, which assists in transporting it across cell membranes. Once in the blood, this hormone signals liver, muscle, fat and other tissues to take up glucose. Insulin also encourages the removal of fat from the blood. If the pancreatic beta cells make too little insulin (as in type 1 diabetes), or if the body's cells can't respond to it (as in type 2 diabetes), the tissues will be short of their essential fuel and will draw on protein and fat stores to make up for the lack. The classic symptoms of diabetes are blurred vision, frequent urination (polyuria), excessive thirst (polydipsia) and weight loss.

Diabetes is usually diagnosed by a blood test done after fasting for 12 hours—the fasting glucose test. A high blood sugar reading confirms the presence of diabetes.

In poorly controlled diabetes, alternate fuel stores are used to the point where the person may lose weight and feel tired most of the time. If blood sugar levels remain out of control, the body can suffer lasting abuse, resulting in complications such as kidney failure, stroke, heart disease, nerve damage and eye problems. Diabetes is a leading cause of blindness in North America and a frequent reason for people to go on dialysis or require kidney transplants.

Type 1 or insulin-dependent diabetes mellitus (IDDM)

Type 1 diabetes, formerly called "juvenile" diabetes but now known as insulin-dependent diabetes mellitus, accounts for about 10 percent of all diabetes and affects 1 in 600 North Americans, mostly children, often showing up in childhood or early adolescence with symptoms such as extreme fatigue, constant thirst and dramatic weight loss.

Type 1 diabetes, or IDDM, is now viewed as a progressive autoimmune disorder in which antibodies attack the body's own insulin-producing beta cells, resulting in insulin deficiency. At diagnosis, 70 to 90 percent of those with IDDM have identifiable anti-insulin and anti-islet antibodies. The triggers that lead to the autoimmune destruction aren't fully understood, but may include genetic and environmental factors. Researchers have identified some genetic markers (HLA or *human leukocyte antigens*) that occur more frequently than usual in people with type 1 diabetes, and they are searching for other markers that may identify those at greatest risk.

Studies of identical twins show that if one has type 1 diabetes there is a 50 percent chance that the other twin will also develop the disorder. But the unpredictability suggests that although the susceptibility to IDDM is inherited, unknown triggers—possibly a virus, toxin or some dietary ingredient—"trip" the autoimmune process into action. Most cases of IDDM occur without a family history of diabetes.

The symptoms of type 1 diabetes—frequent urination, blurred vision, unusual thirst, extreme hunger, tiredness, irritability and nausea—often strike suddenly. Unable to make insulin themselves, people with type 1 diabetes rely on lifelong insulin replacement by injection. The more consistent and regular the timing of insulin shots, the better the control and the easier it is to balance insulin action to activity and diet. People with type 1 diabetes must learn to be consistent in their food intake, exercise regularly and self-administer insulin shots as needed, in correct doses.

Fortunately, people with type 1 diabetes can now be kept alive by lifelong use of insulin —first isolated by the historic Banting and Best research team at the University of Toronto physiology department in 1921. Treatment aims to mimic or duplicate as closely as possible the body's normal control of blood sugar with regular insulin doses to prevent fluctuations in blood sugar. Very recent studies confirm that intensive therapy to keep blood sugar levels as normal as possible *markedly* lowers the risk of diabetic complications such as eye and kidney problems. "These results," notes one researcher "show that more frequent insulin injections, better monitoring and stricter diets can halve the rate of major complications, including blindness, kidney failure and nerve damage."

Insulin is available in short-, medium- or long-acting forms. Thanks to recombinant genetic engineering, besides beef (cow) and pork (pig) insulin, there is now also a human variety that causes fewer skin and allergy problems, although it's shorter acting. However, human insulin is more expensive than animal-based products and provides neither better control nor fewer serious complications.

Managing diabetes is a balancing act involving frequent and diligent blood-sugar monitoring with accurate dosing of insulin to gear treatment to one's own lifestyle and activities. Most manage to lead active, productive lives. The management of diabetes has improved immensely with recent advances, allowing more freedom and easier travel. These improvements include easy-to-use home glucose monitors (small enough to fit into a pocket or purse), less cumbersome injection devices and more versatile forms of insulin allowing it to be more precisely tailored to fluctuating blood sugar readings. Many people with diabetes achieve the best control by using a mixture of fast- and intermediate-acting forms, geared to their particular needs. Insulin requirements increase at times of stress, illness or extra activity and during pregnancy. People with the disease can plan ahead for such events as dining out, a fitness class or an anticipated stress situation, testing their blood sugar levels and injecting insulin accordingly. The injection site should be rotated, and experts caution about the need to watch for nighttime dips or peaks in insulin action, to avoid problems while asleep. As low blood sugar levels (hypoglycemia) can occur during sleep and go unrecognized, it is wise to check nighttime blood sugar from time to time.

Taking care of type 1 diabetes is a daily ritual, not so different (time-wise) from brushing one's teeth twice daily. To get a handle on how well insulin injections are keeping blood sugar at safe levels throughout the day and night, blood must be regularly tested (before and after meals, before and after exercise) for its sugar content. This means using simple test kits, most of which register a color change according to the amount of sugar in a drop of blood. The latest blood-sugar monitors can measure glucose through the skin, avoiding the need for finger pricking. In the near future, there will be "glucowatches" that keep constant tabs on blood glucose levels. People with type 1 diabetes must also know how, when and why to test for the presence of ketones in urine. (If the ketone reading is high, a doctor should always be consulted.) And for an accurate overall picture of blood-sugar control, they need a glycolysated hemoglobin (HbA1c) test every few months, done in a lab.

How new methods facilitate insulin therapy

Fortunately, insulin injections are now more tolerable, as modern devices have very fine needles that are more comfortable to use.

WARNING SIGNS OR SYMPTOMS OF DIABETES INCLUDE:

- extreme or unusual tiredness and lethargy ;
- increased thirst (polydipsia);
- frequent urination, day and night;
- changes in appetite; unexplained, possibly
- dramatic weight loss;
- blurred vision;
- itchy skin, slow healing of cuts and wounds; frequent skin infections;
- abdominal pain, nausea;
- curiously "sweet-

smelling" breath;
- tingling or numbness in the limbs. Anyone with these symptoms—including people known to have diabetes—should promptly consult a physician.

There are also advances in ways to monitor blood glucose, easier calculation of the needed insulin dose and simpler injection devices. Different insulins that peak at varying times allow more flexibility. Long-acting forms designed to last 24 hours and fast-acting forms such as *lispro* (Humalog) that take effect within 15 minutes also improve control.

Modern, easy-to-use home blood glucose monitors have essentially replaced the older dipstick urine tests. Blood glucose monitoring was introduced for home use in the late 1970s. Self-monitoring of blood glucose on a finger prick sample can be done with a visually read paper strip (Chemstrip) or with a small, portable meter—a major advance in diabetic management. Some people with diabetes test once a day at a specific time, others more often.

Portable meters can now read the chemical strips and show exact blood sugar levels. Most blood glucose monitors (e.g., Glucometer, Glucosan, Accucheck, One-touch, EXAC-TECA) are small enough to fit in a purse or a pocket and can be used almost anywhere. Some contain an electronic memory, and more advanced models even have built-in modems for transmitting the test results directly to the physician. It is wise to check the home monitor's accuracy from time to time, by doing a self-test on a blood sample that's also sent for laboratory evaluation.

There are now many innovative, user-friendly self-injection methods, with increasingly simpler devices. Especially popular are the new disposable pre-loaded insulin-injecting "pens," about the size of a large fountain pen, which combine the needle, syringe and a vial of insulin all in one and can be carried in the pocket. The small, lightweight insulin pens (e.g., Novolin Pen and B-

D Pen) are plastic devices with a screw mechanism that dials up the necessary dose and injects the needed insulin through the skin with a simple click. The pens are especially useful for intensive control requiring frequent insulin shots. (Their disadvantage is that pens are costlier and, being preloaded, they don't allow for individual mixing or adjustment of slow- and fast-acting insulins.)

Other new ways to administer insulin include insulin pumps smaller than a cell phone that infuse a steady supply or doses at regular times, either implanted or worn on the belt or inside the clothes, which suit some people but give no better control than multiple daily injections. Researchers are also developing skin patches and inhaled insulin preparations.

On the horizon and being researched are transplants of pancreatic islet cells which may some day help to cure people with certain forms of diabetes, replacing the need for insulin injections. For example, a research team at the University of Alberta has successfully pioneered the use of islet cell transplants in certain patients, and the same is happening at other centers, although not yet available for routine use. Other efforts are concentrating on growing beta cells in the lab or encapsulating them for insertion to prevent their destruction by the body's immune system (antibody) defences when transplanted.

Type 2 or non–insulin-dependent diabetes mellitus (NIDDM)

Once called "maturity" or "adult-onset" diabetes but now labeled type 2 diabetes mellitus, this form tends to develop gradually in later life. By age 65, it affects 10 percent of the North American population, much of it going undiagnosed. Many people with type 2 diabetes have none of the usual symptoms (frequent urination, vision problems, tingling of arms, legs or feet and slow healing) and therefore remain oblivious to the problem for years, until complications begin to appear. Owing to the diuretic effect produced by elevated blood glucose, frequent urination may be an alerting symptom, also sugar in the urine, but the condition is usually diagnosed by a routine blood test.

The strongest factors predisposing people to type 2 diabetes are a family history of diabetes and obesity, the risks being almost directly proportional to body weight. In North America, 80 percent of those diagnosed are overweight (but the condition can also develop in lean individuals). Today, vast numbers of overweight people are increasingly at risk for type 2 diabetes. For instance, Aboriginal people in Canada are now at special risk of the disease, which was virtually unknown in that population 50 years ago.

People most at risk for type 2 diabetes include the following:

- anyone who's overweight or obese, especially with excess abdominal fat
- people with close relatives who have or had diabetes
- people of African, Hispanic, Asian or Aboriginal descent
- people with poor blood lipid (fat) readings (e.g., high LDL-cholesterol or triglycerides)
- the physically inactive or under-exercised
- women who have had gestational diabetes during pregnancy, or who have borne babies weighing more than 4 kilograms (9 pounds)

Diabetes is typically diagnosed with a fasting blood sugar test, done after a 12-hour fast, and repeated if the blood sugar levels are elevated. Some patients are also confirmed with an oral glucose tolerance test, in which a fasting patient is given a sugary drink to see how the body handles it.

Patients who have type 2 diabetes are usually treated in steps, first with dietary and exercise improvement, later with medication if and when needed. Those diagnosed with a pre-diabetic condition (who have a fasting blood sugar of 6–7 mmol/L) or actual type 2 diabetes (a fasting sugar above 7 mmol/L) are typically started on a lifestyle change program, with nutritional and exercise advice to reduce the risks of progression to diabetes proper. Two large trials have shown that if obese patients with pre-diabetes take steps to reduce their saturated fat intake, increase their fiber consumption, reduce their weight by 5 to 7 percent and are active for at least 25 minutes a day, they can halve the chances of their progression to diabetes. This is the good news. The bad news is that type 2 diabetes tends to get worse over time and thus needs oral medications and sometimes even insulin shots in the long run.

Certain oral medications work well while the pancreas still produces some insulin, stimulating it to make more or use it better. First-line medical therapy for type 2 diabetes is *biguanide* (metformin), which increases insulin sensitivity and induces the body's cells to take up glucose faster. Other oral medications traditionally used for type 2 diabetes are the *sulfonylureas* (such as DiaBeta, Glyburide, Dymelor), which stimulate the pancreas to make more insulin. Newer medications include Acarbose and Prandase (an alpha-glucosidase inhibitor), which slows absorption and sugar uptake in the digestive tract. The *thiazolidinediones*, *rosiglitazone* (Avandia), and *pioglitazone* (Actos), act by increasing insulin sensitivity in fat, muscle and liver so that these cells increase their consumption of glucose The *nonsulfonylureas—nateglinide* (Starlix) and *repaglinide* (GlucoNorm)—stimulate insulin production.

The downside of some of these oral antidiabetic agents is possible weight gain as they stimulate appetite and promote fat storage, and they may also trigger a bout of hypoglycemia (low blood sugar). So people with diabetes must be on the lookout for signs of hypoglycemia that include shakiness, trembling, confusion, irritability, sweating, clammy hands, staggering and, possibly, sudden ravenous hunger. To be prepared, they can carry quickly absorbed sugary snacks such as fruit juice or a couple of sugar cubes. After a while, oral antidiabetic agents often lose their effectiveness and insulin injections may be needed. It's a mistake to think of type 2 as "mild" diabetes just because routine insulin injections aren't needed to sustain life. Having type 2 diabetes provides a cardiovascular risk similar to that of already having had a heart attack.

Gestational diabetes (in pregnancy)

Gestational diabetes affects 2 to 5 percent of pregnancies, and in Canada pregnant women are advised to have screening tests—especially those who are obese, or have a family history of diabetes—for the condition during weeks 24 to 28 of gestation. In some pregnant women, diabetes develops for the first (and only) time and seems to differ somewhat from types 1 and 2. In pregnancy, two things may trigger diabetes: first, weight gain, second, the production of certain hormones (such as cortisol and placental lactogen) in quantities that alter the way insulin works, making blood sugar levels rise and perhaps tipping a predisposed woman into a transient diabetic state. Older, overweight diabetic women are at greater risk of producing *macrosomic* (large but immature) infants. A baby born to a diabetic mother, although very large (4.5 kg or 10 lb), may have immature organs and suffer the complications of prematurity.

If blood sugar levels cannot be normalized (and occasionally even if they are), complications may arise during pregnancy. New research suggests that the condition is due to enhanced resistance to insulin rather than to full-fledged diabetes and that the fetal risks may have been overestimated. Gestational diabetes may vanish after delivery but recur in subsequent pregnancies. Statistics from the Canadian Diabetes Association show that, after giving birth, about 30 to 40 percent of women with gestational diabetes eventually develop type 2 diabetes.

Women who already have diabetes and wish to become pregnant should get preconception counseling, plan their pregnancy carefully and make sure to get their diabetes well under control first. With adequate control of blood sugar, they have as good a chance of successful pregnancy outcomes as nondiabetics.

The many possible complications of diabetes

Eye problems in diabetes arise because of bleeding from burst blood vessels in the retina, known as *diabetic retinopathy*, which can occur without warning—so those affected should have regular eye checkups. If caught in time, the blood vessel may be sealed with laser treatment. The vision blurring that happens from time to time is *not* related to retinal blood flow problems, and may vanish on its own with better blood glucose control. Strict attention to blood sugar levels is believed to reduce the danger of eye damage.

The arterial blood vessel changes that commonly accompany diabetes occur for unknown reasons, possibly because high levels of circulating glucose damage the walls of large blood vessels, which develop weak spots that balloon out or build atherosclerotic plaque.

Nephropathy (kidney disease) is another complication of poorly controlled diabetes, resulting in leakage of protein into the urine, buildup of waste products in blood and blood vessel problems. Signs of kidney damage may include protein in the urine and swelling of hands and feet.

Neuropathy (nerve damage) is also a possible complication, perhaps signaled by shooting pains in the legs or feet, or by tingling (numbness) in the limbs and a diminished ability to feel pain—especially in the feet—necessitating meticulous foot care.

Treatment of diabetes

Treatment aims have now changed for people who need to manage their diabetes. In the past, doctors used to focus on keeping blood sugar within acceptable limits through careful attention to diet, exercise and, when needed, through use of medications. Now diabetes is viewed as a major risk factor for heart disease, and so people with the condition are urged to lower their blood pressure and blood cholesterol, in order to reduce the risk of heart problems. Diabetes management includes education about the disease, attention to diet, regulated meal plans, weight control, adequate exercise, adherence to insulin or other medication regimes and help in adjusting to the disorder. Nurse educators, physicians, dietitians, pharmacists and other health professionals work closely with diabetics to improve good management.

One primary goal in managing diabetes is to limit blood sugar swings—preventing either hyperglycemia (high blood sugar) or transient hypoglycemia (low blood sugar). In those taking medications for diabetes, there is always a chance that an occasional excess of insulin or antidiabetic agent will cause "hyperinsulinism" and transient hypoglycemia with symptoms that may include irritability, trembling, faintness, clammy hands, blurred vision, mood swings, personality changes, sweating, ravenous hunger (especially for sweets), headache, dizziness, nausea, as well as a staggering gait, slurred speech and drowsiness. The condition is swiftly remedied by consuming something rich in sugar such as a couple of sugar cubes, a glass of juice, a candy or a spoonful of honey. If the hypoglycemic episodes happen often, see a physician about adjusting doses of insulin or other medications.

When a meal is unavoidably delayed, those on insulin should plan ahead and compensate by "borrowing" from the next meal or snack (perhaps nibbling some cheese and crackers). They must always be prepared for bouts of low blood sugar and carry quickly absorbed sugary snacks. As delays in restaurants are common, those with diabetes are advised to "have a little something" at home first when eating out. If blood sugar seems low, start the meal with juice as an appetizer.

When traveling, people with diabetes may need to compensate with more frequent insulin shots for the extra stress and activity, and going through time zones requires vigilance in timing meals and medication. It's wise to keep food on hand for emergencies (e.g., small cans of juice, crackers, dried fruit) to avoid low blood sugar.

Diet plays a key role in managing diabetes

Diet is critical in managing diabetes and is best prescribed by a qualified dietitian who can tailor the diet to the individual's lifestyle. It entails not just losing weight (for those who are overweight), but also knowing which foods to eat and when. Diabetic diets are fortunately becoming more flexible and relaxed and, given good planning, diabetics are now allowed to eat a wide range of foods. However, meals must be regular and eaten every 4 to 6 hours, without skipping. Current dogma suggests a heart-healthy, low-fat diet rich in complex carbohydrates from whole grains, legumes (peas, beans, lentils) and vegetables, with less than 30 percent of total calories coming from fats. But there's still considerable debate over the best diabetic diet. Some experts feel that, provided meals are regular, it doesn't much matter what is eaten, while others suggest that saturated fats should be radically reduced with an accompanying increase in the intake of complex carbohydrates—to "flatten out" the post-meal rise in blood sugar.

Many specialists argue that diets low in fats and high in complex carbohydrates—once forbidden for diabetics—reduce the levels of LDL ("bad") cholesterol, moderate the post-meal rise in blood sugar and improve glucose tolerance. The latest theory is that complex carbo-hydrates may have beneficial effects in flattening the rise in blood sugar and/or increased sensi-tivity to insulin (so that smaller amounts of insulin are more effective). The Canadian Diabetes Association recommends that carbo-hydrates be eaten primarily in the form of legumes, grains, breads and pastas. Foods to avoid include sugar-laden and fatty items such as cookies, cakes, crackers and processed foods.

It has recently been shown that good life-long blood glucose control can help to prevent many diabetes-linked complications. Therefore, people with diabetes must learn to eat at regu-lar times, with regular snacks, without overeating or skipping meals. It's a difficult regime, and many, especially teenagers, need professional counseling and careful dietary plan-ning. Teachers should be alerted to the disorder and equipped with food and the knowledge to deal with potential problems (especially episodes of low blood sugar). The glycemic index, which is a way of assessing foods by the manner and speed with which they raise blood sugar levels, was recently introduced to help manage diabetic diets.

Overall, the current advice from the Canadian Diabetes Association is that 50 to 60 percent of a diabetic's daily calories come from complex carbohydrates, primarily those in whole grains (oat bran, cracked wheat and the like), legumes and vegetables. In general, people with diabetes can eat what everybody else is supposed to eat—a heart-healthy diet comprised of 55 to 60 percent complex carbo-hydrates, about 12 to 25 percent protein, 30 percent or less of the total calories as fat (only 10 percent of the fat quota being the saturated type, 10 percent polyunsaturated forms, the rest monounsaturated fats) and no more than 300 mg of cholesterol a day. Sucrose (refined sugar) should be kept to a prescribed minimum (usually around 50 g a day). Of the artificial sweeteners, noncalorific aspartame is consid-ered safe, even in generous amounts. To keep this regime, it's a good idea to get practical advice from a dietitian.

Exercise also is crucial for good control of diabetes

Physical activity promotes the sensitivity of tis-sues to both insulin and other antidiabetic agents, and regular exercise can guard against or combat type 2 (obesity-linked) diabetes—which accounts for over three-quarters of all cases. Exercise increases sugar uptake by the muscles and produces a short-term improvement in insulin sensitivity—an improvement that disap-pears within a few days of discontinuing an exercise program. Exercise also helps those who are obese to lose weight, improves the blood lipid (fat) profile and may reduce the risks of car-diovascular disease, a major cause of increased mortality in those with either type 1 or type 2

PRECAUTIONS FOR EXERCISING (WITH DIABETES)

- **Try to fit regular exercise into the daily routine at about the same time each day.**
- **Check blood sugar before and after exer-cising to determine the effect of activity.**
- **Ideally, exercise when blood glucose is within acceptable limits, because when the level is either too high or too low vigor-ous activity can cause problems.**

- **A sensible time to exercise is 30 minutes after a meal, when blood sugar is rising.**
- **Never exercise if blood sugar is above a certain prescribed level, or if ketones are present in blood or urine.**
- **Avoid exercising dur-ing the peak insulin action, as this is the time of greatest risk for hypoglycemia.**
- **Inject insulin into**

muscles that won't be worked (e.g., if cycling, inject into the abdomen rather than the thigh). Injecting insulin into or near a hardwork-ing muscle speeds its absorption and may cause hypoglycemia.
- **Note any signs of low blood glucose during and after exercise— for instance, dizziness, confusion or hunger.**
- **Compensate with**

extra food for extra activity, especially if it's strenuous (for instance, playing hockey, speed-swim-ming or running)—perhaps adding one fruit choice per hour of vigorous activity. Get advice on the best way to compensate for blood-sugar use while exercising.
- **Take extra fluids or skip exercise on par-**

ticularly warm days to avoid the risk of dehydration.
- **Carry sugary snacks—such as hard candies, glucose tablets or some other readily absorbed form of carbohy-drate—to use if signs of low blood glucose appear.**
- **Wear a medical alert card or bracelet to identify yourself as having diabetes.**

FOOT CARE FOR THOSE WITH DIABETES MEANS:

- avoiding injury by not going barefoot;
- washing feet daily and drying well;
- preventing dry skin by use of moisturizing creams;
- wearing clean socks daily;
- changing footwear often;
- checking inside shoes
- for sharp bits or bulges;
- avoiding thongs (which may irritate the foot);
- doing a daily "foot check" for sores, blisters, scratches or any other injury;
- filing or cutting nails straight across, taking care to avoid
- nicks (if unable to see well, get someone else to keep your nails short);
- removing calluses gently with pumice or emery boards;
- consulting a physician about any foot sores, pain or redness.

diabetes. Many individuals are unrealistic about their weight and want to lose over 25 percent, whereas health gains are already realized at 5 to 7 percent loss or even just by maintaining one's current weight.

Canadian and U.S. diabetes associations urge people with diabetes to exercise regularly. But as strenuous exercise can aggravate preexisting health problems (for example, by precipitating episodes of arrhythmia in someone with heart disease or by damaging arthritic knees), a thorough medical examination is advised before embarking on a fitness program. Proper footwear is mandatory, as diabetes can reduce the circulation and sensation in the feet. People with diabetes must wear well-fitting shoes and inspect their feet daily for injury after exercising. Blood sugar levels must also be monitored when planning an exercise routine. Taking a few precautions can make regular physical activity a valuable component of diabetic care and help in managing the disease.

Good foot care is essential for those with diabetes

Neuropathy—nerve degeneration—puts the feet in jeopardy due to reduced circulation, increased risks of infection and loss of sensation, which obscures pain so that blisters, sores and other foot injuries don't hurt. People with diabetes must take special care of their feet, shake the shoes before donning them to remove foreign objects and do a daily inspection of the toes, heels, soles, nails and between the toes for sores, cuts, broken skin and any injuries. Many wear specially made shoes to help prevent foot problems. Rotating the shoes—not wearing the same pair

all the time—is a good idea so that one part of the foot doesn't get constantly rubbed or sore.

Some recent developments

Despite an intensive search for ways to eliminate the need for insulin injections, daily insulin shots continue to be the rule for many with insulin-dependent diabetes. Oral insulin is out of the question, as stomach acids destroy the hormone. Several imaginative attempts have been made to develop insulin suppositories, vaginal and anal forms, nose drops and so on, but so far without great success. For blood sugar monitoring, a machine is being developed to detect glucose levels through the skin, avoiding the need for finger pricking. Current trials are underway to assess the value of inhaled insulin.

Immunosuppressants have been tried for type I diabetes. The autoimmune process resulting in the destruction of beta cells takes several years to appear and suggests that immunosuppressive drugs given early in the disease might halt or at least slow its progress. Cyclosporin (an immunosuppressant widely used in transplant operations), started early in diabetes, can induce remission in 10 to 20 percent of young sufferers. Unfortunately, its potential side effects (kidney damage, for instance) detract from its usefulness.

The ideal situation for those with insulin-dependent diabetes would be to throw away the syringes and acquire transplanted, insulin-producing cells. Since rejection is the major problem with pancreas transplants, researchers are working on ways to protect the transplanted cells by surrounding them with a coating or microencapsulation, to protect them from the host's attacking cells.

For more information, contact the Canadian Diabetes Association.

DIZZINESS

Dizziness is among the top five reasons for doctor visits, especially among the elderly. Reassuringly, however, it seldom signals a life-threatening disorder and in the vast majority of cases, there's no worrisome reason for the dizziness. It is often due to anxiety or other psychological causes. In one clinic, over a third of all dizziness investigated was attributed to stress, lack of sleep and emotional problems. But dizziness can arise from inner-ear problems, neurological or cardiovascular ailments or just standing up too quickly.

Dizzy spells mean different things to different people

People use the term "dizziness" to describe a wide variety of symptoms ranging from mental confusion, lightheadedness, wooziness or imbalance to faintness, weak legs or the spinning sensation known as vertigo. If something goes wrong with the ear's balance system, dizziness may result.

Four main categories of dizziness

- *Vertigo*—a swirling, "merry-go-round" sensation—usually due to peripheral (inner-ear) or central (brain) abnormalities (see below).
- *Near-syncope or presyncope* (a near-faint or sense of an impending faint) without loss of consciousness. This mild form of dizziness is often due to orthostatic hypotension (a momentary drop in blood pressure that lessens blood flow to the brain), sometimes experienced on suddenly rising from a lying position. It can also related to heart problems, diabetic hypoglycemia (low blood sugar), vasovagal attacks (due to anxiety or fear, which affect the circulation) or from certain medications.
- *Dysequilibrium*—imbalance or unsteadiness—most frequent in the elderly, can stem from multiple causes, including ear defects, a recent cataract operation or the deterioration of sensory pathways. Typically, the unsteadiness occurs only when standing or walking and may contribute to falls in older people.
- *Lightheadedness*—a vague, confused sensation that can arise from stress, psychological disturbances or through hyperventilation (rapid breathing that lowers the blood's CO_2 content and constricts cerebral blood vessels).

Vertigo differs from other types of dizziness

Although the terms "dizziness" and "vertigo" are often used interchangeably, they are not the same thing. "While all vertigo is dizziness," notes one specialist, "not all dizziness is vertigo."

DIFFERENT FORMS OF VERTIGO

- *Benign positional paroxysmal vertigo* is the most common form, with attacks lasting 30 to 60 seconds, typically set off when rolling over in bed, moving the head to one side or reaching for something ("top-shelf vertigo"). Sufferers can usually describe specific head movements that trigger it. Although BPPV often occurs for no known reason, it can follow an ear infection, a head or ear injury and is thought to result from disturbance of the inner ear's balance detectors. People with BPPV are often relieved to hear that it's an inner-ear condition and does not signify something serious like a stroke or brain tumor. Dizziness from BPPV usually fades in a few months without any treatment. Special head exercises can help to "fatigue" the response and mute the dizzy spells.
- *Vestibular neuritis (or neuronitis)*, arising from viral infections (perhaps following a cold, flu or middle-ear infection) that affect the eighth cranial nerve may produce sudden vertigo, often accompanied by nausea, but no hearing loss, usually lasting one to three weeks. After recovery, a slight feeling of fullness in the ear and dizziness may persist for weeks to months.
- *Ménière's disease*, due to abnormal fluid accumulation in the inner ear, producing episodic attacks of intense vertigo—perhaps lasting hours—accompanied by fullness in the ear, tinnitus and some hearing loss, usually only on the affected side.
- *A perilymph fistula* or abnormal channel between the middle and inner ear—perhaps due to pressure changes when flying or diving, a head blow, whiplash or other injury—is a rare cause of vertigo.
- *Central nervous system disorders* may include vertigo as a symptom, including multiple sclerosis, epilepsy, certain forms of migraine, acoustic neuroma (benign tumor on the auditory nerve), cerebellar and brainstem tumors, and TIAs (transient ischemic attacks or mini-strokes).

Dizziness means general lightheadedness, imbalance or just feeling faint. Vertigo, from the Latin vertere, "to turn," is a circling sensation or distinct type of dizziness that's a movement hallucination. It is aptly described as a twirling sensation, a feeling that the room is swirling around or that one is spinning in space. It arises from abnormalities in the inner ear's vestibular balance system or from disruption of certain brain pathways (central vertigo).

Most vertigo (about 85 percent) is due to *peripheral* (inner ear) problems and often starts suddenly, can last seconds or hours (as with Ménière's disease) and is frequently accompanied by nausea, hearing loss and tinnitus or ringing in the ears.

In contrast, vertigo arising from central (brain) disorders accounting for 15 percent of

TYPE OF DIZZINESS

Vertigo—a rotational sensation; a spinning or whirling, swaying, room-whirling-around-me feeling

Peripheral (inner ear) causes:
• **Benign positional paroxysmal vertigo**
• **Vestibular neuronitis/labyrinthitis (viral infections)**
• **Ménière's disease**
• **Motion sickness**
• **Medication use (e.g., tranquilizers, heart drugs, aminoglycoids)**
• **Inner-ear dysfunction or trauma (e.g., head blow)**

Central causes:
• **Cerebellar brain disease (e.g., due to excess alcohol intake)**
• **Acoustic neuroma (tumor on the eighth or vestibular nerve)**
• **Multiple sclerosis**
• **Severe migraine headaches**
• **Temporal lobe seizure (epilepsy)—rare**

Presyncope—the sense of an impending faint or faintness
• **Arrhythmias and other heart problems (that reduce blood flow to the brain)**
• **Orthostatic hypotension (brief drop in blood pressure, e.g., if stand up too fast after lying down)**
• **Low cardiac output states**
• **Severe anemia**
• **Hypoglycemia (low blood sugar, as in diabetics)**

Dysequilibrium—loss of balance on standing or walking, unsteadiness
• **TIAs (mini- or pre-stroke signs)**
• **Eye problems (or new glasses)**
• **Dysequilibrium (imbalance) common with aging**
• **Parkinson's disease**
• **Medication use (e.g., streptomycin, gentamicin, ASA, blood pressure drugs, tranquilizers, diuretics)**

Lightheadedness—a vague sensation, giddiness, confusion, befuddlement (not enough to hamper daily activities)
• **Anxiety**
• **Depression**
• **Panic disorders**
• **Hyperventilation (rapid breathing, which lowers the blood's CO_2 content)**
• **Recurrent partial or "absence" seizures**
• **Senile dementia**

To discover the type and cause of dizziness, physicians take a thorough history, paying special attention to its first appearance. "It is not always easy to distinguish organic from psychological dizziness," explains one specialist, "but in general, people with psychogenic [psychological] dizziness tell longer rather rambling stories, while those with an organic cause describe the dizzy spells crisply, pinpointing their onset, duration and precipitating events." Dizzy people may have to repeat their story because the way it started often gives clues to its cause. For example, if turning over in bed sets off the dizziness, it suggests positional vertigo.

The ears, eyes and nervous system are also checked, in particular the ability of the eyes to follow an object (pursuit). The physician may try to reproduce the dizzy attacks—for example, by having the person hyperventilate for 60 seconds (if attacks occur when hyperventilating, psychological causes are suspected).

In those with true vertigo, the physician will test for hearing loss and nervous system dysfunction. If vertigo might arise from an inner-ear problem, a hearing test (audiogram) and a special balance test called the electronystagmogram (ENG) may be done. Dynamic posturography is another test: the dizzy person, attached to recording electrodes, is rotated on a movable platform to try to localize its cause. If there are hints of a neurological abnormality, computerized tomography (CT) and magnetic resonance imaging (MRI) scans may be advised.

Treatment varies, but all dizzy people need reassurance that the problem is usually not serious. For those with psychogenic or anxiety-provoked dizziness, the best remedy is to avoid precipitating factors and possibly try a mild sedative or tranquillizer. Those with stress-related dizziness need encouragement to worry less, perhaps improve sleep habits.

Vestibular neuronitis may respond to antinauseants and drugs such as *meclizine*. Dizziness from inner-ear disorders often has long periods of remission between spells, requiring no treatment. Those with acute attacks of vertigo are advised to rest during the episode and take an appropriate (prescribed) sedative until the attack subsides. For Ménière's disease, salt restriction, diuretics and other

cases—tends to appear gradually, last longer and is frequently accompanied by neurological symptoms such as numbness, swallowing difficulties, clumsiness or speech impairment.

Vertigo may be accompanied by jerky, rhythmic to-and-fro eye movements called *nystagmus*. The direction of these eye jerks can often reveal the cause of vertigo whether it is due to an inner-ear or brain defect.

strategies may help. (See chapter 6 for more on Ménière's disease.)

People with benign positional paroxysmal vertigo, or BPPV, may benefit from either the Epley maneuver—in which special physician-guided head movements are used that try to displace the inner ear's malpositioned crystals— or special head-tilting exercises, done several times daily, that purposely bring on and "fatigue" the vertigo, often making the dizzy spells vanish.

Medications help some forms of dizziness, for instance antinauseants (e.g., Gravol), antihistamines—such as *meclizine* (Antivert), *betahistine dihydrochloride* (Serc) and *dimenhydrinate* (Dramamine)—phenothiazines (such as *chlorpromazine*) and tranquilizers.

Surgery may be considered for serious cases of vertigo and includes operations on the inner ear's balance structures or the more drastic labyrinthectomy (destroying the inner ear's vestibular organs).

Chemical ablation of the inner ear's balance system is occasionally tried, using agents that preferentially destroy the ear's balance system (semicircular canals and otoliths), leaving hearing intact. Great care is needed for the operation.

For more information, consult your family physician, an otolaryngologist, neurologist or dizziness clinic (at some large hospitals).

DRY EYE

Tears are not just for weeping—they are essential for eye health. Dry eye or *keratitis sicca* is an umbrella term covering different disorders in which the eye's natural lubrication or tear film dries up. The eyes look red and feel irritated, gritty, burning, itchy and heavy. Paradoxically, dry eyes may tear excessively (in reaction to the irritation), with an accumulation of sticky mucus. Some sufferers can pull long strings of mucus from their eyes!

Common symptoms of dry eye
- burning (as if there were soap or shampoo in the eyes);
- grittiness (as though there were sand in the eyes);
- itching or scratchiness (like an insect bite);
- photophobia (inability to stand bright light, especially fluorescent);

- occasionally, a sticky, mucus discharge.

Tears are for more than crying
Seemingly watery expressions of sadness or laughter, or a response to peeling onions, tears serve many purposes. They make the eye's surface smooth and optically clear. Tears bathe the eye and allow the lids to slide smoothly over them; they carry oxygen and nutrients to nourish the cells of the cornea (outer transparent covering); they dilute and remove noxious toxins. Tears contain salts (electrolytes), enzymes, protein (albumin), immunoglobulins, peroxidases and protective antibacterials that prevent infection and keep the eye's surface safely sterile.

Treatments for dry eye
Therapy for dry eye aims to preserve the eye's own lubrication, and uses artificial tears to increase moisture and correct any contributing causes. For the very severely dry-eyed, surgery—punctal occlusion—may be tried. It retards tear drainage by occluding or closing the tiny ducts through which tears drain out of the eye. Since blocking these ducts can cause overflow problems, the operation is ideally first done as a trial run, using temporary collagen implants (that slowly dissolve in a week) or removable silicone plugs to block the holes. If the procedure doesn't cause overflow, the ophthalmologist may do a permanent blockage.

Tear-replacement is the mainstay for treating dry eyes, using lubricating ointments or drops to add moisture and reform a tear-like layer. Many tear substitutes are available—both prescribed and over the counter. They include *polyvinyl alcohol*, *cellulose derivatives* and *mucomimetics*. Besides tear replacement, lubricants, mostly used at night, can help to relieve the dryness.

Severe cases may require tear replacement every hour, even every 15 minutes. If artificial tears are needed more than six times daily, a *nonpreserved*, single-dose artificial tear preparation is recommended, to avoid irritation from the preservatives. (The main disadvantage of nonpreserved artificial tears is their slightly higher cost.)

The drawbacks of artificial tears are their short-acting capacity and need for repeat application; and people with very dry eyes may not have enough natural tears to dissolve the preservatives in them—in which case the tear substitutes may provoke rather than alleviate the irritation. Newer nonpreserved solutions are less likely to cause sensitivity.

Sjögren's syndrome (SS)—an autoimmune disorder that involves the body's antibodies attacking its own salivary and lacrimal glands—is a notorious cause of dry mouth, and also dry eyes and a dry vagina. SS affects about one per 2,500 people, women more than men, usually starting in middle age.

For more information contact the Sjögrens Syndrome Foundation, (516) 767-2866.

EMERGING INFECTIOUS DISEASES: A NEW DANGER

The threat of emerging infections lies not only in newly identified diseases but also in the reemergence of old ones that have become resistant to the antibacterial drugs (antibiotics) used against them. Scientists are alarmed at the rapid emergence of bacterial strains resistant to most or all of the antibiotics used to kill them. For example, tuberculosis is now back in a more threatening, multi-drug-resistant form. "This is a huge setback," notes one microbiologist. "We may soon have no drugs to treat this disease, and may even have to resort to surgery and other methods used for TB long ago, in the pre-antibiotic era."

Equally worrisome are drug-resistant strains of *Salmonella, Staphoylococcus aureus* (a threat for wound infections), *Neisseria gonorrhoeae* (responsible for gonorrhea), *Campylobacter* and *Enterococci* (which cause diarrhea), *Shigella* organisms and the *Pneumococci* that cause sinusitis, pneumonia, meningitis and middle ear infections.

Antibiotic resistance spreads fast. For example, a survey by the U.S. Centers for Disease Control showed that whereas in 1987 only 0.02 percent of pneumococcal strains infecting hospital patients were penicillin resistant, today 6.6 percent of pneumococcus strains are resistant. Resistance to common staphylococci and streptococci has also risen astronomically.

Vancomycin resistance is a new and especially worrisome threat because this antibiotic was the antibiotic of last resort for multi-drug-resistant infections. Until now, vancomycin, always worked where other antibacterials failed. Vancomycin-resistant enterococci (VRE), first

reported in Europe in 1987, and detected in a New York hospital in 1989, are rising at a significant pace. Vancomycin resistance is now affecting hard-to-vanquish hospital staphylococcal infections that resist all antibiotics except vancomycin.

Why has this happened? "Drug resistance has arisen partly due to complacency," explains one infectious-disease specialist, "and the false perception that we had licked bacterial infections. Many drug companies stopped working on new antibacterials, turning to other areas. Now, in the late 1990s, we've come to a point where we don't have any agents left for certain infections. Researchers have identified bacteria that resist *all* currently available antibiotics."

Antibiotic resistance develops because in any population of bacteria there are variants with unusual traits that can withstand antibiotics. Technically, the antibiotic does not create resistance, but an *already existing*, drug-combatting variant flourishes, while drug-susceptible bacteria die off.

When someone takes an antibiotic, the drug kills the defenseless bacteria, leaving behind—or "selecting," in biological terms—the sturdy types that resist drug action. Bacteria become resistant to antibiotics when drug-combatting mutants multiply and flourish, while the weaker or less resistant forms die off in the drug-laden environment. The drug-resistant bacteria then multiply and become the predominant form. One specialist explains that "people can develop a drug-resistant infection either by contracting a resistant bug to begin with, or by having a resistant microbe emerge in the body once antibiotic treatment begins. Drug-resistant infections are often associated with prolonged hospital stays. The drug-resisting genes can spread from one type of bacteria to another especially in hospital settings."

"Many consumers assume that antibiotics are the answer to almost all infections," says one expert, "and they pressure physicians to prescribe them even when the illness is viral, for which antibiotics are no use." Another problem is that patients often stop taking the drug too soon—when symptoms abate—allowing resistant microbes to proliferate. The infection may flare up a few weeks later requiring a different drug to treat it. Another key concern is use of low-level antibiotics in animal feeds to prevent disease and speed up weight gain, at the cost of increasing drug resistance.

Researchers fear we may be running out of the seemingly endless flow of antimicrobial drugs and that bacteria are outpacing human ingenuity. When penicillin-resistant microbes surfaced, pharmaceutical companies developed slightly different agents such as *methicillin* and *oxacillin*, later adding new drugs including *chloramphenicol, neomycin, teramycin, tetracycline* and *cephalosporins*. But bacteria have developed resistance to all of them.

Time to say no to antibiotic overuse

The solution, according to many health authorities, is stricter controls on antibiotic use, education of health professionals and the public about proper use, banning vancomycin in livestock (used to promote growth) and recognizing that we live in a global village and must be vigilant. Roughly half of all antibiotics prescribed today are considered unnecessary, or wrongly used, especially for upper-respiratory infections such as colds and bronchitis.

"It's high time," notes one family physician, "to unlearn these bad prescribing habits and distinguish conditions that require antibiotics from the many that don't." Experts believe antibiotics should only be offered to patients who can truly benefit from them. Physicians are urged to rethink the need to prescribe them. And when an antibiotic is required, older, narrow-spectrum antibiotics that only fight a few strains of bacteria should first be tried—for instance, erythromycin or amoxicillin—lessening the chance of multiple resistance. Experts discourage the modern practice of prescribing expensive, multi-attack, broad spectrum antibiotics for simple disorders such as bronchitis or sinusitis (which usually don't require such potent drugs).

Finally, we healthcare consumers must change the mindset that expects an antibiotic for every little sniffle, cold, flu or cough. As patients, we should also make absolutely sure we follow instructions, since taking just part of an antibiotic course and not thoroughly destroying the bacteria also breeds drug resistance.

EPILEPSY (SEIZURE DISORDER)

Anyone who has witnessed someone having an epileptic seizure can understand why the ancients thought that it represented "a visit from the gods." It's high time to set the record straight and replace superstition with science. In fact, epilepsy is a common neurological (brain) disorder, characterized by recurrent seizures, that usually has no impact on intelligence, character or ability. It affects about 1 in 100 people, equal numbers of males and females, three-quarters of whom develop the condition in childhood. Most people with seizures manage to carry on normal, productive lives, but it can be a difficult condition for people of all ages to manage—especially for adolescents, who are simultaneously undergoing hormonal changes and struggling with emerging independence. The management of epilepsy includes correct diagnosis, evaluation and medication, as well as dealing with any associated psychosocial problems.

Understanding epilepsy

Once called the "falling sickness," the term "epilepsy" takes its name from the Greek lepsis meaning "a seizure"—and that's just what the disorder is: a tendency to have recurrent seizures. Epilepsy sometimes called "seizure disorder"—is a neurological condition that predisposes the brain (or parts of it) to bursts or *paroxysms* of abnormal electrical activity.

Brain cells usually communicate in an orderly manner by means of electrochemical signals, mediated by neurochemicals that inhibit some messages, selectively allowing others through, to avoid "cross-talk" or nerve-message overload. But occasionally a group of brain cells simultaneously "fires" or discharges excess electrical signals that produce a temporary rise in electrical activity in certain parts of the brain. A seizure is thus due to a burst of electrical energy that temporarily disturbs normal brain function and may disrupt consciousness and muscular action—much as a lightning storm can disturb the electrical power supply.

The type of seizure reflects the brain areas affected by the electrical paroxysm, and the seizure may spread throughout the brain. A person with epilepsy can have more than one type of seizure. During a seizure, the body some-

AN AURA MAY BE ACCOMPANIED BY:

- distorted perception ("hallucinations") of sound, sight, smell and taste;
- dreamlike experiences, floating sensation;
- distortion of time, space, memory ("*déjà vu*" experiences);
- a curious taste in the mouth, hand tingling and other sensations.

SORTING OUT THE SEIZURES

- *Simple partial seizures* (formerly known as "focal seizures") may involve strange or unusual sensations, including sudden, jerky movements of one body part, distortions in hearing or sight, stomach upsets or a sudden sense of fear. Consciousness is not impaired. If no seizure follows, these sensations may simply be called an aura.
- *Complex partial seizures* (formerly called "psychomotor" or "temporal lobe" epilepsy) are most common in adults, but can occur at any age. They are characterized by complicated "automaton-like" actions and altered consciousness. Complex partial seizures are so termed because they affect complex cerebral functions rather than just muscular actions. In this type of seizure, memory usually fades, there's a loss of awareness and some impairment of learning and perception, but no drop attacks or falling episodes. Typically, the person seems dazed and confused, appears irritable and edgy, with glassy eyes

and ceaseless fidgeting, often performing purposeless actions such as random walking, mumbling, head turning or pulling at clothing. During the seizure some experience numbness of hands or feet, a choking sensation, sweating, strange, "*déjà vu*" dreams or visions. In some people, this seizure may consist merely of staring and a little lip-smacking and can be confused with absence seizures. After the episode, the person often has no memory of it and is usually sleepy. Although not violent, someone with complex partial epilepsy may struggle or fight if impeded during a seizure. This type of epilepsy is renowned because of its use as a defense ploy by some people accused of criminal actions: since the person supposedly had no awareness of what happened, the defense may argue that he or she bears no responsibility for the crime. However, most people with this form of epilepsy are not violent and during a seizure can not perform complicated

actions such as robbing, hitting or killing others.
- *Absence (formerly called "petit mal")* seizures are characterized by 5- to 10-second lapses in consciousness, during which the person stares mindlessly into space with the eyes rolling upwards. Most common in children aged 4 to 12, the seizure has a loss of consciousness, but no aura, no falls or drop attacks, just a lack of awareness during the attack. A child may simply appear momentarily blank, with blinking eyes, facial twitching, odd finger movements, confusion and inattention—as though daydreaming. However, unlike a daydreamer, the child cannot be aroused. Some children have several such brief seizures during the course of a day, without knowing it, with total amnesia (forgetfulness) afterwards. One-third of childhood absence seizures stop in adolescence.
- *Tonic-clonic (formerly "grand mal") seizures,* in which the brain is swamped with "electrical overload,"

involve two phases. In the tonic phase, the Individual loses consciousness, goes stiff and falls. The muscles go into spasm and the body becomes rigid. In the clonic stage, the limbs jerk repeatedly and twitch. Tonic-clonic seizures may just affect part of the body, but more often the entire body goes rigid, shakes and trembles. In this most dramatic of seizures, the person may cry out (not in fear or pain but as a reflex reaction when air is forced out of the lungs), contort the face, lose consciousness and fall to the ground. The person may briefly stop breathing and go blue. There may be some drooling, biting of cheeks or tongue and possibly loss of bladder and bowel control. Tonic-clonic seizures that begin locally (with a partial seizure) are usually preceded by an aura. Tonic-clonic seizures rarely last longer than a minute (averaging 40 seconds) and, although frightening to watch, generally pass without inflicting any harm—unless the

head is hit, the seizure happens while swimming or driving, for example, and leads to some other injury, or if the person chokes on vomit. After the seizure, consciousness slowly returns and the person may become limp and confused, usually falling into a deep sleep.
- *Status epilepticus* represents serial seizures—one after another—without recovery in between, the person coming partly out of one seizure and going into another. This is an emergency situation that risks permanent brain injury or death, and the person must promptly receive medical attention. Besides these main types of epileptic seizure, other subtypes include atonic or "drop attacks," procursive epilepsy (a complex-partial form with a curious, swift running behavior), photogenic epilepsy (triggered by flickering lights such as strobe lights, television or video games) and musicogenic epilepsy (set off by certain types of music).

times loses control of sensory systems (such as sight and hearing), breathing, body temperature and/or blood-pressure regulation, possibly also bowel and bladder action.

The causes of epilepsy

In many cases there is no identifiable cause for epileptic seizures and the condition is termed "idiopathic epilepsy." There may be a familial or genetic link.

When physicians can identify a reason for the disorder, it's called "symptomatic epilepsy," and the reasons include:

- head injury;
- birth trauma (e.g., lack of oxygen, forceps delivery);
- an excess of certain drugs or toxic substances—e.g., lead or theophylline bronchodilators (used for asthma), and illicit drugs (such as cocaine);
- stroke, brain tumors and other conditions that interrupt cerebral blood flow;
- low blood sugar (hypoglycemia);
- diseases that alter the balance of blood or its chemical constituents or those that damage brain cells (such as Tay-Sachs disease, multiple sclerosis);
- high fever in infancy (a rare cause);
- serious infections of the brain (such as encephalitis, meningitis, herpes).

Not all seizures add up to epilepsy

One seizure alone does not an epileptic make. Having had one or two seizures does not mean someone has epilepsy. Eight to 10 percent of people have isolated seizures, usually in infancy or old age. For example, a very high fever will provoke seizures in 2 to 5 percent of children aged 6 months to 5 years. While childhood seizures understandably frighten parents, and may—in a few cases—go on to become epilepsy, a seizure associated with fever does not usually signal epilepsy and does not harm the child. Almost any injury or condition that affects the brain can trigger a seizure—for example, fetal injuries, birth mishaps, newborn infections, anoxia (lack of oxygen). Certain metabolic diseases such as phenylketonuria are also accompanied by seizures. Other seizures not classed as epilepsy are those due to alcohol, drug withdrawal or a result of illnesses such as meningitis or encephalitis.

In contrast to isolated seizures, epilepsy involves *recurrent* seizures, varying from infrequent—occurring once or twice a year or less—to once a month or even several times daily. In some people, certain stimulants or triggers—such as flickering lights or excitement—bring on a seizure.

An "aura" or warning sign may herald a seizure

People with epilepsy often report curious sensations before a seizure. These vary from person to person and can take many forms, including strange smells, abdominal flutters, hallucinations, illusions (distorted perception), musical sounds, a sense of dread, feelings of tension or anxiety. The type of aura may help to pinpoint the abnormally reacting brain site. Odd smells may indicate that the medial temporal lobe is involved; strange sounds may indicate injury to the hearing area of the brain and so on.

The aura may occur far enough in advance to give the person time to lie down, thereby avoiding possible injury. An aura can occur without a seizure following, which may in some cases constitute a simple partial seizure.

Diagnosing epilepsy

Correct diagnosis and evaluation are imperative for the treatment of seizures. Disorders commonly mistaken for epilepsy include hysterical outbursts (psychogenic seizures), transient ischemic attacks (ministrokes) and migraine headaches. Studies show that one-fifth of those referred to epilepsy clinics have pseudoseizures—not true epilepsy. Correct diagnosis depends on careful history-taking—preferably with a description of the seizure by someone who witnessed it—blood tests, and neurological and electroencephalogram (EEG) exams to detect patterns of increased brain activity (The EEG procedure samples brain-wave activity via small electrodes placed on the scalp.) Additional tools for diagnosis include brain imaging with CAT (computerized axial tomography) scans, magnetic resonance imaging, single photon emission, computerized tomography and positron emission tomography.

STAGES OF AN EPILEPTIC SEIZURE

- **The prodome, or altered sensations occurring minutes to hours before a seizure (a rare experience);**
- **the aura—altered sensations or other early signs of a seizure, occurring before consciousness fades, usually seconds before a seizure (often suggesting focal onset);**
- **the ictus—the seizure itself;**
- **the postictal state— often with confusion and lethargy—following a seizure.**

EPILEPSY MEDICATIONS INCLUDE:

- *phenobarbital* **(Luminal);**
- *ethosuximide* **(Zarontin);**
- *primidone* **(Mysoline);**
- *phenytoin* **(Dilantin);**
- *valproic acid* **(Depakene or Epival);**
- *carbamazepine* **(Tegretol);**
- *clonazepam* **(Rivotril).**

New Add-on Drugs
clobazam **(Frisium)**
felbamate **(Felbatol)**
gabapentin **(Neurontin)**
lamotrigine **(Lamictal)**
tiagabine **(Gabitril)**
topiramate **(Topamax)**
vigabatrin **(Sabril)**
levetiracetam **(Keppra)**

FIRST AID—WHAT TO DO FOR SEIZURES

For tonic-clonic ("grand mal") seizures:
• Remain calm.
• Let the seizure run its course. You cannot stop a seizure once it has started. Do not try to revive or restrain the person. People having seizures don't know what they're doing and their body movements can be very powerful.
• Ease the person to the ground; loosen tight clothing.
• Remove glasses.
• Turn the head to one side to allow saliva to drain out. Do not put anything into the person's mouth.
• Remove any hard, sharp or hot objects that might injure the person. If the casualty is in a dangerous position (for example, at the top of a flight of stairs), you may be able to drag him or her a few feet away by the clothing, but be careful.
• After the seizure, allow the person to rest or sleep.
• After resting, most people can carry on as before. If the person is not at home and still seems groggy, weak or confused, it may be best to accompany him or her home.
• If a child has a seizure, contact the parents or guardian; if they are not available, be sure they are notified later.
• Allow the seizure to stop on its own. If it lasts more than 5 or 10 minutes, call for emergency medical services (dial 911).
• If the person starts to bleed from the mouth, do not panic. He or she has probably bitten the tongue and is not bleeding internally.
• Do not be frightened if the person appears to stop breathing for a few seconds only. This is to be expected.

• If the person undergoes a series of seizures, with each new one occurring before consciousness is regained, immediately seek emergency medical assistance.
• Do not attempt resuscitation unless the person fails to start breathing again once the seizure stops. If this happens, begin artificial respiration and call an ambulance.
• When the seizure is over (if not possible before), place the person in the "recovery position" (see Chapter 11) to keep the airway open and prevent the possibility of breathing vomitus or saliva into the lungs.
• After a tonic-clonic ("grand mal") seizure, the person should be checked by a physician so that any injuries may be detected or necessary adjustments made in the medication.
• After the seizure, stay close by and reassure the person once he or she is awake.
• Do not give food or drink until fully awake.
• Record the seizure's duration.

For complex partial ("psychomotor") seizures:
• Do not restrain. Protect from injury by moving away sharp or hot objects.
• If wandering occurs, stay with the person and talk quietly and reassuringly.

For simple partial (focal) seizures:
• No first aid required.

For absence ("petit mal") seizures:
• No first aid required.

New classification of seizures

The frequency and form of seizure vary greatly from person to person. Because there are so many nuances in epilepsy and so many different kinds of seizure (over 30 types), a new classification system has been established by the International League against Epilepsy (ILAE), which aims to replace outdated seizure terminology such as "grand mal" and "petit mal."

According to the new classification, there are two basic types of epilepsy:
• *generalized epilepsy,* where the seizure activity spreads throughout the brain, disabling large areas of consciousness, even if the attack begins as a focal (local) burst of abnormal electrical activity;
• *partial epilepsy,* where specific, localized areas of the brain are affected and the abnormal

electrical activity is confined to a small area—a condition possibly arising from a head blow or injury, birth complications, meningitis, encephalitis, central-nervous-system infection or other identifiable causes.

The distinction between "partial" and "generalized" seizures is the key to the new classification. In focal or partial seizures, the most frequently encountered type, the electrical overstimulation, is confined to a small brain area without any loss of consciousness. But if the seizure activity involves centers of consciousness on both sides of the brain, with loss of consciousness, it is said to be generalized. But even a generalized seizure may produce so minor a change in function that the person having the seizure is unaware of anything wrong, as happens in "absence" (formerly called "petit mal") seizures.

Treatment of epilepsy

Treatment is primarily with anticonvulsant medications that aim to control the seizures and help the person to carry on a normal life—participating in usual activities, including most sports. Many different anticonvulsants are now available. The medications dampen the hyper-excitable areas of the brain, mute nerve conductivity and lessen the frequency and likelihood of seizures. They allow many people to achieve prolonged remission—sometimes just with one medication. (Remission is defined as "freedom from seizures for two to five years.") In 50 to 60 percent of those with epilepsy, correct medication eliminates all seizures, and another 30 percent obtain enough control to work and live normally. The chances that epilepsy will vanish or go into remission are greatest during the first few years after diagnosis. If the seizures have not diminished or disappeared after 5 years, chances of complete remission fade.

Those who have problems with one anti-seizure medication can try another. Finding the right medication and its dosage can take some time. The medication should be taken as prescribed and never stopped abruptly. Typical side effects depend on the drug used and may include unsteadiness, sleepiness/drowsiness, skin rashes and poor concentration. Other side effects, which lessen over time and vary from one medication to another, may include tremor, weight gain and nausea. Side effects may also include vision blurring and dizziness—calling for a change of dose and/or a different drug. About 20 percent of cases of epilepsy resist medication.

People with seizure disorders often need lifelong medication. But neurologists believe that anticonvulsant drugs can be stopped if seizures have vanished and the EEG is normal. If someone goes for about 2 years without a seizure, the medications may be slowly tapered off. But epilepsy drugs should never be suddenly stopped, as this may prompt a series of seizures that could be fatal.

Unfortunately, about a third of those who stop their medication will have repeat seizures during withdrawal, requiring reinstatement of drug therapy. Once the pills are stopped, 30 percent ultimately experience recurrent seizures and must go back on the medication. Emotional stress, drugs, alcohol and lack of sleep can provoke repeat seizures. If medication is stopped and seizures are allowed to continue unhalted, the condition may worsen. New anticonvulsant drugs are appearing all the time, and research has recently produced 17 new medications currently being tested.

Living with seizures

Although medication allows most people with epilepsy to lead normal lives, common sense suggests a few precautions. For example, activities such as contact sports may be risky if there's a chance of hitting the head. Those prone to sudden seizures without warning must be wary while cooking (burns are common in these cases). People with epilepsy must also take care in baths, boating or swimming, as deaths by drowning are a distinct risk. (Many experts promote showers as safer than baths for those with seizure disorder.) Of the many annual bathtub drownings in North America, almost half the victims have a history of seizure disorder. Wearing a lifejacket while boating is a wise precaution for those who have seizures, as for everyone. Driving regulations vary from place to place but have been largely standardized in Canada: people who have been seizure-free for 12 months or more and are under good medical supervision are usually licensed.

People with epilepsy are barred from some activities (such as airplane piloting) and may be well advised to avoid occupations that necessitate the use of dangerous machinery or put themselves or others at risk. But employers should remember that people with seizure disorders do *not* necessarily have more accidents than others on the job, nor do they take more time off work.

CARE OF ADOLESCENTS WITH SEIZURE DISORDERS

- Eliminate myths about epilepsy.
- Reassure the teenager that:
- the condition is not contagious;
- the seizures may disappear or become less frequent with age;
- most seizures can be controlled with medication;
- epilepsy does not lower intelligence;
- it's still possible to participate in most activities;
- there is no need for special schooling.
- Keep an accurate record of seizures.
- Know what to do for a seizure.

For further information on epilepsy, contact your local epilepsy association or the neurology department of a local hospital.

Initially, people diagnosed with epilepsy (and their families) may experience shock or denial. Anger, fear and depression are common. However, given information and support, people with epilepsy can understand the condition and develop coping skills. Family and friends may be overprotective or impose needless restrictions, making the person lose confidence and feel useless. It is important to remember that most people with epilepsy can and do live full, productive lives. Open discussion with friends, family and professional counselors can help people overcome hurdles.

For further information on epilepsy, contact your local Epilepsy Association or the neurology department of a local hospital.

FIBROMYALGIA

Fibromyalgia is a baffling malady with no discernible cause, in which people hurt all over, complaining of diffuse muscle aches, joint pain, exhaustion and disturbed sleep. This ill-defined ailment afflicts about 2 to 3 percent of the general population (compared to 1 percent who suffer from rheumatoid arthritis). Fibromyalgia may surface after some trauma or distressing event, typically in young adults aged 25 to 50, afflicting twice as many women as men. Sufferers tend to be perfectionists, with above-average sensitivity to bodily twinges, generally under-exercised and aerobically unfit, complaining of muscles too sore to withstand exercise. Many feel too weak to work, incurring large disability and compensation costs. Yet standard laboratory tests find no underlying organic abnormalities to explain the demoralizing symptoms. Now, there is a more scientific attempt to classify this chronic pain syndrome.

Historically, the affliction has gone under various names such as fainting paralysis, muscular rheumatism and fibrositis. Much confusion surrounds fibromyalgia, and many medical scientists still question its authenticity. "It is not a disease," notes one University of Toronto rheumatologist, "but a syndrome, a collection of signs and symptoms that have no detectable organic cause to date."

Debate about causes and best therapy for fibromyalgia

Experts are divided in their opinion about the causes and management of fibromyalgia. One group regards it as a physical problem of unknown origin, calling for exhaustive tests and pain management. Others consider it a *somatoform* or psychosomatic illness in which psychological problems—such as anxiety, depression, disappointment or failure to achieve goals—express themselves or *somatize* as physical symptoms such as backache and sore muscles.

One psychiatrist who considers the complaint a stress-related disorder suggests that fibromyalgia may be "the modern equivalent of formerly fashionable maladies, such as hyperglycemia or yuppie flu—illnesses that have no physical reason for the weakness, fatigue and muscle aches." Such ailments exert an immense burden, "not only in terms of human distress, but also in disability and healthcare costs." In focusing on physical reasons for the pain, sufferers and their caregivers may overlook underlying psychological causes, so that the problem remains unsolved. Today there are greater efforts to define this chronic pain syndrome scientifically.

Exhaustive tests reveal no causes

Looking for relief, many sufferers spend years "doctor-shopping," receiving no satisfactory answers. They may undergo blood tests, ultrasound, X-rays and other investigations—only to be told the results are normal, there is nothing physically wrong. Some are referred to mental health specialists, who may likewise find no basis for the pain. (Nonetheless, studies show that depression, anxiety, behavioral and personality disorders occur at above-average rates in fibromyalgia sufferers.)

Sleep disturbance has been a suspected but now discounted cause. Despite the diminished physical energy, there is no evidence of muscular deterioration. Neither morphological, histochemical, biochemical, magnetic resonance, spectroscopy, electromyography, serological or other measurements reveal any physical changes or abnormalities that can explain fibromyalgia symptoms. (Some speculate that the postexertional pain stems from tiny muscular microtrauma.)

One University of Toronto arthritic specialist claims that fibromyalgia arises as referred pain from neck and back problems and that underlying spinal problems need correction. Others suggest the disorder arises from enhanced pain sensitivity (perhaps from elevated levels of substance P, the pain transmitter) or hypervigilance (excessive preoccupation with bodily sensations). More recent speculation attributes it to changes in neurotransmitters or nerve-messengers, perhaps altered serotonin or tryptophan levels.

Others think fibromyalgia stems from psychological disorders. But while sufferers show a high incidence of depression and anxiety, there is no consistent link to psychiatric illnesses. One psychiatrist warns that "too hazy a definition of the ailment and too permissive a compensation system might make healthy people with everyday aches into invalids at an immense cost to society."

So, what is fibromyalgia?
Coined in 1976, the term "fibromyalgia" (fibro for "fibre," myo for "muscle," algos meaning "pain" and ia, "condition") aptly describes its cardinal symptoms: widespread muscular and joint pain, enhanced sensitivity to bodily perceptions, brief morning stiffness, poor sleep, fatigue and specific tender points above and below the waist. In addition, some sufferers report numbness, cold extremities (hands and feet), weakness, exercise aversion (because of muscle pain), restless legs, abdominal upsets, menstrual irregularity and anxiety. Broadly speaking, it's a soft-tissue disorder.

Fibromyalgia (FM) comes in two forms: primary, occurring in the absence of other illnesses, and secondary, accompanying some identified diseases, such as arthritis. The disorder may start as "growing pains" in childhood, and resurface later—perhaps precipitated by some distressing event like bereavement, thwarted career plans, a fall, whiplash injury or other life experiences.

Burgeoning interest has led the American College of Rheumatology to establish diagnostic criteria that require the presence of specific symptoms, particularly the tender points that

hurt if palpated (pushed or squeezed). Diagnosis must exclude other diseases such as anemia, rheumatoid arthritis, ankylosing spondylitis, thyroid disorders, cancer, infections (such as influenza) or use of medications (such as cholesterol-reducing agents). Fibromyalgia should also be differentiated from chronic fatigue syndrome (CFS), with which it shares similarities.

Criteria for classifying fibromyalgia include:
- *pain in at least 11 of 18 tender point sites*, present on digital palpation (pressure), evaluated by pressing with the thumb or first two or three fingers at a pressure of approximately 4 kg;
- *pain all over*, present for at least three months, on the right and left sides of the body, above and below the waist;
- *inability to use muscles* (owing to musculoskeletal pain);
- *sleep disturbances*—nonrefreshing sleep;
- *morning stiffness*.

Treatment means pain management
Education is the cornerstone of treatment for fibromyalgia, starting with reassurance that the condition is not crippling, will not weaken joints or muscles, is not life-threatening and need not hinder a return to work. Restorative sleep is critical in helping to relieve symptoms; therefore, education about sleep hygiene (quiet, darkened room; relaxation exercises or tapes; same retiring and arising times) is important, with the addition of low dose antidepressants or hypnotics if necessary. A meta-analysis of 16 randomized, placebo-controlled trials of tricyclic antidepressants (e.g. 25–50 mg amitriptyline nightly), selective serotonin re-uptake inhibitors (e.g. fluoxetine), and S-adenosylmethionine in fibromyalgia patients revealed improved sleep, less fatigue, reduced pain, and improved well-being, but no alleviation of tender points. Supervised aerobic training improved physical capacity and reduced symptoms. Strength training may also have benefits on some FM symptoms. A non-medical approach often works best with the emphasis on muscle conditioning; exercise programs to improve aerobic fitness; pool therapy; stress management; group,

POLYMYALGIA RHEUMATICA

This uncommon disease, seen mainly in elderly, involves simultaneous pain and stiffness in many parts of the body—hips, back, thighs, shoulders, arms. The entire body seems to ache at once, the discomfort often being so bad that sufferers can barely move or even get up from a chair or out of bed in the morning. Polymyalgia rarely occurs in persons under age 50, and it can strike suddenly for no apparent reason. Its causes are a mystery although it often afflicts people with arthritis, especially rheumatoid arthritis, more women than men.

Diagnosis can be elusive and tricky as the discomfort is so diffuse and the condition relatively rare so that physicians may not easily recognize it. Blood tests and very extensive physical examination (to rule out other disorders) can confirm its presence. Fortunately, polymyalgia responds dramatically to corticosteroid drugs which usually alleviate the pain and stiffness within a few days, doses being gradually reduced as the pain fades. (Sometimes even small steroid doses bring immediate relief.)

behavioral and cognitive therapy; physical therapy and perhaps tender-point injections.

GALLBLADDER PROBLEMS

A normally functioning gallbladder stores bile (digestive juice) produced by the liver: after a meal, the pear-shaped gallbladder contracts to move the bile through the common bile duct into the small intestine, where it mixes with food to help digest fat. Gallbladders can become diseased, resulting in gallstones, which occur in 20 percent of women and 10 percent of men by age 60. The tendency to form gallstones is partly inherited and is more common in the obese or those who lose weight rapidly through extreme diets (which release a flood of fat and cholesterol into the bloodstream). In many people gallstones remain "silent" and undetected, but if the gallstones move into the smaller, funnel-like end of the gallbladder or enter the narrow bile duct, they can block the flow of bile and cause severe and sudden pain.

When gallstones need treatment

If the gallbladder contracts against a stone, it causes biliary colic, a characteristic, severe pain in the upper abdomen or under the breastbone, which may radiate to the right upper abdomen and into the back. Biliary colic is the only specific symptom of uncomplicated gallstones. It often occurs after eating fatty foods and typically awakens people in the middle of the night. While "silent gallstones" are best left alone, even a single episode of biliary colic indicates a stone that may cause complications and must be treated. If a gallstone becomes lodged in the narrow bile duct, the flow of bile from the liver may be blocked, causing jaundice, liver infection or inflammation of the pancreas—illnesses that can occasionally be life-threatening.

The most effective remedy for gallstones is removal of the gallbladder (cholecystectomy). While traditional open surgery is highly successful with minimal risks, most people dread the discomfort of a large abdominal incision, the 6-day hospital stay and the 6-week recuperation period, and so the newer, less invasive laparoscopic cholecystectomy is more popular. This new technology permits a return home the day after surgery, and, in most cases, return to work

in 1 to 2 weeks. The financial benefits are also considerable: about $2,000 less than an open gallbladder operation.

Very few people with gallstones are now considered unsuitable for laparoscopic surgery, but one condition that still makes the operation inadvisable is cholangitis (stones in the bile duct causing inflammation). In some cases, however, stones lodged in the duct can be removed with an endoscope and the gallbladder taken out via laparoscope a day or two later. Open surgery remains the favored choice for people who have more than one of the following: previous abdominal surgery, gallbladder inflammation, disorders that hinder distention of the abdomen, certain liver diseases and portal hypertension (high blood pressure within the liver).

Other treatment options

Other new treatments available for gallstones include dissolution therapy (using drugs) and shock-wave lithotripsy (shock waves that smash the gallstones so that they can be naturally excreted or dissolved with drugs). However, dissolution therapies have not been as successful as hoped, since, if the gallbladder remains, stones often recur. Only 15 to 20 percent of patients have the type of gallstones that qualify for shock-wave lithotripsy—usually a single, small stone 1 to 2 cm (half an inch to an inch) in diameter. Possible complications of the treatment include recurrent pain, and infection and/or inflammation of the pancreas, gallbladder and bile ducts caused by residual fragments.

HALITOSIS: BANISHING BAD BREATH

Bad breath, or as dentists call it, halitosis or oral malodor, is mostly due to gases produced by bacterial action on food remnants in the mouth. Whatever it's called, malodorous breath can be very distressing and a social handicap; it's been known to ruin many a love affair. Millions are spent each year on efforts to freshen the breath with over-the-counter gums, sprays and mouthwashes—most of which do little good. Since bad breath is mostly due to bacterial putrefaction in an unclean mouth, it can often be remedied by better mouth care. But it can also arise from periodontal (gum) disease, lung or sinus infections and occasionally from systemic diseases such as diabetes, liver or kidney disorders.

Many are unaware of their bad breath

According to television commercials, the worst thing about bad breath is not knowing you have it. In many cases, people remain oblivious to their offensive breath through a phenomenon called adaptation. The cells in the nose responsible for smell become unresponsive to the continuous stream of bad odor. Halitosis sufferers may only get the message from the body language of others—who recoil at the smell—or they may realize they have bad breath only when friends or colleagues tell them. People may need to be tactfully told they have bad breath by a concerned friend or relative, or by their dentist. (You can do a self-check by licking your wrist, letting it dry for a few seconds and smelling the area, or by cupping the hands over the mouth and sniffing your own breath.)

Conditions that contribute to bad breath or halitosis:

- periodontal (gum) disease is a common cause producing a characteristic fetid odor); the teeth become loose, creating pockets in the gums, which harbor bacteria that can be impossible to clean with a toothbrush; in advanced periodontal disease, the gums may begin to ooze, adding pus, blood and dead skin to the causes of bad breath.
- Sjögren's syndrome (an autoimmune disease);
- chronic nose, throat and sinus infections;
- mouth breathing—perhaps because of enlarged tonsils or adenoids;
- mouth infections (e.g., candidiasis—with a typically "fruity" smell);
- lung disorders, e.g., tuberculosis;
- general infections with fever, e.g., typhoid fever;
- starvation, fasting, hunger, skipping meals;
- leukemia—with an odor of decaying blood;
- diabetes mellitus—with a sweet or acetone-like smell;
- liver disease—producing breath smelling like rotten eggs;
- kidney disease—with a typically fishy or ammoniacal mouth odor;

- gastrointestinal problems such as heartburn—an occasional cause;
- medications that reduce salivary flow such as antidepressants, antipsychotics, antihistamines, decongestants and some blood-pressure drugs.

HEADACHES

Most headaches are transient annoyances that disappear by themselves or with the help of mild painkillers such as ASA (e.g., Aspirin) or acetaminophen (e.g., Tylenol). But for 1 person in 10, a headache is an excruciating experience, and in a few rare cases a headache may herald some serious disorder. About 15 percent of the population has headaches severe or frequent enough to consult a physician. Even children get headaches, some well before the age of 10. Before puberty, headaches are more common in boys. But in adults, headaches are 4 times more prevalent in women and often linked to menstrual fluctuations. In both sexes the severity and frequency of headaches decline with advancing years. Although many of us call any headache a "migraine," only about a quarter of all headaches are true migraines.

While the vast majority of headaches don't signal serious diseases, some do require prompt medical investigation.

FOOD CHOICES AND HUNGER CAN PRODUCE BAD BREATH

Bad breath is notoriously worsened by certain foods—for instance, garlic, onions and some fish—and by diets rich in fat and meat. When these foods are digested, the smelly metabolites pass to the lungs where they are exhaled. In one study, even rubbing garlic on the feet led to bad breath! Missing meals, hunger, fasting, starvation and low-calorie diets can also cause malodorous "hunger breath," as the breakdown products of body proteins used for energy are exhaled through the lungs.

TIPS FOR BANISHING BAD BREATH

- *brush the teeth* three times a day and floss once daily;
- *clean the tongue* before bedtime by scraping with a plastic tongue cleaner or brushing gently;
- *prevent hunger breath*—avoid fasting;
- *try the baking soda solution:* brush the teeth with baking soda toothpaste (but it can be abrasive to sensitive gums);
- *use a Water Pik™* to help clean the mouth, perhaps with

added baking soda, which changes the pH (acidity) of the mouth and can be especially helpful for gingivitis;
- *keep the nose* and sinuses clean;
- *stimulate saliva flow* with acidic fruits—such as oranges and lemons—or sugarless citric gums and candy;
- *use an oil-and-water mouthwash* made with a mixture of Listerine™ or Cepacol® and olive oil, gargled

and spat out three times a day; or try a mouthwash that's half hydrogen peroxide and half water;
- *chew fibrous vegetables such as parsley and wintergreen*, to stimulate saliva flow;
- *know your medications*—ask whether they dry the mouth (as can happen with antidepressants, antihistamines, diuretics, decongestants and many blood pressure and heart medications).

HEADACHES THAT DEMAND MEDICAL ATTENTION

- Those that come on suddenly in middle age;
- those that strike like a "bolt from the blue" with unbearable intensity;
- those accompanied by seizures, loss of consciousness, mental confusion;
- those accompanied

by fever and/or a stiff neck (which could signal meningitis);
- recurrent headaches;
- those that relentlessly worsen over days or weeks;
- those localized to one spot—ears, eye or one side of the head;
- those accompanied

by impaired function such as imbalance or double vision (which could signify a stroke);
- those at the back of the head;
- those worst early in the morning and lightening during the day (could be due to high blood pressure).

Tension headaches afflict most of us occasionally, particularly when we're overtired, rushed, anxious, emotionally upset or harassed. Tension contracts the muscles of scalp, jaw, neck, shoulder and face, possibly causing the headache. Generally described as pressure or a "dull ache"—usually all over rather than on one side of the head—tension headaches are said to occur in "uptight" people with "uptight" muscles. They can also stem from undue fatigue, eyestrain or sitting for prolonged periods in one position, such as over a computer or behind a steering wheel.

Tension headaches typically appear in the late teens or early twenties, and in contrast to migraines are not hereditary, are not usually one-sided and have no clear-cut onset or ending, one headache merging imperceptibly into the next. Tension headaches are typically worst at the end of the day. Since the reason for them is often obvious, self-treatment—avoiding or eliminating the stressful situation, taking some over-the-counter remedy, relaxing, exercising usually suffices. But if they continue or worsen, medical help is needed.

Sinus headaches usually occur with or following nasal congestion and disappear once the sinusitis is cleared up with antibiotics or other treatment.

"Cluster headaches," an uncommon acute form, far more prevalent in men than women, come on and vanish very quickly. They are typically accompanied by a stuffy nose, tearing eyes, almost unbearable pain, but no nausea. They tend to occur in clusters—over a few days, weeks or months—are nonhereditary and not stress-related, and are often triggered by alcohol. They respond poorly to most medication, although lithium, methysergide and calcium channel blockers help some cases.

"Ice pick" headaches, of unknown cause, are sudden severe headaches that hit at a small, localized spot.

Migraine is no ordinary headache

Migraine, which ranges from mild to severe, often occurs as one-sided head pain but sometimes on both sides, even in those who usually have it on just one side. Its location, intensity and duration vary widely, not only from person to person, but also within each individual. Migraine is no recent affliction—Hippocrates was one of the first to describe it. Many famous people, such as Karl Marx, Charles Darwin and Sigmund Freud, were "migraineurs." About 10 to 12 percent of the population suffers from migraine, half developing it before age 20, some during early childhood. Migraine headaches afflict more women than men, often occurring just before or during menstrual periods and usually waning after the menopause. In about 75 percent of those afflicted there is a clear family connection—parents, siblings, children or other relatives being fellow-sufferers. In fact, a family history of migraine is often the most telling clue to its diagnosis.

Some suffer only the occasional migraine; others have it as often as twice a month or more. Migraine is typically experienced as a pulsating pain on one side of the head, commonly accompanied by other symptoms such as nausea, vomiting and possibly visual disturbances. Each episode lasts 2 to 72 hours—averaging 12 to 18 hours—and may be incapacitating enough to disrupt daily activities. Some people retire to rest in a dark room until it's over.

During a migraine attack the body may swell with retained fluid, and appetite wanes. Sufferers feel wretched and often have a strong aversion to noise, light and certain smells. The end of an attack is marked by a rewarming of the limbs and return of appetite. There are seldom any aftereffects.

Recent investigations have linked migraine to fluctuations in a brain neurotransmitter called serotonin. Other research suggests that many migraineurs also have below-normal amounts of

DIFFERENT HEADACHES HAVE DIFFERENT FEATURES

	Muscle-contraction headache	Common migraine	Classic migraine	Cluster headache
Incidence	very common	common	not common	uncommon
Age of onset	15–40	19–30		20–40
Sex	more females	more females		mostly males
Family history of headache	frequent	very frequent		infrequent
Headache frequency	variable, can be daily	variable, but "never" daily		daily during cluster
Possible triggers	stress or fatigue	stress, fatigue, menstruation, oral contraceptives, certain foods, alcohol, weather changes, bright lights, odors		alcohol if taken during cluster
Exacerbating factors	stress or fatigue	movement, head jarring, low head position		none
Onset during sleep	extremely rare	not uncommon		typical
Warning signs	none	none	visual or sensory aura	none
Location	bilateral (both sides of head)	often unilateral (one side of head), sometimes bilateral		unilateral
Severity	mild to moderate	moderate to severe		extremely severe
Accompaniments	none	nausea, sometimes vomiting, light and noise aversion		redness and tearing in one eye, stuffiness and dripping in one nostril, on same side as affected eye
Duration	hours to days	hours to all day—seldom more than two days		20–90 minutes

endorphin—the body's natural painkiller—making them ultra-sensitive to pain.

Despite the misery of migraine and the new drugs available to relieve it, reports show that over half of the sufferers receive no or inadequate medical counseling; many don't consult or fail to return to their physician for follow-up, instead trying to self-medicate with over-the-counter remedies. Some people endure headaches for many years before seeking medical help, even though there are now many effective medications.

An aura may precede the migraine

About 1 in 7 migraineurs experiences a clear pre-headache stage known as an aura, which lasts about 10 to 30 minutes and typically includes visual disturbances such as jagged blind spots, zigzag flashes, shimmering sparks or size distortion. Some auras also feature a transient tingling or numbness on one side of the face and/or body, speech defects and fleeting incoherence. Normally the aura clears as the

headache starts, but there can be some overlap. Many experience other pre-headache symptoms, such as elation, depression, unusual chattiness, voracious hunger or specific food cravings.

During the aura of classic migraine, blood flow to the brain is decreased, but after about 20 minutes the blood flow rises to above-normal levels, and the increased circulation is associated with the headache phase. However, since the increased blood flow may outlast the headache by days, the headache cannot be due to the raised blood flow alone. Migraine is now seen as a central-brain problem, and the blood-flow changes are considered secondary to the initial events. Pain-causing chemicals such as bradykinin and inflammatory agents like prostaglandins are known to accumulate near the distended vessels and probably play some role.

In the most common forms of migraine there's no real aura, although many have some warning hints that may permit them to take evasive action in time to avert a full-fledged headache. Excitability and mood swings can occur a day or two before migraine appears.

Triggers may provoke migraine attacks

Despite popular misconception, most migraines have no obvious, provocative cause, although some people can cite specific triggers that bring on their headache. The triggers vary from person to person and may not be consistent for the same individual. Reported migraine triggers include weather changes, hunger, certain foods, perfumes, bright lights, intense noise, strong emotions, stress, allergies, menstrual fluctuations and too little sleep. Extreme fatigue can be the reason, as can "sleeping in" on the weekend. While stress is a migraine-provoker, paradoxically relaxation is also a frequent trigger. The headache often appears after the week's stress, producing the weekend migraine typical among busy professionals.

Curiously, migraines tend to disappear temporarily in times of extreme stress or physical duress—during life-threatening illnesses or other crises and in wartime, for example. Migraine is common in general hospital patients but is seldom seen in intensive-care units.

Treatment to relieve migraine

Migraine treatment involves identifying and avoiding any triggers (if possible), and using suitable medication at the first sign of a headache. Black coffee or caffeine can help to offset a migraine headache in some people, provided it's taken as soon as the migraine is felt coming on.

Medications include:

- Pain relievers such as ASA and acetaminophen, which can mute or abort the headache if taken early enough, in high enough doses, possibly together with an antinauseant such as *dimenhydrinate* or *metoclopramide*. (Adding codeine may help.)
- *Ergot alkaloids* such as Cafergot and Migral, which help many if taken soon enough, but are not effective once the headache has taken hold. In excess, especially with poor timing, these medications may exacerbate rather than vanquish a headache.
- *Beta-blockers* such as *propranolol* (Inderal)—commonly used heart medications—which give relief in about 50 percent of cases (by

their effect on cerebral blood vessels).

- *Pizotyline* (Sandomigran), which blocks serotonin and histamine release, has had varying success rates.
- *Methysergide* (Sansert), a potent anti-migraine drug, which must be used with extreme caution, and only with strict medical supervision.
- *Calcium-channel blockers*, which alter narrowing and dilation of blood vessels.
- *Nonsteroidal anti-inflammatory drugs* and low-dose antidepressants (such as amitriptyline), now under investigation. *Triptans* such as *naratriptan* (Amerge), *rizatriptan* (Maxalt), *sumatriptan* (Imitrex), and *zolmitriptan* (Zomig) are the most effective therapy for migraines. They work on the serotonin and 5-HT (5-hydroxytryptamine) neurotransmitter pathways thought to be involved in migraine. The drugs are available by prescription and can be used at any stage of a migraine, either as tablets or by self-injection, apparently bringing relief within half an hour, but they are expensive and may have adverse effects on those with cardiovascular and heart problems. Although claims for this type of drug (*triptan*) suggest it affects only blood vessels in the head (constricting them), new evidence shows that it can produce chest pain or tightness and may pose a danger to people with any cardiac dysfunction.

New guidelines for managing migraine

Although migraine is very common (affecting 5 percent of men and 15 percent of women), it's vastly underrecognized and undertreated—a neglect that has prompted the International Headache Society to establish guidelines for its management.

New criteria for diagnosing migraine (without aura) require that other possible causes be ruled out and that it be distinguished from tension and cluster headaches. (Tension headaches are usually bilateral and occur 2 to 4 times a week; cluster headaches are one-sided, excruciatingly painful—like a hot poker—and usually strike in the middle of the night coming in clusters of several one after another.) In contrast, migraine occurs roughly 5 times a month, each (untreated) attack lasting 2 to 72 hours, sometimes triggered by stress, weather changes, certain foods or menstrual cycles, usually abating with sleep.

To be diagnosed as migraine, each attack should have at least two of the following features:

- predominantly one-sided location (usually over one eye)—although 40 percent are bilateral, or spread to both sides;
- a throbbing or pulsating quality (present in 50 percent of cases);
- moderate to severe intensity;
- pain worsened by walking up and down stairs or similar movements;
- nausea or vomiting accompanying attack;
- photophobia (light aversion) or sound aversion with attacks;
- no other diseases that could explain the symptoms.

Migraine sufferers should seek prompt medical advice if their headaches suddenly worsen or change—for instance, to the worst headache of a lifetime—or if they become more frequent, last longer or are accompanied by jaw pain, fever or muscle aches.

Since most people only have a few migraines per month, the experts warn against overmedication, which can lead to rebound headaches, even ultimately a nonstop headache. The guidelines suggest using different drugs for migraine according to its severity, stressing the need to take medication at the very first hint of an oncoming headache. (Most failures occur because people wait too long before taking the headache remedy.)

Attacks are categorized as "mild" if the person can continue usual activities, as "moderate" if function is disrupted, and as "severe" if the person can't carry on with daily life. Evidence supports the following migraine therapies:

- *For mild attacks*: ASA (Aspirin)—preferably buffered or soluble—ibuprofen and naproxen, all of which have a proven track record. Antinauseants may also be given to quench nausea or vomiting. (Although acetaminophen is widely used, there's no good evidence to support its effectiveness for acute migraine.)
- *For moderate attacks:* nonsteroidal anti-inflammatories (NSAIDs) are useful (for instance, ibuprofen, naproxen, mefenamic acid), as well

as sumatriptan (either injected or as pills—twice in 24 hours, but not during the aura phase), *dihydroergotamine* or DHE (as nasal spray) or *ergotamine* (as pills or under the tongue). (Side effects of several migraine drugs include chest tightness and tingling sensations.)

- *For severe attacks:* first line treatment is *dihydroergotamine* (injected), *sumatriptan* (pills) and metoclopramide; for more severe cases other drugs may help, for instance *chlorpromazine*, *dexamethasone*, *meperidine* and *butorphanol.*
- *For ultra-severe attacks:* guidelines are the same as for severe migraines, making sure to rehydrate if vomiting. DHE is a recommended first-line drug, plus *chlorpromazine* and *dexamethasone.*
- *Prophylactic treatment to prevent attacks* might be considered for people with 3 or more severe migraines a month. The idea is to use the least amount of preventive medication with the fewest side effects to control symptoms, to step up doses gradually and not to use preventives at the same time as headache-remedying drugs. Ideally, people should keep a headache diary to track the success of therapy and do their best to avoid known triggers. One preventive drug only should be taken at a time, and the patient should make sure to try it for long enough (at least 1 month) and go off it slowly to avoid rebound effects. Medications for preventing migraine include beta-blockers (such as *propranolol*, *metoprolol* or *atenolol*), calcium-channel blockers (such as *flunarizine* and *verapamil*), serotonin-receptor antagonists (such as *pizotyline*) and tricyclic analgesics (such as *amitriptyline* and *nortriptyline*). Exactly how they prevent headaches isn't clear.

HEART DISEASE

The heart is a fist-sized, hollow, muscular pump protected by the ribs and breastbone and covered by a thin, double-layered membrane, the pericardium. The heart normally contracts about 70 to 75 times a minute, pumping fresh oxygenated blood around the body, and its muscular wall, the myocardium, is strong enough to propel blood through the entire body. The heart's four chambers are two upper, thin-walled atria (which receive incoming blood) and two stronger-walled lower ventricles (which do the pumping). These four chambers are connected by valves that allow the blood to flow in one direction only. The heartbeat is divided into two main parts—the diastole (the relaxation phase) and the systole (the contraction or pumping phase).

Because it works hard, the heart needs a good oxygen supply, and the coronary arteries, which encircle it like a web, continually supply it. If blood flow in the coronary arteries is impaired, blocked or obstructed in any way, heart tissue is deprived of oxygen, possibly damaging the myocardium (heart muscle). A temporarily blocked coronary artery can cause angina pectoris (chest pain). If the heart's blood flow is severely diminished, or stops altogether oxygen lack (ischemia) results, perhaps causing a myocardial infarction—a heart attack.

What is atherosclerosis or "narrowing of the arteries"?

Arteries can become obstructed through the condition known as atherosclerosis, in which a fatty sludge or "plaque" coats the inner artery walls and obstructs blood flow, forcing the heart to work harder. Atherosclerosis in the heart's own arteries may deprive the heart muscle of oxygen and result in angina or a heart attack. In the legs, atherosclerosis can cause peripheral artery disease, which may lead to phlebitis (thrombosis or clot formation). In the brain, blood-vessel obstruction due to atherosclerosis can cause strokes.

Coronary artery disease

Coronary artery disease (CAD) is the forerunner and prime cause of heart attacks and strokes. The main risk factors are: advancing years, male gender smoking tobacco, lack of exercise, obesity, high blood-cholesterol levels

---

STRUCTURE OF THE HEART AND ITS VESSELS

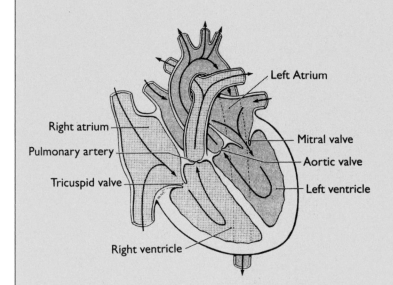

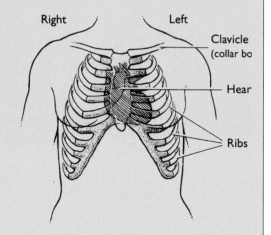

Usual position of the human heart

The heart is made up of four chambers: right atrium, left atrium, right ventricle, left ventricle. The right atrium receives blood (dark bluish, deoxygenated) from the body and passes it through the tricuspid valve to the right ventricle, which pumps blood out through the pulmonary valve to the lungs where it absorbs oxygen. The oxygenated blood returns to the heart's left atrium, then passes via the mitral valve into the left ventricle. The left ventricle pumps oxygenated (bright red) blood out through the aortic valve into the aorta from which it is dis-

tributed to all parts of the body, delivering oxygen to the tissues.
The arteries carry oxygenated blood to the body's cells and the veins collect deoxygenated blood. A network of capillaries connects the veins and arteries and distributes blood to the body's tissues. Arteries, which carry blood under high pressure, have thicker walls than veins, which carry blood back to the heart and lungs for oxygenation. A system of valves in the blood vessels controls the direction of flow.

and atherosclerosis. Middle-aged males have the highest incidence of coronary heart disease, risks increasing with age. Being female is a protector up to menopause, after which (because of waning estrogen levels) women acquire heart-disease rates similar to men's.

Narrowing or blockage of the coronary arteries through atherosclerosis is the most frequent cause of CAD. It diminishes the heart's blood supply so that the heart receives too little oxygen; it may still be able to cope at rest or during minor activities, but not with more exertion—shoveling snow, running for a bus, or enduring stress.

Fortunately, the risk of CAD can be lowered. The most important modifiable activity is cigarette smoking; giving up smoking alone can ameliorate CAD and slash heart-attack risks by 50 to 70 percent. Lowering serum cholesterol levels can also reduce risks, although people with a total cholesterol level below 180 mg/dl should stop worrying and focus on something else, such as getting enough exercise. Regular exercise (done at the right heart rate) may offset heart disease. A lower-fat diet may help to reduce blood cholesterol, reduce weight and lower blood pressure.

Whether or not someone at risk of CAD should take medications (which have side effects) to reduce the dangers depends on individual risk profiles. Many physicians now promote an "Aspirin a day" to keep heart attacks at bay—but not for those with peptic ulcer, gastritis or a tendency to easy bleeding. (See also "Strokes," later in this chapter.)

Diagnosing CAD

Exercise stress tests may be done to find out how efficiently someone's heart can cope with the stress of exertion. In this test, the subject is wired to a machine that records heart patterns as the person works a treadmill. Pulse and blood pressure are also recorded. Changes in an EGG heart tracing during exercise may reveal areas of poor coronary circulation that spell heart trouble.

Radio-isotope scanning (with thallium or persantine) may be done at the same time as exercise stress testing. A radioactive substance injected into a vein is scanned by a computerized

camera that can distinguish normal from damaged cells. The scan can provide details of heart size, capacity, sites of poor blood flow or scars from previous heart attacks. Echocardiograms, that use ultrasound to image the heart and the valves, are another common test.

Coronary angiography is a well-tried and informative test, done under local anesthetic, and is not painful (but momentarily uncomfortable). A dye-like chemical is infused into the body through an arm or groin vessel and X-rays display its progress through the coronary artery network, outlining areas of narrowing that may need bypass graft surgery. (See "Bypass surgery" on page 522.)

Heart attacks (myocardial infarction)

Officially termed a myocardial infarction, a heart attack results from injury to the heart muscle when its blood (and oxygen) supply is cut off or reduced. If only a small amount of heart muscle is damaged, pumping ability may return virtually to normal once healing is complete. More severe injury may leave lasting damage.

Tragically, many heart-attack deaths occur within minutes or hours—often before the person reaches hospital—usually due to disturbance of the heart rhythm (ventricular fibrillation). A heart in ventricular fibrillation does not pump enough blood to keep brain cells alive, so the person may suffer brain death, although the original problem—the heart damage—need not have been fatal. Since ventricular fibrillation is highly responsive to electric shock treatment, ambulance crews are now trained

---

SOME COMMON HEART AND CARDIOVASCULAR DISEASES

- **Atherosclerosis (artery narrowing, popularly called "hardening" of the arteries);**
- **coronary artery disease (leading to angina and heart attack);**
- **congestive heart failure;**
- **heart-valve defects (such as mitral-valve** stenosis);
- **cardiomyopathies (due to a damaged myocardium, or heart muscle);**
- **arrhythmias (irregular heart rhythms);**
- **pericarditis (infection of the pericardium, the heart's outer covering).**

Known risk factors for atherosclerosis and heart disease:
- **male gender;**
- **age (risk increases as people get older);**
- **family history of early heart disease;**
- **tobacco smoking;**
- **diabetes;**
- **high blood pressure;**
- **high blood-cholesterol levels;**
- **lack of exercise;**
- **obesity.**

POSSIBLE SYMPTOMS OF HEART DISEASE

- **Chest pain or discomfort, perhaps radiating to left arm or jaw;**
- **difficulty breathing, shortness of breath;**
- **palpitations;**
- **dizziness/fainting;**
- **swelling of the legs;**
- **excessive fatigue.**

WARNINGS OF HEART ATTACK INCLUDE:

- **persistent chest pain, possibly radiating to the neck, jaw, shoulder or left arm;**
- **tightness ("squeezing") in the chest;**
- **heaviness that may feel like indigestion;**
- **sweating, nausea and vomiting;**
- **pallor;**
- **shortness of breath;**
- **denial—a refusal to believe anything is seriously wrong.**

UPDATE ON HEART PROTECTORS AND THREATENERS

Yet another heart risk factor—a high blood level of homocysteine—now joins the list of other coronary threats, namely tobacco smoking, obesity, inactivity, diabetes mellitus, high blood pressure and a high LDL ("bad") and low HDL ("good") blood cholesterol level. High levels of homocysteine (an amino acid) are thought to damage the blood vessel linings, thereby increasing heart attack and stroke risks. There is also a nutritional connection because high homocysteine levels are linked to low intakes of B vitamins, especially a lack of folic acid, vitamin B 12 and B6 (pyridoxine).

People are urged to consume enough B vitamins to keep homocysteine levels down and reduce cardiovascular risks. To protect against heart disease people need 400 mg of folic acid (folate) daily, to an upper limit of 1,000 mg. To ensure adequate folate intake, flour, breads and cereals are now fortified with this vitamin. (Good natural sources of folate are liver, legumes and green leafy vegetables.) Most multivitamin preparations supply the right amount. In addition, an adequate intake of niacin or vitamin B3 helps to keep down LDL or bad cholesterol

and raise the good or HDL form. However, avoid excess as too much niacin can cause face and neck flushing. (Good natural sources are meat, fish and eggs.)

The overall heart protection message is becoming ever more clear. Avoid tobacco smoking, exercise plenty, maintain body weight at desirable levels, keep blood pressure within normal limits, eat a sensible low-fat diet (preferably Mediterranean type), lower LDL blood cholesterol and raise the HDL or good form.

The most recent advice for adequate exercise from the U.S. National Academy of Sciences, taking into

account the expanding waistlines of many North Americans, suggests people aim for 40 to 60 minutes of moderate daily activity, tailored into their everyday lives, even by just taking the stairs instead of the elevator or walking to the grocery store instead of driving. Also, moderate rather than extreme weight loss is the newest goal: losing even 5 to 10 percent of one's excess weight by small dietary and exercise changes can bring big health benefits by reducing the risks of developing diabetes and cardiovascular disease.

To lower LDL blood cholesterol, more and

more people are taking statin drugs, but the latest advice includes ways to raise HDL or "good" cholesterol by exercising more vigorously, losing weight, and switching to Mediterranean type diets richer in complex carbohydrates and monosaturated fats (such as olive and canola oils). The Mediterranean style diet includes plenty of grains, fresh fruit, vegetables, nuts and legumes, using olive oil as the principal fat, consuming only moderate amounts of cheeses and meats, and drinking red wine in moderation (2 glasses a day for men, 1 glass a day for women).

and equipped to treat it *en route* to hospital, greatly increasing survival rates.

What often happens in a heart attack is that a "thrombus," or blood clot, lodges in one or more coronary arteries and further narrows the passage. Heart attacks may also be caused (less commonly) by sudden oxygen reduction due to a drop in blood pressure during surgery, or when there is a huge increase in oxygen demand, as during extreme exertion. (Cocaine abuse is increasingly implicated in heart attacks.)

The key to successful treatment of heart attacks is to get immediate medical aid and prevent further injury. Since many conditions mimic heart attacks, diagnosis can only be confirmed in hospital with an electrocardiogram. Electronic monitors allow quick diagnosis of the heart's condition, and biochemical tests measure cardiac enzymes released into the bloodstream from dying heart cells to aid in evaluating the damage. Heart catheters give minute-by-minute readings of pressure changes in the heart's chambers and monitor pumping ability. Today,

immediate infusion of a clot-busting drug—such as streptokinase or tPA (a newer genetically engineered product) can save lives and reduce the damage done by a heart attack.

The critical phase in recovery from heart attack is the first week after the attack. About 5 to 10 percent of those admitted die during this time, often while still in hospital. After this, the risk of death falls significantly, but a further 5 to 10 percent perish within the next 6 months to 1 year. Only after that does the risk truly drop. Consequently, current efforts concentrate on improving survival chances in three crisis periods: the first hours after the heart attack, the next week and the following year.

If you suspect a heart attack in yourself or someone else, never delay calling for help in the vain hope that the pain will vanish. Call an ambulance or dial emergency medical services and get to the nearest hospital or medical center at once, not only to avoid sudden death, but to minimize damage to the heart. (See Chapter 17 for first aid for a heart attack.)

TREATMENT OF CAD AND HEART ATTACKS

- *Beta-adrenergic blockers (beta-blockers, for short)* such as *propranolol* (Inderal) and *timolol* (Blocadren) can reduce heart-attack risks by slowing the heartrate and allowing the heart to get along with less oxygen.
- *Blood-thinning medications* such as **ASA** can decrease platelet clumping and blood stickiness (clotting). Aspirin is the mainstay of blood-thinning therapy with the most evidence to support its use. Newer options such as *clopidrogel* (**Plavix**),

or Aspirin combined with a calcium channel blocker (Aggrenox) are also now available.
- *Calcium-channel blockers*, a relatively recent class of drugs, can be used during the first stage of a heart attack, when oxygen-deprived heart cells lose their ability to block out calcium. (Calcium dissolved in the fluid surrounding the heart cells may move inward in excessive amounts and damage the cells.) These drugs block the channels through which

calcium moves into the heart and may combat coronary-artery spasms.
- *Ballooning angioplasty*, increasingly used, involves inserting a thin plastic catheter with an inflatable balloon at its tip to squash any clots or other coronary-artery obstructions. In those deemed suitable, the ballooning works well, usually relieving angina and helping to prevent a heart attack. It has the great advantage of avoiding the need for surgery. Experts have now become so

skilled, with such refined equipment, that they can guide a catheter right to the blockage within a coronary artery and squash it. But time is of the essence.
- *Chemical infusion with clot-buster chemicals* is a promising new procedure for clearing blocked heart arteries during, or right after, a heart attack with an enzyme called streptokinase, or newer agents, such as tPA. New studies show that tPA is more effective in preventing heart attacks, but

more expensive than streptokinase.
- *Bypass surgery*, a dramatic and astonishingly successful method of alleviating **CAD**, replaces blocked coronary arteries with sections of vein—usually taken from the person's leg—reinstating the heart's oxygen supply. Bypass surgery is usually planned ahead, but is occasionally tried on the spot as an emergency operation for life-threatening heart blockages—but success is uncertain under such acute conditions.

It is critical for survival that life-saving treatments be started within hours preferably in the first hour. If only a small portion of the heart muscle is damaged, the heart can limp along, or even do quite well, afterward. Following initial recovery, mortality from a subsequent heart attack remains 6 to 10 percent in the first year. Thus, the goal during that year is to prevent a second attack without encouraging the recovering person to become a "cardiac cripple."

Angina

Angina pectoris—which can be "stable" or "unstable" occurs when the heart's oxygen needs temporarily exceed its supply. A common forerunner of heart attacks, it has similar symptoms—chest pain or heaviness and shortness of breath—often brought on by exercise, emotional upheavals, anger, stress, cold exposure, a big meal or illness. Angina may be mistaken for indigestion. The symptoms are quickly relieved by rest and medication.

Stable angina crops up at predictable and regular intervals and is usually no cause for alarm. Typically the angina symptoms come on with increased heart rate and then dissipate when the heart rate lessens. For example, a per-

son may walk two blocks and feel fine, but walk three blocks and get a predictable chest heaviness that is relieved by rest. But anyone suddenly getting angina for the first time should seek medical advice.

In unstable angina, someone with ongoing,

WAYS TO REDUCE HEART-ATTACK RISKS

- **Quit smoking; within 5 years of cessation, former smokers lower risks by 50 to 70 percent compared to those still smoking.**
- **Reduce blood-cholesterol levels; there is a 2 to 3 percent decline in risk for each 1 percent reduction in serum cholesterol (levels may drop an average of 10 percent with diet therapy and 20 percent with medication).**
- **Exercise more.**
- **Achieve and maintain your desirable weight.**
- **Ask your physician about the usefulness of regular low-dose ASA (e.g., coated Aspirin)—said to achieve a 33 percent lowering of risk.**
- **Consume one alcoholic drink daily: conservative drinkers have 25 to 45 percent lower heart attack risks than non-drinkers (but risk rises again with**

higher consumption).
- **Reduce hypertension (high blood pressure); a decline in heart-attack risk accompanies a lowered diastolic (bottom number) pressure.**
- **If menopausal, consider estrogen-replacement hormone therapy.**
- **If diabetic, try to maintain normal blood-sugar levels, which may lower heart-attack risks.**

chronic angina may find the pain increasingly severe and frequent, or triggered by less and less physical exertion—perhaps just walking across a room, instead of, as previously, running or climbing stairs. Pain control may require more and more nitroglycerin or other medication. Unstable angina of increasing severity and changing pattern calls for immediate medical attention.

Angina is usually treated with drugs that reduce the heart's oxygen demand—for example, by lowering blood pressure and heartrate—or with drugs (beta blockers or calcium channel blockers) that slow the heart rate, or by techniques to improve coronary blood flow (bypass grafts or angioplasty).

Arrhythmias

Arrhythmias are abnormal heart rhythms: the heart may speed up, miss a beat or slow down. They can cause a great deal of anxiety and worry, but are mostly benign. Some people with atrial or ventricular arrhythmias may have more severe palpitations, dizziness or syncope (fainting).

Serious arrhythmias should be investigated and decisions made as to whether or not to treat them. (In some cases, the condition places an individual at risk for sudden death—if, for example, a more serious heart condition already exists—in which case medications may be required.)

Bypass surgery

Today, coronary-bypass surgery is the most common single operation performed in North America. In the United States, surgeons seem ready to operate on almost anyone with coronary-artery disease—a practice now questioned by some cardiac specialists and critics. With low risks and phenomenal results, bypass surgery is now considered no more hazardous for some patients than a gallbladder or hernia operation, with a survival rate of about 98 percent.

Although the risks vary according to age, the severity and extent of cardiovascular disease, and the technical success of the bypass grafts, the chances are high that people will leave hospital with their heart pain reduced or entirely ban-

MAJOR HEART-SAVING MEDICATIONS

- Antiplatelet-clumping agents, e.g., ASA (Aspirin), reduce the "stickiness" of platelets, thereby decreasing blood clotting in arteries (not in veins). Low-dose ASA has been found effective in preventing myocardial infarction, but it also increases hemorrhage risks, so it should be taken regularly only on a physician's advice. *Clopidrogel* (Plavix) or aspirin combined with *dipyridamole*, a calcium channel blocker, are more expensive drugs that may be used for some special circumstances. Plavix, for example, has been shown to be helpful in individuals after a cardiac procedure in which the surgeons have inserted a stent (a special coil placed inside a coronary artery to help keep it unblocked and maintain blood supply to the heart).

- Cholesterol-lowering drugs lower LDL or "bad" cholesterol, and may raise HDL ("good") cholesterol, and are sometimes used if a cholesterol-lowering diet doesn't work. Some cholesterol-lowering drugs have been shown to reduce heart-attack risks, but the drugs have side effects such as bloating and constipation.

- Thrombolytic ("clot-busting") agents, e.g., streptokinase and tPA (tissue plasminogen activator), are given by infusion right after a heart attack, and have revolutionized its management. They prevent widespread heart-muscle damage and possible death, by dissolving coronary blood clots. Since they are most effective before damage is done, it is important to get to the hospital as soon as a heart attack is suspected.

- Antiangina agents, including beta blockers (such as propranolol and timolol), nitrates, calcium-channel blockers (such as *verapamil* and *nifedipine*), relieve angina, palpitations and abnormal heart-beats and decrease the risk of heart attack in people with ischemic (oxygen-depriving) heart disease. Beta blockers are often given to patients who've already had a heart attack, to prevent further attacks. Since smoking decreases the efficacy of propranolol, smokers who cannot quit should take timolol instead.

- Antiarrhythmics to stabilize the heart-beat include *amiodarone, quinidine, disopyramide*, digitalis.

- Anti–heart-failure drugs include diuretics such as *thiazides* (to prevent water retention), inotropic agents (which influence muscle contractions) such as digitalis, digoxin (to increase the force of heart-pumping contractions) and vasodilators such as ACE inhibitors. These drugs relieve the symptoms of congestive heart failure: shortness of breath, and edema. Together they may prolong life in patients with heart failure.

ished, at least for the time being. Many find their quality of life immensely improved and rejoice at the renewed ability to do many activities.

How long does a bypass operation take?

Coronary bypass grafting is used to circumnavigate blocked coronary arteries and revascularize the heart, restoring its blood flow and overcoming the oxygen shortage that causes symptoms such as angina (chest pain). Bypass surgery is a safe, effective and now routine operation, with few procedure-related deaths and low rates of complications (such as stroke). Although coronary bypass operation is cardiac surgery, surgeons don't actually operate inside the heart but rather work on the coronary arteries that lie on the heart's surface.

Before the surgery, an angiogram test with dye injection and X-rays shows which coronary arteries are most badly obstructed, where the blockages are and the general condition of the arteries. Depending on which and how many of the coronary artery branches are blocked, more or fewer bypass grafts will be done. The surgeons construct a detour bypassing the blocked or narrowed parts of the coronary arteries with pieces of saphenous vein (from the patient's leg), or with parts of the thoracic artery (inside the rib cage). These segments or grafts are used to reroute the coronary blood supply, bypassing the worst obstructions. The new grafts take over the function of the blocked vessel(s). So far, there is no artificial substitute that can be used for grafting.

A bypass operation usually takes 3 to 4 hours. While one surgical team opens up the chest and connects the patient to the heart-lung machine, another works on the leg, removing a piece of vein. The heart-lung machine takes over the function of the heart and lungs, circulating and oxygenating the blood while the surgeons work. The body is sometimes cooled during surgery so that the tissues need less oxygen. The heart is stopped while the surgeons operate on tiny vessels only a few millimeters in diameter. A person may need three, four or more bypass grafts. Whether surgeons use all saphenous vein grafts or include thoracic artery grafts depends on the individual case.

Following the operation, there is an immediate resurgence of the blood supply (revascularization) to the heart muscle. Once the operation is completed, the heart is restarted, the heart-lung machine disconnected and the patient taken to the intensive care unit (ICU).

The stay in the ICU is usually 1 day, maybe slightly longer in some cases. The removal of a leg vein rarely presents any long-term problems because other veins take over its function. There may be some postoperative swelling and discomfort, which soon fade. By the end of the first day after surgery, improvement is usually substantial. Many tubes and lines are out, the patient can talk, sit up, move around and drink fluids. By the second to fourth day, patients are taking walks along the corridor. During the rest of the hospital stay, the staff try to start bypass patients on an exercise program. By the time most go home—usually 5 to 7 days after the operation—they can take a shower, shampoo their hair, answer mail and climb a few stairs.

About 6 to 10 weeks after surgery, most patients get a checkup with their cardiologist, perhaps an exercise stress test, before starting a rehabilitation program. Many post-bypass patients find that cardiac rehabilitation programs aid adjustment and help to diminish post-surgical depression, lift flagging spirits and teach people how to strengthen the heart by exercising within safe limits.

Large-scale trials have shown bypass surgery to be very successful in relieving angina and it may improve survival in people with extensive coronary artery disease. However, its efficacy declines after 8 to 10 years, as the grafts often deteriorate or atherosclerosis develops in other parts of the coronary arteries. While women undergoing bypass operations tend to have more surgical complications than men, studies at some hospitals find the procedure equally successful in both sexes.

Angioplasty or "ballooning" to clear artery blockages

Angioplasty—insertion of a thin catheter (tube) with an inflatable balloon at the end to stretch the artery wall and squash the plaque that causes arterial blockage is increasingly tried as a quick and less invasive way to unblock coronary arteries and revascularize the heart. It can restore coronary blood flow, provided there aren't too many blockages and the arteries are suitable for this procedure. Success rates compare well with bypass surgery, and the procedure has similarly low risks of death and complications.

The advantages of angioplasty are that it does not require anesthesia or surgery, and it is less traumatic with a shorter hospital stay. However, angioplasty is less effective than bypass surgery in keeping people angina-free, and up to one-third get recurrent chest pain that requires further treatment. In one study, those who underwent bypass surgery subsequently had less angina, required less heart medication and were less likely to need repeat treatments than those who had angioplasty. Bypass grafting continues to be the preferred method for many people with coronary heart trouble.

Amazing improvement in the quality of life

Many people previously severely disabled by their angina are amazed at their swift post-surgical improvement and the things they can do, including exercise, quite soon after a bypass operation. But for many, a heart operation still seems terrifying. The anxiety that accompanies most surgery is greater with the heart because of its symbolic significance and its image as the "center of life." Tampering with this organ seems worse than operating on other parts of the body, even though the actual risks may not be greater.

Surgery cannot cure atherosclerosis. It's up to those who undergo bypass operations to adopt a lifestyle that helps fight their heart disease: to eat sensibly, exercise regularly, avoid stress and above all to quit smoking. Smoking is the one thing that will definitely cause artery hardening and clog up bypass grafts.

For more information on heart disease, contact the Heart and Stroke Foundation.

BYPASS SURGERY TO REPLACE BLOCKED CORONARY ARTERIES

Bypass surgery doesn't actually cut into the heart; it involves the coronary arteries which lie on the heart's surface and have several branches. Dye injection and X-ray tests (angiograms) prior to surgery show which coronary arteries are most badly blocked. Surgeons then construct a detour, bypassing the narrowed parts of the arteries with a piece of vein from the patient's leg. One end is attached to an opening made in the coronary artery beyond the blockage, and the other end is connected to the aorta, the body's main artery, bringing fresh blood to the heart. So far, there's no reliable, artificial substitute for the use of human vessels in bypass surgery.

Sometimes surgeons circumvent the blocked artery by another technique—connecting the body's mammary artery (inside the rib-cage) to a healthy vessel beyond the obstruction.

Someone with severe blockage of the coronary arteries may need three, four or as many as eight bypass grafts. But until surgeons actually assess conditions inside the body, they cannot decide in advance how many they will do.

The removal of a leg vein rarely presents any long-term problems because other veins take over its function after a few months. There may be some post-operative swelling, numbness and discomfort which soon fade.

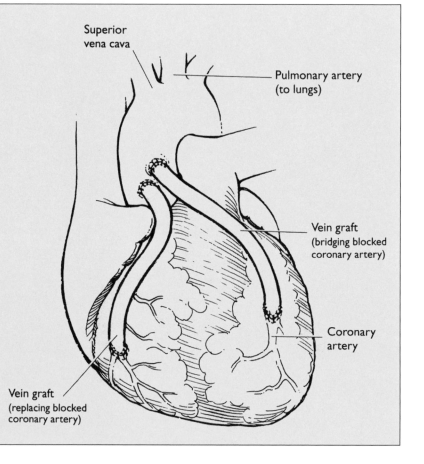

Superior vena cava

Pulmonary artery (to lungs)

Vein graft (bridging blocked coronary artery)

Coronary artery

Vein graft (replacing blocked coronary artery)

MANAGING CHEST PAIN

Many worry that every little twinge in the chest may signal a heart attack, while others ignore symptoms and ascribe them to indigestion. Besides angina (heart pain) and myocardial infarction (heart attack), chest pain can arise from stomach irritation, arthritis in the ribs, heartburn, anxiety or pleurisy (inflammation of the lung's lining tissue). Both doctors and their patients find it hard to distinguish between pain from the heart and other causes. As rough pointers, chest pain from anxiety is usually vague and diffuse; that from the lungs is sharp and worsens with coughing; pain due to angina (lack of oxygen to the heart) is like that due to a heart attack—a tightness or crushing sensation in the middle of the chest, often radiating into the jaw, left shoulder or elbow.

While chest pain from angina usually vanishes in 5 to 10 minutes, or is relieved by taking nitroglycerin, pain due to a heart attack lasts longer (20 minutes or more), doesn't abate with rest or a change in position and is often accompanied by pallor (pale skin), sweating, restlessness, a sense of unease, nausea, maybe vomiting. Anyone with these symptoms should immediately take 1 adult Aspirin (to help dissolve clots in the coronary arteries) and get to a medical facility at once. Arriving at hospital fast may enable thrombolytic (clot-dissolving) therapy to be administered. Given within 3 hours of the onset of chest pain, this therapy unclogs blocked arteries and can prevent damage to the heart muscle; but after 6 hours it's too late for this treatment to work. Note that angina and heart-attack symptoms in women often differ from those in men—rather than a crushing central chest pain, women often have more diffuse pain (in the shoulder and neck). (See Chapter 8.)

Whether taking daily ASA (Aspirin) can prevent heart attacks (and what dose to take) remains a hotly debated issue because studies give divergent results. While taking 325 mgm of ASA a day can significantly reduce fatal heart-attack rates, It also increases the risk of hemorrhagic (bleeding) stroke. Some studies show that far lower amounts of ASA (165 mgm per day or less) are enough to ward off heart attacks. In weighing up the pros and cons of taking ASA, consider the advantages (reduced rate of heart attack and thrombotic stroke) versus drawbacks (possible worsening of hemorrhagic stroke, increased bleeding risks, stomach ulcers).

Heart failure

Technically called congestive heart failure, it's a condition characterized by left ventricular dysfunction—inability of the heart's left ventricle to pump sufficient blood around the body. The condition is increasing because of an aging population and new cardiac treatments that keep people alive, albeit with damaged hearts. Main causes of heart failure are a previous heart attack, damaged heart muscle, long-standing high blood pressure, heart valve problems and alcohol abuse. The failing heart is a weakened pump that works less efficiently than usual, with consequent "congestion" or fluid buildup in many parts of the body, including the lungs, liver and peripheral tissues such as the ankles, which may swell up. As it strives to pump harder, the heart may become enlarged.

Alerting signs may be subtle—no more than some fatigue and slight breathlessness on exertion—slowly worsening and even occurring at night.

Key signs and symptoms of heart failure are:
• shortness of breath on exertion, even when lying down or sleeping;
• swelling of abdomen, ankles;
• distended neck veins;
• fatigue;
• weight gain (from accumulating fluid).

Treatment aims to help the heart pump more efficiently with medications such as *digoxin*, to remove excess fluid with diuretics and to improve blood flow with vasodilators that dilate the blood vessels—such as the angiotensin-converting enzyme (ACE) inhibitors, now first-line drugs for heart failure, with a good track record in reducing hospital stays, improving quality of life and lowering death rates. Other drugs such as beta-blockers may be used as add-ons to improve blood flow and stabilize heart rhythm; in particular, *carvedilol* (Coreg), a newly approved drug for mild to moderate heart failure, helps preserve pumping ability. In addition, lifestyle changes, such as salt-restricted diets, limiting alcohol intake and moderate exercise, can help relieve symptoms.

Palpitations

Many people experience occasional palpitations—felt as a racing heartbeat, disturbed heart rhythm or sensation of extra or missed heartbeats—often described as unpleasant awareness of the heartbeat. Usually, the symptoms signify nothing serious but it's always wise to report palpitations to your doctor. Palpitations are most often due to anxiety or stress. They can be due to heart problems, but may also arise from other causes such as an overactive thyroid. One common type of palpitation is due to sinus tachycardia, where the heart begins to beat extra fast (at 100 to 150 beats per minute) often seen in young, healthy women a few times a year, and more frequently at menopause. While palpitations often occur because of stress, anxiety problems, unaccustomed exercise, a high fever or from fluctuations in female hormones, they may arise from underlying arrhythmias or heart rhythm disturbances (such as atrial fibrillation, supraventricular tachycardia or atrioventricular block), so should be checked out by a cardiologist. Seek immediate medical attention for palpitations felt in the neck or those accompanied by dizziness, chest pain or shortness of breath.

Treatment is geared to the cause(s) and may simply mean reassurance that nothing's wrong with the heart and cutting down on caffeine and stress. Palpitations arising from heart rhythm disorders, especially those described as missed beats may benefit from various antiarrhythmic heart medications including beta-blockers, digoxin and calcium-channel blockers. Beta-blockers (such as *propranolol*, *sotalol*, *esmolol* and *atenolol*) are often the first drugs tried to control the heartbeat and stabilize the rhythm.

Atrial fibrillation (AF), which causes fluttering palpitations or "heart flutters"—sometimes accompanied by shortness of breath—is a common result of long-standing high blood pressure, heart muscle damage, angina, thyroid disorders or rheumatic fever. Uneven contractions in the heart's upper chambers stop the lower compartments from filling properly between beats, producing an irregular heartbeat and a stagnating pool of blood in which clots may form in the heart. Bits of the clot can break off and travel to the brain, causing a stroke. (AF is a major cause of strokes.) Treatment is with beta-blockers or selected calcium-channel blockers (e.g., *diltiazem*) to stabilize the heart and slow down its excitability.

HEART MURMURS

A heart murmur is a vibration or sound other than that of a normal heartbeat, due to unusual turbulence in the cardiac flow. Many heart murmurs are harmless variations from the norm. An estimated 1 in 20 people (especially women) has some kind of heart murmur, frequently of no consequence.

Distinguishing normal from abnormal heart sounds

Normal heart sounds arise from the opening and closing of the heart's four cardiac valves.

- *First heart sound*—closure of the mitral and tricuspid valves.
- *Second heart sound*—closure of the pulmonary and aortic valves.
- *Third heart sound*—early filling of blood into the right and left ventricles, which may be a normal sound in young people, but later in life may signify heart failure.
- *Fourth heart sound*—late ventricular filling, which may denote a non-compliant or "stiff" ventricle.
- *Ejection click*—opening of the aortic and pulmonary valves, often heard after the first heart sound.

Heart murmurs in children, young adults and pregnant women are often innocent. Those that arise later in life may be serious, but many due to sclerosis (thickening) of the heart valve are also considered innocent. Many childhood murmurs fade with time, vanishing before the age of 30. Those that persist longer may warrant further investigation, such as an echocardiogram (ultrasound examination). Some murmurs should be followed and checked every few years. For example, a murmur resulting from a congenitally defective heart valve may be faint in childhood but later become loud due to narrowing or calcification (hardening) of the valve. Athletes often have innocent heart murmurs because their rigorous training increases the heart's size and ability to pump blood with each heartbeat. The extra blood pumped may produce a harmless "flow" murmur that's heard when the athlete is lying down, but tends to disappear when upright.

When is a heart murmur serious?

Innocent heart murmurs usually stem from the systolic (pumping) phase of the heartbeat, due to a slight turbulence in the ejection of blood through the aortic and pulmonary valves. They are often not associated with any disability or medical problem and show no clinical, radiographic or electrocardiographic evidence of anything other than normal blood flow through the heart.

By contrast, diastolic and continuous murmurs are always due to some disease and/or faulty cardiac flow. Serious, noncongenital heart murmurs are usually caused by some degenerative disease or infection, such as rheumatic fever. The long-term consequences of an abnormal cardiac valve can be heart enlargement and eventual heart failure. Some damaged heart valves need to be surgically repaired or replaced.

Treatment of heart murmurs

Innocent murmurs require no treatment. Most organic or pathological murmurs need preventive antibiotics before dental work or surgery to prevent a possible heart infection (pericarditis) caused by a collection of stale blood.

A medically threatening heart murmur may call for medications and/or heart surgery, the urgency depending upon the severity of valve damage. Current medical opinion tends to favor valve repair rather than replacement because there are problems associated with mechanical valves. Nonetheless, artificial valves are needed when valve repair isn't feasible. Close monitoring is necessary for those with valve replacements. Blood-thinners may have to be taken, and artificial valves often develop structural flaws that necessitate repeat surgery.

HEARTBURN: NOT FROM THE HEART

Heartburn, a burning sensation felt beneath the breastbone—frequently after meals, especially large ones—stems *not* from the heart, but from irritation of the lower esophagus or gullet (foodpipe).

About half the world's Western population suffers occasional heartburn, known as reflux esophagitis, and it's particularly prevalent among the elderly. An irritated esophagus may cause not only heartburn, but also occasionally a sharp spasm or crushing pain beneath the breastbone that can be confused with angina or heart pain (see above).

REASONS FOR A HEART MURMUR INCLUDE:

- minor structural irregularities in the heart valves that cause innocent "flow" murmurs due to eddies in the flow of blood through the heart;
- a larger-than-usual amount of blood flowing through the heart, which may cause innocent flow murmurs in pregnant women and athletes;
- a narrowed (stenosed) valve that obstructs the normal amount of blood flowing through it—murmurs due to valvular stenosis can be serious;
- a regurgitant or leaky ("incompetent") valve that causes a murmur as blood backs up through it;
- a fistula (hole or small opening) in the partition between the heart's right and left sides;
- a floppy mitral valve —known as *mitral-valve prolapse*— where valve closure is imperfect and blood slips backward, giving a slight click, murmur or both.

It is obviously crucial to distinguish angina—which could require emergency aid—from a mere bout of esophageal irritation, but it's some-

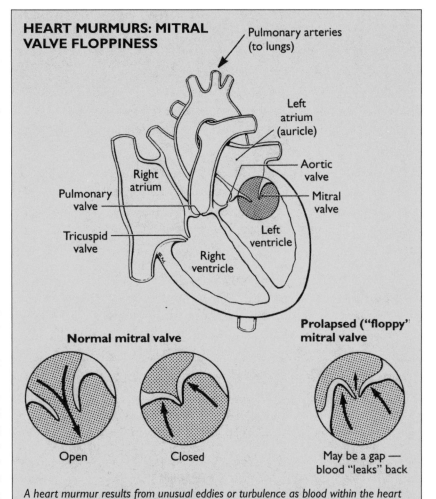

HEART MURMURS: MITRAL VALVE FLOPPINESS

Pulmonary arteries (to lungs)

Left atrium (auricle)

Right atrium

Aortic valve

Pulmonary valve

Mitral valve

Tricuspid valve

Left ventricle

Right ventricle

Normal mitral valve

Open

Closed

Prolapsed ("floppy" mitral valve)

May be a gap — blood "leaks" back

A heart murmur results from unusual eddies or turbulence as blood within the heart flows through its valves.

MEDICATIONS TO RELIEVE HEARTBURN

- *Antacids* (e.g., Maalox, Gelusil, Mylanta, Amphojel, Tums, Pepto-Bismol or Rolaids) may help mild to moderate heartburn by neutralizing stomach acids—these are the traditional mainstays of heartburn therapy.

Liquid forms give speedier relief but are messier and less portable than tablets. (N.B.: Some antacids contain magnesium and aluminum, which can be harmful in large doses. Those on salt-restricted diets must watch the sodium content of antacids.)

- *Alginic acid* (Algicon) and other mucilaginous or foaming agents—taken as tablets to suck, not chew—form a "raft" that floats on top of the stomach, coating its contents and preventing reflux.

- *H2-histamine receptor blockers* (e.g., ranitidine, Zantac), taken as tablets, can ease severe heartburn by inhibiting gastric-acid secretion. These are now available over the counter.

- **Proton Pump Inhibitors:** These medications are used for more severe heartburn and include *rabeprazole* (Pariet), *omeprazole* (Losec), or *pantoprazole* (Pantoloc).

---

times hard to tell the difference. Heartburn usually worsens when lying down or bending over, and lessens on standing, while angina frequently worsens with exercise. If in doubt, get medical assistance—better safe than sorry!

Understanding heartburn

During normal swallowing, food moves down the digestive tract by involuntary smooth-muscle contractions known as peristalsis. At the lower end of the esophagus, the lower esophageal sphincter (LES) opens to let food pass into the stomach and then normally shuts tight once swallowing is finished. Between meals, this sphincter normally stays well closed, keeping down the stomach contents. However, for a variety of reasons, it can become lax and fail to shut tightly enough, allowing the stomach's acidic contents to escape back up (reflux) into the esophagus. This acidic reflux may irritate, inflame and perhaps damage the sensitive lining of the esophagus, producing the burning sensation known as heartburn. As the stomach empties, heartburn wanes.

Heartburn must be differentiated from pain due to stomach or duodenal ulcers, which worsens on an empty stomach, tends to awaken people at night and is often relieved by milk. Tests for heartburn include a barium X-ray to inspect the lower esophagus and stomach, and direct endoscopic examination with a long fiber-optic viewing tube that can visualize the esophagus, stomach and duodenum.

The link to hiatus hernia

Hiatus hernia is one cause of heartburn. It occurs when part of the stomach protrudes past the diaphragm into the chest cavity. Many people (about 10 percent) have unsuspected hiatus hernia with absolutely no symptoms, but by the same token many people with severe heartburn do actually have a hiatus hernia. Pressure from a hiatus hernia can weaken the LES, allowing gastric juices to back up and produce heartburn, causing sufferers to seek medical aid. (See also "Hernias" on page 539.)

People prone to heartburn

The obese tend to have heartburn because a large part of the abdominal cavity is filled with fat, which pushes the stomach against the diaphragm. The increased abdominal pressure may force some acidic stomach contents back into the esophagus.

FACTORS THAT EXACERBATE HEARTBURN

- **Too much stomach acid.**
- **Fatty and fried foods, chocolate, hot spices, citrus juices and tomato products.**
- **Tobacco, alcohol and caffeine—which may** aggravate the stomach, increase acid production and cause esophageal backflow. (Caffeine and alcohol stimulate the production of gastric juices.)
- **Eating large meals,** especially at night.
- **Gas in the stomach;** almost everyone swallows some air, especially if gulping food.
- **Certain drugs that reduce esophageal** sphincter action, such as progesterone; antispasmodics (often taken to relieve indigestion and/or heartburn, they in fact aggravate it); a few antibiotics (especially tetracycline and erythromycin) that may irritate or "burn" the esophageal wall.
- **Stress, nervous tension and anxiety.**

MEASURES TO PREVENT HEARTBURN

- **Avoid dietary fat, which slows gastric emptying.**
- **Do not eat large meals that over-distend the stomach (especially within 3 hours of bedtime); it takes about 4 hours to empty a large meal from the stomach. Small ones are less** burdensome.
- **Chew food well and eat slowly to decrease swallowed air.**
- **Avoid suspected heartburn-inducing foods (e.g., coffee, fried items, citrus juices or tomato products).**
- **Avoid peppermint (which acts directly** on the esophageal sphincter).
- **Abstain from tobacco products, as nicotine lowers esophageal sphincter pressure and impairs stomach action.**
- **Lose weight if obese.**
- **Do not take post-prandial naps or lie down right after meals; a recumbent** posture worsens the discomfort. Instead take a walk, exercise or move about following a large meal, staying upright for 2 to 3 hours.
- **Remove tight-fitting belts and girdles.**
- **Prop up the head of the bed to raise the upper part of the body above the feet** and minimize backup of stomach juices due to gravity.
- **Eliminate or cut back on heartburn-aggravating medications (e.g., some antibiotics and anti-spasmodics—such as Buscopan);**
- **Minimize stress whenever possible.**

Pregnancy may also cause heartburn (in about 25 percent of expectant women). Progesterone, a hormone of pregnancy, tends to decrease sphincter muscle tone, allowing acidic stomach contents to regurgitate. Also, the growing uterus increases intra-abdominal pressure. Progesterone-containing birth-control pills cause heartburn in some women.

The elderly tend to get heartburn because their esophageal sphincters become weak and less efficient.

Surgery is a last resort for heartburn

When heartburn coexists with a hiatus hernia and symptoms resist all efforts at medical therapy, surgical repair of the hernia may relieve the discomfort. Fewer than 5 percent of those with reflux esophagitis qualify for an operation. Those who develop severe bleeding from esophageal ulcers or a critical narrowing of the esophagus are the most likely candidates. Aside from the cost, discomfort and risk, after-effects—such as "trapped gas"—can be more troublesome than the symptoms that prompted surgery. Seeking a second medical opinion about a proposed hiatus hernia operation makes good sense, especially if surgery is suggested before all non-operative measures have been thoroughly exhausted.

HEMOPHILIA

Hemophilia is an inherited, recessive, sex-linked bleeding disease, transmitted from mothers to sons via a genetic mutation or flaw in the X ("sex") chromosome, that leads to the absence of vital clotting factors. It affects about 1 per 5,000 male live-births. By the processes of inheritance, affected males pass the faulty recessive gene (on the long arm of the X-chromosome) to all their daughters but to none of their sons. This recessive condition manifests itself only in males because there is no "normal" or protecting gene in a second X chromosome to mitigate its effect. (The Y sex chromosome of males is shorter and has no matching or normal gene to offset the disease.) Affected women who inherit a hemophilia gene on one of their X chromosomes become "carriers" of a disease that doesn't affect them but endangers half their male offspring. (Statistically, half the sons of a carrier mother will inherit the hemophilia gene.) Hemophilia is renowned for its prevalence among the royal families of Europe who frequently intermarried. Queen Victoria, for instance, a carrier with no sign of the disease, passed hemophilia to her son Leopold and to two daughters, who in turn became carriers and transmitted the disease to the Russian and Spanish royal families.

The most common types of hemophilia involve missing clotting factor VIII (hemophilia A, the predominant form) or absence of clotting factor IX (hemophilia B), but the two forms are virtually identical. (Another milder bleeding disorder, von Willebrandt's disease, is due to a different genetic mechanism.) Hemophilia can be severe or mild according to the exact type of mutation and the molecular makeup of the missing clotting factors. Mild hemophilia may produce bleeds only after serious injury, but those with the severe form may have 20 to 30 bleeds a year.

Hemophilia is often detected in affected males by their tendency to bruise easily, or by nonstop hemorrhaging of cuts and wounds, or after tooth extractions. Internal or joint bleeds may produce pain and other symptoms. In severe cases, it is usually detected in early childhood, but milder cases may go unnoticed until a severe injury or surgery brings it to light. Hemophilia is diagnosed by a blood clotting test that reveals low or absent coagulation activity. Tests can now also determine whether a woman is a hemophilia gene carrier, and if pregnant, whether her fetus is affected.

Whereas, half a decade ago, many hemophiliacs didn't survive into adulthood, and children may have had several hospitalizations and been seen by many doctors for hemorrhages by age 10, treatments are now available to stop or prevent bleeds with special blood-clotting products. Since the 1970s, plasma products have been produced to supply the missing clotting factors VIII or IX. Affected people can even administer the blood products themselves by home infusion to stop or prevent bleeding episodes, although serious hemorrhages still require hospital treatment. In some cases, antibodies, inhibitors or allergies develop that diminish the effectiveness of clotting factors.

While the provision of new plasma products greatly improved the quality of life for those with hemophilia, it also brought great problems and much heartbreak by transmitting infections such as HIV and hepatitis alongside the life-saving clotting agents. During the 1980s, factor VIII products were made from pooled donor blood obtained from many people that, despite screening procedures, still often contained viruses, even lethal ones such as HIV. Before effective screening was established, thousands of hemophiliac men and their sexual partners developed and died of AIDS and hepatitis B and C.

Better screening methods, more purification and heat treatment of clotting factor products (to 80° F or higher) to inactivate viruses, as well as the development of new recombinant or genetically engineered antihemophilia agents have greatly improved treatment and reduced infection risks. Treatment "on demand" as bleeds occur may be the chosen management, or prophylactic therapy, using clotting factors regularly to avoid hemorrhages. Recombinant clotting factors are becoming the treatment of choice for hemophilia as they eliminate the risk of transmitted infections. A new recombinant clotting factor (rFVIIa) has now been FDA-approved (not yet approved in Canada) to help people with hemophilia who develop antibodies that inhibit the usefulness of other clotting products.

Children with hemophilia are still encouraged to avoid high-injury activities (such as hockey and football). Female relatives of people with the disorder can get genetic counseling before starting a family, although genetic testing of girls is not advised until they are 14 to 16 years old and can fully comprehend the implications.

In future, gene therapy may be the solution for treating hemophilia, as DNA-analysis can now determine exactly what gene mutations are causing the disease and which molecular abnormalities deter clotting. Trials with gene replacement for hemophilia A and B are currently under way, but although the results have been encouraging so far, this therapy hasn't succeeded in producing enough blood clotting to avoid the need for additional coagulation products. While researchers confidently predict that affordable gene therapy will be the ultimate method of banishing hemophilia, thousands of hemophilia sufferers around the world still remain undiagnosed and untreated.

HEMORRHOIDS

An estimated 50 percent of North American men and women have hemorrhoids—formerly known as "piles"—at some time in their lives. Hemorrhoids are rare before age 30, frequent over age 50. Although many people are reluctant to discuss anal problems, it is vital to report any rectal discomfort, bleeding or change in bowel habits to a physician as it may herald some more serious disorder.

The term "hemorrhoid" is often mistakenly applied to any minor anal or rectal problem, itching or irritation, but anal discomfort may arise from any number of other causes—such as *pruritis ani* (skin itchiness). Hemorrhoids are enlarged, blood-filled pads in the anal region. Humans are prone to them because their erect posture exerts a lot of pressure on blood vessels around the anus. While some hemorrhoids give little or no discomfort, others cause burning during bowel movements, itchiness and a sense of incomplete emptying. The most common symptom is bleeding from small vessels in the anal area.

Differentiating internal from external hemorrhoids

There are both "internal" and "external" hemorrhoids. Internal hemorrhoids are distended blood vessels in the moist bowel lining above the transition line. Visible only through a special viewing instrument, they usually produce no symptoms other than bleeding in their early stages and are generally painless unless thrombosed (clotted) or strangulated (causing muscle spasms at the anus). Spongy, swollen internal hemorrhoids sometimes prolapse—protrude through the anus—and can be difficult to ease back up, at which stage they often hurt. Although they usually go back spontaneously to their inner position, protruding internal hemorrhoids may need to be pushed back into the canal after defecating. As they develop further,

---

OTHER ANORECTAL PROBLEMS (SOMETIMES MISTAKEN FOR HEMORRHOIDS)

- **Pruritus ani:** relatively common anal itching due to irritation from various causes, which responds well to hemorrhoidal ointments and scrupulous cleansing with moistened pads or "baby wipes."
- **Anusitis:** inflammation of the lining in the anal canal—treated with steroidal anti-inflammatories or Anurex.
- **Anal fissures:** thin, slit-like tears in the anal tissue, which cause itching, pain and bleeding during bowel movements. They usually respond to stool-softening agents, emollients or bulk laxatives and local application of a steroid cream. (Seek a physician's advice before proceeding with these measures.)
- **External skin** tags: not usually painful, they are leftover tissue from external hemorrhoids, which may interfere with anal hygiene, a problem usually overcome by emollient cleansers.

---

they may bleed more and cause greater discomfort, especially if they protrude during bowel movements. In their late stages, internal hemorrhoids may permanently hang down (although they don't block defecation), be quite uncomfortable and bleed a lot.

External hemorrhoids (also called para-anal lesions) include a variety of bluish swellings, hematomas (small pea-sized lumps) and skin tags (loose skin flaps) that occur outside the anus or opening of the rectum below the transition line. The small bumps can be seen using a hand-held mirror. They are swollen skin-covered vessels, which some experts do not regard as real hemorrhoids. External hemorrhoids may be itchy and tender, worsened by scratching and imperfect or overvigorous cleaning. Bleeding is rarely a sign of external lesions unless the area is injured or ulcerated.

Diagnosis and medical examination

Medical examination will include a visual and manual (gloved) inspection of the rectal area and use of viewing instruments—a rigid or flexible sigmoidoscope or the longer, farther-reaching colonoscope—to look varying distances up the colon. Some physicians suggest that all men and women over 45 should have a sigmoidoscopy every year or two and a more extensive bowel examination when indicated.

Treatment of hemorrhoids

Most hemorrhoids can be controlled by home treatment with warm sitz baths, soothing ointments and suppositories, as well as avoidance of

---

HEMORRHOIDS: ANATOMY OF THE ANAL REGION

- Rectum
- Moist mucus membrane
- Transition line
- Internal hemorrhoid
- Protrusion into canal
- Skin
- Anus
- External hemorrhoid (blood clot)

MAIN CAUSES OF HEMORRHOIDS

- Anything that increases intra-abdominal pressure, such as forcing or straining at stool, heavy physical effort, prolonged sitting or standing.
- Pregnancy—in the last trimester—as the enlarged uterus presses on anal blood vessels. Sometimes the strain of child-birth leads to post-partum hemorrhoids.
- Faulty diet—eating foods low in fiber (roughage) and fluid may produce hard stools that irritate the bowel. Hemorrhoids are less common in those who eat high-fiber diets.
- Poor bowel habits such as "holding back."
- Reading on the toilet may contribute, as sitting there too long exerts undue strain, without support for anal structures.
- Explosive diarrhea and chronic coughing may increase the risks.

ALERTING SIGNS AND SYMPTOMS

- An external hemorrhoid may be felt as a lump, perhaps due to a sizable blood clot.
- Itching, discomfort and difficulty in cleansing are most typical of external hemorrhoids.
- Bleeding from internal hemorrhoids may produce:
  - a smudge on the toilet tissue;
  - blood in the toilet bowl;
  - streaks of blood on the stool;
  - blood-stained underwear.
- Protrusion of internal hemorrhoids may be noticed after a bowel movement (they should be pushed back to avoid discomfort).
  N.B.: The first sight of rectal bleeding should trigger a prompt visit to the doctor. One cannot assume that rectal bleeding is due to hemorrhoids until other more serious causes (such as colitis or bowel cancer) have been ruled out. Any new rectal bleeding should be reported at once.

HOME HEMORRHOID REMEDIES

- Cold compresses to reduce the pain.
- Avoiding constipation. Relieve constipation with increased fiber and fluid intake, or gentle stool softeners such as Surfak or laxatives (such as milk of magnesia) if needed. (See also section in this chapter on constipation.)
- Witch hazel or other soothing lotions to alleviate the itching.
- Over-the-counter preparations such as Anusol ointment or suppositories, or Preparation H.
- Sitz (sitting) baths that soak the anal area in warm water two or three times a day.
- Anurex-R, an over-the-counter, reusable device—a thin, short probe containing a gel that is cooled in the freezer before insertion into the anal canal. Used twice daily, it provides soothing relief and can stop bleeding from internal hemorrhoids.
- Good anal hygiene—best achieved by wiping with moist pads rather than dry toilet tissue.
- ASA or acetaminophen to relieve pain (but avoid codeine, which only increases constipation).
- Loose cotton underwear rather than tight synthetics.
- Avoiding prolonged sitting or standing when hemorrhoids act up.

Medical treatments:
- Always seek medical advice about acute hemorrhoids that are large, hard, swollen and uncomfortable.
- Early excision and evacuation of a thrombosed (clotted) external hemorrhoid is a simple doctor's-office procedure done under a local anesthetic that sometimes gives immediate relief. Healing is speedy and helped along by warm sitz baths.
- Rubber-band ligation is a common treatment for eliminating internal hemorrhoids—done in the doctor's office with a high success rate. An elastic band is wrapped around the hemorrhoid with a special instrument that chokes off the blood supply, so that the rubber band and hemorrhoid slough off in 2 to 14 days. The procedure is performed without anesthetic since there are no pain endings in the mucosal tissue where internal hemorrhoids occur. It is quick, relatively painless and inexpensive.
- Rubber-banding is occasionally combined with cryotherapy (freezing). After the hemorrhoid is wrapped with an elastic band, the tissue is frozen. Since the rubber band is then snipped off, the patient may experience less discomfort than with rubber-banding alone.
- Injection sclerotherapy—injecting the hemorrhoid with certain solutions—is rarely used any more.
- Laser therapy is expensive and still experimental.
- Surgery in hospital is now rarely used, although occasionally needed for internal hemorrhoids that resist other therapy.

constipation. Both internal and external hemorrhoids generally clear up within 2 weeks, but if not, medical treatment is needed. Office procedures (ligation, injection, freezing) can usually cure hemorrhoids, although persistent and/or particularly painful ones may require surgery in hospital.

HEPATITIS

Viral hepatitis endangers millions around the world, and is responsible for more than 2 million deaths a year—far more than those affected by the HIV virus that causes AIDS. Some forms of viral hepatitis can lead to cirrhosis and liver cancer years after people contracted the infection. Governments and health professionals are striving to cut the toll by better blood screening, educating people about ways to avoid catching or spreading this infection, and, above all, by vaccination whenever possible.

It's not so much the acute or initial attack of infectious hepatitis, but its long-term consequences that pose the greatest danger. What's new in the war against hepatitis is an effective vaccine for hepatitis A, global immunization programs against hepatitis B and screening of blood donations for hepatitis C. Nonetheless, healthcare officials fear the global impact of viral hepatitis due to the many undiscovered carriers who spread the infection via shared drug equipment, unclean vaccination needles, contaminated blood products, mother–child transmission, promiscuous sex, tattooing and body piercing. While hepatitis B has been a long-recognized health threat, hepatitis C is a newly emerging danger. About 3.5 million North Americans carry the hepatitis C virus (an estimated 15 percent of those were supposedly infected through blood products, before testing began). The Krever Commission of Inquiry on the Blood System in Canada revealed that thousands of Canadians may have contracted hepatitis C through blood transfusions received before 1990 (when blood testing for this virus first started).

Although it often goes unnoticed, hepatitis C can smolder for decades, perhaps ultimately producing liver cirrhosis or cancer. Testing has reduced blood-transfusion risks, but still in high danger of this infection are needle-sharing drug users, those who share contaminated medical equipment, vaccination needles, household or hygiene articles, and—to a lesser extent—organ transplant recipients. Even a trace of contaminated blood on a tattoo needle, toothbrush or razor can transmit the virus.

Recapping the ABCs of viral hepatitis

To date, several different hepatitis-causing viruses have been isolated and named alphabetically: A, B, C, D and E. (Two further forms, F and G, have been identified but little is yet known about them.)

The different forms spread differently. Hepatitis A and E are waterborne and spread mainly via sewage-contaminated food and water—rare in Canada, although outbreaks occur in areas of poor sanitation. Hepatitis B is transmitted much like AIDS—through sexual activity and contact with infected semen, blood and vaginal secretions and from mother to newborn baby. Hepatitis C spreads almost exclusively via direct blood-to-blood contact, as with shared (blood-contaminated) drug-injection needles or other articles and through blood transfusions. The D virus cannot cause illness on its own, only in combination with hepatitis B.

Few warning signs of infectious hepatitis

The hepatitis viruses attack and inflame the liver by invading hepatocytes (liver cells), but the acute phase often produces few or no symptoms—other than tiredness, perhaps a slight fever and nausea—sometimes taken for a bout of flu, or passing unnoticed. There may be some jaundice (yellowing of skin and whites of the eyes). But the initial infection is rarely serious or life-endangering, although occasionally a so-called fulminant or fast-progressing form is rapidly fatal. The chief concern is not so much the acute illness but its lasting effects in those who harbor the virus and become carriers. The fact that someone has viral hepatitis is often discovered accidentally when routine blood tests are done.

Different types of hepatitis have different effects

After the initial or acute stage, the course of viral hepatitis distinguishes the different types. Once hepatitis A and E infection fades, after a few weeks, the viruses are cleared from the body and the person develops lifelong immunity to that particular form. In contrast, with hepatitis B, C and D, viral particles can linger on in the body, producing a chronic infection that lasts for life and may lead to liver cirrhosis and perhaps liver cancer.

Hepatitis A (HAV): One travel souvenir better left behind

Worldwide, almost 2 million cases of hepatitis A are reported each year, but the incidence is likely higher as many cases go unreported. Although much more rare, hepatitis A can also occasionally be found in Canada, typically transmitted in restaurants or other places where infected individuals are handling food. Hepatitis A spreads primarily through water and fecally contaminated food, especially raw or undercooked shellfish. Food handlers and healthcare workers easily pass on the disease. Homosexual men are at risk as the A virus spreads via anal contact.

Hepatitis A is a generally mild illness, perhaps signaled by diarrhea, stomach cramps, headache and low fever—possibly also jaundice. But many don't realize they have the illness,

which usually disappears in 1 to 3 months, although it can last up to 6 months. About one quarter of adult cases need hospital treatment. Occasionally a severe, fulminant form—rare in young people—is rapidly fatal, mostly in the over-50 age group; seniors have a 3 percent mortality rate (compared with 0.1 percent for younger groups). There's no known treatment for hepatitis A, but once over it the person is immune for life. In endemic areas, where the disease is widespread, most people are exposed as children and therefore immune.

This infection is an escalating threat to vacationers who venture into endemic or hepatitis A–ridden areas such as Asia, Africa, Latin America, the Middle East, Mexico, the Caribbean and Mediterranean (southern) Europe. But travelers can now protect themselves from hepatitis A by immunization with safe, effective vaccines (such as Havrix, Vaqta, or Twinrix—a combined hepatitis A and B vaccine). Two intramuscular shots one month apart, and a booster 6 to 12 months later, can protect people for up to 10 years. Most of those vaccinated are 90 percent protected 1 month later. Since the incubation period for hepatitis A is about 4 weeks, even a last-minute shot offers some protection.

As a rule of thumb, all travelers, even those who go just once off-trail, should all be vaccinated. "Yet," bemoans one tropical disease expert, "although hepatitis A is 100 times more common than typhoid fever, and 1,000 times more prevalent than cholera, too few vacationers bother to get immunized; some don't even take the most elementary precautions—such as washing hands before eating, drinking only bottled or sterile water (no ice!), eating well-cooked food and avoiding raw or steamed shellfish."

Hepatitis B (HBV)

Hepatitis B infects 300 million people globally, with almost 2 million deaths per year. In Canada, about 3,000 new cases are reported annually (thousands more probably going unreported). Hepatitis B is particularly widespread in some aboriginal communities and among immigrants from highly endemic countries (e.g., Asia, Africa, southern Europe). It can be acquired at birth by contact with the mother's contaminated body

RISKS OF GETTING HEPATITIS FROM BLOOD TRANSFUSION GOING DOWN

Now that all donated blood is screened for hepatitis B and C, the risk has fallen considerably, although it varies from place to place. Canadian Red Cross officials put the odds of contracting hepatitis B from blood transfusion at approximately 1 per 250,000 units, and for hepatitis C at 1 in 60,000—compared to an estimated risk of getting the human immunodeficiency virus (HIV) that causes AIDS (from blood transfusion) of 1

per 913,000. "But," notes one official, "hepatitis C risks are still only a guesstimate, as the tests are only 90 to 95 percent accurate, compared with a 99 percent plus accuracy for HIV." Tests on donated blood are not foolproof because the tests are not 100 percent accurate and there is a "window" when someone newly infected with hepatitis has not yet developed detectable antibodies. The current risks for

hepatitis C from transfusion is estimated at 1 in 100,000. Transmission of hepatitis A by transfusion is very rare because the virus is not usually found in blood. However, about 4 weeks after infection, when the virus is at peak production, it may spill over into the blood, If blood is donated during this short window of time—usually a few days—the A virus may enter the blood supply.

fluids. About 90 percent of babies and young children infected with hepatitis B, but fewer adults (5 percent), become lifelong carriers.

As with other types of viral hepatitis, the B form often shows few obvious signs of illness, but infected carriers can pass the disease to others, even if they feel perfectly well. The chief danger of hepatitis B is not the acute illness, which isn't usually severe, but its long-term consequences. About 20 percent of carriers eventually die of the disease—due to liver cirrhosis or liver cancer often decades after being infected. In a few instances (about 0.1 percent), hepatitis B is a swiftly progressing, rapidly fatal disease.

Hepatitis B is primarily a sexually transmitted disease that spreads through contact with blood, semen or vaginal secretions; sexual activity causes over half the adult cases. Injection drug use is also a major transmission route. All it takes to be infected with hepatitis B is one use—for any purpose—of a needle or other shared equipment bearing even traces of infected blood. Few realize that hepatitis B spreads far more easily than HIV. Being hardier, hepatitis B viruses survive on razors, needles and other instruments and are also transmitted through saliva, easily infecting household contacts. Traces of infected blood left on household items such as toothbrushes, manicure tools and hairbrushes spread the virus. But unlike AIDS, it is preventable by a reliable, safe vaccine. Simple blood tests can detect antibodies showing that someone carries hepatitis B viruses and can infect others. Family members and companions of infected carriers should all be immunized. All persons with chronic hepatitis B not immune to hepatitis A should receive 2 doses of hepatitis A vaccine 6 to 18 months apart.

For patients with chronically elevated liver enzymes, some may benefit from anti-viral medication such as *interferon alpha* (IFNα) and *lamuvidine* (a drug that's still being evaluated). These drugs are expensive and have side effects (muscle aches, chills, cough), and many relapse once treatment ends.

Universal hepatitis B immunization strongly promoted

A safe, effective hepatitis B vaccine, given in 3 doses over a 6-month period, provides immunity lasting at least 10 years, probably longer. Since 1995, many countries have introduced maternal screening and newborn immunization for newborns of infected mothers, as well as routine, population-wide immunization. In Canada, all provinces and territories except Manitoba immunize schoolchildren or teenagers at various ages. Officials estimate that 90 percent of Canadian students are getting their shots.

Besides immunization, many health agencies promote needle-exchange programs and encourage use of sterile, disposable equipment for all skin-piercing situations—such as tattooing, body piercing and acupuncture. Transfusion risks for hepatitis B are now minimal, as all blood and blood products are screened for the virus (since 1973). (See also page 305.)

Hepatitis C (HCV): thousands at risk

First identified in 1989, the C form of hepatitis has become a pressing health concern. Worldwide, 50 to 300 million people are infected, including 1 percent of Canadians and 4 percent in some European countries (such as Spain and Italy). At highest risk are people who received blood products before 1990 (when testing began for this virus), dialysis patients, needle-sharing injection drug users and transplant recipients. Hemophiliacs and others who received blood components during the 1980s now have infection rates of 40 to 70 percent.

While the Krever Inquiry highlighted the spread of hepatitis C via transfusion, it emphasized that this blood-borne pathogen is transmitted mainly through injection drug use. (Up to 90 percent of past or present intravenous drug users are infected.) Sharing injection drug needles or other drug equipment even once is enough to transmit the virus.

When first contracted, hepatitis C often passes unnoticed, causing nothing more than some fatigue, perhaps skin itching and transient jaundice. In contrast to the B form, where only a small proportion of adults become carriers, 70 to 90 percent of those infected with hepatitis C become lifelong carriers—facing possible liver cirrhosis or cancer. One Health Canada official puts the risk of hepatitis C–induced cirrhosis at "25 percent after 20 years of infection, some progressing to liver cancer."

HIGH-RISK PEOPLE WHO NEED HEPATITIS B SHOTS

- **Those frequently exposed to blood products—such as healthcare workers and embalmers;**
- **residents and staff of institutions for the developmentally handicapped;**
- **sexually active homosexual and bisexual males;**
- **people with multiple sex partners;**
- **injection-drug users;**
- **household contacts of hepatitis B carriers;**
- **travelers to areas where hepatitis B is rampant, such as Southeast Asia and tropical Africa.**

N.B.: For those not included in universal immunization or high-risk programs, vaccination can be arranged with a family physician. Today in Canada, authorities advise universal hepatitis B vaccination for all school-age children.

THE ABCs OF VIRAL HEPATITIS AT A GLANCE

Virus Type	How it's spread—transmission routes	Symptoms	Disease/illness features
Hepatitis A (HAV) (waterborne)	• from feces (fecal-oral route) in sewage-polluted water, food; on cooking utensils, dirty hands, soiled diapers (daycare centers); • to travelers in endemic areas; • via raw or undercooked shellfish such as clams, mussels, oysters; • blood-transfusion risks minimal, but some concern regarding pooled blood products.	• often none, especially in children under 2 years; • may include appetite loss, diarrhea, vomiting, dull abdominal pain and flu-like symptoms (fever, headache); • jaundice (yellowed eye whites and skin) in some; • severity increases with age; • raised levels of liver enzyme in blood.	• short incubation, one month (most infectious for 3 to 5 days at end of this period); • virus cleared in 1 to 3 months (6 months at most); • does not produce chronic infection; • 0.1 percent are fulminant (rapid, intense) cases possibly fatal—overall, 0.1–1 percent mortality rate, rising to 3% over age 50.
Hepatitis B (HBV) (in body fluids)	• through intimate and sexual contact, via blood and other body fluids; • by shared injection drug use, tattooing, body piercing, needle-stick injuries; • by sharing razors, toothbrushes and other household items; • from mother to newborn at birth, possibly also through breastmilk; • blood transfusion risk now about 1 per 250,000 units.	• often subclinical with few or no symptoms; • possibly flu-like malaise, diarrhea, abdominal pain and jaundice (yellowed eye whites and skin); • dark urine, pale stools; • detected by blood tests for viral markers.	• long incubation period (3 months or more); • acute phase lasts 1 to 3 months with about 1 percent mortality (from fatal, fulminant, rapid course); • 60 to 90 percent of infected infants and 6 to 10 percent infected adults become persistent chronic B carriers, at risk of later cirrhosis and liver cancer; • asymptomatic carriers can unknowingly infect others.
Hepatitis C (HCV) (blood borne)	• via blood-to-blood contact; • mainly by shared-injection drug use; • tattooing, body piercing and household items; • before blood screening began, 2 percent of donated blood units infected, but transfusion risks now down to about 1 in 60,000 units; • sexual transmission doubtful in absence of sores, menstrual blood; • not transmitted from infected mother to baby in womb but possible risk of infection at birth, also perhaps through breastmilk (uncertain).	• usually subclinical, with few or no signs of infection; • may produce fatigue, jaundice, itchy skin; • detected by blood tests for viral markers.	• incubation at least 50 days; • fatal, acute and fulminant cases rare; • 60 to 90 percent become chronic carriers at risk of liver cirrhosis and liver cancer; • disease worsened by excessive alcohol consumption.
Hepatitis D (HDV) (delta agent)	• mainly by same routes as HBV, but not via infected mothers to newborns; • primarily via shared injection drug use/equipment.	• in combination with B causes severe liver disease with swifter progression to cirrhosis, liver cancer; • high fatality rate.	• defective virus can usually only infect liver together with B form; • high mortality rates in acute phase; • virus rarely cleared—almost all progress to chronic disease.
Hepatitis E (HEV) (waterborne)	• fecal-oral route (like A form) in sewage-polluted water and food; • via shellfish such as clams, mussels, oysters.	• incubation period 45 days; • possible diarrhea, abdominal pain, flu-like symptoms, jaundice (yellowed eye whites and skin); • often no symptoms, especially in children.	• as for HAV, no chronic infection; • mortality rate from 0.1 to 4 percent; • very dangerous to pregnant women especially in third trimester (high mortality rate).

Prevalence, where and in whom

• found everywhere, but most common in Asia, Africa, Mexico, Central and
  Eastern Europe;
• rare in Canada but can be acquired in endemic areas;
• also pockets of high prevalence in poverty-stricken, crowded areas; "outbreaks" in institutions (prisons, homes for disabled, crowded daycare
  centers).

• worldwide causes 2 million deaths per year;
• commonest in tropical Africa, Latin America, S.E. Asia, Southern Europe;
• groups at high risk: injection-sharing drug users, homosexuals, people with
  many sex partners; newborns of infected mothers, family members of
  infected individuals, travelers to endemic areas; health and emergency
  response workers, police, embalmers.

• worldwide, 150 to 300 million infected;
• in North America, estimated 1 percent infected;
• most common in S.E. Asia, China, Japan, Middle East, Mediterranean areas
  (e.g., Italy);
• equipment-sharing drug users at high risk; also those who share razors,
  combs, and other household items.

• most common in Mediterranean countries (e.g., Italy, Greece), South
  America and parts of Middle East and Africa;
• in Canada and U.S., mostly among injection drug users.

• outbreaks reported in parts of Africa, Middle East, Asia, Mexico;
• rarely encountered in Canada but can infect travellers to endemic areas.

Treatment and/or prevention

• safe, effective vaccines available, good for travelers;
• vaccination advised for frequent or "off-trail" travel (even once) to
  endemic areas;
• wash hands after toilet, and before meals;
• drink boiled or bottled water/drinks (no ice);
• don't eat raw or undercooked shellfish in endemic areas;
• avoid salads and non-peelable fruit and vegetables.

• safe, effective vaccine available;
• universal vaccination promoted for all children and adolescents, and high-
  risk groups;
• newborns of hepatitis B-carrying mothers receive immune-globulin and
  vaccine;
• use disposable, sterile needles for all injections, tattooing, body piercing;
• no effective cure; some respond to interferon-a and other antivirals, but
  one-third relapse.

• no effective therapy;
• interferon-a gives sustained remission in some and is becoming more popular in its new form that is more tolerable;
• liver transplants can help HCV-induced end-stage liver disease;
• no vaccine available;
• use only disposable, sterile needles for injections, tattooing, body piercing,
  acupuncture;
• consider use of condoms, especially for new or unknown sex partners.

• no effective treatment to date;
• poor response to antivirals;
• hepatitis B vaccination protects against infection and disease spread
  because of the dependence on HBV.

• no effective therapy;
• no vaccine yet;
• hand-washing and better hygiene may cut spread;
• use same precautions as for hepatitis A.

However, carriers may remain healthy for decades, with no signs to indicate the silent liver destruction. Unaware of being carriers, they may spread the disease to others for years to come. As the disease gives no clues to its presence, many discover they have it only through a routine blood test. Tests on donated blood have now reduced the risk of transfusion-acquired hepatitis C to 1 per 60,000 units—not to zero, as the test is not completely accurate and some hepatitis C–infected blood slips through the screening net.

Whether hepatitis C can be sexually transmitted remains questionable, although those with multiple sex partners could be at risk, especially if they have open sores on the genitals. Hepatitis C–infected women should refrain from sexual intercourse when menstruating.

Pregnant women rarely transmit hepatitis C to the fetus unless they are also HIV-positive, but there is some danger to newborns at delivery. The hepatitis C virus is not thought to be present in breastmilk, but infected mothers with cracked nipples could infect their babies.

There is no cure or vaccine for hepatitis C, however new antiviral medications have reduced the impact of the virus on liver inflammation. Interferon alpha (interferon alfa-2a [Roferon-A] or interferon alfa-2b [Intron A]) has been used for the treatment of chronic active hepatitis C. "Pegylated Interferon," which requires fewer injections and provides more stable levels of drug, has become a popular choice for treatment. Combination treatment with oral Ribavirin is still more effective and the choice is based on patient factors and results of genetic testing. Combination treatment has been shown to completely eradicate markers of disease in up to 70 percent of patients. Liver transplants offer hope, and hepatitis C is now the second leading reason for liver transplants in Canada. (The new liver is also likely to become infected, but not necessarily harmed.)

Hepatitis D (HDV): Worsens hepatitis B infections

The D virus cannot infect liver cells on its own but only in combination with active B viruses— a deadly duo. Those infected with both hepatitis B and D simultaneously face ravaging complications. Fatality rates for acute hepatitis D plus B infection are far higher than for hepatitis B alone. Moreover, even those who survive the immediate D plus B infection rapidly develop severe liver disease. Hepatitis D is rare in North America (although IV drug users are a high-risk group); the D form is most common in Italy, South America and parts of the Middle East. There is no treatment for hepatitis D, but since it requires the B virus to produce illness, hepatitis B vaccination also protects against HDV.

Hepatitis E (HEV) now surfacing in Canada

Hepatitis E is a waterborne virus that causes acute, self-limited hepatitis, especially common among children. Like the A form, it's transmitted via fecally contaminated food and water but doesn't produce long-term disease. It is particularly prevalent in India, with over 2 million cases recorded per year. The mortality rate for hepatitis E averages 4 percent, but is higher in pregnant women, especially in the third trimester. More than one-third of women infected late in pregnancy get a fulminant form, with death rates reaching 20 percent. Pregnant women should avoid travel to endemic areas, or at least take strict food and water precautions. Hepatitis E is less preventable than hepatitis A as there is no vaccine, and immune globulin shots are ineffective.

How to "think" hepatitis and stand on guard against it

To avoid hepatitis A:

- *Wash hands well* before eating and after using any washroom—infected feces can linger on toilet flushers and doorknobs.
- *Get protective vaccination* before traveling to hepatitis A–ridden places such as Mexico, Eastern Europe and most of the developing world.
- *Drink only commercially bottled (or boiled) water* in endemic areas—wipe lids first—and avoid ice cubes.
- *Eat only well-cooked foods*, avoiding raw or steamed shellfish.
- *Avoid non-peelable raw* fruit and vegetables.
- *Eat no salads* (they might be washed in contaminated water).

To protect against hepatitis B:

- *Remember that this virus spreads primarily through sexual contact*—practise safer sex, use latex condoms plus recommended spermicide.
- *Tell your sex partners if you're a carrier*, and urge them to be tested and perhaps vaccinated. Don't donate blood or semen.
- *Get immunized* and make sure your sex partners and children are vaccinated—universal immunization programs now exist across Canada.
- *If pregnant*, or planning to have a baby, get a hepatitis B test so that if you're a carrier your baby can be vaccinated at birth.
- *Don't share equipment or personal care items*— IV drug needles, razors, toothbrushes, manicure tools or other items that could bear traces of infected blood.
- *Do not allow yourself to be* tattooed, have a body part pierced or undergo acupuncture with anything other than sterile, disposable, once-only-use needles.
- *Make sure tattoo ink bottles* are fresh (not already used).

To minimize risk of hepatitis C infection:

- *Never share IV drug needles* or other drug equipment; use only disposable, once-only-use needles and sterile body-piercing equipment.
- *If living with a carrier*, do not share household items such as razors, combs, toothbrushes.
- *Practice safer sex.* While the risk of sexually transmitting hepatitis C is low in monogamous couples, people with new or multiple partners could be at risk. Inform sex partners if infected.
- *If you are a carrier beware of infecting others with your blood.* Cover open wounds, don't share razors, manicure tools or anything else that could harbor even traces of blood.
- *Protect your liver.* Limit alcohol intake. (There's some evidence that alcohol increases liver injury.) Consult a physician before taking non-prescription drugs or alternative medicines. Consider vaccination against other forms of hepatitis (A and B).

As protection against hepatitis D:

- Since this virus cannot infect without piggy-backing on the B form, taking steps to prevent hepatitis B will also protect against D.

To combat hepatitis E:

- *Follow the same precautions* as for hepatitis A, although there is no vaccine against the E virus.
- *If pregnant, be aware of the very serious risk* from this infection, especially in the last trimester.

For more information, contact the Canadian Liver Foundation at (800) 563-5483 (website: http://www.liver.ca); The Hepatitis Society at (800) 652–HEPC (website: http://web.idirect.com/hepc): Hepatitis C Counsel at (800) 229–5323.

HERNIAS

Theoretically, any soft part of the body can herniate (bulge into or penetrate surrounding areas), but in fact hernias occur most commonly in the abdominal area—from the thorax to the groin.

Hiatus hernia

A hiatus, or diaphragmatic, hernia occurs when the abdominal contents protrude up through the hiatus—the space in the diaphragm through which the esophagus (food tube) passes into the stomach.

There are two main types of hiatus hernia: the more common "sliding" hiatus hernia and the less prevalent but more serious "paraesophageal" hernia. Pregnant women and the obese commonly suffer hiatus hernias from the extra load on the abdomen.

An estimated 10 percent of Canadians have hiatus hernia, climbing to 30 percent by age 60. The majority of people with this abdominal defect have no symptoms but when symptoms do arise, it's usually because the sphincter muscles around the lower end of the esophagus have become weakened. The esophagus runs from the mouth to the stomach, with a valve between the stomach and the gullet that remains tightly shut between swallows. If the valve's controlling muscles don't function properly, the valve won't stay closed, and stomach acids may spill into the esophagus.

Since the lining of the esophagus is sensitive to acid, unlike the tough lining of the stomach, heartburn, sharp pain, regurgitation, belching and sometimes bleeding may result. There may

SYMPTOMS OF GROIN HERNIA

Groin hernias may produce a small, egg-like lump that often does not hurt at first, tends to vanish on lying down but becomes prominent with certain activities such as coughing. There may be constant or intermittent pain on exertion, or no symptoms at all. Wearing a truss to remedy an inguinal hernia—a formerly common practice—is now discouraged and can even worsen the condition by weakening tissues. Children with inguinal hernias may have fever and vomiting. If the bulge in the groin is strangulated—squeezed at the neck—the blood circulation can be cut off and an infection can then cause a crisis. Symptoms of a strangulated hernia include pain, swelling, discolored, bluish or red skin, inflammation, vomiting and an inability to urinate—requiring emergency measures.

also be breathlessness and a choking sensation if regurgitated stomach contents are breathed in at night. Some people with symptomatic hiatus hernia have been wrongly diagnosed with asthma. About one-third of those with hiatus hernia eventually develop esophagitis, or heartburn, as the acids damage the esophageal lining, which may irritate the channel and make swallowing difficult. The gullet can even be perforated.

Diagnosis of a hiatus hernia depends on X-rays and diagnostic tests such as endoscopy (looking at the stomach via a fiberoptic tube); esophageal manometry (using a special instrument to measure sphincter pressure); and tests to measure esophageal acidity.

In the vast majority of cases (85 to 90 percent), therapy for hiatus hernia is simply treatment of heartburn. Losing weight may be recommended to relieve pressure. At night, sleeping with the upper part of the body propped up on pillows, or with the head of the bed raised 15–20 cm (6–8 in), relieves nocturnal acid reflux, and standing straight rather than slouching should also relieve the problem. (See the section on heartburn for drugs used to relieve it.)

Surgery to reinforce the malfunctioning sphincter muscle is now uncommon, but remains an option in severe cases if medical and dietary management don't succeed.

Paraesophageal hernia

A paraesophageal hernia, fortunately very rare, can be life-threatening because the hole enlarges and, in some cases, can allow the entire stomach (which may perforate) to slip into the chest cavity. Many sufferers have no symptoms, but if they do occur, the most common are pain, indigestion, nausea and retching. Heartburn and regurgitation are unusual with this problem. There is no medical treatment for paraesophageal hernia, and surgery is usually needed.

Inguinal (groin) hernias

A groin or inguinal hernia, often wrongly called a rupture, is a bulge of tissue that occurs when some abdominal contents, usually part of the intestine or a piece of bowel, protrude into the groin area through a tear or weakness in the

abdominal wall. Groin hernias affect 3 to 8 percent of the population, 10 times more men than women, often occurring after age 50 (on one side of the groin or both), accounting for 10 percent of all hospital admissions for surgery.

Groin hernias include both direct and indirect forms and the uncommon but risky *femoral hernias*, in the lower groin. Femoral hernias are a possibly life-threatening condition with the blood supply cut off, affecting more women than men, requiring immediate care. Groin hernias usually appear in middle life but can occur in infancy because of a congenital weakness in the abdominal wall, affecting as many as 5 percent of full-term infants and up to 30 percent of premature babies. However, the flaw may not show up until adulthood.

Quite often an incipient groin hernia does not reveal itself until, with aging and years of strain, the abdominal wall becomes weaker because of straining during bowel movements or from heavy coughing. (Heavily coughing smokers are prone to groin hernias.) Physical exertion, such as lifting, may bring on a hernia by suddenly causing the weakened abdominal lining to give way.

While not generally life-threatening, groin hernias can be dangerous because of strangulation or incarceration when a piece of protruding intestine (or bowel) is caught or strangled, cutting off the blood supply. The result can be putrefaction in the "dead" piece of bowel, leading to infection, inflammation, gangrene and life-threatening abdominal infection.

Treatment for groin hernias is surgical repair to bundle the protruding mass back where it belongs and reinforce the weakened area often a simple operation, sometimes done under local anesthetic. Unfortunately about 10 percent require another hernia repair at some later date. Complications after surgery include neuralgia (from a trapped nerve) and urinary problems (particularly in older men), so regular medical follow-up is recommended.

The latest method of laparoscopic hernia repair, done through a tiny incision (with the help of fiberoptic viewing instruments) avoids the need for open surgery, hastening postoperative healing. The surgeon conducts the operation by watching what is happening inside the patient on a TV viewing screen, moving the instruments accordingly. Its advantages are less postoperative pain and disability than with open surgery, often permitting a return to work within a few days. Studies also suggest less likelihood of recurrence.

While some surgeons favor a swift postoperative return to activity, others restrict exercise for many weeks after the operation. Toronto's Shouldice Clinic, a world leader in surgery for groin hernias, favors a speedy return to activity. Hospital stays average 2 to 3 days, and activity is resumed soon, if not immediately, after surgery, with special exercise programs to reduce pain and swelling.

HYPERTENSION (HIGH BLOOD PRESSURE)

A leading cause of heart attacks and strokes, hypertension afflicts one-tenth of North America's population. It may be linked to obesity, faulty diet and lack of exercise, but often arises for unknown reasons. High blood pressure weakens the walls of small arteries, which can lead to strokes, heart attacks, kidney damage and vision loss (due to injured blood vessels in the eyes). Because it is a "silent killer" usually symptomless until the blood vessels have suffered considerable damage and damage to the heart or other organs has already occurred, the only way to know if you've got high blood pressure is to have it checked regularly. Even after diagnosis, people often don't take their prescribed medication. It's a dangerous mistake, increasing the risk of unexpected death.

A decade or so ago, over half of those with hypertension were unaware of its presence, and of those who knew they had high blood pressure, only half got sufficient treatment. Today, many more people are aware of hypertension and the importance of getting proper treatment for it. Blood pressure should be measured every year or so, especially after the age of 30. This is one routine medical test that can really save lives, provided that those with unacceptably high readings take steps to redress the problem.

How high is high?

Blood pressure is measured using an inflatable cuff on the upper arm and a stethoscope to detect heart sounds. The cuff is inflated until the point where the pulse disappears, which gives the approximate systolic pressure in the arteries as the heart contracts and pumps blood. The cuff is then slowly deflated and, as the heart rests between beats and fills with blood, the diastolic pressure is measured. Blood pressure is recorded as systolic over diastolic, expressed in millimeters of mercury (Hg). Normal readings range from 100/60 to 130/80, and an average normal reading is 120/80 mm Hg. When someone is thought to be hypertensive, physicians usually do several readings, maybe a few weeks, even months, apart, to get an accurate picture before initiating treatment; one high reading alone does not prove hypertension. External influences such as a heavy meal, exercise, anxiety—even the sight of a white lab coat—may alter readings.

The dividing line between normal and high

RISK FACTORS FOR HYPERTENSION

Although the underlying mechanism is not fully understood, known risk factors include:
- a genetic predisposition;
- obesity—weight loss alone often lowers blood pressure;
- smoking—a high-risk factor (nicotine both constricts blood vessels and speeds up the heartrate, raising blood pressure);
- pregnancy, which can temporarily elevate blood pressure;
- contraceptive drugs, especially in those prone to hypertension; women on the Pill should get regular medical checkups;
- lack of exercise (but while physical activity may lower blood pressure in some borderline cases, there is no guarantee of lasting effects);
- stress—long considered an accompaniment to hypertension—may activate the sympathetic nervous system and enhance adrenaline release, raising blood pressure;
- insufficient potassium or an imbalanced ratio of sodium to potassium—another possible cause that needs clarification. Researchers are investigating whether a potassium-rich diet can counteract high blood pressure;
- high alcohol consumption (three or more drinks per day), which seems to raise blood pressure, possibly by altering kidney function. Some experts consider this alcohol-related rise to be reversible if excess drinking ceases.

BLOOD-PRESSURE DRUGS

The choice of blood-pressure drugs depends on the type and causes of hypertension and the person's individual health profile.

- *Diuretics* (such as thiazides), which flush water out of the body and reduce the blood volume pumped by the heart, are widely used, inexpensive and easy to tolerate. But because they tend to raise blood-lipid (cholesterol) levels and deplete the body's potassium and magnesium stores, they are sometimes replaced by other drugs such as beta-blockers as the first line of attack.
- *Beta-blockers* mute the heart's activity, dilate blood vessels, slow the heartbeat and reduce the pressure in blood vessels. Newer forms such as *atenolol* (Tenormin) and *acebutolol* (Monitan or Sectral) now complement older types such as *propranolol*.
- *Angiotensin-converting inhibitors* such as *captopril* (Capotec) and *enalapril* (Vasotec) relax blood vessel walls by blocking the vessel-constricting (pressure-raising) action of the kidney's angiotensin hormone. ACE-inhibitors are well tolerated but may produce an irritating cough and lower white-blood-cell counts.
- *Angiotensin-receptor blockers*—e.g., *losartan* (Ozocor, Cozaar)—overcome some of the side effects (cough and lowered white-cell count) of ACE inhibitors.
- *Calcium-channel blockers*—such as *diltiazem* (Cardizem), *bepridil* (Vascor), *mibefradil* (Posicor)—dilate the blood vessels decreasing resistance and lowering pressure. Short-acting forms may cause cardiac problems, so are no longer advised for treating blood pressure.

---

blood pressure (hypertension) is somewhat arbitrary. But the World Health Organization designates "normal" blood pressure as below 140/90 and calls it "high" if it is 160/95 or more. "Borderline" hypertension is the area in-between (diastolic readings from 90 to 95 mm Hg). People with diabetes or kidney problems require lower readings of under 130/80. People with mild hypertension can often lower it by lifestyle changes such as losing weight, getting more exercise, quitting smoking and (maybe) by lowering salt (sodium) intake.

New guidelines for blood-pressure management

While blood-pressure measurement is one of the simplest, cheapest and most worthwhile of medical tests, far too few have their pressure measured and the readings aren't always accurate. For example, so-called white-coat syndrome—a pressure rise due to anxiety about having it measured and the clinical atmosphere—can throw off readings; even chatting to a doctor or nurse can raise the pressure. New guidelines developed in the U.S. and Canada call for more careful pressure measurement. People should avoid caffeine and cigarettes for at least half an hour beforehand and rest for 5 minutes before having blood pressure read. Measurement is best done with the person seated in a chair, the arm at roughly heart level. To confirm a diagnosis of hypertension, several high readings should be recorded at different times.

Healthy adults under age 55 need a blood-pressure check every 2 years (or at each medical checkup), more often if they have cardiac risk factors such as diabetes, high blood cholesterol or a family history of early heart disease. Older people should have blood pressure measured at least yearly. In some cases, a personal 24-hour ambulatory monitor is the surest way to get an accurate fix on someone's blood pressure. A specially designed cuff is worn to sample the wearer's pressure at regular intervals through the day, recording it on a microchip for later analysis. Experts do not recommend the automated machines in drugstores and shopping malls as there's no proper follow-up and the machines may give inaccurate readings.

TO LOWER BLOOD PRESSURE:

- keep weight down to a desirable level;
- exercise regularly (20 to 30 minutes at least 3 times weekly);
- limit alcohol intake to 2 (women) or 3 (men) daily drinks;
- do not smoke;
- moderate salt (sodium) intake;
- eat a varied low-fat diet, rich in magnesium, potassium and calcium;
- continue taking any prescribed blood-pressure medication(s);
- get regular checkups.

Individualized treatment to control blood pressure

The guidelines divide hypertension into three stages of severity: pressures from 140/90 to 159/99 are stage 1, those from 160/100 to 179/109 are stage 2, and pressures above 180/110 are called stage 3 hypertension. Treatment aims to bring blood pressure down as close as possible to the optimal—that is, to 135/90 or lower. (Ideally, blood pressure is 120/80 or less.) For those who need them, there are now many different blood-pressure-lowering drugs to choose from.

For mild to moderate hypertension, if there are no other heart risk factors (such as smoking, obesity, high blood cholesterol), the guidelines suggest starting with lifestyle changes—which may bring blood pressure down enough to postpone or avoid the need for medication. Such changes may include losing weight (if over the desired level), limiting alcohol intake, doing regular exercise—e.g., a brisk daily 2-mile (40-minute) walk—and the new DASH (Dietary Approach to Stop Hypertension) diet. Low in fat and high in fiber—from 7 to 8 daily servings of grain and 5 or more servings of fruit and vegetables—this study shows that a healthy diet helps many lower blood pressure.

Authorities now recommend diuretics (water-loss pills) and beta-blockers (such as propranolol) as first-line drugs for treating uncomplicated hypertension, followed by the angiotensin-converting enzyme (ACE) inhibitors (e.g., *captopril* or *enalapril*), and the latest class of blood pressure drugs the angiotensin-receptor blockers.

Calcium-channel blockers (e.g., *nifedipine*, *diltiazem* or the newer, *mibefradil*) should be used with caution, as evidence shows that short-acting forms such as *nifedipine* (Adalat) and *verapamil* (Isoptin, Calan) increase heart-attack risks; they are no longer recommended for blood-pressure control. Instead, people might switch to a long-acting form or an ACE-inhibitor.

The guidelines also spell out which drugs are best for specific types of hypertension. For instance, someone who's had a heart attack and remains hypertensive may do best with beta-blockers plus an ACE inhibitor; someone with diabetes may need ACE drugs. People react differently and experience more or less troublesome side effects with one or other of these medications. For example, the beta-blockers (and the latest addition, the alpha-beta-blockers) may cause drowsiness and a lowered sex drive; ACE inhibitors can cause a nagging cough. It's best to choose a suitable drug regimen in collaboration with your healthcare advisors. Make sure your blood pressure stays well controlled as it's a key risk factor for heart attack and stroke.

Treatment can control but not cure hypertension

The correct therapy for the 10 percent of the population with mild high blood pressure—a diastolic reading between 90 and 99—remains a much-debated question. In the absence of other risk factors, this level of hypertension probably poses few health hazards. But accompanied by smoking, obesity, high blood cholesterol or a family history of heart disease, even slightly elevated blood pressure can be a health threat.

INFLUENZA

Although we loosely apply the term "flu" to anything from the common cold to a stomach upset, real flu or influenza is a specific and sometimes serious infection. Influenza is a self-limiting viral infection lasting a week to 10 days, its severity dependant on the particular virus strain and the individual's overall health, age and vulnerability. Influenza can be deadly, especially for the very young and elderly, mainly owing to complications such as pneumonia, and it is the cause of many hospitalizations (and possible deaths) in each flu season. Occasionally, about 3 to 4 times in each century, a new and particularly virulent strain of flu virus emerges causing widespread global pandemics that kill millions around the world. Examples of large global outbreaks include the notorious 1918–1919 Spanish influenza pandemic that killed 30 to 40 million people worldwide, the 1957 Asian flu responsible for 80,000 deaths in the U.S. alone, and the 1968 Hong Kong flu responsible for an estimated 1.5 million deaths around the world. Currently, influenza leads infectious diseases as a cause of death among the elderly and debilitated

WHO NEEDS FLU SHOTS?

• **Canada's Advisory Committee on Immunization lists** special groups of people most in need of annual flu shots, but increasingly health authorities advise most people to be vaccinated. Current campaigns in Canada suggest that everyone over 6 months old should have a yearly flu shot. Previously only people over age 65 were targeted (because of the risk of serious lung complications). Today, many experts believe young children also need to be protected as they tend to be the vectors (carriers or transmitters) of viral infections. in communities. Those with an allergy to eggs (the virus is grown in chick eggs) or who have had a previous adverse reaction to the flu vaccine should abstain. From an individual perspective, getting a flu shot is worthwhile given the high likelihood of avoiding a bout of influenza. From a societal viewpoint, mass influenza vaccination can reduce losses due to flu epidemics in terms of work hours, parenting time and other endeavors, as well as reducing use of emergency rooms and hospital beds.

This is especially true for people looking after ill or infirm people.

Common myths regarding the flu shot: "I will get influenza from the flu shot": The flu shot is a vaccine made from dead (inactivated) virus particles, so it is impossible to get flu from the shot. Many people tend to get colds anyway in the fall and might blame it on the flu shot. After a flu shot most people notice nothing except maybe slight redness or a little soreness at the injection site for a day or two.

"Influenza is the same as a cold and it is not worth preventing": Influenza is a much more severe infection than the common cold (*see below*). People who rarely miss work often miss a week or more with influenza, feel very ill with it and may remain tired and weak for weeks afterwards.

Special groups that definitely require annual flu shots include:
• anyone 65 years of age or older;
• adults with chronic heart or lung conditions (severe enough to merit frequent medical care), kidney disease, severe anemia, diabetes, immunosuppression, HIV infection, and

nonmalignant tumors;
• residents of nursing homes or other chronic-care facilities (where close, confined quarters may enhance viral spread);
• children with recurrent (chronic) lung disorders, such as bronchopulmonary dysplasia (found in those who were premature babies with respiratory distress at birth); cystic fibrosis; asthma (bad enough to require frequent medical supervision); significant heart disease; cancer; immunodeficiency; sickle cell disease; and conditions requiring long-term ASA (e.g., Aspirin) therapy;
• those who might transmit influenza to high-risk individuals, e.g., all healthcare personnel, those working in nursing homes, hospitals or some other institutions, or those caring for elderly relatives;
• possibly those who provide essential services, e.g., the military, firefighters, police (controversial);
• family and household members of those living with people at high risk of getting influenza;
• providers of essential and emergency or community services.

(weak), often owing to secondary infections. Annual vaccination is the best way to avoid or lessen the severity of flu outbreaks.

Influenza is caused by A, B or C viruses which constantly mutate or change their structure slightly—undergoing small alterations in the proteins on their surface membranes producing "antigenic drift." Because of these mutations or changes in the viral coat, each year's crop requires a slightly different vaccine to confer protection. But when there is a major reshuffling of the genetic material (antigenic shift), thought to occur through the exchange of genetic material between animal and human influenza viruses, it produces a radically new influenza strain that causes especially severe illness—and perhaps a major pandemic. Since humans develop antibody defenses only against viruses they have already encountered, a large new viral change leaves the population unprotected and produces severe epidemics. (Experts surmise that the reason why over 30 million died in the 1919 epidemic after World War I was that a particularly virulent flu strain struck populations malnourished and weakened by years of war.)

Of the three known types of influenza viruses, the A strain produces the most severe illness, and so far only mutations in type A have given rise to severe global outbreaks. An example of the genetic exchange between human and animal viruses is the so-called "bird flu" (first detected in Hong Kong in 1997, but now also found elsewhere) in which a completely new type A influenza strain killed several people. Fortunately, mass chicken slaughter halted the outbreaks and so far bird flu viruses have not been easily transmitted between humans. However, should a strain freely transmissible between humans emerge, it could trigger a huge pandemic. The possibility is a wake-up call to the urgent need for pandemic planning. Unfortunately, big genetic changes in flu viruses are unpredictable and sudden, so no one knows just when and where a pandemic strain will hit. However, global flu watchers are on the alert and, under guidance of the World Health Organization (WHO), more than 80 countries track annual viral variants that could spell trouble.

Influenza-B strains, more stable than the A forms, usually cause only mild flu but can produce severe illness in children and the elderly, while type C usually causes only sporadic, local outbreaks of mild illness.

The symptoms of influenza, usually begin with fever, chills, headache, muscle and joint aches, and a dry cough. The nasal involvement or sniffles are usually absent or less pronounced than with a common cold, but with influenza—unlike a typical cold—the fever may be quite high. The cough may become irritating, with consequent chest soreness and interrupted sleep. Secondary infection of the lungs with Pneumococci, the bacteria responsible for pneumonia, can follow influenza, requiring prompt medical attention.

Treatment for a mild bout of influenza is bed rest, plenty of fluids and antipyretics (fever reducers) such as acetaminophen or salicylates (e.g., ASA or Aspirin). However, Aspirin should not be used in children or adolescents because of the possible danger of Reye's syndrome (a serious condition affecting the liver and brain), which is linked to ASA-treated influenza B. Antibiotics do not help influenza since they're ineffective against viral illnesses, but they may be required for a secondary bacterial infection, such as pneumonia. Taken within 2 days of the appearance of flu symptoms, antiviral drugs such as *oseltamivir* (Tamiflu) and *zanamivir* (Relenza) can alleviate the illness and shorten its duration. However, side effects limit the usefulness of these antivirals.

New influenza vaccines created yearly

Vaccination is the best way to prevent or lessen the risk of influenza. Although it's never entirely certain which particular flu viruses are most likely to hit in a given season, vaccines can be prepared with a fair degree of accuracy. The decision as to which strains should be included in the year's vaccine is taken in the spring (according to the year's probably predominant flu strains) and the manufacturing process takes about 6 months, so batches are usually ready by late September. The new "split-virus" vaccines are now generally recommended, especially for children under 13 years, because they produce fewer side effects. Immunization is best done in September or October before the start of the flu season in late October or early November; it

takes roughly 1 month after vaccination for the body to build adequate antibody defenses.

Some Key Flu Facts and Figures

- Influenza is a viral illness that affects as many as 1 in 6 to 10 adults (more children)
- Flu viruses are transmitted through the air in droplets shed by infected persons ("coughs and sneezes") and by surface contact, for instance by touching objects such as doorknobs or telephones that have been handled by an infected person
- Seasonal flu outbreaks occur in different parts of the world at different times
- Global pandemics (which occur roughly every 30 years) arise from large changes in A strain influenza viruses, likely through exchange of genetic material between human and animal viruses (e.g., from pigs or birds)
- In Canada, influenza (and consequent pneumonia) result in approximately 500 to 1,500 deaths annually, and 70,000 to 75,000 hospitalizations
- Most deaths from flu occur among the elderly, very young children and those with serious heart or lung conditions
- The incubation period or time taken to develop symptoms after being infected is 2 days
- People with flu stay contagious for 5 to 7 days after symptoms begin
- Yearly immunization (with vaccine containing inactivated viral particles) is the best protection.
- Annual re-vaccination is necessary because flu viruses constantly change and each year's vaccine contains slightly different strains.
- Flu shots are 70 percent effective in preventing infection in young healthy adults; the vaccine is less effective in the elderly, but reduces risk of complications, hospitalization and death.
- Antiviral drugs can help to shorten the duration and lessen the severity of uncomplicated influenza.

Is it a cold or flu? Distinguishing influenza from the common cold

Many of us mistakenly refer to a common cold as "the flu," although these ailments are quite different. The common cold, caused by a variety of *rhinoviruses*, rarely causes fever or muscle aches and is a generally mild infection lasting about a week. Influenza is far more serious, with possibly life-threatening complications. As one sufferer puts it: "With a cold one may enjoy a few days of pampering without feeling really sick, but influenza makes one feel truly ill, too lousy to do anything but stay put." A cold usually comes on gradually with a sore throat and sneezing, typically involving no more than a runny nose and stuffy head. Colds just need symptom relief—keeping warm, plenty of fluids (to thin out the secretions), perhaps decongestants.

COLD VS. INFLUENZA ("FLU")

Symptom	Cold	Influenza or real flu
Fever	none or low—around 38°C (100°F)—mostly in children	almost always, often high, sudden onset, lasts 3–5 days
Chills	rare	almost always
Headache	absent or mild	common
Muscle aches	uncommon	frequently, often severe, usually in legs and back
Fatigue/weakness	absent, mild or none; doesn't prevent daily activities	often extreme, may linger on for 2–3 or more weeks
Cough	sometimes, often after runny nose stage passes	usual, may become severe with phlegm
Runny, stuffy nose	common, often only (local) symptom	rarely, may come on later
Sore throat	common	occasional, perhaps just "dry" feeling
Sneezing	common, specially at start	rare
Prevention	handwashing, don't rub nose, eyes (cold viruses enter body via nasal passages)	annual vaccination; frequent handwashing; antiviral medication (only for adults or older children)
Treatment	symptomatic relief with cough/cold medications (e.g., decongestants), plenty of fluids	fever-reducers (but no ASA for children); prescribed antiviral medication only in adults and children over age 12 (e.g., *amantadine, oseltamivir, zanamivir*)
Complications	sinus congestion, earache, bronchitis, may trigger asthma (in those prone to it)	pneumonia, bronchitis, exacerbation of heart, lung and other disorders

By contrast, real influenza hits abruptly with sudden chills, an often high fever, dry cough, headache, muscle pains, fatigue and weakness. (Unlike the common cold, there is generally no runny nose.) Although influenza is usually self-limiting and over in a week or two, it often leaves lingering weakness and has a high rate of complications. If there is a high fever or severe coughing, seek prompt medical attention. (You might suspect pneumonia if, after seeming to recover, the temperature rises again and there is a lot of coughing with thick sputum.)

For more information contact:
CDC's voice information service at 888–232–3223, or their website: www.cdc.gov/incidod/diseases/flu/weekly.htm; or the WHO fluwatch website at: http://oms2.b3e.jussieu.fr/flunet/ or Health Canada's website at: www.hc-sc.gc.ca or the LCDC website at: www.hc-sc.gc.ca.hpb-lcdc/bid/respdis/fluwatch/index.html

ITCHING OR PRURITUS
Itching, or pruritus in medical terms, is a protective mechanism that likely evolved as a signal to alert animals to the presence of parasites and other skin irritants. Not only is itching a symptom of many skin disorders and infestations, but it can also herald the presence of systemic diseases such as thyroid problems, diabetes and kidney failure. Interestingly, itching can also reflect inner thoughts and emotions. An itch can start in the mind—even a conversation about itching can set people scratching. Some people only itch when they are stressed or depressed. Some scratch their heads when deep in thought. It's easy to make jokes about itching, but itchiness can drive people to distraction. It's defined as an "unpleasant skin sensation that creates an intense desire to scratch." An itch differs from pain, although it can burn and tingle unbearably. A poison-ivy itch or shingles doesn't feel like a cut or a stubbed toe. Itching is a different sensation.

Breaking the itch–scratch cycle
Scratching goes with itching and is characteristic animal behavior. Scratching momentarily relieves the itch, but scientists are not sure why. Maybe scratching overwhelms the itch message, replac-

ing one nerve signal with another. While scratching may feel good, it irritates the skin and perpetuates the itch–scratch cycle. One expert at the University of Massachusetts Medical School says, "With certain itches, one scratch is too many, and a thousand are not enough." Ironically, scratching often causes more damage than relief. Too much scratching creates skin abrasions, tears and cuts that allow a bacterial infection to develop.

Why we itch: tracking the causes

The first step in dealing with pruritus is to determine whether the itching is general or localized—affects the entire skin or just certain sites such as the groin, legs or pressure points (elbows and knees)—and whether it stems from a disorder such dermatitis, shingles, eczema, psoriasis, hives (urticaria), lichen planus or fungal infections (such as candidiasis or athlete's foot).

ITCHING IN PREGNANCY NEEDS CAREFUL ATTENTION

Itching in late pregnancy should be taken seriously as it could signal a liver problem known as intrahepatic cholestasis of pregnancy (ICP), also called jaundice of late pregnancy, which can endanger the birth. Itching is its chief alerting symptom, usually starting in the palms and soles and extending to the trunk, often worst at night. The itching may be followed by signs of jaundice (yellowing skin or eyes). ICP tends to run in families, and is more common in twin or multiple than single pregnancies. Specific testing for ICP takes time and is not readily available in many centers, making the diagnosis a clinical one and sometimes hard to obtain. Risks of ICP include preterm delivery, and because there is a 3 percent risk of stillbirth at term, treatment generally involves induction of the baby's birth at 38 weeks' gestation. Steroids such as *dexamethasone* can be used to relieve the itching.

- *Localized itching* can often be diagnosed by the location of the itch and the skin lesions—blisters, crusting, rash, sores or redness. For instance, a scalp itch may be due to psoriasis, folliculitis (bacterial infection of the hair folli-

---

TIPS TO REDUCE ITCHING

- *Pat, don't rub,* the skin dry after bathing.
- *Add baking soda or bath oil, mineral or vegetable oils, hydrolyzed cornstarch, bran or colloidal oatmeal* (Aveeno) to bath water. But beware—oils can make the tub slippery!
- *Try sitz baths* to relieve anal and vulvar (female genital) itching.
- *Apply rich, oil-based, non-perfumed moisturizers* immediately after bathing, showering or swimming.
- *Use a humidifier* in winter.
- *Wear loose clothing,* preferably cotton; avoid wearing synthetics and scratchy fabrics. Permanent press and wrinkle-resistant clothes may contain formaldehyde and other skin irritants.
- *Wash new clothing and towels* before use; wash clothing and bedding in mild, unscented detergents, such as those recommended for infant clothing, and rinse many times.
- *Avoid* bleaches, fabric softeners and other laundry additives.
- *Keep pets free of fleas* and other parasites.
- *Trim fingernails* to lower the risk of injury from scratching. If you scratch in your sleep, wear cotton gloves to bed.
- *Apply a cold compress* or cool washcloth, or pressure, to relieve itching.
- *Apply Burrow's solution (aluminum acetate), milk of magnesia (unflavored), or milk* to dry out oozing eruptions.
- *Do not put alcohol solutions on the skin.* Although they soothe initially, they dry the skin and ultimately aggravate the itch.
- *Try anti-itch medications, which include:*
- *Antihistamines,* such as *hydroxyzine* (Atarax) and *diphenhydramine* (Benadryl)—good for itching due to histamine release, particularly hives. (Non-sedating, second-generation antihistamines, such as *terfenadine, loratadine* and *astemizole,* don't work as well.)
- *Skin-hydrating lotions*—applied while the skin is still damp.
- *Corticosteroid ointments*—a major standby. Low- to medium-potency topical hydrocortisone, such as *triamcolone* or *betamethasone* can be helpful, but long-term use produces skin thinning and striae (marks).
- *Topical phenol* (0.5 percent) and *menthol* (0.25 percent) added to creams.
- *Pramoxine* (as in Prame gel)—a topical anesthetic that helps relieve itching.
- *Capsaicin,* or red-pepper cream—containing the hot ingredient in chili peppers—can reduce itching from mastectomy, hepatitis, renal failure or psoriasis, but use is limited by the stinging and burning that occurs on initial application (although the stinging fades with continued use).
- *Naloxone,* an opiate antagonist, helpful against itching in liver disease, hives and atopic dermatitis (eczema).
- *Doxepin* (Zonalon), a new topical anti-itch cream that blocks histamine receptors, is proving useful for many itchy conditions, including eczema, lichen simplex and contact dermatitis. But it has to be applied 4 times a day and can cause drowsiness.

SUBTLE SYMPTOMS OF KIDNEY FAILURE

Ideally, declining kidney function should be spotted *before* symptoms become troublesome. Occasionally, however, even advanced kidney disease may be asymptomatic, detected only by blood tests.

Possible symptoms of kidney failure include:

- **changes in urination; nighttime urination;**
- **puffy eyes;**
- **swollen feet and ankles;**
- **pain in the side or back**
- **protein in the urine;**
- **blood in urine, making it tea- or cola-colored;**
- **uremia, in end-stage renal disease—literally "urine leaking into the blood"—a toxic condition characterized by fatigue, listlessness, nausea, vomiting, appetite loss, shortness of breath, rising blood pressure, headaches, itchiness and perhaps tingling of toes and fingers; sleep problems and sexual disturbances may also arise.**

cles) or seborrheic dermatitis (scalp greasiness). On the hands, it can arise from an irritant or allergic reaction. The legs may itch from insect bites, the feet because of fungal infections, the groin because of pubic lice or scabies (a mite infestation).

- *Skin problems* are a common cause—for instance, *eczema* (hard, crusty or weepy skin lesions), *hives* (with raised red skin weals), *psoriasis* (excessive skin turnover) and various infections, such as athlete's foot, herpes, chickenpox, shingles and vaginitis.
- *Allergies* are another common reason for itchiness—persistent itching is a prime symptom or accompaniment of many allergies.
- Insect bites from ants, bedbugs, fleas, lice, mites, pinworms and the like—cause big itches. Scabies—due to the female mite, *Sarcoptes scabiei*—is a common cause of generalized itching. The condition can be diagnosed by spotting the mite's S-shaped or linear burrows, or by small inflammatory papules. When several members of a household all itch, scabies or fleas might be suspected.
- *Aquagenic pruritus* is severe itching brought on by jets of water (e.g., when taking showers).
- *Lichen simplex chronicus* is a condition with patches of lichenified, bark-like skin due to repeated scratching that itch, exacerbated by stress.
- *Generalized*, body-wide itching may arise from xerosis (skin dryness), from an allergy or from systemic illnesses such as kidney failure, thyroid disorders, Hodgkin's disease (which can start with leg itchiness), lymphoma, liver disorders, HIV infection, infestations (e.g., with lice, fleas, giardia parasites), drug abuse and some psychiatric disturbances.
- *Psychiatric and neurological conditions* that cause itchiness include depression, eating disorders and parasitosis (delusions of insect infestation or the obsessive belief that insects are crawling all over one's body).

Treating itchiness

Given the long list of possible causes of itching, the first step is to try to trace the trigger and remove or mute it. For example, scabies can be treated by killing the mites with *permethrin* or

lindane (but the itch can persist long after the mites are dead).

Xerosis, or dry skin, can be relieved by frequent application of moisturizing emollients, bathing less often and using mild soaps (such as Dove or Neutrogena).

KIDNEY FAILURE

Kidney or renal failure can occur gradually or suddenly when the kidneys can no longer carry out their task of purifying blood and eliminating wastes. People don't generally give much thought to their kidneys, an unglamorous but marvelously efficient pair of bean-shaped organs tucked into the small of the back, on either side of the spine. Healthy kidneys have excess functional capacity and can suffer considerable damage before producing symptoms. In fact, people can lead a healthy life with only one functioning kidney. But complete shutdown or failure of *both* kidneys is a medical emergency—without prompt treatment (dialysis or a transplant), people can only survive about a week to 10 days.

As recently as the 1960s, total kidney failure spelled certain death. Today, however, such a diagnosis, while still severe, is no longer a death sentence. Thanks to modern dialysis with artificial kidney machines, home dialysis methods and transplants, even those with renal shutdown can now survive, travel, work and continue productive lives.

Kidneys vital to health

Kidneys purify and excrete the body's fluids and cleanse the blood of normal metabolic products that become toxic if allowed to accumulate. They also regulate the body's acid-base balance, ensuring that our tissues don't get too acidic or alkaline; they maintain the body's delicate balance of minerals—levels of potassium, sodium, calcium and phosphorus—and they control the amount of water excreted so that the tissues don't become waterlogged or dehydrated. If the kidneys no longer purify blood, it becomes a "sewer" full of metabolic byproducts.

Why kidneys sometimes falter or fail

Kidney failure can be sudden and acute, as happens with poisonings, people hurt in traffic mishaps or soldiers wounded in battle (due to blood loss and shock), or it can develop gradually from chronic conditions such as diabetes (responsible for almost 25 percent of kidney failure) and high blood pressure. Disorders that affect human kidney function include kidney diseases such as glomerulonephritis (inflammation), polycystic kidney disease (an inherited condition) and urinary-tract obstructions. Kidneys can also be damaged by autoimmune disorders such as lupus and scleroderma, certain drugs (such as *gentamycin*) and snake venoms.

During its early stages, kidney failure may be reversible, but when kidney function dwindles to about 10 percent of normal—so-called end-stage renal disease—one of two life-saving therapies becomes essential: either dialysis (blood purification by artificial means) or kidney transplant.

Dialysis saves lives

Dialysis, which means "purification through a membrane," replaces normal kidney filtration, removing accumulated wastes from the blood, getting rid of surplus fluid and restoring a healthy acid-base balance.

Hemodialysis—in which the person is hooked up to a machine—circulates blood through a purifying dialyzer or filter and then returns it (cleansed) to the body. Wastes, excess potassium and other minerals diffuse out into the rinsing fluid. Hemodialysis takes 3 to 4 hours per session, done 3 times a week. The person is attached to the dialysis machine through an arteriovenous fistula (a surgically joined artery and vein), permanently placed in the wrist, providing a large, strong arterialized vein for the insertion of dialysis needles. Alternatively, an internal shunt or short piece of plastic tubing may be used to connect an artery to a vein. About 4 percent of blood is drawn out and circulated through the dialyzer at any one time, avoiding drastic side effects.

The dialyzer consists of numerous fibers containing tiny pores through which small molecules diffuse out of the blood, leaving in proteins and blood cells, which cannot pass through the tiny pores. During hemodialysis, an anti-clotting substance (such as heparin) must be added to stop the blood from clotting in the machine. While the process is not painful, there may be

SPECIAL DIETS FOR HEMODIALYSIS PATIENTS

Although dialysis cleanses the blood, patients must follow a special renal diet, with several restrictions:

• *Fluid and salt intake*—because surplus fluid and excess salt strain the heart. Salt (sodium) intake must be limited—salt substitutes are also forbidden because they contain potassium.

• *Potassium*—because if the body's potassium balance is out of kilter, it can lead to cardiovascular problems and disrupted nerve conduction. Potassium-rich foods such as nuts, potatoes, bananas, oranges, potatoes and some other vegetables are forbidden.

• *Phosphorus*—because excess can cause painful joint and bone disease and itchy skin. High-phosphate foods to be avoided include seeds, nuts, dried beans, peas, colas and milk products. Phosphate binders, such as Tums, which contain calcium carbonate, are often prescribed.

• *Protein*—because it breaks down into urea and other toxins that cause uremic syndrome at high levels. Foods rich in protein such as meat, fish and cheese are usually restricted, although dialysis patients need enough to offset muscle wasting, and those who lose protein into the solution need extra.

some discomfort from the rapid weight loss that occurs as dialysis removes excess fluid. Someone who eats or drinks too much between dialysis sessions and gains excess weight may find its removal during hemodialysis causes a sudden drop in blood pressure.

Peritoneal dialysis—an increasingly favored method—is now used by almost 40 percent of Canadian dialysis patients. It involves insertion of a catheter (tube) just below the navel into the peritoneal or abdominal cavity, through which dialysis fluid is inserted to flush out wastes 3 to 4 times daily. The fluid exchange takes 30 to 45 minutes, usually done first thing in the morning, at lunchtime, late afternoon and before bed. In practice, about 2 liters of fresh dialysis fluid is put into the abdomen every 6 hours, flowing into the peritoneal cavity from a bag held above the abdomen while sitting or lying down. The old fluid is drained out into another bag.

Deciding on the preferred dialysis method

In choosing between hemodialysis and peritoneal dialysis, people and their caretakers must consider age, overall health, the facilities available and whether or not a fistula (insertion point for dialysis needles) can be put into the body and retained.

With peritoneal dialysis, the advantages are: no need to hook into a machine, no need for hospital facilities, permits a flexible schedule (can do it at home) and is easier on the body—avoids the chemical swings and rapid fluid loss of hemodialysis; also diets are less stringent, there's less risk of hyperkalemia (potassium overload) and, not being tied to a machine, a person can travel more easily. Its drawbacks are: fluid swilling inside the abdomen, the need to do it 4 times daily—a schedule that some find more grueling than the thrice-weekly hemodialysis sessions—weight gain (owing to the high sugar content of the dialysis solution) and a high risk of infection. Bacterial peritonitis occurs an *average* once every 18 to 24 months in those on hemodialysis, but antibiotics cure most episodes.

With hemodialysis advantages include swift relief of uremia (blood toxicity), and only three brief (3- to 4-hour) dialysis treatments a week. Its drawbacks are the reliance on machines, strict dietary rules, the need to take several medications and to plan social life around dialysis times.

Kidney transplants

A kidney transplant is the best solution for those with kidney failure, providing relief from the relentless dictates of dialysis. A kidney transplant from an identical twin donor survives in almost all cases, even without immunosuppressants. Kidneys donated by matched close relatives, such as siblings, have a 5-year survival rate of 85 percent. But usually the transplanted kidney comes from an unknown accident victim, in which case the 5-year transplanted kidney's survival averages 65 to 70 percent in most units.

Not everyone with kidney failure is eligible for a transplant. In general, although there are no absolute rules, kidney transplants are a declining option with advancing age—mainly because of increased risks and reduced survival chances. The major risks of kidney transplant are rejection, infection and (in the long term) cancer—due to the immunosuppressants used. Unless there is a good tissue match between donor and recipient, the body tries to reject or cast off the foreign organ. Signs of rejection include pain, fever decreasing urine output, ankle swelling and increasing blood creatinine levels.

Efforts to prevent rejection include match-ing the donor kidney as closely as possible to the recipient's tissues and use of strong immunosuppressants to help the body accept the foreign kidney. Most transplantees take a "cocktail" of immunosuppressives, including corticosteroids (e.g., *prednisone*), *cyclosporine* and *azathioprine*—usually for the rest of their lives. Cyclosporine, a potent immunosuppressant derived from a fungus, has markedly improved survival for transplantees. But immunosuppressants have undesirable side effects. Prednisone, for example, causes weight gain, a rise in blood pressure, facial changes, acne and perhaps depression—effects that generally disappear once the dose comes down. Azathioprine might cause bone-marrow suppression and leukopenia (low white blood cell counts). Cyclosporine increases body hair produces mild tremors, gum enlargement, blood-pressure elevation, nephrotoxicity (which may damage the transplanted kidney) and, uncommonly, lymphoma (lymph gland cancer).

Living with kidney disease

People with chronic renal failure become partners with a team of surgeons, renal specialist, nurses, dieticians and counselors. Adapting to a chronic disease and its treatment takes great courage, and different people cope in different ways. Some go on working, traveling, playing sports, enjoying family life; some choose to become invalids; a few opt out of dialysis therapy and prefer to die. Yet dialysis patients can now travel all over the world, although it takes some advance planning. Hemodialysis units are available almost everywhere across North America, Europe, Asia and South America.

For further information, contact your local chapter of the Kidney Foundation of Canada, or (in Toronto) the Renal Education and Support Group, tel.: (416) 360–4000.

KIDNEY STONES

Anyone who has ever experienced it knows that passing a kidney stone—even one smaller than a grain of sand—through slender urinary channels can be excruciating. Although the passage of some stones causes little or no pain, most stones send people rushing in agony to the nearest hospital. The symptoms and severity depend on the location, type and size of the stones: whether they're smooth or spiky, whether they stay put, start moving or get stuck somewhere *en route* from kidney to bladder.

Stones may form either in the bladder or inside the kidney, from where they can move down to the bladder and pass out through the urethra. In Western society, kidney stones are the common type and bladder stones are a rarity. But in developing countries, and in Europe up to the 1900s, bladder stones predominated, probably owing to inadequate diets.

About 70 percent of kidney stones (more precisely known as renal calculi) pass out spontaneously in the urine given enough time, often causing extreme pain while doing so. The remaining 30 percent create trouble by getting stuck inside the kidney or in the ureter leading from the kidney to the bladder. When they obstruct the flow of urine, stones must be removed, since blockage can damage the kidney. The lifetime incidence of kidney stones is 15 percent for men and 7 percent for women. The incidence increases with age, peaking at 65. Half of all patients who have experienced a bout of kidney stones will have a subsequent episode within 10 years.

Different stones afflict different folks

Stones are more prevalent in men than women and usually occur between the ages of 30 and 50. Certain races and ethnic populations are more prone to kidney stones than others, and more likely to have one kind of stone than another.

There are four main types of stones: calcium-containing; uric-acid; struvite; and cystine. About 40 to 70 percent of urinary-tract stones in Anglo-Saxon populations contain calcium (as calcium oxalate or as an insoluble phosphate salt, or a combination of both).

Apparently, uric-acid stones tend to form in Mediterranean races owing to a genetic propensity toward acidic urine, which favors uric-acid crystallization. Only 5 percent of kidney stones in Anglo-Saxons contain uric acid.

Struvite stones are large accretions accounting for about 10 to 20 percent of all renal stones. They involve the kidney's whole collecting system, accumulating in a branched structure known as a staghorn.

Cystine stones are relatively rare (about 2 percent of all stones). They form in people with cystinuria, a genetic defect in which an excess of cystine, an amino acid and normal body constituent, accumulates in the urine.

How do you know if you have kidney stones?

Symptoms of a kidney stone range from none at all, blood in the urine or a dull ache in the side or back, to intense pain radiating into the groin accompanied by nausea and vomiting. The worst pain usually occurs as a stone passes from the kidney along the ureter to the bladder. The presence of stones is confirmed by different tests. These include X-ray, an intravenous pyelogram—X-rays taken with iodine-containing dye injected into the bloodstream to outline the kidney and its collecting system—and CT scan (helical).

Treatment for kidney stones

Some uric-acid stones, and occasionally the cystine types inside the kidney, can be dissolved and then passed without difficulty. Small, uninfected stones in the kidney that cause no serious symptoms may be left alone.

The vast majority of stones in the ureter normally pass out with time. Should they fail to pass within a reasonable period, or cause unbearable pain or endanger the kidney, they're removed by surgical or other means. Fortunately, there are new nonsurgical ways to get some stones out.

- *Endoscopic basket extraction* is done under general or local anesthetic, for small stones stuck in the lower section of a ureter. Using a cystoscope, through which the surgeon can see, a fine tube is passed via the urethra and the bladder into the ureter and a basket is then passed up the tube to ensnare and pull out the stones.
- *Ultrasound lithotripsy* is another way to avoid surgery. Under epidural (spinal) anesthesia an optical scope is used to "see" the stone, and then high-frequency ultrasound vibrations strike and crumble it into pieces small enough to be passed out or removed with a basket.
- *Nephroscopy* allows the stone to be seen inside the kidney through a nephroscope passed through a small puncture in the side.

The opening is gradually widened to allow entry of the scope and instruments that search for grab and retrieve the stone. An ultrasound probe may be used through the same instrument to break up stones too large to be removed whole.

- *Extracorporeal lithotripsy*, another new method, blasts stones from outside the body and allows the fragments to pass out normally. Guided by X-ray technology, special "shock waves" shatter the kidney stones into fine sand. The procedure is done under epidural anesthesia while the patient is immersed in a water bath. Hard stones break up and pass without harming any tissues.

Surgery, involving a general anesthetic and abdominal incision, is still sometimes necessary for ureter stones caught in an awkward spot (high up in the ureter) or too large for basket removal or resistant to ultrasound crushing. Stones caught in the kidney that are infected, or cause bad pain or urine blockage, must come out and in some cases still require open surgery.

Preventing kidney stones—possible or not?

Chemical analysis of any stones passed and caught may improve the chances of finding out the underlying metabolic quirks that lead to stones, and possibly help to prevent their recurrence. Uric-acid and cystine stones can be dissolved by alkalinizing the urine, by either appropriate diet or taking chemicals—a strategy that may prevent recurrence of stones or stop existing ones from getting bigger.

In the days of Hippocrates, stone formers were urged to drink plenty of fluids to "flush out the pipes and dilute the salts." The advice still holds; stone formers should drink 3 or more liters or quarts a day.

Dietary means of reducing stone formation may work for stones resulting from underlying metabolic defects, particularly those due to elevated blood calcium. People with calcium-metabolizing problems, detectable by blood and urine tests, may reduce kidney-stone formation by going easy on calcium-rich foods such as dairy products, and reducing intake of items high in oxalate, such as rhubarb, spinach, tea, chocolate and colas.

People prone to high uric-acid levels (as in gout) may benefit by cutting down on foods high in purine—a precursor of uric acid found in meats, fish, organ meats, poultry and legumes.

For more information, contact the Kidney Foundation of Canada.

LEUKEMIA

Leukemia is a rare cancer of the bone marrow that destroys the body's normal hemopoiesis, or blood-formation, taking over the bone marrow. The disease can be acute, with sudden onset, or chronic, developing slowly over several years. While leukemia remains a serious disease, some forms are now curable. Whereas 20 years ago a child diagnosed with acute leukemia could expect to survive just a few months, nowadays not only can many children be cured of the disease but even the once-dismal outlook for adults is improving. The increased survival has come about through treatment administered in specialized centers, use of new drug combinations, better support measures (such as blood transfusions) and bone-marrow transplants.

Of the approximately 3,200 new Canadian cases of leukemia diagnosed every year about 250 are in children (usually aged 2 to 6). Although it's thought of as a childhood illness, leukemia is actually more frequent in adults, who tend to get different forms and generally do less well in treatment.

What goes wrong in leukemia?

Leukemia is a disease of uncontrolled blood-cell proliferation. It is really a group of related diseases involving destruction of the bone marrow's blood-forming compartment. Each form of leukemia has varying signs and symptoms, requiring different treatment. Some types are curable, others less so.

What happens is that abnormal cells within bone marrow (the spongy substance at the center of bone) become malignant, remain immature and rapidly fill up the bone marrow, impeding normal blood production. "The disease is always advanced when we find it," notes one specialist. "We never catch leukemia early. By the time it produces symptoms, the bone marrow is already in serious trouble, with normal blood cells squeezed out." Deprived of red

DIAGNOSING LEUKEMIA: POSSIBLE SYMPTOMS

In its early stages, leukemia may cause no symptoms other than a pale complexion and listless manner. Anemia—with a low red-blood-cell count and shortage of hemoglobin (the oxygen-carrying pigment)—can be the first alerting sign, making people weak and weary. Lack of platelets impairs clotting and leads to small hemorrhages, so the person bruises and bleeds easily. The depletion of normal white blood cells weakens the body's defenses, increasing vulnerability to infections—often the cause of death in those with leukemia. Expansion of the bone marrow may produce joint and bone pain.

A typical case is Johnny, aged 5, whose rosy cheeks paled and habitual energy faded as he became increasingly listless, also complaining of leg pain. The doctor, on examination noticing the child's striking pallor and numerous bruises, ordered blood tests that revealed the abnormal blood picture—the raised white-cell count, depleted red cells and reduced clotting power typical of acute lymphoblastic leukemia or ALL.

A bone-marrow biopsy confirms diagnosis by examining a small piece removed from the back of the pelvic bone with a needle, under local anesthetic. Analysis of the bone marrow sample identifies the type of leukemia—whether it is lymphoid in origin (and if it involves B- or T-cells), or myeloid. A spinal tap may be done to see if there are any leukemic cells detectable in the central nervous system.

Newly developed immunophenotyping can identify genetic and immunological markers—for example, chromosome and gene changes within leukemic cells, helping to predict prognosis (probable outlook) and choose the right treatment.

Alerting signs and symptoms of acute leukemia
- pallor (extremely pale complexion);
- anemia (with low hemoglobin);
- constant fatigue, weakness;
- fevers (especially in children);
- frequent bleeding—e.g., repeat nose and gum bleeds;
- easy bruising (because of impaired clotting mechanisms);
- non-healing cuts and mouth sores (in adults);
- bone pain, especially in the legs, perhaps a limp;
- abnormal white-blood-cell count (unusually high);
- possibly enlarged spleen and lymph nodes.

---

blood cells and platelets (little cells that aid clotting), the blood can no longer do its job of carrying oxygen to the tissues.

Various forms of leukemia—more than one disease

The leukemias are named according to the origin of the abnormal cells, whether they are lymphoid (also termed lymphoblastic or lymphocytic) or myeloid (also termed non-lymphoblastic, myelogenous or myelocytic). Both lymphoblastic and myeloid leukemia can be acute or chronic.

In the acute form, the type most common in children, rapidly dividing, immature white blood cells quickly invade bone marrow, producing illness in a few weeks. The acute forms include acute lymphoblastic leukemia (ALL) and acute myelogenous leukemia (AML), each with several subtypes. Acute leukemia requires prompt treatment with chemotherapy (cancer-killing drugs) and blood transfusions. Modern cure rates are generally good for children and improving for adults.

In the chronic leukemias, which affect mainly adults, cancerous cells gradually invade the bone marrow, and symptoms may take several years to evolve. The major types are chronic lympho-cytic leukemia (CLL) and chronic myeloid or myelogenous leukemia (CML). Less common forms include hairy cell leukemia and adult T-cell leukemia. Chronic leukemia can smolder for years, with no or few symptoms—other than perhaps some malaise, fatigue and increased infections—allowing those affected to live in harmony with the disease and carry on as usual. Chronic leukemia can go undiagnosed for years, often being discovered by chance through a routine blood test. But ultimately chronic leukemia will progress to an acute or blastic phase with symptoms such as weight loss, fevers, fatigue, night sweats and spleen enlargement. Although they take longer to surface, the chronic leukemias are harder to treat or cure.

Causes of leukemia still a puzzle

There are genetic clues and environmental clues, but so far nobody knows how to fit them together and the reasons for leukemia remain obscure. The disease is not inherited; rarely is there more than one case in a family, except for identical twins who may both be afflicted. It is not contagious. About 3 percent of leukemia is linked to congenital disorders present at birth, such as Down syndrome and Fanconi's anemia. Radiation is known to trigger it. For example,

REMISSION IS NOT CURE

Intense, multidrug therapy can now often put acute leukemia into remission within a month or so, especially in children. Remission is defined as the disappearance of all disease signs and symptoms, with no detectable leukemic cells in bone marrow and the apparent restoration of normal blood formation. "But remission does not guarantee cure," warns one hematologist, "and even when chemotherapy seemingly manages to put the disease into remission and the bone marrow normalizes, residual leukemic cells may linger undetected in parts of the body and cause a relapse." Even for those in remission, treatment must continue to consolidate it.

"Cure" is medically defined as 5 years with all evidence of leukemia gone and for low-risk acute lymphoblastic leukemia, standard therapy now achieves cure in 70 to 80 percent of cases, with few long-term after effects. For acute myeloid leukemia in children, cure rates are somewhat lower and even less in adults. Chronic leukemias are harder to cure but bone-marrow transplants can improve the chances.

Despite everything possible done to prevent them, relapses do occur, both during treatment, or soon after its completion. A relapse may be heralded by a repeat of the original symptoms—fatigue, anemia, leg pain, bleeding and fevers. Depending on the type of leukemia, there may be signs of brain and nervous system invasion. "There is no such thing as a slight relapse," comments one specialist from Toronto's Hospital for Sick Children. "Relapse at any site, any time, is a grave event and second or subsequent remissions are harder to maintain." Rescue therapy for relapses may involve different drugs in different doses, or a bone-marrow transplant for suitable candidates.

after the atomic bombs were dropped on Hiroshima and Nagasaki, the incidence of leukemia among Japanese survivors rose 10- to 20-fold. X-rays of the pelvis taken during pregnancy are a previously well-documented cause of leukemia in the fetus. However, ordinary chest and other X-rays do *not* increase the risk of leukemia. Altogether the known causes only account for 10 percent of all cases. No explanation can yet be found for the remaining 90 percent of leukemia.

Treatment of leukemia

Therapy for leukemia is given in stages over a period of months to years, using cancer-killing drugs, perhaps also radiation and possibly a bone marrow transplant. The goal is to clear the bone marrow and blood of all leukemic cells, allowing blood-producing cells to repopulate the marrow and reinstate normal blood production—putting the disease into remission. Treatment is best obtained in specialist centers.

Therapy often begins with blood transfusions to help reconstitute the blood, plus chemotherapy. For some forms, giving several combined cancer-killing agents at once is more effective than using one. The drugs may be injected, infused into the spine or taken by mouth. In order to facilitate intravenous drug administration and blood sampling (to test how well treatment is progressing) a central indwelling venous catheter (tube) or a subcutaneous device may be inserted for use as and when needed. High-dose antibiotics and transfusions are also given by this route. Growth factors may also be used to stimulate blood production. In lymphoblastic forms, leukemic cells may hide in the brain and spinal cord, or sometimes in the testicles, requiring special treatment. The head may be irradiated in those over age 10.

Although remission can be achieved and the blood revitalized within a month or so of starting treatment, stray leukemic cells can lurk undetected in the body's nooks and crannies. So consolidation treatment is often needed, with repeat bouts of chemotherapy in hospital. For some types of leukemia, maintenance therapy may continue for months or even years with anti-cancer medications taken at home, plus periodic visits to the clinic for bursts of high-dose chemotherapy. Spinal taps may be done from time to time to test for lingering leukemic cells, or to instill preventive medication.

One hematologist warns of the pitfalls if people stop the maintenance therapy too soon. "Feeling perfectly well, people may forget that the bone marrow is still in danger and neglect to take the life-saving medication, risking relapses that are harder to treat."

Side effects of chemotherapy vary according to the drugs and doses used, some patients tolerating them better than others. Side effects can include nausea and vomiting, hair loss, skin blisters, gut bleeds, heart disturbances and frequent infections that demand strong antibiotics.

Bone-marrow transplants offer hope for some cases

Bone-marrow transplants, although no panacea, are dramatically improving survival chances for leukemia. The transplants may be allografts, using

RUNDOWN OF THE DIFFERENT LEUKEMIAS

The acute leukemias

- **Acute lymphoblastic** or **lymphocytic leukemia** (ALL) affects primarily children aged 2 to 6. It is divided into three subgroups, each with different features; chromosome changes help predict outlook and determine treatment. Treatment lasts 3 years, starting with high-intensity, multidrug chemotherapy in hospital for 1 to 2 weeks to achieve remission, and spinal infusion (or irradiation) to eradicate cells in the brain, thereafter continuing with pills (such as *methotrexate* and *mercaptopurine*) at home, plus blood transfusions and antibiotics if needed. Initial remission rates for ALL average 90 percent, with 70 to 80 percent of children (and about 30 percent of adults) "cured"— alive and well 5 to 10 years after diagnosis.
- **Acute myeloid** or **myelogenous leukemia** (AML), also called acute *nonlymphoblastic leukemia* (ANLL), responsible for 15 to 20 percent of childhood cases (mainly older children and adolescents) is primarily an adult form, average onset age 55. Alerting symptoms are anemia, fevers, easy bruising, gum or nose bleeds and fatigue. AML has a worse outlook than ALL. About 70 percent go into remission but only about 25 percent stay cured. Treatment is with blood transfusions and very intense chemotherapy given for 3 to 6 months.

The chronic leukemias

- **Chronic lymphocytic** or **lymphoblastic leukemia** (CLL), not seen in children, is the most common adult form, rarely occurring before age 40, affecting slightly more men than women. CLL may take many years to develop, often goes unnoticed, and is generally not treated until it becomes acute with symptoms such as fever, breathlessness, swollen lymph nodes, bleeding episodes, spleen enlargement, diminished appetite, weight loss and frequent infections.
- **Chronic myeloid leukemia** (accounts for only 2 percent of childhood leukemia) affects mainly adults aged 55 and up. Characterized by leukemic cells possessing the Philadelphia chromosome (a 9;22 translocation), CML develops slowly, often over 3 to 5 years, eventually reaching crisis with weight loss, bleeds, fevers, spleen enlargement and night sweats. The crisis stage is hard to treat, but drugs such as *bisulfan* may prolong life by months to years, although they cannot offer cure. Bone-marrow transplants, given soon after diagnosis (during the chronic phase), can achieve long-term survival in younger sufferers. Treatment with *alpha interferon* (which eradicates cells with the Philadelphia chromosome) offers new hope.

marrow donated by a relative or by a matched (unrelated) donor, or autologous, using the patient's own marrow, taken during remission. For donor transplants, the bone marrow is harvested (taken by needle) from a sibling or an unrelated donor and infused into the patient to regenerate the blood supply. Before receiving the marrow transplant, the patient must undergo massive chemotherapy to destroy all traces of the "bad" (malfunctioning) bone marrow. With an autologous (self) transplant, some of the patient's *own* bone marrow is removed, stored and later reinfused. A recent development is the use of stem cells—blood-forming cells taken from the peripheral (circulating) bloodstream to restore blood production. Growth factors may be given to stimulate blood formation.

Since transplant procedures pose considerable dangers, especially by depressing the immune defenses (which exposes people to life-threatening infections) the probable benefits must be carefully weighed against possible risks. Graft-versus-host disease is a serious complication in which the donor cells reject the host's body cells, provoking an immune response that attacks the patient's organs. The most successful candidates for bone-marrow transplants are young adults with chronic myeloid leukemia who have a sibling donor and adults with acute myeloid leukemia in first remission who also have a sibling donor.

LIVER CIRRHOSIS

Liver cirrhosis is a pressing global health problem and a major cause of death in men aged 25 to 64. It is twice as common in men as in women; however, *susceptibility* to alcohol-related liver injury appears to be greater in women than men, even though women drink less.

Cirrhosis is an insidious condition that often reaches an advanced stage without giving any hint of its presence. Among the causes of liver cirrhosis—such as some forms of viral hepatitis, inherited disorders of iron and copper metabolism, certain drugs and bile-duct obstruction— excess alcohol intake is by far the most frequent. Cirrhosis is about 30 times more common among heavy drinkers than among nondrinkers.

Anyone who drinks heavily for many years will almost certainly end up with a damaged liver.

How alcohol harms the liver

There are three major types of liver injury related to alcohol: fatty liver, alcoholic hepatitis and cirrhosis. The first two are potentially reversible, but full-blown cirrhosis is not.

- *Fatty liver* is common in obese people. The liver is enlarged and full of fat droplets, but the condition usually has few overt symptoms, except perhaps some abdominal pain and possibly some jaundice. Most do not have any negative effects, although if combined with other liver disease processes, such as hepatitis or heavy drinking, it can be damaging.

- *Alcohol-induced hepatitis* may also go completely unnoticed. However, in severe alcoholic hepatitis the drinker has malaise (unwellness), perhaps also some vomiting, appetite loss, upper abdominal pain, sometimes jaundice and spider nevi (enlarged surface or skin blood vessels that look like a red spider's web). Approximately 30 percent of people who have alcoholic hepatitis go on to develop cirrhosis if alcohol intake does not cease.

- *Cirrhosis* is a form of liver damage whose main feature is breakdown of the liver's normal architecture, with the formation of scar (fibrous) tissue and nodules (the liver's attempt to regenerate its injured cells).

    Extensive liver scarring develops over many years, generally giving little or no sign of its progress until the disease is advanced and complications occur—such as bleeding from enlarged veins (varices) that may burst and hemorrhage (the most common cause of death in cirrhotics). In addition, ascites may form, corresponding to the biblical description of the dropsy—a huge accumulation of fluid in the abdomen that greatly expands its girth. Owing to the blockage and diversion of normal blood routes, nutrients may bypass the liver, resulting in malnutrition. Toxins from the gut that accumulate because liver cells can no longer detoxify them may disturb brain chemistry, creating apathy, confusion, drowsiness and ultimately coma.

    There are no effective treatments for established liver cirrhosis, which is essentially irreversible. But impairment due to a fatty liver and "portal hypertension" (high blood pressure within the liver) can be greatly reduced by abstinence from alcohol. Various drugs for cirrhosis are currently under investigation.

LUNG CANCER

Lung cancer causes more deaths among men than any other cancer in North America, and in women it's overtaken breast cancer as the leading cancer killer. Almost one-third of all cancer deaths in industrialized nations is due to lung cancer—largely blamed on tobacco smoking. In Canada, this cancer claims about 17,000 lives annually. It has dismal cure rates, with death rates undiminished in 50 years. Overall, only 10 to 13 percent of those affected survive 5 years after diagnosis, and 95 percent of lung cancer victims are dead within 2 years.

Cigarette smoking is the chief (preventable) cause

Few nonsmokers develop lung cancer. Worldwide, 98 percent of men and 85 percent of women who develop lung cancer have been or are tobacco smokers. (Recent studies show that smoking marijuana may potentiate risks.) Smoking even a pack a day increases lung cancer risks tenfold. Giving up smoking gradually lessens the risk with a significant decline 10 to 15 years after quitting. The U.S. Environmental Protection Agency (EPA) estimates that in the U.S. 3,000 (and in Canada 300) lung cancer deaths annually are due to "secondhand" or passive smoking.

    Other possible causes of lung cancer include family history (a genetic susceptibility to the disease) and work exposure to certain carcinogens, including asbestos, arsenic, chromium, coke oven emissions (polycyclic hydrocarbons) and ionizing radiation (from coal and radon gas, a uranium breakdown product).

    N.B.: The extent of risk from these agents under modern working conditions is much debated.

Different types of lung cancer, all more or less lethal

Lung cancer occurs as small-cell carcinoma, which accounts for about 25 percent of cases, and as non-small-cell carcinoma (which includes squamous cell carcinoma, adenocarcinoma and large or giant cell carcinoma). People with very early, well-differentiated, localized non-small-cell (squamous) cancers have the best chances of survival. In contrast, small-cell carcinoma, which has often spread to other organs by the time it is found, has a less hopeful outlook and many are dead within 2 months of diagnosis.

Few warning signs until an advanced stage

Lung cancer rarely causes symptoms until it is advanced, so it often goes undetected until it's beyond the stage of effective treatment. It is often found incidentally during a routine physical checkup, or when people consult their physician about a persistent cough, shortness of breath or spitting up blood. (Chest X-rays are not considered a useful screening tool since the cancer usually shows up radiographically only at an advanced stage.) Diagnosis requires bronchoscopy, with a fiberoptic viewing instrument to examine the lungs, perhaps also a biopsy, done under local anaesthetic, and CAT scans to look for malignancies beyond the lung.

The treatment of lung cancer includes surgery, chemotherapy and radiation, depending on the tumor type and stage and the person's overall health. If the cancer is small and localized, surgery is the usual treatment. It may be curative in the small group of patients with localized non-small-cell (squamous) lung cancers.

Surgery is rarely indicated for those with small-cell lung cancer because by the time it's found, the cancer has often already spread beyond the lungs (to the bones, lymph glands, liver kidneys, adrenal glands and, particularly, the brain). At diagnosis, 85 percent of those with small-cell lung cancer already have metastases. Most people with this type of lung cancer receive chemotherapy with anti-cancer drugs—such as *cyclophosphamide*, *doxyrubicin* and *vincristine*—and perhaps also radiation. Radiation may be used in late-stage lung cancer to shrink the tumor stop blood-spitting, clear the airways and alleviate pain.

LUPUS

Popularly known as lupus, *systemic lupus erythematosus* or SLE, is a chronic rheumatoid or autoimmune condition affecting primarily the skin and joints, although it can spread to other organs such as the heart, kidneys and nervous system. Its name comes from the 19th-century observation of a prominent, red "butterfly" rash across the nose and cheeks of many sufferers—resembling the attack of a wolf or "lupus." Lupus affects about 1 per 1,000 people, 90 percent of them women—striking mainly in the reproductive years from age 18 to 40. Being an unpredictable disease of many faces, lupus can be difficult to recognize, and it may take several years to connect the sporadic symptoms with the illness. Lupus flares periodically, followed by remissions that can last for years.

Lupus is an autoimmune disease in which the body's immune system—normally directed against foreign bacteria and viruses—fails to recognize "self" substances and makes antibodies that attack the body's own tissues. People with lupus also fail to clear antigens (foreign particles) from the body, and certain white blood cells behave abnormally, gobbling up one another's cell nuclei. These changes are the basis of a diagnostic test for lupus, as almost all sufferers have elevated blood levels of antinuclear antibodies and other strange auto-antibodies.

Although its causes remain a mystery, certain triggers such as sunlight, viral infections or some medications can set off lupus in susceptible people. Sunlight typically makes symptoms flare. Other environmental factors such as extreme cold and stress can bring on the illness. The condition also worsens after viral or bacterial infections and in response to certain drugs such as *isopiazid*, *hydralazine* or *methyldopa* (Aldomet). But drug-induced lupus tends to be less severe than other forms, and vanishes once the medication is discontinued.

Lupus has varied signs and symptoms

Lupus comes in many disguises, mild or severe, with a range of complaints such as pervasive fatigue, weakness, occasional low-grade fever poor appetite, weight loss and sometimes the butterfly face rash. Arthritic complaints are its hallmark, with painful, sometimes swollen joints—mainly in the hands and wrists, but also in the elbows, hips, knees and ankles.

The American College of Rheumatology has compiled a list of signs and symptoms, among which four must be present to establish a diagnosis of lupus. They include:

- skin rashes, perhaps a malar (cheek) rash;
- *discoid* bumps and "plaques" (especially on the ears);
- photosensitivity—redness or rash on sun-exposure;
- arthritic joint aches (with morning stiffness);
- ulcers or sores in the mouth, nose and vagina;
- dry and puffy eyes;
- blood disorders such as hemolytic anemia;
- immune system abnormalities (e.g., DNA changes, antinuclear antibodies);
- swollen lymph glands;
- signs of kidney malfunction (e.g., protein in the urine);
- neurological disorders (such as headaches, severe depression, seizures, psychosis);
- diffuse hair loss (all over the head);
- coughing, inflamed linings of lungs.

Raynaud's phenomenon affects 40 percent of lupus sufferers—an episodic condition in which fingers and toes go white in the cold (from arterial spasms), and then red and throbbing in the warmth (as blood flow returns). Stress can aggravate it and produce fingertip sores.

The inflammatory processes may spread to internal organs, such as the kidneys, central nervous system and heart. These more severe complications usually appear within the first few years of diagnosis. Over half of those with lupus have some kidney inflammation—usually mild with few or no symptoms, and sufferers may not notice the problem until an advanced stage. However, once it progresses, there may be signs of kidney trouble such as bloating, ankle swelling and abnormal blood and urine tests.

Medications for treating lupus

- *Nonsteroidal anti-inflammatories or NSAIDs* are the first line of attack. People with mild lupus require only simple NSAIDs, such as ASA (for joint pain, headaches and chest pains).
- *Antimalarials,* medications commonly used to treat malaria, are highly effective in controlling lupus. Such drugs as the older *chloroquine* and the newer *hydroxychloroquine* help to reduce fever fatigue and joint pain, as well as clear skin rashes. These drugs are generally non-toxic, but some cases of eye damage have been reported. People embarking on anti-malarials should have their eyes checked before starting on the drugs and receive regular medical supervision.

- *Corticosteroids* (such as *prednisolone* and *prednisone*) may be taken orally for more serious cases. Corticosteroids improve energy and appetite. Short-term side effects may include facial and body swelling, easy bruising, mood changes and raised blood pressure. Over the long haul, corticosteroids can increase susceptibility to diabetes, cataracts, infections and osteoporosis, so they are used for the shortest possible time to control flare-ups, then tapered off—never suddenly withdrawn.

- *Immunosuppressive agents* for severe lupus include *azathioprine, methotrexate* or *cyclophosphamide* to calm the immune system overreaction. Since people on these drugs have diminished immune defenses, they must be closely monitored for infection.

Tips for people with lupus

- Managing fatigue means accepting it as a chronic, lifelong condition and learning to live with it—getting enough rest.
- It's best *not* to take over-the-counter medications other than those suggested by the consulting physicians—lupus sufferers are especially prone to adverse drug reactions.
- Those on corticosteroids and other immune-suppressing drugs must watch for infections.
- Avoiding sunlight is a must. All people with lupus should use PABA-free, high SPF (30) sunscreens, wear long-sleeved clothing and hats when sun exposure is unavoidable.
- Although kidney failure is rare, there may be some kidney inflammation, so lupus sufferers need regular monitoring.
- During pregnancy, lupus needs carefully tailored drug therapy to keep the disease under control while avoiding damage to the fetus. Consult a physician if contemplating pregnancy.
- Self-help and support groups can be useful.

For more information, contact Lupus Canada, tel.: (800) 661-1468; the Ontario Lupus Association, tel.: (416) 979-7228; or Lupus Québec, tel.: (514) 849-0955.

LYME DISEASE

Lyme disease—now the number one insect-borne disease in North America, exceeding Rocky Mountain spotted fever (a bacterial disease carried by dog ticks)—is caused by bacteria carried by tiny, wingless, eight-legged Ixodid ticks.

The U.S. Centers for Disease Control report some 1,500 new cases annually, and the numbers increase each year. Lyme disease is also prevalent in Northern and Central Europe. The real number of cases may be considerably higher because many people know little about the disease and may be totally unaware of having been bitten by a tick. In addition, some health professionals still have trouble identifying this unfamiliar illness. It tends to remit and flare up, but gradually improves with time in most cases. It is identified by a skin rash, neurological (nerve) and heart disturbances, and if left untreated, can cause serious arthritis.

Lyme disease got its name from two small New England townships—Lyme and Old Lyme in Connecticut. Juvenile arthritis is very rare, and its incidence among children in the Lyme area in the mid-1970s was many times the national average: 1 in 100 compared to 1 in 100,000 nationwide. Also, parents noticed that children aged 5 to 16 developed a curious ring-shaped rash and severe headaches as well as swollen joints.

Many of the initial juvenile Connecticut sufferers lived near heavily wooded regions and caught the disease in summertime. At first, scientists suspected some environmental pollutant. But some children remembered having a tick bite, and all clues pointed to the small woodland biting tick, of the *Ixodes* genus. Yale University researchers ultimately confirmed the link to tick bites and to a similar condition already identified in Europe during the early 1900s.

A corkscrew-shaped bacterium (a spirochete) was extracted from the gut of one biting tick in 1982, and later identified in the blood, spinal fluid and inflamed skin of some humans. The spirochete was named *Borrelia burgdorferi* in 1982, for its discoverer, Dr. Willy Burgdorfer.

The ticks that transmit Lyme disease include *Ixodes dammini* in eastern areas of this continent, *Ixodes pacificus* in the west and *Ixodes ricinus* in Europe. The tick measures 1 to 4 millimeters across—not much larger than a sesame

THE THREE STAGES OF LYME DISEASE

- *Stage one:* a rash that appears within 3 days to 3 weeks (but usually within a week) of the tick bite, starting as a small red pimple at the bite site and gradually expanding to form a ring-shaped "bull's eye"—red at the edges, clear in the middle—which can get as large as a dime or a dinner plate. While the strange rash (which fades within 3 to 4 weeks) appears in only about half of those infected, other skin rashes may appear anywhere on the body (usually the chest, back, thigh, groin and armpit). The rash fades in a few weeks even if untreated. Some people never experience the rash and don't notice a tick bite, yet go on to develop more advanced stages, months, perhaps years, later. Other symptoms include a flu-like illness (with fever, chills, headache, malaise, stiff muscles, an aching neck), extreme fatigue and swollen lymph nodes.

- *Stage two:* Temporary neurological (nervous system) problems appear in about 8 to 10 percent of those with untreated Lyme disease—usually starting 2 to 11 weeks after the tick bite, signalled by violent headaches (similar to those experienced with meningitis), neuritis (inflammation of the neck nerves) and sensory disturbances (such as transient deafness). A condition similar to Bell's palsy (paralysis of the face muscles) is a common but temporary complication. In most cases the neurological symptoms vanish with appropriate treatment, or spontaneously in a few weeks to months. Heart problems, from blockage of the heart's electrical-conducting system, also develop in 5 to 8 percent of untreated people with Lyme disease, producing dizziness, palpitations, shortness of breath and irregular heartbeats. The cardiac difficulties may last from a week to a couple of months, and a temporary pacemaker may be needed.

- *Stage three:* Months or even years after the tick bite (but typically within 6 to 24 months), this stage strikes 60 to 80 percent of untreated patients, beginning with hot, painful joint swelling, especially in the knees, ankles, elbows, wrists and shoulders. If not promptly treated with antibiotics, this arthritic condition can lead to permanent disability. The third stage may also include demyelinating problems involving nerve-coat degeneration, limb numbness, memory lapses and overpowering fatigue.

seed or small ant, and roughly half the size of the common dog tick. It is tiny enough to be overlooked or mistaken for a freckle or a fleck of dirt. Many of those who develop Lyme disease don't remember having seen any such creature, nor do they recall being bitten.

Between hosts, the ticks usually inhabit tall grasslands and wooded areas. The likelihood of people becoming infected is greatest when the feet and legs come in contact with long grass or shrubs; the hungry ticks linger low down on the vegetation with their front legs up, poised in a

HOW TO AVOID LYME DISEASE

- **Find out whether any area you inhabit or plan to visit is known to harbor ticks. (In Canada, so far, only Long Point, Ontario, is a clearly defined risk area.)**
- **If in tick-infested areas, especially woodlands or fields, practice a daily skin inspection, not omitting hairy areas. Since a tick may take 2 or more days to attach and feed, the risk of infection can be reduced by frequent body checks and prompt tick removal.**
- **Immediately remove any ticks detected, brushing off those unattached and removing those already affixed by gently using tweezers to grasp head and mouth parts as close to skin level as possible, pulling slowly to detach the entire tick Try not to squash them as this releases bacteria, which may enter the body.**
- **Avoid handling the ticks, as the infective spirochetes could pierce the body through a scratch or cut in the skin.**
- **Disinfect with soap and water (or with alcohol or Betadine) after tick removal.**

- **If gardening, hiking, playing or romping in a known tick-infested area, wear long-sleeved and long-legged clothing that fits tightly around wrists and ankles (tucking pants into socks or boots).**
- **Walk along the center of trail paths to reduce contact with underbrush.**
- **Favor light-colored clothes on which a black tick shows up.**
- **Use insect repellents containing diethyl m-toluamide (DEET).**
- **Apply the tick-repellent *permethrin* (Permanone) to clothing.**
- **Be sure to apply repellent to shoes, socks and pantlegs to protect the vulnerable feet and legs.**
- **Check pets and remove ticks before they enter the house.**

N.B.: Contrary to popular belief, getting rid of ticks with nail polish, salt, mineral oil, matches or cigarettes is not as effective as removal with tweezers or forceps.

"questing" position, ready to attach themselves to animals or humans that brush against them. While most common in tall vegetation, they have been detected on well-trimmed suburban lawns and found crawling amid the foliage of England's famous parks. The ticks are especially numerous in places where deer thrive.

In their habitual hosts (mice and deer) the ticks cause no illness, but when infected ticks take a meal from other warm-blooded animals, they may cause disease. Ixodes ticks have been found on animals ranging from dogs, horses, sheep and cats to birds (e.g., wrens and yellowthroats). In Canada, Ixodes ticks infected with Lyme-disease spirochetes were first detected in Ontario's Long Point Wildlife Sanctuary and Provincial Park on Lake Erie, a popular tourist resort and stopover point for many migrating birds. (It is theorized that birds carrying infected ticks imported Lyme disease to this Ontario site, but the ticks may have been introduced when the area was purposely repopulated with deer during the early 1900s.)

Diagnosis of Lyme disease remains tricky

Physicians sometimes have difficulty in identifying Lyme disease, which may become clear only when its later manifestations—the neurological

complications and cardiovascular symptoms—emerge. The characteristic bull's-eye rash appears in only some of those infected, but "satellite" skin lesions away from the original bite site may be telltale clues. Confirmation of diagnosis depends on culturing the organism from the skin lesions, blood or cerebrospinal fluid. A high white-blood-cell count (denoting infection), muscle aches and general flulike malaise may be preliminary hints. A blood test for antibodies to the causative agent (present 3 to 6 weeks after the infecting tick bite) may help to confirm the disease. But serological (blood) tests lack specificity and many labs aren't set up to do them. Several different tests may have to be done for accurate diagnosis. Some people who experience no rash and no cardiac or nerve problems may become aware of having Lyme disease only when arthritis surfaces 2 or more years after the tick bite. New research is investigating the use of DNA probes for diagnosing Lyme disease.

Treatment of Lyme disease

Fortunately, Lyme disease responds well to antibiotic therapy. Treatment with antibiotics such as amoxicillin, ceftriaxone, penicillin, doxycycline or others prevents most serious complications of this bacterial illness. Even if Lyme disease has advanced to stage 2 or 3, antibiotics are still effective in most cases.

LYMPHOMA, NON-HODGKIN'S TYPE

Non-Hodgkin's lymphoma is a cancer of the lymphatic system, lymph nodes and spleen — part of the body's immune system—in which the lymphocytes (white blood cells) multiply abnormally. There are several different types of the disease, one of the most common being diffuse large B-cell lymphoma. The likelihood of getting non-Hodgkin's lymphoma increases with age, and for unknown reasons its incidence has been rising steadily in the past few decades, especially in North America. It currently accounts for about 3 percent of all cancer deaths. Its causes remain unknown, but it is especially common in the immunosuppressed (for instance transplant recipients) and in people with AIDS and leukemia. The severity of the disease varies according to the nature and aggressiveness of the malignant cells.

Symptoms of lymphoma include unexplained weight loss, fatigue, night sweats, fever, aching bones and pain in the area affected. Swollen or enlarged lymph nodes (especially in the armpit, neck or groin) may be an alerting sign, particularly if they are hard, bigger than a dime, rubbery or matted. The spleen may be obviously enlarged and palpable (easily felt). People with lymphoma may present with lumps and pain almost anywhere— in the head, neck, skin, armpit, abdomen, gastrointestinal tract or back. Virtually any organ or tissue can be involved. Affected people may suddenly become very ill without any early warning signs, other than weight loss and tiredness.

Diagnosis and staging depend on tests such as ultrasound imaging, CT-scans and other X-rays, MRIs and biopsy of enlarged lymph nodes to determine the cancer's type. It should be controlled as soon as possible to prevent spread. Since the bone marrow is often affected, bone marrow sampling may be done at the spine or some other site. Indolent forms of the disease may come and go, wax and wane, with few acute symptoms.

Treatment of non-Hodgkin's lymphoma typically includes radiation, chemotherapy and perhaps use of new monoclonal antibodies— depending on the site(s), extent and stage of the disease. Radiation may be used before or after chemotherapy. Chemotherapy usually involves the CHOP regimen using a cocktail of cancer-killing drugs that includes *cyclophosphamide, doxorubicin and vincristine*, along with steroids to boost energy and appetite, and anti-nauseants to counter the ill effects of chemotherapy. In addition, white-cell boosters may be given to offset the neutrophil depletion (neutropenia) due to chemotherapy, which undermines the immune system.

Nowadays, monoclonal antibodies that specifically target cancerous lymphocytes, for example *rituximab* (Rituxan), are often used together with chemotherapy. This strategy gives high (80 percent) remission rates. Unlike chemotherapy drugs that destroy healthy as well as cancerous tissue, designer monoclonal antibodies seek out and inactivate or eliminate only those cells or proteins responsible for the disease, leaving healthy cells untouched.

The prognosis or outlook for recovery varies according to the type and stage of the lymphoma and the affected person's age. Given optimal treatment, about 15 percent of those with low-grade non-Hodgkin's lymphoma recover fully and three-quarters achieve remission and survive for 5 years or more. For aggressive lymphoma that relapses, high-dose chemotherapy followed by bone marrow transplants or autologous (self) stem cell transplants are an option.

New radioactive or radio-labeled monoclonal antibody products are also coming on stream for treating lymphoma, for instance *yttrium-90 labeled* or *Y-ibritumomab* (Zevalin) and iodine-131 *tositumomab* (Bexxar), recently approved by the FDA (but not in Canada) for use in people who are resistant to Rituxan. These products give promising results, although they can cause serious side effects such as drastically reduced blood cell counts and thyroid problems. So far, their use is approved only for relapsed patients in whom all other lymphoma treatments have failed. More studies are needed to assess their safety, efficacy and long-term effects.

MULTIPLE SCLEROSIS

Multiple sclerosis (MS) is a chronic, often progressive, degenerative and debilitating disease that attacks the central nervous system by destroying scattered patches of *myelin*, the protective fatty coating around nerves in the brain and spinal cord. Although classically described as an inflammatory disease that injures the myelin nerve sheath, axonal damage to the nerves themselves can also occur, worsening the disability.

Multiple sclerosis is the most common acquired disease of the nervous system in young adults, affecting about one per 1,000 persons, more women than men, symptoms usually first surfacing in their 30s to 40s. (In 90 percent of cases, MS begins between the ages of 20 and 50, and its incidence seems to be rising.) Its causes remain unknown although there is a genetic component to MS as it is 8 times more common in those with affected relatives. The lifetime risk for a child whose mother has MS is 3 to 5 percent but less if it's the father who has MS. Environment also plays a role as the disease is more common among those living in northern or temperate zones such as Europe or North America than those inhabiting the tropics. (Canada has one of the world's highest MS incidence.) Recent evidence suggests that besides a genetic susceptibility, MS may be linked to certain infections.

Basically, MS is thought to be an auto-immune disease in which the body falsely regards myelin as a "foreign substance" to be attacked by the person's own immune system, destroying its protective effect on nerve fibres in the brain, optic nerves and spinal cord. One analogy is to regard myelin as similar to the insulation on your stereo or other wiring. If this protective insulating sheath is compromised, it ruins the wire's performance. The same holds true for your body; the damaged myelin may form scar tissue (sclerosis) that undermines or diminishes the nerve's function or might even permanently damage the nerve fibre. When part of the myelin sheath is damaged or destroyed, nerve impulses to and from the brain or spinal cord are distorted, altering the body's ability to control such activities as walking, vision, balance and bladder function.

The severity of MS varies markedly among sufferers according to the parts of brain and spinal cord affected, ranging from mild—perhaps with long periods of remission between attacks—to progressive and severely disabling. MS often runs an unpredictable course, with huge variations in severity from one affected person to another. In some, the disease consists of mild attacks interspersed with long and completely symptom-free remissions while others with MS experience series of severe flare-ups that leave them progressively disabled. Those with severe MS may need help with walking, becoming incontinent and perhaps ultimately bedridden. However, MS is not a fatal disease and affected individuals generally have near-normal life expectancies; most of those afflicted learn to cope with the disease and continue to lead productive lives.

Early heralding symptoms may include tingling, numbness or a sense of heaviness in the extremities (hands, feet), face pain, slurred speech and blurred or double vision. The four most common initial symptoms are visual problems, numbness, weakness and gait imbalance. Many people with MS experience impaired co-ordination, muscle rigidity and tremors which may be temporary or permanent. Problems with bladder, bowel or sexual function are common. MS can produce forgetfulness or difficulty concentrating, and frequently, mood swings. Depression, weakness and fatigue are common problems in those with MS. Symptoms can appear singly or together. They are most severe if the myelin destruction happens in the brain, producing paralysis, clumsiness, trouble walking, loss of vision and urinary problems. Attacks may last weeks to months, then disappear or persist and worsen. Relapses can be triggered by stress or injury. The progress, severity and specific symptoms of MS in any one person cannot be predicted.

MS is often called "the great masquerader" as some of its symptoms occasionally occur in all of us.

Diagnosis is tricky and there is no single easy confirmatory test. Magnetic Resonance Imaging (MRI) is the investigation of choice for diagnosing MS when it is suspected clinically, revealing patchy damage to the white matter of the central nervous system. However, MRIs are negative in up to

10 percent of cases. Nerve conduction studies, analysis of cerebrospinal fluid (to detect inflammatory changes) and optic nerve tests are also sometimes used to delineate MS. Prognosis or outlook for MS is highly variable and it usually has a relapsing or remitting course.

There are several basic forms of MS:

- *relapsing and remitting MS* (RRMS) seen in about 80 percent of cases, with self-limiting attacks and often full recovery between episodes. About 10 to 20 percent of those with MS experience benign relapsing-remitting disease with little progression or serious disability after 10 years. Several factors influence the prognosis of relapsing-remitting MS. The prognosis or outlook is better in younger patients, in females and those in whom only a limited number of neuro-anatomical areas are affected, or those who have primarily sensory symptoms, experience a complete first remission and have few deficits after 5 years.
- *secondary progressive MS* which starts out as RRMS but progresses to a steadier deterioration and certain amount of disability after 15 years or so. In over half of those with relapsing-remitting MS, secondary progressive disease eventually develops.
- *Primary progressive MS*, which occurs in 10 to 15 percent of cases, where the course of MS is progressive and disabling from its onset, with gradually declining abilities from the start, but no acute attacks. Primary progressive MS tends to involve only one part of the nervous system, usually the spinal cord, and has a poor prognosis, sometimes producing serious disabilities within 5 years of diagnosis.

Overall, 10 years after the onset of MS, 50 percent of those affected can no longer work, and after 15 years 50 percent cannot walk unassisted; after 25 years of living with MS, 50 percent cannot walk at all.

Treatment for MS aims to prevent relapses and diminish the disabilities that hamper the activities of daily living. This complex illness wears people down with its unpredictability and variable symptoms. Treatment entails significant support, mental fortitude and help in maintaining a positive outlook. Getting plenty of rest is essential to offset the fatigue. As co-existing depression rates are high, those affected may require ongoing antidepressant therapy. Diet with supplements of sunflower and evening primrose oil may help. Corticosteroid medication can alleviate acute inflammatory episodes.

Disease-modifying agents for relapsing-remitting MS that may lengthen remission rates or prevent relapses include *beta interferons* such as *interferon beta-1b* (Betaseron) and *interferon beta-1a* (Avonex, Rebif) and *glatiramer acetate*. Interferons can reduce MS flare-ups by blocking the migration of immune system cells into the brain. Both interferon beta-1a and interferon beta-1b decrease the number of relapses and the number of plaques found on MRI scans in patients with relapsing-remitting MS. However, beta-1b interferon, given by subcutaneous injection, has recently been shown to be somewhat more effective than other forms. On the other hand, interferon-1a when given after the first demyelinating event may delay the onset of clinically definite MS. The evidence is inconsistent regarding the role and benefits of interferon in secondary progressive MS. *Glatiramer* (Copaxone) reduces the relapse rates over a 2-year period, but does not slow the onset of disability. (Its side effects include flushing, anxiety and chest-tightness.) Newer drugs like *mitoxantrone* (Novanthrone) have been shown to delay the progression of disability in relapsing-remitting or progressive MS by inhibiting immune system activity, but there are significant side effects such as bone marrow suppression which increases risks of infection. Other drugs currently being investigated include *natalizumab*, a recombinant monoclonal antibody, *alemtuzumab*, an antileucocyte (CD52) antibody and *statins* (cholesterol-lowering agents). There is no evidence so far that drugs such as Azathrioprine, IV Ig and methotrexate have any benefit in treating MS. Reliable trials have shown hyperbaric oxygen therapy, previously thought to be helpful, to be ineffective for MS. Given the complexities of drug management for multiple sclerosis, experts are often needed to guide individual therapy decisions.

PEPTIC ULCERS: DIGESTING MORE THAN FOOD

One of the world's most common maladies, peptic ulcers make life miserable for 10 percent

THE NSAIDs LINK

Aspirin (ASA) and other nonsteroidal anti-inflammatory drugs (NSAIDs) have recently emerged as a significant risk factor in peptic ulcer formation, especially gastric ulcers. Regular consumption of NSAIDs such as *ibuprofen* (Advil, Motrin), *naproxen* (Naprosyn) or *piroxicam* (Feldene) ranks high as a cause of peptic ulcers. The incidence of ulcer increases by 5 to 10 percent in those who take NSAIDs—the dangers of complications, especially bleeding and perforation being greater with gastric ulcers than duodenal. (Note that taking one coated ASA/Aspirin pill daily to guard against heart disease and stroke poses little extra risk of gastric ulcer). Serious NSAID-induced ulcers affected about 1 to 2 percent of heavy NSAID users each year, but it usually takes months to a year or more for an ulcer to develop from these medications. In general, the higher the NSAID dose and the longer the treatment, the greater the risk of peptic ulcer. Taking misoprostol (Cytotec) or a proton pump inhibitor (e.g. Pariet, Pantoloc) with the anti-inflammatories may decrease ulcer risks. Finally, newer medications such as celecoxib (Celebrex), which are special anti-inflammatories called Cox-2 inhibitors, may reduce risk in those who need to take anti-inflammatories but are at high risk (e.g., previous ulcer bleed). One of these new medications, called Vioxx, was recently pulled off the market because of increased heart risks. Celebrex is also under investigation for its safety profile.

of Canadians at some point in their lives. While ulcers can also occur in other parts of the body, we use the term "ulcer" to describe peptic ulcers in the duodenum (first part of the small intestine leading out of the stomach) and in the stomach itself.

Recapping what ulcers are and who gets them

"Peptic ulcer" is an umbrella term for certain lesions—little pits or "craters" (sores)—in the mucous membranes or lining of the stomach and duodenum (top part of the small intestine). Peptic ulcers occur most often in the duodenum (duodenal ulcers), less commonly in the stomach itself (gastric ulcers). The word "peptic" comes from *pepsin*, the enzyme that helps to break down food in the presence of stomach acid and contributes to the erosion that produces an ulcer. Ulcers often appear as white or pale yellow spots due to surrounding inflammation. Occasionally ulcers arise in the esophagus or in the small bowel. In the past, peptic ulcer disease afflicted mainly men, but nowadays

women are equally affected—particularly the elderly. Ulcers are also common among those who take ASA (Aspirin) and other nonsteroidal anti-inflammatory drugs (NSAIDs), which irritate the stomach.

Although ulcers vary in size from a pinhead size to one inch (2.5 cm) or more across, size has little to do with the intensity of the pain or distress. While some ulcers heal spontaneously on their own, others persist for months or recur and some cause serious complications such as bleeding or perforation.

The discovery that a specific bacterial infection is largely to blame for peptic ulcers has revolutionized the diagnosis and treatment of these common disorders. "Triple therapy," using two antibiotics and an acid suppressant, can now cure most bacterially caused duodenal and gastric ulcers, dramatically reducing the risks of recurrence and serious complications.

Bacteria to blame

The old adage of "no acid, no ulcer" is being dispelled, with the realization that not acid but bacteria are primarily to blame. Peptic ulcers were previously attributed mainly to stress, diet, or "too much acid." This view has been supplanted by the realization that acid plays second fiddle to bacteria in causing peptic ulcers. Recent studies implicate a spiral bacterium, Helicobacter pylon (H. pylori).

Australian researchers demonstrated its presence in 60 percent of those with peptic ulcers and 50 percent of stomach cancer patients. Today we know that about 95 percent of duodenal ulcers and 70 to 80 percent of the gastric variety are linked to the H. pylori bacteria and that they respond to antibacterial treatment (the remainder are largely caused by medications, mainly ASA and other nonsteroidal anti-inflammatories). Antibiotics that eradicate the stomach-dwelling microbe can now cure most peptic ulcers and—most importantly prevent recurrences.

The exact link between H. pylori and ulcers is slowly becoming clear. At the onset of H. pylori infection, mild gastritis (gastrointestinal irritation) produces pain, and a transient hypochlorhydria (acid depletion) may facilitate bacterial colonization. The flagella and spiral

ADDITIONAL ULCER MEDICATIONS INCLUDE:

- **Histamine H2-receptor blockers, taken as tablets, which act on the stomach's "receptor" and prevent release of histamine, a substance that stimulates hydrochloric acid secretion. H2-blocker treatment decreases stomach acid and speeds ulcer healing. These drugs, which can reduce ulcer pain within hours of the first dose, include cimetidine (Tagamet), introduced in the 1970s—the first of the H2-blockers, which revolutionized peptic ulcer treatment, ranitidine (Zantac), famotidine (Pepcid) and nizatidine (Axid). However, this class of drugs is no longer considered top-of-the-line therapy for ulcers.**
- **Proton-pump Inhibitors (PPIs) are potent acid suppressors that include omeprazole (Losec) and lansoprazole (Prevacid). These drugs suppress stomach acid production for hours, and antagonize but do not kill H. pylori. About 10 times more powerful than H2-blockers in suppressing stomach acid production, the PPIs suppress about 95 percent of stomach acid production and heal duodenal ulcers, but are less effective for gastric ulcers.**
- **Bismuth compounds such as Pepto Bismol have some antimicrobial action and are still used for ulcer treatment, in combination with antibiotics.**
- **Antacids. Still of value in ulcer treatment (mostly for duodenal ulcers), antacids neutralize the acid, relieve pain and promote mucosal healing. Antacids come in tablet or liquid form—liquids being the most effective. They are best taken 1 to 3 hours after meals and at bedtime. Calcium carbonate (found in Tums and Rolaids) gives rapid relief but is apt to trigger "acid rebound"—a surge of acid after 2 or 3 hours. One big problem with antacids is failure to take the right amount people often self-medicate without advice and stop taking the medication as soon as the pain vanishes, rather than continuing until the ulcer heals.**
- **Gut-lining protectors or barrier shields (ulcer-coating, "cytoprotective" agents)—such as sucralfate (Sulcrate or Carafate), an aluminum salt of sucrose—do not alter stomach acid levels but coat the ulcer (crater), permitting it to heal. Taken 2 to 4 times a day and at bedtime, sucralfate has fewer side effects than H2-blockers. However, about 5 percent of those on it report nausea, constipation or a metallic taste in the month.**
- **Prostaglandin-like medications (synthetic prostaglandin with potent anti-ulcer properties) include misoprostol (Cytotec), especially valuable for people who take ASA/Aspirin or other NSAIDs that suppress natural prostaglandin production. Misoprostol decreases acid production and enhances mucosal defenses, combatting some of the damaging effects of NSAIDs. (Misoprostol is highly effective in healing Aspirin-induced ulcers.) Misoprostol may be prescribed together with NSAIDs, but side effects—diarrhea, abdominal cramps and menstrual disturbances—limit its usefulness.**

shape of the H. pylori help it to penetrate the mucous layer of the digestive tract. In many cases, the body's immune system clears up the infection. But in others the bacteria linger in the system and lead to ulcers.

The way in which H. pylori spreads is unknown, but it's probably from person to person, as no animal reservoir has been found. There is mounting evidence that spread is by fecal-oral transmission, especially in conditions of poor sanitation and among lower socioeconomic groups. Left untreated, the infection is likely lifelong, but only a small percentage (10 to 15 percent) of those infected develop ulcers. Why some people carrying these bacteria develop ulcers while others don't remains a mystery, but smoking and toxins produced by some H. pylori strains increase the risk.

Diagnosis: How to tell if you have an ulcer
The symptoms of peptic ulcer disease include stomach discomfort, abdominal pain (which tends to vanish on eating), vomiting and blood in the stool. Most peptic ulcers herald their presence by abdominal pain—sometimes described as "bad indigestion." A peptic ulcer typically produces a dull, gnawing ache or hunger pain in the pit of the stomach, particularly in the middle of the night often relieved in short order by eating, drinking or taking an antacid.

COMPLICATIONS OF UNTREATED ULCERS CAN BE SEVERE

- *A bleeding ulcer*—found in 15 to 20 percent of ulcer patients—may be undetected until it signals its presence with bloody vomit and/or black, tarry stools. Slow-bleeding ulcers may cause anemia (with dizziness and fatigue) due to internal blood loss, but ulcer bleeding stops spontaneously in 90 percent of cases. The rest may need surgery, although injection therapy and laser treatment show promise in halting ulcer bleeds.
- *A perforated ulcer*—which eats into and penetrates the stomach or duodenal wall—affects 5 to 10 percent of ulcer sufferers, more commonly men than women.
- *An obstructive ulcer*—perhaps due to gastric-scar formation—blocks the passage of food through the stomach outlet and may cause sudden nausea and vomiting, typically late in the day.

Tests for H. pylori infection include non-invasive blood and breath tests, and examination of the digestive tract with a long, flexible tube called an endoscope.

The urease breath test is done in hospital using nonradioactive C_{13} or radioactively labeled C_{14} urea swallowed by the person, and subsequent breath analysis. Detection of C_{13} or radioactive CO_2 confirms presence of the bacteria. The breath test takes about 1 hour, is accurate and specific for H. pylori, but not yet widely available.

Rapid finger-prick blood tests with special kits (such as FlexPack and Helisal) now available for use in physicians' offices are simple to do and 80 percent accurate in detecting H. pylori infection but are unable to confirm its eradication.

Endoscopy, done with a fiberoptic tube or endoscope inserted via the mouth to look inside the gastrointestinal tract, can detect the presence of an ulcer. The endoscope permits physicians to directly view the gut lining, revealing any small changes in its surface—not generally visible by X-ray. An endoscopic exam also allows a biopsy to be done, collecting small tissue samples for microscope examination by a pathologist.

If the examination reveals a duodenal ulcer, the person is generally treated with medication (antibiotics plus acid-suppressing drugs). However, if the examination indicates a gastric ulcer further tests may be suggested, as about 4 percent of gastric ulcers are cancerous.

New treatment for ulcers

In the past few years, peptic ulcer treatment has changed radically. Traditional treatment was with medications to decrease stomach acid production, but although previous acid-reducing treatment managed to control peptic ulcers, about three-quarters of those with duodenal ulcers had a relapse or repeat ulcer within a year of having one treated.

Modern treatment is with antibiotics, acid suppressors and bismuth salts to eliminate H. pylori infections. The latest method is "triple therapy" with two antibiotics plus acid suppressor for 1 week, or two antibiotics with bismuth subsalicylate for 2 weeks. After H. pylori eradication, subsequent reinfection is rare—less than 1 percent a year.

The experts stress that no single antibacterial agent alone can extinguish H. pylori infection. For successful treatment or cure, two antibiotics must be given as joint therapy. More than one antibiotic is necessary to avoid drug resistance.

In general, the specialists agree that anyone infected with H. pylori who has a diagnosed peptic ulcer should have antibiotic therapy. But those with dyspepsia (no ulcer) are not currently given antibiotics. Whether everyone infected with H. pylori should ultimately receive antibiotic treatment—rather than just people with detectable ulcers—remains a debated question. One argument about such widespread antibiotic treatment is drug resistance, an increasingly worrisome problem.

The antibiotics used to eradicate H. pylori include a choice of clarithromycin, metronidazole, tetracycline and amoxicillin, used in pairs, usually at high doses.

STROKES

A stroke typically strikes unexpectedly, out of the blue, with symptoms such as speech-slurring, unsteadiness, dimmed vision and perhaps one-sided paralysis. Strokes are not unavoidable, not restricted to the elderly and not a distinct disease but a symptom of many different disorders. The third leading killer disease in Canada, after heart attacks and cancer, stroke is also a leading cause of disability (ahead of car accidents).

The modern approach is early identification and prompt remedial steps to prevent worse trouble. Everyone should learn the warning signs of a stroke and seek medical advice if they occur, however fleeting they may seem.

A stroke damages brain cells

A stroke is a constellation of symptoms due to any of several possible disorders that disrupt blood flow to parts of the brain, cutting off its oxygen supply and impairing its function. The former medical term for stroke, "cerebrovascular accident," is now considered outdated and has been replaced by the World Health Organization definition, "a rapidly developing focal (localized) disturbance of cerebral (brain) function, lasting more than 24 hours or leading to death, with no apparent cause other than vascular." Sudden symptoms such as speech difficulties, visual loss, limb tingling and weakness are presumed to stem from a blood-supply problem unless other causes are found. In essence, a stroke arises because a blood clot or ruptured blood vessel limits blood flow to parts of the brain.

About 20 percent of the blood pumped by the heart goes to the brain, which is extremely sensitive to any disruption in its oxygen supplies. Even a few seconds of oxygen depletion can impair delicate neuron (brain cell) function. If the brain's blood (and oxygen) is cut off for 2 to 8 minutes, some brain cells will inevitably die. The ischemia, or oxygen lack, causes different disabilities according to the location and severity of the brain injury. Those parts of the body controlled by the damaged parts of the brain can no longer operate properly.

Besides the oxygen lack, a cascade of chemical reactions triggered by the oxygen starvation contributes to the death of brain cells. An excess of glutamate and other nerve transmitters, released by the oxygen-deprived tissues, accelerates cell destruction. Impairment of nerve function appears before brain tissue is irreparably damaged, and if blood flow is swiftly restored, normal function may return.

New approaches to stroke management

The modern management of stroke is more vigorous in order to reduce the brain damage as much as possible, adopting a far more urgent approach than in the past to the acute stage when stroke symptoms first appear. "It's high time," says one expert, "to abandon the former fatalistic and 'low priority' attitude toward stroke the hopelessness, the belief that nothing can be done, or that there's no rush." A stroke is a "brain attack" requiring immediate emergency action, just like a heart attack. Treating a stroke with special clot-busters within the first 3 to 6 hours of onset can dramatically reduce the amount of brain damage due to the infarct (blood clot), saving people from death or disability.

Once the attack is past the acute stage, modern stroke management aims to prevent further strokes with antiplatelet therapy (using ASA/Aspirin or other agents) to reduce platelet clumping, and anticoagulants to reduce blood clotting. New antiplatelet agents such as *ticlopidine*, *dipyridamole* and *clopidogrel* may replace or be given alongside ASA to enhance stroke prevention. In prescribing ASA, physicians must weigh its antithrombitic power (protection against clot formation) versus the extra risk of bleeding—especially in the stomach (leading to peptic ulcers). New ways to manage carotid artery blockages—with stents and angioplasty (ballooning)—are another part of modern stroke prevention.

Acute stroke is an emergency needing swift attention

As with a heart attack—when chest pain and other alerting signs send people rushing to the emergency department—symptoms of stroke should trigger equally rapid action. At the first sign of stroke, people should call an ambulance and get to a specialized stroke unit where the problem can be analyzed and swift action taken to prevent disability and death. Reaching hospital within 3 to 6 hours of developing stroke symptoms allows time for brain-saving steps that prevent the condition from worsening. Within the so-called therapeutic window or first 6 hours after symptoms appear, administration of neuroprotective agents (such as ASA) and clot-dissolving therapy can greatly reduce the brain damage.

New imaging methods (such as magnetic

resonance imaging and CT scans) quickly reveal the brain area in danger of ischemia (oxygen lack) at a stage when the amount of irreversible damage is still small. While the "core" hit by a stroke (blood clot) might be irrevocably injured in minutes, the "penumbra," or surrounding area, can be saved from the "ischemic cascade"—creeping oxygen depletion—that occurs during the next few hours. The technique of thrombolysis—infusing special clot-dissolving substances such as recombinant tissue plasminogen activator or rTPA—can speedily disintegrate or dissolve a clot. Experts stress the urgency of giving this clot-busting treatment at once, with the shortest possible delay.

Other tactics to lessen brain damage from oxygen depletion are to prevent fever (as heat harms the brain), keep the person cool, stop blood pressure from dropping too low and prevent hyperglycemia (high blood sugar).

Refinements of the technique are on the way, with new clot-busting substances, use of "drug cocktails" and better methods of drug delivery.

What are the signs and symptoms of stroke?

Stroke symptoms vary according to the causes (clots versus bleeding) and the location and severity of brain damage. They range from momentary slurring, brief visual loss and transient dizziness to complete paralysis. Since many functions, including movement, sight and sensation, are controlled by the *opposite* side of the brain, damage to the brain's left side will impair (perhaps paralyze) the body's right side and vice versa.

Specialized skills such as language, mathematical ability and space perception may be located on one or other side of the brain, so damage to the brain's left side will produce different disabilities from those of right-side injury. For example, language centers are usually situated in the brain's left hemisphere, so left-sided brain damage may abolish the ability to speak or understand speech. Right-sided brain (stroke) injury may leave speech untouched but ruin artistic or constructional capacities.

Heed the warning signs, however brief

Do not ignore the signs of stroke, however transient or seemingly insignificant, and even though the symptoms vanish completely. Symptoms may last only 10 to 15 minutes, but heeding even brief warning signals and obtaining swift medical advice can prevent more devastating future consequences.

Transient ischemic attacks may be a warning

Transient ischemic attacks, or TIAs—popularly called incomplete, "mini" or "threatened" strokes—precede about 30 percent of all strokes. They involve a sudden, temporary loss of brain function, lasting less than 24 hours and leaving no residual ill effects. People who survive TIAs have a 10 to 20 percent higher-than-average risk of a repeat and worse attack within the next 2 years. Any unexplained fainting of an older person should be investigated as a possible TIA.

RISK FACTORS FOR STROKE

- *Increasing age*—stroke risks double for each decade after age 55. The incidence of stroke at ages 55 to 64 years is about 150 per 100,000 population per year, compared to 600 per 100,000 population per year in those over 80.
- *Male gender*—men are 30 percent more likely than women to suffer strokes, especially before age 65.
- *Race*—blacks are twice as likely as whites to suffer strokes, perhaps because they're more prone to high blood pressure.
- *Family* history—stroke is not inherited, but risk factors such as atherosclerosis and hypertension run in families.
- *Smoking*—an avoidable risk factor.
- *Hypertension* (high blood pressure)—one of the main modifiable risk factors. Studies confirm that the higher the blood pressure is, the greater the chance of stroke.
- *Diabetes mellitus*—diabetics have stroke risks 2 to 3 times above average. Controlling diabetes can diminish the risk.
- *Certain drugs*—such as crack/cocaine and amphetamines ("speed")—can induce hemorrhagic strokes.
- *Cardioembolic heart problems*—blood clots originating in the heart—trigger 15 to 25 percent of strokes. One particular heart disorder, *atrial fibrillation* (AF)—a "quivering" upper heart chamber that produces an irregular heartbeat, which affects about 5 percent of those over 60—greatly increases stroke risks. The Framingham Heart Study found a sixfold rise in strokes among those with AF compared to others. AF may arise from rheumatic heart-valve (e.g., mitral valve) flaws, coronary-artery disease, an enlarged heart, thyroid disorders and some lung diseases.

Those with TIAs due to severe carotid (neck) artery obstruction may consider surgery to prevent a subsequent stroke. Those at suspected risk due to blood clots can start on anti–platelet-clumping drugs such as ASA or the newer ticlopidine (Ticlid). People with cardiogenic (from the heart) stroke symptoms may be put on anticoagulants such as warfarin (Coumadin).

Sadly, the TIA danger signs can be so brief and faint that they are ignored. Yet those who experience TIAs have the good fortune to be warned; they have time to take preventive action and avoid lasting disability. Take the case of a 40-year-old advertising manager who, in the middle of a planning session, suddenly felt her right arm go inexplicably numb, her vision dim, her words—usually so crisp and clear—come out jumbled. Within half an hour the symptoms vanished, and she thought no more of them until the weekend, when she gave the perplexing episode a passing mention to her skiing companion. He advised her to tell her physician, and at her next checkup she was promptly sent for a full investigation. Her heart was thoroughly checked, the carotid artery in her neck was examined by ultrasound, a CT (brain) X-ray scan was ordered, a battery of blood tests was done for her "clotting index" (platelet count, blood-fat profile) and her thyroid function was tested. A mild heart-valve condition seemed to have caused the fleeting symptoms and she was put on ASA therapy to avoid a possible future stroke.

Diagnosing the cause is essential

A stroke always originates from a vascular (blood supply) disorder. Conditions that mimic stroke and are commonly misdiagnosed as stroke include Bell's palsy (transient facial paralysis due to an inflamed nerve), seizures, psychiatric disorders (such as hysteria) and confusion due to previous strokes.

Where a true stroke is involved, modern practice tends to classify it not only by cause and location but also by why it arose. It's essential not to accept a stroke as an unavoidable happening from which to recover as well as possible, but to discover why and how it occurred, track down the causes and prevent any future, possibly worse, episode. *Prevention is the essence of today's therapy.*

Tests may include CAT scans (special brain X-rays), magnetic resonance imaging (MRI), carotid-artery soundings, echocardiograms (to visualize the heart's chambers), a spinal puncture to detect blood in the cerebrospinal fluid (from a brain bleed) and other investigations. The tests check for cardiac causes—for instance, a faulty heart valve or a heartbeat irregularity—and for atherosclerotic narrowing

WARNING SIGNS OF STROKE

- **Sudden weakness, numbness or paralysis in face or limbs;**
- **sudden vision blurring or double vision, especially in one eye;**
- **an unbearably severe headache (out of the blue);**
- **difficulty talking or understanding speech;**
- **sudden loss of balance, dizziness;**
- **difficulty swallowing.**

STROKES ARISE FROM CEREBRAL BLOOD FLOW PROBLEMS

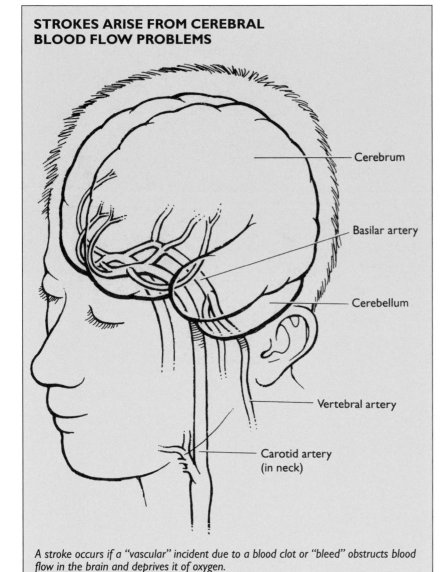

- Cerebrum
- Basilar artery
- Cerebellum
- Vertebral artery
- Carotid artery (in neck)

A stroke occurs if a "vascular" incident due to a blood clot or "bleed" obstructs blood flow in the brain and deprives it of oxygen.

THE MAIN WARNING SIGNS OF STROKE

- Sudden weakness or numbness, or even paralysis, on one side of the body (face, arm and/or leg);
- sudden speech loss, trouble speaking or difficulty in understanding spoken words or reading. The person may simply slur words, be unable to find the "right" word, experience a weakness in the jaw or a lack of tongue coordination;
- sudden blurring or partial visual loss, sometimes in one eye only;
- severe, unusual headache (the "worst ever experienced"), often accompanied by nausea and drowsiness;
- dizziness or vertigo ("room spinning");
- sudden falls, unsteadiness, clumsy movements;
- unexplained unconsciousness or falls (drop attacks);
- gait unsteadiness, imbalance;
- tingling on one side, one arm, one leg;
- difficulty swallowing;
- diminution in touch and feeling.

of the neck arteries that supply blood to the brain. Physicians listen for a special sound or "bruit" in the neck to show whether or how badly the carotid arteries are obstructed.

Hemorrhages (bleeds) into the brain may arise because of:

- the bursting of a small, deep brain artery due to longstanding hypertension (high blood pressure), accounting for 10 percent of strokes;
- a subarachnoid hemorrhage or ruptured aneurysm (outpouching) that spills blood into the space between the brain and skull. An aneurysm is a tiny sac or ballooning of a cerebral artery, more common in women than men. It may form because of a congenital (inherited) blood-vessel weakness, or due to head blows, atherosclerosis or inflammation. Responsible for 10 percent of all strokes, aneurysms account for half of all fatal strokes in people under age 45. An aneurysm rarely announces its presence until the bubble "bursts" and produces severe symptoms. Rupture can occur during sleep or if blood pressure suddenly increases (for instance during physical exertion, emotional stress, arguments, sex). If an aneurysm ruptures (not all do), blood rushes out at enormous pressure and can cause an excruciating headache ("as if hit on the back of the head"), nausea, vomiting, hallucinations, photophobia (light aversion), a stiff neck and perhaps confusion, lethargy and unconsciousness.

Serious consequences may be headed off by rapid diagnosis and treatment to stop the bleed. Neurosurgeons stress the importance of so-called warning leaks experienced by many people with aneurysms—producing symptoms such as double vision, a searing headache, pain at the base of the neck—in the days, weeks or months before a devastating attack. Treating the warning leak may avoid a full cerebral bleed—but the early signs are often confused with migraine, flu or sinus headaches.

Infarcts (clots that block blood flow) may arise because of:

- *atherosclerosis*—where arteries are narrowed by fatty deposits. Blood clots form easily in arteries scarred by atherosclerosis. Pieces of plaque may travel from wider to narrower brain blood vessels and obstruct blood flow Blockages in small cerebral vessels account for 20 percent of strokes due to infarcts;

- *a narrowing or blockage* in one or more of the four large blood vessels supplying blood to the brain—the *carotids* in front of the neck and the *vertebral* arteries at the back—blamed for 20 to 25 percent of infarct-caused strokes;
- *cardiogenic embolisms*—breakaway clots from the heart—which account for another 25 percent of clot-caused strokes. A heart attack can trigger a stroke if a freshly damaged heart wall doesn't pump properly and forms a *mural thrombosis* (wall clot) that travels to the brain. Clots formed in malfunctioning heart valves may also break away and reach the brain; artificial replacement heart valves are especially prone to form clots;
- *atrial fibrillation*—(a heart flutter) described above;
- *blood coagulation problems* and rare blood disorders;
- *unknown causes.*

Surgery can unclog blocked carotid arteries

The operation known as *carotid endarterectomy*, which removes plaque from carotid (neck) arteries, has proved highly successful for preventing stroke in those with badly clogged carotid arteries. The American National Institutes of Health issued a 1991 medical alert suggesting that carotid endarterectomy be "considered standard treatment in those with severely blocked carotid arteries."

The presence of carotid-artery obstruction is suspected when a "bruit" or whooshing sound is heard in the neck. But surgery is advised only after extensive tests by ultrasound and angiography (X-rays after dye injection) confirm at least a 70 percent carotid narrowing. The surgery entails opening up the artery in the neck (under general anesthetic), scraping out the diseased portion, then sewing the artery up again: a piece of leg vein is sometimes inserted to patch the artery. Researchers stress that, although low, the surgical risks are not negligible: about 2 percent are disabled or suffer a stroke

during or soon after carotid surgery. Thus it's wise to seek out a specialized center for the procedure.

For those with mildly (less than 30 percent) obstructed carotid arteries, surgery doesn't help. Patients who haven't had a TIA but have a carotid bruit are generally advised to take ASA (such as Aspirin) and "watch and wait."

The stroke-prevention message

It's estimated that half of all strokes could be avoided by correct preventive measures. Those who smoke should quit, those with high blood pressure can try to get it down. People who experience TIAs or minor strokes should be thoroughly examined to track down any underlying disorders that increase stroke risks. They may be advised to adopt a preventive program, which can avoid serious disability or death. Rapid, appropriate treatment promises good stroke recovery, particularly in younger people (under age 60 to 65)—and more crucially can prevent subsequent and worse attacks.

Preventive steps:

- Have blood pressure regularly measured and, if it's high, try to lower it.
- Check for and correct cardiac disorders such as heartbeat irregularities, mitral-valve and other heart abnormalities.
- Women (especially those with migraine headaches) who take contraceptive pills and also smoke may be at increased risk of stroke and should try to reduce the danger (e.g., stop smoking).
- Heed mild signs of stroke and get immediate medical advice.

Can an "Aspirin a day" keep strokes away?

Even after 100 years of use, we do not know exactly how acetylsalicylic acid or ASA (such as Aspirin) works. Nevertheless, the results of a U.S. Physicians' Health Study released in 1989 showed that regular ASA use almost halved the incidence of stroke and heart attacks, especially in men (allegedly less so in women). While ASA diminishes platelet stickiness, clumping and clot formation, not all medical trials show that it can prevent strokes.

Nonetheless, many clinicians now prescribe

enteric-coated brands of Aspirin as standard therapy after a TIA or mini-stroke—in doses of about 650 mg per day. Recent research suggests that "baby Aspirins" (75–81 mg daily) are just as effective in preventing clot formation, with less stomach irritation.

How ASA reduces stroke risks isn't fully understood. One theory is that it blocks the release of thromboxane-A2—a substance that promotes blood clotting. While the best dose for stroke prevention isn't conclusively known, it's important to remember that ASA is a powerful drug that should only be taken under medical supervision. In the Physicians' Health Study, Aspirin-takers were 33 percent more likely than average to suffer nosebleeds, bruising, vomited blood, bleeding ulcers, oozing from cuts and other anticoagulant effects.

Disabilities from stroke

The degree of recovery from stroke varies greatly: some people make a good recovery with little or no lasting impairment, others suffer minor but permanent handicaps and yet others are left virtually helpless. Although rehabilitation from stroke may take a long time (up to a year or more) full function may ultimately return.

The treatment and rehabilitation of stroke sufferers depends on the severity of the stroke and its effects. Nondamaged areas of the brain may continue to function efficiently, so that many intellectual and physical tasks can be carried on as before, making the person appear as capable as ever. However, even minor brain injury may make it hard to perform other seemingly comparable tasks. Damage to either side of the brain tends to affect the *opposite* side of the body, with severity ranging from weakness and/or clumsiness to complete paralysis.

Damage to the brain's left side often produces aphasia (language loss), one of the most devastating consequences. Different aspects of language—reading, writing, naming objects, word meaning, the ability to repeat words—can be affected. Aphasics may "get stuck" and repeat the same word (maybe a swear word) over and over or use nonsense words and bizarre phrases to express desires. Caregivers must learn to respond to the new modes of communication and use simple, clear language in a normal tone of voice. Treating stroke sufferers as though they don't understand is a mistake.

Damage to the brain's right hemisphere may undermine the ability to convey emotions and to judge distance, space and time. People with right-sided cerebral damage may also have trouble finding their way, knock into things or be unable to button up their clothes or recognize familiar faces and places. (In most left-handers and some right-handers, language function is situated in the brain's *right* hemisphere, so aphasia may also follow right-sided brain injury.)

Articulation and swallowing abnormalities are common in stroke sufferers, whichever side of the brain is injured. Strokes that affect nerve fibers controlling movement of the face, lips, mouth, throat and tongue can make speech sound different and hard to understand (dysarthria).

Hearing is rarely affected by a stroke, but if there was a prior hearing problem, the stroke may further diminish hearing ability as well as comprehension. Hearing aids can help.

Visual pathways may be affected and cause double vision or the sensation that objects are oscillating. With right-sided brain injury, left-sided vision may be impaired, and vice versa. Some stroke sufferers miss certain parts of the visual field; most learn to compensate for these cuts by turning their heads, but some cannot make the adjustment. Such "neglect" can involve signals from all senses on one side, so the person may not recognize his or her own arm or leg as a part of the body. Neglect on one side may make someone divide things at the midline (viewing only half the field): for example, eating from one side of the plate and leaving the rest, unless the plate is then turned around. Sufferers may ignore those who speak to them from the impaired side and the speaker's appearance on the "good" side may elicit surprise—as if he or she had just arrived. Or they may become confused when traveling; if wheeled down and back an unfamiliar corridor, they may see one side going the other coming back, as if there were two separate corridors.

While intellectual abilities often remain untouched or return within a few months, there may be startling alterations in behavior. The previously garrulous person may become uncom-

LEFT-BRAINED STROKES AND THEIR MANAGEMENT

Left-brain injury may produce:
- right-sided paralysis or weakness;
- slow, cautious manner and hesitant, anxious approach (perhaps in sharp contrast to former confident style);
- dysarthria—difficulty in clearly articulating words;
- swallowing problems;
- disorganized way of doing familiar actions;
- aphasia—language, reading and writing difficulties. Some people with left-brain damage may be unable to speak but still understand more than is apparent; others are better at saying things than understanding them. In a society so dependent on verbal communication, the inability to speak seems catastrophic. But just because people can't communicate verbally does not mean that they can't communicate at all. A lot of day-to-day communication can be carried on without speech—with hand gestures, body language, music, writing on a board, drawing pictures or using computers.

Tips for dealing with left-brain strokes
- Never underestimate the ability to communicate, even if normal language modes cannot be used.
- Try other forms of communication—such as pantomime, drawing, demonstration and writing. Computers and "communication" boards can improve interaction. Use whatever works best for the individual situation.
- Don't over- or underestimate residual speech comprehension.
- Don't overload the person with too many words—use simple, brief statements.
- Don't shout—keep messages simple and short. (But watch for possible hearing problems.)
- Don't be patronizing or use "special" voices.
- Divide tasks into simple steps.
- Give plenty of feedback for tasks well done and applaud/reward progress.

RIGHT-BRAINED STROKES AND THEIR MANAGEMENT

Injury to the brain's right side may produce:
- difficulty with dressing, spatial tasks (throwing, catching, tooth-brushing), inability to judge distance, space, position, rate of movement;
- perceptual deficits (poor understanding of what's seen);
- quick, impulsive behavior (perhaps in sharp contrast to former deliberate manner);
- memory flaws, problems in remembering dates, appointments, difficulty learning new tasks, impaired performance of music, math, many motor skills;
- problems in positioning hands, feet (e.g., misses buttons, applies lipstick crookedly);
- frequent stumbling, inability to steer wheelchair through door;
- inability to tell whether leaning or standing upright;
- unsafe driving or crossing of streets;
- poor judgment about own actions; a sufferer may wildly overestimate remaining capacities, ignore defects, display overconfidence;
- understanding of oral commands but not visual cues;
- a need for feedback for success in relearning tasks—encouragement to "go slow," "take your time," "try again."

Tips for dealing with right-brain strokes
- Anticipate poor spatial judgment, impulsiveness, clumsiness, over-rapid movements.
- Put good lighting in rooms, halls, stairwells.
- Don't overestimate abilities. Spatial-perceptual deficits are easy to miss.
- Use spoken cues if visual demonstrations seem hard to grasp.
- Break tasks into small steps and give much positive feedback.
- Make sure that tasks are done safely rather than taking safety for granted.
- Minimize clutter and remove obstacles to trip over.
- Avoid over-rapid movements.

For more information, contact the Heart and Stroke Foundation; social workers from any large rehabilitation center or hospital rehabilitation department; speech-recovery clinics—e.g., the Ontario Speech Centre.

municative, the meticulous become sloppy, the energetic become lazy or the lazy become hyperactive. Right-sided strokes may make people impulsive, while left-sided brain injury often leaves people passive. These behavior changes make enormous demands on caregivers.

It can take weeks or longer just to assess the full impact of a stroke. Although destroyed brain tissue cannot regenerate itself, other parts of the brain may develop new connecting pathways and take over the functions of damaged areas. Post-stroke management strategies must

USUALLY STARTS IN CHILDHOOD

Stuttering generally begins between the ages of 2 and 7 years, peaking at age 3 to 4. It tends to come on gradually, although it can happen suddenly. Most children stutter occasionally as they master the art of speaking; many repeat words and use a lot of "ers" as they talk, or they hurry along, tripping over words. While most children who stutter before the age of 6 outgrow the habit, some continue with the speech hesitations, and for them prompt speech-language therapy can help to avoid a permanent speech problem.

be individually tailored by rehabilitation experts for maximum results.

Rehabilitation is a multidisciplinary process

Therapy for stroke involves the joint help of physicians, occupational, physical and speech therapists, nurses, psychologists, social workers and other experts to help stroke victims adapt to their handicaps. The patient and caregivers must be "active" members of the rehab team and participate in the recovery process, not just accept advice. With good rehabilitation methods and time, many can return to near-normal activities.

STUTTERING

Whatever its elusive causes, stuttering—which interrupts the normal flow of speech with involuntary repetitions and hesitations—is a universal problem with historic roots. Renowned stutterers date back to biblical times and include Moses, Sir Isaac Newton, Charles Darwin, Winston Churchill and Marilyn Monroe. Stuttering—or stammering, as it's sometimes called—spans the whole range of personality types and professions. It has nothing to do with character intelligence or talent.

Roughly 4 percent of children and 1 percent of Canadian adults stutter to some extent, about 4 times more males than females, and more left-handers than right-handers. Stuttering is the subject of many a joke; to those afflicted, it's no laughing matter but a source of immense tension and misery. Luckily, early professional attention to a childhood stutter can often head off this speech problem.

A problem of "dysfluency"

In modern terms, stuttering is regarded as an interpersonal communication problem in which dysfluency interrupts the natural flow of spoken communication. The disorder involves physical, psychological and central nervous system (brain) components. Stutterers prolong sounds and syllables—usually the first syllable of a word, particularly those beginning with consonants—perhaps accompanied by signs of a struggle, tension and facial contortions as people try desperately to "get the words out."

Mysteriously, most (even severe) stutterers speak quite fluently when whispering (which doesn't tax the vocal system), and when singing or speaking in unison. Many also speak without trouble when talking to themselves, to pets, to young children or to certain individuals. Some can read aloud fluently but not converse; some can give public lectures but stutter badly in private conversation. Others can talk fluently one to one but stutter when speaking in public. Stuttering tends to be episodic, coming and going unpredictably, with days or weeks going by with little or no difficulty speaking, followed by a reappearance or worsening of the stutter. Improving the person's self-confidence often relieves the stutter.

How to tell if your child has a real stutter

It is not easy to pick out an incipient stutterer from a normal child who's just learning to speak, especially as some stutterers become astonishingly adept at hiding their stutter with avoidance tactics. Stuttering children are often unaware of doing anything different at first—simply concentrating on *communicating*, never mind the odd sound prolongation. But once a child realizes there's something "funny" about the way he or she speaks, the hesitancies increase along with a fear of using difficult words. Children (and stuttering adults) go to extraordinary lengths to avoid using certain words.

Neurological (brain) differences may cause stuttering

Despite numerous theories, the reason that people stutter defies explanation. Parents should not blame themselves for a child's stutter; while parental attitudes, stress, anxiety and

SOME TELLTALE CLUES AND ALERTING SIGNS

- Frequent hesitations and unusual trouble getting words out;
- many sound repetitions, especially on the initial word or phrase—worse with words that start with a consonant (m-m-m-mummy,

d-d-d-dog);
- prolonging sounds for more than a second (s-s-s-s soup);
- breathlessness in mid-sentence;
- galloping speech, or overuse of "filler" words—"you know" or "um";

- beginning then stopping and restarting sentences with gaps or silences between;
- signs of anxiety or fear when trying to speak;
- self-consciousness, shying away from talking.

TIPS FOR DEALING WITH A STUTTERER

- *Try to create a relaxed, accepting atmosphere that encourages talking—stuttering is usually worse under stress.*
- *Do not make stuttering a taboo topic. If the child is aware of the speech defect and obviously struggling, it's best to communicate concern and understanding, without exaggerating its importance. A simple comment such as "It's hard for you, isn't it?" can help.*
- *Replace the word "stuttering" with terms like "hesita-*tion" or "difficulty." If the child calls it stuttering, then don't avoid the word (which would seem phony).*
- *Try not to show worry, embarrassment, rejection or disapproval—but do not pamper! Expect usual responsibilities and rear like siblings.*
- *Encourage talking; spontaneous conversation and expression of feelings, both verbal and nonverbal—wait silently for speech to continue.*
- *Look directly at the stutterer while talking* and show by your expression that you are interested in what is said, not how it's said or how long it takes.*
- *Never jump in and speak for a stutterer.*
- *Do everything possible to be a good listener.*
- *Feed back or repeat the message to show attentiveness.*
- *Praise fluency and all episodes of trouble-free speech.*
- *Expect ups and downs.*
- *Try not to show impatience or annoyance—which might trigger attempts at faster speech.*
- *Set a good example by speaking calmly and slowly, in an unhurried manner—use short sentences and easy words.*
- *Never suggest the stutterer stop and start again.*
- *When a stutter seems especially frustrating, point out that everyone has occasional fluency problems. Do not press for conversation on a bad day.*
- *Try to stop any teasing. Intervene (out of the child's sight and hearing); if siblings and friends have an* accepting attitude, others tend to respond similarly.*
- *Do everything possible to make speaking fun. Organize games that involve rhymes and speaking in unison (easier for stutterers).*
- *Emphasize that people who stutter are no different from others, except for trouble with words.*
- *Explain that the dysfunction results from factors over which the person has little or no control.*

psychological factors influence its severity, they do not cause stuttering.

The latest theory is that although stuttering involves the speech muscles and vocal tract, its underlying cause is neurological. Stutterers tend to use the right side of the brain rather than the left (more usual) side to process language. The new PET scan (Positron Emission Tomography) X-ray technique shows that people who stutter employ mainly the brain's right side when speaking. "It's possible," says one expert at Toronto's Clarke Institute of Psychiatry, "that stutterers are born with a predisposition to process speech on the brain's right side, which is less efficient than the left for this function." (A fair proportion of stutterers are also left-handed.)

How parents can help improve a child's fluency

Although they're in no way to blame for causing the stutter, parents, siblings, teachers and the home atmosphere can greatly influence its severity. The first step is to seek professional help and find ways to create a "fluency-promoting" atmosphere. While some physicians and pediatricians might advise parents to forget it, as it will disappear on its own, a stutter is rarely outgrown after age 8. Speech and language specialists advise parents to err on the side of caution, and get therapy for a suspected stutter.

Parents must also face their own feelings about a stuttering child—sadness, anger annoyance, guilt or hoping it will go away. Some parents and teachers try to correct a stutter by

FLUENCY-ENHANCING THERAPY MAY HELP

Fluency programs teach stutterers some steps and rules to reconstruct phonation (voice production), breathing and articulation. "Since there's nothing organically amiss with the voice-producing apparatus, and as it only goes wrong sporadically," explains one speech pathologist, "stutterers can and often do talk normally." One fluency-shaping program at Toronto's Clarke Institute of Psychiatry is an intense 3-week course in which stutterers are immersed in full-day sessions, with homework, first in a clinical setting, then practising in the outside world under supervision.

Overall, 90 percent find their fluency improved and follow-up sessions help consolidate the gains. But to retain fluency, stutterers must stick to the rules. Unfortunately, 25 to 30 percent lose the speaking skills learned, usually because of insufficient practice. However, participants are taught to expect and overcome relapses, and refresher courses help maintain communication skills.

telling the child to slow down, but this is asking the impossible, as the speech pattern is beyond control. The best way to slow down speech—reduce the stumbling over words—is for parents to model a relaxed, unhurried speaking manner themselves.

The home atmosphere should foster open communication, with non-pressured attention to a stuttering child. "Make the child feel comfortable," advises one speech therapist, "stimulate lots of talk, read stories aloud, encourage the child to speak, even if it takes time—praise all bouts of fluency." If stuttering is treated as a taboo topic—ignored or never discussed—the child may feel it's something bad. Open acknowledgment of the problem is best, with reassurance that what's said is more important than how it is said.

For more information, contact the Canadian Association for People Who Stutter (CAPS), tel.: (888) 788–8837; local speech-language or speech pathology units at hospitals or universities; the Ontario Association of Speech-Language Pathologists and Audiologists, tel.: (416) 920–3676; the National Stuttering Project in San Francisco, tel.: (800) 364–1677.

THYROID DISORDERS

The thyroid gland can produce health problems through changes within its own tissues or changes in its hormone output. Severe thyroid disease can cause dramatic symptoms, but milder more subtle thyroid problems may take years to develop. However, once thyroid disease is accurately diagnosed, treatment is generally simple and effective.

The thyroid gland is part of the body's endocrine system, which encompasses the lymph glands, which fight infection, and the endocrine glands, which make and release hormones—biochemical messengers that target specific organs and tissues.

What the thyroid does

A well-functioning thyroid is essential to normal growth and development. The gland stores and secretes two hormones—thyroxine (T4), and triiodothyronine (T3)—both of which circulate in the bloodstream and act on specific target cells or organs. T3 and T4 hormones are vital cell accelerators that speed up the metabolism. In order for the body to maintain a healthy metabolic rate, the thyroid must release the correct amount of hormones into the blood. Its balance is constantly adjusted by a feedback process similar to the thermostatic control of room temperature.

The rate at which the thyroid gland produces T3 and T4 hormones is regulated by yet another hormone—thyrotropin, or thyroid-stimulating hormone (TSH)—secreted by the *pituitary gland* in the floor of the brain. And TSH production is controlled by yet another hormone, thyrotropin-releasing-hormone (TRH), from the *hypothalamus*, within the brain.

Once a certain level of thyroxine in the blood is reached, TSH and TRH production drop, shutting off thyroid-hormone release, achieving just the right balance for the body's needs.

Too much or too little thyroid hormone can cause health problems. If the thyroid gland is low in hormone output, cellular processes slow down; "hypothyroidism" can reduce the basal metabolic rate—the body's rate of oxygen use and energy production—by as much as 40 percent. If, on the other hand, thyroid hormones are produced in excess, the basal metabolic rate may rise 60- to 100-fold, leading to "hyperthyroidism"—the target cells and tissues working too hard. For unknown reasons, thyroid dysfunction affects more women than men.

Hyperthyroidism—too much thyroid hormone

Hyperthyroidism, due to an excess of T4 hormone or thyroxine, affects mainly women aged 20 to 45, with an estimated incidence of 2 per 1,000 men and 19 per 1,000 women. Thyroxine increases the rate at which fats and carbohydrates are used by the body's cells, also increasing rates of protein synthesis. Someone with T4 overproduction may have an accelerated metabolic rate and lose weight despite a normal or large food intake, may also have an increased respiration rate and is apt to pant or perspire with the least exertion.

Thyroxine also stimulates cardiovascular activity, so people with overactive thyroid glands may have an increased heart rate and experience palpitations. Robert Graves, the

TREATMENT OF HYPERTHYROIDISM

- *Antithyroid drugs*, such as *propylthiouracil* and *methimazole*;
- *radioactive iodine*;
- *surgical removal* of part of the thyroid gland.

The most usual treatment is with antithyroid drugs to block the formation of thyroid hormones. These drugs are relatively safe and effective, although it may take several weeks before thyroid hormone levels revert to normal, as some hormone lingers in tissue stores. Methimazole is fairly cheap, administered only once a day and tastes better than propylthiouracil. (Propylthiouracil may be preferable for pregnant and lactating women.) Those who require antithyroid medication usually stay on it for about a year. About 20 percent go into permanent remission with drug therapy alone, requiring no further treatment. Those with mild hyperthyroidism and small goiters usually go into remission with drug therapy. (The antithyroid medication somehow tips the person's immune system back toward normal.) The remainder may suffer relapses once antithyroid medication is stopped. Adverse effects are rare, but about 1 to 5 percent of people on these drugs develop allergic reactions, and one serious side effect is a decreased white-blood-cell count, perhaps signaled by a severe sore throat. If this happens, the thyroid sufferer may need to stop the drug for a while.

Beta-blockers such as propranolol may also be used to manage accompanying heart palpitations and cardiac irritability. Although beta-blockers don't affect thyroid hormone levels to a significant extent, they calm people awaiting the benefits of drug therapy.

Radioactive iodine therapy has been used since the mid-1940s for those who don't respond to drugs. The iodine is absorbed almost entirely by the thyroid gland, without harming other body tissues. It is administered after drugs have rendered the patient euthyroid (back to normal hormone outputs). Some studies suggest—but don't prove—that radioiodine may worsen eye disorders linked to hyperthyroidism unless antithyroid drugs are used first.

Radioiodine therapy means taking a tiny amount (about a millionth of a milligram) of radioactive iodine as a liquid or capsule. Over the years, this therapy has proven safe and effective; it alleviates Graves' disease in 90 percent of cases, and despite earlier fears, it does not produce birth defects or cancer. Its main drawback is that, as the years go by, the likelihood of *hypothyroidism* (lack of thyroid hormone) increases by about 3 percent per year to almost 100 percent in 10 years. Thus hyperthyroid patients treated with radioactive iodine may ultimately also require hormone replacement therapy.

Thyroid surgery—subtotal *thyroidectomy*, or partial removal of the thyroid gland—is not often done anymore, although it still has a place for those with very large, cosmetically unattractive goiters, in whom the amount of radioactive iodine needed to reduce the swelling would be dangerously high, or for those who prefer surgery to taking radioactive substances. Hypothyroidism following surgery is a risk, but less so than with radioactive iodine therapy.

19th-century Irish physician who originally described hyperthyroidism, was struck by its cardiac manifestations: "I could distinctly hear the heart beating when my ear was distant at least four feet from the chest," he said. In addition, an excess of thyroxine can affect the central nervous system, making people anxious, jumpy, irritable and generally "hyper." Those with thyroid overproduction often sleep badly. In extreme cases, hyperthyroidism can result in mental illness and psychosis.

Graves' disease

Graves' disease is now regarded as an autoimmune disorder in which the body produces an antibody that attacks its own thyroid cells, tricking the thyroid gland into producing excess T3 and T4 hormones. Since the antibody is not subject to the normal feedback mechanisms that inhibit excess thyroid activity, even if the level of thyroid hormone in the bloodstream rises dramatically, T3 and T4 thyroid hormones continue to be overproduced. In Graves' disease, the thyroid gland can secrete as much as 15 times above-normal amounts of T4 hormone.

Although not invariably present, a goiter or painless thyroid enlargement—a lump in the lower front of the throat—is a classic sign of the disease. Graves' disease may also be associated with bulging eyes, retraction of the eyelids and a

THE THYROID GLAND NEEDS IODINE

In order to form thyroxine (T4 hormone), the thyroid gland must obtain at least a trace of iodine—about 1 mg a week. Iodine deficiency during early childhood development can lead to goiter and possible mental retardation. Good natural sources of iodine are fish and other seafood, but some inland areas are low in iodine. Iodine-poor areas in North America include the Great Lakes region from the Appalachians to Washington—formerly called the "goiter belt"—where thyroid-deficiency problems used to be widespread.

To offset the possibility of iodine-deficiency, ordinary table salt is now iodized in North America. However, many developing countries don't iodize their salt, and international agencies still list iodine deficiency as one of the world's most pressing health problems. Millions in China, India, Africa, Latin America and other countries are at risk of thyroid disorders through iodine lack.

staring "pop-eyed" look known as exophthalmos. The eye complications in Graves' disease can be severe, with thickened eye muscles producing double vision. If the optic nerve is compressed, blindness may follow. Whether Graves' disease and exophthalmos are both manifestations of the same underlying autoimmune disease, or whether they are closely related but different disorders, remains debatable. Mild eye problems are dealt with symptomatically, using lubricating eyedrops, or eye patches at night, or raising the head of the bed to prevent fluid accumulation. Severe cases require corticosteroids or immunosuppressants to reduce inflammation. Very severe cases may require eye surgery.

Tests for hyperthyroidism

A suspicion of thyroid dysfunction is followed up by tests to measure thyroid-hormone levels in the blood. Thyroid function may also be assessed by a radioactive iodine scan, a test used to determine the underlying cause(s) of hyperthyroidism and look for possible triggers other than Graves' disease.

"Thyroid storm"—a rare occurrence

Very occasionally, exacerbation of a preexisting thyroid problem gives rise to a "thyroid storm." A sudden excess of thyroid hormones leads to burning fever, racing heart, severe sweating and restlessness—a medical emergency. Thyroid storm can result in dehydration, shock and death. It sometimes arises in those with an untreated hyperthyroid problem, or after sudden withdrawal of an antithyroid drug, infection, surgery or trauma (damage) to the thyroid. A thyroid storm is generally treated with propylthiouracil, sodium iodide, propranolol and steroid drugs to halt the hormone overproduction.

Hypothyroidism

In contrast to the restless energy of people with excess thyroid activity, those with a low thyroxine output are generally slow, sluggish and perpetually fatigued. An estimated 0.5 percent of adults—mainly women—have hypothyroidism, its prevalence increasing to about 10 percent among the elderly. Full-blown hypothyroidism, known as myxedema is characterized by laziness, apathy, sleepiness and a bloated, puffy face. People with hypothyroidism tend to gain weight, are constipated, have noticeably slow speech, can't stand the cold and may develop coarse dry skin, a hoarse voice and a goiter (neck swelling). Milder cases, perhaps

DIFFERENT FORMS OF HYPERTHYROIDISM

- *Graves' disease*, the most common example of hyperthyroidism, especially in those under age 40.
- *Toxic multinodular goiter*—an enlarged, benign thyroid with hyperthyroidism, most common in people over age 50.
- *Pituitary or hypothalamic tumors*, which increase thyroid hormone production (rare).
- *Hyperthyroidism due to certain drugs* such as amiodarone (an antiarrhythmic heart drug containing iodine).
- *Transient hyperthyroidism due to thyroiditis* (see below)—possibly accompanied by the release of stored thyroid hormone.

SYMPTOMS OF GRAVES' DISEASE (THYROXINE OVERPRODUCTION)

- Sweating;
- palpitations, racing heart;
- heat intolerance;
- fine tremor of outstretched hand;
- diarrhea, weight loss (despite good nutrition);
- extreme nervousness, irritability; if severe, the hyperthyroidism (rarely) causes mental illness and psychosis.
- *In children*—retarded sexual maturation. During pregnancy, Graves' disease tends to remit spontaneously—a result of the auto-immune suppression that often occurs in pregnancy so that a woman's body won't reject the fetus as "foreign." However, Graves' disease tends to recur following the birth.

THYROIDITIS

Thyroiditis is a term for inflammation of the thyroid gland, with consequent depletion of thyroid hormone. Infections or the formation of specific autoimmune antibodies can cause thyroiditis. Some types of thyroiditis involve both hyperthyroid (overactive) and hypothyroid (underactive) phases.

- *Hashimoto's thyroiditis*, an autoimmune condition that runs in families, affects 3 to 4 percent of the population. Treatment is with thyroxine. In fact, many patients and their physicians are highly relieved when a diagnosis of hypothyroidism is confirmed, since treatment is both easy and harmless.

- *Painful thyroiditis* is due to infective organisms that destroy thyroid tissue. Infectious thyroiditis usually causes an enlarged, tender thyroid, severe neck and ear pain and a high fever. Bacterial forms are called acute or bacterial thyroiditis, viral forms subacute thyroiditis or de Quervain's disease. Antibiotics are used to treat the bacterial forms.
  Viral thyroiditis occurs in sporadic epidemics, often preceded by upper-respiratory-tract infections, and possibly followed by hypothyroidism due to destruction of thyroid tissue. Treatment is with analgesics (such as ASA or acetaminophen), plus corticosteroids to reduce inflammation. Thyroid function almost always returns to normal after a few months.

- *Postpartum thyroiditis*—after pregnancy and childbirth—is more common than once imagined. Postpartum thyroiditis seems to occur if the stress of pregnancy uncovers a latent but transient autoimmune abnormality, most episodes resolving spontaneously. It affects 2 to 5 percent of pregnant women. Painless postpartum thyroiditis usually appears as a brief period of hyperthyroidism, followed by hypothyroidism. The condition may appear 2 to 4 months after delivery—with mothers feeling tired, anxious and irritable, experiencing palpitations and sweating. The hyperthyroidism phase may last for four months or so, followed by hypothyroid lethargy, fatigue, weight gain, depression and cold-intolerance. While the disorder usually resolves itself within months, a small goiter may remain. Women who have one bout of pregnancy thyroid trouble usually have repeat bouts after subsequent pregnancies. Treatment of postpartum thyroiditis is with propranolol during the hyperthyroid phase, followed by thyroid replacement during the temporary (6 to 12 months) of ensuing hypothyroidism.

- *"Hamburger" thyroiditis* (or epidemic thyroiditis)—due to consumption of thyroid tissue accidentally ground up in products such as hamburger meat and sausages—has been reported in both the United States and Europe as a very unusual form of thyroiditis.

- *Congenital hypothyroidism*, or "cretinism," occurs in about one birth per 4,000, resulting in permanent mental retardation and growth defects. The condition is not associated with maternal thyroid disease. In Canada all newborns are screened for hypothyroidism, and early thyroid replacement therapy has virtually eradicated the disorder. (In iodine-poor developing countries, cretinism remains a serious problem.)
  Hypothyroidism may also accompany irradiation of the head and neck (for cancer or some other disease); hypothalamic and pituitary tumors; and treatment with certain drugs (such as lithium, amiodarone and antithyroid drugs).

experiencing just some fatigue, a slowed heart rate and depressed mood, are more common than full-blown hypothyroidism. Thyroid hormone deficiency may also follow destruction of the gland by surgery or radioiodine therapy.

Congenital hypothyroidism is a serious cause of mental retardation that used to go unnoticed and unchecked. But today in Canada all newborns are screened for thyroid function within five days of birth. Giving thyroxine replacement to those in need by 1 month of age can prevent cretinism due to thyroid deficiency (still a widespread problem in many developing areas).

Treatment of hypothyroidism

Whatever its causes, the treatment of hypothyroidism is with hormone replacement. In Hashimoto's disease and hypothyroidism, due to radioactive iodine treatment, or after surgery for Graves' disease, the gland can never function normally again, necessitating lifelong thyroxine replacement. In the elderly and those with heart problems, thyroxine

A THYROID NODULE MAY BE MALIGNANT IF:

- it's in a child, adolescent or male (thyroid nodules are less common in these groups, thus more likely to be malignant);
- there has been excessive head and neck irradiation (a formerly common treatment for enlarged tonsils, adenoids or an enlarged newborn thymus, halted in the 1960s);
- a thyroid nodule is rapidly expanding;
- there is hoarseness (although this can also be associated with nonmalignant thyroid nodules).

  While many of the above factors increase the suspicion that a thyroid nodule is cancerous, full investigation is required before surgery is recommended.

doses must be kept low, as too much can trigger cardiac problems. Thyroid sufferers over age 60 should consult physicians about lowering their drug dosages.

Experts caution against overtreating hypothyroidism, an error less likely to occur nowadays as hypothyroidism can be accurately detected by blood tests. (Before blood tests were widespread, many people with transient hypothyroidism or nonthyroid-related disorders were needlessly given thyroxine.)

There is considerable debate as to whether people with *subclinical* hypothyroidism—without symptoms, where the condition shows up only in blood tests—should be treated. Although taking thyroxine is relatively safe, treatment is usually lifelong. In addition, recent research suggests that even slightly too much thyroxine may predispose to loss of bone mass and osteoporosis. On the other hand, subclinical hypothyroidism may predispose to lipid abnormalities and coronary heart disease, therefore perhaps meriting correction.

Thyroid nodules and thyroid cancer

Sometimes the thyroid gland develops small, painless lumps or nodules—often discovered incidentally during a medical examination. While under 1 percent of children have thyroid nodules, 6 percent of North American adults have palpable (easily felt) lumpy thyroids—and, as with other thyroid disorders, women are likelier to have them than men. Although the overwhelming majority of nodules are benign—often just a variant of normal—some 5 to 10 percent are malignant.

Owing to the possibility of cancer, doctors must differentiate between nodules that are premalignant or frankly malignant (requiring removal) and those that are benign and require conservative management. In the past, all nodules were removed, because there was no way to tell which were cancerous and which harmless. However, diagnostic advances make it far less likely that a malignant nodule will be missed, and somewhat less likely that a benign nodule will be needlessly treated with surgery. In some cases, for example, a very large goiter or one that impinges on the voicebox or windpipe—a benign nodule may also be surgically removed. Thyroxine treatment shuts off the growth-stimulating effect of thyrotropin and may be given to decrease the size of multi-nodular goiters before surgery.

In the last few years several new techniques have been developed to improve the diagnosis of thyroid cancer including radioisotope imaging. This procedure measures iodine uptake to determine how well the nodular area of the gland is functioning, helping to confirm or allay the suspicion that a nodule may be malignant and indicating whether the patient needs more tests. Fine-needle-aspiration biopsy (FNAB), another innovation pioneered by University of Toronto researchers, is now standard technique for diagnosing malignancy in thyroid nodules. The procedure involves insertion of a very thin needle into the suspicious nodule to obtain cells for direct examination. The combination of radioisotope imaging and FNAB has considerably improved thyroid-nodule diagnosis, so that it is less likely that a thyroid malignancy will be missed.

A final reassuring note: although certain types of thyroid cancer are highly lethal, death from cancer of the thyroid is extremely rare.

TUBERCULOSIS: BACK WITH A VENGEANCE

A bacterial disease thought to be vanquished, tuberculosis, or TB, is making an ominous comeback. Health authorities warn of a post-antibiotic resurgence of drug-resistant forms. A potentially fatal and formerly much-feared disease, TB was a recurring theme in 18th- and 19th-century literature. It cut short the lives of such notables as Frédéric Chopin, John Keats and Anton Chekhov. With the advent of antibiotics in the 1950s, TB rates dwindled to negligible numbers in developed countries. By the 1970s it was no longer considered a major health concern—in fact, it was popularly regarded as history. Climbing TB rates are now forcing physicians to rethink TB.

Reversal of fortune: TB back in epidemic numbers

Globally, tuberculosis always was, and still is, a leading cause of death, and it was a huge killer during the Industrial Revolution. Although better hygiene, nutrition and housing have reduced its impact, without proper antibiotic treatment, half of those who develop symptoms die of the disease. The World Health Organization (WHO) estimates that about one-third of the world's population, almost 2 billion people, are currently infected, of whom 20 million have active tuberculosis. The annual death toll is predicted to reach 3.5 million annually by the year 2000. Particularly worrisome is the emergence of bacterial strains resistant to some or all of the medications that cure TB. The director general of WHO calls this "an unnecessary tragedy," adding that "we have the tools to control this disease. There is no rational reason why tuberculosis deaths should continue to rise."

In the U.S., an estimated 10 to 15 million people carry dormant TB bacilli, and 10 percent of them are likely to develop active disease. An incidence exceeding 15 per 100,000 people has been defined as an epidemic and, by that standard, TB is already epidemic in New York, New Jersey, Georgia, Florida and California.

In Canada, TB rates run at around eight cases per 100,000, except among Native populations and recent immigrants from areas where the disease is far more widespread. Given Canada's healthcare system and less urban poverty than in the U.S., we do not yet have the same inner-city health problems, but wherever there is poverty, homelessness and poor health, TB is likely to flourish.

Multidrug-resistant TB is the problem

The resurgence of TB is largely due to bacterial strains resistant to one or more of the drugs used to treat it. In the early days of antibiotic therapy, TB patients were hospitalized and supervised to make sure they completed their full antibiotic course. With the closing of sanatoria, patients were no longer closely monitored but sent home with their drugs; all too often, once they felt better, many decided they were "cured" and stopped taking the medication. Lingering in the body, drug-resistant bacteria, impervious to the drug(s) used, multiplied and went on to infect others. By the early 1990s, many people were carrying TB strains resistant to the most powerful anti-TB medications known (*isoniazid* and *rifampin*).

Understanding tuberculosis

Names such as "consumption" and "the white plague" aptly describe the wasting effects of classical TB. The bacterial organism responsible, *Mycobacterium tuberculosis* (also called the tubercle bacillus) was first identified by the German scientist Robert Koch at the end of the 19th century. TB bacteria typically attack the lungs, and those infected spew bacteria into the air as they cough and sneeze. While people who repeatedly breathe in TB-contaminated droplets can become infected, healthy, well-nourished and immunologically strong people, may not become ill. Nine out of 10 people infected with TB never develop symptoms.

TB bacteria cause active disease in those with a weakened immune system, malnutrition, old age, alcoholism, poverty or illnesses such as cancer, diabetes and AIDS. Active TB usually affects the lungs first—causing cavities that show up on chest X-rays—although any body system, including kidneys, spine, lymph nodes and bone can be affected. Active TB is transmissible until treated with appropriate antibiotics.

Symptoms of tuberculosis
- persistent cough;
- unexplained weight loss;
- low-grade fever;
- night sweats;
- blood in the sputum;
- chest pain;
- extreme weakness and wasting;
- swollen neck glands.

Tests for TB include a chest X-ray, analysis of sputum, urine and tissue samples and a skin test—in which purified *tuberculin* (protein from the TB bacteria) is injected under the skin. A

TUBERCULOSIS SPREADS PRIMARILY THROUGH CLOSE CONTACT

Fortunately, TB bacteria are not easily transmitted through casual everyday contact—as in an elevator or bus, via a single cough or ordinary conversation. TB bacilli spread via bacteria-laden sputum and generally only cause disease among people living in close quarters or working with an infected person for an extended time. Lengthy, intimate contact with someone who has active TB poses the greatest threat, although sometimes brief contact with a highly infectious person can transmit the disease.

red weal or bump developing in 48 to 72 hours usually means that the person carries TB organisms but does not necessarily denote active disease. In fact, most people who have positive skin tests never develop active disease. If the skin test is positive, further tests such as sputum culture are done.

Treatment of TB

The first-line of treatment is usually a three-drug regimen, using the antibiotics *rifampin, isoniazid* and *pyrazinamide* for 2 months, then isoniazid and rifampin for at least 6 months. If these agents fail, others such as *ethionamide, ethambutol* and *streptomycin* may be added. Drug-resistant cases may require further medications such as *ofloxacin* and *ciprofloxacin*. Once people have been on the appropriate antibiotics for a few weeks, they usually cease to be infectious to others. Provided people stick to and finish the complete course of prescribed drugs, all the bacteria will probably be eliminated and the disease cured. But if people stop taking the medications too soon, not only may they relapse but drug-resistant strains of bacteria can develop in their bodies and spread to others.

Halting the rising tide of TB

Those with a positive TB skin test may be considered for preventive drug therapy with *isoniazid* for 6 to 12 months, to reduce the risk of developing active tuberculosis. BCG vaccination is another preventive measure used in some high risk areas such as Asia and the Philippines. But the vaccine is not 100 percent effective, and in low-risk populations, it obscures screening results of TB skin tests.

To stem the tide, physicians are urged to watch for signs of TB such as a persistent cough, fever night sweats or weight loss, order tests and follow up. The Canadian Thoracic Society and Canadian Lung Association have set up a Tuberculosis Speakers' Bureau to update health-care providers about TB and its prevention.

URINARY TRACT INFECTIONS

Urinary tract infections or UTIs, often popularly called cystitis or bladder infections, are very common bacterial infections of the urinary tract, especially in women. The most common

VARIOUS TYPES OF UTI

Urinary tract infections are named according to their location.

• **Cystitis** affects primarily the bladder.

• **Urethritis** is confined to the urethra, or urinary-outlet duct. Although the symptoms may resemble those of cystitis—i.e., frequency, urgency and burning—there's no suprapubic pain (over the bladder area) and the bladder is free of bacteria. Sexually transmitted microorganisms such as herpes, chlamydia and gonococci often cause urethritis in

both men and women,

• **Prostatitis** (prostate-gland inflammation), prostatic enlargement or other male prostate problems can cause symptoms similar to UTI—frequency, urgency and burning—but may require altogether different treatment.

• **Pyelonephritis**—kidney infection and inflammation—can occur if an otherwise uncomplicated bladder infection extends to and affects the kidneys. Acute pyelonephritis—signaled by fever and

flank pain—may permanently damage the kidneys if not promptly treated. UTI generally remains localized in the lower tract, only threatening the kidneys in about 2 to 5 percent of cases. However, the possibility of kidney involvement is greater in diabetics, pregnant women, people with indwelling catheters (plastic voiding tubes), those with stones or other urinary-tract obstructions and/or congenital anomalies

and people with **ureteral reflux** (where a little urine flows back upward toward the kidneys). Other conditions can also give rise to pyelonephritis—such as septicemia (blood infection) or post-surgical complications.

• **Asymptomatic bacteriuria** is diagnosed when urine tests reveal the presence of bacteria in the bladder, even if there are no alerting signs. Asymptomatic bacteriuria poses an ever-present problem in the bed-ridden and incontinent.

Catheters, initially sterile, tend to attract bacteria, and studies indicate that up to 80 percent of the catheterized elderly have infected urinary tracts. While some specialists promote treatment to eliminate the bacteria even when the condition gives little discomfort, others suggest treating bacteriuria only if it's bothersome, rather than risking the emergence of untreatable drug-resistant bacterial strains.

form of UTI is bladder infection or cystitis. If the urethra is also infected it produces urethritis. UTIs occur more often in women than in men because women have a shorter urethra (tube carrying urine from the bladder to the exterior), making it easier for bacteria to enter the bladder where urine is stored. Common symptoms of UTI include discomfort or a burning sensation while urinating, pelvic pain and difficulty passing urine. "Frequency" or an urgent need to go to the washroom frequently can be another sign. However, a recent University of Toronto study showed that there are many causes for the need to urinate frequently, including consumption of drinks like coffee, tea and colas, and anxiety. So the usefulness of a need to urinate frequently as a sign of bladder infection is not overly reliable.

UTIs in women can result from a variety of factors, including sexual intercourse, use of a diaphragm, use of spermicides (including from a partner's use of spermicide-coated condoms), delayed post-intercourse urination, entry of bacteria (such as *Escerichia coli* or *E. coli*) from the nearby rectum. Introduction of a catheter into the bladder for the treatment of various diseases also increases the risk of urinary tract infection. Another risk factor is delaying emptying of the bladder and reduced fluid intake. Women who have had a previous UTI infection are at increased risk for future episodes. During pregnancy, UTIs are a special concern and often missed because of other changes associated with being pregnant. Men also do get UTIs, albeit less frequently, sometimes because of obstructed urine flow.

Treated promptly and properly, UTIs are generally curable and rarely pose a health threat. But if they are left unrecognized, or diagnosis and treatment are delayed, they can lead to serious complications such as *pyelonephritis* or infection of the kidneys. Usually, pyelonephritis presents with UTI symptoms as well as flank pain, maybe blood in the urine, and a high fever, often with chills,

UTIs are diagnosed clinically by a urine dipstick in the clinic. The urine sample is sometimes sent for "culture" to identify the infecting bacteria—typically E. coli—to help determine what antibiotic treatments will be most effective. In such cases, you might get a call from the doctor's office saying that the type of bacteria found in your urine sample was resistant to the first-line medication that was prescribed and that you should likely try another one.

When people get repeat urinary tract infections, or UTIs that are resistant to treatment, further investigations are usually required, especially if they occur in men and children. Further tests typically involve ultrasound imaging of the bladder and urine collecting systems. A cystoscopy—a procedure in which a very small fiberoptic tube is inserted through the urethra to look inside the urethra and view the bladder—may also be suggested.

Treatment of UTIs is generally uncomplicated, typically with a short course of antibiotics, usually for 3 days, along with increased fluid intake. Typical antibiotics used for UTIs include *trimethoprim-sulfamethoxazole* (Bactrim, Septra), *nitrofurantoin* (MacroBid) and amoxicillin. If there is a great deal of pain, some clinicians will also prescribe pyridium, a bladder anesthetic that turns the urine quite orange. More complicated or recurrent cases need longer term antibiotics. Pyelonephritis occasionally requires intravenous antibiotics. A study of elderly women found that those who drank 300 ml of cranberry juice daily had a decreased incidence of bacteriuria with pyuria compared with control subjects given placebo. However, whether drinking cranberry or blueberry juice will prevent UTIs in young women is unknown.

Elderly individuals can occasionally have bacteria in their urine without experiencing any symptoms. The Canadian Task Force on Preventive Health Care has concluded that no evidence has shown that the treatment of asymptomatic bacteriuria in the elderly is beneficial.

Some women are more prone to UTIs than others.

Many otherwise healthy women are particularly susceptible to UTI, possibly because of receptivity to the attachment of harmful bacteria. Lactobacilli—bacteria normally present in the vaginal flora (a natural mix of microorganisms living harmoniously in the female tract)—are believed to ward off harmful bacteria. But some women have unusually low amounts of lactobacilli, while others have less after a menstrual

SYMPTOMS OF UTI

- **Urgent need to urinate;**
- **frequent need to urinate;**
- **need to urinate at night;**
- **burning/painful sensation when urinating;**
- **cloudy or foul-smelling urine;**
- **bladder spasms;**
- **sense of incomplete bladder emptying;**
- **pain over bladder area;**
- **blood in the urine.**

In addition (if the kidneys are also involved):
- **lower back and/or flank pain;**
- **fever and chills (rare with lower-tract UTI). While cystitis alone rarely elevates the temperature, a fever and flank pain may indicate kidney involvement;**
- **weakness, fatigue, nausea.**

SOME PRACTICAL ADVICE ON URINARY TRACT INFECTIONS

Once a UTI has set in, and for those prone to recurrences, try a few preventive measures:

- Drink lots of water, to encourage frequent urination and flush bacteria out of the urinary tract.
- Pay careful attention to personal hygiene.
- Always wipe from front to back after going to the toilet, or use separate tissues for front and back—a practice that may curb the transfer of bacteria from rectum (anus) to urinary opening.
- Avoid tight underwear, pantyhose and jeans—which create a warm, damp environment ideal for bacterial growth.
- Wear cotton undergarments that "breathe," to discourage bacteria from growing on undergarments. Panty liners should be frequently changed.
- Void promptly—at least every three to four hours; do not delay urination until "time permits."
- Avoid douching, which tends to wash away beneficial bacterial strains that help to maintain a healthy urinary tract.

Those prone to post-sex cystitis can try:
- Cleaning the genitals before having sex—which may remove harmful bacteria.
- Urinating after intercourse—to help flush bacteria out of the urinary tract.
- Temporarily halting use of spermicidals—recent research suggests that spermicides may disturb the vagina's normal balance.

---

period. Studies suggest that a lack of lactobacilli allows overgrowth of harmful organisms, increasing the chances of UTI.

Sexual activity may also aggravate UTI problems. In some women, bacteria seem to be easily swept up the urethra during intercourse, although post sex symptoms can simply be due to urethral irritation (not real infection). Urinating immediately after sex may help to dispel the bacteria. Some women seem to be most susceptible to UTI in the early phase of the menstrual cycle, when estrogen levels are higher than at the end of the cycle. Use of a diaphragm for contraception may increase the likelihood of UTIs in some women

Diagnosis and treatment of UTI

Physicians usually establish the presence of UTI by testing an uncontaminated midstream urine sample for bacteria. To collect the sample, the genitals are washed well with soap and water. The first third of the urine sample is discarded into the toilet and a sample of the remaining urine is collected into a sterile bottle.

New dipstick (Multistix) kits are available for home urine testing, but anyone with recurrent UTI should see a physician to make sure the problem is not something else. Long-term, stubbornly persistent cases may require further diagnostic tests such as ultrasound, X-rays, cystoscopy (bladder examination) and an intravenous pyelogram (dye test) to rule out underlying structural abnormalities.

Treatment with antibiotics usually brings swift relief

Many urinary tract infections vanish even without treatment, but today's approach is to treat symptomatic cases with antibiotics. Most cases clear up quickly with a short course of antibiotics such as amoxicillin, *trimethoprimsulfamethoxazole* (Bactrim or Septra), *nitrofurantoin* (Furadantin) and/or the newer quinolone products, such as *norfloxacin* (Noroxin), and *ciprofloxacin*. The drugs are taken either as a single large dose, or as a 3- to 7-day course. Treatment is ideally continued until all symptoms are gone and a midstream urine sample is free of bacteria. A repeat infection requires another course of antibiotics. If an infection persists, more of the same antibiotic or a different drug may be tried, as bacteria easily mutate and resistant forms may surface. If the UTI is associated with sexual activity, an antibiotic pill taken directly after intercourse may prevent cystitis.

Experimental treatments for UTI

Some experts promote cranberry juice, lactobacilli, (e.g., in yogurt) and vitamin C as possible dietary aids that acidify urine and may help in preventing UTI. Trials have given mixed results as to whether these remedies are truly effective. Perhaps the key message is "the more fluid the better."

VARICOSE VEINS

Varicose veins (from the Greek for "grape-like") are bulging, twisted or knotted bluish veins—usually seen in the veins of the legs and backs of the calves, near the skin surface. They are a common but generally harmless complaint, affecting people of all ages, roughly 5 times more women than men.

In technical terms, varicose veins arise because of a flaw or malfunction in small valves within the veins, often in the upper leg, calves or groin area. They may bulge because of vein-valve incompetence—a breakdown or loosening of valves in the veins so they no longer close properly.

For those who desire it, the distorted veins can be removed by a variety of modern techniques. While some people with varicose veins hardly notice them, others detest the cosmetic blemish and want them gone. "However," notes one vascular surgeon, "if they aren't troublesome, there's often no need to treat them."

Varicose veins do not endanger health

Many people with varicose veins have few or no symptoms, other than displeasure at their gnarled appearance. But others develop pain sometimes described as a dull ache, a burning or feeling of heavy tiredness in the legs—which can be troublesome when standing for long periods, or in hot weather. About 18 percent of people with varicose veins have leg pain, and some develop an itchiness. Skin ulcers, which can be severe and incapacitating, are an occasional complication.

Even those who hardly notice or feel them often worry about the possible health risks of varicose veins, and whether the swollen veins might do harm. "The answer," explains one vascular expert, "is that varicose veins are virtually never a health risk, and nothing bad will happen from them. The swelling does *not* travel to other parts of the body or pose any threat to the lungs."

Most varicose veins are harmless and will never cause any serious problems, but because they're distended and near the skin surface, they are prone to injury. Sometimes, a thrombosis (clot) may develop and produce superficial phlebitis—inflammation—that's painful, red and hot, but no health danger. Treatment is with ice and painkillers. The clot usually resolves and vanishes on its own, occasionally requiring surgical removal.

Treatment choices for getting rid of varicose veins

Those who consider varicose veins a minor cosmetic problem often need no treatment other than reassurance that the condition is not harmful or likely to become a danger. But for people who hate the varicosities and want them removed, there are various options.

Conservative therapy is often enough. It includes:

- regular exercise, especially walking;
- avoidance of prolonged standing:
- if job necessitates long hours of standing, doing squeeze-and-relax calf-muscle exercises to encourage blood flow;
- taking regular rest periods, putting the legs up on a chair or stool so they are higher than the knee, at least for a few minutes now and then;
- raising the foot of the bed at night:
- wearing compression stockings; these garments, which are usually quite comfortable, gently compress the vein evenly up the leg and relieve pressure; incorporated into a regular regimen of rest and leg elevation, compression may relieve and prevent the condition from worsening.

Sclerotherapy, already used in Europe for years, is an injection technique especially suitable for small or spidery varicose veins. It means injecting parts of the varicose vein with a chemical called a *sclerosant* (such as sodium tetradecyl sulphate or ethanolamine oleate), which creates an inflammatory reaction that seals or "glues" the vein shut. Immediately after the injection, the leg is tightly bandaged with compression stockings, which must be worn continuously for three to 6 weeks so the vein seals up. Tight compression following sclerotherapy is essential for the vein to close completely and to offset recurrences.

Before offering sclerotherapy, surgeons explain that varicose veins tend to reappear; in which case the procedure might need to be repeated, or surgery can follow to remove the vein. Not everyone with varicose veins can be considered for sclerotherapy. "For example," explains a surgeon, "it's not suitable for those

POSSIBLE CAUSES AND AGGRAVATING FACTORS

There's no clear reason why varicose veins occur, although they tend to run in families, so there may be a genetic link. Many a daughter desperately hopes she won't have her mother's or grandma's knotty blue leg veins!

The vein swellings often tend to pop up during pregnancy, owing to increased pelvic pressure. During pregnancy, the female hormones

cause relaxation of the smooth muscles (including those in the blood vessel linings), which may add to the development of varicose veins and explain why more women than men suffer from them. In addition, they may arise because of fistulas (tiny connections formed between veins and arteries).

Classically, varicose veins have also been blamed on factors such

as obesity, jobs that involve prolonged standing and sports injuries (like being hit in the groin by a cricket ball). However, besides pregnancy—known to bring out varicose veins—there's considerable debate about the other alleged causes. Many experts believe that being overweight or standing for long periods has little to do with it.

with an incompetent or leaky sapheno-femoral valve in the groin." Sclerotherapy is generally most effective for uncomplicated, relatively small varices below the knees in people who can do follow-up walking exercises and who can wear the necessary compression bandages. The advantages are that it can be done quickly, on an outpatient basis; the person can walk right afterward, needs no time off work and the procedure doesn't disturb ordinary activities. One drawback is the necessity (and sometimes difficulty) of compressing the vein after the procedure.

Surgery for varicose veins. Varicose veins can be surgically stripped out under local or general anesthetic, using carefully placed incisions. (There are many veins in the legs, and removing some of them does no harm: the blood is rerouted into another set of veins.) After freezing the groin area and vein, the surgeon makes a tiny incision and pulls out as much of the vein as possible using "microscopic loops." The patient goes home the same day and can be back to work in a day or two. Recovery is good, and the scar usually small, often hardly visible afterward. (Compared with older surgical methods, which often damaged the nerve and left the lower leg numb, today's techniques for removing varicose veins are minimally disruptive.)

Choosing between doing nothing, conservative therapy alone, sclerotherapy or surgery involves information and a solid understanding

of the type of vein problem and options available. Very often there's no medical reason to remove varicose veins; those who opt for therapy must understand the pros and cons of each procedure. Both surgery and sclerotherapy can usually be done on an outpatient basis. For most, there is little pain after either procedure, although some experience discomfort for a few days.

Rare complications with sclerotherapy include allergic reactions to the chemicals used and minor, not uncommon but annoying aftereffects such as skin discoloration over the sclerosing vein, where the "ghost of the vein" might be seen under the skin for 6 to 12 months (or can be permanent). On the other hand, surgery may leave some scars—usually small, and the legs can be temporarily disfigured with eccymosis (bruising).

Following either surgery or sclerotherapy, the veins may re-varicose, requiring repeat treatment. Some varicose vein surgeons think sclerotherapy is less likely to result in a permanent cure, and that retreatment is more likely to be required, perhaps surgical. Another consideration with sclerotherapy is that it usually requires several sessions, and after it the person must have the leg bandaged for several weeks.

VOICE ABUSE: REMARKABLY COMMON!

Far more prevalent than many realize, voice abuse inflames the vocal cords and produces a hoarse, breathy, raspy speaking style. Many a potentially good, natural voice is spoiled by overuse or abuse. Like a fingerprint, a voice is a unique personal trademark allowing us to express emotions—without it we cannot sing, laugh, cry out, or indeed, speak. An unappealing voice can have a drastic impact, undermining someone's image and communication skills.

Some people unknowingly abuse their voices simply by the way they speak or sing, needlessly straining their vocal cords by breathing incorrectly. Others harm their voices by shouting too often or by phonating (speaking) in an unnatural pitch. Other common voice abuses are perpetual throat clearing, persistent coughing, singing incorrectly and excess yelling. Voice problems are aggravated by smoking tobacco and/or stress. Under stress, people often hold their breath, stiffening the laryngeal muscles that control the vocal cords. People can improve their voices by correcting their breathing, learning to relax the vocal cords while speaking and improving the pitch, resonance and intonation (melody) of speech.

Common ways to abuse your voice

Excessive *throat clearing*, often done more from nervous habit than necessity, strains the vocal cords. When clearing the throat, a little mucus may be expelled, but the action presses the vocal cords together violently and can irritate throat tissues. Habitual throat clearers should make a conscious effort to break the habit. One way to do it is to sniff intensely instead of clearing the throat. The "quick sniff" can rid the vocal cords of some mucus, and what is sniffed can then be swallowed.

Continuous heavy coughing is very hard on the vocal cords. High-speed photography during a cough shows that the vocal cords are slammed together and then blown apart suddenly by the outgoing air. Continued heavy coughing can produce swollen, irritated vocal cords, distorting the speaking voice, making normal vocalization almost impossible. Try "silent coughing," which is easier on the vocal cords.

Talking repeatedly against a very noisy background can seriously strain the voice. Many bars and restaurants not only have on a television set but also play loud background music. After prolonged attempts to converse in noisy settings, a person will experience vocal fatigue, throat discomfort and hoarseness—aggravated by cigarette smoke and dehydration from alcohol intake.

Warning signs of voice overuse

Signs of voice abuse include continuous hoarseness, breathy, halting or raspy speech, tightness in the throat and involuntary pitch changes or breaks in the voice. The typical voice abuser may have thickened vocal cords, a sore throat, a swollen larynx and possibly benign (noncancerous) nodules or polyps on the vocal cords. Larger polyps and nodules may develop in those who consistently misuse their voices, such as singers, aerobics teachers or hockey coaches. Voice disorders can also arise or be aggravated by stress, anxiety or fear of public (or other) speaking situations.

Some common voice disorders

- *Vocal abuse in speaking and singing*—speaking in loud environments, teaching, cheerleading, other activities that tax the voice and improper voice or singing lessons—can greatly abuse the human voice. With proper training, such activities can be done safely, but many people (even singers) have little or no voice training. Abuse of the voice during singing is a particularly complex problem that may require referral to an otolaryngologist.

- *Voice nodules and polyps*—often due to voice abuse—may not obviously interfere with voice production. Some famous singers have had untreated vocal nodules. If the nodules are asymptomatic, they should be left alone. However, in many cases, nodules produce hoarseness, breathiness, a reduced vocal range and voice fatigue. Speech therapy is the first line of treatment. Even apparently large nodules may regress, disappear or become asymptomatic with 6 to 12 weeks of voice therapy. Some nodules eventually need surgical removal, but voice therapy can help prevent recurrences. Polyps are usually single lesions that regress spontaneously; some require excision. A trial of speech therapy, low-dose steroids and reevaluation in 4 weeks have surprisingly resolved some cases.

- *Laryngitis*—a common source of voice distortion—usually treated with antibiotics; sinusitis (often accompanying a laryngeal infection) also responds to antibiotics. Cigarette smoke should be avoided as it worsens throat and voice problems. (Friars balsam and other menthol inhalants may be soothing.)

- *Gastroesophageal reflux laryngitis*—laryngitis due to heartburn—is a common cause of voice disturbance. Its typical symptoms are: morning hoarseness, halitosis (bad breath), a bitter taste in the mouth, a feeling of having a "lump in the throat," frequent throat clearing, coughing and airway inflammation. The problem tends to disappear once the reflux disorder is treated.

- *Tonsillitis* gives a painful, red, inflamed throat that can alter the speaking or singing voice. In professional singers and other voice users, it can pose treatment dilemmas. On one hand, physicians hesitate to remove the tonsils in voice professionals (in case the voice deteriorates as a result), on the other hand, a singer or lecturer cannot afford to be off sick several times a year. In general, a conservative approach is advised.

• *Anxiety or fear of public speaking* can be a special problem in voice-troubled people who wish to communicate or speak in public. It often shows itself as shallow breathing during speech, producing a quiet, breathy, tense voice—sometimes even aphonia (no speech emerging). If the voice problem stems mainly from anxiety, reassurance that it's not due to a physical abnormality, diagnosing anxiety as the reason and perhaps a short session of speech therapy may be all that's needed.

Finding the source of voice problems

Modern, sophisticated tools can now assist physicians and speech-language pathologists in diagnosing the cause of a voice problem. Otolaryngologists can observe vocal-cord function (and malfunction) using a laryngoscope or stroboscope inserted into the throat. Multidimensional Voice Programs (computerized voice analyzers) can trace and pinpoint the exact symptoms and types of voice abuse, giving an instant analysis, readout and sound reproduction of the voice pitch, intensity and speed. On-the-spot feedback and visualization show people the right and wrong way to vocalize. Videostroboscopy can be used to film a voice abnormality while the vocal cords are in motion.

New equipment and better understanding of laryngeal function have increased awareness of subtle problems in the head and neck (or elsewhere in the body) that can affect voice. Many advances have come from research into the problems of professional singers and actors.

Speech-language therapy can remedy many voice flaws

Voice therapy, which can take 12 to 24 weeks of consistent practice, works on the mechanical voice system and teaches people to make it operate as well as possible—aiming to give them back the good voice they were probably born with. Therapists teach breath control, abdominothoracic breathing and ways to relax the laryngeal muscles. People learn proper breathing and to open the throat correctly when speaking (perhaps starting with a yawn—Nature's way!).

Voice training can improve or reverse voice problems such as faulty breathing, poor delivery or a jarring quality, monotonous intonation, pitch and pronunciation errors, hypernasality (due to habit or a structural abnormality), hyponasality (from blocked nasal passages), aphonia (no or "small" voice), spasmodic dysphonia (weak voice possibly from a paralyzed vocal cord) and flawed acting or singing styles. A competent speech-language therapist will analyze the voice and evaluate emotional issues that could underlie the voice problem. But it takes patience, time and understanding to acquire a more desirable voice. In some cases, training the speaking voice, even when there's no sign of vocal abuse, can benefit teachers, politicians, actors and public speakers.

Tips to keep your voice natural and healthy

Cut down on needless throat clearing and coughing. Never hold the breath while speaking.
Don't yell. Yelling is very hard on the vocal cords.

Develop an easy voice attack. "Voice attack" means the degree of abruptness with which we say words. In music, an easy attack is called *legato*, with no discernible breaks between notes. The soft, legato-like voice, or an easy attack, that blends words and sounds together gently, as in Southern speech, is much easier on the vocal cords—and on the listener's ears.

Use a pitch that is natural for you. Many men try to express authority by speaking at the bottom of their pitch range, and some professional women try to sound more in command by speaking with an exaggeratedly low pitch. The best pitch level is the one that's easy and natural, usually several notes above the person's lowest note.

Don't use the same pitch (a dull monotone) all the time—varying the pitch up and down as particular words or syllables are stressed makes speech livelier and pleasanter.

Renew the breath often by pausing, to keep

the voice natural and avoid strain. Trying to speak without adequate air, by muscle exertion alone, strains the vocal tract. The best breath for speaking comes from good diaphragm control.

Learn when to pause, using natural breaks—for instance, at the ends of phrases and sentences.

Reduce demands on the voice—avoid excessive talking. Many people get voice trouble because they talk non-stop. "Friendly chattiness and being the life of the party are fine," warns one speech therapist, "but overdoing it can produce a hoarse, weak voice."

Develop an open vocal tract. Many voices are destroyed by tightening the vocal tract, shutting down the larynx, the throat and the mouth while speaking, making the voice sound tense and lacking resonance.

Avoid smoke-filled rooms and excessive use of alcohol. Cigarette smoke irritates the vocal cords. (Incidentally, marijuana smoke is hotter than tobacco smoke, and even more irritating.) Excess alcohol intake can produce a lowered pitch and hoarseness—a "whisky voice."

Drink enough liquid. Excessive dryness is hard on the voice—a healthy voice is a wet one; humidify your home. Singers favor nose breathing because air passing through the nose and throat becomes moister.

WEST NILE VIRUS INFECTION

Infection by the mosquito-borne West Nile Virus (WNV) can cause fever, flu-like symptoms, meningitis, encephalitis and a polio-like illness. Long-term consequences of the illness can include lingering fatigue, memory loss, trouble walking and muscle weakness. The disease, first recognized in Uganda's West Nile region in 1937, has since caused epidemics in France, Israel and South Africa, spreading to North America in 1979 and attracting attention in 1999. Although the virus infects primarily birds, it spreads to humans via the bite of infected *Culex pipiens* mosquitoes. Since the virus persists in the blood for several days after someone is bitten by an infected mosquito, there are rising concerns about its possible transmission via blood transfusion and scientists are working to develop screening tests for WNV.

Although many people infected with West Nile Virus may have either no symptoms or just a headache or mild fever, others can be very ill or even die from the infection. Symptoms of WNV typically appear 2 to 6 days after the infected mosquito bite, starting with headache, fever and muscle or joint pain, perhaps accompanied by stomach upsets or abdominal discomfort. A rash and swollen lymph nodes may follow. The symptoms usually last about a week

A small minority of those affected (about 1 percent), especially people over age 50, become severely ill with WNV, developing meningitis or encephalitis (brain inflammation and swelling) with high fever, bad headache, stiff neck, disorientation and even convulsions, paralysis and coma. (In this group, mortality ranges from 10 to 15 percent.) The cerebral effects may not be noticed, or may be overlooked, and only detected later by a lumbar (spinal) tap.

To protect yourself from WNV infection, take the following precautions:

- *Eliminate pools of stagnant* water from your surroundings (to remove mosquito breeding grounds);
- *Stay away from* insect-infested outdoor areas, especially from dusk to dawn (when mosquitoes are most active); keep screens in good repair;
- *Keep mosquitoes off your skin* by wearing light-colored, tightly-woven protective clothes that cover your neck, shoulders, arms, legs and feet;
- *Apply effective insect repellant*, favoring products that contain DEET (N.N-diethyl-3-methylbenzamine). More concentrated DEET products give better protection, but do not use those over 30 percent strength because of health concerns, avoid putting the repellant on the mouth or eyes and wash it off every day, re-applying it as needed. Use DEET repellants sparingly on children—do not use it at all on those under 6 months old—and apply repellant to their clothing rather than directly onto their skin, not more than 3 times a day. Products containing Citronella or lavender oil are less effective than DEET and are currently being re-evaluated. Eating garlic or taking thiamine (Vitamin B1) does *not* repel mosquitoes.

DOES YOUR WORK ENVIRONMENT MAKE YOU SICK?

In our society, work underlies self-esteem and identity. On the other hand, monotonous, soulless jobs can erode self-identity, stifle initiative and impair mental health, leading to injuries, absenteeism and staff turnover. Job satisfaction depends on both the work and the "work culture" or environment. Managers are increasingly encouraged to humanize workplaces—giving employees a greater voice in the planning and organization.

Stress-related worker health complaints on the rise

In the past, workplace health concerns centered mainly on safety and physical conditions. But the U.S. National Institute for Occupational Safety and Health (NIOSH) reports that stress-related disorders are fast becoming the most prevalent reason for worker disability claims. In Canada, as in the rest of the industrial world, there is a dramatic rise in workdays missed for "family-related" and "stress" reasons. Over 60 percent of Canadians claim to have experienced "negative job stress" during the past year. Distressed employees are more likely to be involved in accidents, make mistakes and miss work.

Stress-related disorders typically stem from task monotony, boredom, authoritarian supervision, time pressure, tight schedules, lack of stimulation, coercion, harassment and poor employee-to-employee interaction. The more stressful the work atmosphere, the greater the likelihood of symptoms such as fatigue, anxiety, insomnia, headaches, dizziness, panic attacks, depression, cardiac symptoms, muscular strain syndromes and substance abuse.

High pressure and low control—the deadliest twin job stressors

Unremitting job demands, coupled with little or no control, can grind people into illness. The combination is a deadly duo that produces not only mental strain, but also elevates blood pressure and increases heart risks. Authoritarian practices that allow employees little or no influence over the pace and execution of tasks can make them ill. Employees who feel more in command of their work are likelier to gain mastery over other aspects of life, including their health. Employees who take part in the decision-making are likely to be more cooperative, less prone to sabotage, errors and illness.

"Learned helplessness" can carry over into everyday life

While some react to stress by trying to alter circumstances, many adopt a helpless, passive attitude, withdraw stop trying and just take sick leave. Poor work conditions may make employees with minor workplace injuries become helplessly incapacitated and take prolonged disability leave. Even if there is no medical evidence of organic impairment and employees are deemed fit enough to resume work, the injury may take over their lives so they just can't face going back to work.

Lack of power over decision-making induces depression, a sense of losing control, aptly called "learned helplessness." Learned helplessness can arise as the cumulative endpoint of being treated like a subordinate. It may spill over into everyday life, undermining the will to make decisions, causing apathy and lack of interest in community affairs. Feeling helpless at work, people believe they cannot alter any aspect of life. If the distress is not recognized and tackled, the sense of helplessness may become entrenched and lead to sickness. "Instead of facing and dealing with mental health problems," explains one therapist, "ailing workers who feel helpless exhibit signs of dependency and become unable to work."

Anxiety, depression or other stress-related disorders often express themselves or "somatize" as physical ailments such as backache and other muscular pain syndromes, headaches, digestive upsets, sleeplessness and cardiovascular (heart) symptoms. People may unconsciously label emotional problems as physical ailments, calling for medical treatment, thus avoiding the stigma of mental illness. Taking on the sick role because of organic ailments, they seek medical solutions—instead of getting the needed psychosocial counseling.

Supportive relationships can help to mute the ill effects of job distress. Sharing and discussing problems can lessen the strain. For example, a study of more than 1,000 male workers showed that support from supervisors

POSSIBLE REASONS FOR THE RISE IN WORK STRESS

Part of the increase in stress-linked illness is blamed on computerization, monotony, restrictive supervision and employees' underutilized abilities as well as the separation of "conceivers" from "executors." Workplace stress, sometimes coupled with home stressors such as family problems, can undermine health.

The "psychotoxic workplace"
A hierarchical, non-participatory, authoritarian organization is stressful for employees. Conflicts or disagreement with a boss or workmates, and uncertainty about responsibilities are also powerful stressors. The latest trend to Total Quality Management emphasizing "customer satisfaction" and "zero defects" can place enormous stress on employees trying to deliver flawless goods. For example, telephone operators feel stressed by being monitored for their voice and client approach, while also being bombarded with consumer questions they can't answer—about weather conditions, road reports, restaurants or movies. Teachers experience high stress when, besides uninterested pupils, they face extra administrative chores.

Specific workplace stressors include:
• unrelieved task overload, high pressure;
• needlessly intimidating supervision—"rule by fear";
• bullying, discrimination, harassment;
• monotony, boredom, underused capabilities;
• little control and low decision-making influence;
• changes—even those meant to "humanize" and improve conditions; being "shunted around";
• ambiguous roles, blurred lines of authority;
• conflicts, not getting along with supervisors, workmates;
• social isolation, lack of support, poor communication;
• no feedback, lack of encouragement;
• few learning, career or promotional opportunities;
• shift work that disturbs body's circadian rhythm (daily biological clock);
• competing responsibilities from personal life;
• competition and job insecurity.

and co-workers diminished rates of depression, helplessness and absenteeism.

Links discovered between job stress and heart disease

Many studies now link job stress to elevated blood pressure and cardiovascular risks. Workers who describe their jobs as "overly demanding" especially with little say in what they do are likelier than others to develop cardiovascular disease. Studies of Finnish industry workers demonstrated clear links between low decision-making influence and elevated risks of *angina pectoris* (heart pain) and heart attacks. A Swedish study showed that young men working in non-learning occupations that underutilized their abilities were more likely than others to have physical signs of stress—high levels of blood adrenaline and elevated blood pressure. Other investigators found that men who had heart attacks before age 45 described less skill requirements and less influence over their tasks than men without heart problems. job monotony was a significant discriminator between "cases" (men with heart attacks) and "controls" (those without heart attack).

Moreover, high-level positions don't carry the most stress. Although executives, bureau chiefs and medical officers bear heavy responsibilities, they also possess the authority to carry through their plans. Bosses who run the ship tend to be less stressed than subordinates who lack control. Assistants, secretaries and nurses, who often take the brunt if things don't run smoothly, without authority to make decisions, are most highly prone to job-related illness. The lower the job rank, the higher the illness and death rate for virtually every disease.

The renowned British Whitehall study, which tracked 10,000 civil servants for nearly 20 years, found a striking difference in heart disease rates between those at the top and bottom of the job scale. Lower-rank civil servants (mainly unskilled manual workers) had coronary disease rates almost 4 times greater than those in top (administrative) positions. One explanation is that since low job status is also associated with poor workplace support, those in lower rank jobs may be short on all three stress-reducing factors: a sense of control, decision-making influence *and* social support.

Humanizing workplace design and organization

Work stress can be reduced by changing people's responsibilities or altering the work situation. Although poor work conditions produce stress and illness, many organizations still focus on changing employee behavior rather than correcting workplace problems.

SIGNS OF STRESS-LINKED HEALTH PROBLEMS ON THE JOB

- memory lapses, distracted, "daydreaming";
- diminished concentration, wandering attention;
- withdrawal, avoidance of peers, supervisors;
- inability to do job, declining performance;
- unexplained lateness, long lunch hours, absences, quitting work early, frequent sick leave
- sloppy appearance, change in attire;
- borrowing money from colleagues;
- waning interest in workmates, family, friends;
- perpetual fatigue;
- agitated, nervously restless, emotional outbursts;
- thought preoccupa-

tion (overriding usual interests, sociability, friendliness);
- unexplained anxiety, "jitters," irrational fears;
- unusual sensitivity to others, expressed sense of helplessness, personal problems;
- complaints of "heart pounding," sweating, dizziness;
- sleep disturbances, insomnia;
- dismal outlook, negative thoughts— nothing working out "as it should," expressions of unworthiness, guilt (signs of depression).

Consequences of stress reactions:
- deteriorating performance;
- tasks undone or poorly done;

- increased accidents, injuries, illness;
- disciplinary/corrective action;
- absenteeism;
- disturbing to colleagues;
- medical attention needed for stress-related symptoms.

Possible obstacles to seeking professional help:
- denial, avoidance, stigma of mental illness;
- ignoring the problem, hoping it will just vanish;
- belief that one should solve one's own problems, that seeking help signifies weakness;
- conviction that nothing can help.

Modern experts believe the solution lies in humanizing and democratizing the workplace, altering the work culture, and targeting what needs change. It may mean restructuring jobs to give workers more control, better incentives and a voice in planning changes. The essential steps are to listen to complaints, identify stressors, define responsibilities, increase employee autonomy, promote social interaction, give positive feedback and allow opportunities for career development no mean feat! "Yet," bemoans one corporate consultant, "the current system, and especially labor laws, are set up to hinder rather than encourage a collaborative process."

Therapy can alleviate stress-linked disorders

Therapy can often ferret out the sources of stress and help to relieve it. Even brief counseling may do wonders and markedly diminish

stress, perhaps short-circuiting illness behavior getting workers back on the job, with huge savings—both to the individual, in terms of self-esteem and to employers in terms of productivity (See Chapter 14 for more on stress-reduction techniques.)

Employee Assistance Programs (EAPs), available in many companies, give confidential advice and assistance for mental, emotional or other problems. Many programs are run offsite, available free to employees and their families, offering assistance not only with emotional, relationship, anxiety, mental and other problems, but also with legal, financial, child and eldercare concerns. Some have a 1–800 number and many also offer trauma response services around the clock.

For more Information, consult your local Health and Safety Committee, Employee Assistance Programs (if available); Ontario Ministry of Labour Office of the Worker Advisor: (416) 325–8570; WIALT (Workers Information Organization on Labour Relations): (416) 392–1203; Institute for Work and Health: (416) 927–2027; health and safety organizations or private corporate health consultants.

ERGONOMIC WORKPLACE HEALTH

Ergonomics—a term barely heard until recently—has become a trendy catchword used to sell products such as car seats ("ergonomically perfect for human backs") or office chairs ("with optimal ergonomic comfort"). The science of ergonomics deals with "human factors" and work environments—the relationship between humans and their equipment and environment. For example, keyboards and other fine hand tools are best used with *straight wrists*, which lessens injury risks. Additional ergonomic features to consider include back posture, head tilt, the heights and types of work surfaces, seating arrangements, visual angles, illumination and wrist supports or footrests. (Tools for women should have different dimensions from those used by men.)

Ergonomic concerns about VDT use surfaced in the 1970s because of a dramatic increase in operator complaints of muscle strain, particularly in the back, neck, shoulders and wrists. Such health problems are blamed on the incredibly fast tempo of today's keyboarding. Rapid action of fingers on keyboards for hours on end can inflame parts of the hand and/or wrist.

"Repetitive strain injury": a modern worker's nightmare

Musculoskeletal ailments rank high among job-related injuries and compensation claims. The National Institute for Occupational Safety and Health found the incidence of repetitive strain injury (RSI) in some occupations, particularly among newspaper reporters, exceedingly high.

RSI describes musculoskeletal disorders in which pain, discomfort and muscular weakness develop, sometimes with tissue swelling. (Alternative names include overuse syndrome and cumulative trauma disorder or CTD.) The rise in RSI is attributed to repetitive movements (as in keyboarding or assembling small parts). Physicians attribute the problem to poor posture, inefficient work habits, and lack of ergonomic planning. Prevention is a must because many of those afflicted take ages—weeks or months—to recover and the condition often worsens or improves without rhyme or reason.

Therapy for RSI includes physiotherapy, biofeedback, movement retraining and electromyography, but some sufferers can never return to their previous occupations. People with RSI must also take care not to re-injure themselves. Work-hardening programs conducted by qualified physiotherapists may lessen risks of recurrence.

Keyboarders need frequent mobility breaks

Frequent breaks are vital for VDT users, not only to move the muscles but also to reduce fatigue and promote social interaction. Short, frequent breaks are better than occasional long ones. Although there are no rules, many ergonomists suggest a 5-to-10-minute break after each hour of computer work. Studies show that even 10 percent of VDT working time can be spent in rest periods *without* lowering productivity. On the contrary, frequent breaks increase efficiency. Pauses are best individually negotiated rather than by strict protocol.

Good workplace design is crucial to ergonomic health

Although immobility is one factor in muscular strain, badly placed equipment and poor design contribute. Good workstation layout can help to avoid musculoskeletal discomfort. There's no need to spend a fortune on improvements: simply ensuring good *adjustability* and reorganizing existing furniture, perhaps purchasing a few inexpensive items (such as footrests, lamps or document holders) may suffice to make the VDT station ergonomically sound. The idea is to arrange things so that the body works in a biomechanically healthy manner least likely to cause muscular strain. VDT tables and chairs should be easily adjustable, as operators differ in size and shape. Seats should support the lower back and be comfortably padded. Arm and wrist supports may relieve the keyboarding load. Document holders and viewing screen should also be adjustable.

Protect hands and wrists to avoid keyboard grief

For keyboarding, elbows should be away from body, with wrists kept straight, not bent too much up, down or sideways. Prolonged wrist extension (palm down, back of hand turned upward) can cause pain and musculoskeletal disorders such as carpal tunnel syndrome. While activating keys does not usually stress the hands unduly, uninterrupted, long-term, rapid keying, done in awkward positions, may cause RSIs in susceptible individuals.

Sit right at your VDT

Sitting, especially for hours on end, is very hard on human backs and exerts a far greater load on the spine than standing or walking, straining the back, neck and shoulders. The intervertebral disc pressure while seated can be twice that of standing at ease.

The right chair is a key element for ergonomic well-being. The seating position can damage or protect the back, alter the effort required and pressure on the spine. Seat height is a key factor in avoiding muscle trouble. Thighs should be roughly parallel to the floor, feet flat on the floor or on a footrest. Seating too low puts pressure on the thighs, but having the seat too high puts pressure on the back of the knees.

ERGONOMIC CHECKLIST FOR HEALTHY VDT/COMPUTER USE

Workstation layout

- Make sure all parts of the workstation are easily reachable to avoid undue twisting of neck or trunk.
- Try to make workstation design suit all tasks done.
- Adjust workstations to fit the body, not vice versa.
- Arrange working surfaces at correct height/position for eyes and posture, with no sharp edges.

Posture

- Try to keep head and neck in one line, head not jutting forward, chin down.
- If using the telephone while at the VDT, use a headset or speaker phone to avoid neck strain (from cradling the receiver against the shoulder).
- Support the back.
- Distribute body weight as evenly as possible.
- Take frequent pauses to stand up, move about, stretch the muscles.

Arms

- Use correct movements to minimize strain, keeping wrists and hands as straight as possible while working.
- Place forearms parallel with the floor or angled slightly downward. (This can be achieved by lowering the desk to suit the user or, with a fixed-height desk, by raising the chair.)
- Padded arm and wrist supports can help.

Legs and leg room

- Keep feet flat on floor or on a footrest (big enough for both feet).
- Knees should be at about a 90-degree angle, thighs parallel to floor, body weight not restricting circulation, with ample leg room.
- Legs should be able to move without hitting furniture.

Chair

- Be sure chairs are easily adjustable when seated, and well padded.
- Seats should allow clearance for the thigh muscle; the back of the knee should not touch the seat.
- Seat pan height is adjusted to put user's weight on the buttocks, *not* the thighs.
- Seat tilt is best *horizontal* or a little backward, to prevent sliding forward.
- Seats should be firm and upholstered (preferably in material that absorbs perspiration).
- Backrests should adjust up, down, backwards and forward for good lumbar support, and fit the small of the back to support the spine, with users sitting upright while keying—but ergonomists disagree about the best type.
- For chair mobility; wheels or castors can be fitted on (hard castors for soft floors, soft for hard floors).
- For tasks involving lateral movements, seats should swivel.

Keyboard

- Should be near the table edge and fully movable in any direction, detachable from screen to ensure comfortable working position.
- Tilt slightly forward to avoid awkward wrist/hand positions.
- Be sure the keyboard is thick enough for comfortable arm positioning (less than 30 mm thick at the home row of keys).
- Use a document holder (adjustable and detachable).

Screen

- Put the screen at a comfortable reading distance.
- When looking straight ahead, be sure you're looking at the top edge of the screen.
- Ensure that all characters are easily legible.
- Adjust screen contrast and brightness as needed.

Light right to avoid eyestrain

The visually taxing nature of VDT work may reveal a previously unnoticed eye problem. (About 30 percent of the population have uncorrected or misdiagnosed eye-focusing problems, whether or not they use VDTs.) Corrective lenses different from those for everyday activities may be needed. For instance, wearers of bifocals who use the reading portion of their lenses to view the screen may force their necks into awkward positions that strain the neck and shoulder muscles.

Poor illumination, illegible manuscripts and screen glare (from reflected lights, incorrect lighting or shiny surfaces) are common reasons for eyestrain. VDT screens should be positioned to minimize glare, and the brightness knob used to control brightness. Correct contrast between characters and background is also crucial to avoid eyestrain. The screen image should not flicker but should be sharp, without blurred edges. Since VDT users constantly glance from document to screen to keyboard, all three should be on the same plane of focus to reduce the need for focusing changes.

For more information, consult a practicing ergonomist; the Canadian Center for Occupational Health and Safety (800) 263–8466. Read *Voluntary Office Guidelines*, published by the private-sector Canadian Standards Association.

ZOONOSES: DISEASE FROM PETS

Our pets provide comfort and amusement and may even promote good health by their friendly presence, which can alleviate stress and counter loneliness. The wag of a tail, a quiet purr or the song of a bird comforts many. But while pets provide unconditional love and companionship, they can also transmit diseases and provoke allergies in susceptible individuals.

Worldwide, there are more than 200 zoonoses (animal diseases transmissible to humans), of which at least 150 occur in Canada and the United States—including diseases caused by viruses, bacteria, fungi and parasites. Among city dwellers in industrialized countries, animal diseases are most likely to spread via house pets, usually dogs, cats, birds, mice, rabbits and hamsters. Cat-scratch fever, rabies and a variety of skin and stomach ailments are among the animal-transmitted illnesses that afflict millions of North Americans every year. Children who play in areas where animals have deposited infected feces are especially at risk.

The most common zoonoses cause just mild discomforts, perhaps a skin irritation, upset stomach, headache or slight chill, but in a few cases they can be serious, even fatal. For instance, in 1992 a 31-year-old Colorado man died of pneumonic plague after rescuing a cat from under his house. The man picked up the disease agents by inhaling bacteria directly into his lungs from the cat, which was sneezing and coughing. Pneumonic plague is endemic among wild animals in several southwestern U.S. states, but not in Canada's cooler climate.

Untreated animal bites frequently cause trouble

Animal bites are the commonest way in which animal diseases are transmitted to humans, as the wounds are liable to become infected—especially cat bites (or scratches). Thousands of people in North America are bitten or mauled each year by animals, particularly dogs. Health authorities view the bites as a preventable consequence of irresponsible pet ownership. Besides leaving permanent and disfiguring scars, the bites may spread rabies, tetanus and other infections. Nine out of 10 animal bites are caused by dogs, male dogs being more dangerous than females, large dogs inflicting worse wounds than small ones. Men are evidently twice as likely as women to be bitten by a dog, but women are twice as likely to be bitten or scratched by cats. (For first aid for animal bites see "Animal bites" under "Bites and stings," in Chapter 17.)

Some diseases from pets

- *Rabies*: Of the viral and bacterial diseases transmitted to humans from animals, rabies—although not the most common—is the most dreaded because, left untreated, it is virtually 100 percent fatal. Rabies, derived from the Latin *rabere*, "to rave or be mad," is spread by a virus transferred from the saliva of the biter that invades the nervous system and travels to the brain. Almost any warm-blooded animal can become rabid, but since the disease is transmitted through saliva, it's usually spread by bites or licks, particularly those of carnivores (meat eaters). Animals living in the wild may bite pets, who pass on the disease to their owners. Southern Ontario has the highest reservoir of rabies in North America, carried mainly by foxes, bats, raccoons, dogs, skunks and cats.

The incubation period (time within which the disease may reach the brain and show itself) is 10 days to 8 months after the bite. The onset of the disease (in humans as well as animals) is heralded by pain around the wound, general malaise, behavior changes, a feeling of anxiety, perhaps a mild fever, unusual excitability (snapping and biting in a pet) or unusual docility (in a wolf or fox who approaches humans). Muscle spasms, especially in the throat, produce gagging and hydrophobia (fear of water), a dramatic aversion to fluids due to the inability to drink, followed by vomiting, salivation to the point of drooling and ultimate paralysis and death. An animal with paralyzed limbs should be examined for the disease. Pet owners should make sure that their animals are annually inoculated against rabies.

The life of someone bitten by a rabid animal can be saved only by injecting rabies vaccine soon after exposure, *before* symptoms appear. The sooner the vaccine is given, the faster antibodies build up. Rabies vaccination, first developed by Louis Pasteur, the "father of immunology," previously consisted of 14 daily abdominal injections that were both painful and risky. A vaccine prepared from duck embryos superseded the Pasteur vaccine, although the injections were still painful. However, a new, safe vaccine grown in human

TO PREVENT ANIMAL DISEASES, PRACTISE SENSIBLE HYGIENE

- **Keep pets' living quarters clean at all times and examine animals regularly for ticks and fleas.**
- **Wash your hands thoroughly after playing with your pets and teach your children to do likewise.**
- **If your pet is sick, take it to the veterinarian—don't wait.**
- **Be sure your animal is vaccinated properly against rabies**

and other diseases.
- **Get puppies and kittens dewormed as early as possible—some experts say 2 weeks old is not too soon.**
- **Never approach wild animals, especially in rabies-ridden areas such as southern Ontario; beware of any animal that seems to be behaving oddly, is excessively friendly or very aggressive.**

- **Teach children not to tease, overexcite or irritate animals, since it could provoke an attack, and tell them not to approach strange dogs, cats or other animals.**
- **Don't touch dead animals, as corpses can still pass on infections.**
- **Don't leave animals out alone overnight, as they may easily socialize with infected wild ones.**

diploid cells can now be administered as 5 (rather than 14) relatively painless injections.

- *Cat-scratch fever:* A mysterious malady, possibly due to the *Pasteurella* organism, this mild ailment afflicts many who are scratched or bitten by cats. Young children, liable to tease cats and get scratched, are more frequently affected than adults. The infected cats themselves show no signs of illness but carry the disease-causing pathogen on their claws or teeth. In its mild form it produces merely local swelling and soreness, but if full-blown it may lead to an abscess, swollen lymph nodes, appetite loss, fever, long-lasting malaise and other symptoms. Treatment is bed rest and fever antidotes. A team at the Centers for Disease Control in Atlanta has just isolated the bacterium that causes cat-scratch fever and is attempting to find an appropriate antibiotic.
- *Salmonellosis:* Due to *Salmonella* bacteria, a common cause of food poisoning, the disease can also be carried by many mammals, birds and reptiles, and infects about 50 percent of pet dogs. But the most notorious sources of pet-transmitted salmonellosis are imported baby turtles. During the heyday of the pet turtle business, cases of human salmonellosis acquired from touching these reptiles or their feces were a serious problem. In the United States, for instance, there were an estimated 280,000 cases of salmonellosis associated with

pet turtles during the early 1970s. Although the Canadian government banned the importation of these creatures, some Montreal dealers circumvented the regulations in 1984 and imported and hatched turtle eggs, with a consequent salmonellosis outbreak.

The symptoms of salmonellosis include diarrhea, cramps, nausea, fever and septicemia (blood poisoning). The disease is seldom serious in healthy adults, but it can be life-threatening in young children or the elderly.

- *Psittacosis* (parrot fever or ornithosis): Previously viewed as a viral infection, this is now known to be due to a rickettsial microorganism that infects birds—especially parrots, canaries, parakeets, pigeons and others of the parrot variety, as well as some small mammals. Birds infected with psittacosis may seem droopy, off their food and unkempt and should be promptly treated by a vet. In humans, the disease attacks the lungs, and symptoms often resemble influenza, with chills, coughing, headaches and fever. If severe, it can lead to chronic respiratory illness that requires antibiotic therapy.
- *Fish-tank disease:* This curious disorder, caused by a type of marine bacteria that occasionally grow in fish tanks, may spread to humans if the bacteria get into open cuts or lesions, triggering a local inflammation. The problem is easily avoided by wearing rubber gloves when cleaning fish tanks.
- *Ringworm:* Unsightly and disfiguring but not dangerous, ringworm infections stem not from worms but from a fungus that grows in a ring-shaped formation on the skin and scalp. Infected kittens, puppies, dogs, cats, and occasionally monkeys and horses, can transmit ringworm to humans. Children are at higher risk than adults, and boys more than girls. The disease is also contagious between humans. The fungal spores easily spread from person to person through inanimate objects such as toys, barber's instruments, towels and floor coverings.

Cats with ringworm often have round, sore, scaly, hairless patches on face and head. Humans who get the infection from their pets may develop small local sores and itchy swellings especially on the hands, arms and abdomen. The condition is short-lived and readily treated with antifungal creams.

- *Roundworms:* Roundworm eggs from the intestines of puppies, dogs and cats can be swallowed by humans, causing toxocariasis. After ingestion, the roundworm embryos hatch and travel to various organs, including the lungs, liver, spleen, heart, muscles and intestines, causing inflammation, flulike symptoms, diarrhea, perhaps reddened eyes. Occasionally the larvae of these worms migrate through the body to the eyes, where they can cause blindness if left untreated.

  Health authorities believe that human roundworm infections are more prevalent than previously believed, especially among toddlers. Roundworm eggs, passed out with feces, may survive for months, even a year, and infect children who play in sandboxes, gardens and playgrounds. Youngsters may ingest roundworm eggs when licking fingers or swallowing contaminated dirt or soil. Roundworm infections are particularly frequent in children with the disorder called pica (a behavioral aberration with compulsive ingestion of soil and grit).

- *Toxoplasmosis:* Caused by *Toxoplasma gondii*, a crescent-shaped microscopic parasite, this flu-like ailment goes unnoticed in most people or is mistaken for another illness such as influenza. Toxoplasmosis can be contracted by consuming undercooked, contaminated meat (especially pork) or unpasteurized milk. Cat feces can also infect humans, but only for a short period, since the infective cysts are not infective when freshly excreted, but only 3 to 5 days later. Recent studies show that almost 50 percent of North Americans show some evidence (in blood tests) of previous toxoplasma infections.

  Toxoplasmosis is a widespread parasitic disease and usually causes no symptoms. Public interest in this animal-transferred disease arises from the fact that it may attack those with weakened immune systems, such as AIDS patients, and may also endanger unborn babies. An acute toxoplasma infection in pregnancy may produce fetal brain damage, seizures, eye and skin defects, jaundice and an impaired liver and spleen. As a precaution, pregnant women should wash their hands thoroughly after preparing raw meat, not eat undercooked meat or unpasteurized milk and avoid emptying the cat's litter box if possible.

Emergency first aid

How to help in an emergency • General principles of first aid • The ABCs of AR and CPR • Allergic shock • Asphyxiation • Asthma • Bites and stings • Bleeding • Burns and scalds • Choking • Choking infants • Convulsions • Dressings and bandages • Ear injuries • Electric shock • Eye injuries • Fainting • Fractures • Frostbite and freezing • Head injuries • Heart attack • Hyperthermia • Hypothermia • Mouth injuries • Nosebleeds • Poisonings • Seizures • Shock • Sports injuries • Teeth (knocked out) • Unconsciousness • Water accidents • Where to learn first aid and CPR

17

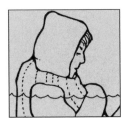

HOW TO HELP IN AN EMERGENCY

The prime necessity in helping injured people in an emergency is to *recognize* the situation as an emergency, and to know the local emergency phone number. Although the 911 number has been widely publicized, there are many areas where it is not yet operational. Know your emergency numbers at home, cottage and other regions you frequent. Post the emergency telephone number clearly on every phone in the house, and carry the appropriate emer-

gency number with you if traveling away from home. Know how to reach your provincial police or RCMP in case of a highway accident.

When calling for emergency services, clearly state what the problem seems to be—a possible heart attack, drowning or broken bone—so that the dispatcher can estimate its urgency. Also provide precise information about your location, giving the address, and stating whether it is a house, apartment or office building, the floor and room number. Always put your home address on or near the telephone(s) so that strangers such as babysitters, housecleaners and workmen can quickly find it. If you have helpers available, get someone to stay by

FIRST-AID PROVIDERS SHOULD:

- assess the situation, stay calm, take confident charge and ensure that no further harm befalls the casualty, rescuer, or bystanders; too often, a would-be rescuer becomes the next casualty;
- reassure the casualty, and urge him or her to accept necessary assistance (people sometimes deny real problems, out of

embarrassment or fear);
- summon emergency medical services quickly—speed may be of the essence;
- keep the injured warm and at rest, if possible covered and on soft ground (clothes, blankets);
- check for consciousness, breathing, pulse and bleeding;
- look for injuries—

ask the casualty whether it hurts and where;
- try to find out what happened—it may give clues to possible injuries (ask the casualty and/or onlookers what went wrong);
- prevent the condition from worsening: cover wounds, try to immobilize possible fractures, handle gently.

Do not:
- attempt more than you are able or qualified to do;
- move the casualty unless you are *certain* the injuries are minor, or unless it is absolutely necessary;
- allow people to crowd around;
- touch the casualty's body or remove the casualty's clothing unnecessarily;
- give anything by

mouth to people with a suspected internal injury, those going unconscious or those who may need an anesthetic;
- administer any medications (although you may assist a conscious casualty to take necessary medications—e.g., heart pills, insulin, etc;
- force first aid on anyone who refuses it.

FIRST AID IN THE AGE OF AIDS

Today's health-conscious good Samaritan may pause before attempting to render assistance to an injured person. The AIDS (HIV) and hepatitis B (HBV) viruses have been identified in the blood, breastmilk, sputum, tears and urine of infected people. Has first aid become risky? How can the risk be minimized?

Fortunately, there is a safe and effective vaccine against hepatitis B. All healthcare workers, those living with HBV carriers and others at risk should be immunized. For healthcare workers such as surgeons, dentists, nurses, emergency-care workers, ambulance drivers and laboratory staff who routinely come into contact with people carrying infectious diseases, there remains the risk—albeit slight—of becoming infected with HIM The likeliest way to become infected is via a cut with an infected needle or scalpel that pierces the protective gloves. It is estimated that about one person in every 200 to 250 punctured by an HIV-contaminated needle or scalpel will develop HIV infection. However, so far in Canada only one healthcare worker has reportedly developed AIDS through an occupational mishap since the epidemic began.

All healthcare professionals are encouraged to "think AIDS" and protect themselves. Very precise guidelines have been laid out for those handling body fluids and looking after sick people. In its "Universal Precautions," published in 1988, the American Centers for Disease Control (CDC) set out precise rules to make the minimal risk of contracting AIDS or hepatitis B even smaller.

Professional emergency workers and trained volunteers, such as the St. John Ambulance personnel who give first aid to the injured, are equipped with "pocket masks" for mouth-to-mouth resuscitation, as well as gloves and other protective devices. However, casual first-aiders, teachers, daycare workers and bystanders at the scene—who may be called upon to give mouth-to-mouth resuscitation or to stem bleeding—do not usually carry protective equipment.

So what is the risk to an unmasked, ungloved layperson attempting to give mouth-to-mouth rescue breaths? It's estimated to be immeasurably small—zero or close to it. True, HIV and HBV viruses have been isolated from saliva, but neither HIV nor HBV infection has ever been documented following mouth-to-mouth resuscitation given by casual first-aiders. Similarly, the risk of contracting these infections by being splashed even with contaminated blood is minimal. No case of infection by this means has ever been reported in a first-aid provider—whereas the risk to a casualty of not receiving first aid may well be tragic. Still, it is up to the rescuer to assess the situation and make the decision.

Committees of the American Heart Association (AHA) and the World Health Organization (WHO) and, most recently, the 1992 Conference on Cardiopulmonary Resuscitation and Emergency Cardiac Care, have closely examined the risks of acquiring infectious diseases through giving first aid. The AHA concluded that "the average layperson who responds in an emergency should be guided by individual moral and ethical values." That is, you do what you think is right. The WHO is even less compromising, concluding that "mouth-to-mouth resuscitation is a life-saving procedure and should not be withheld through fear of contracting HIV or other infections." It adds that "people who are bleeding require immediate attention. The first-aider must not hesitate to help them as some wounds may be life-threatening." But ultimately it is the first-aider's decision. You are never *obliged* to begin first aid unless (like a police officer or an ambulance driver) you have a special responsibility to do so.

For those who are still anxious about administering first aid, especially in situations where there is a considerable likelihood that the casualty may harbor HBV or HIV infection, various national and international agencies recommend the following procedures:

- wipe blood and saliva from the casualty's mouth with a handkerchief before attempting mouth-to-mouth resuscitation;
- try to avoid touching blood by wearing latex gloves or using a thick cloth or clothing to prevent skin contact with the injured person;
- take particular care to prevent blood from coming in direct contact with your own broken skin, abrasions, a sore or mucous membranes (mouth, nose);
- wash the hands thoroughly with soap and water after giving first aid;
- if you are bleeding yourself while performing first aid (the most likely, indeed probably the only way of contacting a blood-borne disease), encourage the wound to bleed and then wash it well;
- if you believe you have been cut or splashed in the eye or mouth with the blood of an injured person, wash promptly and consult a physician.

the front door to open it and guide the emergency personnel to the injury scene.

GENERAL PRINCIPLES OF FIRST AID

First aid is defined as "things to do until medical help arrives," not ways to replace medical procedures. Its aims are

- to sustain life;
- to relieve pain and distress;
- to prevent the condition from worsening;
- to promote recovery;
- to obtain medical care as fast as possible.

Stocking a first-aid kit

Your first-aid kit should be tailored to your family and environment—a cottage kit will need more medications than a city kit, and a car kit should have ample dressings to stop bleeding on multiple casualties. The following is a list of basics:

- absorbent cotton;
- adhesive strip plasters—assorted sizes;
- adhesive tape;
- calamine lotion;
- cotton-tipped swabs;
- painkillers such as acetaminophen or ASA (do not give ASA products such as Aspirin to children because of the risk of Reye's syndrome);
- disinfectant;
- rubbing alcohol;
- "triangular bandages" for tying splints and securing dressings;
- safety pins;
- sharp needles and tweezers to remove splinters (sterilize first);
- scissors;
- sterile eye pads;
- sterile gauze bandages—25 mm and 50 mm;
- sterile gauze pads—50 mm and 100 mm square;
- thermometer;
- tongue depressors—wooden;
- antihistamine tablets of choice;
- antibiotic cream;
- pad and pencil;
- latex gloves.

THE ABCs OF AR AND CPR

The two processes of breathing and circulation (blood being pumped by the heart) combine to supply oxygen to the cells of the body. If breathing stops, either because the air passages are blocked by a foreign object (choking) or for some other reason, the heart will be pumping blood without adequate oxygen. Soon two things will happen—brain cells will begin to die, and the heart itself will stop.

Artificial respiration (AR) refers to first-aid techniques to replace breathing—the most common and effective method being mouth-to-mouth breathing. The principle is simple—first the rescuer checks whether the airway (air passages) is blocked by a foreign body, and clears them if they are (see "Choking" in this chapter for the Heimlich maneuver); then the rescuer breathes into the casualty's lungs, supplying enough residual oxygen to keep the brain cells alive and prevent the heart from stopping. Often AR will cause natural breathing to resume.

If the heart has stopped beating too—through a heart attack, drowning, poisoning, electrocution or any other cause—AR alone is not enough, because the oxygen put into the lungs will not be pumped to the cells that need it. In this case, the further step in cardiopulmonary resuscitation (CPR)—chest compressions—is required. This is a simple process of rhythmically squeezing the heart between the breastbone and the backbone to mimic the heart's natural pumping action. The combination of rescue breathing and chest compressions may not restart the heart, but it is designed to keep oxygenated blood flowing to the brain, preventing irreversible brain damage and death, until medical help can reach the scene.

The Heimlich maneuver, AR and CPR are vital techniques for laypeople, because brain damage can begin in as little as four to six minutes—often sooner than an ambulance can arrive, even in the best of circumstances. Too many people—the diner who chokes in a restaurant, the child who slips in a wading pool, the grandparent who climbs the stairs a little too quickly—die unnecessarily, just because no one on the scene knows how to bridge that gap of a few minutes!

All these first-aid techniques are taught together in a single course under the general heading of "CPR." The methods for adult casualties can be learned in a few hours, and the

AIRWAY

It's possible that the casualty's tongue is blocking the airway. Sometimes just tilting the head and dislodging the tongue allows the unconscious person to breathe again. Gently roll the person onto his or her back (supporting the head). Then tilt the casualty's head by simultaneously lifting up on the chin and pushing down on the forehead. With the airway open, place your ear close to the victim's mouth and again try to detect breathing:

- *look—at the chest and stomach for movement;*
- *listen—for sounds of breathing;*
- *feel—for exhaled breath on your cheek.*

  If none of these signs is present, the victim is not breathing and AR is needed. If the person is breathing, and you have to go for help, first place him or her in the recovery position.

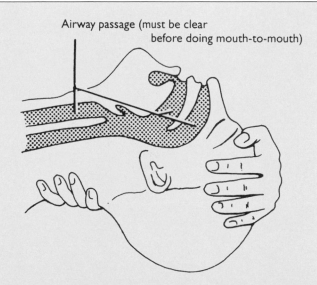

Airway passage (must be clear before doing mouth-to-mouth)

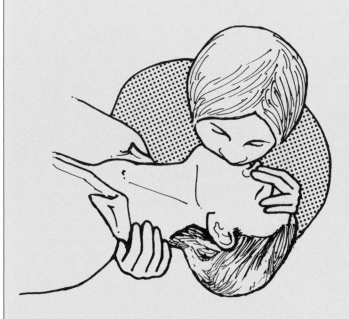

CIRCULATION

If there is no pulse, and you are trained in CPR, begin external chest compressions for artificial circulation, kneeling beside the casualty, near the chest. The chest compressions should be a straight up-and-down movement, avoiding rocking while exerting rhythmic pressure on the breastbone with one hand atop the other (see diagram) and avoiding the xiphoid process (the posterior segment of the sternum). The arms are kept straight, with relaxation between the downward pushes. A solo rescuer with a pulseless, non-breathing casualty must alternate rescue breathing with chest compressions—giving two full mouth-to-mouth breaths and then 12–15 compressions per minute—until help arrives. CPR for a child is done with one hand only, alternating one breath and five compressions. CPR on an infant alternates one puff of air with five chest thrusts done with two fingers—see infant Heimlich, "Choking infants," in this chapter. Remember that CPR must never be done on a casualty with any detectable pulse.

BREATHING

Place your mouth over the casualty's mouth, sealing well. Pinch the nostrils closed but continue to hold the head gently tilted. Breathe in two full breaths (each held for about 1–2 seconds), allowing time for the casualty to exhale in between. Watch the chest—if it does not rise, the air is not going in, and you should reposition the head and try again. If air still doesn't go in, the airway is obstructed—see "Choking." Then check for a pulse by putting two fingers gently over the carotid artery at the side of the neck for ten seconds. (The carotid is used because it's an accessible, strong pulse.) If there's a pulse but no breathing, continue rescue breathing at a rate of one mouth-to-mouth breath per five seconds (four seconds for a child). Keep watching the chest, to be sure that the breaths are going in. (If the casualty is an infant, place your mouth over the mouth and nose, and blow in light puffs only—1 every 3 seconds. Check the brachial pulse—on the inside upper arm—as the carotid is hard to find on infants.)

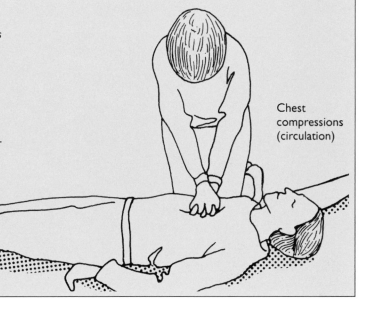

Chest compressions (circulation)

RECOVERY POSITION

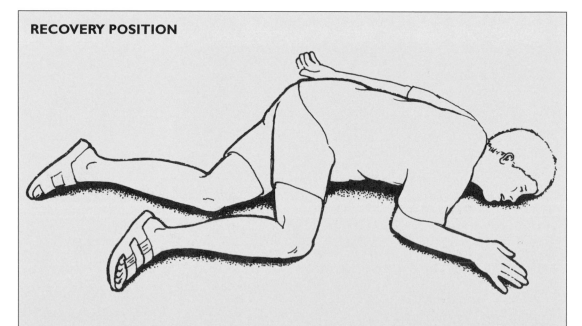

An unconscious casualty who is lying on his or her back may easily choke on the tongue or on inhaled vomit. If you are with a casualty you can watch for this and be prepared to act, but if you have to leave an unconscious person, or someone who may become unconscious—or if you have been injured yourself and are concerned about becoming unconscious—the safest position is the "recovery" position. The one knee forward and one arm back serve to prop the person securely, the bent arm should be forward near the face. The gently tilted head holds the airway open, with the mouth downward so any blood or vomit can drain out.

WHAT TO DO FOR ANAPHYLACTIC SHOCK

- **Help the casualty inject adrenalin (epinephrine) if available. Rub the site vigorously afterward to increase the absorption rate.**
- **If leaving an unconscious casualty to get help, place in recovery position.**
- **Call emergency medical services immediately.**
- **Be prepared to give artificial respiration or CPR (if qualified) if this becomes necessary.**
- **Get the casualty to hospital as fast as possible.**

techniques for children and infants take a few hours more. And the breathing and compressions are practised on mannequins, not on strangers! (See "Where to learn first aid and CPR," at the end of this chapter.)

Although basic information on the Heimlich maneuver, AR and CPR is presented below, it is no substitute for an instructor and hands-on practice. CPR (chest compressions) in particular should not be attempted without training.

Before starting first aid on someone who has collapsed, the rescuer determines whether the casualty is conscious by gently shaking his or her shoulders, asking loudly, "Are you okay?" If there's no response, it is assumed that the casualty is unconscious. After shouting out for help, and sending anyone available to call for medical aid, the rescuer kneels over the casualty—placing the cheek above the casualty's mouth and nose, and looking at the chest—and spends five seconds trying to feel or hear breathing, and to see the chest move. If there is no sign of breathing, the rescuer begins the sequence known as ABC—Airway, Breathing, Circulation.

ALLERGIC SHOCK (ANAPHYLAXIS)

Environmental pollutants, plant components, food ingredients, insect stings and other specific agents can occasionally provoke a drastic response in those allergic to them. Anaphylactic shock is an emergency indicated by one or more of the following:
- swelling of eyes, throat, tongue;
- face flushing;
- widespread hives (red weals or rash);
- difficulty breathing;
- vomiting, diarrhea;
- irregular heartbeat;
- faintness;
- loss of consciousness.

All or some symptoms can occur at the same time, often within minutes of exposure. Death can result unless the person is immediately given a shot of adrenalin (epinephrine) and taken to the nearest medical facility. People who know they are severely allergic to certain substances should wear an identification bracelet. (For details on allergic reactions, see Chapter 13, allergies section, and Chapter 11, childhood allergies section.)

ASPHYXIATION (SUFFOCATION)

Asphyxiation occurs when the airway is blocked due to any number of causes, such as strangulation, smothering or near-drowning. Airway blockage may occur from choking on foreign bodies, food, teeth, vomit and even the tongue. It also follows other conditions that prevent oxygen from entering the body, such as airway spasms due to food, water smoke, irritant gases, asthma and some chest infections. It may be caused by pillows and plastic bags that block breathing, smoke and gas fumes that displace the oxygen in the air.

Its symptoms are:
- heartbeat fast and faint, perhaps irregular;
- noisy labored breathing, with froth on the mouth;
- head, neck, face, lips and whites of eyes turning red, purple and then blue;
- drowsiness, person becoming unconscious.

ASTHMA

Asthma is a chronic breathing disorder marked by recurrent attacks of wheezing, coughing, shortness of breath, inflammation and thickened secretions (mucus). The symptoms may come on quickly or may slowly worsen over days.

Signs and symptoms of a severe asthma attack
- Tight, difficult breathing;
- wheezing (whistling) sound;
- pale, clammy skin;
- rapid pulse;
- blueness around mouth, earlobes.

What to do for a severe asthma attack
- Call 911 or relevant number for emergency medical services. Never delay seeking help—most asthma deaths are preventable with prompt medical assistance.
- Stop any activities and remove any known triggers.
- Place person leaning forward comfortably, back upright.
- Calm and reassure the sufferer.
- Check if usual medication was taken—which and how much; help casualty take more if appropriate.

- Allow plenty of fresh air—no cigarette smoke, dust.
- Be prepared to give artificial respiration or CPR (if qualified) if necessary.

BITES AND STINGS

Animal bites
Animal bites, by a bat, skunk, raccoon, fox, cat or dog, always carry some danger of infection, especially if the bite is deep. They may also carry some risks of rabies, and the animal should be kept under observation for signs of the affliction, such as agitation, viciousness, drooling, water-aversion, and paralysis.

What to do for animal bites:
- Allow some bleeding, to help cleanse the wound.
- Wash wound site thoroughly with soap and water (preferably antiseptic soap) for several minutes to remove the animal's saliva.
- Rinse well with running water or salt solution.
- If wound is on arm or leg, apply a firm bandage.
- Get medical attention even for a small cat or dog bite to see if further care is warranted, and whether there is a need for tetanus and/or rabies vaccination.
- Try to catch and restrain the animal, while taking care no one else is bitten.
- Contact animal control or police to collect the animal for observation if necessary.
For human bites that cause bleeding:
- Wash wound thoroughly with soap and water.
- Seek medical care—human bites that bleed can easily become infected.
- Notify the local-public health agency (see sections on hepatitis B and HIV infections in this chapter and Chapter 16).

Snake bites
A snake bite will show one or more puncture wounds, with swelling and discoloration in the area. Reactions may include pain and swelling, nausea, vomiting, weakness, vision blurring, sweating, difficulty breathing, speech slurring, paralysis and convulsions. But remember that the vast majority of snakes are harmless to people; unnecessary panic will only make matters worse.

WHAT TO DO FOR ASPHYXIATION
- **Move casualty to open, fresh air.**
- **Call emergency medical services.**
- **Clear airway—make sure that nothing is obstructing the air flow.**
- **Begin artificial respiration if casualty is not breathing.**
- **If no pulse can be felt, begin CPR, if qualified.**

WHAT TO DO FOR SNAKE BITES
- **Stay calm, reassure the casualty and have him or her lie down.**
- **If the snake is known to be poisonous, seek immediate medical attention. Do *not* attempt to suck out venom.**
- **Move affected part as little as possible.**
- **Do not apply ice.**
- **If bite is on a limb, splint to immobilize completely.**
- **Call the local poison control center.**
- **Be prepared to do artificial respiration or CPR (if qualified) if necessary.**
- **Transport the victim to the nearest medical center, moving the bitten part as little as possible. Bring the snake (dead); pick it up by the tail and place in a bag or sack.**

WHAT TO DO FOR STINGS BY BEES, WASPS, HORNETS, YELLOW-JACKETS OR FIRE ANTS

- **If the sting is from a bee, remove the stinger. Don't pull at it with fingers because it has a sack that can pump in more venom. Instead, scrape away cleanly with a sharp blade or credit card held against the skin.**
- **Do not squeeze or rub the skin.**
- **Wash sting site with soap and water.**
- **Apply rubbing alcohol, ice, calamine lotion or a paste of water and baking soda, unless the sting is near the eyes; if nothing else is available, cover sting with a cold compress.**
- **If the sting is in the mouth, rinse well with mouthwash made up of 1 tsp (5 ml) of bicarbonate of soda in a tumbler of cold water.**
- **Call emergency medical services if there are any signs of a severe allergic reaction (hives, pallor, weakness, nausea, vomiting, breathing problems or collapse).**
- **For allergic shock see "Allergic shock."**

Insect bites and stings

The venom of bees, wasps, hornets, yellow-jackets and fire ants produces a fierce burning, swelling and redness, as well as local swelling and itching around the sting.

What to do for bedbug, sand-fly and mosquito bites

- Wash affected area with soap and water; apply cold compresses or ice if swollen.
- Apply calamine lotion, eau de cologne or cheap perfume.
- Use antihistamine tablets if the bites are very itchy.
- For mosquito bites in malaria-infested areas, seek immediate medical advice if not protected by antimalarial tablets.

Tick bites

Wingless creatures about the size of a tiny ant, ticks range in color from brown to gray and are usually picked up in woodsy underbrush or tall grass or from the fur of free-ranging deer. The tick embeds its head in the skin to feed on animal blood. Tick bites are relatively painless, and the chief danger comes from the disease-causing organisms they may carry, such as Rocky Mountain spotted fever, Colorado tick fever tularemia or Lyme disease.

What to do for tick bites

- Remove ticks with care—don't detach with bare fingers as it may increase penetration by tick-borne microorganisms. Preferably remove tick with fine-tipped tweezers (or a gloved finger), grasping the tick near the head, as close to the skin as possible, and pulling away in a straight line. This may be painful, as the tick glues itself into the skin. Pull until tick releases its hold. Don't twist as you pull, and don't squeeze its bloated body—that may inject more bacteria into the skin. Ensure that the head of the tick is removed. (If the head stays in, seek immediate medical care.)
- Do not apply petroleum jelly, a burning cigarette or other popular methods touted for tick removal; these methods do not work.
- Thoroughly wash hands and bitten area with soap and water and apply antiseptic (such as rubbing alcohol). If you must touch the tick,

cover fingers with tissue before doing so. Wash hands thoroughly.
- Save the tick in a small container labeled with the date, the bite site and where you think the tick came from. Tell the attending physician.

Stings from marine creatures

These need emergency medical assistance, as they are often very severe and some can be fatal. Adhere carefully to local guidelines for swimming and water safety as a preventive safeguard to avoid trouble. Get local advice on whether protective wear (such as a lightweight bodysuit) is advisable. Never harass marine creatures or touch underwater life.

Marine stingers include jellyfish, sea anemones, Portuguese men-of-war and some corals. On contact with the skin, they discharge a small barb and toxin. Some sea urchins, which live on the sea bottom but may show up in shallow water have poisonous spines that can puncture the skin even through thongs or sneakers. If vacationing in places with exotic marine life, pack a small first-aid kit with needles and tweezers, rubbing alcohol, calamine lotion and baking soda.

What to do for specific marine creature attacks

- For stings by lionfish, catfish, stingrays and stonefish: place affected area in warm water (to deactivate the toxin).
- For jellyfish stings by translucent, bell-shaped creatures, of which about one in 10 produces a severe reaction with burning and stinging, possibly long red weals that look like whip marks:
  - pull off the tentacles, protecting hands with cloth or gloves to keep the stingers off the skin;
  - deactivate the jellyfish sting by washing with seawater then apply rubbing alcohol, vinegar or witch hazel.
- For Portuguese man-of-war stings (these are bright blue or purplish-red creatures that are easy to spot but have tentacles that can trail invisibly for up to 18 m or 60 ft and can provoke red weals, a severe burning pain, shortness of breath, nausea, stomach cramps and shock):

- seek immediate medical aid:
- meanwhile, treat similarly to jellyfish stings—described above (you can also try ammonia).
- For injury from coral—which on contact may release toxins, or fragments that become embedded in the skin—seek immediate medical attention as it's a potentially life-threatening situation, but meanwhile:
  - apply calamine lotion or rubbing alcohol;
  - remove coral fragments with anything at hand—a handkerchief, tweezers or needle;
  - wash with soap and water;
  - splint if possible to immobilize limb.
- For sea-anemone stings—follow same measures as for jellyfish (do not rub and do not rinse with fresh water), seek medical advice.
- For sea-urchin barbs, where the toxic spines may cause infection if not promptly removed:
  - scrub with soap and water (gets rid of some barbs);
  - extract spines with sterilized needle or tweezers—ask a physician to pull out remainder;
  - apply hot compresses or immerse in hot seawater to increase blood flow, which helps remove toxins (since the punctured part may be numb, check the water temperature with your hand or uninjured foot).
- For attacks by blue-ringed octopus, which may cause weakness of the muscles, numbness and labored breathing: be prepared to give artificial respiration or CPR (if qualified) as necessary; this may have to be maintained until the paralysis wears off. Summon medical aid.
- For stingray attacks, which may cause sudden pain, swelling, redness around wound, nausea and vomiting, muscle spasms, convulsions and breathing difficulties:
  - carefully remove stinger if possible;
  - watch the breathing; if it stops, give artificial respiration or CPR as above;
  - watch for signs of allergic shock and, if necessary, give appropriate treatment (see "Allergic shock").

BLEEDING
Any blood looks alarming, but most small wounds stop bleeding after a minute or so or with slight local pressure. Minor cuts, scrapes and abrasions do best if kept dry and open to some air. The loss of large amounts of blood causes pallor weakness, possible collapse and unconsciousness, requiring swift medical aid.

What to do for external (visible) bleeding
For minor bleeding and small cuts:
- wash with soap and warm water; apply sterile gauze dressing.
  For deeper cuts:
- apply firm, direct pressure with a gauze pad for 10 to 15 minutes (use disposable latex gloves if available, to reduce risks of picking up an infection from the casualty's blood). Apply more pressure if bleeding doesn't stop; maintain pressure and call for medical aid. (See "Dressings and bandages" in this chapter.)
- Elevate the part if possible, to drain blood back toward the heart.
- Keep person comfortable, lying down, reassure, give no drink or food.
- Call emergency medical services immediately if bleeding is severe, or if casualty vomits blood or passes blood through the rectum (blood by rectum may be black or tar-like in appearance).

BURNS AND SCALDS
For a minor burn, do not, as folklore suggests, apply butter—it won't relieve pain and may cause infection if blisters form and then break. Instead, use cold (not iced) water—by far the most effective first-aid burn treatment—which eases the pain as it cleanses.

What to do for minor (first-degree) burns
- Place the burned part in cold water or cover with cold, wet cloths, for 10–15 minutes or until the pain subsides.
- Do not apply pressure over burned skin, or try to remove clothing which has become stuck to the skin.
- Try a local anesthetic cream if skin is not broken—to minimize the discomfort.
- Apply light, dry dressing for comfort (burn ointments are not necessary). See "Dressings and bandages" in this chapter.

BLEEDING NEEDS MEDICAL AID IN THE FOLLOWING SITUATIONS:

- if blood comes in spurts (an artery may have been cut);
- if bleeding won't stop with pressure. Cover the wound with a large soft cloth and, if possible, elevate above heart level. Press directly on the wound to stop blood flow; apply an additional compress *on top* of the first, if necessary (do not remove blood-soaked dressings, as clotting may be disturbed);
- if scrape is very large (for example, the whole length of an arm or leg);

- if the face is cut, which may need plastic surgery to avoid scarring;
- if a wound seems to have dirt or debris in it;
- if there are any signs of infection—redness, pus (meanwhile, soak the wound in salty water to encourage draining);
- for cuts that look deep, with gaping edges, or jagged cuts, particularly from broken glass. If a cut seems to need stitches, do not wait more than six hours

to get them;
- for a deep puncture wound, especially one made with a dirty object (gardening toot, for example), if a tetanus booster shot hasn't been given within the past five years. Any puncture wound carries a potential threat of tetanus and calls for protective vaccination—not just clearly "dirty" ones. Arrange for a tetanus shot as soon as possible if unable to remember the date of the last one.

THE DISTRESS SIGNALS OF CHOKING

- A hand clutching the throat;
- a weak, ineffective cough;
- inability to speak or make sounds;
- increasing difficulty breathing—high-pitched wheeze;
- blue color of lips and earlobes;
- extreme efforts by the choking person to move air into the lungs, possibly with thrashing movements.

Second-degree burns and what to do for them

Signs of a second-degree burn are blistering, pain and swelling. Sunburn that causes blisters, swelling and oozing is also a second-degree burn. For second-degree burns:

- do the same as for minor burns.
- don't put on creams or lotions, they may hamper medical treatment.
- don't break blisters or peel damaged skin—you will only encourage infection.
- seek physician care.

Third-degree, or serious, burns need prompt medical attention

A deep or extensive burn, especially one caused by hot liquids or contact with fire, electricity or corrosive chemicals, requires immediate medical aid. Signs of a third-degree burn are lack of immediate pain (nerve endings have been destroyed), whiteness and or charring. These burns create severe shock, which can be life-threatening in itself. For serious burns:

- call emergency medical services.
- remove any tight clothing that is not stuck, such as rings, bangles, belts and shoes, before

tissues swell. Do not try to remove damaged tissue or break blisters.
- cover loosely with a clean dry dressing, such as gauze, handkerchief, pillowcase or strip of sheet; do not apply any home remedies such as ointments and antiseptics.
- elevate and support injured arms or legs higher than the chest.
- do not apply cold water.
- Be prepared to give artificial respiration or CPR (if qualified) if needed.
- cover casualty with a clean sheet and blanket to keep casualty warm.
- if medical help is delayed, give frequent small cold drinks if burns are extensive to replace fluid loss.

CHOKING: THE HEIMLICH MANEUVER

Choking often occurs in the pleasantest of surroundings—enjoying Christmas dinner, talking with friends over coffee and cookies or cheering at a ball game while munching popcorn. Usually a good strong cough releases whatever has stuck in the throat and the person is left somewhat red-faced, teary-eyed, possibly with a sore throat and perhaps a trifle embarrassed. But respiratory distress and oxygen lack can quickly ensue if a small object, such as a piece of food or the tab of a pop can, becomes lodged in the throat (windpipe), partially or totally cutting off air to the lungs. If coughing can't dislodge the object, death can quickly follow. Within one or two minutes the choking person can become unconscious and suffer cardiac arrest.

A large proportion of choking deaths occur because—prompted by good manners and social conditioning—the choking person seeks privacy while trying to clear the airway. Many people die locked in the bathroom. A choking person should never leave a room where others are present. If the person does leave, the potential rescuer should follow and offer to help if necessary.

Until 1976, there were two medically recommended ways to help a choking person—"washing down" the object stuck in the throat or slapping the back to dislodge it. Although today's experts consider both these older methods ineffective and even dangerous, many

THE HEIMLICH MANEUVER

Before performing any lifesaving technique on a conscious person, the rescuer must obtain consent. Ask the victim: "Are you OK? Can I help you?" Once consent is received (a nod will do), the Heimlich maneuver can be performed.

The four basic Heimlich steps used to clear the airway in adults, and in children over age one, are:

• From behind, place your arms around the victim's waist.
• Make a fist with one hand (thumb outside, not tucked in) and place the thumb side of the fist against the choking person's abdomen, well below the rib cage and just above the navel.

• Grasp your fist with the other hand and press into the victim's abdomen (just above the navel) with quick upward thrusts. (Remember, you are simulating a forceful cough.)
• Repeat thrusts until the object is expelled.

If the casualty becomes unconscious, try to make the person's fall to the ground as gentle as possible to prevent injury, especially to the head. An ambulance should be called at once, since brain and heart damage can quickly follow loss of consciousness.

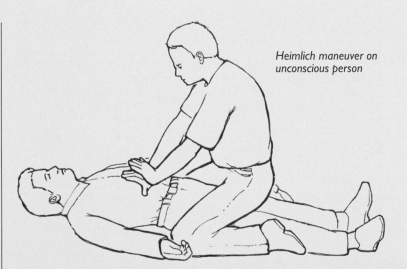

Heimlich maneuver on unconscious person

While awaiting emergency medical help, a trained rescuer can perform the Heimlich technique on an unconscious choking person, placed on his or her back. Although the principle is the same when the casualty is lying down, the technique varies slightly—the rescuer kneels astride the person, using body weight to produce upward thrusts—and several additional steps are required.

If the choker is seated, you may be able to save time by doing the maneuver in that position—depending on the chair. If the choker is a young child, you can kneel rather than stand behind. If the choker is so pregnant or obese that abdominal thrusts are impossible, pass your arms beneath the armpits and do the maneuver on the *upper* chest.

Any casualty who receives the Heimlich maneuver should seek medical attention as soon as possible, as the maneuver can cause unavoidable internal damage.

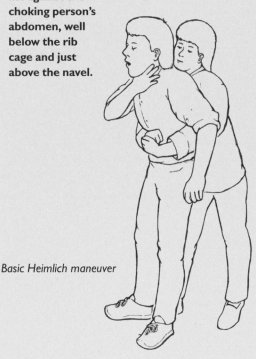

Basic Heimlich maneuver

People who choke while alone can perform steps two to four of the standard Heimlich technique on themselves, applying upward thrusts with their hands, or they can lean over a fixed horizontal object, such as a table edge, chair back or railing, pressing the upper abdomen against the edge with quick, upward thrusts.

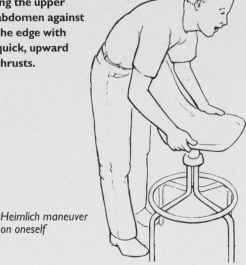

Heimlich maneuver on oneself

people still give choking persons a vigorous back blow or encourage them to take a drink or eat a piece of bread. These well-meaning techniques can push the object further down or create a bigger and more dangerous blockage.

The Heimlich maneuver, a quick, upward thrust below the diaphragm which simulates the effects of coughing, is now widely recognized as the safest and most effective way to help a choking adult or child over age one. A series of abdominal thrusts forces objects up and out of the airway. But proper training is necessary to perform the technique safely. Everyone should learn this life-saving measure.

Anyone who is choking but can still speak or cough with reasonable force should be encouraged and reassured (but *not* subjected to the Heimlich maneuver which may do unnecessary damage). But anyone who has little or no ability to breathe needs help *immediately*. Lack of oxygen does damage to the brain within minutes, so it is *not safe* to wait for an ambulance.

On children aged 1 to 8 a modified version of the Heimlich maneuver is used (see below). On infants under 12 months, use back blows and chest thrusts (see below).

Call for emergency help as soon as any choking victim can't speak, becomes unconscious or begins to turn blue.

What to do for choking

- Ask the person, "Are you choking?" If the person can still breathe and make sounds, just reassure and stay with him or her and encourage vigorous coughing.
- If the person has little or no ability to cough, speak or breathe, offer to perform the Heimlich maneuver. If consent is obtained (a nod will do), go ahead (see above).
- Summon immediate emergency help if the blockage can't be dislodged within one minute or by doing the Heimlich maneuver or if the choker can't cough or speak or is losing consciousness. (Get someone else to call, while you stay with the choking person.)

CHOKING INFANTS NEED BACK BLOWS AND CHEST THRUSTS

The Heimlich method is not recommended for infants under one year old. Instead, Canada's Red Cross Society, Heart and Stroke Foundation and St. John Ambulance advise use of back blows and chest thrusts. Always call emergency medical services at once if a choking infant becomes limp or unconscious.

First aid for choking infants

- Test whether the infant is breathing by looking for chest movements, listening (placing ear near nose and mouth) and feeling for breath on the cheek. An infant who can still breathe and cry should be reassured and allowed to cough naturally. Do *not* pound the child on the back.
- Have someone call for emergency medical services if the infant has little or no ability to breathe, cough or cry, and/or if the child is turning blue or limp.
- Meanwhile try first aid: place the infant face down—hold by the legs or straddle over the arm with *head lower* than the trunk. Deliver four blows with the heel of the hand between

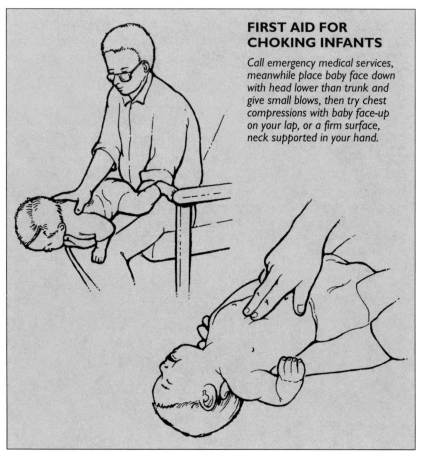

FIRST AID FOR CHOKING INFANTS

Call emergency medical services, meanwhile place baby face down with head lower than trunk and give small blows, then try chest compressions with baby face-up on your lap, or a firm surface, neck supported in your hand.

the infant's shoulder blades. (A larger infant can be lain down across your lap.)

- If the blockage is not relieved, roll the infant face up on your arm or on a firm surface, still keeping the head lower than the trunk. Give four rapid chest compressions (thrusts) over the breastbone, using two fingers only (The fingers should be centered between the nipples, and about one finger-width *below* the nipple-line.)
- If the blockage is still there after backslaps and chest thrusts, open the baby's mouth (place your thumb over the tongue and wrap your fingers around the lower jaw). If the foreign body can be seen, gently and carefully remove it with a sideways sweep of the finger (For an infant, never poke a finger into the throat or do "blind" finger sweeps for an obstruction you can't see, as this may push the object farther down.)

CONVULSIONS

During a convulsion, people may fall to the ground, stiffen, arch backward, froth at the mouth, have uncontrollable jerking movements and become unconscious. There may be a high temperature.

What to do for convulsions

- Do not try to restrain the person, or put anything between the teeth.
- Offer nothing to drink during the attack.
- Clear the surroundings of hard or sharp objects.
- Loosen any tight clothing, especially around the neck, chest or waist.
- When the convulsion has stopped, place the person in the recovery position. Cover with a warm blanket or coat if cold.
- If hot, remove excess clothing or covers and sponge with tepid water.
- Be prepared to give artificial respiration or CPR (if qualified) if necessary.
- Call for emergency medical services.

DRESSINGS AND BANDAGES

A dressing should be germ-free (sterile) and act as a filter—restricting entry of germs but allowing air to reach the wound. If sweat cannot evaporate, an infection can set in. It should also be of nonadherent material so that it will not damage the repairing wound.

Adhesive dressings (e.g., Band-Aids) consist of an absorbent pad of gauze or cellulose with an adhesive backing, which, if perforated, allows sweat to evaporate. The surrounding skin should be dry before application.

Sterile dressings are layers of gauze covered by a pad of cotton wool. They come with a roller bandage to tie them in position.

Plain gauze dressings come in a variety of sizes. They tend to stick to wounds and assist clotting. There are specialized commercial dressings for burns, eye injuries and so on. But dressings may be improvised from clean hankies, freshly laundered towels or linen, or any other clean absorbent material.

Bandages are used to hold dressings and other protections in place, and to immobilize injured areas. It is not essential that they be clean as they do not touch the wound—ties, plastic bags or even used socks can be employed, in a pinch!

Wash the hands before handling dressings, and avoid touching wounds with fingers or breathing on them. In general, minor wounds are best cleaned with soap and water—creams and ointments should be avoided. Infected wounds need physician attention.

EAR INJURIES

Ear injuries are commonly due to cuts, foreign bodies and infection. If they are associated with possible head injuries, or if blood or clear fluid is escaping from *inside* the ear seek immediate medical aid.

What to do for ear injuries

- Control bleeding from cuts by pressing gauze or a clean cloth directly over the wound and elevate the head.
- If bleeding is from *within* the ear bandage loosely and keep head elevated but with injured side tilted slightly down, to encourage drainage. (Blocking the bleeding may cause pressure inside the ear.)
- Remove insects by gently flooding the ear with tepid water or olive oil. Beads, beans, nuts and other solid objects should be removed by a doctor.

- Never stick sharp objects such as a Q-tip in the ear; if the ear feels blocked, see a doctor or instill a little warm mineral oil (a few drops) nightly and then flush well with warm water.

ELECTRIC SHOCK

Injuries due to low-voltage electrical contact are not usually severe, but can be serious for very young children or the elderly, who may go into shock. Higher-voltage shock is a major emergency causing severe burns and life-threatening shock, and requires immediate medical assistance. In *any* case of electrical shock, be careful not to touch the casualty until the source of the current has been removed.

What to do for electric shock

- Break the contact by switching off the current, removing the plug or wrenching the cable free.
- If the power is hard to disconnect, stand on something dry (blanket, rubber mat, newspapers) and break the contact by pushing the person free with a wooden pole or board, or pulling with a loop of rope around an arm or leg—or pull away a rug or carpet the person is lying on.
- Start artificial respiration or CPR (if qualified) if necessary.
- Give first aid for any burns (see "Burns and scalds" in this chapter).
- Summon emergency medical services.

EYE INJURIES

All eye injuries are potentially serious and require medical attention. Do not attempt to remove a foreign body which is on the pupil of the eye. Do not rub the eye.

WHAT TO DO FOR EYE INJURIES

For chemicals in the eye:

- Hold the eyelid open and flush with gently running tepid water for at least 15 minutes. (Make sure that the flow of water is away from the unhurt eye.)
- Don't press on the eye.
- Cover the eye with gauze loosely held in place with a bandage and seek medical aid.
  For penetrating eye injuries:
- Lay the person down.

- Give comfort and reassurance.
- If the penetrating object is still embedded, *do not remove it.* Immobilize the head to prevent movement and cover the eye and object with a paper cup or cone, secured with tape. Be sure there is no pressure on the eye or the object.
- Cover the eye with gauze padding held in place with a light bandage around the head.
- Transport to hospital immediately.
  For foreign body on the eye:
- Remove from white of eye with the corner of a clean handkerchief or a moistened wisp of cotton wool.
- If under the lower lid, pull the lid down and remove foreign body.
- If this is unsuccessful or the object is under the upper lid, try blinking with the eye under water.
- If still not removed, seek medical help.

FAINTING

Fainting is caused by a temporary shortage of oxygen to the brain. It is often due to fatigue, long periods of standing still or such stresses as fear, pain or distress. But it may also signal a more serious condition, especially in older people. If the cause of fainting is not clear, a physician should be consulted.

What to do for unusual, single episodes of fainting

- Don't allow someone who feels faint to go off alone. Help the person into fresh air if possible, and to lie down with feet up. If a standing person starts to faint, allow him or her to fall to the ground gently—do not keep sitting upright.
- Loosen tight clothing. Sponge face lightly with cold water and keep person warm. If casualty does not respond in a short time, summon medical help.
- Once consciousness returns, the person should remain lying down quietly for 10 or 15 minutes.

FRACTURES

Anyone with a suspected fracture or joint dislocation needs prompt medical attention. Suspect a fracture if an injured part is very painful, swollen or deformed, or if movement causes pain. If in doubt, treat as a fracture. Try not to move until the injury is splinted. If a neck or back injury is sus-

---

SYMPTOMS OF FRACTURES AND DISLOCATIONS

- **Pain at or near the site of injury, made worse by movement of the part;**
- **tenderness when gentle pressure is applied to affected part;**
- **swelling due to internal bleeding around fracture;**
- **loss of control of limb, deformity of limb, inability to move, unnatural movement of part;**
- **coarse, grating sound of broken ends of fractured bone;**
- **shock due to blood loss—internal or external.**

pected, do not move the casualty; summon emergency medical services. Moving someone with a spinal injury can cause paralysis or death.

What to do for fractures

- Attend to bleeding of severe wounds before dealing with fracture (see "Bleeding" in this chapter).
- Move the person as little as possible from the site of accident—only if life (the casualty's or your own) is endangered. Move by pulling the person along, holding underneath the armpits.
- Cover with blanket or clothes; give reassurance.
- Immobilize injured part as soon as possible, using other limbs and bandages as emergency support, or with makeshift splint and bandages. Raise the injured part after immobilization to reduce pain and swelling.
- Splints can be improvised from walking sticks, umbrellas, broom handles, pieces of wood, cardboard, firmly folded newspapers, folded pillows, magazines, etc.
- Splints should be sufficiently rigid, long enough to immobilize the joint above and the joint below fracture, well padded, wide enough to immobilize the part and applied over clothing.
- Bandages must be tight enough to immobilize the part but not so tight as to interfere with the circulation. Check the tightness of bandaging every 10 minutes—if distal parts of limb such as fingers or toes become pale or blue, or feel cooler than on the other limb, bandages may be too tight—and in case of swelling (especially important in elbow injuries) loosen slightly.

FROSTBITE AND FREEZING

The body areas most vulnerable to frostbite are those most exposed—the toes, fingers, ears, cheeks, nose, neck. To avoid frostbite, use the old mountaineer's adage: "Keep warm, moving and dry." Most frostbite damage occurs during the freezing and thawing process, so people who are frostbitten should be left cold until they can be completely thawed out and remain so— a repeated thawing and freezing will only increase the damage. A few hours or an extra day of frostbite causes no further damage to already frozen human tissue.

What to do for frostbite

- Shelter from further cold exposure.
- Handle and rewarm the frostbitten area gradually, but only if there is a chance of refreezing.
- For mild frostbite (tingling, slight white patches), warm extremities by holding in own (or someone else's) armpits. Warm ears and nose with palm of hand.
- Give warm drinks, not hot and *no alcohol*.
- Remove constrictive clothes, rings, boots, bracelets.
- Do not rub the affected part. Do not apply snow, cold water or any kind of direct heat.
- Do not break any blisters formed.
- For deeper frostbite, put frozen part in warm (not hot) water (41 to 43°C or 106 to 110°F) for 20 minutes or more.
- Protect frozen part from further damage. Apply sterile gauze and elevate the injured area.

HEAD INJURIES

Any moderate to severe blow on the head will likely cause some concussion (temporary brain disturbance), even if there is no damage to the underlying bone. If the blow has been severe enough that spinal injury is possible, keep the person still, do not move, and call for emergency medical services. For lesser injuries that are anything more than a small superficial cut or knock to the head, remove the person to the nearest medical aid. Any tear or cut to the scalp or face tends to bleed heavily. Most are not serious, although they look bad. Severe injury to the head can cause fracture of the underlying bones and in some cases injury to the brain.

Emergency care for head injuries

- Keep casualty lying down.
- Give warmth and comfort.
- Do not give any drinks.
- Apply a cold compress to the location of the blow or injury, but do not put pressure on the skull.
- If bleeding, clean with soap and water compress wound to stop bleeding. (Do not, however, put pressure on the skull if you suspect a fracture there, as this might put pressure on the brain.)

FIRST AID FOR FREEZING TO METAL OBJECTS

If someone has frozen his or her tongue or hand to a metal object:

- try to prevent pulling away from the metal;
- blow hot breath onto the stuck area or pour warm water onto the object. Then gently release the person;
- if bleeding occurs, as on the tongue, grasp with folded sterile gauze and apply direct pressure.

SIGNS OF FROSTBITE

- Grayish color, or whitening of skin;
- heavy numbness;
- loss of touch, sensation;
- sharp pricking, stinging, itchiness.

- If unconscious, place casualty in the recovery position (see "Recovery position," earlier in this chapter) and call emergency medical services.
- Watch the casualty in case unconsciousness sets in later even if this means half-waking the person once or twice during the night to check responsiveness (for the first 24 hours).

Call emergency medical aid if the person is:

- unconscious or drowsy;
- twitching or having convulsions;
- experiencing weakness or inability to move any body part;
- vomiting;
- oozing blood or fluid from ears or nose;
- complaining of persistent headache or double vision;
- less than 1 year old.

HEART ATTACK

A heart attack, otherwise known as a myocardial infarction, results from a small clot in one of the coronary arteries that supply the heart muscle itself with oxygen. Some heart-attack deaths are instant and likely could not be prevented by first aid; others could be averted by quicker recognition of a life-threatening situation. All too many victims of a heart attack—or those who witness one—mistake it for something else, perhaps indigestion or a muscular twinge. Lacking a sense of urgency, or denying a suspicion they are afraid to accept, many wait too long before seeking help. Waiting to "see what happens next time" often has fatal consequences. It is crucial to understand that such denial is one of the signs of heart attack; if the casualty will not respond to the situation, someone else must take charge.

Recognizing the signals of heart attack, knowing the emergency telephone number and applying CPR—an easily learned procedure—can save lives. (See "The ABC's of AR and CPR" and also Chapter 16.)

What to do for a heart attack

- Recognize the signals. Expect denial. Take charge.
- Have the person sit or lie down (semi-sitting is usually most comfortable).

- Offer reassurance; loosen tight clothing.
- If the person has known heart disease, assist in taking the usual medication, if appropriate. Maybe suggest taking an Aspirin tablet. This is especially true if the person they haven't has not taken(or been taking) their his or her daily aspirin.
- Call emergency medical services *immediately*, or go to the nearest emergency room. When calling for emergency help, identify the problem as a possible heart attack.
- Be prepared to begin CPR (if qualified) if cardiac arrest occurs.

HYPERTHERMIA (HEAT ILLNESSES)

The degree of heat-related illness ranges from mild to severe, and its onset often goes unnoticed—producing only irritability, confusion and slowed reactions. A severe rise in body heat impairs coordination, hindering the ability to focus or think clearly. Hot, confused people may further endanger themselves by failing to don hats, losing sunglasses, forgetting to take off excess clothes and not drinking enough fluids. Huge swings in blood volume and pressure may produce sudden collapse, even death.

General first aid for heat illness

- Cool down in the shade with legs and feet elevated.
- Apply wet towels or tepid water spray over the body.
- Put ice packs in groin, neck and underarms.
- Slowly sip cool (not ice-cold), noncaffeinated fluids.
- Summon medical help if serious.

Signs of different stages of heat illness

Heat cramps:
- pallor;
- sweaty skin;
- weakness and nausea;
- tingling in arms or legs.

  What to do for heat cramps:
- Massage the cramped muscle.
- Cool the body with tepid water and wet towels.
- Sip plain, cool water (don't use salt tablets). Solutions such as Gatorade aren't as good as plain water.

Heat syncope (fainting):
Typically seen in outdoor summer workers, travelers unaccustomed to hot, humid conditions and those who stand a lot in one position (e.g., military personnel), its symptoms are dizziness fainting, light-headedness, clammy skin.

What to do for heat syncope:
- Get away from the heat.
- Lie down with legs raised.
- Apply wet towels all over.

Heat exhaustion:
This stage of heat illness may build slowly over several days or weeks. Its symptoms are profuse perspiration; vague flulike malaise; fatigue, extreme listlessness; rapid pulse; pale, clammy skin.

What to do for heat exhaustion:
- Stay in a cool place, lying down with feet elevated.
- Replace body fluids.
- Apply wet towels to the body.

Heatstroke

The most serious stage of heat illness, and a potentially fatal condition, heatstroke calls for emergency medical aid. In heatstroke, the sweat glands stop working, resulting in a dangerously high body temperature—possibly above 41 (106°F) or rectally, even as high as 44°C (111°F).

The symptoms are:
- cessation of sweating;
- agitation, restlessness, bizarre behavior (the most telltale sign);
- rapid pulse;
- hot, dry, reddened look;
- drop in blood pressure, dizziness;
- headache;
- staggering gait;
- seizures, unconsciousness.

N.B.: A cool skin may hide a deceptively high core body temperature.

What to do for heatstroke (while awaiting medical aid):
- Remove casualty to a cool place.
- Remove as much clothing as possible.
- Cool the body by fanning, spraying or sponging with cool, not cold, water. (Even if clothes can't be removed, water-cool the casualty.)
- Give small amounts of fluids.

- Monitor the casualty. Be prepared to do artificial respiration or CPR (if qualified) if necessary.

HYPOTHERMIA (COLD INJURY)

Hypothermia is a dangerous cooling of the body's interior or "core." Mild hypothermia occurs with a body temperature drop to between 33 and 35°C (91–95°F); below 30°C (86°F), hypothermia is life-threatening. Hypothermia may result from cold weather or from prolonged exposure to chilly water.

In *mild hypothermia*, shivering is intense (the body's effort to produce heat); the person has slow reactions, stumbles, has slurred speech and acts as if intoxicated.

In *moderate hypothermia*, shivering lessens; the person is very tired, seems withdrawn and irritable, may act strangely—even undress despite the cold—due to a deceptively warm sensation. The pulse is slow and weak. Breathing can be slow and shallow.

In *severe hypothermia* (core body temperature under 30°C or 86°F), shivering ceases, the pupils have a fixed stare, the person may hallucinate and lose consciousness; heartbeat and breathing become slow, almost undetectable.

What to do

For mild to moderate hypothermia (person still shivering and coherent):
- Prevent further heat loss, get to shelter.
- Put on extra clothes, replace wet clothing with dry.
- Gradually rewarm by placing between blankets, cuddling against others, sharing a sleeping bag.
- Give tepid water sweets (sugar) if still conscious.
- Do not give alcohol; it dilates the blood vessels and gives a false sense of warmth.
- Check pulse—if slow, condition is worsening.
- If person doesn't recover within 30 minutes, summon emergency medical services.

For severe hypothermia:
- Get medical aid as fast as possible. Correct rewarming of someone with severe hypothermia can make the difference between life and death. (It's often safest to leave severely hypothermic people cold until reaching medical assistance.)

WARNING SIGNS OF HEAT-RELATED ILLNESS

- **Red, dry skin (later turning pale and clammy);**
- **decreased sweating;**
- **confusion;**
- **rapid pulse;**
- **dizziness;**
- **headache;**
- **nausea.**

- Rewarming must not be fast, as it may harm the heart. Below 30°C (86°F) the heart is in danger of fibrillating (producing irregular beats) and needs constant monitoring.
- While transporting to hospital, keep the hypothermic person horizontal with as little jolting as possible. With a slowed metabolic rate, the body is in a "metabolic icebox" that may protect it from more damage.

MOUTH INJURIES

- Clear the mouth of any broken teeth. For first-aid action if whole teeth have been knocked out, see "Teeth (knocked out)," later in this chapter.
- Lean the casualty slightly forward. Provide a bowl for the person to spit into.
- Apply direct pressure to tooth socket or wound by placing thick gauze or cotton-wool pad firmly in position.
  For tongue, cheek or lip:
- Compress the bleeding part between finger and thumb, using a clean handkerchief or gauze dressing until bleeding stops. Have the casualty bite on the pad for five to ten minutes, supporting the chin with the hand.
- Do not wash the mouth out, as this can disturb the clotting. Do not attempt to plug the sockets of lost teeth.

NOSEBLEEDS

Bleeding from the nose is very common and does not usually denote anything serious. It is generally due to a ruptured blood vessel in the septum, which divides the nostrils. However, severe head injuries may cause blood to trickle from the nose (see "Head injuries" in this chapter).

What to do for nosebleeds

- Sit up and do not lean forward tilt the head slightly back.
- Loosen any tight clothing around the neck.
- Pinch the lower end of the nose to close the nostrils continuously for 5 to 10 minutes. (Do not press on the bony part of the nose because this does not work.)
- Apply cold compress to forehead and bridge of nose.
- Don't blow nose for several hours afterward.
- If bleeding doesn't stop within 15 to 20 minutes, seek prompt medical advice.

POISONINGS

There are nearly three million cases of poisonings each year in North America, almost 70 percent of them in children under age six. Poisons may enter the body by being swallowed, inhaled, absorbed through the skin or injected under the skin. Children mistake household cleaners for beverages, or medications for candy, sometimes playfully emulating adult drug-taking, with possibly serious, even fatal, results. Nearly half of all accidental poisonings are caused by ASA, acetaminophen (such as Tylenol), insecticides, household bleach, detergents, fragrances, cleaners, furniture polish, kerosene, iron and vitamin compounds, disinfectants, deodorizers, lye, other corrosives or laxatives. To be prepared for poisonings, post the number of the local Poison Control Center near every phone.

Poisoning can cause a variety of effects on breathing and the central nervous system, and may lead to collapse, unconsciousness and death. The following early signs may help to identify the nature of the poison.

- *Swallowed*: nausea, cramps, vomiting; burning or discoloration around mouth; odor of poison on breath.
- *Inhaled*: coughing, chest pain, disturbed breathing; some gases cause dizziness and headache.
- *Injected or absorbed through the skin*: irritation at point of entry. Injected poisons usually act more quickly than those absorbed through the skin, and have more widespread effects.

What to do for poisonings

- Call your local poison control center. Give the age of the person, what was ingested, how much, when ingested, how the casualty is feeling or acting, your name and phone number. If you are directed to go to an emergency department, take the container of poison or a sample with you. Save any vomit for later analysis.
- Keep a bottle of syrup of ipecac (available over the counter at pharmacies) on hand to induce vomiting if needed. But *do not use it* unless instructed to do so by the Poison Control Center or a physician. Some corrosive chemicals and petroleum products cause even more harm if they are brought up. If in doubt, treat the poison as a corrosive substance.

- If using syrup of ipecac, give 5–10 ml (1–2 tsp) every 15 minutes.
- Never make someone vomit if he or she:
  - is drowsy, sleepy or unconscious;
  - has swallowed a petroleum product (such as furniture polish, Varsol, kerosene, gasoline) or corrosives (such as lye or bleach).

What to do for specific poisonings

- *For swallowed poisons*, give plenty of milk or water if so instructed by a physician or Poison Control Center loosen clothes, allow plenty of fresh air.
- *For splashes in the eye*, flood the eye with luke-warm water for at least 15 minutes. Encourage blinking while flushing the eye, but do not force the eyelid open. (See "Eye injuries" in this chapter.)
- *For liquid poisons on the skin*, remove contaminated clothing and flood the area with water, then follow with mild soap wash and a final rinse.
- *For corrosive powders on the skin*, brush off powder using a cloth or tissue (not the bare hand), then treat as for liquid poisons on the skin.
- *For inhaled poisons*, move casualty to fresh air immediately or open all doors and windows. Be prepared to do artificial respiration or CPR (if qualified) if necessary.
- *For injected poisons*, keep casualty at rest and keep limb at heart level to slow absorption. Seek medical aid immediately. Be prepared to do artificial respiration or CPR (if qualified) if necessary.
- *If the casualty is unconscious*, place in recovery position (see "Recovery position" in this chapter).
- *As a rescuer*, take care not to get contaminated while decontaminating someone else.

SEIZURES

Seizures, or convulsions, are characterized by a stiffening of the body, eyes rolling upwards and jerky movements of face and limbs. They are usually very brief, lasting one to two minutes, but occasionally up to 15 minutes. Most seizures, especially in young children, are due to high fever—known as febrile seizures, these occur in 2 to 5 percent of children aged five months to five years of age. Other seizures are due to epilepsy. (See "Childhood fever" in Chapter 11, and "Epilepsy" in Chapters 11 and 16.) But seizures can also indicate serious medical problems such as stroke.

What to do for seizures

- Remain calm.
- Protect the person from injury.
- Lie the casualty on the side, with head lower than hips, or on the stomach.
- Put nothing in the mouth.
- Summon emergency medical help if the seizure lasts more than five minutes, or if it is the person's first seizure.

SHOCK

The medical condition known as "shock" results from inadequate blood circulation to body tissues. It accompanies all injuries and illnesses, to some degree, and when severe it can lead to unconsciousness or death. It should certainly never be underestimated and dismissed as "just shock"!

Signs of shock are:
- pale or bluish complexion;
- cold, clammy, sweaty skin;
- possible giddiness, blurring of vision and vomiting;
- pulse at first rapid, perhaps later becoming very faint, almost undetectable;
- drowsiness and possibly unconsciousness;
- rapid and shallow breathing.

What to do for shock

- Sit or lay the person down and deal with the immediate causes of shock (bleeding, pain, despair, fear, etc.). Move as little as possible.
- Do not overheat, as warmth draws blood into skin and away from vital organs.
- Do not give drinks.
- Loosen any tight clothing and allow plenty of fresh air.
- If injuries permit, keep the person's head flat and support the legs in an elevated position—this encourages blood flow to the brain.
- If vomiting seems likely or the person is unconscious, place in the recovery position (see "Recovery position," on page 559).
- Summon medical aid as soon as possible.
- Be prepared to give artificial respiration or CPR (if qualified) if necessary.

SPORTS INJURIES

Sports injuries range from simple bruises and strains to dislocated joints and broken bones. They can be sudden and acute or occur slowly due to overuse. A few, such as spine or skull fractures, hyperthermia (heat stress), abdominal bleeds or organ rupture can threaten life. Given the importance now placed on physical fitness, the management of sports injuries has become a prime sphere of emergency medicine.

Main types of sports injury

Acute sports injuries can happen in several ways:

- by a hard force, blow or jolt—including overstretching (such as a pulled hamstring muscle);
- through friction or repetitive mechanical irritation (such as friction tenosynovitis—inflammation of the sheath around the tendon);
- by twisting (such as ligament or tendon tears and fractures);
- via shearing/sliding forces (such as abrasions, cuts, fractures);
- from consistent overuse—repeated, long-term abuse of the musculoskeletal system—through intrinsic factors (such as muscle imbalance or malalignment of the leg/foot during activity) or extrinsic factors (such as faulty training techniques, improper equipment or poor surfaces).

Key steps in managing sports injuries

- Use the PRICE principle: protect, rest, ice, compression and elevation, plus limited motion as soon as possible after injury. The primary goal is to reduce the inflammation that follows injury in the first 72 hours as blood and tissue fluids accumulate at the injured site.
- Rapid swelling suggests damage to blood vessels. Once the swelling goes down, gentle controlled movement should begin, with gradual return of the injured area to full function. Experts strongly promote prudent, limited movement during recovery.
- Consult a physician about any but the mildest of sprains, strains or other injuries.
- Never disregard pain.
- Wrap the injured part in well-crushed ice or a package of frozen peas (wrapped in a towel or old woolen sock to prevent frostbite) and apply for 15 to 20 minutes every two hours for severe injuries, every six hours for less severe injuries. Deep-seated injuries will require the full 20 minutes, one to four times daily. Apply ice for briefer periods if the injury is close to the skin. (Do not use ice if you have circulatory problems.)
- Apply pressure (compression) with an elastic bandage that's moderately tight but does not press on nerves or reduce blood circulation. Always wrap from the point farthest away from the heart toward the heart (e.g., wrist to elbow). The tensor bandage should not usually be worn at night, to prevent circulation problems. Tip: if the far end of the injured limb turns blue, the bandage is too tight!
- Elevate the injured part to prevent pooling of the fluid accumulated by inflamed tissues. The goal is to let gravity direct blood back to the heart. Injured legs should be propped at rest above hip level. Injured hands and forearms can be supported in a sling with hands at shoulder level. For upper-arm injuries, raise the arm above the head at regular intervals.
- To combat pain, use painkillers.
- To reduce swelling/inflammation, take ASA or other nonsteroidal anti-inflammatories—such as naproxen (Naprosyn or Aputex) or ibuprofen (Advil)—as advised by a physician.
- Beware of prolonged inactivity—begin limited gentle exercise during recovery to regain strength and flexibility, preferably guided by a trained physiotherapist.
- Return to full activity only when well healed and pain-free—usually 10 days to 8 weeks for a sprain or fracture, depending on severity.
- Beware of heat, often improperly used to treat exercise-induced injuries. Never apply heat to any bruise, strain or soft-tissue injury. (That means no hot baths and no heating pads following such injuries.) It's generally best to opt for ice. Heat may make the injury feel better, but will also increase local inflammation and worsen the swelling. Heat should only be used, if at all, once the swelling has gone down. Contrast baths alternating cold with hot water—may be useful for stimulating blood circulation to the injury, but only several days after the acute injury phase.

COMMON SPORTS INJURIES AND THEIR TREATMENT

- *Skeletal injuries* are fractures that involve the breaking of bone(s) and are potentially serious. If the skin remains intact, the broken bone is a simple or closed fracture. If the skin is pierced by the broken bone, the break is an open fracture. Skeletal injuries result mainly from falls and blows in cycling and contact sports such as football, hockey, soccer and rugby. Consequently, sport authorities ban potential sources of severe fracture injuries, such as "boarding" in hockey and "collapsing the scrum" in rugby. Bicycling accidents and careless diving into shallow or rocky waters are common causes of severe head and spinal injuries.

Treatment of bone fractures involves:
- consultation with a trained physician;
- cleaning and covering up any open wound(s) to avoid infection;
- elevating the limb/part at first if possible;
- immobilizing the affected limb by splinting;
- applying a supportive cast, and sometimes surgery to fix the bone by a plate or nail

- *Soft-tissue injuries/bruises* usually include blood-vessel damage, muscle spasm, pain and swelling.

Treatment of soft-tissue injuries aims to reduce swelling, relieve pain and prevent further damage (allowing a return to activity as swiftly as possible) by applying ice and compression (pressure), elevating the damaged part and ensuring limited motion only, until healed. (Heat is not the best treatment for acute bruises or other soft-tissue damage in the first 72 hours.) Medications can be helpful for pain, but in the long run active physiotherapy and a graded return to activity are most helpful.

- *Muscle strains*—among the mildest and commonest of sports injuries—usually arise from a direct or indirect blow, or from overuse when muscle fibers are overstretched or torn, causing bleeding and an acute inflammatory response with pain, tenderness, swelling and reduced mobility.

The basic treatment for strains is:
- application of ice or cooling packs;
- elevation of the affected area;
- an elastic support bandage (between ice treatments);
- alleviating the load on the affected part while it heals with crutches, canes, walkers or slings;
- rest—but usually not total disuse. Limited movement is often best during recovery.

- *Sprains* are joint injuries involving the partial or complete tearing of ligaments (which join bone to bone), such as ankle, knee, shoulder and elbow sprains. They occur when a joint is forced beyond its normal range of motion. Quick diagnosis and speedy treatment hasten recovery.

Treatment for sprains includes a thorough examination by a physician, physiotherapist, or athletic therapist to diagnose the severity of the ligament tear plus prompt measures to reduce the swelling with ice, compression and elevation. Usually it is very difficult to tell the extent of the injury at the beginning and this becomes more apparent with time. The sooner ice is applied, the more it diminishes swelling due to fluid accumulation. Ice also acts as a local anesthetic and may relieve muscle spasm. Apply ice three to four times a day to the injured area, for 20 minutes each time. A flexible elastic bandage will stabilize the joint, help to reduce swelling and aid recovery. Depending on their severity, sprains require complete rest (and sometimes immobilization in a cast) for 72 hours or longer and perhaps also temporary use of crutches for ankle and knee sprains. Controlled motion is usually advocated (to avoid prolonged joint immobility) after the first 72 hours, avoiding twisting or full weight-bearing, slowly progressing to more movement—using pain as the guide. The return to full activity should be gradual, with only limited movement until the sprain is completely healed. Serious sprains may need surgical repair.

- *Joint dislocation* occurs if the joint capsule and its surrounding ligaments are torn by an extreme movement exceeding the joint's normal range of motion. Dislocations can be total (joint parts no longer in contact with each other) or partial (bone ends still partly in contact).

Treatment of dislocations is by application of cooling packs and immediate transportation to a physician or hospital for assessment and treatment to reposition the dislocated bones. *Do not* try to replace a dislocated joint by home methods.

- *Tendon injuries* involve the complete or partial rupture of a tendon (which attaches bone to muscle). Tendon tears may be acute (sudden) or chronic (from continual overuse), and are especially frequent in people who take up a new sport, in those who exercise after a sedentary life and in athletes who increase their training volume too quickly.

Treatment of tendon injuries requires the usual—rest, ice, elevation—and perhaps also a supportive bandage or immobilizing cast, a mild exercise regime during recovery (especially stretching exercises) and anti-inflammatory drugs. Complete tendon tears need the attention of an orthopedic surgeon, immobilization in a brace, sling or cast, and occasionally surgical repair. Athletes should not return to full training until complete tendon strength is regained. Stretching exercises and gentle movement aid recovery.

- *Nerve or neurological injuries* involving the brain and spinal cord are mostly due to the impact of the head, neck or back against a solid structure (such as the boards in hockey, the cement bottom of a swimming pool or an icy surface)—even at a slow pace. Head and spine injuries—most frequent in young males—can be catastrophic, producing lifelong disability or death. Sport and recreational activities are the second-commonest cause of spine and head injuries in Canada (following auto crashes).

Treatment of head and spinal injuries requires extreme caution. The spine must be completely immobilized to prevent additional damage from the movement of an unstable vertebral column. Return to some sports may be impossible after severe injuries; even mild spinal injury may hamper the resumption of usual sporting activities.

- *Eye injuries* are particularly common in racquet sports such as squash, tennis and badminton (among adults) and in hockey, baseball, football and soccer (among children). Many can be prevented by enforcing game rules, better supervision, wearing suitable eye protectors endorsed by the Canadian Standards Association—types with polycarbonate lenses mounted in a sturdy frame. Lensless eye protectors are no longer recommended for racquet sports and hockey. (See "Eye injuries" in this chapter.)

WATER SAFETY TIPS (ESPECIALLY FOR CHILDREN)

- Teach children to swim as soon as possible.
- Don't leave unsupervised young children near water deeper than 5 cm (2 in).
- Never leave a baby alone near water or in the bathtub even for a moment—drowning can happen in seconds.
- If the telephone rings while bathing baby, wrap in towel and carry with you to the telephone—also when answering the doorbell.
- Never let young children play around cesspools, puddles, ditches or wells.
- Keep swimming pools covered with a hardtop during months when not in use.
- Forbid young children to enter neighbors' swimming pools without permission.
- Never let a toddler run loose near a pool.
- Know the depth of a pool before letting a child enter the water.
- Encourage children to use inflated tubes, rafts or armbands under supervision.
- Never let your child go swimming alone.
- Never allow a child to get out of his or her depth unless well able to swim.
- Keep all children out of boats unless supervised.
- Supervise all fishing expeditions—never let a child go fishing alone.
- Insist that everyone wear life-jackets or PFDs when boating or canoeing.

When to seek medical advice for sports injuries

One person's ache is another's agony. Pain is an individual matter, but even minor delays in consulting a physician can allow serious, longstanding problems to develop. Never hesitate to seek expert help if the injury is more than a simple bump or bruise. Consult a physician or sports-medicine specialist within 48 hours if the injury does not seem to be getting better, to check for fractures and other damage. Sports-medicine specialists can discuss the right shoes and equipment, and the safest training techniques.

TEETH (KNOCKED OUT)

Baby (primary) teeth are not usually replaced if knocked out or broken, but adult (permanent) teeth may recover if carefully replanted.

What to do for knocked-out teeth

- Rinse mouth gently in running water.
- Do not rub or scrub mouth.
- Do not handle the tooth by its roots.
- Gently insert the tooth into its socket and hold it there.
- If it's not possible to reinsert the tooth, place it in cool water or milk or in damp gauze. Do *not* store the tooth in antiseptic.
- Get to dentist as fast as possible preferably within 30 minutes.

UNCONSCIOUSNESS

The first stage of unconsciousness is often drowsiness, from which the casualty may be easily aroused; the next stage may be stupor, from which arousal is difficult; the most serious and advanced stage is coma, from which the person cannot be aroused. Unless the person is fully alert, or can be roused, treat as if unconscious.

What to do for unconsciousness

- Ensure that the airway is open and that the person is breathing.
- Summon emergency medical services immediately.
- Loosen clothing around neck, chest and waist.
- Ensure that plenty of fresh air is available.
- If injuries permit, lay in recovery position—preferably with the lower part of the body slightly raised above the head. This will ensure that vomit or saliva does not flow into the lungs. (See "Recovery position" in this chapter.)
- Cover with a blanket and stay with casualty until medical help arrives. Never leave an unconscious person unattended for even a moment unless it is absolutely necessary.
- Speak reassuringly even while the casualty appears to be unconscious.
- If consciousness returns, moisten the lips and keep the person calm and quiet. Never try to give a drink to an unconscious person.

WATER ACCIDENTS

Personal flotation devices (PFDs) should be worn at all times when boating—not just in rough or cold weather. The type to choose is a CSA-approved one. Standard kapok and loose foam vests give little protection; close-fitting foam vests or garment-type, insulated plastic flotation jackets or suits are better. The newer survival body suits—hooded and with shorts—are best for extending survival time.

What to do in a water accident

- If submerged in water or fallen overboard, don't remove clothes (except large, loose boots). Although clothing feels heavy, it retards body-cooling by over 50 percent. The heavier the clothing, the better the insulation.
- Given a choice in a boating mishap, don't dive

but jump feet first into water. Lower yourself in gently if possible.

- Keep as much of the body as possible above water and hang on to any available floating object, such as an overturned boat or log.
- Reduce movement to a minimum. Exercise increases core heat loss—by over 30 percent—compared to holding still and shivering in cold water.
- Treading water is best (if not wearing a PFD), keeping the head above water.
- Adopt the HELP (Heat Escape Lessening Posture—see diagram), a tucked-up or fetal position, with arms tight against chest, elbows bent, knees tucked up to protect the groin. This posture lessens heat loss and increases survival time.
- Unless in warm water, never adopt the "drownproofing" position (floating with arms wide open, face down, coming up occasionally for air). Although "drownproofing" uses less energy than treading waters, much heat is lost from the open arms and immersed head. In cold Canadian waters, drownproofing is a fast route to hypothermia, exhaustion and drowning.
- Several people who are immersed can preserve body heat by huddling together pressing their chests together.
- Sandwich children between adults or place them on top of a flotation device.
- After the rescue, wrap up in warm, dry blankets topped by a waterproof cover (even a plastic garbage bag). Later get into a warm bath. Have hot, nonalcoholic drinks and calorie-rich snacks.

Scuba-diving complications

Scuba divers learn to recognize dive-related disorders (barotrauma) in their training, but often react to their symptoms with denial; also, some people dive without proper training. Dive-related disorders require intensive oxygen administration and frequently need treatment in a hyperbaric (pressure) chamber as well.

Anyone who shows any of the following signs of barotrauma after scuba diving—regardless of the length or depth of the dive—should contact a physician knowledgeable about diving without delay:

- dizziness, visual blurring;

"HELP" POSITION IN WATER

A "tucked-up" position lessens heat loss in cold water, increasing survival time.

- pain in chest or limbs;
- disorientation or personality change;
- numbness, tingling;
- unusual fatigue, weakness or paralysis;
- bloody froth from nose or mouth;
- skin itching or blotchy rash;
- shortness of breath or coughing spasms;
- staggering;
- convulsions or collapse.

If a "diving doctor" is not available, call the Divers Alert Network (DAN) 24-hour emergency hotline: (919) 684-8111.

WHERE TO LEARN FIRST AID AND CPR

You can learn first aid—including the Heimlich maneuver and artificial respirations, with or without CPR—in a weekend or a few evenings. Courses are run regularly by local branches of the Red Cross and the St. John Ambulance Society.

Courses in artificial respiration and CPR (as well as the Heimlich maneuver) are also taught by the Red Cross and St. John Ambulance, as well as the Heart and Stroke Foundation, the Royal Life Saving Society, and many other educational and community organizations. Courses range from a few hours to a full weekend or several evenings.

Specially tailored courses are available for people with particular needs and interests—such as babysitters, new parents and those giving extended healthcare in the home. Courses in first aid and CPR for children are also offered by the Canadian Pediatric

IN CASE OF DROWNING

- **Once on land, immediately hold children hanging over the knee for five to ten seconds to encourage free drainage of water from lungs.**
- **Summon emergency services.**
- **If necessary, commence artificial respiration or CPR (if qualified).**
- **Be sure *anyone* who has aspirated (breathed in) water—fresh or salt—gets medical attention. Even someone who feels fine may have suffered lung damage which, if not treated immediately, can lead to acute respiratory distress within hours.**

Sensible use of medications

Use and abuse of prescribed drugs • Use nonprescription medications wisely

 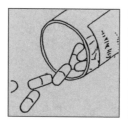

MEDICATIONS ARE AN essential part of modern healthcare, but they can bring harm if used unwisely. Today's medications fall under two broad headings: prescribed drugs available only with a physician's prescription, and nonprescription or over-the-counter (OTC) medications. Prescription medications are usually dispensed for more serious or ongoing chronic conditions and include those most likely to be misused or to cause dangerous side effects. Some products available as over-the-counter preparations in one form need a prescription in another. The amount of active drug in the medication usually determines whether a prescription is required. Examples: "222s" (containing 8 mg codeine) can be purchased over-the-counter *without* a prescription, but "Tylenol No. 3s" (containing 30 mg codeine) need a prescription; Advil (containing 200 mg ibuprofen) is available OTC, while Motrin (tablets containing 300 mg ibuprofen) needs a prescription.

When and how to take medications

Always follow instructions about how and when to take medications. Although we may leave the doctor's office clutching a prescription we hope will cure us, many of us collect the medication from the pharmacy but fail to follow the instructions, or perhaps never even start on what was prescribed. On average, only half of us complete the course or take all the pills as commanded. We may skip pills or just stop taking the medication as soon as we feel better or seem to recover from whatever ails us. In some cases, not completing the course or skipping medication may do no harm, but for many conditions such as diabetes, high blood pressure, depression and heart disease, failure to adhere to the prescribed treatment plan can have serious consequences. For example, taking too much or too little insulin can be life threatening for those with diabetes; suddenly giving up antidepressants (instead of tapering them off slowly) can precipitate withdrawal symptoms such as nausea, headaches and overwhelming anxiety; and stopping antibiotics before finishing the whole course can create antibiotic-resistant bacterial strains that make people very ill. The key to better adherence is better doctor-patient relationships in which the caregiver takes time to explain what the problem is and why and how certain medications can help, how they work and why it's necessary to stick with it. (Many people only adhere to instructions once they have had a fright or experienced complications from failing to take medications properly.) For complex medication regimes involving several different drugs to be taken at different times, marking each container with the medicine's name and what it's for, getting a pillbox with compartments and making a calendar can help. Also, getting to know and asking about possible

HOW GRAPEFRUIT JUICE ALTERS MEDICATION EFFECTS

Grapefruit juice boosts the serum (blood) concentrations of many medications. It contains *furanaocoumarin* substances that bind to and inhibit the activity of certain *cytochrome* enzymes (such as cytochrome **P450** and **CYP3A4**) in the small intestine. Usually, the cytochrome enzymes metabolize or partially break down many medications before they are absorbed into the bloodstream. Owing to its particular make-up, grapefruit juice blocks or hand- cuffs the enzymatic breakdown of many medications, thereby allowing blood levels of the drug to build to greater-than-normal concentrations, with possibly toxic effects.

The ability of grapefruit juice to increase drug absorption was first discovered during trials with *felodipine* (**Plendil**), a calcium channel blocker used for heart disease, in which blood levels of Plendil shot up after people drank grapefruit juice. Since then, the list of drugs affected by grapefruit juice has grown to include many familiar and widely used medications such as the cholesterol-lowering statins (including **Lipitor, Zocor, Crestor** and others), some benzodiazepines (tranquilizers), budesonide, cyclosporine and erythromycin antibiotics, some estrogens, nifedipine (**Adalat**), sertraline (**Zoloft**), fluoxetine (**Prozac**), verapamil and the anticoagulant, warfarin (**Coumadin**).

Since the drug-boosting effects of grapefruit juice can last several hours, even up to 24 hours, people should be wary when taking medications affected by this citrus fruit. The effect varies according to the type and amount of grapefruit juice swallowed. For example, 1 daily glass of normal-strength white grapefruit juice for 3 days doubled blood levels of some statin drugs (lovastatin and simvastatin); and 3 full glasses a day gave up to fifteenfold increases in these medications.

Most other citrus juices (sweet orange and tangerine) don't contain furanocoumarins and therefore have no effect on drug concentrations although **Seville** oranges, tangelos and Indian pomelos can affect medication levels. So it's best to check with the pharmacist or doctor about possible interactions, especially when blood concentrations need to be carefully controlled.

side effects, and telling your doctor about any experienced is a good idea. In some cases, simply taking an alternative medication may solve the problem.

Finding out how and when best to take medications, and what may interact adversely with them helps people obtain their best effect. For instance, some medications should never be taken with or soon after milk or other dairy products, while others are powerfully affected by acidic or citrus foods such as grapefruit. To aid absorption, some drugs should be taken on an empty stomach (one hour before or two hours after meals) with a full glass of *cold* water. It is sometimes unwise to take medications with acidic juices, milk, fizzy pop or food unless advised by a pharmacist or doctor that it's okay to do so. For example, the (prescription) antibiotic tetracycline does not work nearly as well when accompanied by milk products, antacids or calcium supplements, as they bind to the drug and reduce its effectiveness. Laxatives containing bisacodyl (found in Dulcolax) may cause severe cramping if taken with milk or antacids. Many antibiotics and the bone-building anti-osteoporotic drugs (such as Fosamax, Actonel) are best taken on an empty stomach. On the other hand, some medications should be consumed with food. For example, ASA (Aspirin), especially non-coated preparations, commonly cause some stomach bleeding and are best consumed with light food, milk or a full glass of water. Certain substances, such as the cholesterol-lowering statin drugs (e.g., Lipitor, Zocor), work best if taken in the evening as the body's cholesterol production rises during the night and their inhibiting presence is needed then.

Watch for adverse drug reactions with alcohol

Alcohol interacts with many medications. Itself a potent drug, alcohol reduces coordination, depresses central-nervous-system function, diminishes alertness and impairs judgment These effects are easily exacerbatedby various prescription and OTC drugs, which increase central nervous system depression, perhaps even leading to respiratory failure. For instance, with antihistamines, tranquilizers or sedatives, alcohol greatly increases drowsiness, further depresses brain function and may cause dizziness, impairing coordination and driving ability, undermining the capacity to handle any complex machinery. Medications that should *not* be taken with alcohol include: muscle relaxants, codeine, antihistamines, tranquilizers, blood-pressure-lowering drugs and sleep-aids. The caution

SOME COMMON ADVERSE DRUG COMBINATIONS

- *Antibiotics and the blood-thinner, warfarin (Coumadin,) because the drugs compete for binding sites, allowing blood concentrations of Coumadin to soar dangerously. Antibiotics that interact with Coumadin are mainly the "sulfa" types (such as Septra, Bactrim), and if taken together, blood clotting capacity should be carefully monitored.*
- *NSAIDs and ACE inhibitors also make a bad mix. ACE inhibitors used to lower blood pressure become less effective in combination with some NSAID anti-*

inflammatories such as ASA/Aspirin, ibuprofen (e.g., Advil, Motrin) and COX-2 inhibitors like Celebrex.
- *Digoxin with the antibiotics azithromycin, clarithromycin and erythromycin may cause ill effects because these antibiotics raise blood digoxin levels too high.*
- *Potassium supplements with potassium-sparing diuretics (such as Aldactone, Dyrenium) may cause trouble by elevating blood potassium to levels that endanger the heart.*

- *Nitrates with erectile dysfunction drugs such as Viagra. Levitra and Cialis may be dangerous because the erectile dysfuction products can interact with nitrate drugs (such as nitroglycerin for angina) to cause a sudden drop in blood pressure.*
- *Statins together with some antifungals (such as ketgoconazole, fluconazole and itraconazole) can also be a bad combination because taken together these antifungals may allow statins to shoot up to levels that produce serious muscle pain.*

against using drugs with alcohol is usually marked on the label and should be heeded. (Note that some OTC products themselves also contain alcohol.)

Know about and watch for drug interactions

Different drugs interact with each other and can intensify or decrease, perhaps block, efficacy. Whenever two medications are taken at the same time, there's a possibility of adverse interaction. For instance, some sedatives (such as Sleep-Eze) may render blood-thinners (anticoagulants) less effective or on the other hand, they could increase the sedating effect of antihistamines. Taken together ASA/Aspirin and the blood-thinner warfarin—both of which act on blood platelets—can cause excessive bleeding. According to one estimate, people taking more than five medications have a 7 percent chance of developing a serious problem; the probability rising to 24 percent in those on more than 10 medications. The additive effect

of two drugs can sometimes be beneficial, as when ASA/Aspirin and codeine together increase painkilling efficacy. But their joint action can also produce unwanted side effects—such as confusion, blood pressure changes and impaired coordination. Cough and cold medications often contain antihistamines and cough-suppressants which increase drowsiness if used together or with other antihistamines, antidepressants or anti-Parkinsonian drugs. By contrast, some drugs block the absorption of another. For example, antacids block the absorption of many drugs (such as tetracycline and propranolol) and can lead to phosphate depletion and vitamin-D deficiency. Mineral-oil laxatives hinder absorption of the oil-soluble vitamins (A, D, F, K) and of certain elements such as calcium.

Almost half of all North Americans over age 65 take several different medications, and 1 in 8 take 6 to 8 different types, some of which can interact to threaten health. Several high-profile drugs have been taken off the market because of bad interactions such as cerivastatin (Baycol) and the antihistamine, terfenadine (Seldane).

USE AND ABUSE OF PRESCRIBED DRUGS

Prescription-drug misuse results in more North American injuries and deaths than *all* illegal drugs combined. Adverse drug reactions account for 15 percent of hospital admissions in those over age 50. Hypnotics (sleep medications) result in almost 60 percent of drug-related emergency-room visits and 70 percent of all drug-related deaths. Prescription drugs may be misused even if taken in moderate amounts for the wrong reason—for example, codeine in cold/cough remedies taken to solve psychological distress rather than to suppress a cough or mute pain.

There is no exact dividing line between moderate and excessive drug use. If drug use begins to disrupt social and family life, damages the user's health, reduces work performance or causes financial burdens, use becomes "abuse." CAMH (Centre for Addiction and Mental Health) states that "addiction or dependence exists when a drug is so central to someone's thoughts, emotions and activities that there's a compulsive need to obtain and use it." Physical dependence can occur without the addictive component, as happens with severe or chronic pain sufferers who hardly ever become addicted to their narcotic (opiate) medications and readily give them up once the pain goes away.

According to one University of Toronto expert, "many substances are over-prescribed, especially antibiotics, blood pressure medications, hypnotics (sleep-inducers) and narcotic analgesics (painkillers)." Among today's most misused medications are the opiates, such as codeine. The 1989 National Alcohol and Other Drugs Survey, conducted by Health Canada, reported that one in 20 adult Canadians regularly uses opiate painkillers. When correctly used these medications are invaluable pain relievers, but they're sometimes inappropriately used in wrong doses and for too long.

Opiate misuse widespread

The opiates include natural poppy derivatives such as codeine and morphine and related synthetics such as oxycodone, and meperidine (Demerol). Some are contained in combination products, for instance: Percocet (a mixture of oxycodone and acetaminophen), Percodan (with oxycodone and ASA), Tylenol No. 3 (containing codeine, acetaminophen and caffeine) and Fiorinal-C (containing codeine, ASA, caffeine and barbiturates).

Canada is currently one of the world's top codeine consumers with a per-capita consumption twice that of the United States. Codeine is *not* an innocuous substance. Those who habitually use it are apt to have impaired concentration and diminished performance skills—risky when on the job, operating machinery or driving a car. Studies show that drivers who take codeine have more collisions in simulated tests than those who took tranquilizers (e.g., diazepam) or alcohol (0.5 mg per kg body weight).

Physician misprescribing

The prescription pad has become as much a part of the modern physician's paraphernalia as the stethoscope. A 1987 Canadian literature review, entitled *Drug Utilization*, concluded that prescribers (physicians) and consumers are both to blame for prescription-drug misuse. The report states that "physicians know too little about the correct use of the medications they prescribe, and what they do know comes primarily from biased sources: the pharmaceutical companies." Practicing physicians are often inadequately prepared for good medicine prescribing. They may prescribe the wrong drug or faulty doses because of failure to keep up with new scientific evidence, unfamiliarity with new medications and over reliance on the promotional material of pharmaceutical companies. It may seem easier (but is not safer) to rely on material put out by pharmaceutical companies instead of consulting scientific journals or research surveys of contemporary trial results such as the Cochrane Review, now easily available on the Internet..

To improve matters, more ongoing physician education in applied pharmacology (how to utilize drugs to best advantage) might help. Pharmacology courses in modern medical schools often pay too little attention to the clinical (practical) aspect of prescribing. There's an ongoing need to update physicians' knowledge about new products, whether genuine breakthroughs or copy drugs. Some new drugs offer few or no advantages over established products. Some even prove dangerous, such as Vioxx (the COX-2 inhibitor) commonly prescribed for arthritis which has now been shown to cause heart problems and been taken off the market. (Other COX-2 inhibitors such as Celebrex and Bextra are also currently under FDA investiagation for their safety.) There's an equal call for consumers to become more knowledgeable and well informed medication-takers.

Consumer expectations compound drug misuse

In a society that believes "there's a pill for every ill," and that demands medication for the slightest pain , some people seek a remedy for every little twinge, expecting every doctor visit to terminate with a prescription, whether or not they need one. Having got the prescription, some may not properly follow directions, discontinue the medication too soon, take wrong amounts, skip or forget a pill and then take two or three to "make up." Some go on the mistaken theory that "if one dose is good, two or three must be better." Conversely, some carry a treasured prescription around without ever getting it filled, as a talisman or symbol of recovery. Not knowing (or checking) the patient's failure to follow drug-taking instructions, physicians may be misled into believing that the medication didn't work and prescribe more of the same or other drugs.

Physicians like to appear "actively helpful," and sometimes handing out a prescription seems a satisfactory way to end the visit. "The act of transmitting a prescription from doctor to patient," comments one expert, "has nonpharmacological dimensions. It symbolizes an act of healing and the psychological reaction can facilitate recovery." In many cases, the mere anticipation of relief, the sense of "help on the way," exerts a beneficial neurohormonal effect on the mind. Recent trials show that over one-third of patients respond with a placebo effect by feeling better, even if no actual medication is or was taken. But if used as a coping mechanism for unresolved or everyday problems, medications may expose people to needless risks. The

dangers may arise not only from the drugs (chemicals) themselves but because reliance upon them undermines coping skills.

Doctors may feel pressured to prescribe drugs even when non-drug interventions without adverse side effects—such as a diet change, relaxation therapy, biofeedback, exercise, a vacation or counseling—might be as good or better. Trying to find out what's causing a problem and discussing both medication and non-drug alternatives can help people decide which to choose. For example, while some might opt for sedatives to combat insomnia, others may decide to try relaxation therapy or take some exercise, maybe just a walk around the block, before bedtime.

"Multiple doctoring"
Popularly called "double doctoring," the practice of visiting several physicians to obtain multiple prescriptions for the same problem is quite widespread. Yet people are legally obligated to inform physicians of any controlled drug, especially narcotics (opiate drugs, such as codeine) obtained from another doctor within the same month. Getting a prescription for a narcotic or controlled substance from more than one physician within a 30-day period is a criminal offense under the Narcotic Control Act. It can lead to a fine or jail sentence. Health Canada reports that nearly 90 percent of prescription-drug abuse convictions in the past decade were for opiates—codeine accounting for most of it, followed by oxycodone, Percocet and Percodan.

The elderly are particularly "endangered" by drug misuse
Adverse drug reactions among the elderly account for many hospital admissions, especially as they often take several different medications, sometimes prescribed by different physicians. Older people are at special risk of harmful drug reactions because doses suitable for younger adults may be too high for aging bodies that absorb, metabolize and eliminate drugs differently. The elderly require specialized prescribing tactics, better supervision and accurate records of all drugs taken. On medical visits they're encouraged to "brown bag" it—to put *all* med-

USE YOUR PRESCRIBED MEDICATIONS WISELY

- **Be sure to tell the prescribing physician about all other medications being taken, including OTC products and those prescribed by other doctors.**
- **Write down both the generic and brand names of each medicine prescribed.**
- **Ask the doctor about the purpose of each medication ordered—is it for symptom relief or disease-cure? How soon will improvement occur?**
- **Ask the physician or pharmacist exactly how, when and for**

- **how long to take each medicine. Should the medication be taken with or between meals?**
- **Discard unused and outdated medications—they can deteriorate over time.**
- **Keep all medicines correctly labeled in original containers.**
- **Ask about possible side effects from a particular medication (e.g., drowsiness, difficulty in concentrating, mood, appetite or sex-drive alterations).**
- **Find out what to do if any listed, unpleasant**

- **or seemingly harmful side effects occur.**
- **Store medicines properly. A bathroom medicine chest may be a poor location because of high humidity or easy access for children. Likewise, unless directed to do so, don't put medication in the refrigerator, as the cold may affect it and household members can take it by mistake. A locked cabinet in the bedroom is a good place to store medications, well beyond the reach and sight of children.**

ications (including over-the-counter products) in a bag to show the physician everything being taken. Older people should beware of taking drugs that are only marginally useful. They can ask their doctor(s) what the medication is for and whether there's any nondrug alternative or a substitute with fewer side effects.

Ways to improve prescription-drug use

Responsible use of prescribed medication ideally involves a partnership between the consumer with a problem (bodily discomfort, pain, stress, anxiety or illness) and the physician who diagnoses and treats the disorder. In the Hippocratic tradition and to the best of their ability, physicians follow the tenet of *primum non nocere*—"above all, do no harm." But the safe administration of substances considered too dangerous for over-the-counter availability is no easy matter. Prescribing today's vast array of medications requires considerable pharmacological knowledge. What's needed is more continuing education for physicians about new products and better-educated consumers who follow drug-taking instructions.

Consumers need to ask about their medicines—whether they are supposed to relieve symptoms (e.g., remove pain) or cure disease (e.g., kill the bacteria causing infection). Informed consumers use their medication correctly, know when and how to take it, for how long and possible side effects to watch for. In some cases, medications may do little good, and sometimes the potential harm outdoes any possible benefits. In all cases, both consumers and their caregivers should carefully evaluate the possible benefits versus potential harm of drugs taken and evaluate the pros and cons from time to time. The key is to weigh the benefits against possible risks and keep tabs on what's being taken and why.

USE NONPRESCRIPTION MEDICATIONS WISELY

Nonprescription medications, available without a doctor's prescription, are generally considered safe, with little potential for damaging health at recommended doses. Some are "public access" products that can be sold in grocery stores as well as pharmacies. Others—considered potentially harmful—are obtainable only "behind the counter" by asking the pharmacist. They include, for example, products containing the narcotic

TIPS FOR SENSIBLE USE OF NONPRESCRIPTION OVER-THE-COUNTER MEDICATIONS

- **When buying an OTC medication ask yourself: Why am I taking it? What type of drug is it? How soon will it work? What's the right dose? How and when should it be taken? Are there any restrictions on who should use it, or with what?**
- **Remember that OTC medications are meant for brief, intermittent use, not for extended periods (except under physician guidance). If symptoms increase even when using a medication—if a headache becomes worse despite use of painkillers, or a stomachache doesn't get better with antacids—seek medical advice.**
- **Don't take OTC preparations for continuing or worsening pain, which usually signals something wrong. Taking pills to mask symptoms will not cure a serious illness. For instance, habitually taking painkillers or antacids for a stomachache can mask an underlying condition that needs medical attention.**
- **Keep track of what you're taking and how much.**
- **Always take single-ingredient medications rather than combination products.**
- **Those with diabetes, epilepsy, heart conditions, bleeding disorders, high blood pressure or asthma should consult a physician before taking any OTC products.**
- **Always read the label and/or package insert—noting when and for how long the medicine should be taken and which drugs or foods it may interact with. (Ideally, read the inserts while in the pharmacy and ask the pharmacist about whatever is unclear.)**
- **Follow package instructions. People often do not comply with them. It is a common mistake to think that if one dose is good, two will be better. With many nonprescription medications (e.g., acetaminophen, ASA) there is a "ceiling" beyond which more is not only useless but possibly harmful.**
- **Always store medications well out of the reach of children.**
- **Don't reach for medicines in the dark: you may take the wrong thing.**
- **Tell the physician about any medications you're taking—especially before lab tests are done—as some can interfere with the results.**
- **If pregnant, do not use any medication without consulting your physician.**
- **Consult the pharmacist about medications—the pharmacist is a trained professional who can be very helpful, sometimes more so than a physician. Asking the advice of both may be a good idea.**
- **Make the pharmacist your ally. Choose a pharmacy close to home with a pharmacist who is helpful, especially as you get older and may need several medications or have a chronic health problem.**
- **Home delivery of medications is a definite plus if your mobility is restricted. To attract and keep customers, some pharmacies also offer private areas for counseling about medications.**

codeine—such as 222s or Tylenol No. 1. Because they contain codeine—a potent and addictive substance—these medications must be specifically requested. Similarly, the antihistamine Hismanal has been placed "behind the counter," because it can cause problems in people with heart ailments.

With such a variety of drugs on the pharmacy shelves, how does one choose which to buy? Cost is one factor: choose the cheapest generic brands. For instance, "Swiss Herbal" vitamins are the same chemicals as other, cheaper brands. Once inside your body the cells don't discriminate about the name, origin or cost of a vitamin or other substance. Similarly, one type of acetaminophen is like any other of the same strength. When possible, choose longer-acting medications that need to be taken only once a day (to increase compliance and reduce the possibility of forgetting to take a pill). People with digestive problems can try coated pills. Check whether the medication will make you sleepy; look for nondrowsy forms. Drugs have different effects on different people: if one drug doesn't work for you, consult a health professional or a pharmacist for advice about choosing another. Pharmacists are knowledgeable, know how drugs interact and can help you to use OTC products wisely. Try to avoid combination products: choose a different medicine for each symptom.

Generic versus brand-name medications

When a drug is first developed, it's given a generic name and a patent granting the discovering company the sole right to sell the drug while the patent remains in effect. Once the patent has expired, the drug becomes public property and other companies are free to manufacture and market it under either its generic or a brand name. Generic drugs cost 30 to 50 percent less than brand-name products, and buying generics is one way to reduce medication costs. Generic products must contain precisely the same active ingredients, in the same form and strength, as the brand-name drug. Ask the pharmacist for advice when deciding between generic versus brand-name products.

Not all nonprescription medicines are entirely safe

Today's most popular over-the-counter medications include analgesics (painkillers), laxatives, cough and cold products and allergy remedies. Since it wastes everybody's time and money to dash off to the doctor for every bellyache or muscle twinge, OTC drugs are useful for minor ailments. However, successful self-medication depends on good judgment, common sense and reading the labels. Self-medicating with OTC products should never delay or deter you from seeking medical advice for a persistent or serious problem. It is foolish to mask a severe headache (that may signal a stroke) with ASA or to treat the symptoms of bowel cancer with Milk of Magnesia.

Since nonprescription medications—for example, painkillers (such as acetaminophen or Tylenol), antihistamines (such as chlorpheniramine or Chlor-Tripolon) and laxatives (such as phenolphthalein or Ex-Lax)—are sold in supermarkets alongside cat food and soap, many assume that they and other OTC medications are harmless. While over-the-counter drugs are used by millions of people and generally considered safe, they are still chemicals that affect the body's metabolism. Even nonprescription drugs can be toxic and cause adverse side effects in some people. All medications, even those bought at the corner variety store, must be treated with cautious respect.

Read the labels!

When selecting OTC medications, look for the following information: the name of the medication, directions for use, special precautions, the suggested dosage and the list of possible (main) adverse effects. The package inserts and labels usually contain information about the purpose of the medication, its proper dosage, precautions, warnings about when not to take it and a mention of possible drug interactions. As the print may be small, you can ask the pharmacist to read or explain it to you.

A recent survey revealed that many people don't read labels or seek medical advice before popping pills. Most OTC drug users consult neither a physician or pharmacist about the medications they're taking, nor about mixing them with each other. Yet it can be potentially risky to mix drugs—either OTC or prescription types. For instance, the survey found that one-third of allergy sufferers take their allergy medication along with several other products, perhaps causing drug interactions that compound drowsiness. In addition, 70 percent of allergy sufferers wrongly thought that the allergy drugs lose their effectiveness after a while, 40 percent mistakenly believing that all allergy drugs are much the same. Adding OTC to prescription medications can make a dangerous cocktail. U.S. statistics show that almost 10 percent of emergency-room poisonings involve OTC drugs, mostly analgesics (painkillers) and sedatives.

To obtain maximum benefits while minimizing harmful effects, people should find out as much as possible about their medicines. Don't hesitate to question your physician and/or pharmacist. While some OTC drug side effects are mild and relatively harmless such as feeling slightly "hyper" or restless (as with some decongestants) or somewhat constipated (as with codeine-containing products)—other side effects may be serious and warrant a call or visit to the physician. Examples of potentially hazardous side effects are dizziness (e.g., from decongestants), allergies, excessive drowsiness (e.g., from antihistamines) and stomach bleeds (e.g., from ASA or other NSAIDs).

GUIDE TO SOME COMMONLY USED NONPRESCRIPTION MEDICATIONS

Drug name	Uses	When or why to choose	Warning: Don't choose	Adverse interaction with:
ANALGESICS (Painkillers) • acetylsalicylic acid (ASA) —e.g., Aspirin, Anacin, Midol; • acetaminophen—e.g., Tylenol, Panadol, Tempra; • ibuprofen—e.g., Motrin, Advil; • products with codeine —e.g., 222s, Tylenol #1, some cough syrups.	• fever-reduction; to ease minor pains (e.g., headache, menstrual cramps, muscle aches).	• for pain relief; • for reducing fever; • to reduce inflammation—ASA (but not acetaminophen).	• if pain/problem is persistent—in which case seek medical advice.	• other painkillers; • sedatives; • alcohol; • antihistamines.
Acetylsalicylic acid (ASA) (e.g., Aspirin, Arthrisin, Entrophen, Percodan)	• to reduce fever, ease pain, lessen inflammation; • blood-thinning (anti-clotting) properties may help to prevent cardiovascular (heart) disease (but also increase wound-bleeding).	• cheap, well tolerated by most; • very effective anti-inflammatory (e.g., for arthritis); • preventive for cardiovascular disease, heart attack, stroke; ask about right dose and safety.	• if you have asthma (ASA can trigger attack); • if you have ulcers (ASA can worsen them); • in children or teens (because of link to Reye's syndrome—a deadly liver/brain condition); • if diabetic (ASA may lower blood sugar and alter insulin needs); • if on anticoagulants (unless medically advised); • before surgery.	• zidovudine; • oral antidiabetic agents, e.g., sulfonylureas (ASA prolongs action); • acetazolamide, methotrexate, valproic acid, alcohol; • anticoagulants (ASA increases risks); • other painkillers (excess may dampen breathing); • other NSAIDs (ASA decreases their efficacy).
Acetaminophen (e.g., Tylenol, Panadol, 222s).	• reduce fever, ease pain.	• if allergic to ASA (allergic reactions rare with acetaminophen); • in children (who shouldn't use ASA).	• if liver problems or alcohol abuser (as may increase liver damage).	• alcohol; • phenobarbital, other sleep-aids; • other painkillers.

GUIDE TO SOME COMMONLY USED NONPRESCRIPTION MEDICATIONS (continued)

Drug name	Uses	When or why to choose	Warning: Don't choose	Adverse interaction with:
Ibuprofen (e.g., Advil, Motrin, Apotex)	• painkiller.	• if effective, although relatively expensive.	• don't use if allergic to ASA.	• oral anticoagulants, diuretics, lithium, methotrexate.
Codeine-containing products (e.g., Tylenol # 1, Coryphen)	• narcotic painkillers; • cough suppressants.	• for severe pain (stronger than ASA); • for nighttime cough (codeine suppresses cough).	• if need to stay alert (it is very sedating, disturbs coordination); • if pregnant; • if constipated (it is constipating); • overuse causes pinpoint pupils, respiratory distress.	• oral anticoagulants; • alcohol (avoid combination); • other sedating products.
LAXATIVES	• to alleviate constipation, facilitate passage and elimination of stool, to stimulate bowel action.	• never use for too long—if no relief after 10–14 days, consult a doctor.	• if severe cramps, diarrhea, electrolyte losses, calcium loss (osteoporosis), fatty stools, liver disease.	• other laxatives; • overuse can produce lazy, flaccid, nonfunctioning colon/bowel.
Bulk-forming laxatives e.g., Metamucil, Prodiem, psyllium, Fibyrax.	• absorb water; good for initial constipation relief, also for elderly, those with irritable bowels, postpartum; • facilitate passage of stool, stimulate bowel action—may take two to three days.	• inexpensive, more "natural," mild; • not absorbed into bloodstream, few side effects (although some allergies); • take with full glass of water.	• with intestinal ulcers (because can cause fecal impaction/obstruction); • for fast relief, because take some days to work; • unless you follow product instructions exactly.	• other bulk-formers.
Stimulant laxatives e.g., phenolphthalein (Ex-Lax, Feen-A-Mint), bisacodyl (Dulcolax), senna glycosides (Senokot, Glysenid), cascara, castor oil.	• speed intestinal movements; • powerful purgatives, act quicker than bulk formers (three to eight hours).	• for fast relief, occasional use; • work quickly (but unpredictably); • can cause severe cramps, diarrhea, fluid loss, electrolyte imbalance.	• when pregnant or breastfeeding (can cause diarrhea in babies); • castor oil not generally recommended (can lead to excess fluid and electrolyte losses).	• antacids; • some blood pressure medications; • cimetidine, ranitidine (stomach ulcer remedies).
Stool-softening laxatives e.g., docusate sodium (Colace, Doss), docusate calcium (Surfak).	• short-term occasional relief for constipation; • increase stool wetness, take 24–48 hours to work.	• only on physician recommendation; • for elderly, infirm, postsurgery, or if have very hard stools.	• don't use if have abdominal pain, cramps, diarrhea.	• danthron, digoxin; • mineral oil; • phenolphthalein.
Osmotic and saline laxatives e.g., magnesium hydroxide (Milk of Magnesia), magnesium citrate (Citro-Mag), magnesium sulfate, sodium phosphate (Fleet-enemas).	• powerful forms used to evacuate bowel before medical tests/surgery; • use with care; • draw water into gut and increase intestinal motility.	• with physician advice as they are potent agents; • not in the infirm, heart patients.	• without medical advice; • don't use if have kidney disorders, heart disease, high blood pressure; • risk of dehydration, electrolyte imbalance, cramps, gas.	• digoxin; • tetracycline; • diuretics.

Drug name	Uses	When or why to choose	Warning: Don't choose	Adverse interaction with:
Lubricant laxatives e.g., liquid petrolatum (Mineral oil), olive oil, Agarol.	• coat and soften stools; • take six to eight hours to work; • emulsified oils more effective than nonemulsified forms; • only for occasional use.	• best to use on doctor's recommendation; • after surgery or hemorrhoid treatment to avoid danger of "straining" (e.g., with hernia, aneurysm, postsurgery).	• if elderly, debilitated, very young (inhalation of oil may cause pneumonia); may delay gastric (stomach) emptying; • in pregnancy (may decrease absorption of vitamin K by fetus).	• possibly decrease effect of anticoagulants; • hinder absorption of fat-soluble vitamins (A, D, E, K).
ANTACIDS (e.g., Tums, Rolaids, Amphojel)	• to neutralize stomach acidity, heartburn, gastritis, indigestion; • liquid forms act better than tablets (chew well, with full glass of water); • contain various ingredients—e.g., calcium carbonate, magnesium, aluminum; • promote healing of gastric mucosa (lining).	• choose types least likely to disturb electrolyte balance; • for mild heartburn, indigestion; • best taken one to three hours after meals to prolong effects—up to three hours; • if no relief after two weeks or if problem recurs—see doctor; • select most suitable type—not indiscriminately.	• interchangeably—differ in action; • avoid calcium-rich types for long-term use (upset bone turnover); • aluminum and magnesium products offer best results with least toxicity; • if on low-salt diet, choose forms without sodium; • if have persistent stomach pain or indigestion—need medical investigation.	• may enhance action of ephedrine and some antidepressants; • decrease absorption of tetracyclines, digoxin, corticosteroids, levodopa, diazepam, valproic acid, ketoconazole (Nizoral), ranitidine (Zantac); • increase clearance of ASA and phenobarbital (Luminal); • interfere with warfarin, anticonvulsants.
Sodium bicarbonate e.g., Alka Seltzer, Eno.	• good for fast, short-term relief of overeating, indigestion, heartburn, gastritis (acid stomach); • not for too long—may produce sodium overload.	• for most transient digestive upsets (N.B.: baking soda and water—cheaper than Alka Seltzer and equally effective).	• if have peptic ulcer or gastric bleeding; • if pregnant; • if on low-sodium diet or diuretics; • not with milk or calcium—can cause milk-alkali syndrome (nausea, vomiting, mental confusion).	• iron supplements; • ketoconazole (antifungal); • evodopa; • lithium; • some antibiotics; • salicylates (e.g., ASA).
Calcium carbonate e.g., Tums, Os-Cal, Caltrate.	• potent acid neutralizer.	• for occasional heartburn, gastritis; • for gas or bloating.	• for prolonged time, as may cause hypercalcemia (which may lead to kidney stones).	• anticoagulants, corticosteroids, diuretics, iron supplements.
Aluminum e.g., Amphojel, Basaljel.	• good acid-neutralizing ability (but less than calcium carbonate).	• choose for occasional use; • avoid if have kidney problems.	• if constipated (as is constipating); • if family history of Alzheimer's.	• can bind to and prevent absorption of phosphate.

GUIDE TO SOME COMMONLY USED NONPRESCRIPTION MEDICATIONS (continued)

Drug name	Uses	When or why to choose	Warning: Don't choose	Adverse interaction with
VITAMINS Popular OTC drugs—many people believe vitamins give extra energy, ward off colds and make one "smarter" — but no scientific validity.	• needed for all body functions but well-balanced diets supply plenty; • most don't need supplements, but preschoolers, pregnant or breastfeeding women, the elderly, alcoholic and malnourished may need extra vitamins; also vegetarians lacking vitamin B_2 (riboflavin) and B_{12}.	• choose only products with DIN numbers (federal drug permits); • never take in excess of recommended daily allowances.	• never take megadoses; • keep out of children's reach (excess can be toxic).	
Vitamin C	• some people take megadoses in mistaken belief vitamin C will prevent colds or other ills.	• remarkably safe even at high doses, but megadoses can decrease vitamin B_{12} absorption; side effects include diarrhea, nausea, urinary-tract stones.	• in pregnancy—large doses may cause "rebound" scurvy in newborns; • if prone to kidney stones.	• amphetamines; • some antidepressants; • ASA.
Vitamin A, Vitamin D (Fat-soluble vitamins)	• for health of bones, skin, teeth and eyes.	• with calcium (1000 mg per day) for prevention of osteoporosis—after menopause, in women (vitamin D).	• high doses can lead to hypervitaminosis A (fatigue, malaise, lethargy, scaly skin, loss of hair or hyper-vitaminosis D (anorexia, nausea, wakefulness, weight loss, kidney damage).	• cholestyramine; • mineral oil (decreases vitamin absorption); • isotretinoin (for skin problems).
Iron	• if iron-deficient (e.g., anemic).	• use if anemic (low iron stores); • if on vegetarian diets low in iron; • watch for toxicity (even 15 tablets of ferrous sulfate may be lethal).	• in children or elderly for long time as may develop iron poisoning which can cause acute illness; • not if have fever (iron alters body reaction to fever).	• interacts with ASA, may cause excess bleeding; • don't take with antacids (which decrease iron absorption); • tetracycline reduces absorption.
COLD MEDICATIONS	• to relieve runny nose, nasal congestion; • often sold in combination, perhaps with vitamin C, antihistamines; • single-ingredient types best.	• select single-ingredient medicines—e.g., pseudo-ephedrine for decongestion; ASA (Aspirin) for muscle aches and fever; DM or codeine for cough; antihistamine for allergy symptoms.	• not in pregnancy without medical advice (especially forms containing pseudoephedrine); • if have asthma, diabetes, heart condition.	• may alter effect of oral antidiabetic pills (e.g., DiaBeta).
Oral decongestants e.g., pseudoephedrine (e.g., Actifed, Novahistex, Slnutab, Benylin, Sudafed), phenylpropanolamine, (Sucrets), phenylephrine (Neo-Synephrine, Novahistine).	• to reduce congestion, nasal stuffiness, shrink nasal tissues; • peak effect three to four hours after taken.	• if don't need sleep (decongestants are stimulating, perk one up), may transiently raise blood pressure.	• if need sleep; • if have hypertension, thyroid or heart condition, diabetes, glaucoma; • if taking MOAI anti-depressants.	• certain blood-pressure pills.

Drug name	Uses	When or why to choose	Warning: Don't choose	Adverse interaction with:
Nasal decongestant sprays e.g., naphazoline (Privine, Rhino-Mex-N), xylometa-zoline (Otrivin), oxymeta-zoline (Afrin, Dristan Mist).	• for temporary relief of nasal stuffiness; • shrink nasal tissues.	• if desire fast local relief rather than slower systemic effect; • impair ciliary action in clearing mucus.	• for long periods of time— more than three to five days—as causes rebound congestion if overused; • if have diabetes, thyroid trouble, heart disease, glaucoma.	• may irritate nasal tissues; • interact with CNS stimulants (cause jitteriness).
COUGH MEDICINES DM/dextromethorphan e.g., Balminil DM syrup, Delsym, Benylin.	• DM is nondrowsy, doesn't cause jitteriness; best choice for children; • nonaddictive (in contrast to codeine).	• for dry cough or if cough prevents sleep.	• for too long, if need to expel phlegm, mucus.	• MAOI antidepressants.
Codeine (e.g., Benylin-codeine, D.E.)	• acts on brain's cough center and is sedating (with abuse potential— can be addictive).	• for those nonresponsive to DM, e.g., for whooping cough; • effect lasts three to six hours.	• for long periods, if tendency to addiction— not without medical advice; • not in children under age 12.	• alcohol, other painkillers, sedatives, antihistamines (enhanced depression of brain and breathing).
ANTIHISTAMINES e.g., ethanolamines (such as Benadryl, Tavist), ethylenediamines (e.g., Pyribenzamine), alkylamines (e.g., Chlor-Tripolon, Dimetane, Actifed), piperazines (e.g., Atarax).	• for hay fever, hives, skin rashes and other allergies; • very sedating, can have other side effects.	• ethanalomines most sedating but give least gastrointestinal side effects; • alkylamine, piperazines (less sedating); • phenothiazines and piperazines for motion sickness, skin allergies, rashes.	• for stuffy nose; • if must stay awake, drive a car, operate machinery; • if have narrow-angle glaucoma; • during pregnancy (without medical advice); • if have prostate trouble (may worsen it).	• MAOI antidepressants; • narcotics (e.g., codeine); • sedatives; • alcohol (bad mix); • muscle relaxants.
New (nondrowsy) antihistamines terfenadine (Seldane), astemizole (Hismanal), loratadine (Claritin).	• nonsedating, longer-acting	• useful if other anti-histamines put you to sleep; some find them good, but adverse cardiovascular effects reported if taken in excess.	• if have heart, blood-pressure, liver problems; • without medical advice— too much can produce health-harming cardiovascular effects.	• sleep-aids, alcohol, barbiturates; • erythromycin; • ketoconazole (but not loratadine).

Web Resources

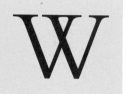

NIH Medline Plus

http://medlineplus.gov

Put out by the National Institutes of Health in the U.S. This service has a very large database and thus is great for searches on a specific health topics.

Canadian Health Network

http://www.canadian-health-network.ca

Obviously, a Canadian product that represents a network of services and resources. The database is not as large as medlinePlus but often the best resource for a variety of local tools to help manage health problems.

HealthyOntario.com

http://www.healthyontario.com

The HealthyOntario.com website, was created to provide Ontarians with a web destination for trusted health information, services and advice for healthier living. It includes:

• Telehealth Ontario (1-866-797-0000)
• Information on medications
• Local health priorities (such as West Nile Virus info)

Hitting the Headlines

http://www.nelh.nhs.uk

This link takes you the NHS (National Health Service) in the U.K. At the top right hand of the page you will see "Hitting the Headlines." Simply click on "Archives." You will then see a list of recent headlines and if you follow the links, you will find unbiased analysis of those headlines to better put the information into perspective.

NIH Senior Health

http://nihseniorhealth.gov

This website is "senior-friendly"…a talking website with formats and topics tailored to the needs of older people.

Center for Disease Control

http://www.cdc.gov/az.do

This is the consumer site for the Center for Disease Control in Atlanta. Here you will find an alphabetical list of topics. The emphasis is on infectious disease and public health problems, but the list is quite extensive. (Hint: Hold down the control key and punch the letter "F" and it will produce a box to find a topic on the page.)

familydoctor.org

http://familydoctor.org

A simple, but well done, resource base developed by the American Academy of Family Physicians.

Cochrane Consumer (What's New Digest)

http://www.informedhealthonline.org

This organization is the consumer face of an international collaboration in systematic reviews of various health topics. The database is still quite limited but the quality is excellent.

Google

http://www.google.ca

Google is a very quick and effective search engine. However, caution should be used, as it is very difficult to discern quality, bias and sources of funding.

Herbal Medicine

http://www.herbmed.org

This is a high-quality service that outlines various trials done on most herbal products. It does not summarize the evidence but rather you have to look at the individual trials.

CV Risk Score

http://www.riskscore.org.uk

This is a user-friendly site out of the U.K. that allows you to estimate your personal cardiac risk.

Motherisk

http://www.motherisk.org

Motherisk is a Canadian resource for pregnant and breastfeeding mothers. You can also access this service by phone. It is especially useful when you are considering taking a medication while you are pregnant or breastfeeding.

Web MD

http://www.webmd.com

A commercial site that makes it difficult to assure quality but has lots of resources.

Index

Page citations in **boldface** here signal either direct primary references or citations that might profitably be consulted first.

For **First Aid information** see **page 598** in this index

AA. See Alcoholics Anonymous
abdominal pain. See pain, abdominal
abscesses, 128, 178, 192, 334, 596
absence-of-disease concept, 20
accessory apartments for seniors, 434
accidents. See also safety, 50, 54–55, 87, **299–300**, 392, 436, 509, 592, 611, 618
    tips for preventing, 57, **300–302**
acetaminophen, 49, 86–87, 303, 305, 307, 319, 333, 464, 478, 489, 513, 516, 600, 614, **623**, **627**
acetylsalicylic acid. See ASA
acne, 121–23, 127–28, 133–34, 200, 227, 350–51, 550
acupuncture, 20, 30, 32, 82–83, **84**, 88, 171, 535, 539
acute glaucoma, 161
acute retention (of urine). See urination
acyclovir tablets, 131, 193, 195, 279–80, 314
addiction. See also drugs, abuse of
    to coffee, 28, 62, 108
    to smoking, 24–32
Addison's disease, 214, 414, 417
adenoids, 52, 165, 513, 580
    removal of, 334
ADHD (attention-deficit hyperactivity disorder), 473–76
adolescence. See also puberty
    as a biopsychosocial process, 337
    and depression, 343, 346–47, 349–50, **355–57**
    developmental tasks of, 349
    psychosocial development during, 348
    school problems during, 351
    stages of, 338–40
    suicide during, 355–58
adrenaline. See also epinephrine; EpiPen, 309, 363, 367, 541, 591
aging. See also geriatrics; menopause, 164, 430–55
    in the brain, 430

mental changes of, 431
myths about, 430
senile dementia and. See senile dementia
sex and, 186
agoraphobia. See phobias
AIDS. See also HIV infection, 189–97, 417, **456–60**, 561, 581, 597, **599**
    precautions against, 191, 194, 599
    risks from encounters with, 189–91
air bags, 56–57
air-flow rates and asthma, 467, 469, 471
airborne microorganisms, 373, 375–76
air quality. See indoor air contaminants
alcohol. See also liver cirrhosis; Fetal Alcohol Syndrome
    abuse of, 64–65, 69, 360
    accidents/injuries and, 55, 56–57, 68, 189
    dependency See also alcoholism, 61–65, 69
    the diuretic action of, 93, 95, 120, 480
    erectile failure and, 254–55
    exercise and, 43, 48
    the "French paradox" and, 68, 70
    headaches and, 514–16
    heart disease and, 70, 98, 521, 525
    medications and, 44, 72, 81, 86, 113, 218, 364–65, 621–23, 627–28, 631
    pregnancy and, 260–61, 264, 266, 278–79
    sensible vs. problem drinking, 71, 73, 90, 93, 100, 241, 244, 446, 451, 521, 539, 541–42
    sleep and, 49–51, 53
    women and, 69, 206
Alcoholics Anonymous, 72–73
alcoholism, 63, **68–72**, 255, 347, 356, 397, 398, 419, 436, 462, 581
allergic reactions. See also asthma; hay fever; hypoallergenic states; itching; total allergy syndrome, **362–78**
    anaphylaxis. See allergic shock
    to animals, 595–96

in childhood. See also in infancy, 308–10, 362
    delayed, 363, 367
    diagnoses of, 363
    eczema and, 296, 319
    eggs and, 326, 468
    eyes and, 158
    to foods, 369–73
    headaches and, 516
    hives and, 124, 295–97, 308–9, 362–63, 367, 370–72, 547–48
    as immunological reactions, 363–64
    in infancy, 293–97
    to insect stings or bites, 366–67
    management and treatment of, 364–65, 387, 631
    to medicines and pharmaceuticals, 29, 85, 177, 199, 203, 483, 544, 547, 577, 586, 627–28, 630
    to dust mites, 300, 311, 332, 362, 365, 468, 471
    to milk types, 292, 296–97, 372
    to peanuts, 309–10
    to poison ivy, 368
    and "tight-building syndrome," **373–74**, 377–78, 415–16, 471
    and the skin, 123–25, 139
allergic rhinitis. See also hay fever, 365, 376
allergic shock (anaphylaxis), 363, **602**, **604–5**
alopecia, 141–42, 144
alpha blockers, 249
alphafetoprotein, 269, 272
alpha-hydroxy acid creams, 132, 134
alpha-linolenic acid, 115
alpha-tocopherol. See Vitamin E
ALS. See amyotrophic lateral sclerosis
"alternative" medicine, 12, **82–85**, **378**, 539
aluminum, 126, 378, 447, 454, 480, 528, 629
Alzheimer's disease, 431, 451–55
    risk factors for, 378, 454
amenorrhea, 215, 217, 343–44
amino acids, essential, 106–7
amniocentesis, 268–70
amphetamines, 61–63, 66, 420, 569, 630
amyotrophic lateral sclerosis (ALS), 460
analgesics, 67, 86–87, 489–90, 517, 579, 623, 626–27

anaphylaxis. See allergic shock
anecdotal evidence, cautions about, 19–20
anemia, 91, 117, 118, 171, 207, 271–72, 278, 342, 372, 383, 417, **460–63**, 482, 484, 502, 511, 553–55, 566
    during pregnancy, 113, 462
    pernicious. See pernicious anemia
    sickle cell, 80, 243, 264, 269, 308, 321, 462
anencephaly, 113, 268, 278
aneurysms, 570, 629
angel dust, 63, 66
angel's kiss, 312
angina. See also chest pain; heartburn, 233–36, 257, 392, 518–19, **521–28**, 591, 622
angiogram, 233–34, 523–24
angioplasty, 234–36, 521–24, 567
animal diseases, 333, 389, 544–45, 595–97
ankylosing spondylitis, 463, 466–67, 511
anogen effluvium, 141
anorectal problems, 530–533
anorexia nervosa See also bulimia, 48, 91, 209, **342–47**, 357, 416, 444–47, 630
anorgasmia, 213–14
antacids, 446–47, 480, 528, 565, 621–22, 625, 628–30
anthrocyanins, 108–9
anti-allergy products. See also allergic reactions, management of, 86
antibiotic(s), 128, 163, 173–74, 192, 247–48, 286, 304, 318–19, 324–31, 333–35, 387, 390–91, 438, **487**, **504–5**, 527, 550, 554, 560–61, 564–66, 580–84, 587, 596
    creams, 86, 158
    in interaction with other meds, 198, 203, 218, 364, 470, 621–22
    the overuse of, 219, 291, 315, 487–88, 623
    resistance to, 191, 504–5, 580, 582, **620**
    side effects from, 218
    and STIs, 195
antibodies. See also autoimmune disorders; vaccines, 266, 279, 290, 292–93, 452, 459, 494, 496, 530, 544–45, 563, 595

and allergic reactions, 308, **363**, 367–68, 370–72
lack of sufficient, 189
monoclonal, 561
testing for, 264, 329, 388, 417, 457, 534–35, 560
anticoagulants, 141, 235, 567, 569, 572, 621–22, 627–29
anticonvulsants, 169, 197–98, 278, 323, 414, 454, 509, 629
antidepressants, 32, 52, 131, 169, 216, 320, 346, 348, 356, 402, **404–11**, 414–15, 418, 420–24, 439, 443, 454, 474, 482, 511
in interaction with other meds, 364, 393, 410, 622, 629–31
side effects from, 50, 254–55, 410, 436, 438, 513, 620, 622
SNRIs. See SNRIs
SSRIs. See SSRIs
tricyclics as, 406–7, 410, 423, 439, 474, 511
antidiuretic, 320–21
anti-estrogens. See also breast cancer; 226–27, 242, 245
antifungals, 85, 141, 220, 292, 334, 472–73, 597
in interaction with other meds, 364, 622, 629
antihistamines, 86, 124, 126, 158, 165, **364–65**, 367–68, 371, 387, 418, **489–90**, 503, 547, 600, 604
in interaction with other meds, 56, 66–67, **364**, 438, 621–22, 626
side effects of, 207, 255, 279, 308, **364–65**, 436, 513, 627, 630–31
anti-inflammatory agents, 86, 126, 227, 311, 319, **464–68, 470**, 479, 617
nonsteroidal (NSAIDs), 248, 414, 438, 465, 470, 516–17, 558, 564, 616
antinauseants, 86, 163, 171, 200, 387, 502–3, 516–17, 561
side effects of, **278**, 441
antioxidants, 90, 92, 102, **108–9**, 112–13, 115, 442
antiperspirants, 125–27
antipsychotic medications, 414, **426–28**
side effects of, 255, 438, 441, 513
antipyretic medication, 86–87, 308, 330, 490, 545
anti-rheumatic drugs. See DMARDs
antiseptic agents, 86, 121, 126, 131, 291, 331, 375, 387, 603–4, 606, 618

antispasmodic drugs, 230, 320, 439, 482, 528
anxiety. See also burnout; depression; stress; worry, 74, 169, 287–88, 333, 338, 348, 350, **395–96**
disorders, 171, 356, 358, 395–97, 408, 418, **419–24**, 475
about health matters, 22, 51, 82, 179, 229–30, 236, 238, 244, 250, 254, 263, 432, 541–42
incorrect self-diagnoses of, 233
about medical treatments and outcomes, 164, 201, 271, 524
influencing medical outcomes, 262
as a symptom or side effect, 25, 29, 48, 65–67, 76, 105, 164, 170, 185–8, 206–7, 211–12, 216–17, 234, 242, 247, 254, 302, 321, 343, 356, 404, 407, 412, 417, 419, **420–21**, 436, 452, 481, 501, 507, 510–11, 522, 525–26, 563, 574, 587–88, 590, 595, 620
treatments (good & bad) for, 40, 51–52, 61, 64, 71, 88, 217, 408, 418, **420–24**, 592
Apgar score, 278, 284
aphakic cataract spectacles, 163
aphasia, 572–73
apnea, 33, 52–53, 329, 332–34, 416–17
apolipoproteins, 97
Apparent Life-Threatening Episodes, 333
appendix, rupture of, 266
arrhythmias, 72, 235, 500, 502, 519, **522**, 526, 578
arsenic, 141, 378–80, 556
arteries. See also angiogram; angioplasty; bypass surgery; coronary artery disease; strokes, 235, 254, 541
blockages of, 97, 99, 233, **518–25**, 570
arthritis. See also pain, 17, 41, 76, 82–83, 130, 149–50, 207, 386, 404, 430, **463–67**, 525, 559–60
contraindicated foods or medicines with, 394, 623
and obesity, 210
and omega-3 fatty acids, 106
osteoarthritis, 463-64
remedies or treatments for, 86, 123, **465–66**
risks with, 436, 482
rheumatoid, 156, **463–67**, 510–11
artificial insemination, 268, 457

artificial respiration, 324, 508, **601**, 602–3, 605–6, 610, 613, 615, **619**
contraindications for, 324, 508
atrial fibrillations (AF), 526, 569, 571
ASA (aspirin) 49, **86–87**, 158, 235, 464–67, 478, 487, 489, 513, 516–17, 544–45, 558, 579, **600**, **614**
contraindications for or with, 88, 161, 305, 307, 314, 331, 333, 546, **600, 614, 622, 626–30**
and heart attack & stroke prevention, 521–22, 525, 567, 569, **571–72**
possible side effects of, 167, 414, 462, 525, 564, **621–22**, 625, **627–30**
asbestos, 379, 556
ascorbic acid. See vitamin C
asphyxiation, 58, 273, **603**
aspiration(s), 162, 239, 251, 258, 580
aspirin. See ASA
asthma, 76, 302, **310–11**, 420, **467–71**, 540, **603**
contraindicated foods or medicines with, 507, 625, 627, 630
dangers with and from, **471**
predisposing conditions for and by, 24, 124, 296, 319, **362–63**, 372, 374, 376, 467, **471**, 546
treatments (good & bad) for, 106, 157, 161, **311**, **364–65**, **468–71**, 487, 507, 544, **603**
astigmatism, 156–57
astringents, 121–22, 126, 133
the ATBC Study, 109
atherosclerosis, 26, **97**, 233, 254–55, 430, 497, **518–19**, 523–24, 569–70
athletes. See also sport injuries; sport safety, 43, 100, 119, 149, 217–18, 445–46, 464, 526, **617**
and nutrition, **95–96**
athlete's foot, **471–73**, 547–48
atopic dermatitis, **124**, 547
atrial fibrillation, 526, 569, 571
attention-deficit hyperactivity disorder. See ADHD
autism, **311–12**, 475
autoimmune disorders, 158, 206, 394, 461, 494, 504, 549, 557, 562, 577–79
treatments of, 500
AZT (AIDS treatment), 459

babies. See also Apgar score; baby formulas; breastfeeding; childbirth; newborns; pregnancy; Sudden Infant Death Syndrome

choking in, 58, 295, **300–301**, **608–9**
illness in, **302–8**
injuries to, **299–301**
mortality in, 280, 285
poisonings in, 56, **59**, 300, **614**
baby formulas. See also breastfeeding, 113, **293–97**, 317, 319, 384
back problems. See also muscle spasms, 247, 400, 405, **476–79**, 510, 590
"failed backs," 478
bacteremia, 306
bacterial meningitis, 325, 327–28
bacterial tracheitis, 325
baldness, 139, 141, **142–44**, 323
basal cell cancers. See cancers
baths (tub), dangers or risks of, 49, 122, 150, 218, 219, 253, 307, 319, 509, 616
bearberry, 88
bedwetting. See enuresis
bee stings, 367, 604
behavior therapy, 37–38, 415, 420–21, 424, 435, 439
Bell's palsy, 158, 569
beta blockers, 130, 144, 161, 207, 235, 422, 438, 470, 516–17, 521–22, 525–26, 542–43, 577
beta-carotene, 92, 109
biofeedback, 169, 439, 593, 624
biomedical model of health, 15
biopsies, 130, 137–38, 141, 154, 223–24, 226, **239–40**, 240, 242, 250–51, 485, 553, 557, 561, 566, 580
biopsychosocial model of health, 16, 61, 337, 404
biotin, 109, **111**
bipolar disorder. See also depression; manic episodes, 349, 355, 401, **412–15**
treatment of, 406, 413
birth. See childbirth
birth control. See contraception; morning-after pill
birth defects, 278, 312–14, 323, 332, 553, 570, 579
promoting avoidance of, 264, 268
risks of and for, 113, 128, 195, 278, 380, 553
birthmarks, 137, **312–13**
bites,
animal and reptile, 333, 595, **603**
insect, 367–69, 389–90, 559–60, 589, **604**
B-K moles, 137
bladder infections. See also urinary tract infection, 248–49, 332

bladder surgery, 439

bleeding. See also hemorrhages

emergency treatment for, **605–6**

blindness, 132, 159–60, 163, 191, 195, 285, 369, 490, 493–94, 578, 597

    vitamin A deficiency and, 110, 112

blisters, 123–24, 131–32, 135–36, 153–54, 195, 279, 314, 326, 368–69, 472, 500, 554, 605–6, 611

blood. See also anticoagulants; bleeding; diabetes; hypertension; Rh blood problems

    coagulation problems of the, 70, 110, 112, 199, 529–30, 571

blood pressure tests and monitors. See also hypertension, 80–82, 235, 272, **541–42**

blood sugar tests and monitors, 494–96

BMI. See body mass index

body fat, 41, 105, 119, 217, 341, 483

body lice, 146

body mass index, 33–34

body-image, 338, **341–42**, 348

bone. See also fractures;

    osteoporosis

    spurs, 477

marrow transplants, 552–55

bottle feeding, 295

    formulas for. See baby formulas

borderline personality disorder, 408, 414–15

bovine spongiform encephalopathy. See "Creutzfeldt-Jakob disease; "mad cow" disease

bowel problems. See cancers, bowel; colitis; constipation; Crohn's disease; diarrhea; diverticulitis; inflammatory bowel disease; irritable bowel syndrome; spastic colon

brain cancers. See cancers

brain damage or injury, 45, 57, 63, 69, 313, 323, 327, 440–41, 567, 597, 600

Brazelton's Neonatal Scale, 285

BRCA (breast cancer) genes, 224–25, 238, 241, 243–45, 258

breast cancer. See also chemotherapy; lumpectomy; mammograms; mastectomy, **236–43**

    anti-estrogens and, 242, 245

    and hormone replacement therapy, 231–32, 241

    male, 237, 244, **258–59**

    postoperative treatments for, **241–42**

    risk factors for, 69, 199, 207, 224, 230, **241**, 259

    self-examinations for, 236–38

breastfeeding, 118, 224, **288–92**

breastmilk, 285, 288, 290–91, **292–93**

    undesirable contaminates of, 410, 457, 536

breast reconstruction, 242–43

breathing difficulties. See also asthma; choking, 233, 308 314, 322, 362, 420, 519, 522, 602–3, 606

brief therapy (psychotherapy), 70–72, **408**, 592

broccoli, 115

bronchitis, 67, 468, **486–87**, 505, 546

bruises and bruising, 49, 206, 239, 253, 530, 553, 558, 572, **616–18**

BSE. See "mad cow" disease; Creutzfeldt-Jakob disease

bulimia, 209, 342, **343**, **347–48**

Bureau of Nonprescription Drugs (Canada), 114

burnout, 397, **399–401**, 590–92

burns and scalds. See also sunburns, 54–55, **58**, 59, 299–300, 488, 509, **605–6**, 609–10

Burow's solution, 126, 131, 172, 368, 473

bypass surgery, 233–34, 236, **521–24**

café-au-lait patches, 312

caffeine, 48, 53, 60–62, **67**, 90, 93, 95, **107–8**, 120, 186, 322, 420, 447, 490, 516, 528, 542

calcium, 107, 113–16, 210, 233, 379, 628–30

    bone strength and, 58, 93–95, 434, **444**

    iron absorption and, 119

    requirements for, 90–91, 95, **118**, **277–78**, **446–51**

    stones, 249, 551–52

calcium channel blockers, 235, 439, 514, 516–17, **521–22**, 526, 542–43, 621

CAMH. See Centre for Addiction and Mental Health (Clarke Institute)

Canada ETHIC, 257

the Canadian Lung Association, 40, 471, 582

cancers. See also tumors

    basal cell, 135

    brain, 169–70, 414, 425, 452, 501, 507

    breast. See breast cancer

    cervical. See cervical cancer

    colon, 26, 33–34, 80, 109, 115, 258, **483–86**, 532, 626

    endometrial. See cancers, uterine

    genetic/DNA risk testing for. See BRCA

    leukemia. See leukemia

    lung. See lung cancer

    lymphoma, 521

    malignant melanoma. See melanomas

    ovarian, 197, 199, **223–25**, 241, 243–45

    prostate, 80–82, 246, **249–52**, 258

    thyroid. See thyroid gland, disorders of

    uterine, 33–34, 197, 199, 220, **225–27**, 232, 450

candida. See also yeast infections

cannabis. See marijuana

carbohydrates, 38, 46–48, 89–93, **96**, **104–5**, 220, 295, 297, 316, 409, 485, 498–99, 520

carbon monoxide, 32, **374–75**, 436, 442

cardiac rehabilitation programs, 235, **523**

cardioembolic heart problems, 569

cardiologists, **79**, 233, 523, **526**

cardiomyopathies, 519

cardiopulmonary resuscitation. See CPR

cardiovascular disease. See also coronary artery disease; heart disease; stroke, **519**

    risk factors for, 22, 34, 94–95, 97, 113, 499, 519, 591

    in women, 206, 208, 233

cardiovascular endurance, 41, 209

carditis, 67, 329, 519, 527

caregiving. See also midwives, 205, **210**, 235, **432**, 453–54, **455**, 572–73

carotid endarterectomy, 571

carpal tunnel syndrome, **487–88**, 593

case-control study, definition of, 19

castration, 251–53, 259, 419

cat-scratch fever, 595–96

cataracts, 80, **161–64**, 430, 435–36, 501

    risk factors for, 24, 156, 558

catheterization, 248, 437, 582

CATMAT, 394

CDC National STD Hotline, 280

celiac disease, 372

cellulitis, 324

Center for Disease Control (U.S.), 387

central nervous system disorders, 440, **501**

Centre for Addiction and Mental Health (Clarke Institute), 70, 622

cephalopelvic disproportion, 287

cerebral palsy, 281, **313–14**, 323–24

cervical cancer. See also cervix; genital warts; human papilloma virus; Pap testing, 80, 190, 194, 202, **220–23**

    risk factors for and with, 24, 26, 151–52, 203, **221**

    and smoking, 194

    vaccine for reducing, 223

cervical caps, 198–99

cervix. See also cervical cancer, 192–94, 198–99, **220–21**, 252, 280, 284, 354

    dilation of, 280, 282–83

Cesarean births, 195, 261, 271–72, 279, 281–84, **285–87**

    vaginal births after, 286–87

chancroid, 193

checkups (medical), 41, 48, 76, **79–82**, 99, 173, 194, 200, 221–22, 236, 238, 319, **350–51**, **434–35**, 497, 541–42

    fetal, 261

chelation therapy, 84, 384

chemotherapy, 224–25, 258, 553–54, 557, 561

    drugs used in, 85, 224, 242

    reasons for using, 241

    side effects from, 141–42, **242**, 461

    systemic (total-body), 259, 555

chest pain. See also angina; heartburn, 18, 43, **233–34**, 419–20, 486–87, 516, **525**, 581, 614

chickenpox See also shingles, 132, 303

childbirth. See also birth defects; circumcision; epidurals; labor; newborn(s), **260–63**

    Cesarean. See Cesarean births

    complications during, 82, 261, **281**, 283

    episiotomy during. See episiotomy

    as a family affair, 262

    planning for, **272–75**, **281–83**

    and post-partum depression, 287, 409–11

    predicting the date of, 274

    premature, 166, 267, 270, 278, **280–81**, 284, 332

    vaginal, 261, 271, 285–86

childhood. See specific aspects thereof, e.g. (bedwetting; etc.). See also babies

chiropodists, 149

chiropractic methods, 82, 84, 478

chlamydia, 80, 82, 152, 190, **191–92 195**, 219, 247, 272, 354

chloasma, 276

chlorine, 116, 377, 379–82, 391

chocolate, 62, 67, 93, 108, 319, 371–72, 516, 528, 552

choking. See also babies, choking in; Heimlich maneuver, 58, 299–300, 302, 324, 420, 506, **606–8**

cholecalciferol. See Vitamin D

cholera, **388–89**, 392, 534

cholesterol, 34, 68, 70, **97–102**, 109, 498

    "bad". See LDL (low-density lipoprotein)

    content of foods, 68, 92–94, 98, **100–104**, 112, 115, 229, 499

    and coronary risks, 98–99, **518–21**

    gender differences and, 205, 230, 233, 236, 292

    "good". See HDL (high-density lipoprotein)

    screening for blood levels of, **82**, **98**, 435

cholesterol-free labels, **100**

cholesterol-lowering drugs. See also statin drugs, **522**, 563

chorionic villus sampling, 268–69

chromosomes. See also DNA testing, 181, 224, 243, 259, 267, 269, 316, 452, 454, 479, 529, 555

chronic fatigue syndrome, 207, **415–18**, 511

chronic liver disease, 259

cialis, 257

    risks associated with, 622

circadian rhythms. See also jet lag; melatonin, **50**, 53, **388**, 392–93, 403, 591

circumcision, 257–58

cirrhosis. See liver cirrhosis

CJD. See Creutzfeldt-Jakob disease

clitoris, 181, 211, 213–14

cloning, 269

club foot, 323–24

cocaine, 60–66, 151, 420, 520, 569

Cochrane collaboration, 20, 623

codeine, 60, **67**, 87, 401, 480, 489, 516, 532, 620–22, **623–24**, 626–28, **631**

coffee. See caffeine

cognitive behavioral therapy, 208, **346**, 356, 408, 418, **420**, 512

cold remedies. See also common colds, **87**, 278, **488–90**

colic, 291, 296–97, **315**

    biliary, 512

colitis. See also Crohn's disease; irritable bowel syndrome, 124, 466, 481–84, 485–86, 532

collagen, 122, 133, 440, 444, 503

colons. See also bowel problems; cancers, colon, 480–86, 531

colonoscopy, 80, 82, **483–86**

colostrum, 289–90

comas. See unconsciousness

common colds. See also cold remedies, 173, 302, **314–15**, 329–31, 486–87, **488–90**, **545–46**

    and vitamin C, 112

communication gap, 22, 349

Computerized Lifestyle Assessment program, 23

computer assisted symptoms and illness, **592–94**

conception, 265

concussion, 611–12

condoms **196**, **202–3**, 352, 354, 373, 457

    female, 199–200

    and HPV, 222

    and STDs, 189–91, 193–94, 458, 539

    and travel, 387

    use of, 189–91, 196–97, **201**

congenital disorders. See birth defects

congestive heart failure, 519, 522, 525

conjunctival hemorrhage, 158

conjunctivitis, 158, 192, 328

constipation, 92, 94–95, 104, 276, 347, 438, **480**, 481–82, 532, 628

    as a side effect, 406–7, 463, 522, 565

contact dermatitis, **123**, 124, 368

contact lenses. See vision, contact lenses and

contraception methods. See also emergency contraceptives; tubal ligation; vasectomy, 190, **196–203**, 222, 352–53

    oral contraceptives, 189, 196–204, 220, 225–27, 230

    "rhythm method" and, 204

convulsions. See also epilepsy; seizures, **609**, 612

    potential triggers of, 64, 66–67, 308, 335, 589, 603, 605, 619

corneal ulceration and scratches, 157–58

coronary artery disease. See also atherosclerosis; heart disease, 80, 233, **234**, 236, 493, **518–19**, 522–23

    risk factors for, 34, 68, 236, 580

cough medicines, **87**, 279, 489, **631**

counseling. See also psychotherapy; websites, 78–80, 167, 187–88, 201, 214, 224, 244, 253, 256, 261–64, 266, 321, 333, 351,

358–60, 406, 409, 418, 420, **428–29**, 473, 482, 492, 497, 592, **624**

    about drugs, 68, 70, **72**

cowper's glands, 247

CPR (resuscitation), 235, **600–602**, 612

Creutzfeldt-Jakob disease, 442, 454, **479**, **490**

cramps. See also menstruation, cramps during; muscle spasm; pain, abdominal

    abdominal [non-menstrual] and stomach, 44, 111, 225, 316, 367, 370, 372, 390, 417, 466, 480–82, 534, 565, 596, 604, 614, 621, 628

    muscle, 72, 116, 443, 450, 460, 612

crib death. See Sudden Infant Death Syndrome

Crohn's disease, 461–62, 482–83, **484**, 485

croup, 310, **315–16**, 322

crying. See also tears, 166, 285, 287, 291, **308**, **315**, 335, 403, 410, 608

cryotherapy. See also liquid nitrogen treatment, 151–54, 222–23

cumulative trauma disorder (CTD). See repetitive strain injury

cystic fibrosis, 243, 261, 264, 269, **491–92**, 544

cystitis, 248–49, **582–84**

cystoscopy, 247, 250, 551, 583–84

cysts, 127–28, 225, 239

    ovarian, 202, 225

Dalkon Shield. See also contraception, 197

dandruff, 126, **144–145**, 147

deafness. See hearing loss

decongestants, 53, **87**, 158, **165–67**, **314**, **365**, **489–90**, 546, **630–31**

    possible side effects from, 438, 513, 627

dehydration, 43–46, 48, 63, **95–96**, **119**, 122, 290, 295, 302, 306, 317, 347, 488, 493, 499, 628

dengue fever, 387, 390–91

dentin sensitivity. See teeth, sensitivity in

deodorants, 121, **125–26**, 133, 219

depilatories, 144

Depo-Provera, 200

depression. See also bipolar disorder; manic episodes; puerperal psychosis, 112, 453

    causes of, **404–5**, 431, 590

    and exercise, 40, 209, 433, 479

    and insomnia, 51, 393

pharmacotherapy and. See also antidepressants, 402, **406**, 620

    postpartum. See childbirth, and post-partum depression

    psychotherapy for, **408**

    risk factors for, 33—34, 61, 95, 161, 206–7, 215–16, 228–30, 243, 343, 346–47, 351, 393–94, 397–98, **402–4**, 418, 421–22, 430, 437, 443, 475, 481, 483, 510–11, 523, 562, 621

    risk factors with, See also suicide, 61, 64–67, 72, 94, 141–42, 200, 207, 212, 216, 247, 255, 280, 410, 414–15, 548, 590

    symptoms of, **357**, 395, **401–4**

dermatitis, **122–24**, 130, 148, 162, **368**, 547–48

dermatologists **79**, 121–26, 130, 133, 136, 222

diabetes, 76, 435, **492–500**

    gestational, 262, 272, **497**

    nutrition and, 103–5, **498–99**

    risk factors for, 33, 82, 99, 117, 235–36, 321, 558

    risk factors with, 41, 97, 141, 162, 202–3, 209, 212, 219, 232, 254–55, 267, 280–81, 446–47, 472, **497–98**, 519–20, 542, 549, **569**, 581, 625, 630–31

    symptoms of, **316**, **495**, 546

    and travel, 495, 498

    testing for, 82, 98

    treatment of, **498–500**, 620

    type I, **315–16**, **494–96**

    type II, **496–97**

dialysis, 53, 494, 535, **548–50**

diaper rash, 333–34

diaphragm. See also contraception, 196, 198, **202–3**, 583, 584

    hernia (abdominal) and, 528–29

diarrhea. See also dehydration; irritable bowel syndrome, 39, 292, 296, **316**, 333, **371–73**, **378**, **390–92**, 394, 628, 630

    dangers of, 116, 214, 302

    as a side effect or symptom, 18, 67, 111–12, 115, 161, 173, 251, 297, 308–9, 318, 324, 347, 367, 370, 406, 413–14, 419, 457, 463, 470, 484, 504, 534, 536, 565, 578, 596–97, 602

    treatments for, 86, **317**, 387, **390–91**, 482

Dietary Reference Intakes (DRIs), 89–90, 112–14

dieting **38–39, 92–93**
  consequences of, 36–37
  difficulties during, 36–37
  eating disorders and, 208–10, 343–46
  as a false concept, 37
  and nutritional deficiencies, 342
  pills and, 38
  relapse rates following "set-points" and, 35, 209, 342
  successful, 39–40
diets (nutritional). See also Mediterranean diet; vitamins, 19
  blood pressure lowering, 542–43
  for children, 295, 309, 448
  cholesterol and, **97–100**
  crash, 37
  and diabetes, 316, 493–94, **498**
  "elemental," 484–85
  fat and, 90, 97–99, **102–3**, 241, 244, 249, 519, **520**
  healthy, 16, 34, **37–38, 89–96, 103–7**
  heart health and, 68, 113, 235, 499
  for hemodialysis patients, 549
  importance of proper, 16, 77, 81
  low-carbohydrate high-fat (Atkins), 17, 38
  low-fat high-carbohydrate, 38
  minerals in, **115–19**, 215
  obesity and. See obesity
  for pregnancy, 264, **277–78**
  for seniors, 444, 447, 449, 466
  vegetarian, 106–7
diet therapy, 34, 521
diffuse alopecia, 144
digital thermometers, 306
diphtheria, **316**, 330, 334
  inoculations against, 80, 303–4, 388
disease-modifying anti-rheumatic drugs (DMARDs). See DMARDs
dissolved radon gas, 379
diuretics, 48, 88, 93, 116, 120, 167, 171, 216, 255, 347, 438, 480, 496, 502, 513, 522, 525, 542–43, 622, 628–29
diurnal enuresis, 321
diverticulitis, 480
dizziness. See vertigo
DMARDs, 464–66
DNA testing, 243, 269, 530
doctors (physicians). See also walk-in clinics
  choosing among (or referral to), **75–78**, 351, 440
  continuing education of, 20, 75
  double-doctoring, 624

  expectations of, 74, **78**
  family physicians. See family physician
  hospital affiliation and, 76–77
  and patient relationships, 11–12, 22, **74–75**, 77–78, 81, 134, 333, 468, 510, 623–24
  patient supervision by, 37
  payments to, 79, 429
  selection of, 76–77
  specialists, **79**
  when to consult a, 57, 65, 79–81, 86, 102, 124, 138, 279, 307–8, 317, 323, 329, 335, 350, 358, 388, 390, 486, 488, 495, 532, 609–10
double vision, 110, 162, 323, 514, 562, 569–70, 572, 578, 612
double-blind studies, 19
the "doula", 263
Down syndrome, 141, 269, 312, **316–17**, 454, 553
  risks for, 267–68, 317
drinking. See alcohol; hydration (body)
drownings, 44, 54, 56, **59–60**, 299–300, 355, 509, 603, 618–19
Drug Identification Numbers (DIN), 85, 114
Drug Information Line, 68
drugs
  abuse of, 30, 60–62, 65, 397, 414, 419, 425, 548, 624
  "designer," 63
  dependency, 51, 62–64
dynamic posturography, 502
dysmenorrhea, 215, 225
dyspareunia, **213**, 226, 254, 284
dysplastic nevi, 135, 137
dysthymia, **408**

ears. See also hearing loss; tinnitus
aches, 166, 172–73, 314, 319, 486, 546
  infections of, 24, 166, 169, **172–74**, 302, 306, **315–19**, 326, 330, 334, 501, 504
  injuries involving, 501, **609–10**
  fluids in the, **165**, 173, 319
  and flying, 165
  structure of, 165
  tubing of, 174, 319
  wax and, 164
ear-piercing, 124
eating disorders. See anorexia; bulimia
echocardiography, 234, 519, 526, 569
eclampsia, 270, **277**, 280–81, 284
ecstasy (drug). See also drugs, abuse of, 63

ectopic pregnancy. See also pregnancy, 265
eczema, **122–23**, 296, **319**, 370, 373, 472, 547–48
eldercare. See also geriatric care and problems; seniors, 210, **436**, 455, 592
  home-support services and, 433, 436
ejaculation, 187, **197**, 247–49, **252–54**, 265, 341, 407
  premature, 188, 252–54, 266
electrocardiograms, 79, 234, 413, 520, 527
electrocautery, 152, 154, 222–23
electroconvulsive shock therapy (ECT), 408
electrolysis, 144
electronic fetal monitoring, 283–84
electronystagmogram, 502
elephantiasis, 369
"embryo suicide," 267
embolisms, 113, 198, 231, **568, 571**
emergency contraceptives, 200–201
emotional problems. See also specific exemplars (e.g. anxiety); and psychiatric medicine; psychotherapy; stress, **395–429**
  difficulties of recognizing, 78, 395, 590
  importance of recognizing and disclosing, 11–12, 16–17, 23–24, 76, 81, 208, 256, 356
  reassurance available for, 78
  reluctances to acknowledge or disclose, 15, 271, 402
  as risk factors for medical problems, 51, 54, 124, 130, 142, 161, 184, 204, 207, 209, 215, 321, 356–57, 417, 509, 514, 521
  as side effects of other problems, 62, 173, 216, 318, **395**
  therapies for, **428–29**
encephalitis 304, 314, 326, 332, 389, **391**, 440, 442, 507–8, 589
encephalomyelitis, 415
endocrine function, 142, 144, 217, 255, **340**, 414, 417, 438, 576
endolymphatic hydrops, 170
endometriosis, 213–15, **225–27**, 266
endorphins, 40, 84, 217, 515
endoscopy, 512, 528, 540, 551, **566**
enemas, 19, 263, 271, **483–84**, 628
  barium, 82, 485
enucleation, 153
enuresis, 49, **320–22**, 333, 439
the environment, **362–94**
  noise in, 168, 396

pollution of and toxins in, 24, 264, 362, 373–74, 377, 441–42, 454, 460, 468, 556
Environment Canada, 381, 384
epidemiological research, 19, 190
epididymis, 247
epidural, 263, 286, 551–52
epiglottitis, 304, **322–24**
epilepsy, 67, 202–3, 278, 308, 321, **323–24**, 425, 501–2, **505–10**, 615, 625
epinephrine (adrenaline). See also asthma, anaphylaxis, 39, 161, 308–9, 363, 365, 411, 602
EpiPen, 364–65, 371
episcleritis, 158
episiotomy, 19, 213, 261, 263, 273, 282, 284
epsom salts, 86, 126
Epstein-Barr virus, 330, 415, 417
erectile problems, 22, 186, 247, 249–51, **253–57**, 622
ergonomics. See computer-assisted symptoms and illness
erythromycin, 102, 128, 191, 257, 285, 331, 364, 487, 528, 621–22, 631
estradiol, 144, 200, 229, **231**, 340
estrogen. See also phytochemicals, 212–13, 228, 237, 240, 255, 258–59, 448
  in birth control pills, 198–99, **202–3**, 224, 241
  protective or desirable potentials of, 94, 144, 217, 224, 227–28, 232, 439, 444–45, 449–51, 521
  risks associated with, 69, **202–3**, 219, 225, 228, 230–32, 241, 259, 444–45, 450
  menopause and, **229–31**
estrogen receptor modulators, 242, 450
etretinate, 129, 134
evidence-based medicine, 11–12, **19–20**, 75, **76**
exercise. See also fitness; pain
  athletes and, 95–96, 217–18, 226
  benefits of and needs for, 16, 23, **40–43**, 53, 71, 95, 98–99, **209**, 226, 232, 235, 241, 244, 405, 417, 430, 433, 439, 442–43, 446, 464, 499–500, 520, 525, 542–43, 585
  how best to, **40–45, 48–49**, 387, 418, 451, 542–43
  compulsive, 343–44, 398, 416, 444
  during pregnancy, **280**, 281, 283

safety and, **44–49**, **96**, 366, 369, 385–86, 446, 468, 499–500
  for seniors, 433, 436, 446
  for weight control, 17, 32, 34, 38–39, 90, **209**, 343
expectorants, 87, 487, **489**
exposure therapy (for phobias), 420, 422
external otitis. See also otitis media, 172
extracapsular surgery (cataracts), 164
eye(s). See also cataracts; glaucoma; macular degeneration; vision, **155–58**
  aging and, 157–62
  cosmetics/lotions and the, 121, 126, 128
  drops or ointments applied to the, 157
  injuries to the, **610**, 615, 617
  risks to the, 132, 156, 191–92, 195, 257, 375, 482, 494, 558, 577–78, 594, 597, 617
  specialists for, 156
  strain and, 514, 594
  symptoms and disorders of the, 157–58, 328, 366, 374, 502–3, 558–60
  testing of, 80, 155, 157, 312, 435, 497
eyelid problems, 123, 125, 158, 313, 363

fainting or feeling faint. See also vertigo, 43, 367, 371, 422, 498, 501–2, 519, 522, 568, 602, **610**, **613**
falling sickness. See epilepsy
falls
  dangers of, 46, 54–56, **57–59**, 299–300, **434**, **436–37**, 451, 501
  first aid for. See fractures
fallopian tubes, 190, 192, 201–2, 215, 225, 243, 252, **265–68**. See also ectopic pregnancy, 190, 191, 195, 198, 203
family physician(s), 21, 68, **74–77**
  choosing among, **76**
  consultations with and referrals by, 130, 149, 167, 188, 196, 222, 238, 255, 352, 373, 378, 402, 406, 429 435, 465, 487
fatigue. See also chronic fatigue syndrome; sleep, 66–67, 206, **207**, 323, **395**, 558
  potential causes of, 91, 108, 110–11, 114, 117, 173, 195, **207**, 210, 215–16, 204, 230, 242, 249, 251, 255, 342, 344,

347, 357, 365, 374, 385, 388–89, 396, 400–404, 409, 411–12, 422, 461, 464, 482, 494, 511, 514–16, 519, 525, 535, 546, 548, 553, 557, 561, 562, 566, 578, 583, 589, 590, 592, 613, 630
  overexertion and, 45–46
fat (body). See body fat
fat (nutritional)
  contents of in foods, 94, 96, 99, 101–3, 106, 292
  dietary choices among, 90–94,102–3, 107, 520
  monounsaturated. See monounsaturated fats
  polyunsaturated. See polyunsaturated fats
  recommended amounts of, **89–93**
  saturated. See saturated fats
  trans fatty acids. See trans fatty acids
favism. See hemolysis
feet. See foot problems
fertility. See contraception; infertility
fertilization, **181**, **215**, 252, **264–65**, 270
  in vitro, **266–67**, 269
fetal. See also childbirth; pregnancy
  activity, 275–76
  distress, 284, 286–87
  growth and development, **274–78**
fetal alcohol syndrome, 69–70, 279
fever, 72, 125, 130, 142, 173, 192, 195, 314, 316–19, 322–23, 325–28, 329–31, 333, 372–77, 390–92, 440, 457, 487–90, 507, 513, 517, 526, 545–46, 550, 553–55, 557–59, 578, 582, 589, 596, 615
  "beaver." See giardiasis
  "Dengue," 387, 390–91
  hay. See hay fever
  in infants and children, **304–8**
  "Lassa," 387, 391
  parrot, 596
  "Pontiac," 376
  rheumatic. See rheumatic fever
  "spotted," 327, 559, 604
  tick, 604
  travel and, 390, 394
  treatments for. See also
    antipyretic medications, **86**, 173, **307–8**, 314, 331, 487, 489, **627**
  trench, 146
  typhoid, 389, 513, 534
  yellow, 388
  when to call a doctor about, **173**, **307–8**, 486, 517

fiber (dietary), 90, **92**, 95, 99, **103–4**, 105–6, 235, 249, 344, 379, 440, 480–83, 485, 496, 532, 543
fibromyalgia, 206, 416, **510–11**
fifth disease, 323
fine-needle aspiration, 239, 251, 491, 580
fire ants, 369, 604
fire safety, 45, 54, **57–58**, 59, 80, 436
firearms, dangers of, 54, 56, 355, 358, 360, 383
first aid, 598–619
  for **allergy related emergencies.** See first aid, for **shock (allergic)**
  for **bleeding** and **wounds**, **605–6**, 609
  for **burns** and **scalds**, **605–6**
  caution required while giving, **599**
  for **choking**, **606–9**
  for **convulsions**, **609**
  for **ear injuries**, **609–10**
  for **eye injuries**, **610**
  for **fainting**, **610**, **613**
  for **fractures** or suspected fractures, **610–11**
  for **frostbite** or **freezing** or **hypothermia**, 385, **611**, **613–14**
  for **head injuries**, **611–12**
  for **heart attack** or **stroke**, 520, **612**
  for **heat exhaustion**, 385, **612–13**
  kits for, 45–46, 301, 309, **600**
  for severe **mouth** and/or **tooth injury**, **614**, **618**
  for **nosebleeds**, 614
  for **poisonings**, **614–15**
  for **poisonous stings** or **bites**, 369, **603–5**
  the **recovery position** during, **602**
  and **resuscitation AR & CPR**, **600–602**, 619
  for **shock (allergic)**, 309, **602–3**
  for **shock (electric)**, **610**
  for **shock (traumatic)**, **606**, **615**
  for **seizures**, 508, **615**
  for **sports injuries**, **616–18**
  for **suffocation**, **asphyxiation**, **drowning**, **603**
  training in and **readiness** for, 59, 387, **598–600**, **619**
  for **unconsciousness**, **618**

for accidents in or on the **water**, **618–19**
fitness. See also exercise, 17, **40–43**, 48, 209, **385–87**, 397, 443, 479, 495, 500, 511
flat feet, 324
fleas, 367, **369**, 391, 548, 596
fluids. See hydration (body)
fluoride, 90, 113, **117**, 175, 177–78, **379–81**
  osteoporosis and, **449–51**
fluorouracil cream, 154, 222
folic acid 109, 114, 264, 520
  importance of, 91, 93–94, **95**, **113**, 278, **461**
  at conception and during pregnancy, **113**, **264**, **278**
  and seniors, 94
  sources of, **111**
food allergies, 295, **296**, **310**, 315, **369–72**
food intolerances, **296**, **371–72**
food poisoning. See also diarrhea; salmonella poisoning, **371–73**, 436
foot problems, **148–150**, 472, 500
formula (baby), 113, 292–94, **295–97**, 317, 319, **384**
foster care (for seniors), 434
foxglove, 85
fractures, 69, 437–38
  crush, 447
  first aid for, **610–11**
  of the hip, 446
  osteoporosis related, 82, 94, 210, 217, **444–49**
  preventive and safety measures against, 46, 48, 57, **118**, 230–32, **449–51**
  stress, 45, 149, 217
Framingham study, 34, 234, 569
free radicals, 108, 471
friction alopecia, 141
frostbite, 46–47, 49, 126, **611**, 616
functional bowel disorder. See irritable bowel syndrome

gallbladder problems, 232, **512**
gallstones, 210, **512**
gamma globulin, 325–26, 417
garlic, 108, **115**, 372, 513, 589
gastroenterologists, **79**
gender identity and development, **179–83**, **181**, 185, 210
generalized anxiety disorder, 419, **422**
genes. See DNA testing
genetic counseling, **243–44**, 261, 263–64, 492, 530
genetic screening, 261, **263**, 268–69

geneticists, **79**

genital herpes, 192–93, 221–22, 272, **279**

genital warts. See also cervical cancer; human papilloma virus, 151–52, 191

removal of, 154, 223

gentian violet, 220, 292

geriatric care and problems. See also seniors, 432–33, 435–36

german measles. See Rubella

Gerson method, 84

giardiasis, **324–25**, 378, 548

gingivitis, **175–77**, 513

glasses. See vision, glasses and

glaucoma. See also diabetes, **159–61**, 435–36

risk factors for, 156, 158, 312

risk factors with, 157, 161, 364, 630–31

glucose (blood; dietary), 89, **96**, **104–5**, 116, 272, 316, 396, 431, **493**, **495–500**

glucose intolerance. See also diabetes; insulin, 33, 82, 316

glycogen stores, 46, **96**, 105, 218

gnats, 369

gonadotropin, 217, 227, 259, 269, 340

gonads, 181, 340

gonorrhea, **190–91**, **195**, 202, 264–65, 285, 354, 504

gout, 112, 150, 383, 463, **465–66**, 488, **552**

grains (dietary), 35, 38, 89, 91, **92–93**, 94, 100, 104, 106–7, 109, 112–13, 116–17, 235, 498–99, 520

grand mal seizures, **323–24**, 506, **508**

granny flats, 434

grapefruit juice, 92, 345

medicines and, **621**

graves disease, 577–79

grommits, 174, 319

group homes, 428, 434

guided tissue regeneration, 178

gum inflammation. See also gingivitis, 174–75

gynecological exams and status, 212, 214, 217–18, **221–23**, 225–26, 440

gynecomastia, 258–59

haemophilus influenze type b. See Hib

hair, 106, 122, **139–40**, 145

hair loss. See also baldness, **141–44**

hair products, 123, 125, **144–45**, 364

halitosis, 234, **512–13**, 587

hammertoes, 150

hand and nail care, 129, **148**

Hashimoto's thyroiditis, 579

hashish, 62, 67

hay fever. See also allergic rhinitis, 365–66

HDL (high-density lipoprotein), 27, 70, **97**, **99–100**, 102, 235–36, 520, 522

HDL/LDL ratio, 97, 100

headache, 270, 349–50, 388, **513–17**

as one element of a syndrome, 131, 170, 215–16, 327–28, 357, 371–72, 374–77, 389, 393, 395, 397–98, 400, 416–18, 422, 461, 488, 498, 534, 536, 545–46, 548, 558–59, **569–70**, 589–90, 595–96, 612–14

migraine, 232, 371, 501–2, 507, **513–17**, 571

as a side effect, 72, 108, 110, 112, 120, 128, 143, 160–61, 197, 200, 203, 257, 323, 406–7, 459, 470, 474, 483

treatments for, 86, 106, 232, 489, **513**, **516**, **625–27**

as a withdrawal symptom, 25, 66–67, 620

head injuries. See also concussion, 507, 609, **611–12**, 614

prevention of, 44, 57, 332, 617

head lice, 145–48

health. See also fitness; healthcare; hygiene; nutrition

basics about, 15–16

contributing factors to, 15–16, 24

and exercise. See exercise, benefits of and needs for

mental. See mental health

news about, 21–22

validity assessments for studies relating to, 12, 18, 250, 284, 630

Health Canada

behavior advised by, 80, 104, 179, 326, 388

conclusions reached by, 62

substances banned or controlled by, 85, 114, 227

toll free telephone number and website of, **32**, **546**

healthcare, 16, 20–21, 75–78, 261

Health Protection Branch (Canada), 114

hearing aids, **167–69**, 572

hearing impairments, 164, 166, 436

hearing loss, 166–68, 326, 328, 369

age-related, 164, **167**

noise-induced, **168**

sudden, 167

heart attack (myocardial infarction),

early warning signs of, 43, 48, 519, 612

first aid for, **612**

mortality from, 233, 521

physiology of, 233–34, 518

risk factors for and with, 32–33, 40, 66–68, 97–98, 101, 109, 112–13, 196, 206, 210, **235–36**, 383, 497, 519, **520–21**, 541, 543, 571, 591

treatment of, 235, 519, **521–24, 627**

in women, **233–35**

heartburn. See also chest pain; hiatus hernia, 22, 234, **527–29**

as one element of a syndrome, 276, 484

discriminated from heart problems, 525, **527**

treatments for, 86, **528–29**, **629**

heart disease. See primarily angina; cardiovascular disease; congestive heart failure heart attack; hypertension, **519**

diagnosis of, **234**

heart failure. See congestive heart failure

heart murmurs, 234, **526–27**

heart palpitations, 372, 421–22, 461, 519, **522**, **525–26**, 559, 576–79

heart-rate, "training range," 41–42

heart-valve defects, 324, 329, 519, 525–27, 571

heat-sensitive fever strips, 306

heatstroke, 43–44, 133, 391, **613**

the Heimlich maneuver, 600–602, **606–8**, 619

hematologists, 79

hemlock, 85

hemoccult test, 80

hemoglobin. See also anemia; iron, 107, 264, 271, 375, 383, **460–63**, 553

hemolysis, 372, 461, 558

hemophilia, 79, 243, 264, **529–30**, 535

hemorrhages. See also hemophilia; stroke, 110, 158, 163, 272–73, 280, 287, 289, 553, 556, **605–6**

aspirin and, 522, 525

hemorrhoids, 485, **530–33**, 629

as one element of a syndrome, 484

factors predisposing to, 103

remedies for, **532**

hepatitis. See also liver cirrhosis, 66, 68, **389**, **533–39**, 547, 556, 599

hepatitis A, 304–5, **325**, **389**, **533–39**

hepatitis B, 190, 194, **195**, 263, 272, 292, 294, **304–5**, **325–26**, **533–39**

hepatitis C, 64, **533–39**

hepatitis D, 533–34, **536–37**

hepatitis E, 533, **536–38**

infectious, **533**

protection from, 191, 194, 263, 272, **303–5**, **389**, 392, **533–39**

risk factors for, 85, **389**, 474, 530, 534, **538–39**

symptoms of, **533–37**

transmission of, 292, 294, 389, **533–37**

vaccines against the various types of, **533–37**

herbalism, 85, 88, 411

herbal remedies, 84, 411, 464, 489, 626

hernias (abdominal). See also hiatus hernias, 259, 315, **539–41**, 629

herniated disc, 477

herpes infections, 141, 148, 158, **189–95**, 329, 417, 457, 459, 487, 507, 548, 582

facial (simplex), 132, 156, 327

genital (simplex II), **192–95**, 221–22, 272, **279–80**

zoster. See also shingles, 131–32, 158

hiatus hernias, 528–29, **539–40**

Hib infection. See also vaccine, 80, **304**, 322, **324–25**, 327–28

high-density lipoprotein. See HDL

hip fractures, 18, 231–32

hirsutism, 144, 227

hives, **124**, 295–97, 308–9, 362–63, 367, 370–72, 483, 547–48, 602, 604, 631

HIV infection. See also AIDS; sexually transmitted diseases, 193, **456–60**, **599**

mortality from, 206, **457–59**

prevalence of, 61, 189, **457–58**

risks for, 64, 189, 190–91, 197, 257, 392, **457**, 530, 534, **599**

risks with, 219, 221, 272, 292, 303, **456**, 538, 544

symptoms of, **457**

tests for, **457**, 530

treatment for, **457–60**

home-sharing, 434

homeopathy, 82, **84**

home remedies for the medicine cabinet, 86

home visits, 76–77, 435, 455

homocysteine, 109, **113**, 235, 462, **520**

homosexuality. *See also* sexual, orientation, 182–83, 188, 190–91, 458, 534–35, 537

hormones, 89, 97, 117–18, 133, 268, 280, 283–84, 289, 297, 393, 444–45, **449**, 479, 529, 542, 586

  disorders of, 107, 259, 315–16, 321, 417, 419, 446, 493, 497, 576

    glands producing, 37, 50, 252, **340**, 393, 450, 576

    imbalances of, 50, 67, 85, 215, 217, 254, 344, 388, 393, 409–10, 438, 576–78

    sex, 38, 67, 69, 141–42, 181, 213–19, 225, 227, 233, 239, 252–53, 276, 337, **339–40**, 446

    stress, 38, 396–97, 624

    suppressors of, 249, 251

    therapy with, 215, 217, 227, 242, 251, 255, 259, 266, 320, 449–50, 459, 500, 521, 577–79

hormone replacement therapy. *See also* breast cancer; menopause, 18, 95, 206, 219, 228, **230–32**, 450, 577, 579.

hot flashes, 115, **227–30**, 232, 450

HPV. *See* human papilloma virus

HRT. *See* hormone replacement therapy

human chorionic gonadotropin, 269

human papilloma virus (HPV) *See also* genital warts, cervical cancer, 151, 190–91, **193–95, 221–23**, 354

humidity and humidifiers, 81, 122–23, 126, **315**, 362, **374–77**, 392, 547, 589, **624**

Huntington's disease, 243, 414, 442

hydration (body). *See also* dehydration; water, 95, **119**, 128, 385, 480, 552, 584

  importance of, 43, 46, 48

  oral rehydration solution (ORS) and, 317, 373, 390

hydrocortisone creams, 86, 123–24, 126, 472, 547

hygiene, 16, 80, 174, 193, 219–20, 257–58, **298**, 384, 426, **433, 436**, 437, 453, 472, 531–33, 581, 584, 596

hymenal tags, 213

hyperlipidemia, 97–98, 466

hyperopia, 156

hypersensitivity pneumonitis, 376

hypertension (high blood pressure). *See also* blood pressure, 41, 210, 232, 267, 391, 465–66, 514, **625**, **628**

monitoring of, **541–43**

"portal," 512, 556

potential causes of, 33–34, 48, 93, 379, 396–98, 407, **541**, 620

as a risk factor for heart disease and stroke, 48, 68, 97–99, 202, 236, 519–21, 525–26, **541, 568–71**

as a risk factor for other problems, 156, 158–59, 262, 273, **541**

treatments (good and bad) for, 106, 112, 236, **542–43, 620, 630**

hyperthermia. *See also* heatstroke, 384, 612, 616

hyperthyroidism, 447, **576–79**

hypnosis, 25, **30**, 32, 84, 439, 482

hypoallergenic states, 296, 319

hypoglycemia. *See also* diabetes, **105**, 171, 415, 495, **497–99**, 501–2, 507

hypoparathyroidism, 162

hypothalamus, 38, 65, 217, 252, 340, 385, 576, 578–79

hypothermia. *See also* frostbite, 44, 46–48, **385, 613–14**, 619

hypothyroidism, 98, 403–4, 416–17, **576–80**

hysterectomy, 227–28, 231

hysteria, 374, 569

ibuprofen, 173, 216, 227, 307, 319, 464, 489, 517, 564, 616, 620, **622**, **627–28**

ice. *See also* methamphetamine

  contaminating drinks, 391–92, 534, 537–38

  as a safety danger, 46–47, 59, 436

  for treating sprains or inflammation, 45, 48–49, 465, 616–17

  for use treating other conditions, 230, 239, 253, 307, 367–68, 585, 603–4, 612

illness, basics regarding, 15–17, 20

immune globulin. *See also* gamma globulin, 304, 325, 534, 537–38

immunization. *See also* vaccines

  for health maintenance, **80**, 194, 261, 264, **302–5**, 316, 325–26, 328–30, 332–35, 433, 435, 487, 533–35, 539, 544–45, 599

  for travel, **387–89**

immuno-augmentation therapy, 85

immunological reactions. *See* allergic reactions

impetigo, **124**, 148, 319, **326**

impotence, 66, 69, 161, 186–87, 201, 203, 251, 254, 256, 266, 343

incontinence. *See also* bedwetting; enuresis; stress incontinence, **438**, **440**, 582

  in adults, 228, 248–51, 263, 284, 562

  in children, 321–22

  in seniors, 430, **435**, **437–40**

indoles, 115

indoor air contaminants, 375

infancy. *See* babies; newborns

infarcts. *See also* heart attack; stroke, 567–68, 570

infertility

  causes of, 24, 82, 191–92, 195, 226, 266, 382

  in men, **252–53**

  reversal of in women, **265–68**

inflammation. *See* swellings

inflammatory bowel disease, 482–83

influenza(s). *See also* Hib, 167, 305, 307, 322, 330, 436, 468, 486–87, 489, 511, **543–46**,

anti-viral drugs for, 490, 545

  distinguished from a common cold, **545–46**

  immunization against, 80, 82, 433, **544**

inhibited orgasm, 187

injuries. *See also* burns and scalds; ears; eyes; falls; **first aid**; fractures; head injuries; hemorrhages; mouth injuries; sports injuries

  prevention of, 16, **23, 43–49, 54–60, 299–302**

insects. *See also* mosquitoes, ticks, 146, **366**, 389–90, **604**

  allergies and, 308, 363, **366–67, 369**

  symptoms and diseases caused by, 123, 326, 330, **362, 369, 391**, 548, 559, 589, 602

insomnia, **51–52**, 216, 349, 357, 393, 397, 403, 420, 422–23, 453, 590, 592, 624

  as a side-effect, 29, 66–67, 227–28, 242, 345, 364, 407, 442, 459, 470, 474

institutionalization. *See also* caregiving, 80, 432, 434

insulin. *See also* diabetes; glucose (blood), 117, 444, 494

  as a hormone, 106, 315, 340, 493

  obesity and, 33, 37–38

  as a therapy, 316, **493–95**, 500

intercytoplasmic injection, 267–68

interferons, therapy with, 131, 153, 222, 459, 490, 535, 537–38, 555, 563

internists, 79

interpersonal therapy (IPT), 405, 408–9

in-toeing, 324

intraocular lens. *See also* cataracts, 163

intraocular pressure, 156, 159–60

inverted nipples, 291

in-vitro fertilization, 266–67

iodine (as an antiseptic or diagnostic tool or therapy), 86, 391, 551, 561, 577, 579–80

iodine (dietary or environmental), 107, 115, **117–18, 578**

iron (dietary). *See also* anemia; hemoglobin, **117–18, 630**

  absorption of, 90, 112, **114, 118–19**, 292, 449

  excess, 441

  importance of, 91, 93, 113, 296

  requirements for, 91, 93–94, 107, 115, 118, 210, 215, 277–78, 292–93, 296–97

  sources of, **118–19**, 296–97

  supplements and, 91, 94, 119, 215, 629, **630**

irritable bowel syndrome, 18, 416, 462, **481–82**

ischemia, 233, 235, 518, 567–68

isolation (social), 94, 164, 205, 207, 236, 343, 350, 355, 358, 397, 412, 426, 434, 437, 453, 475, 591

itching, 18, 29, 138, 503, **546–48**

  causes of, 112, **123–24**, 129, 131, 133, 147, 172, 219, 308–9, 336, 362, 373, 472, 530–32, 535, **547–48**, 604, 619

  genital, 195, 219, 221, 279, 373

  as a side effect, 143

  treatments for, **124–26**, 364, 367–68, **547**

IUDs. *See also* contraception methods, 190–91, 194, **196–99, 202–3**

Japanese B encephalitis vaccine, 389

jaundice, in newborns, 291; as alerting sign of hepatitis, 195, 325, 533–536

jet lag, 50–51, 391–93

  "occupational," 388

Kegel exercises, 213–14, 280, **439**

keratinization, 133

kidney failure, **548–50**

  associated causes of, 63, 248, 258, 378, 465, **548–49**, 558

  dialysis for, **549–50**

  risk factors with, 98, 414, 493–94

kidney stones, **550–52**

prevention of, 552
risk factors for, 90, 111–12, 115–16, 465–66, 482, 629–30
symptoms of, 550–51
treatment of, 551–52
kidney transplants, 494, 549, **550**
killer cells, 85, 417
"kissing tonsils," 334
Klinefelter's syndrome, **259**

labor. See also Cesarean births; childbirth, 193, **281–84**
lactation. See breastfeeding
lactic acid, 41, 87, 126, 134, 152–53, 459
lactose intolerances, 296–97, 371–72, 485
La Leche League, 292
Lamaze system, 281–82
laparoscopy and laparoscopic treatments, 224, **226**, 267, 512, 540
laryngitis, 315, 488, 587
laser use
by alternative medicine, 30, 32
for improving vision, 156, 158–61, 164, 497
in surgery, 226, 267–68, 532, 566
for treating skin problems, 133, 152, 154, 194–95, 220–23, 312–13
LASIK eye surgery, 156
lassa fever, 387, 391
latex, sensitivity to, 196, 203, 364, **373–74**
laxatives, 86, 209, 278–79, 341, 347, **480**, 490, 531–32, 614, 622, 626, **628–29**
LDL (low-density lipoprotein). See also cholesterol, **97–102**, 109, 112, 115, 236, 450, 496, 498, 520, 522
lead poisoning, 362, **382–84**
Lea's shield, 196
Legionnaire's disease, 375, 377
legumes, 38, 89–90, 92–94, 101, 104–7, 110–11, 113, 117, 235, 264, 277, 363, 461, 498–99, 520, 552
leishmaniasis, 391
leukemia, 513, **552–55**, 561
risks and cautions with, 303, 308, 314, 462
leukotriene. See also asthma, 106, 311, 363, 365, 377, 467, 470
Levitra, 257, 622
lice, **145–48**, 367, 548
lifestyles. See Computerized Lifestyle Assessment
lily of the valley, 85
lipoproteins, 97, 236

liquid nitrogen treatment, 133, 141, 151–54, 194, 223
liver cirrhosis, 23, 66, 68, 195, 255, 259, 533–36, **555–56**
liver spots, 137
lockjaw. See tetanus
loneliness, 65, 71, 94, 236, 349–50, 412, 436, 594
Lou Gehrig's disease, 460
low-density lipoprotein. See LDL
LSD, 61–64, **66**
lumpectomy, 240–41, 258–59
lung cancer, 379, **556–57**
in men, 246
risks and cautions with, 109
and smoking , 23–24, 26–27, 67, 208, **556**
in women, 206, 208, 236
lungs, 42, 124, 304, **468–69**, 486, 545, 557, 581, 600
lupus, 141, 206, 463, 549, **557–58**
lutein, 109, 159
luteinizing hormone-releasing hormones, 227, 242, 340
lycopene, 108–9
lyme disease, 362, **559–61**, 604
lymphoma. See cancers
lysine, 106–7

macular degeneration. See also eye(s), 109, **158–59**, 436
"mad cow" disease, 106, 479, **490–91**. See "mad cow" disease; Creutzfeldt-Jakob disease
magnesium, 86, 90, 115, **116**, 342, 379–80, 528, 542, **628–29**
malaria, 369, **389–90**, **394**, 461, 604
medications for, 130, 387, 390, 466, 558
mammograms, 80, 82, **236–42**, 244–45
manganese, 115, **117**, 379, 442, 460
manic depression. See bipolar disorder
manic episodes, 412–14
MAOIs. See also antidepressants, **407**, 423, 442, 630–31
marijuana, 60–62, 64, **67**, 253, 255, 266, 360–61, 420, 556, 589
mastectomy, **240–43**, 245, 258–59, 547
mastitis, 291
mastoiditis, 173
masturbation, 183, **185**, 187–88, 214, 253–54, 258
measles, 166–67, 264, **326**, **329–30**, 388
immunization for, 80, **302–4**, 328
meat. See also proteins, 92–94, 96,

99, 101, **106–7**, 116–19, 215, 272, 277–78, 370–73, 520, 597
mechanical bladder dysfunction, 247
meconium, 290
medical technology, 261
medications. See also analgesics; antacids; antihistamines; antipyretic medication; codeine; cold remedies; cough medicines; laxatives; malaria, drugs for
adverse reactions to, 78, 83, 85, 99, 232, 261, 303, 370, 390, 408, 410, **435–36**, 459, 463, 466, 516, 544, 558, 577, **621–22, 624–31**
generic, 81, **626**
instructions on taking, **620**, **624–27**
for and in the medicine cabinet, 81, 86–87, **627–31**
for pain, 49, 85–87, 131, 153, 173, 226, 314, 319, 387, 466, **600, 622–23, 627–28**
safe control and management of, **56**, 60–61, 67, **622–28**
the Mediterranean diet, **38**, **520**
megavitamins, 109, 114
melanomas, 135–38
melatonin, **393–94**, 409
melilot, 85
menarche, 189, 214–15, 217, 224, 241, **340–41**
Ménière's disease, 169, **170–71**, 501–3
meningitis, 173, 292, 303–4, 306–8, 324–25, **327–28**, 332, 504, 507–8, 514, 589
meningococcal, 305, 308, **327–28**, 389
menopause. See also hormone replacement therapy, 144, **227–30**
altered health risks following, 33, 69, 82, 219, 223–25, 233, 241, 438, 444–45, 465, 514, 519
hot flashes and. See hot flashes and libido, **212–13**, **228**
nutrition and, 91, 93–95, 115–17, 446–49, 451, 630
remedies for the discomforts of, **230**
side effects during, **228**, 526
menstruation. See also amenorrhea; contraception; menopause; premenstrual syndrome; spotting (menstrual), **214–32**, 457, 515, 538
cramps during, 198–200, 202–3, 215, 218, 225, 627
and excessive exercise, 217–18

conception during, 214
heavy periods during, 113, 199–200, 215, 227, 231, 462
pain during, 215, 225, 227
mental health. See also self-esteem; stress; worry, 15–16, 61, 78, 350, **358–59**, **395**, **419**, 429, 590
meta-analysis, **19–20**, 198, 511
metabisulfite, 372
metabolic therapies, 84
methamphetamine, 61, 63
middle-ear infections. See otitis media
Midwifery Act, 275
midwives, 261–62, 271–72, **273–75**
migraine. See headache, migraine
milk sensitivity. See lactose intolerances
mineral oil, 86, 121, 125, 133, 145, 547, 560, 610, 622, 628–30
minerals (dietary). See also specific exemplars (e.g. calcium), 89, 93–94, 107, 113–14, **115–20**, 159, 277–78, 347, **380**, 444, 548
miotics, 161
miscarriage, 195, 203, 222, 267, 269–70, 278, 280, 383
moles. See also melanoma, 135–38
mongolian spots, 312
mongolism. See Down syndrome
monoamine oxidase inhibitors, 407, 411
monoclonal antibodies. See antibodies, monoclonal
mononucleosis, 167, 330, 415
monosaccharides, 105
monosodium glutamate (MSG), 372
monoterpenes, 115
monounsaturated fats, 102, 520
morning-after pills. See Yuzpe
morning sickness. See pregnancy
morphine, 60, 67, 85, 441, 623
mosquitoes, 362, 366–67, **369**, **388–91**, 457, **589**, 604
mouth care, 174–76, 512
mouth injuries, 614
moxybustion, 84
MRI scans, 226, 238, 502, 507, 510, 561–63, 569
mucous colitis, 481
multiple chemical sensitivity. See allergic reactions; "total allergy syndrome"
multiple sclerosis (MS), 169, 171, 214, 255, 414, 501–2, 507, **562–63**
mumps, 167, 253, 259, 266, 327, **328**
immunization for, 80, 303–4, 329, 388
muscle spasm. See also cramps, 66, 169, 213, 310, 477, 531, 605, 617

muscular dystrophy, 264
muscular (isotonic) endurance, 41
muscular (isometric) strength, 17,
40–41, 43
musculoskeletal complaints, 50, 84,
511, **593**, 616
myalgic encephalomyelitis. See
encephalomyelitis
myocardial infarction. See heart
attack
myocardial perfusion imaging, 234
myoclonus, 52, 479
myopia, **156**, 161, 350
myringotomy, **173**, 319

narcolepsy, 52
narcotic (opioid) analgesics, 67,
623–24, 628, 631
Narcotics Anonymous, 68, 70
natural family planning, 202, 204
naturopathic medicine. See also
"alternative" medicine, 84–85
neck. See stiff neck
Neisseria bacteria, 191, 327–28, 504
nephropathy. See also kidney failure,
498
nervous bowel. See irritable bowel
syndrome
neural tube defects, 93, 111, **113**,
210, 264, 268–69, 272, **278**, 461
neurofibromatosis, 312
neuroleptic medications, 426,
441–42
neurologists, 79, 444, 503
neuropathy, 112, 498, 500
nevi, 135–37, 556
newborn(s). See also birthmarks;
breastfeeding; childbirth; circumcision; colic, 119, 137, **284–85**
abilities and reflexes of, 287–88
assessments of, 80, 166, 278,
281, 284–85, 323–24, 579
bonding by and with, 262–63,
287
care of, 262–63, 273, 275, 280,
283, 285, 288–93
crying in, 166, 287, 291, 335
fever in, **306–7**
safety measures for, 55, 138,
191, 194, 535
niacin. See vitamin B₃
nicotine. See also tobacco, **24–32**,
60, **67**, 132, 255, 278, 529, 541
substitution therapy for, 25, 28–30
withdrawal from, 24–29
night terrors, 52, **53–54**
nipples. See also inverted nipples
nits. See head lice
soreness of, 291–92
nocturnal emissions, 341
noise. See hearing loss

noise maskers. See also tinnitus, 169,
171
non-hydrogenated fats. See polyunsaturated fats
nosebleeds, 67, 572, **614**
NSAIDs. See anti-inflammatory
agents
nutrient-dense foods, 94
nutrients. See also nutrition, 89,
104, 107–8, 114, 460
recommended intakes of, **90**,
96, 113, 119
nutrition. See also athletes; breastfeeding; diabetes; dieting;
menopause; obesity; osteoporosis;
prenatal; Recommended Nutrient
Intakes (RNIs), **89–90**
at different stages of life, **91, 94**,
277–79
"sensible," **92–109**, 208, 342

obesity. See also dieting; weight
(body), 448
contributing causes of, **34–35**,
105, 210, 342
definitions for, **33–34**
effect of diets on, **34–35**
the importance of controlling,
32–33
risk factors due to, **33–34**, 82,
98–99, 130, 236, 241, 259,
280, 286, 416, 438, 465, 493,
496–97, 512, 518, 520, 528,
539, 541, 543, 556
treatments for, **35, 37–40**, 209
obsessive-compulsive disorder, 346,
419, **423–24**
obstructive sleep syndrome, 334
occupational burnout or stress. See
burnout; stress
oils, essential, 177
oligomenorrhea, 217
omega-3 fatty acids, 93, 99, 102,
106, 235
oophorectomy, 225, 245
open-angle glaucoma, 160–61
opiates, 40, 60, 63–64, 66, 84, 547,
623–24
opium, 60, 67, 402
ophthalmologists, 156, 503
opticians, 156
optometrists, 156
oral contraceptives. See contraception methods
oral rehydration solution (ORS).
See hydration (body)
oral steroids (systemic), 142,
470–71
orchidectomy, 252
organic chemicals. See also vitamins,
375, **379**, 381

orthopedic surgeons, 149, 617
osteoarthritis, 463–64
osteoporosis, **444–51**
and calcium. See calcium
diagnosis of, 82, **448**
estrogen and, 69, 94, 229,
445–46
fractures with, **444–45**, **447**
hormone replacement therapy
and, 18, 230
nutrition and, 58, 94, 118, 210,
379–80, 434, **446–49**
prevention of, 40, 58, 69, 94,
229, 379–80, 433–34, 436,
451, 630
risk factors for, 108, 200, 207,
210, 217, 227, 344, 346,
446–47, 483, 558, 580
treatments for, **449–51**
otitis media See also ears, infections
of; external otitis, 172–74, 317–19
ototoxicity, 166
Ottawa Charter for Health
Promotion, 16
out-toeing, 324
ovarian cancer. See cancers

PABA, 139, 558
pain. See also angina; bronchitis;
chest pain; childbirth; circumcision; fractures; headache;
hemorrhoids; injuries; kidney
stones; medications; menstruation; mouth care; peptic ulcers;
pharyngitis; premenstrual syndrome; retrosternal pain;
pregnancy; prostatitis; sunburn;
teething; urination, 17, 49–51
abdominal, 190–92, 194–95,
221, 225, 246–48, 324, 480,
482–85, 495, 512, 528, 536,
539–40, 548, 556, 565,
581–83
arm and shoulder, 48, 233
arthritic, 463–66
back. See also back problems,
84, 249, 276, 395, 397, 444,
448, **476–78**, 548
bone and joint. See also pain,
arthritic, 250–51, 323, 416,
444, 450, 510–11, 553,
557–59, 561, 589–90, 610
chronic whole body, 510–11
in an ear, 165–66, 173, 318, 579
from exercise, 41, 45, 49
eye, 157–58, 328
foot or leg, 151, 472, 477, 498,
500, 553–54, 585
the importance of, **49, 173, 616**
during intercourse, 211–13, 226,
228, 247–48, 254, 284

lung and throat, 233, 581, 587
management of, 84, 131, 135,
173, 226–27, 319, 330, 418,
451, 466, 478, 511, 600,
605–6, 622–23, 625, 627
muscle. See also muscle spasm,
357, 376, 395, 397, 418, 477,
546, 590, 593
as a side effect of treatments,
101, 110–12, 128, 152–54,
156, 541
skin or nerve, 128, 131–32, 329,
562, 604–6
palpitations. See heart
palpitations
panic attacks, 63, 66–67, 105, 187,
234, 377, 414, 418, 590
as a side effect, 256, 420
panic disorder, 419, **420–21**, 502
pantothenic acid, 111
papilloma viruses. See human papilloma viruses (HPV)
Pap testing, 221–23
paraphilias, 183
parathyroid (gland and hormone),
118, 162, 444–45, 449–50
parenteral streptomycin, 171
parents. See also adolescence; caregiving; newborns; safety, home;
seniors,
as accepting advisors, 182–83
knowledge or training of, 55, 80,
184, 263, 294
as role models, 180, 182, 184,
229
role comfort and preparedness
of, 262–63
support groups for. See also
websites, 359
Parkinson's disease, 63, 255, 404,
427, 435, **440–44**, 502
possible causes of, **442**
treatments for, 414, 438,
441–43, 622
parvovirus B, 323
patients (medical). See also doctors
(physicians), and patient relationships
as therapy partners, 20, 74
PCP, 61, 63–64, 66
peak expiratory flow rates, 469
peak-flow meter (for asthma), 311,
469
peanut products, 58, 92–93,
100–102, 105, 107, 110–11,
300–301
allergies to, **308–10**, 363,
369–70
pediculicide shampoos, 147
pedophilia, 183
pellagra, 111–12

pelvic inflammatory disease, 82, **190–92**, 195, 199, 202, 265–66

penile blood vessel disorders, 255

penile prostheses, 256

penis, See also circumcision; contraception; erectile problems; genital warts; human papilloma virus (HPV); syphilis, 180, 247, **252–58**, 338, **340–41**, 350

peptic ulcers, 397, **563–66**
    risk factors for, 467, **564–65**, 567
    risk factors with, 451, 462, 519, **566**, 629

perilymph fistula, 501

periodontal disease, **174–178,** 513

periodontitis, **175–77**

pernicious anemia, 93, 108, 111, 117, 141, 461

pertussis. See whooping cough

Pervasive Development Disorder (PDD). See autism

pets. See also bites; rabies, 29, 384, 574
    allergic responses to, 363–64, 366
    diseases and, 147, 336, 368, 546, 560, **594–97**
    "therapy" from, 436, 594

PET scans, 452, 473, 575

phacoemulsification. See also cataracts, 162, 164

pharyngitis, 330–31

phenolic compounds, 115

phenylketonuria, 264, 507

phosphorus, 90, 115–16, 548–49

phobias. See agoraphobia; exposure therapy; photophobia; simple phobia; social phobia

photophobia, 157–58, 327, 421, 503, 517, 570

photosensitization, 126

physiatrist, 79, 465

physical fitness. See fitness

physical therapy, 79, 84–85, 314, 512

physicians. See doctors

phytochemicals, 92, 108–9, 115

"ping-pong" reinfection, 195, 215

pinkeye, 158, **328**

pinworms, 335, 548

pituitary gland, 227, 252, 259, 576

the placebo effect, **17–19**, 624

placebo treatments in research, **19**, 30–31, 39, 84, 112, 143, 159, 213, 216, 231–32, 393, 511, 583

the placenta, 273–74, 276–78, **280–81**, 282–87, 289, 497

placental
    blood, 269
    extracts, 133

plaques
    arterial, 97, 99, 233, 236, 497, 518, 523, 571
    dental, 174–77
    neuronal (brain), 452, 479, 490
    skin, 129–30, 134, 558

plastic lens implants, 162–63

plastic surgery, 79, 606

PMS. See premenstrual syndrome

pneumonia, 376–77, 459, 486–87, 546, 595
    immunization against, 80, 292, 304, 433, 435
    risk factors for, 192, 195, 293, 314–15, 324, 326, 329, 336, 457, 490, 504, 543, 545, 629
    risk factors with, 191

podiatrists, **149**, 473

Poison Control Centers, 59, 86, 603, 614

poisonings, **59**, 375, 378, 382–83, 442, 454, 548, 596, 604
    first aid for, 86, **614–15**
    from food, 75, 371, **372–73**, 596
    risks of, 54, 56, 80, 85, 627

poison ivy, 86, 123, **368**, 546

polio (poliomyelitis), 21, 80, 292, **302–3,** 316, 327, **328–29**, 388, 589

polymyalgia, 206, **511**

polyps, 52, 80, 483, **485–86**, 491, 587

polysaccharides, 105, 303

polyunsaturated fats, 99–100, 102, 106

Pontiac fever, 375–76

"port wine stains," 312

postpartum depression, 287, **409–11**

postpartum hair loss, 141

post-traumatic stress disorder, 206, 415, 419, **422–23**

potassium, 115–16, 170–71, 178, 218, 345, 347, 385, 480, 541–42, **548–50**, 622

poverty, as a health risk factor, 15, 205, 207, 236, 360, 396, 402, 434, 537, 581

pre-eclampsia, 277, **281**

pregnancy. See also anemia; contraception; eclampsia; ectopic; fetal; infertility; Kegel exercises; labor; miscarriage; Rh blood problems; risk scoring
    health changes during, 141, 214, 219, 226, **276**, 312, 314, 461, 488, 493, 495, 497, 529, 532, 538–39, 541, 547, 578–79, 582, 586
    morning sickness during, 276, 279

nutrition during, 91, 93–94, 110, 118, **277–79**, 448, 461, 630

prenatal and maternal care during, 76, 260–61, **270–71**

testing before or during, 82, 194, **268–69**, **271–72**, **280**, 304, 325, 329, 458, 492, 530, 538–39

things to avoid before and during, 29, **70**, 84, 128, 134, 143, 154, 156, 195, 200, 216–18, 220, **261**, **263–64**, **278–80**, **303**, 364, 394–95, 450, 554, 577, **625**, **628–31**

premature ejaculation, 188, 252, **254**, 266

premenstrual syndrome, 112, 200, **215–17**

prenatal. See also miscarriage; pregnancy
    care, 261, 263–64, **271–73**
    classes, 262, 280, **281–83**, 289
    nutrition, **277–79**

presbycusis, 166–67

presbyopia, 156

prescriptions. See medications

primigravida, 270

progesterone, 69, 198, 200, 215–16, **231**, 240, 258, 276, 340, 353, 528–29

prolapsed disc, 477

prostaglandins, 106, 226, 515

prostate cancer. See cancers

prostatectomy, 248, 251

prostate gland, 142, **246–50**, 255

prostate specific antigen (PSA), 80, 82, **249–51**

prostatic hyperplasia, 246, 250

prostatitis. See also psychogenic prostatitis, 195, **246–48**, 250, 582

proteins. See also meat, 93, **105–7**, 119, 444
    allergies to, 296, 370, 373–74
    as antibodies and cellular "gates," 457, 544, 561
    in vaccines, 303–4

PSA blood test. See prostate specific antigen

pseudogout, 463, 465–66

psittacosis, 596

psoriasis, 123, **128–30**, 133–34, 141, 145, 148, 368, 472, 547–48

psychiatric medicine, 79, 187, 359, 399, 402, 404, 406, 418, 428–29

psychodynamic therapy, 408

psychogenic prostatitis, 427

psychotherapy. See also behavior therapy; brief therapy; cognitive behavioral therapy; counseling; exposure therapy; interpersonal therapy, **405**, **408–9**, **428–29**

potentially helpful uses of, 52, 54, 188, 254, 346, 356, 377, 401, 406, 413, 415, 418, 421–24, 426, 482

psychotoxic workplace, 591

puberty. See also adolescence, 141, 147, 181–83, 248, **337**, **340–41**, 350, 491

puerperium, 273

puerperal psychosis, 410–11

punch-graft surgery for baldness, 143

pustular psoriasis, 130

pyridoxine. See vitamin B₆

quinsy, 334

rabies, **389**, **595**, 596, 603

radiation
    diagnosis using, 79, 238, 448
    possible harm from, 132, 134–35, 138, 141–42, 161, 266, 446, 461, 553, 579–80
    protection from. See UV rays, protection from
    therapy with, 79, 225, **240–42**, 248, **251**, 259, 554–57, 561

randomized control procedures, 18

rashes, 631
    as an allergic symptom, 86, 123, 297, 319, 371, 373, 375, **602**
    diaper. See diaper rash
    as a disease symptom, 131, 173, 190, 192, 194–95, 314, 319, 323, 326–27, 329–30, 335–36, 368, 373, 391, 394, 437, 463, 482, 557–60, 589, 619
    as a side effect, 29, 111, 126–27, 173, 390, 459, 466, 483, 509

Raynaud's phenomenon, 558

Recommended Daily Allowances (RDAs), 90, 113

Recommended Nutrient Intakes (RNIs), 90, **110–11**, 113, **116–17**

the recovery position. See first aid, the recovery position

Reference Dietary Intake report, 112

repetitive strain injury, 593

reproduction. See fertilization; infertility; pregnancy

reproductive technologies, 268–70

respiratory distress, 66, 281, 544, 606, 619, 628

respiratory syncytial virus, 329

restless leg syndrome, 53, 511

retinal detachment, 162–64

retinoic acid, 133–34
    cis-retinoic acid (Accutane), 128, 133–34

retinoid products, 128–29, **133**, 134, 152

retinol carotene. *See* vitamin A

retinopathy, 156, 158, 497

retrograde ejaculation, 249

retrosternal pain, 234

revascularization, 234–35, 523

reversible ischemic neurological deficit, 568

Reye's syndrome, 545

Rh blood problems, 166, 272

rheumatic fever, 124, **329**, 331, 334, 526–27

rheumatoid arthritis. *See* arthritis

rhythm method. *See* contraception

riboflavin. *See* vitamin B₂

ringworm, 141, **335–36**, 472, 596

risk scoring (pregnancy), 280

roseola, 302, **329**

roundworms, 335–36, 597

"Royal Free" disease, 415

rubella, 80, 166, 261, 264, 272, 293, 303–4, **328–30**, 388

ruptured disc, 477

safety. *See also* Recommended Nutrient Intakes, **54–60**, **87**, **301**, **618**
   while exercising, **44–47**

St. John's Ambulance, 599, 608, 619

St. John's wort, 88, **411**

St. Vitus dance, 329

salicylic acid, 125, 129, **152–53**

salmonellosis, 596

salt, 86, 90, 93, 107, 116–17, 171, 277–78, 292, 379, 385, 491, 502, 525, 528, 542, 549, 578, 612

sand flies, 369, 391

saturated fats, 92, 99–100, 102–3, 106, 496

scabies, **330**, 548

scalding. *See* burns and scalds

Schilling's test, 461

schistosomiasis, 259, 392

schizophrenia, 66, 355–56, 358, 395, 403, 413, 419, 428, 475
   symptoms of, **425**
   treatment of, **426–27**

sciatica, 477–78

scientific research, 18–22

scuba diving, 165–66, 280, 619

scurvy, 111–12, 115, 630

seasonal affective disorder (SAD), 408

sebaceous glands, **122**, 127–28, 140, 164

seborrheic dermatitis, 130, 548

seborrheic keratoses, 135

sebum, 122, 127–28, 133, 140

sedatives, 49–53, 56, 66, 71, 171,

364, 436, 438, 489, 502, 621–22, 624, 627, 631

seizures. *See also* convulsions; epilepsy; grand mal seizures
   first aid for, 508, **615**

selective serotonin reuptake inhibitors. *See* SSRIs

self-esteem (low). *See also* depression, 61, 127, 206, **207–8**, 280, 288, **298–99**, 342, 344, **348**, 350, 356, 360, 409, 474–75

seminal vesicles, 247, 251

seniors. *See also* eldercare; geriatric care and problems; loneliness, 149, 167, 186, 430–31, **436**, 534
   care of, 432–34
   immunizations for, 304, 433
   nutrition for, 94–95, 108, 434
   safety for, 122, 434–35

sentinel node biopsy, 240

septic shock, 327

seronegative arthritis, 466

serotonin. *See also* SSRIs, 39, 105–6, 216, 356, 404, 408, 411, 424, 427, 511, 514, 516–17

serum screening, 269, 457, 462, 519, 521, 621

sex. *See also* gender identity and development; sexual; sexually transmitted diseases;
   aging and, 186
   education about, 179–80, 183–85, 341, 349, 352–54
   therapy and, 187–88, 213–14, 254, 256–57
   women and, 211–14

sexual. *See also* hormones; pregnancy; sex; sexually transmitted diseases
   abuse, 184–85, 187, 206, 214, 344, 348, 356, 415
   development, 180–83, 340–41, 344
   dysfunction, 185–87, 206, 211–12, 248, 253–54, 407
   health, 179–80, 182, 211–13
   orientation. *See also* homosexuality, 183

sexually transmitted diseases (STDs), 82, 146, 151, **189–96**, 197, 202, 221, 249, 257, 457, 535, 539

shingles, **131–32**, 141, 158, 314, 457, 546–48

shock therapy. *See* electroconvulsive shock therapy

shoes, 47–48, 59, 129, 148, **149–50**, 324, 386, 436, 472–3, 500, 560, 606, 618

sickle cell anemia. *See* anemia, sickle cell

sick mother syndrome, 288

SIDs, 331–33

sigmoidoscopy, 80, 82, 481, 531

sildenafil. *See* Viagra

silver-nitrate drops, 191, 285

simple phobia, 421–22

Sjögren's syndrome, 158, 206, **504**, 513

skin. *See also* dermatitis; itching; sunburn
   aging of, 132–34
   cancers of. *See also* melanomas, 135
   discolorations. *See also* birthmarks, 133, 138, 586
   dry. *See also* skin creams, 66, 87, 121, **122–23**, 125, 148, 345, 500, 548, 578, 613

skin creams and moisturizers, 124–26, 133, 606
   allergic reactions to, 125

sleep. *See also* insomnia, **49–54**, 402

sleep apnea, 33, **52**, 334, 416–17

sleep deprivation therapy, 51

sleeping sickness, 391, 440

sleepwalking, 53–54

smoking. *See also* nicotine; tobacco
   risks from, 19, **23–24**, 58, 63, 97, 99, 159, 175, 203, **208**, 221, **235–36**, 255, **278**, 380, 440, 444, 447, **518–21**, 524, 543, **556–57**, 565, **569**, 586–87
   stopping of, **24–32**, 264, 386, 407, 524, 542

SNRIs. *See also* antidepressants, 356, **406–7**, 410

social phobia, 422

sodium (dietary). *See also* salt, 84, 90, 93, **116**, 120, 171, 278, 379–80, 480, 541, 549, 629

solvents (industrial), 67, 126, 375–77, 380

somatization, 206, 357, 377, 395, 405, 417–18

sore throats. *See* pharyngitis

spastic colon, 481

speech-language therapy, 433, 574, 576, 587–89

sperm. *See also* fertilization; spermicide, 197–202, 204, 246–48, 383
   counts of, 192, 252–53, **265–66**

spermicide, 189, 194, **196–99**, 201–2, **203**, 266, 457, 539, 583–84

spider angiomas, 312

spina bifida. *See* neural tube defects

spinal "crush" fractures, 450

spinal stenosis, 438, 477

the spine. *See also* back problems;

neural tube defects; osteoporosis, 150, **476**, 593–94

sport injuries, 17, **48–49**, **616–18**

sport safety, **44–47**, **618**

spotted fever, 327, 559, 604

spotting (menstrual), 200, 226, 231

SSRIs (selective serotonin reuptake inhibitors), *See also* antidepressants, 216, 254, 356, **406–7**, 408, **410–11**, 511

staphylococcal bacteria and medications, 124, 292, 326, 504

statin drugs, 520, 621

status epilepticus, 506

STDs. *See* sexually transmitted diseases

sterilization. *See* tubal ligation; vasectomy

stiff neck, 308, 325, **327**, 514, 570, 589

STIs. *See* sexually transmitted diseases

stomach. *See also* hiatus hernia, 39, 43–44, 340, 528, 567, 621, 627–29
   cancer, 24, 379, 564
   ulcers, 26, 66–67, 467, 525, **563–66**, 628
   upset, 18, 29, 316, 333, 349, 370, 372, 400, 405, 417, 466–67, 489, 525, 534, 589, 625

strabismus, 155

strain (psychological). *See also* stress, 432, 590

strain injuries. *See also* back problems, 49, 84, 123, 150, 477, 587, 589–90, **592–94**, **616–17**

strawberry mark, 312–13

strength (muscle). *See* muscular (isometric) strength; muscular (isotonic) endurance

strep throat, 306, **329–331**

streptococcus, 124, 130, 292, 304, 326–31, 504

stress. *See also* anxiety; burnout; post-traumatic stress disorder, 206, **396–99**
   coping with, 16, 24, 70, 399, 433
   emotional, 124, 188, 412, 433, 570
   and exercise, 40, 207, 209
   and genetic makeup, 397
   and heart problems, 233, 521, 526, 541, **591–92**
   and other problems, 130, 132, 141, 169, 215, 416, 443, 452; 473, 476, 481, 495, 500–501, 509–10, 515–16, 528, 548, 557–58, 562, 574, **592**